Nobel Prizes Awarded for Research in Genetics or Genetics-Related Areas

Year	Recipients	Nobel Prize	Discovery/Research Topic
2012	J. B. Gurdon S. Yamanaka	Physiology or Medicine	Differentiated cells can be reprogrammed to become pluripotent
2009	E. H. Blackburn C. W. Greider J. W. Szostak	Physiology or Medicine	The nature and replication of the DNA of telomeres, and the discovery of the telomere-replenishing ribonucleoprotein enzyme telomerase
2007	M. R. Capecchi M. J. Evans O. Smithies	Physiology or Medicine	Gene-targeting technology essential to the creation of knockout mice serving as animal models of human disease
2006	R. Kornberg	Chemistry	Molecular basis of eukaryotic transcription
2006	A. Z. Fire C. C. Mello	Physiology or Medicine	Gene silencing using RNA interference (RNAi)
2002	S. Brenner H. R. Horvitz J. E. Sulston	Physiology or Medicine	Genetic regulation of organ development and programmed cell death (apoptosis)
2001	L. Hartwell T. Hunt P. Nurse	Physiology or Medicine	Genes and regulatory molecules controlling the cell cycle
1999	G. Blobel	Physiology or Medicine	Genetically encoded amino acid sequences in proteins that guide their cellular transport
1997	S. Prusiner	Physiology or Medicine	Prions—a new biological principle of infection
1995	E. B. Lewis C. Nusslein-Volhard E. Wieschaus	Physiology or Medicine	Genetic control of early development in *Drosophila*
1993	R. Roberts P. Sharp	Physiology or Medicine	RNA processing of split genes
	K. Mullis M. Smith	Chemistry	Development of polymerase chain reaction (PCR) and site-directed mutagenesis (SDM)
1989	J. M. Bishop H. E. Varmus	Physiology or Medicine	Role of retroviruses and oncogenes in cancer
	T. R. Cech S. Altman	Chemistry	Ribozyme function during RNA splicing
1987	S. Tonegawa	Physiology or Medicine	Genetic basis of antibody diversity
1985	M. S. Brown J. L. Goldstein	Physiology or Medicine	Genetic regulation of cholesterol metabolism
1983	B. McClintock	Physiology or Medicine	Mobile genetic elements in maize
1982	A. Klug	Chemistry	Crystalline structure analysis of significant complexes, including tRNA and nucleosomes
1980	P. Berg W. Gilbert F. Sanger	Chemistry	Development of recombinant DNA and DNA sequencing technology
1978	W. Arber D. Nathans H. O. Smith	Physiology or Medicine	Recombinant DNA technology using restriction endonuclease technology
1976	B. S. Blumberg D. C. Gajdusek	Physiology or Medicine	Elucidation of the human prion-based diseases, kuru and Creutzfeldt-Jakob disease
1975	D. Baltimore R. Dulbecco H. Temin	Physiology or Medicine	Molecular genetics of tumor viruses

Year	Recipients	Nobel Prize	Research Topic
1972	G. M. Edelman R. R. Porter	Physiology or Medicine	Chemical structure of immunoglobulins
	C. Anfinsen	Chemistry	Relationship between primary and tertiary structure of proteins
1970	N. Borlaug	Peace Prize	Genetic improvement of Mexican wheat
1969	M. Delbrück A. D. Hershey S. E. Luria	Physiology or Medicine	Replication mechanisms and genetic structure of bacteriophages
1968	H. G. Khorana M. W. Nirenberg	Physiology or Medicine	Deciphering the genetic code
	R. W. Holley	Physiology or Medicine	Structure and nucleotide sequence of transfer RNA
1966	P. F. Rous	Physiology or Medicine	Viral induction of cancer in chickens
1965	F. Jacob A. M. Lwoff J. L. Monod	Physiology or Medicine	Genetic regulation of enzyme synthesis in bacteria
1962	F. H. C. Crick J. D. Watson M. H. F. Wilkins	Physiology or Medicine	Double helical model of DNA
	J. C. Kendrew M. F. Perutz	Chemistry	Three-dimensional structure of globular proteins
1959	A. Kornberg S. Ochoa	Physiology or Medicine	Biological synthesis of DNA and RNA
1958	G. W. Beadle E. L. Tatum	Physiology or Medicine	Genetic control of biochemical processes
	J. Lederberg	Physiology or Medicine	Genetic recombination in bacteria
	F. Sanger	Chemistry	Primary structure of proteins
1954	L. Pauling	Chemistry	Alpha helical structure of proteins
1946	H. J. Muller	Physiology or Medicine	X-ray induction of mutations in *Drosophila*
1933	T. H. Morgan	Physiology or Medicine	Chromosomal theory of inheritance
1930	K. Landsteiner	Physiology or Medicine	Discovery of human blood groups

CONCEPTS OF
GENETICS

CONCEPTS OF
GENETICS

ELEVENTH EDITION

William S. Klug
THE COLLEGE OF NEW JERSEY

Michael R. Cummings
ILLINOIS INSTITUTE OF TECHNOLOGY

Charlotte A. Spencer
UNIVERSITY OF ALBERTA

Michael A. Palladino
MONMOUTH UNIVERSITY

With contributions by
Darrell Killian
COLORADO COLLEGE

PEARSON

Boston Columbus Indianapolis New York San Francisco Upper Saddle River
Amsterdam Cape Town Dubai London Madrid Milan Munich Paris Montréal Toronto
Delhi Mexico City São Paulo Sydney Hong Kong Seoul Singapore Taipei Tokyo

Library of Congress Cataloging-in-Publication Data
Klug, William S., author.
Concepts of genetics / William S. Klug, Michael R. Cummings, Charlotte
A. Spencer, Michael A. Palladino.–Eleventh edition.
    p. ; cm.
Preceded by Concepts of genetics / William S. Klug . . . [et al.].
    10th ed. c2012.
Includes bibliographical references and index.
ISBN 978-0-321-94891-5 (student edition)–ISBN 0-321-94891-2
    (student edition)–ISBN 978-0-13-386536-3 (books a la carte
    edition)–ISBN 0-13-386536-3 (books a la carte edition)
I. Cummings, Michael R., author. II. Spencer, Charlotte A., author.
III. Palladino, Michael Angelo, author. IV. Title.
    [DNLM: 1. Genetic Phenomena. QU 500]
QH430
576.5–dc23
                                           2014019403
ISBN 10: 0-321-94891-2; ISBN 13: 978-0-321-94891-5 (Student
Edition)

Editor-in-Chief: Beth Wilbur
Senior Acquisitions Editor: Michael Gillespie
Executive Director of Development: Deborah Gale
Executive Editorial Manager: Ginnie Simione-Jutson
Project Editor: Dusty Friedman
Editorial Assistant: Chloe Veylit
Text Permissions Project Manager: Timothy Nicholls
Text Permissions Specialist: PreMedia Global USA, Inc.
Program Manager Team Lead: Michael Early
Program Manager: Anna Amato
Project Manager Team Lead: David Zielonka
Project Manager: Lori Newman
Project Manager—Instructor Media: Edward Lee
Production Management and Composition: Cenveo
    Publisher Services
Copyeditor: Betty Pessagno
Proofreader: Joanna Dinsmore
Design Manager: Marilyn Perry
Interior Designer: Cenveo Publisher Services
Cover Designer: Tandem Creative
Illustrators: Imagineeringart.com, Inc.
Image Lead: Donna Kalal
Photo Researcher and Permissions Management: PreMedia Global
    USA, Inc.
Manufacturing Buyer: Jeffrey Sargent
Cover/Text Printer: Courier Kendallville
Director of Marketing: Christy Lesko
Executive Marketing Manager: Lauren Harp
Executive Media Producer: Laura Tommasi
Associate Content Producer: Daniel Ross

Cover Photo Credit: Dr. Gopal Murti / Science Source

www.pearsonhighered.com

ISBN 10: 0-321-94891-2; ISBN 13: 978-0-321-94891-5 (Student Edition)
ISBN 10: 0-133-97147-3; ISBN 13: 978-0-133-97147-7 (Instructor's Review Copy)
ISBN 10: 0-133-86536-3; ISBN 13: 978-0-133-86536-3 (Books a la Carte Edition)
1 2 3 4 5 6 7 8 9 10—CRK—18 17 16 15 14

Dedication

To Kathy, Lee Ann, Bob, and Cindy, who mean the very most to us, and serve as our respective foundations when we are writing, and when we are not.

WSK, MRC, CAS, and MAP

William S. Klug is an Emeritus Professor of Biology at The College of New Jersey (formerly Trenton State College) in Ewing, New Jersey, where he served as Chair of the Biology Department for 17 years. He received his B.A. degree in Biology from Wabash College in Crawfordsville, Indiana, and his Ph.D. from Northwestern University in Evanston, Illinois. Prior to coming to The College of New Jersey, he was on the faculty of Wabash College as an Assistant Professor, where he first taught genetics, as well as general biology and electron microscopy. His research interests have involved ultrastructural and molecular genetic studies of development, utilizing oogenesis in *Drosophila* as a model system. He has taught the genetics course as well as the senior capstone seminar course in Human and Molecular Genetics to undergraduate biology majors for over four decades. He was the recipient in 2001 of the first annual teaching award given at The College of New Jersey, granted to the faculty member who "most challenges students to achieve high standards." He also received the 2004 Outstanding Professor Award from Sigma Pi International, and in the same year, he was nominated as the Educator of the Year, an award given by the Research and Development Council of New Jersey.

Michael R. Cummings is Research Professor in the Department of Biological, Chemical, and Physical Sciences at Illinois Institute of Technology, Chicago, Illinois. For more than 25 years, he was a faculty member in the Department of Biological Sciences and in the Department of Molecular Genetics at the University of Illinois at Chicago. He has also served on the faculties of Northwestern University and Florida State University. He received his B.A. from St. Mary's College in Winona, Minnesota, and his M.S. and Ph.D. from Northwestern University in Evanston, Illinois. In addition to this text and its companion volumes, he has also written textbooks in human genetics and general biology for nonmajors. His research interests center on the molecular organization and physical mapping of the heterochromatic regions of human acrocentric chromosomes. At the undergraduate level, he teaches courses in Mendelian and molecular genetics, human genetics, and general biology, and has received numerous awards for teaching excellence given by university faculty, student organizations, and graduating seniors.

Charlotte A. Spencer is a retired Associate Professor from the Department of Oncology at the University of Alberta in Edmonton, Alberta, Canada. She has also served as a faculty member in the Department of Biochemistry at the University of Alberta. She received her B.Sc. in Microbiology from the University of British Columbia and her Ph.D. in Genetics from the University of Alberta, followed by postdoctoral training at the Fred Hutchinson Cancer Research Center in Seattle, Washington. Her research interests involve the regulation of RNA polymerase II transcription in cancer cells, cells infected with DNA viruses, and cells traversing the mitotic phase of the cell cycle. She has taught courses in biochemistry, genetics, molecular biology, and oncology, at both undergraduate and graduate levels. In addition, she has written booklets in the Prentice Hall Exploring Biology series, which are aimed at the undergraduate nonmajor level.

Michael A. Palladino is Dean of the School of Science and Professor of Biology at Monmouth University in West Long Branch, New Jersey. He received his B.S. degree in Biology from Trenton State College (now known as The College of New Jersey) and his Ph.D. in Anatomy and Cell Biology from the University of Virginia. He directs an active laboratory of undergraduate student researchers studying molecular mechanisms involved in innate immunity of mammalian male reproductive organs and genes involved in oxygen homeostasis and ischemic injury of the testis. He has taught a wide range of courses for both majors and nonmajors and currently teaches genetics, biotechnology, endocrinology, and laboratory in cell and molecular biology. He has received several awards for research and teaching, including the 2009 Young Investigator Award of the American Society of Andrology, the 2005 Distinguished Teacher Award from Monmouth University, and the 2005 Caring Heart Award from the New Jersey Association for Biomedical Research. He is co-author of the undergraduate textbook *Introduction to Biotechnology*, Series Editor for the Benjamin Cummings *Special Topics in Biology* booklet series, and author of the first booklet in the series, *Understanding the Human Genome Project*.

Brief Contents

Explore Cutting Edge Topics

Six Special Topics

in **Modern Genetics** mini-chapters concisely explore cutting-edge, engaging, relevant topics, and three are new to the Eleventh Edition:

- Epigenetics
- *New!* Emerging Roles of RNA
- DNA Forensics
- Genomics and Personalized Medicine
- *New!* Genetically Modified Foods
- *New!* Gene Therapy

End-of-Chapter

Questions are provided for each Special Topic chapter to help students review key ideas and to facilitate class discussions. Questions are assignable through MasteringGenetics

New! Photos and illustrations have been added throughout the text.

Genetically Modified Foods

SPECIAL TOPIC 5

Throughout the ages, humans have used selective breeding techniques to create plants and animals with desirable genetic traits. By selecting organisms with naturally occurring or mutagen-induced variations and breeding them to establish the phenotype, we have evolved varieties that now feed our growing populations and support our complex civilizations.

Although we have had tremendous success shuffling genes through selective breeding, the process is a slow one. When recombinant DNA technologies emerged in the 1970s and 1980s, scientists realized that they could modify agriculturally significant organisms in a more precise and rapid way—by identifying and cloning genes that confer desirable traits, then introducing these genes into organisms. Genetic engineering of animals and plants promised an exciting new phase in scientific agriculture, with increased productivity, reduced pesticide use, and enhanced flavor and nutrition.

> "Genetic engineering of animals and plants promised an exciting new phase in scientific agriculture, with increased productivity, reduced pesticide use, and enhanced flavor and nutrition."

Beginning in the 1990s, scientists created a large number of genetically modified (GM) food varieties. The first one, approved for sale in 1994, was the Flavr Savr tomato—a tomato that stayed firm and ripe longer than non-GM tomatoes. Soon afterward, other GM foods were developed: papaya and zucchini with resistance to virus infection, canola containing the tropical oil laurate, corn and cotton plants with resistance to insects, and soybeans and sugar beets with tolerance to agricultural herbicides. By 2012, more than 200 different GM crop varieties had been created. Worldwide, GM crops are planted on 170 million hectares of arable land, with a global value of $15 billion for GM seeds.

Although many people see great potential for GM foods—to help address malnutrition in a world with a growing human population and climate change—others question

violence. On August 8, 2013, 400 protesters broke through security fences surrounding a field trial of Golden Rice in the Bicol region of the Philippines (**ST Figure 5–1**). Within 15 minutes, they had uprooted and trampled most of the GM rice plants. The attackers argued that Golden Rice was a threat to human health and biodiversity and would lead to Western corporate control of local food crops.

Opposition to GM foods is not unique to Golden Rice. In 2013, approximately two million people marched against GM foods in rallies held in 52 countries. Some countries have outright bans on all GM foods, whereas others embrace the technologies. Opponents cite safety and environmental concerns, while some scientists and commercial interests extol the almost limitless virtues of GM foods. The topic of GM food attracts hyperbole and exaggerated rhetoric, information, and misinformation—on both sides of the debate.

So, what are the truths about GM foods? In this Special Topic chapter, we will introduce the science behind GM foods and examine the promises and problems

ST Figure 5–1 Anti-GM protesters attacking Golden Rice. On August 8, 2013, protesters in the Philippines broke through a security fence and destroyed an experimental field of GM rice plants.

Philippine Department of Agriculture Regional Field Unit 5)

Review Questions

1. How do genetically modified organisms compare with organisms created through selective breeding?
2. Can current GM crops be considered as transgenic or cisgenic? Why?
3. Of the approximately 200 GM crop varieties that have been developed, only a few are widely used. What are these varieties, and how prevalent are they?
4. How does glyphosate work, and how has it been used with GM crops to increase agricultural yields?
5. Describe the mechanisms by which the Cry proteins from *Bacillus thuringiensis* act as insecticides.
6. What measures have been taken to alleviate vitamin A deficiencies in developing countries? To date, how successful have these strategies been?
7. What is Golden Rice 2, and how was it created?
8. Describe how plants can be transformed using biolistic methods. How does this method compare with *Agrobacterium tumefaciens*-mediated transformation?
9. How do positive and negative selection techniques contribute to the development of GM crops?
10. Describe how the Roundup-Ready soybean variety was developed, and what genes were used to transform the soybean plants.

Discussion Questions

1. What are the laws regulating the development, approval, and use of GM foods in your region and nationally?
2. Do you think that foods containing GM ingredients should be labeled as such? What would be the advantages and disadvantages to such a strategy?
3. One of the major objections to GM foods is that they may be harmful to human health. Do you agree or disagree, and why?

Explore Classic and Modern Approaches

Evolving Concept of the Gene sections, integrated in key chapters, highlight how scientists' understanding of the gene has changed over time.

Chapters 3, 4, 5, 6, 10, 12, 14, 16, 21

Chapter 10

EVOLVING CONCEPT OF THE GENE

Based on the model of DNA put forward by Watson and Crick in 1953, the gene was viewed for the first time in molecular terms as a sequence of nucleotides in a DNA helix that encodes genetic information. ■

Chapter 21

EVOLVING CONCEPT OF A GENE

Based on the work of the ENCODE project, we now know that DNA sequences that have previously been thought of as "junk DNA", which do not encode proteins, are nonetheless often transcribed into what we call noncoding RNA (ncRNA). Since the function of some these RNAs is now being determined, we must consider whether the concept of the gene should be expanded to include DNA sequences that encode ncRNAs. At this writing, there is no consensus, but it is important for you to be aware of these current findings as you develop your final interpretation of a gene. ■

NEW!

Modern Approaches to Understanding Gene Function feature introduces the impact of modern gene targeting approaches on our understanding of gene function. Each entry explores experimental approaches, analyzes data, and relates to a concept discussed in the chapter. Includes discussion questions.

MODERN APPROACHES TO UNDERSTANDING GENE FUNCTION

Mouse Models of Down Syndrome

The underlying hypothesis concerning the genetic basis of Down syndrome is that the presence of three copies of chromosome 21 leads to the overexpression of some portion of the genes on that chromosome and that the resulting gene products are responsible for the multiple characteristics associated with the complete phenotype. It is possible that, even though Down syndrome is not caused by a single gene, individual genes may be responsible for specific characteristics making up the syndrome. Elucidation of which genes are involved has long

of the same content and arrangement of *orthologs*, genes with similar sequences that are present in different species. One of the earliest models created (Ts16) has an extra copy of mouse chromosome 16, and indeed it displays some, but not all, human Down syndrome characteristics. Therefore Ts16 mice are missing some of the critical orthologs present on Hsa21. Ts16 mice also have extra copies of other genes not present on Hsa21.

Further investigation has established that mouse chromosomes 10 and 17 also contain orthologs for

hydrocephalus, accumulation of cerebrospinal fluid in the brain, and a resulting rounded and enlarged cranium. There are no known genes on Hsa21 that are directly associated with hydrocephalus in humans, so this condition is likely caused by expressing multiple copies of several orthologs.

Conclusion:

Research with mouse models has demonstrated that no single gene is responsible for all phenotypes associated with Down syndrome, but instead that overexpression of many genes is necessary to produce the full human syndrome. The creation of new models such as the Mmu 10, 16, 17 animals demonstrates

Topics include:

- Identifying Mendel's Gene for Regulating White Flower Color in Peas (Ch. 3)
- *Drosophila Sxl* Gene Induces Female Development (Ch. 7)
- Mouse Models of Down Syndrome (Ch. 8)
- Lethal Knockouts of DNA Ligase Genes (Ch. 11)
- Transposon-Mediated Mutations Reveal Genes Involved in Colorectal Cancer (Ch. 15)

- MicroRNAs Regulate Ovulation in Female Mice (Ch. 17)
- Single-Gene Signaling Mechanism Reveals Secrets to Head Regeneration in Planaria (Ch. 18)
- *RbAp48* and a Potential Molecular Mechanism for Age-Related Memory Loss (Ch.24)

NOW SOLVE THIS

13–3 The following represent deoxyribonucleotide sequences in the template strand of DNA:

Sequence 1:	5'-CTTTTTTGCCAT-3'
Sequence 2:	5'-ACATCAATAACT-3'
Sequence 3:	5'-TACAAGGGTTCT-3'

(a) For each strand, determine the mRNA sequence that would be derived from transcription.

(b) Using Figure 13–7, determine the amino acid sequence that is encoded by these mRNAs.

(c) For Sequence 1, what is the sequence of the partner DNA strand?

■ **HINT:** *This problem asks you to consider the outcome of the transfer of complementary information from DNA to RNA and to determine the amino acids encoded by this information. The key to its solution is to remember that in RNA, uracil is complementary to adenine, and that while DNA stores genetic information in the cell, the code that is translated is contained in the RNA complementary to the template strand of DNA making up a gene.*

Learn problem-solving skills by pausing to complete integrated *Now Solve This* problems.

Apply problem-solving strategies by studying hints, and checking your work against the Answers Appendix.

INSIGHTS AND SOLUTIONS

As a student, you will be asked to demonstrate your knowledge of transmission genetics by solving various problems. Success at this task requires not only comprehension of theory but also its application to more practical genetic situations. Most students find problem solving in genetics to be both challenging and rewarding. This section is designed to provide basic insights into the reasoning essential to this process.

Genetics problems are in many ways similar to word problems in algebra. The approach to solving them is identical: (1) analyze the problem carefully; (2) translate words into symbols and define each symbol precisely; and (3) choose and apply a specific technique to solve the problem. The first two steps are the most critical. The third step is largely mechanical.

The simplest problems state all necessary information about a P₁ generation and ask you to find the expected ratios of the F₁ and F₂ genotypes and/or phenotypes. Always follow these steps when you encounter this type of problem:

(a) Determine insofar as possible the genotypes of the individuals in the P₁ generation.

(b) Determine what gametes may be formed by the P₁ parents.

(c) Recombine the gametes either by the Punnett square or the forked-line method, or if the situation is very simple, by inspection. From the genotypes of the F₁ generation, determine the phenotypes. Read the F₁ phenotypes.

(d) Repeat the process to obtain information about the F₂ generation.

Determining the genotypes from the given information requires that you understand the basic theory of transmission genetics. Consider this problem: *A recessive mutant allele, black, causes a very dark body in Drosophila when homozygous. The normal wild-type color is described as gray. What F₁ phenotypic ratio is predicted when a black female is crossed to a gray male whose father was black?*

To work out this problem, you must understand dominance and recessiveness, as well as the principle of segregation. Furthermore, you must use the information about the male parent's father. Here is one logical approach to solving this problem:

The female parent is black, so she must be homozygous for the mutant allele (*bb*). The male parent is gray and must therefore have at least one dominant allele (*B*). His father was

Apply the approach we just studied to the following problems.

1. Mendel found that full pea pods are dominant over constricted pods, while seeds are dominant over wrinkled seeds. One of his crosses was between full, round plants and constricted, wrinkled plants. From this cross, he obtained an F₁ generation that was all full and round. In the F₂ generation, Mendel obtained his classic 9:3:3:1 ratio. Using this information, determine the expected F₁ and F₂ results of a cross between homozygous constricted, round and full, wrinkled plants.

Solution: First, assign gene symbols to each pair of contrasting traits. Use the lowercase first letter of each recessive trait to designate that trait, and use the same letter in uppercase to designate the dominant trait. Thus, C and c indicate full and constricted pods, respectively, and W and w indicate the round and wrinkled phenotypes, respectively.

Determine the genotypes of the P₁ generation, form the gametes, combine them in the F₁ generation, and read off the phenotype(s):

P₁:	*ccWW* constricted, round		×	*CCww* full, wrinkled
Gametes:	*cW*			*Cw*
F₁:		*CcWw* full, round		

You can immediately see that the F₁ generation expresses both dominant phenotypes and is heterozygous for both gene pairs. Thus, you expect that the F₂ generation will yield the classic Mendelian ratio of 9:3:3:1. Let's work it out anyway, just to confirm this expectation, using the forked-line method. Both gene pairs are heterozygous and can be expected to assort independently, so we can predict the F₂ outcomes from each gene pair separately and then proceed with the forked-line method. The F₂ offspring should exhibit the individual traits in the following proportions:

Strengthen your problem-solving strategies by studying the step-by-step solutions and rationales modeled in *Insights and Solutions.*

Mastering Genetics™

MasteringGenetics helps students master key genetics concepts while reinforcing problem solving skills with hints and feedback specific to their misconceptions.

Tutorial topics include:

- Pedigree analysis
- Sex linkage
- Gene interactions
- DNA replication
- RNA processing
- Genomics

"How Do We Know?" questions
ask students to identify and examine the experimental basis underlying important concepts.

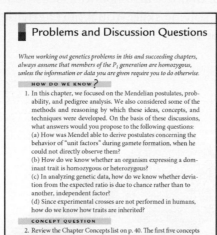

Problems and Discussion Questions

When working out genetics problems in this and succeeding chapters, always assume that members of the P_1 generation are homozygous, unless the information or data you are given require you to do otherwise.

HOW DO WE KNOW?

1. In this chapter, we focused on the Mendelian postulates, probability, and pedigree analysis. We also considered some of the methods and reasoning by which these ideas, concepts, and techniques were developed. On the basis of these discussions, what answers would you propose to the following questions:
(a) How was Mendel able to derive postulates concerning the behavior of "unit factors" during gamete formation, when he could not directly observe them?
(b) How do we know whether an organism expressing a dominant trait is homozygous or heterozygous?
(c) In analyzing genetic data, how do we know whether deviation from the expected ratio is due to chance rather than to another, independent factor?
(d) Since experimental crosses are not performed in humans, how do we know how traits are inherited?

CONCEPT QUESTION

2. Review the Chapter Concepts list on p. 40. The first five concepts provide a modern interpretation of Mendelian postulates. Based on these concepts, write a short essay that correlates Mendel's

NEW! **Concept Questions** ask students to check their understanding of Key Concepts.

Extra-Spicy Problems

22. During the analysis of seven *rII* mutations in phage T4, mutants *1*, *2*, and *6* were in cistron A, while mutants *3*, *4*, and *5* were in cistron B. Of these, mutant *4* was a deletion overlapping mutant *5*. The remainder were point mutations. Nothing was known about mutant *7*. Predict the results of complementation (+ or –) between *1* and *2*; *1* and *3*; *2* and *4*; and *4* and *5*.
23. In studies of recombination between mutants *1* and *2* from the previous problem, the results shown in the following table were obtained.

Strain	Dilution	Plaques	Phenotypes
E. coli B	10^{-7}	4	*r*
E. coli K12	10^{-2}	8	1

(a) Calculate the recombination frequency.
(b) When mutant 6 was tested for recombination with mutant *1*, the data were the same as those shown above for strain B, but not for K12. The researcher lost the K12 data, but remembered that recombination was ten times more frequent than when mutants *1* and *2* were tested. What were the lost values (dilution and colony numbers)?
(c) Mutant 7 (Problem 22) failed to complement any of the other mutants (*1–6*). Define the nature of mutant 7.
24. In *Bacillus subtilis*, linkage analysis of two mutant genes affect-

Extra-Spicy Problems challenge students to solve complex problems, many based on data derived from primary genetics literature.

MasteringGenetics™

NEW! **140 Additional Practice Problems** offer more opportunities to develop problem solving skills. These questions appear only in MasteringGenetics, and they include targeted wrong answer feedback to help students learn from their mistakes.

Prepare students for the challenging problems they will see on tests and exams: question types include sorting, labeling, entering numerical information, multiple choice, and fill-in-the-blank.

Complete the **Problems and Discussion Questions** at the end of each chapter. 90% of questions are now available in MasteringGenetics

Succeed with MasteringGenetics

MasteringGenetics is a powerful online learning and assessment system proven to help students learn problem-solving skills. You'll find activities for use **before class, during class, and after class.**

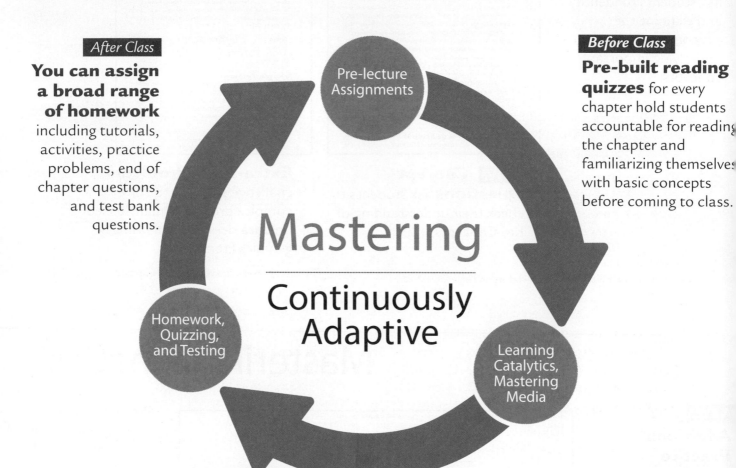

After Class

You can assign a broad range of homework including tutorials, activities, practice problems, end of chapter questions, and test bank questions.

Pre-lecture Assignments

Homework, Quizzing, and Testing

Learning Catalytics, Mastering Media

Mastering
Continuously Adaptive

Before Class

Pre-built reading quizzes for every chapter hold students accountable for reading the chapter and familiarizing themselves with basic concepts before coming to class.

During Class

NEW! **Learning Catalytics** is a "bring your own device" (smartphone, tablet, or laptop) assessment active classroom system that expands the possibilities for student engagement. Using Learning Catalytics, genetics instructors can deliver a wide range of auto-gradable or open-ended questions that test content knowledge and build critical thinking skills.

Instructors can create their own questions, draw from community content shared by colleagues, or access Pearson's new library of question clusters that explore challenging topics through a series of 2-5 questions that focus on a single scenario or data set, build in difficulty and require higher-level thinking.

Contents

5   Chromosome Mapping in Eukaryotes   *104*

PART TWO
DNA: STRUCTURE, REPLICATION, AND VARIATION

10 DNA Structure and Analysis   *231*

22 Applications and Ethics of Genetic Engineering and Biotechnology *569*

GENETICS, TECHNOLOGY, AND SOCIETY

PART FIVE
GENETICS OF ORGANISMS AND POPULATIONS

23 Quantitative Genetics and Multifactorial Traits   604

GENETICS, TECHNOLOGY, AND SOCIETY

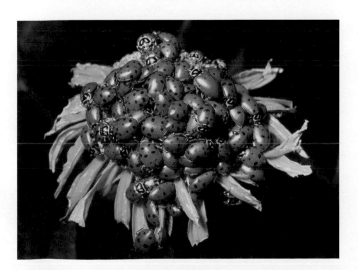

Preface

It is essential that textbook authors step back and look with fresh eyes as each edition of their work is planned. In doing so, two main questions must be posed: (1) How has the body of information in their field—in this case Genetics—grown and shifted since the last edition; and (2) What pedagogic innovations might be devised and incorporated into the text that will unquestionably enhance students' learning? The preparation of the 11th edition of *Concepts of Genetics*, a text now entering its fourth decade of providing support for students studying in this field, has occasioned still another fresh look. And what we focused on in this new edition, in addition to the normal updating that is inevitably required, were two things: (1) the need to increase the opportunities for instructors and students to engage in **active and cooperative learning approaches**, either within or outside of the classroom; and (2) the need to provide more **comprehensive coverage of important, emerging topics** that do not yet warrant their own traditional chapters.

Regarding the first point, and as discussed in further detail below, we have added a new feature called **Modern Understanding of Gene Function**, which appears within many chapters. In addition, we have retained the very popular **Genetics, Technology, and Society** essays that appear at the end of many chapters. This feature includes an active learning format called *Your Turn*, which directly engages the student with provocative assignments. These features are in addition to **Exploring Genomics** entries, and together, these all may serve as the basis for interactions between small groups of students, either in or out of the classroom. Regarding emerging topics, we continue to include a unique approach in genetics textbooks that offers readers a set of abbreviated, highly focused chapters that we label **Special Topics in Modern Genetics**. In this edition, these provide uniquely cohesive coverage of six important topics: *Epigenetics, Emerging Roles of RNA, Genomics and Personalized Medicine, DNA Forensics, Genetically Modified Foods,* and *Gene Therapy*. Three of these (*RNA, GM Foods,* and *Gene Therapy*) are new to this edition.

Goals

In the 11th edition of *Concepts of Genetics*, as in all past editions, we have five major goals. Specifically, we have sought to:

- Emphasize the basic concepts of genetics.

- Write clearly and directly to students in order to provide understandable explanations of complex, analytical topics.

- Maintain our strong emphasis on and provide multiple approaches to problem solving.

- Propagate the rich history of genetics, which so beautifully illustrates how information is acquired during scientific investigation.

- Create inviting, engaging, and pedagogically useful full-color figures enhanced by equally helpful photographs to support concept development.

These goals collectively serve as the cornerstone of *Concepts of Genetics*. This pedagogic foundation allows the book to be used in courses with many different approaches and lecture formats.

Writing a textbook that achieves these goals and having the opportunity to continually improve on each new edition has been a labor of love for us. The creation of each of the eleven editions is a reflection not only of our passion for teaching genetics, but also of the constructive feedback and encouragement provided by adopters, reviewers, and our students over the past three decades.

New to This Edition

- **Special Topics in Modern Genetics**—We have been pleased with the popular reception that the Special Topics in Modern Genetics chapters has received. First introduced in the tenth edition, our goal has been to provide abbreviated, cohesive coverage of important topics in genetics that are not always easily located in textbooks. Professors have used these focused, flexible chapters as the backbone of lectures, as inspiration for student assignments outside of class, and as the basis of group assignments and presentations.

  New to this edition are chapters on topics of great significance in genetics: Emerging Roles of RNA, Genetically Modified Foods, and Gene Therapy. For all Special Topic chapters, we have added a series of questions that send the student back into the chapter to review key ideas or provide the basis of personal contemplations and group discussions.

- **Modern Approaches to Understanding Gene Function** This new feature highlights how advances in genetic technology have led to our modern understanding of gene function. Appearing in many chapters, this feature also prompts students to apply their analytical thinking skills, linking the experimental technology to the findings that enhance our understanding of gene function.

- **Evolving Concept of the Gene** Also new to this edition is a short feature, integrated in appropriate chapters, that highlights how scientists' understanding of what a gene is has changed over time. Since we cannot see genes, we must infer just what this unit of heredity is, based on experimental findings. By highlighting how scientists' conceptualization of the gene has advanced over time, we aim to help students appreciate the process of discovery that has led to an ever more sophisticated understanding of hereditary information.

- **Concept Question** A new feature, found as the second question in the Problems and Discussion Questions at the end of each chapter, asks the student to review and comment on common aspects of the Chapter Concepts, listed at the beginning of each chapter. This feature places added emphasis on our pedagogic approach of conceptual learning.

- **Neurogenetics** A major change that is evident in the Table of Contents involves Chapter 24. Previously entitled Behavior Genetics, this chapter has been reworked and redefined to reflect the wealth of information regarding the impact of genetics on the field of neurobiology, linking genetic analysis to brain function and brain disorders. Thus, the fully revised Chapter 24 is now entitled Neurogenetics.

- **MasteringGenetics** This robust online homework and assessment program guides students through complex topics in genetics, using in-depth tutorials that coach students to correct answers with hints and feedback specific to their misconceptions. New content for *Concepts of Genetics 11e* includes a library of Practice Problems that are like end of chapter questions and only appear in MasteringGenetics. These problems are not included in the Student Solution Manual and offer a valuable extension of questions available for assignments. These questions include wrong answer feedback to help students learn from their mistakes.

New and Updated Topics

While we have revised each chapter in the text to present the most current findings in genetics, below is a list of some of the most significant new and updated topics present in this edition.

Ch. 1: Introduction to Genetics
- New chapter introduction vignette emphasizing translational medicine

Ch. 3: Mendelian Genetics
- New Understanding Gene Function section: Identifying Mendel's Gene for Regulating White Flower Color in Peas
- New end-of-chapter problems based on Migaloo, the albino hump-backed whale

Ch. 7: Sex Determination and Sex Chromosomes
- New coverage on paternal age effects (PAEs) in humans
- New Understanding Gene Function section: *Drosophila Sxl* Gene Induces Female Development

Ch. 8: Chromosome Mutations: Variation in Number and Arrangement
- Updated coverage of fragile-X syndrome
- New Understanding Gene Function section: Mouse Models of Down Syndrome

Ch. 9: Extranuclear Inheritance
- New coverage on mitochondrial swapping and the prevention of mtDNA-based disorders

Ch. 11: DNA Replication and Recombination
- Updated coverage of DNA Pol III holoenzyme
- Revised figures involving DNA synthesis
- New coverage of the initiation of bacterial DNA synthesis
- New coverage of homologous recombination and gene conversion
- New coverage of replication of telomeric DNA
- New Understanding Gene Function section: Lethal Knockouts of DNA Ligase Genes

Ch. 12: DNA Organization in Chromosomes
- New coverage of kinetochore structure and function

Ch. 14: Translation and Proteins
- Revision of all ribosome figures

Ch. 15: Gene Mutation, DNA Repair, and Transposition
- New data on spontaneous mutation rates in humans.
- Reorganization and updates for mutation classification
- Updated coverage of xeroderma pigmentosum and DNA repair mechanisms
- New Understanding Gene Function section: Transposon-Mediated Mutations Reveal Genes Involved in Colorectal Cancer

Ch. 16: Regulation of Gene Expression in Prokaryotes
- Updated coverage of gene regulation by riboswitches

Ch. 17: Regulation of Gene Expression in Eukaryotes

- Expanded coverage of chromatin modifications
- Introduction of Weintraub and Groudine's experiments involving chromatin structure and transcription regulation
- Updated coverage of promoter and enhancer structures and functions
- Updated coverage of the mechanisms of transcription activation and repression
- Updated section on RNA silencing
- New section: ENCODE Data Are Transforming Our Concepts of Eukaryotic Gene Regulation
- New Understanding Gene Function section: MicroRNAs Regulate Ovulation in Female Mice

Ch. 18: Developmental Genetics

- New section: Binary Switch Genes and Signaling Pathways, including four new figures
- New Understanding Gene Function section: Single-Gene Signaling Mechanism Reveals Secrets to Head Regeneration in Planaria

Ch. 19: Cancer and Regulation of the Cell Cycle

- New coverage of the progressive nature of colorectal cancers
- Revised and updated coverage of driver and passenger mutations
- Expanded coverage of the role of viruses in human cancers

Ch. 20: Recombinant DNA Technology

- Expanded coverage and new figure on third-generation DNA sequencing
- New section on gene targeting that includes content and figures on gene knockout animals, conditional knockouts, and transgenic animals

Ch. 21: Genomics, Bioinformatics, and Proteomics

- Updated coverage of the Human Microbiome Project
- New content introducing exome sequencing
- Updated coverage of personal genome projects
- Revised and expanded coverage of the Encyclopedia of DNA Elements (ENCODE) Project
- New content and figure covering chromatin-immunoprecipitation (ChIP) and ChIP-sequencing (ChIPSeq)
- New Case Study discussing the microbiome as a risk factor for disease

Ch. 22: Applications and Ethics of Genetic Engineering and Biotechnology

- New section and figure on Synthetic Biology for Bioengineering Applications

- New coverage and figure on deducing fetal genome sequences from maternal blood
- Updated coverage of prenatal genetic testing
- Updated coverage of the minimal genome
- New coverage involving genetic analysis by sequencing individual genomes for clinical purposes and single-cell sequencing
- Revised ethics section to include additional discussion on the analysis of whole genome sequences, preconception testing, DNA patents, and destiny predictions
- Major revision of PDQ content and additional new questions
- New Genetics, Technology, and Society essay: Privacy and Anonymity of Genomic Data
- New Case Study on cancer-killing bacteria

Ch. 23: Quantitative Genetics and Multifactorial Traits

- Updated coverage of quantitative trait loci (QTL) in studying multifactorial phenotypes

Ch. 24: Neurogenetics

- Conversion of the Behavior Genetics chapter to one entitled Neurogenetics, with emphasis on molecular events in the brain and nervous system related to behavior. Includes 10 new figures and 3 new tables.
- New Understanding Gene Function section: *RbAp48* and a Potential Molecular Mechanism for Age-Related Memory Loss

Ch. 25: Population and Evolutionary Genetics

- New coverage on macroevolution and the rate of speciation
- Revision of the discussion of the molecular clock
- Two new sections: The Complex Origins of Our Genome and Our Genome Is a Mosaic

Special Topic Chapter 1: Epigenetics

- New section: MicroRNAs and Long Non-Coding RNAs

Special Topic Chapter 2: Emerging Roles of RNA

- New chapter on the newly discovered emerging roles of RNA—focuses on the diverse functions of RNAs with an emphasis on noncoding RNA

Special Topic Chapter 3: DNA Forensics

- New coverage describing how DNA can be inadvertently transferred to a crime scene, leading to false arrests
- New coverage of DNA phenotyping

Special Topic Chapter 4: Genomics and Personalized Medicine
- New coverage on personal genomics and cancer, including new story of one person's successful experience using "omics" profiling to select a personalized cancer treatment
- Updated coverage of personalized medicine and disease diagnostics
- Updated coverage of recent studies using "omics" profiles to predict and monitor disease states

Special Topic Chapter 5: Genetically Modified Foods
- New chapter on genetically modified foods—the genetic technology behind them, the promises, debates, and controversies

Special Topic Chapter 6: Gene Therapy
- New chapter on the modern aspects of gene therapy—provides up-to-date applications of gene therapy in humans

Glossary
- Many definitions refined
- Approximately two dozen new terms

Emphasis on Concepts

The title of our textbook—*Concepts of Genetics*—was purposefully chosen, reflecting our fundamental pedagogic approach to teaching and writing about genetics. However, the word "concept" is not as easy to define as one might think. Most simply put, we consider a concept to be a cognitive unit of meaning—an abstract representation that encompasses a related set of scientifically derived findings and ideas. Thus, a concept provides a broad mental image which, for example, might reflect a straightforward snapshot in your mind's eye of what constitutes a chromosome, a dynamic vision of the detailed processes of replication, transcription, and translation of genetic information, or just an abstract perception of varying modes of inheritance.

We think that creating such mental imagery is the very best way to teach science, in this case, genetics. Details that might be memorized, but soon forgotten, are instead subsumed within a conceptual framework that is easily retained. Such a framework may be expanded in content as new information is acquired and may interface with other concepts, providing a useful mechanism to integrate and better understand related processes and ideas. An extensive set of concepts may be devised and conveyed to eventually encompass and represent an entire discipline—and this is our goal in this genetics textbook.

To aid students in identifying the conceptual aspects of a major topic, each chapter begins with a section called *Chapter Concepts*, which identifies the most important ideas about to be presented. Each chapter ends with a section called *Summary Points*, which enumerates the five to ten key points that have been discussed. And in the *How Do We Know?* question that starts each chapter's problem set, students are asked to connect concepts to experimental findings. This question is then followed by a feature new to this edition called *Concept Question*, which, asks the student to review and comment on common aspects of the Chapter Concepts. Collectively, these features help to ensure that students easily become aware of and understand the major conceptual issues as they confront the extensive vocabulary and the many important details of genetics. Carefully designed figures also support this approach throughout the book.

Strengths of This Edition

- **Organization**—We have continued to attend to the organization of material by arranging chapters within major sections to reflect changing trends in genetics. Of particular note is Part IV, which combines the chapter providing foundational coverage of Recombinant DNA Technology with two chapters involving Genomics.

- **Pedagogy**—As discussed above, one of the major pedagogic goals of this edition is to provide features within each chapter that small groups of students can use either in the classroom or as assignments outside of class. Pedagogic research continues to support the value and effectiveness of such *active and cooperative learning experiences*. To this end, there are five features that greatly strengthen this edition.
  - **Case Study** This feature, at the end of each chapter, introduces a short vignette (a "Case") of an everyday encounter related to genetics, followed by a series of discussion questions. Use of the Case Study should prompt students to relate their newly acquired information in genetics to issues that they may encounter away from the course.
  - **Genetics, Technology, and Society** This feature provides a synopsis of a topic related to a current finding in genetics that impacts directly on our current society. It now includes a new section called *Your Turn*, which directs students to related resources of short readings and Web sites to support deeper investigation and discussion of the main topic of each essay.
  - **Exploring Genomics** This feature extends the discussion of selected topics present in the chapter by exploring new findings resulting from genomic studies. Students are directed to Web sites that provide the "tools" that research scientists around the world rely on for current genomic information.

Whether instructors use these activities as active learning in the classroom or as assigned interactions outside of class, the above features will stimulate the use of current pedagogic approaches to students' learning. The activities help engage students, and the content of each feature ensures that they will become knowledgeable about cutting-edge topics in genetics.

Emphasis on Problem Solving

As authors and teachers, we have always recognized the importance of teaching students how to become effective problem solvers. Students need guidance and practice if they are to develop strong analytical thinking skills. To that end, we present a suite of features in every chapter to optimize opportunities for student growth in the important areas of problem solving and analytical thinking.

- **Now Solve This** Found several times within the text of each chapter, each entry provides a problem similar to those found at the end of the chapter that is closely related to the current text discussion. In each case, a pedagogic hint is provided to offer insight and to aid in solving the problem. This feature closely links the text discussion to the problem.

- **Insights and Solutions** As an aid to the student in learning to solve problems, the *Problems and Discussion Questions* section of each chapter is preceded by what has become an extremely popular and successful section. *Insights and Solutions* poses problems or questions and provides detailed solutions or analytical insights as answers are provided. The questions and their solutions are designed to stress problem solving, quantitative analysis, analytical thinking, and experimental rationale. Collectively, these constitute the cornerstone of scientific inquiry and discovery.

- **Problems and Discussion Questions** Each chapter ends with an extensive collection of *Problems and Discussion Questions*. These include several levels of difficulty, with the most challenging (*Extra-Spicy Problems*) located at the end of each section. Often, Extra-Spicy Problems are derived from the current literature of genetic research, with citations. Brief answers to all even-numbered problems are presented in Appendix B. The *Student Handbook and Solutions Manual* answers every problem and is available to students whenever faculty decide that it is appropriate.

- **How Do We Know?** Appearing as the first entry in the *Problems and Discussion Questions* section, this question asks the student to identify and examine the experimental basis underlying important concepts and conclusions that have been presented in the chapter. Addressing these questions will aid the student in more fully understanding, rather than memorizing, the end-point of each body of research. This feature is an extension of the learning approach in biology first formally descibed by John A. Moore in his 1999 book *Science as a Way of Knowing—The Foundation of Modern Biology*.

- **MasteringGenetics** Tutorials in MasteringGenetics help students strengthen their problem-solving skills while exploring challenging activities about key genetics content. In addition, end-of-chapter problems are also available for instructors to assign as online homework. Students will also be able to access materials in the Study Area that help them assess their understanding and prepare for exams.

For the Instructor

MasteringGenetics— http://www.masteringgenetics.com

MasteringGenetics engages and motivates students to learn and allows you to easily assign automatically graded activities. Tutorials provide students with personalized coaching and feedback. Using the gradebook, you can quickly monitor and display student results. MasteringGenetics easily captures data to demonstrate assessment outcomes. Resources include:

- In-depth tutorials that coach students with hints and feedback specific to their misconceptions

- An item library of thousands of assignable questions including end of chapter problems, reading quizzes, and test bank items. You can use publisher-created prebuilt assignments to get started quickly. Each question can be easily edited to match the precise language you use.

- A new category of Practice Problems are like end of chapter questions in scope and level of difficulty and are found only in MasteringGenetics. Solutions are not available in the Student Solutions Manual, and the bank of questions extends your options for assigning challenging problems. Each problem includes specific wrong answer feedback to help students learn from their mistakes and to guide them toward the correct answer.

- A gradebook that provides you with quick results and easy-to-interpret insights into student performance

Instructor Resource DVD
(032175400X)

The Instructor Resource DVD for the 10th edition offers adopters of the text convenient access to the most comprehensive and innovative set of lecture presentation and teaching tools offered by any genetics textbook. Developed to meet the needs of veteran and newer instructors alike, these resources include:

- The JPEG files of all text line drawings with labels individually enhanced for optimal projection results (as well as unlabeled versions) and all text tables.

- Most of the text photos, including all photos with pedagogical significance, as JPEG files.

- The JPEG files of line drawings, photos, and tables preloaded into comprehensive PowerPoint® presentations for each chapter.

- A second set of PowerPoint® presentations consisting of a thorough lecture outline for each chapter augmented by key text illustrations.

- An impressive series of concise instructor animations adding depth and visual clarity to the most important topics and dynamic processes described in the text.

- The instructor animations preloaded into PowerPoint® presentation files for each chapter.

- PowerPoint® presentations containing a comprehensive set of in-class Classroom Response System (CRS) questions for each chapter.

- In Word files, a complete set of the assessment materials and study questions and answers from the testbank.

TestGen EQ Computerized Testing Software
(0321754344)

Test questions are available as part of the TestGen EQ Testing Software, a text-specific testing program that is networkable for administering tests. It also allows instructors to view and edit questions, export the questions as tests, and print them out in a variety of formats.

For the Student

Student Handbook and Solutions Manual
Authored by Harry Nickla, Creighton University (Emeritus) (0321754425)

This valuable handbook provides a detailed step-by-step solution or lengthy discussion for every problem in the text. The handbook also features additional study aids, including extra study problems, chapter outlines, vocabulary exercises, and an overview of how to study genetics.

MasteringGenetics—
http://www.masteringgenetics.com
Used by over one million science students, the Mastering platform is the most effective and widely used online tutorial, homework, and assessment system for the sciences; it helps students perform better on homework and exams. As an instructor-assigned homework system, MasteringGenetics is designed to provide students with a variety of assessment tools to help them understand key topics and concepts and to build problem-solving skills. MasteringGenetics tutorials guide students through the toughest topics in genetics with self-paced tutorials that provide individualized coaching with hints and feedback specific to a student's individual misconceptions. Students can also explore the MasteringGenetics Study Area, which includes animations, the eText, *Exploring Genomics* exercises, and other study aids. The interactive eText allows students to highlight text, add study notes, review instructor's notes, and search throughout the text.

Acknowledgments
Contributors
We begin with special acknowledgments to those who have made direct contributions to this text. Foremost, we are pleased to thank Dr. Darrell Killian of Colorado College for writing the Special Topic chapter on Emerging Roles of RNA. We much appreciate this important contribution. We also thank Jutta Heller of the University of Washington—Tacoma, Christopher Halweg of North Carolina State University, Pamela Osenkowski of Loyola University—Chicago, and John Osterman of the University of Nebraska—Lincoln for their work on the media program. Virginia McDonough of Hope College provided invaluable feedback on our new feature, Modern Approaches to Understanding Gene Function, as well as contributing to the instructor resources along with Cindy Malone of California State University—Northridge. We also express special thanks to Harry Nickla, recently retired from Creighton University. In his role as author of the *Student Handbook and Solutions Manual* and the test bank, he has reviewed and edited the problems at the end of each chapter and has written many of the new entries as well. He also provided the brief answers to selected problems that appear in Appendix B.

We are grateful to all of these contributors not only for sharing their genetic expertise, but for their dedication to this project as well as the pleasant interactions they provided.

Proofreaders and Accuracy Checking
Reading the manuscript of an 800+ page textbook deserves more thanks than words can offer. Our utmost appreciation is extended to Mary Colavito, *Santa Monica College*; David Kass, *Eastern Michigan University*; Kirkwood Land, *University of the Pacific*; Te-Wen Lo, *Ithaca College*; Pamela Osenkowski, *Loyola University—Chicago*; John Osterman, *University of Nebraska—Lincoln*; and Adam Sowalsky, *Northeastern University*, who provided accuracy checking of many chapters, and to Joanna Dinsmore, who proofread the entire manuscript. They confronted this task with patience and diligence, contributing greatly to the quality of this text.

Reviewers

All comprehensive texts are dependent on the valuable input provided by many reviewers. While we take full responsibility for any errors in this book, we gratefully acknowledge the help provided by those individuals who reviewed the content and pedagogy of this edition:

Soochin Cho, *Creighton University*
Mary Colavito, *Santa Monica College*
Edison Fowlks, *Hampton University*
Yvette Gardner, *Clayton State University*
Theresa Geiman, *Loyola University—Maryland*
Christopher Harendza, *Montgomery County Community College*
Lucinda Jack, *University of Maryland*
David Kass, *Eastern Michigan University*
Kirkwood Land, *University of the Pacific*
Te-Wen Lo, *Ithaca College*
Virginia McDonough, *Hope College*
Amy McMIllan, *SUNY Buffalo State*
Sanghamitra Mohanty, *University of Texas—Austin*
Sudhir Nayak, *The College of the New Jersey*
Pamela Osenkowski, *Loyola University—Chicago*
John Osterman, *University of Nebraska—Lincoln*
Pamela Sandstrom, *Unviersity of Nevada—Reno*
Adam Sowalsky, *Northeastern University*
James D. Tucker, *Wayne State University*
Jonathan Visick, *North Central College*
Fang-Sheng Wu, *Virginia Commonwealth University*

Special thanks go to Mike Guidry of LightCone Interactive and Karen Hughes of the University of Tennessee for their original contributions to the media program.

As these acknowledgments make clear, a text such as this is a collective enterprise. All of the above individuals deserve to share in any success this text enjoys. We want them to know that our gratitude is equaled only by the extreme dedication evident in their efforts. Many, many thanks to them all.

Editorial and Production Input

At Pearson, we express appreciation and high praise for the editorial guidance of Michael Gillespie, whose ideas and efforts have helped to shape and refine the features of this edition of the text. Dusty Friedman, our Project Editor, has worked tirelessly to keep the project on schedule and to maintain our standards of high quality. In addition, our editorial team—Deborah Gale, Executive Director of Development, Daniel Ross, Senior Media Producer, and Tania Mlawer, Director of Editorial Content for MasteringGenetics—have provided valuable input into the current edition. They have worked creatively to ensure that the pedagogy and design of the book and media package are at the cutting edge of a rapidly changing discipline. Sudhir Nayak of The College of New Jersey provided outstanding work for the MasteringGenetics program and his input regarding genomics is much appreciated. Lori Newman and Rose Kernan supervised all of the production intricacies with great attention to detail and perseverance. Outstanding copyediting was performed by Betty Pessagno, for which we are most grateful. Lauren Harp has professionally and enthusiastically managed the marketing of the text. Finally, the beauty and consistent presentation of the art work are the product of Imagineering of Toronto. Without the work ethic and dedication of the above individuals, the text would never have come to fruition.

Newer model organisms in genetics include the roundworm *Caenorhabditis elegans*, the zebrafish, *Danio rerio*, and the mustard plant *Arabidopsis thaliana*.

1 Introduction to Genetics

CHAPTER CONCEPTS

- Genetics in the twenty-first century is built on a rich tradition of discovery and experimentation stretching from the ancient world through the nineteenth century to the present day.

- Transmission genetics is the general process by which traits controlled by genes are transmitted through gametes from generation to generation.

- Mutant strains can be used in genetic crosses to map the location and distance between genes on chromosomes.

- The Watson–Crick model of DNA structure explains how genetic information is stored and expressed. This discovery is the foundation of molecular genetics.

- Recombinant DNA technology revolutionized genetics, was the foundation for the Human Genome Project, and has generated new fields that combine genetics with information technology.

- Biotechnology provides genetically modified organisms and their products that are used across a wide range of fields including agriculture, medicine, and industry.

- Model organisms used in genetics research are now utilized in combination with recombinant DNA technology and genomics to study human diseases.

- Genetic technology is developing faster than the policies, laws, and conventions that govern its use.

Information from the Human Genome Project and other areas of genetics is beginning to have far-reaching effects on our daily lives. For example, researchers and clinicians are using this information to improve the quality of medical care via **translational medicine,** a process in which genetic findings are directly "translated" into new and improved methods of diagnosis and treatment. An important area of focus is cardiovascular disease, which is the leading cause of death worldwide. One of the key risk factors for development of this condition is the presence of elevated blood levels of "bad" cholesterol (low-density lipoprotein cholesterol, or LDL cholesterol). Although statin drugs are effective in lowering the blood levels of LDL cholesterol and reducing the risk of heart disease, up to 50 percent of treated individuals remain at risk, and serious side-effects prevent others from using these drugs.

To gain a share of the estimated $25 billion market for treatment of elevated LDL levels, major pharmaceutical firms are developing a new generation of more effective cholesterol-lowering drugs. However, bringing a new drug to market is risky. Costs can run over $1 billion, and many drugs (up to 1 in 3) fail clinical trials and are withdrawn. In the search for a new strategy in drug development, human genetics is playing an increasingly vital role. Blood levels of LDL in a population vary over a threefold range, and about 50 percent of this variation is genetic. Although many genes are involved, the role of one gene, *PCSK9*, in controlling LDL levels is an outstanding example of how a genetic approach has been successful in identifying drug targets and improving the chance that a new drug will be successful. The rapid transfer of basic research on *PCSK9* to drug development and its use in treating patients is a pioneering example of translational medicine.

Soon after the *PCSK9* gene was identified, mutant forms of this gene were found to be associated with extremely high levels of LDL cholesterol, resulting in a condition called familial hypercholesterolemia (FH). When this work came to the attention of researchers in Texas, they wondered whether other mutations in *PCSK9* might have the opposite effect and drastically lower LDL cholesterol levels. To test this idea, they turned to data from the Dallas Heart Study, which collected detailed clinical information, including LDL levels and DNA samples, from 3500 individuals. DNA sequencing of *PSCK9* from participants with extremely low LDL levels identified two mutations that reduced blood levels of LDL by 40 percent. Other work showed that carriers of these mutations had an 88 percent lower risk of heart disease.

Research established that the PCSK9 protein binds to LDL receptors on liver cells, moving the receptors into the cell where they are broken down. Carriers of either of the two mutations have much lower PCSK9 protein levels. As a result, liver cells in these individuals have many more LDL receptors, which, in turn, remove more LDL from the blood. Using this information, pharmaceutical firms developed an antibody-based drug that binds to the PCKS9 protein and prevents its interaction with LDL receptors, which, in turn, lowers LDL cholesterol levels. Successful clinical trials show that this drug reduces LDL blood levels up to 70 percent in the test population; if further rounds of testing are successful, the drug will be on the market in the near future.

Whatever the outcome in the case of *PCKS9*, it is clear that coupling genetic research with drug development will play a critical and exciting role in speeding the movement of research findings into medical practice.

This introductory chapter provides an overview of genetics and a survey of the high points in its history and gives a preliminary description of its central principles and emerging developments. All the topics discussed in this chapter will be explored in far greater detail elsewhere in the book. This text will enable you to achieve a thorough understanding of modern-day genetics and its underlying principles. Along the way, enjoy your studies, but take your responsibilities as a novice geneticist very seriously.

1.1 Genetics Has a Rich and Interesting History

We don't know when people first recognized the hereditary nature of certain traits, but archaeological evidence (e.g., pictorial representations, preserved bones and skulls,

and dried seeds) documents the successful domestication of animals and the cultivation of plants thousands of years ago by the artificial selection of genetic variants from wild populations. Between 8000 and 1000 B.C., horses, camels, oxen, and wolves were domesticated, and selective breeding of these species soon followed. Cultivation of many plants, including maize, wheat, rice, and the date palm, began around 5000 B.C. Such evidence documents our ancestors' successful attempts to manipulate the genetic composition of species.

During the Golden Age of Greek culture, the writings of the Hippocratic School of Medicine (500–400 B.C.) and of the philosopher and naturalist Aristotle (384–322 B.C.) discussed heredity as it relates to humans. The Hippocratic treatise *On the Seed* argued that active "humors" in various parts of the body served as the bearers of hereditary traits. Drawn from various parts of the male body to the semen and passed on to offspring, these humors could be healthy or diseased, with the diseased humors accounting for the appearance of newborns with congenital disorders or deformities. It was also believed that these humors could be altered in individuals before they were passed on to offspring, explaining how newborns could "inherit" traits that their parents had "acquired" in response to their environment.

Aristotle extended Hippocrates' thinking and proposed that the male semen contained a "vital heat" with the capacity to produce offspring of the same "form" (i.e., basic structure and capacities) as the parent. Aristotle believed that this heat cooked and shaped the menstrual blood produced by the female, which was the "physical substance" that gave rise to an offspring. The embryo developed not because it already contained the parts of an adult in miniature form (as some Hippocratics had thought) but because of the shaping power of the vital heat. Although the ideas of Hippocrates and Aristotle sound primitive and naive today, we should recall that prior to the 1800s neither sperm nor eggs had been observed in mammals.

1600–1850: The Dawn of Modern Biology

Between about 300 B.C. and 1600 A.D., there were few significant new ideas about genetics. However, between 1600 and 1850, major strides provided insight into the biological basis of life. In the 1600s, William Harvey studied reproduction and development and proposed the theory of **epigenesis**, which states that an organism develops from the fertilized egg by a succession of developmental events that eventually transform the egg into an adult. The theory of epigenesis directly conflicted with the theory of **preformation**, which stated that the fertilized egg contains a complete miniature adult, called a **homunculus (Figure 1–1)**. Around 1830, Matthias Schleiden and Theodor Schwann proposed the **cell theory**, stating that all organisms are composed of

© 1964 National Library of Medicine

FIGURE 1–1 Depiction of the *homunculus,* a sperm containing a miniature adult, perfect in proportion and fully formed.
(Hartsoeker, N. Essay de dioptrique Paris, 1694, p. 230. National Library of Medicine)

basic structural units called cells, which are derived from preexisting cells. The idea of **spontaneous generation,** the creation of living organisms from nonliving components, was disproved by Louis Pasteur later in the century, and living organisms were then considered to be derived from preexisting organisms and to consist of cells.

In the mid-1800s the revolutionary work of Charles Darwin and Gregor Mendel set the stage for the rapid development of genetics in the twentieth and twenty-first centuries.

Charles Darwin and Evolution

With this background, we turn to a brief discussion of the work of Charles Darwin, who published *The Origin of Species*, in 1859, describing his ideas about evolution. Darwin's geological, geographical, and biological observations convinced him that existing species arose by descent with modification from ancestral species. Greatly influenced by his voyage on the HMS *Beagle* (1831–1836), Darwin's thinking led him to formulate the theory of **natural selection,** which presented an explanation of the mechanism of evolutionary change. Formulated and proposed independently by Alfred Russel Wallace, natural selection is based on the observation that populations tend to contain more offspring than the environment can support, leading to a struggle for survival among individuals. Those individuals with heritable traits that allow them to adapt to their environment are better able to survive and reproduce than those with less adaptive traits. Over a long period of time, advantageous variations, even very slight ones, will accumulate. If a population carrying these inherited variations becomes reproductively isolated, a new species may result.

Darwin, however, lacked an understanding of the genetic basis of variation and inheritance, a gap that left his theory open to reasonable criticism well into the twentieth century. Shortly after Darwin published his book, Gregor Johann Mendel published a paper in 1866 showing how traits were passed from generation to generation in pea plants and offering a general model of how traits are inherited. His research was little known until it was partially duplicated and brought to light by Carl Correns, Hugo de Vries, and Erich Tschermak around 1900.

By the early part of the twentieth century, it became clear that heredity and development were dependent on genetic information residing in genes contained in chromosomes, which were then contributed to each individual by gametes—the so-called **chromosomal theory of inheritance.** The gap in Darwin's theory was closed, and Mendel's research has continued to serve as the foundation of genetics.

1.2 Genetics Progressed from Mendel to DNA in Less Than a Century

Because genetic processes are fundamental to life itself, the science of genetics unifies biology and serves as its core. The starting point for this branch of science was a monastery garden in central Europe in the late 1850s.

Mendel's Work on Transmission of Traits

Gregor Mendel, an Augustinian monk, conducted a decade-long series of experiments using pea plants. He applied quantitative data analysis to his results and showed that traits are passed from parents to offspring in predictable ways. He further concluded that each trait in the plant is controlled by a pair of factors (which we now call genes) and that during gamete formation (the formation of egg cells and sperm), members of a gene pair separate from each other. His work was published in 1866 but was largely unknown until it was cited in papers published by others around 1900. Once confirmed, Mendel's findings became recognized as explaining the transmission of traits in pea plants and all other higher organisms. His work forms the foundation for **genetics,** which is defined as the branch of biology concerned with the study of heredity and variation. Mendelian genetics will be discussed later in the text (see Chapters 3 and 4).

FIGURE 1–2 A colorized image of human chromosomes that have duplicated in preparation for cell division, as visualized under the scanning electron microscope.

The Chromosome Theory of Inheritance: Uniting Mendel and Meiosis

Mendel did his experiments before the structure and role of chromosomes were known. About 20 years after his work was published, advances in microscopy allowed researchers to identify chromosomes (**Figure 1–2**) and establish that, in most eukaryotes, members of each species have a characteristic number of chromosomes called the **diploid number (2n)** in most of their cells. For example, humans have a diploid number of 46 (**Figure 1–3**). Chromosomes in diploid cells exist in pairs, called **homologous chromosomes.**

Researchers in the last decades of the nineteenth century also described chromosome behavior during two forms of cell division, **mitosis** and **meiosis.** In mitosis (**Figure 1–4**), chromosomes are copied and distributed so that each daughter cell receives a diploid set of chromosomes identical to those in the parental cell. Meiosis is associated with gamete formation. Cells produced by meiosis receive only one chromosome from each chromosome pair, and the resulting number of chromosomes is called the **haploid (n) number.** This reduction in chromosome number is essential if the offspring arising from the fusion of egg and sperm are to maintain the constant number of chromosomes characteristic of their parents and other members of their species.

Early in the twentieth century, Walter Sutton and Theodor Boveri independently noted that the behavior of chromosomes during meiosis is identical to the behavior of genes during gamete formation described by Mendel. For example, genes and chromosomes exist in pairs, and members of a gene pair and members of a chromosome pair separate from each other during gamete formation. Based on these parallels, Sutton and Boveri each proposed that genes are carried on chromosomes (**Figure 1–5**). They independently formulated the **chromosome theory of inheritance,** which states that inherited traits are controlled by genes residing on chromosomes

FIGURE 1–3 A colorized image of the human male chromosome set. Arranged in this way, the set is called a karyotype.

faithfully transmitted through gametes, maintaining genetic continuity from generation to generation.

Genetic Variation

About the same time that the chromosome theory of inheritance was proposed, scientists began studying the inheritance of traits in the fruit fly, *Drosophila melanogaster.* Early

FIGURE 1–4 A late stage in mitosis after the chromosomes (stained blue) have separated.

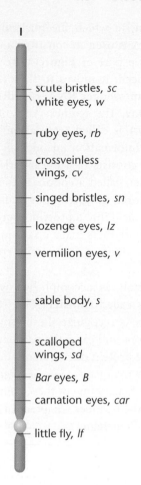

scute bristles, *sc*
white eyes, *w*

ruby eyes, *rb*

crossveinless
wings, *cv*

singed bristles, *sn*

lozenge eyes, *lz*

vermilion eyes, *v*

sable body, *s*

scalloped
wings, *sd*

Bar eyes, *B*

carnation eyes, *car*

little fly, *lf*

FIGURE 1–5 A drawing of chromosome I (the X chromosome, one of the sex-determining chromosomes) of *D. melanogaster,* showing the location of several genes. Chromosomes can contain hundreds of genes.

in this work, a white-eyed fly **(Figure 1–6)** was discovered among normal (wild-type) red-eyed flies. This variation was produced by a **mutation** in one of the genes controlling eye color. Mutations are defined as any heritable change in the DNA sequence and are the source of all genetic variation.

The white-eye variant discovered in *Drosophila* is an **allele** of a gene controlling eye color. Alleles are defined as alternative forms of a gene. Different alleles may produce differences in the observable features, or **phenotype,** of an organism. The set of alleles for a given trait carried by an organism is called the **genotype.** Using mutant genes as markers, geneticists can map the location of genes on chromosomes (Figure 1–5).

The Search for the Chemical Nature of Genes: DNA or Protein?

Work on white-eyed *Drosophila* showed that the mutant trait could be traced to a single chromosome, confirming the idea that genes are carried on chromosomes. Once this relationship was established, investigators turned their attention to identifying which chemical component of chromosomes

FIGURE 1–6 The white-eyed mutation in *D. melanogaster* (top) and the normal red eye color (bottom).

carries genetic information. By the 1920s, scientists knew that proteins and DNA were the major chemical components of chromosomes. There are a large number of different proteins, and because of their universal distribution in the nucleus and cytoplasm, many researchers thought proteins were the carriers of genetic information.

In 1944, Oswald Avery, Colin MacLeod, and Maclyn McCarty, researchers at the Rockefeller Institute in New York, published experiments showing that DNA was the carrier of genetic information in bacteria. This evidence, though clear-cut, failed to convince many influential scientists. Additional evidence for the role of DNA as a carrier of genetic information came from other researchers who worked with viruses. This evidence that DNA carries genetic information, along with other research over the next few years, provided solid proof that DNA, not protein, is the genetic material, setting the stage for work to establish the structure of DNA.

1.3 Discovery of the Double Helix Launched the Era of Molecular Genetics

Once it was accepted that DNA carries genetic information, efforts were focused on deciphering the structure of the DNA molecule and the mechanism by which information stored in it produces a phenotype.

- Sugar (deoxyribose)
- Nucleotide
- Phosphate

Complementary base pair (thymine-adenine)

FIGURE 1–7 Summary of the structure of DNA, illustrating the arrangement of the double helix (on the left) and the chemical components making up each strand (on the right). The dotted lines on the right represent weak chemical bonds, called hydrogen bonds, which hold together the two strands of the DNA helix.

The Structure of DNA and RNA

One of the great discoveries of the twentieth century was made in 1953 by James Watson and Francis Crick, who described the structure of DNA. DNA is a long, ladder-like macromolecule that twists to form a double helix (**Figure 1–7**). Each linear strand of the helix is made up of subunits called **nucleotides.** In DNA, there are four different nucleotides, each of which contains a nitrogenous base, abbreviated A (adenine), G (guanine), T (thymine), or C (cytosine). These four bases, in various sequence combinations, ultimately encode genetic information. The two strands of DNA are exact complements of one another, so that the rungs of the ladder in the double helix always consist of A=T and G=C base pairs. Along with Maurice Wilkins, Watson and Crick were awarded a Nobel Prize in 1962 for their work on the structure of DNA. We will discuss the structure of DNA later in the text (see Chapter 9).

Another nucleic acid, RNA, is chemically similar to DNA but contains a different sugar (ribose rather than deoxyribose) in its nucleotides and contains the nitrogenous base uracil in place of thymine. RNA, however, is generally a single-stranded molecule.

Gene Expression: From DNA to Phenotype

The genetic information encoded in the order of nucleotides in DNA is expressed in a series of steps that results in the formation of a functional gene product. In the majority of cases, this product is a protein. In eukaryotic cells, the process leading to protein production begins in the nucleus

with **transcription,** in which the nucleotide sequence in one strand of DNA is used to construct a complementary RNA sequence (top part of **Figure 1–8**). Once an RNA molecule is produced, it moves to the cytoplasm, where the RNA—called **messenger RNA,** or **mRNA** for short—binds to a **ribosome.** The synthesis of proteins under the direction of mRNA is called **translation** (center part of Figure 1–8). The information encoded in mRNA (called the **genetic code**) consists of a linear series of nucleotide triplets. Each triplet, called a **codon,** is complementary to the information stored in DNA and specifies the insertion of a specific amino acid into a protein. Proteins (lower part of Figure 1–8) are polymers made up of amino acid monomers. There are 20 different amino acids commonly found in proteins.

Protein assembly is accomplished with the aid of adapter molecules called **transfer RNA (tRNA).** Within the ribosome, tRNAs recognize the information encoded in the mRNA codons and carry the proper amino acids for construction of the protein during translation.

We now know that gene expression can be more complex than outlined here. Some of these complexities will be discussed later in the text (see Chapters 14, 17, and Special Topic Chapter 1—Epigenetics).

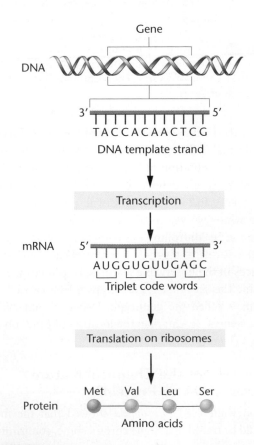

FIGURE 1–8 Gene expression consists of transcription of DNA into mRNA (top) and the translation (center) of mRNA (with the help of a ribosome) into a protein (bottom).

Proteins and Biological Function

In most cases, proteins are the end products of gene expression. The diversity of proteins and the biological functions they perform—the diversity of life itself—arises from the fact that proteins are made from combinations of 20 different amino acids. Consider that a protein chain containing 100 amino acids can have at each position any one of 20 amino acids; the number of possible different 100 amino acid proteins, each with a unique sequence, is therefore equal to

$$20^{100}$$

Obviously, proteins are molecules with the potential for enormous structural diversity and serve as the mainstay of biological systems.

Enzymes form the largest category of proteins. These molecules serve as biological catalysts, lowering the energy of activation in reactions and allowing cellular metabolism to proceed at body temperature.

Proteins other than enzymes are critical components of cells and organisms. These include hemoglobin, the oxygen-binding molecule in red blood cells; insulin, a pancreatic hormone; collagen, a connective tissue molecule; and actin and myosin, the contractile muscle proteins. A protein's shape and chemical behavior are determined by its linear sequence of amino acids, which in turn are dictated by the stored information in the DNA of a gene that is transferred to RNA, which then directs the protein's synthesis.

Linking Genotype to Phenotype: Sickle-Cell Anemia

Once a protein is made, its biochemical or structural properties play a role in producing a phenotype. When mutation alters a gene, it may modify or even eliminate the encoded protein's usual function and cause an altered phenotype. To trace this chain of events, we will examine sickle-cell anemia, a human genetic disorder.

Sickle-cell anemia is caused by a mutant form of hemoglobin, the protein that transports oxygen from the lungs to cells in the body. Hemoglobin is a composite molecule made up of two different proteins, α-globin and β-globin, each encoded by a different gene. In sickle-cell anemia, a mutation in the gene encoding β-globin causes an amino acid substitution in 1 of the 146 amino acids in the protein. **Figure 1–9** shows the DNA sequence, the corresponding mRNA codons, and the amino acids occupying positions 4–7 for the normal and mutant forms of β-globin. Notice that the mutation in sickle-cell anemia consists of a change in one DNA nucleotide, which leads to a change in codon 6 in mRNA from GAG to GUG, which in turn changes amino acid number 6 in β-globin from glutamic acid to valine. The other 145 amino acids in the protein are not changed by this mutation.

FIGURE 1–9 A single-nucleotide change in the DNA encoding β-globin (CTC→CAC) leads to an altered mRNA codon (GAG→GUG) and the insertion of a different amino acid (Glu→Val), producing the altered version of the β-globin protein that is responsible for sickle-cell anemia.

Individuals with two mutant copies of the β-globin gene have sickle-cell anemia. Their mutant β-globin proteins cause hemoglobin molecules in red blood cells to polymerize when the blood's oxygen concentration is low, forming long chains of hemoglobin that distort the shape of red blood cells (**Figure 1–10**). The deformed cells are fragile and break easily, reducing the number of red blood cells in circulation (anemia is an insufficiency of red blood cells). Sickle-shaped blood cells block blood flow in capillaries and small blood vessels, causing severe pain and damage to the heart, brain, muscles, and kidneys. All the symptoms of this disorder are caused by a change in a single nucleotide in a gene that changes one amino acid out of 146 in the β-globin molecule, demonstrating the close relationship between genotype and phenotype.

FIGURE 1–10 Normal red blood cells (round) and sickled red blood cells. The sickled cells block capillaries and small blood vessels.

1.4 Development of Recombinant DNA Technology Began the Era of DNA Cloning

The era of recombinant DNA began in the early 1970s, when researchers discovered that **restriction enzymes,** used by bacteria to cut the DNA of invading viruses, could be used to cut any organism's DNA at specific nucleotide sequences, producing a reproducible set of fragments.

Soon after, researchers discovered ways to insert the DNA fragments produced by the action of restriction enzymes into carrier DNA molecules called **vectors** to form **recombinant DNA** molecules. When transferred into bacterial cells, thousands of copies, or **clones,** of the combined vector and DNA fragments are produced during bacterial reproduction. Large amounts of cloned DNA fragments can be isolated from these bacterial host cells. These DNA fragments can be used to isolate genes, to study their organization and expression, and to study their nucleotide sequence and evolution.

Collections of clones that represent an organism's **genome,** defined as the complete haploid DNA content of a specific organism, are called genomic libraries. Genomic libraries are now available for hundreds of species.

Recombinant DNA technology has not only accelerated the pace of research but also given rise to the biotechnology industry, which has grown to become a major contributor to the U.S. economy.

FIGURE 1–11 Dolly, a Finn Dorset sheep cloned from the genetic material of an adult mammary cell, shown next to her first-born lamb, Bonnie.

1.5 The Impact of Biotechnology Is Continually Expanding

The use of recombinant DNA technology and other molecular techniques to make products is called **biotechnology.** In the United States, biotechnology has quietly revolutionized many aspects of everyday life; products made by biotechnology are now found in the supermarket, in health care, in agriculture, and in the court system. A later chapter (see Chapter 19) contains a detailed discussion of biotechnology, but for now, let's look at some everyday examples of biotechnology's impact.

Plants, Animals, and the Food Supply

The use of recombinant DNA technology to genetically modify crop plants has revolutionized agriculture. Genes for traits including resistance to herbicides, insects, and genes for nutritional enhancement have been introduced into crop plants. The transfer of heritable traits across species using recombinant DNA technology creates **transgenic** organisms. Herbicide-resistant corn and soybeans were first planted in the mid-1990s, and transgenic strains now represent about 88 percent of the U.S. corn crop and 93 percent of the U.S. soybean crop. It is estimated that more than 70 percent of the processed food in the United States contains ingredients from transgenic crops.

We will discuss the most recent findings involving genetically modified organisms later in the text. (Special Topic Chapter 5—Genetically Modified Organisms).

New methods of cloning livestock such as sheep and cattle have also changed the way we use these animals. In 1996, Dolly the sheep (**Figure 1–11**) was cloned by nuclear transfer, a method in which the nucleus of an adult cell is transferred into an egg that has had its nucleus removed. This method makes it possible to produce dozens or hundreds of genetically identical offspring with desirable traits and has many applications in agriculture, sports, and medicine.

Biotechnology has also changed the way human proteins for medical use are produced. Through use of gene transfer, transgenic animals now synthesize these therapeutic proteins. In 2009, an anticlotting protein derived from the milk of transgenic goats was approved by the U.S. Food and Drug Administration for use in the United States. Other human proteins from transgenic animals are now being used in clinical trials to treat several diseases. The biotechnology revolution will continue to expand as new methods are developed to make an increasing array of products.

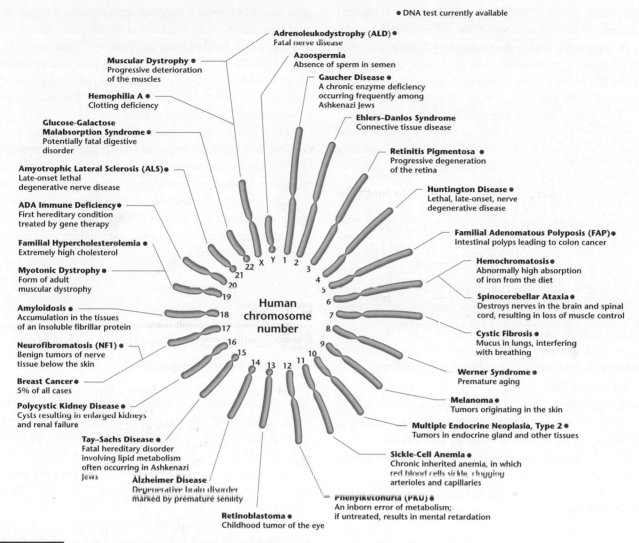

● DNA test currently available

Adrenoleukodystrophy (ALD) ●
Fatal nerve disease

Azoospermia
Absence of sperm in semen

Gaucher Disease ●
A chronic enzyme deficiency
occurring frequently among
Ashkenazi Jews

Ehlers–Danlos Syndrome ●
Connective tissue disease

Retinitis Pigmentosa ●
Progressive degeneration
of the retina

Huntington Disease ●
Lethal, late-onset, nerve
degenerative disease

Familial Adenomatous Polyposis (FAP) ●
Intestinal polyps leading to colon cancer

Hemochromatosis ●
Abnormally high absorption
of iron from the diet

Spinocerebellar Ataxia ●
Destroys nerves in the brain and spinal
cord, resulting in loss of muscle control

Cystic Fibrosis ●
Mucus in lungs, interfering
with breathing

Werner Syndrome ●
Premature aging

Melanoma ●
Tumors originating in the skin

Multiple Endocrine Neoplasia, Type 2 ●
Tumors in endocrine gland and other tissues

Sickle-Cell Anemia ●
Chronic inherited anemia, in which
red blood cells sickle, clogging
arterioles and capillaries

Phenylketonuria (PKU) ●
An inborn error of metabolism;
if untreated, results in mental retardation

Retinoblastoma ●
Childhood tumor of the eye

Alzheimer Disease
Degenerative brain disorder
marked by premature senility

Tay–Sachs Disease ●
Fatal hereditary disorder
involving lipid metabolism
often occurring in Ashkenazi
Jews

Polycystic Kidney Disease ●
Cysts resulting in enlarged kidneys
and renal failure

Breast Cancer ●
5% of all cases

Neurofibromatosis (NF1) ●
Benign tumors of nerve
tissue below the skin

Amyloidosis ●
Accumulation in the tissues
of an insoluble fibrillar protein

Myotonic Dystrophy ●
Form of adult
muscular dystrophy

Familial Hypercholesterolemia ●
Extremely high cholesterol

ADA Immune Deficiency ●
First hereditary condition
treated by gene therapy

Amyotrophic Lateral Sclerosis (ALS) ●
Late-onset lethal
degenerative nerve disease

**Glucose-Galactose
Malabsorption Syndrome** ●
Potentially fatal digestive
disorder

Hemophilia A ●
Clotting deficiency

Muscular Dystrophy ●
Progressive deterioration
of the muscles

Human chromosome number

FIGURE 1–12 The human chromosome set, showing the location of some genes whose mutant forms cause hereditary diseases. Conditions that can be diagnosed using genetic testing are indicated by a red dot.

Biotechnology in Genetics and Medicine

More than 10 million children or adults in the United States suffer from some form of genetic disorder, and every childbearing couple faces an approximately 3 percent risk of having a child with a genetic anomaly. The molecular basis for hundreds of genetic disorders is now known, and many of these genes have been mapped, isolated, and cloned (**Figure 1–12**). Biotechnology-derived genetic testing is now available to perform prenatal diagnosis of heritable disorders and to test parents for their status as "carriers" of more than 100 inherited disorders. Newer methods now under development offer the possibility of scanning an entire genome to establish an individual's risk of developing a genetic disorder or having an affected child. The use of genetic testing and related technologies raises ethical concerns that have yet to be resolved.

1.6 Genomics, Proteomics, and Bioinformatics Are New and Expanding Fields

The use of recombinant DNA technology to create genomic libraries prompted scientists to consider sequencing all the clones in a library to derive the nucleotide sequence of an organism's genome. This sequence information would be used to identify each gene in the genome and establish its function.

One such project, the Human Genome Project, began in 1990 as an international effort to sequence the human genome. By 2003, the publicly funded Human Genome Project and a private, industry-funded genome project completed sequencing of the gene-containing portion of the genome.

As more genome sequences were acquired, several new biological disciplines arose. One, called **genomics** (the study of genomes), studies the structure, function, and evolution of genes and genomes. A second field, **proteomics**, identifies the set of proteins present in a cell under a given set of conditions, and studies their functions and interactions. To store, retrieve, and analyze the massive amount of data generated by genomics and proteomics, a specialized subfield of information technology called **bioinformatics** was created to develop hardware and software for processing nucleotide and protein data.

Geneticists and other biologists now use information in databases containing nucleic acid sequences, protein sequences, and gene-interaction networks to answer experimental questions in a matter of minutes instead of months and years. A feature called "Exploring Genomics," located at the end of many of the chapters in this textbook, gives you the opportunity to explore these databases for yourself while completing an interactive genetics exercise.

Modern Approaches to Understanding Gene Function

New to this edition of *Concepts of Genetics* is "Modern Approaches to Understanding Gene Function." This feature appears in eight chapters and its purpose is to introduce you to examples of current experimental approaches that geneticists use to study gene function. Its location in selected chapters links experimental examples of understanding gene function to the concepts that have just been presented.

Historically, an approach referred to as **classical** or **forward genetics** was essential for studying and understanding gene function. In this approach geneticists relied on the use of naturally occurring mutations or they intentionally induced mutations (using chemicals, X-rays or UV light as examples) to cause altered phenotypes in model organisms, and then worked through the lab-intensive and time-consuming process of identifying the genes that caused these new phenotypes. Such characterization often led to the identification of the gene or genes of interest, and once the technology advanced, the gene sequence could be determined.

Classical genetics approaches are still used, but as whole genome sequencing has become routine, molecular approaches to understanding gene function have changed considerably in genetic research. These modern approaches are what we will highlight in this feature.

For the past two decades or so, geneticists have relied on the use of molecular techniques incorporating an approach referred to as **reverse genetics**. In reverse genetics, the DNA sequence for a particular gene of interest is known, but the role and function of the gene are typically not well understood. For example, molecular biology techniques such as **gene knockout** render targeted genes nonfunctional in a model organism or in cultured cells, allowing scientists to investigate the fundamental question of "what happens if this gene is disrupted?" After making a knockout organism, scientists look for both apparent phenotype changes, as well as those at the cellular and molecular level. The ultimate goal is to determine the function of the gene.

In "Modern Approaches to Understanding Gene Function" we will highlight experimental examples of how gene function has been revealed through modern applications of molecular techniques involving reverse genetics. You will learn about gene knockout, transgenic animals, transposon-mediated mutagenesis, gene overexpression, and RNA interference-based methods for interrupting genes, among other approaches. Our hope is to bring you to the "cutting edge" of genetic studies.

1.7 Genetic Studies Rely on the Use of Model Organisms

After the rediscovery of Mendel's work in 1900, research using a wide range of organisms confirmed that the principles of inheritance he described were of universal significance among plants and animals. Geneticists gradually came to focus attention on a small number of organisms, including the fruit fly (*Drosophila melanogaster*) and the mouse (*Mus musculus*) **(Figure 1–13)**. This trend developed for two main reasons: first, it was clear that genetic mechanisms were the same in most organisms, and second, these organisms had characteristics that made them especially suitable for genetic research. They were easy to grow, had relatively short life cycles, produced many offspring, and their genetic analysis was fairly straightforward. Over time, researchers

(a)

(b)

FIGURE 1–13 The first generation of model organisms in genetic analysis included (a) the mouse, *Mus musculus* and (b) the fruit fly, *Drosophila melanogaster*.

(a)

(b)

FIGURE 1–14 Microbes that have become model organisms for genetic studies include (a) the yeast *Saccharomyces cerevisiae* and (b) the bacterium *Escherichia coli.*

TABLE 1.1	Model Organisms Used to Study Some Human Diseases
Organism	**Human Diseases**
E. coli	Colon cancer and other cancers
S. cerevisiae	Cancer, Werner syndrome
D. melanogaster	Disorders of the nervous system, cancer
C. elegans	Diabetes
D. rerio	Cardiovascular disease
M. musculus	Lesch–Nyhan disease, cystic fibrosis, fragile-X syndrome, and many other diseases

created a large catalog of mutant strains for these species, and the mutations were carefully studied, characterized, and mapped. Because of their well-characterized genetics, these species became **model organisms,** defined as organisms used for the study of basic biological processes. In later chapters, we will see how discoveries in model organisms are shedding light on many aspects of biology, including aging, cancer, the immune system, and behavior.

The Modern Set of Genetic Model Organisms

Gradually, geneticists added other species to their collection of model organisms: viruses (such as the T phages and lambda phage) and microorganisms (the bacterium *Escherichia coli* and the yeast *Saccharomyces cerevisiae*) **(Figure 1–14)**.

More recently, additional species have been developed as model organisms, three of which are shown in the chapter opening photograph. Each species was chosen to allow study of some aspect of embryonic development. The nematode *Caenorhabditis elegans* was chosen as a model system to study the development and function of the nervous system because its nervous system contains only a few hundred cells and the developmental fate of these and all other cells in the body has been mapped out. *Arabidopsis thaliana,* a small plant with a short life cycle, has become a model organism for the study of many aspects of plant biology. The zebrafish, *Danio rerio,* is used to study vertebrate development: it is small, it reproduces rapidly, and its egg, embryo, and larvae are all transparent.

Model Organisms and Human Diseases

The development of recombinant DNA technology and the results of genome sequencing have confirmed that all life has a common origin. Because of this, genes with similar functions in different organisms tend to be similar or identical in structure and nucleotide sequence. Much of what

scientists learn by studying the genetics of model organisms can therefore be applied to humans as the basis for understanding and treating human diseases. In addition, the ability to create transgenic organisms by transferring genes between species has enabled scientists to develop models of human diseases in organisms ranging from bacteria to fungi, plants, and animals (Table 1.1).

The idea of studying a human disease such as colon cancer by using *E. coli* may strike you as strange, but the basic steps of DNA repair (a process that is defective in some forms of colon cancer) are the same in both organisms, and a gene involved (*mutL* in *E. coli* and *MLH1* in humans) is found in both organisms. More importantly, *E. coli* has the advantage of being easier to grow (the cells divide every 20 minutes), and researchers can easily create and study new mutations in the bacterial *mutL* gene in order to figure out how it works. This knowledge may eventually lead to the development of drugs and other therapies to treat colon cancer in humans.

The fruit fly, *Drosophila melanogaster,* is also being used to study a number of human diseases. Mutant genes have been identified in *D. melanogaster* that produce phenotypes with structural abnormalities of the nervous system and adult-onset degeneration of the nervous system. The information from genome-sequencing projects indicates that almost all these genes have human counterparts. For example, genes involved in a complex human disease of the retina called retinitis pigmentosa are identical to *Drosophila* genes involved in retinal degeneration. Study of these mutations in *Drosophila* is helping to dissect this complex disease and identify the function of the genes involved.

Another approach to studying diseases of the human nervous system is to transfer mutant human disease genes into *Drosophila* using recombinant DNA technology. The transgenic flies are then used for studying the mutant human genes themselves, other genes that affect the expression of the human disease genes, and the effects of therapeutic drugs on the action of those genes—all studies that are difficult or impossible to perform in humans. This gene transfer approach is being used to study almost a dozen human neurodegenerative disorders, including Huntington disease, Machado–Joseph disease, myotonic dystrophy, and Alzheimer disease.

Throughout the following chapters, you will encounter these model organisms again and again. Remember each time you meet them that they not only have a rich history in basic genetics research but are also at the forefront in the study of human genetic disorders and infectious diseases. As discussed in the next section, however, we have yet to reach a consensus on how and when some of this technology will be accepted as safe and ethically acceptable.

1.8 We Live in the Age of Genetics

Mendel described his decade-long project on inheritance in pea plants in an 1865 paper presented at a meeting of the Natural History Society of Brünn in Moravia. Less than 100 years later, the 1962 Nobel Prize was awarded to James Watson, Francis Crick, and Maurice Wilkins for their work on the structure of DNA. This time span encompassed the years leading up to the acceptance of Mendel's work, the discovery that genes are on chromosomes, the experiments that proved DNA encodes genetic information, and the elucidation of the molecular basis for DNA replication. The rapid development of genetics from Mendel's monastery garden to the Human Genome Project and beyond is summarized in a timeline in **Figure 1–15**.

The Nobel Prize and Genetics

No other scientific discipline has experienced the explosion of information and the level of excitement generated by the discoveries in genetics. This impact is especially apparent in the list of Nobel Prizes related to genetics, beginning with those awarded in the early and mid-twentieth century and continuing into the present (see inside front cover). Nobel Prizes in Medicine or Physiology and Chemistry have been consistently awarded for work in genetics and related fields. The first Nobel Prize awarded for such work was given to Thomas Morgan in 1933 for his research on the chromosome theory of inheritance. That award was followed by many others, including prizes for the discovery of genetic recombination, the relationship between genes and proteins, the structure of DNA, and the genetic code. In this century, geneticists continue to be recognized for their impact on biology in the current millennium, including Nobel Prizes awarded in 2002, 2006, 2007, and 2009. In 2010, the prize in Physiology or Medicine was given to Robert Edwards for the development of *in vitro* fertilization, and the 2012 prize was awarded to John Gurdon and Shinya Yamanaka for their work showing that mature cells can be reprogrammed to direct embryonic development and to form stem cells.

Genetics and Society

Just as there has never been a more exciting time to study genetics, the impact of this discipline on society has never been more profound. Genetics and its applications in biotechnology are developing much faster than the social conventions, public policies, and laws required to regulate their use. As a society, we are grappling with a host of sensitive genetics-related issues, including concerns about prenatal testing, genetic discrimination, ownership of genes, access to and safety of gene therapy, and genetic privacy. By the time you finish this course, you will have seen more than enough evidence to convince yourself that the present is the Age of Genetics, and you will understand the need to think about and become a participant in the dialogue concerning genetic science and its use.

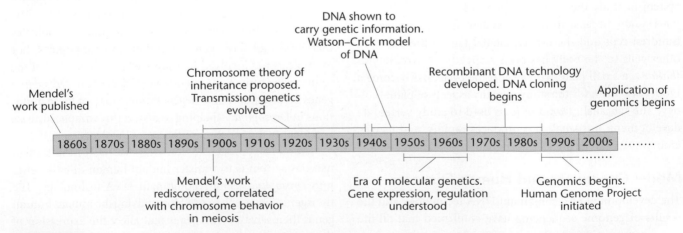

FIGURE 1–15 A timeline showing the development of genetics from Gregor Mendel's work on pea plants to the current era of genomics and its many applications in research, medicine, and society. Having a sense of the history of discovery in genetics should provide you with a useful framework as you proceed through this textbook.

GENETICS, TECHNOLOGY, AND SOCIETY

The Scientific and Ethical Implications of Modern Genetics

One of the special features of this text is the series of essays called *Genetics, Technology, and Society* that you will find at the conclusion of many chapters. These essays explore genetics-related topics that have an impact on the lives of each of us and on society in general.

Today, genetics touches all aspects of life, bringing rapid changes in medicine, agriculture, law, biotechnology, and the pharmaceutical industry. Physicians use hundreds of genetic tests to diagnose and predict the course of disease and to detect genetic defects *in utero*. Scientists employ DNA-based methods to trace the path of evolution taken by many species, including our own. Farmers grow disease-resistant and drought-resistant crops, and raise more productive farm animals, created by gene transfer techniques. Law enforcement agencies apply DNA profiling methods to paternity, rape, and murder investigations. The biotechnology industry itself generates over 700,000 jobs and $50 billion in revenue each year and doubles in size every decade.

Along with these rapidly changing gene-based technologies comes a challenging array of ethical dilemmas. Who owns and controls genetic information? Are gene-enhanced agricultural plants and animals safe for humans and the environment? How can we ensure that genomic technologies will be available to all and not just to the wealthy? What are the likely social consequences of the new reproductive technologies? It is a time when everyone needs to understand genetics in order to make complex personal and societal decisions.

Each *Genetics, Technology, and Society* essay is presented in an interactive format. In the *Your Turn* section at the end of each essay, you will find several thought-provoking questions along with resources to help you explore each question. These questions are designed to act as entry points for individual investigations and as topics to explore in a classroom or group learning setting.

We hope that you will find the *Genetics, Technology, and Society* essays interesting, challenging, and an effective way to begin your lifelong studies in modern genetics. Good reading!

EXPLORING GENOMICS

Internet Resources for Learning about Genomics, Bioinformatics, and Proteomics

MasteringGenetics™ Visit the Study Area: Exploring Genomics

Genomics is one of the most rapidly changing disciplines of genetics. As new information in this field accumulates at an astounding rate, keeping up with current developments in genomics, proteomics, bioinformatics, and other examples of the "omics" era of modern genetics is a challenging task indeed. As a result, geneticists, molecular biologists, and other scientists rely on online databases to share and compare new information.

The purpose of the "Exploring Genomics" feature, which appears at the end of many chapters, is to introduce you to a range of Internet databases that scientists around the world depend on for sharing, analyzing, organizing, comparing, and storing data from studies in genomics, proteomics, and related fields. We will explore this incredible pool of new information—comprising some of the best publicly available resources in the world—and show you how to use bioinformatics approaches to analyze the sequence and structural data that are found there. Each set of Exploring Genomics exercises will provide a basic introduction to one or more especially relevant or useful databases or programs and then guide you through exercises that use the databases to expand on or reinforce important concepts discussed in the chapter. The exercises are designed to help you learn to navigate the databases, but your explorations need not be limited to these experiences. Part of the fun of learning about genomics is exploring these outstanding databases on your own, so that you can get the latest information on any topic that interests you. Enjoy your explorations!

In this chapter, we discussed the importance of model organisms to both classic and modern experimental approaches

(continued)

Exploring Genomics—continued

in genetics. In our first set of Exploring Genomics exercises, we introduce you to a number of Internet sites that are excellent resources for finding up-to-date information on a wide range of completed and ongoing genomics projects involving model organisms.

■ **Exercise I – Genome News Network**

Since 1995, when scientists unveiled the genome for *Haemophilus influenzae,* making this bacterium the first organism to have its genome sequenced, the sequences for more than 500 organisms have been completed. Genome News Network is a site that provides access to basic information about recently completed genome sequences.

1. Visit the Genome News Network at www.genomenewsnetwork.org.

2. Click on the "Quick Guide to Sequenced Genomes" link. Scroll down the page; click on the appropriate links to find information about the genomes for *Anopheles gambiae,*

Lactococcus lactis, and *Pan troglodytes*; and answer the following questions for each organism:

a. Who sequenced this organism's genome, and in what year was it completed?

b. What is the size of each organism's genome in base pairs?

c. Approximately how many genes are in each genome?

d. Briefly describe why geneticists are interested in studying this organism's genome.

■ **Exercise II – Exploring the Genomes of Model Organisms**

A tremendous amount of information is available about the genomes of the many model organisms that have played invaluable roles in advancing our understanding of genetics. Following are links to several sites that are excellent resources for you as you study genetics. Visit the site for links to information about your favorite

model organism to learn more about its genome!

• Ensembl Genome Browser: www .ensembl.org/index.html. Outstanding site for genome information on many model organisms.

• FlyBase: flybase.org. Great database on *Drosophila* genes and genomes.

• Gold™ Genomes OnLine Database: www.genomesonline.org. Comprehensive access to completed and ongoing genome projects worldwide.

• Model Organisms for Biomedical Research: www.nih.gov/science/ models. National Institutes of Health site with a wealth of resources on model organisms.

• The *Arabidopsis* Information Resource: www.arabidopsis.org. Genetic database for the model plant *Arabidopsis thaliana.*

• WormBase: www.wormbase.org. Genome database for the nematode roundworm *Caenorhabditis elegans.*

Summary Points

1. Mendel's work on pea plants established the principles of gene transmission from parents to offspring that form the foundation for the science of genetics.

2. Genes and chromosomes are the fundamental units in the chromosomal theory of inheritance. This theory explains that inherited traits are controlled by genes located on chromosomes and shows how the transmission of genetic information maintains genetic continuity from generation to generation.

3. Molecular genetics—based on the central dogma that DNA is a template for making RNA, which encodes the order of amino acids in proteins—explains the phenomena described by Mendelian genetics, referred to as transmission genetics.

4. Recombinant DNA technology, a far-reaching methodology used in molecular genetics, allows genes from one organism to be spliced into vectors and cloned, producing many copies of specific DNA sequences.

5. Biotechnology has revolutionized agriculture, the pharmaceutical industry, and medicine. It has made possible the mass production of medically important gene products. Genetic testing allows detection of individuals with genetic disorders and those at risk of having affected children, and gene therapy offers hope for the treatment of serious genetic disorders.

6. Genomics, proteomics, and bioinformatics are new fields derived from recombinant DNA technology. These fields combine genetics with information technology and allow scientists to explore genome sequences, the structure and function of genes, the protein set within cells, and the evolution of genomes. The Human Genome Project is one example of genomics.

7. The use of model organisms has advanced the understanding of genetic mechanisms and, coupled with recombinant DNA technology, has produced models of human genetic diseases.

8. The effects of genetic technology on society are profound, and the development of policy and legislation to deal with issues derived from the use of this technology is lagging behind the resulting innovations.

CASE STUDY | Extending essential ideas of genetics beyond the classroom

To make genetics relevant to situations that you may encounter outside the classroom, each chapter will contain a short case study accompanied by questions. Each case is designed to draw attention to one of the basic concepts covered in the chapter. The case is designed to draw attention to one of the basic concepts covered in the chapter. The case uses examples and scenarios to illustrate how this concept can be applied to genetic issues in everyday life.

Many of the case studies and their accompanying questions can serve as the basis of classroom discussions, group projects, or as starting points for papers and presentations. Use these resources to enhance your learning experience and to bring genetics out of the book and into your life.

Problems and Discussion Questions

MasteringGenetics™ Visit for instructor-assigned tutorials and problems.

1. Describe Mendel's conclusions about how traits are passed from generation to generation.

CONCEPT QUESTION

2. Review the Chapter Concepts list on p. 1. Most of these are related to the discovery of DNA as the genetic material and the subsequent development of recombinant DNA technology. Write a brief essay that discusses the impact of recombinant DNA technology on genetics as we perceive the discipline today.
3. What is the chromosome theory of inheritance, and how is it related to Mendel's findings?
4. Define genotype and phenotype. Describe how they are related and how alleles fit into your definitions.
5. Given the state of knowledge at the time of the Avery, MacLeod, and McCarty experiment, why was it difficult for some scientists to accept that DNA is the carrier of genetic information?
6. Contrast chromosomes and genes.
7. How is genetic information encoded in a DNA molecule?
8. Describe the central dogma of molecular genetics and how it serves as the basis of modern genetics.
9. How many different proteins, each with a unique amino acid sequence, can be constructed with a length of five amino acids?
10. Outline the roles played by restriction enzymes and vectors in cloning DNA.
11. What are some of the impacts of biotechnology on crop plants in the United States?
12. Summarize the arguments for and against patenting genetically modified organisms.
13. We all carry about 20,000 genes in our genome. So far, patents have been issued for more than 6000 of these genes. Do you think that companies or individuals should be able to patent human genes? Why or why not?
14. How has the use of model organisms advanced our knowledge of the genes that control human diseases?
15. If you knew that a devastating late-onset inherited disease runs in your family (in other words, a disease that does not appear until later in life) and you could be tested for it at the age of 20, would you want to know whether you are a carrier? Would your answer be likely to change when you reach age 40?
16. Why do you think discoveries in genetics have been recognized with so many Nobel Prizes?
17. The Age of Genetics was created by remarkable advances in the use of biotechnology to manipulate plant and animal genomes. Given that the world population has topped 6 billion and is expected to reach 9.2 billion by 2050, some scientists have proposed that only the worldwide introduction of genetically modified (GM) foods will increase crop yields enough to meet future nutritional demands. Pest resistance, herbicide, cold, drought, and salinity tolerance, along with increased nutrition, are seen as positive attributes of GM foods. However, others caution that unintended harm to other organisms, reduced effectiveness to pesticides, gene transfer to nontarget species, allergenicity, and as yet unknown effects on human health are potential concerns regarding GM foods. If you were in a position to control the introduction of a GM primary food product (rice, for example), what criteria would you establish before allowing such introduction?
18. The BIO (Biotechnology Industry Organization) meeting held in Philadelphia in June 2005 brought together worldwide leaders from the biotechnology and pharmaceutical industries. Concurrently, BioDemocracy 2005, a group composed of people seeking to highlight hazards from widespread applications of biotechnology, also met in Philadelphia. The benefits of biotechnology are outlined in your text. Predict some of the risks that were no doubt discussed at the BioDemocracy meeting.

Chromosomes in the prometaphase stage of mitosis, derived from a cell in the flower of *Haemanthus*.

2 Mitosis and Meiosis

CHAPTER CONCEPTS

- Genetic continuity between generations of cells and between generations of sexually reproducing organisms is maintained through the processes of mitosis and meiosis, respectively.

- Diploid eukaryotic cells contain their genetic information in pairs of homologous chromosomes, with one member of each pair being derived from the maternal parent and one from the paternal parent.

- Mitosis provides a mechanism by which chromosomes, having been duplicated, are distributed into progeny cells during cell reproduction.

- Mitosis converts a diploid cell into two diploid daughter cells.

- The process of meiosis distributes one member of each homologous pair of chromosomes into each gamete or spore, thus reducing the diploid chromosome number to the haploid chromosome number.

- Meiosis generates genetic variability by distributing various combinations of maternal and paternal members of each homologous pair of chromosomes into gametes or spores.

- During the stages of mitosis and meiosis, the genetic material is condensed into discrete structures called chromosomes.

Every living thing contains a substance described as the genetic material. Except in certain viruses, this material is composed of the nucleic acid DNA. DNA has an underlying linear structure possessing segments called genes, the products of which direct the metabolic activities of cells. An organism's DNA, with its arrays of genes, is organized into structures called **chromosomes**, which serve as vehicles for transmitting genetic information. The manner in which chromosomes are transmitted from one generation of cells to the next and from organisms to their descendants must be exceedingly precise. In this chapter we consider exactly how genetic continuity is maintained between cells and organisms.

Two major processes are involved in the genetic continuity of nucleated cells: **mitosis** and **meiosis**. Although the mechanisms of the two processes are similar in many ways, the outcomes are quite different. Mitosis leads to the production of two cells, each with the same number of chromosomes as the parent cell. In contrast, meiosis reduces the genetic content and the number of chromosomes by precisely half. This reduction is essential if sexual reproduction is to occur without doubling the amount of genetic material in each new generation. Strictly speaking, mitosis is that portion of the cell cycle during which the hereditary components are equally partitioned into daughter cells. Meiosis is part of a special type of cell division that leads to the production of sex cells: **gametes** or **spores**. This process is an essential step in the transmission of genetic information from an organism to its offspring.

Normally, chromosomes are visible only during mitosis and meiosis. When cells are not undergoing division, the genetic material making up chromosomes unfolds and uncoils into a diffuse network within the nucleus, generally referred to as **chromatin**. Before describing mitosis and meiosis, we will briefly review the structure of cells, emphasizing components that are of particular significance to genetic function. We will also compare the structural differences between the prokaryotic (nonnucleated) cells of bacteria and the eukaryotic cells of higher organisms. We then devote the remainder of the chapter to the behavior of chromosomes during cell division.

2.1 Cell Structure Is Closely Tied to Genetic Function

Before 1940, our knowledge of cell structure was limited to what we could see with the light microscope. Around 1940, the transmission electron microscope was in its early stages of development, and by 1950, many details of cell ultrastructure had emerged. Under the electron microscope, cells were seen as highly varied, highly organized structures whose form and function are dependent on specific genetic expression by each cell type. A new world of whorled membranes, organelles, microtubules, granules, and filaments was revealed. These discoveries revolutionized thinking in the entire field of biology. Many cell components, such as the nucleolus, ribosome, and centriole, are involved directly or indirectly with genetic processes. Other components—the mitochondria and chloroplasts—contain their own unique genetic information. Here, we will focus primarily on those aspects of cell structure that relate to genetic study. The generalized animal cell shown in **Figure 2–1** illustrates most of the structures we will discuss.

All cells are surrounded by a **plasma membrane**, an outer covering that defines the cell boundary and delimits the cell from its immediate external environment. This membrane is not passive but instead actively controls the movement of materials into and out of the cell. In addition to this membrane, plant cells have an outer covering called the **cell wall** whose major component is a polysaccharide called *cellulose*.

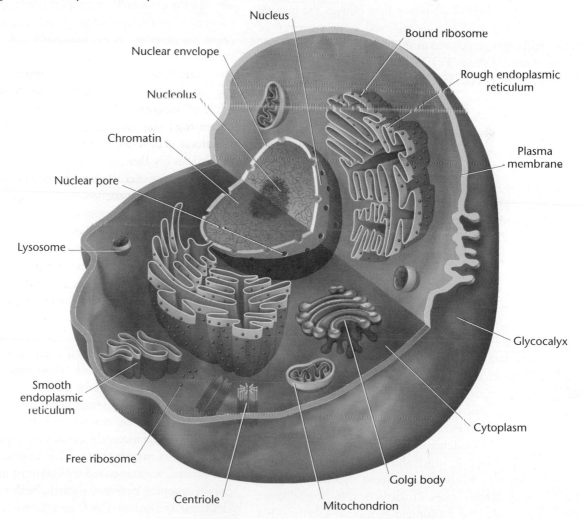

FIGURE 2–1 A generalized animal cell. The cellular components discussed in the text are emphasized here.

Many, if not most, animal cells have a covering over the plasma membrane, referred to as the **glycocalyx**, or **cell coat**. Consisting of glycoproteins and polysaccharides, this covering has a chemical composition that differs from comparable structures in either plants or bacteria. The glycocalyx, among other functions, provides biochemical identity at the surface of cells, and the components of the coat that establish cellular identity are under genetic control. For example, various cell-identity markers that you may have heard of—the AB, Rh, and MN antigens—are found on the surface of red blood cells, among other cell types. On the surface of other cells, histocompatibility antigens, which elicit an immune response during tissue and organ transplants, are present. Various **receptor molecules** are also found on the surfaces of cells. These molecules act as recognition sites that transfer specific chemical signals across the cell membrane into the cell.

Living organisms are categorized into two major groups depending on whether or not their cells contain a nucleus. The presence of a nucleus and other membranous organelles is the defining characteristic of **eukaryotic organisms**. The **nucleus** in eukaryotic cells is a membrane-bound structure that houses the genetic material, DNA, which is complexed with an array of acidic and basic proteins into thin fibers. During nondivisional phases of the cell cycle, the fibers are uncoiled and dispersed into chromatin (as mentioned above). During mitosis and meiosis, chromatin fibers coil and condense into chromosomes. Also present in the nucleus is the **nucleolus**, an amorphous component where ribosomal RNA (rRNA) is synthesized and where the initial stages of ribosomal assembly occur. The portions of DNA that encode rRNA are collectively referred to as the **nucleolus organizer region**, or the **NOR**.

Prokaryotic organisms, of which there are two major groups, lack a nuclear envelope and membranous organelles. For the purpose of our brief discussion here, we will consider the *eubacteria*, the other group being the more ancient bacteria referred to as *archaea*. In eubacteria, such as *Escherichia coli*, the genetic material is present as a long, circular DNA molecule that is compacted into an unenclosed region called the **nucleoid**. Part of the DNA may be attached to the cell membrane, but in general the nucleoid extends through a large part of the cell. Although the DNA is compacted, it does not undergo the extensive coiling characteristic of the stages of mitosis, during which the chromosomes of eukaryotes become visible. Nor is the DNA associated as extensively with proteins as is eukaryotic DNA. **Figure 2–2**, which shows two bacteria forming by cell division, illustrates the nucleoid regions containing the bacterial chromosomes. Prokaryotic cells do not have a distinct nucleolus but do contain genes that specify rRNA molecules.

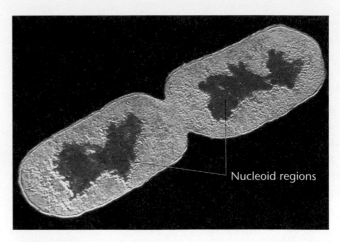

Nucleoid regions

FIGURE 2–2 Color-enhanced electron micrograph of *E. coli* undergoing cell division. Particularly prominent are the two chromosomal areas (shown in red), called nucleoids, that have been partitioned into the daughter cells.

The remainder of the eukaryotic cell within the plasma membrane, excluding the nucleus, is referred to as **cytoplasm** and includes a variety of extranuclear cellular organelles. In the cytoplasm, a nonparticulate, colloidal material referred to as the **cytosol** surrounds and encompasses the cellular organelles. The cytoplasm also includes an extensive system of tubules and filaments, comprising the cytoskeleton, which provides a lattice of support structures within the cell. Consisting primarily of **microtubules**, which are made of the protein **tubulin**, and **microfilaments**, which derive from the protein **actin**, this structural framework maintains cell shape, facilitates cell mobility, and anchors the various organelles.

One organelle, the membranous **endoplasmic reticulum (ER)**, compartmentalizes the cytoplasm, greatly increasing the surface area available for biochemical synthesis. The ER appears smooth in places where it serves as the site for synthesizing fatty acids and phospholipids; in other places, it appears rough because it is studded with ribosomes. **Ribosomes** serve as sites where genetic information contained in messenger RNA (mRNA) is translated into proteins.

Three other cytoplasmic structures are very important in the eukaryotic cell's activities: mitochondria, chloroplasts, and centrioles. **Mitochondria** are found in most eukaryotes, including both animal and plant cells, and are the sites of the oxidative phases of cell respiration. These chemical reactions generate large amounts of the energy-rich molecule adenosine triphosphate (ATP). **Chloroplasts**, which are found in plants, algae, and some protozoans, are associated with photosynthesis, the major energy-trapping process on Earth. Both mitochondria and chloroplasts contain DNA in a form distinct from that found in the nucleus. They are able to duplicate themselves and transcribe and translate their own genetic information. It is interesting to note that the genetic machinery of mitochondria and chloroplasts closely resembles that of prokaryotic cells. This and other observations have led to the proposal that these organelles were once primitive free-living organisms that established symbiotic relationships with primitive eukaryotic cells. This theory concerning the evolutionary origin of these organelles is called the **endosymbiont hypothesis**.

Animal cells and some plant cells also contain a pair of complex structures called **centrioles**. These cytoplasmic bodies, each located in a specialized region called the **centrosome**, are associated with the organization of spindle fibers that function in mitosis and meiosis. In some organisms, the centriole is derived from another structure, the basal body, which is associated with the formation of cilia and flagella (hair-like and whip-like structures for propelling cells or moving materials).

The organization of **spindle fibers** by the centrioles occurs during the early phases of mitosis and meiosis. These fibers play an important role in the movement of chromosomes as they separate during cell division. They are composed of arrays of microtubules consisting of polymers of the protein tubulin.

arm ratios are produced. As Figure 2–3 illustrates, chromosomes are classified as **metacentric**, **submetacentric**, **acrocentric**, or **telocentric** on the basis of the centromere location. The shorter arm, by convention, is shown above the centromere and is called the **p arm** (p, for "petite"). The longer arm is shown below the centromere and is called the **q arm** (q because it is the next letter in the alphabet).

In the study of mitosis, several other observations are of particular relevance. First, all somatic cells derived from members of the same species contain an identical number of chromosomes. In most cases, this represents the **diploid number (2n)**, whose meaning will become clearer below. When the lengths and centromere placements of all such chromosomes are examined, a second general feature is apparent. With the exception of sex chromosomes, they exist in pairs with regard to these two properties, and the members of each pair are called **homologous chromosomes**. So, for each chromosome exhibiting a specific length and centromere placement, another exists with identical features.

There are exceptions to this rule. Many bacteria and viruses have but one chromosome, and organisms such as yeasts and molds, and certain plants such as bryophytes (mosses), spend the predominant phase of their life cycle in the haploid stage. That is, they contain only one member

2.2 Chromosomes Exist in Homologous Pairs in Diploid Organisms

As we discuss the processes of mitosis and meiosis, it is important that you understand the concept of homologous chromosomes. Such an understanding will also be of critical importance in our future discussions of Mendelian genetics. Chromosomes are most easily visualized during mitosis. When they are examined carefully, distinctive lengths and shapes are apparent. Each chromosome contains a constricted region called the **centromere**, whose location establishes the general appearance of each chromosome. **Figure 2–3** shows chromosomes with centromere placements at different distances along their length. Extending from either side of the centromere are the arms of the chromosome. Depending on the position of the centromere, different

Centromere location	Designation	Metaphase shape	Anaphase shape
Middle	Metacentric	Sister chromatids — Centromere	← Migration →
Between middle and end	Submetacentric	p arm — q arm	
Close to end	Acrocentric		
At end	Telocentric		

FIGURE 2–3 Centromere locations and the chromosome designations that are based on them. Note that the shape of the chromosome during anaphase is determined by the position of the centromere during metaphase.

FIGURE 2–4 A metaphase preparation of chromosomes derived from a dividing cell of a human male (left), and the karyotype derived from the metaphase preparation (right). All but the X and Y chromosomes are present in homologous pairs. Each chromosome is clearly a double structure consisting of a pair of sister chromatids joined by a common centromere.

of each homologous pair of chromosomes during most of their lives.

Figure 2–4 illustrates the physical appearance of different pairs of homologous chromosomes. There, the human mitotic chromosomes have been photographed, cut out of the print, and matched up, creating a display called a **karyotype**. As you can see, humans have a $2n$ number of 46 chromosomes, which on close examination exhibit a diversity of sizes and centromere placements. Note also that each of the 46 chromosomes in this karyotype is clearly a double structure consisting of two parallel *sister chromatids* connected by a common centromere. Had these chromosomes been allowed to continue dividing, the sister chromatids, which are replicas of one another, would have separated into the two new cells as division continued.

The **haploid number (n)** of chromosomes is equal to one-half the diploid number. Collectively, the genetic information contained in a haploid set of chromosomes constitutes the **genome** of the species. This, of course, includes copies of all genes as well as a large amount of noncoding DNA. The examples listed in Table 2.1 demonstrate the wide range of n values found in plants and animals.

Homologous chromosomes have important genetic similarities. They contain identical gene sites along their lengths; each site is called a **locus** (pl. loci). Thus, they are identical in the traits that they influence and in their genetic potential. In sexually reproducing organisms, one member of each pair is derived from the maternal parent (through the ovum) and the other member is derived from the paternal parent (through the sperm). Therefore, each diploid organism contains two copies of each gene as a consequence of **biparental inheritance**, inheritance from two parents. As we shall see in the chapters on transmission genetics, the members of each pair of genes, while influencing the same characteristic or trait, need not be identical. In a population of members of the same species, many different alternative forms of the same gene, called **alleles**, can exist.

The concepts of haploid number, diploid number, and homologous chromosomes are important for understanding the process of meiosis. During the formation of gametes or spores, meiosis converts the diploid number of chromosomes to the haploid number. As a result, haploid gametes or spores contain precisely one member of each homologous pair of chromosomes—that is, one complete haploid set. Following fusion of two gametes at fertilization, the diploid number is reestablished; that is, the zygote contains two complete haploid sets of chromosomes. The constancy of genetic material is thus maintained from generation to generation.

There is one important exception to the concept of homologous pairs of chromosomes. In many species, one pair, consisting of the **sex-determining chromosomes**, is often not homologous in size, centromere placement, arm ratio, or genetic content. For example, in humans, while females carry two homologous X chromosomes, males carry one Y chromosome in addition to one X chromosome (Figure 2–4). These X and Y chromosomes are not strictly homologous. The Y is considerably smaller and lacks most of the gene loci contained on the X. Nevertheless, they contain homologous regions and behave as homologs in meiosis so that gametes produced by males receive either one X or one Y chromosome.

TABLE 2.1 The Haploid Number of Chromosomes for a Variety of Organisms

Common Name	Scientific Name	Haploid Number
Black bread mold	*Aspergillus nidulans*	8
Broad bean	*Vicia faba*	6
Cat	*Felis domesticus*	19
Cattle	*Bos taurus*	30
Chicken	*Gallus domesticus*	39
Chimpanzee	*Pan troglodytes*	24
Corn	*Zea mays*	10
Cotton	*Gossypium hirsutum*	26
Dog	*Canis familiaris*	39
Evening primrose	*Oenothera biennis*	7
Frog	*Rana pipiens*	13
Fruit fly	*Drosophila melanogaster*	4
Garden onion	*Allium cepa*	8
Garden pea	*Pisum sativum*	7
Grasshopper	*Melanoplus differentialis*	12
Green alga	*Chlamydomonas reinhardtii*	18
Horse	*Equus caballus*	32
House fly	*Musca domestica*	6
House mouse	*Mus musculus*	20
Human	*Homo sapiens*	23
Jimson weed	*Datura stramonium*	12
Mosquito	*Culex pipiens*	3
Mustard plant	*Arabidopsis thaliana*	5
Pink bread mold	*Neurospora crassa*	7
Potato	*Solanum tuberosum*	24
Rhesus monkey	*Macaca mulatta*	21
Roundworm	*Caenorhabditis elegans*	6
Silkworm	*Bombyx mori*	28
Slime mold	*Dictyostelium discoideum*	7
Snapdragon	*Antirrhinum majus*	8
Tobacco	*Nicotiana tabacum*	24
Tomato	*Lycopersicon esculentum*	12
Water fly	*Nymphaea alba*	80
Wheat	*Triticum aestivum*	21
Yeast	*Saccharomyces cerevisiae*	16
Zebrafish	*Danio rerio*	25

2.3 Mitosis Partitions Chromosomes into Dividing Cells

The process of mitosis is critical to all eukaryotic organisms. In some single-celled organisms, such as protozoans and some fungi and algae, mitosis (as a part of cell division) provides the basis for asexual reproduction. Multicellular diploid organisms begin life as single-celled fertilized eggs called **zygotes**. The mitotic activity of the zygote and the subsequent daughter cells is the foundation for the development and growth of the organism. In adult organisms, mitotic activity is the basis for wound healing and other forms of cell replacement in certain tissues. For example, the epidermal cells of the skin and

the intestinal lining of humans are continuously sloughed off and replaced. Cell division also results in the continuous production of reticulocytes that eventually shed their nuclei and replenish the supply of red blood cells in vertebrates. In abnormal situations, somatic cells may lose control of cell division, and form a tumor.

The genetic material is partitioned into daughter cells during nuclear division, or **karyokinesis**. This process is quite complex and requires great precision. The chromosomes must first be exactly replicated and then accurately partitioned. The end result is the production of two daughter nuclei, each with a chromosome composition identical to that of the parent cell.

Karyokinesis is followed by cytoplasmic division, or **cytokinesis**. This less complex process requires a mechanism that partitions the volume into two parts, then encloses each new cell in a distinct plasma membrane. As the cytoplasm is reconstituted, organelles replicate themselves, arise from existing membrane structures, or are synthesized *de novo* (anew) in each cell.

Following cell division, the initial size of each new daughter cell is approximately one-half the size of the parent cell. However, the nucleus of each new cell is not appreciably smaller than the nucleus of the original cell. Quantitative measurements of DNA confirm that there is an amount of genetic material in the daughter nuclei equivalent to that in the parent cell.

Interphase and the Cell Cycle

Many cells undergo a continuous alternation between division and nondivision. The events that occur from the completion of one division until the completion of the next division constitute the **cell cycle** (**Figure 2–5**).

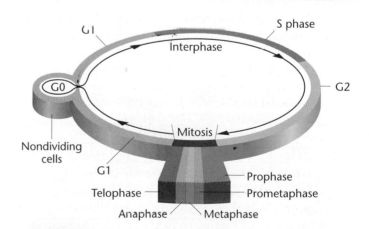

FIGURE 2–5 The stages comprising an arbitrary cell cycle. Following mitosis, cells enter the G1 stage of interphase, initiating a new cycle. Cells may become nondividing (G0) or continue through G1, where they become committed to begin DNA synthesis (S) and complete the cycle (G2 and mitosis). Following mitosis, two daughter cells are produced, and the cycle begins anew for both of them.

We will consider **interphase**, the initial stage of the cell cycle, as the interval between divisions. It was once thought that the biochemical activity during interphase was devoted solely to the cell's growth and its normal function. However, we now know that another biochemical step critical to the ensuing mitosis occurs during interphase: *the replication of the DNA of each chromosome*. This period, during which DNA is synthesized, occurs before the cell enters mitosis and is called the **S phase**. The initiation and completion of synthesis can be detected by monitoring the incorporation of radioactive precursors into DNA.

Investigations of this nature demonstrate two periods during interphase when no DNA synthesis occurs, one before and one after the S phase. These are designated **G1 (gap I)** and **G2 (gap II)**, respectively. During both of these intervals, as well as during S, intensive metabolic activity, cell growth, and cell differentiation are evident. By the end of G2, the volume of the cell has roughly doubled, DNA has been replicated, and mitosis (M) is initiated. Following mitosis, continuously dividing cells then repeat this cycle (G1, S, G2, M) over and over, as shown in Figure 2–5.

Much is known about the cell cycle based on *in vitro* (literally, "in glass") studies. When grown in culture, many cell types in different organisms traverse the complete cycle in about 16 hours. The actual process of mitosis occupies only a small part of the overall cycle, often less than an hour. The lengths of the S and G2 phases of interphase are fairly consistent in different cell types. Most variation is seen in the length of time spent in the G1 stage. **Figure 2–6** shows the relative length of these intervals as well as the length of the stages of mitosis in a human cell in culture.

G1 is of great interest in the study of cell proliferation and its control. At a point during G1, all cells follow one of two paths. They either withdraw from the cycle, become quiescent, and enter the **G0 stage** (see Figure 2–5), or they become committed to proceed through G1, initiating DNA synthesis, and completing the cycle. Cells that enter G0 remain viable and metabolically active but are not proliferative. Cancer cells apparently avoid entering G0 or pass through it very quickly. Other cells enter G0 and never reenter the cell cycle. Still other cells in G0 can be stimulated to return to G1 and thereby reenter the cell cycle.

Cytologically, interphase is characterized by the absence of visible chromosomes. Instead, the nucleus is filled with chromatin fibers that are formed as the chromosomes uncoil and disperse after the previous mitosis [**Figure 2–7(a)**]. Once G1, S, and G2 are completed, mitosis is initiated. Mitosis is a dynamic period of vigorous and continual activity. For discussion purposes, the entire process is subdivided into discrete stages, and specific events are assigned to each one. These stages, in order of occurrence, are prophase, prometaphase, metaphase, anaphase, and telophase. They are diagrammed with corresponding photomicrographs in Figure 2–7.

Prophase

Often, over half of mitosis is spent in **prophase** [**Figure 2–7(b)**], a stage characterized by several significant occurrences. One of the early events in prophase of all animal cells is the migration of two pairs of centrioles to opposite ends of the cell. These structures are found just outside the nuclear envelope in an area of differentiated cytoplasm called the centrosome (introduced in Section 2.1). It is believed that each pair of centrioles consists of one mature unit and a smaller, newly formed daughter centriole.

The centrioles migrate and establish poles at opposite ends of the cell. After migration, the centrosomes, in which the centrioles are localized, are responsible for organizing cytoplasmic microtubules into the spindle fibers that run between these poles, creating an axis along which chromosomal separation occurs. Interestingly, the cells of most plants (there are a few exceptions), fungi, and certain algae seem to lack centrioles. Spindle fibers are nevertheless apparent during mitosis.

As the centrioles migrate, the nuclear envelope begins to break down and gradually disappears. In a similar fashion, the nucleolus disintegrates within the nucleus. While these events are taking place, the diffuse chromatin fibers have begun to condense, until distinct threadlike structures, the chromosomes, become visible. It becomes apparent near the end of prophase that each chromosome is actually a double structure split longitudinally except at a single point of constriction, the centromere. The two parts of each chromosome are called **sister chromatids** because the DNA contained in each of them is genetically

Interphase			Mitosis
G1	S	G2	M
5	7	3	1
Hours			

Pro	Met	Ana	Tel
36	3	3	18
Minutes			

FIGURE 2–6 The time spent in each interval of one complete cell cycle of a human cell in culture. Times vary according to cell types and conditions.

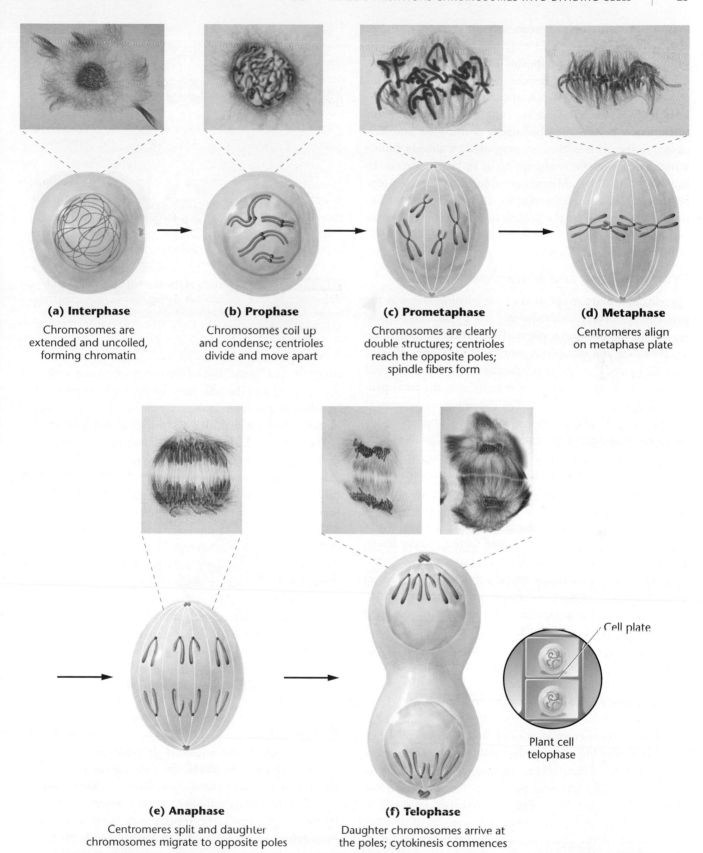

(a) Interphase
Chromosomes are extended and uncoiled, forming chromatin

(b) Prophase
Chromosomes coil up and condense; centrioles divide and move apart

(c) Prometaphase
Chromosomes are clearly double structures; centrioles reach the opposite poles; spindle fibers form

(d) Metaphase
Centromeres align on metaphase plate

(e) Anaphase
Centromeres split and daughter chromosomes migrate to opposite poles

(f) Telophase
Daughter chromosomes arrive at the poles; cytokinesis commences

Cell plate

Plant cell telophase

FIGURE 2–7 Drawings depicting mitosis in an animal cell with a diploid number of 4. The events occurring in each stage are described in the text. Of the two homologous pairs of chromosomes, one pair consists of longer, metacentric members and the other of shorter, submetacentric members. The maternal chromosome and the paternal chromosome of each pair are shown in different colors. In (f), a drawing of late telophase in a plant cell shows the formation of the cell plate and lack of centrioles. The cells shown in the light micrographs came from the flower of *Haemanthus,* a plant that has a diploid number of 8.

identical, having formed from a single replicative event. Sister chromatids are held together by a multi-subunit protein complex called **cohesin**. This molecular complex is originally formed between them during the S phase of the cell cycle when the DNA of each chromosome is replicated. Thus, even though we cannot see chromatids in interphase because the chromatin is uncoiled and dispersed in the nucleus, the chromosomes are already double structures, which becomes apparent in late prophase. In humans, with a diploid number of 46, a cytological preparation of late prophase reveals 46 chromosomes randomly distributed in the area formerly occupied by the nucleus.

Prometaphase and Metaphase

The distinguishing event of the two ensuing stages is the migration of every chromosome, led by its centromeric region, to the equatorial plane. The equatorial plane, also referred to as the *metaphase plate,* is the midline region of the cell, a plane that lies perpendicular to the axis established by the spindle fibers. In some descriptions, the term **prometaphase** refers to the period of chromosome movement [**Figure 2–7(c)**], and the term **metaphase** is applied strictly to the chromosome configuration following migration.

Migration is made possible by the binding of spindle fibers to the chromosome's **kinetochore**, an assembly of multilayered plates of proteins associated with the centromere. This structure forms on opposite sides of each paired centromere, in intimate association with the two sister chromatids. Once properly attached to the spindle fibers, cohesin is degraded by an enzyme, appropriately named *separase,* and the sister chromatid arms disjoin, except at the centromere region. A unique protein family called **shugoshin** (from the Japanese meaning guardian spirit) protects cohesin from being degraded by separase at the centromeric regions. The involvement of the cohesin and shugoshin complexes with a pair of sister chromatids during mitosis is depicted in **Figure 2–8**.

We know a great deal about the molecular interactions involved in kinetechore assembly along the centromere. This is of great interest because of the consequences when mutations alter the proteins that make up the kinetechore complex. Altered kinetochore function potentially leads to errors during chromosome migration, altering the diploid content of daughter cells. A more detailed account will be presented later in the text, once we have provided more information about DNA and the proteins that make up chromatin (see Chapter 12).

We also know a great deal about spindle fibers. They consist of microtubules, which themselves consist of molecular subunits of the protein tubulin. Microtubules seem to

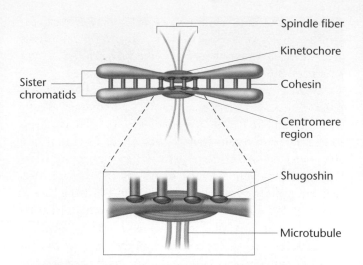

FIGURE 2–8 The depiction of the alignment, pairing, and disjunction of sister chromatids during mitosis, involving the molecular complexes cohesin and shugoshin and the enzyme separase.

originate and "grow" out of the two centrosome regions at opposite poles of the cell. They are dynamic structures that lengthen and shorten as a result of the addition or loss of polarized tubulin subunits. The microtubules most directly responsible for chromosome migration make contact with, and adhere to, kinetochores as they grow from the centrosome region. They are referred to as **kinetochore microtubules** and have one end near the centrosome region (at one of the poles of the cell) and the other end anchored to the kinetochore. The number of microtubules that bind to the kinetochore varies greatly between organisms. Yeast (*Saccharomyces*) has only a single microtubule bound to each plate-like structure of the kinetochore. Mitotic cells of mammals, at the other extreme, reveal 30 to 40 microtubules bound to each portion of the kinetochore.

At the completion of metaphase, each centromere is aligned at the metaphase plate with the chromosome arms extending outward in a random array. This configuration is shown in **Figure 2–7(d)**.

Anaphase

Events critical to chromosome distribution during mitosis occur during **anaphase**, the shortest stage of mitosis. During this phase, sister chromatids of each chromosome, held together only at their centromere regions, *disjoin* (separate) from one another—an event described as **disjunction**—and are pulled to opposite ends of the cell. For complete disjunction to occur: (1) shugoshin must be degraded, reversing its protective role; (2) the cohesin complex holding the centromere region of each sister chromosome is then cleaved by separase; and (3) sister chromatids of each chromosome are pulled toward the opposite poles of the cell (Figure 2–8). As these events proceed, each migrating chromatid is now referred to as a **daughter chromosome**.

Movement of daughter chromosomes to the opposite poles of the cell is dependent on the kinetechore–spindle fiber attachment. Recent investigations reveal that chromosome migration results from the activity of a series of specific molecules called *motor proteins* found at several locations within the dividing cell. These proteins, described as **molecular motors**, use the energy generated by the hydrolysis of ATP. Their effect on the activity of microtubules serves ultimately to shorten the spindle fibers, drawing the chromosomes to opposite ends of the cell. The centromeres of each chromosome *appear* to lead the way during migration, with the chromosome arms trailing behind. Several models have been proposed to account for the shortening of spindle fibers. They share in common the selective removal of tubulin subunits at the ends of the spindle fibers. The removal process is accomplished by the molecular motor proteins described above.

The location of the centromere determines the shape of the chromosome during separation, as you saw in Figure 2–3. The steps that occur during anaphase are critical in providing each subsequent daughter cell with an identical set of chromosomes. In human cells, there would now be 46 chromosomes at each pole, one from each original sister pair. Figure 2–7(e) shows anaphase prior to its completion.

Telophase

Telophase is the final stage of mitosis and is depicted in **Figure 2–7(f)**. At its beginning, two complete sets of chromosomes are present, one set at each pole. The most significant event of this stage is cytokinesis, the division or partitioning of the cytoplasm. Cytokinesis is essential if two new cells are to be produced from one cell. The mechanism of cytokinesis differs greatly in plant and animal cells, but the end result is the same: two new cells are produced. In plant cells, a **cell plate** is synthesized and laid down across the region of the metaphase plate. Animal cells, however, undergo a constriction of the cytoplasm, much as a loop of string might be tightened around the middle of a balloon.

It is not surprising that the process of cytokinesis varies in different organisms. Plant cells, which are more regularly shaped and structurally rigid, require a mechanism for depositing new cell wall material around the plasma membrane. The cell plate laid down during telophase becomes a structure called the **middle lamella**. Subsequently, the primary and secondary layers of the cell wall are deposited between the cell membrane and middle lamella in each of the resulting daughter cells. In animals, complete constriction of the cell membrane produces the **cell furrow** characteristic of newly divided cells.

Other events necessary for the transition from mitosis to interphase are initiated during late telophase. They generally constitute a reversal of events that occurred during prophase. In each new cell, the chromosomes begin to uncoil and become diffuse chromatin once again, while the nuclear envelope reforms around them, the spindle fibers disappear, and the nucleolus gradually reforms and becomes visible in the nucleus during early interphase. At the completion of telophase, the cell enters interphase.

Cell-Cycle Regulation and Checkpoints

The cell cycle, culminating in mitosis, is fundamentally the same in all eukaryotic organisms. This similarity in many diverse organisms suggests that the cell cycle is governed by a genetically regulated program that has been conserved throughout evolution. Because disruption of this regulation may underlie the uncontrolled cell division characterizing malignancy, interest in how genes regulate the cell cycle is particularly strong.

A mammoth research effort over the past 20 years has paid high dividends, and we now have knowledge of many genes involved in the control of the cell cycle. This work was recognized by the awarding of the 2001 Nobel Prize in Medicine or Physiology to Lee Hartwell, Paul Nurse, and Tim Hunt. As with other studies of genetic control over essential biological processes, investigation has focused on the discovery of mutations that interrupt the cell cycle and on the effects of those mutations. As we shall return to this subject in much greater detail later in the text during our consideration of the molecular basis of cancer (see Chapter 19), what follows is a very brief overview .

Many mutations are now known that exert an effect at one or another stage of the cell cycle. First discovered in yeast, but now evident in all organisms, including humans, such mutations were originally designated as *cell division cycle (cdc) mutations*. The normal products of many of the mutated genes are enzymes called **kinases** that can add phosphates to other proteins. They serve as "master control" molecules functioning in conjunction with proteins called **cyclins**. Cyclins bind to these kinases (creating *cyclin-dependent kinases*), activating them at appropriate times during the cell cycle. Activated kinases then phosphorylate other target proteins that regulate the progress of the cell cycle. The study of *cdc* mutations has established that the cell cycle contains at least three major *checkpoints,* where the processes culminating in normal mitosis are monitored, or "checked," by these master control molecules before the next stage of the cycle is allowed to commence.

Checkpoints are named according to where in the cell cycle monitoring occurs (Figure 2–5). The first of three (sometimes considered as two separate checkpoints), the **G1/S checkpoint**, monitors the size the cell has achieved since its previous mitosis and also evaluates the condition of the DNA. If the cell has not reached an adequate size or if the DNA has been damaged, further progress through the cycle is arrested until these conditions are "corrected." If both conditions are "normal" at G1/S, then the cell is allowed to proceed from G1 to the S phase of the cycle. The second checkpoint is the **G2/M checkpoint**, where DNA is monitored prior to the start of mitosis. If DNA replication is incomplete or any DNA damage is detected and has not been repaired, the cell cycle is arrested. The final checkpoint occurs during mitosis and is called the **M checkpoint** (sometimes referred to as the *Spindle Assembly checkpoint*). Here, both the successful formation of the spindle fiber system and the attachment of spindle fibers to the kinetochores associated with the centromeres are monitored. If spindle fibers are not properly formed or if attachment is inadequate, mitosis is arrested.

The importance of cell-cycle control and these checkpoints can be demonstrated by considering what happens when this regulatory system is impaired. Let's assume, for example, that the DNA of a cell has incurred damage leading to one or more mutations impairing cell-cycle control. If allowed to proceed through the cell cycle as one of the population of dividing cells, this genetically altered cell would divide uncontrollably—a key step in the development of a cancer cell. If instead the cell cycle is arrested at one of the checkpoints, the cell can repair the DNA damage or permanently stop the cell from dividing, thereby preventing its potential malignancy.

NOW SOLVE THIS

2–1 With the initial appearance of the feature we call "Now Solve This," a short introduction is in order. The feature occurs several times in this and all ensuing chapters, each time providing a problem related to the discussion just presented. A "Hint" is then offered that may help you solve the problem. Here is the first problem:

(a) If an organism has a diploid number of 16, how many chromatids are visible at the end of mitotic prophase?

(b) How many chromosomes are moving to each pole during anaphase of mitosis?

■ **HINT:** *This problem involves an understanding of what happens to each pair of homologous chromosomes during mitosis, asking you to apply your understanding of chromosome behavior to an organism with a diploid number of 16. The key to its solution is your awareness that throughout mitosis, the members of each homologous pair do not pair up, but instead behave independently.*

2.4 Meiosis Reduces the Chromosome Number from Diploid to Haploid in Germ Cells and Spores

The process of meiosis, unlike mitosis, reduces the amount of genetic material by one-half. Whereas in diploids mitosis produces daughter cells with a full diploid complement, meiosis produces gametes or spores with only one haploid set of chromosomes. During sexual reproduction, gametes then combine through fertilization to reconstitute the diploid complement found in parental cells. **Figure 2–9** compares the two processes by following two pairs of homologous chromosomes.

The events of meiosis must be highly specific since by definition, haploid gametes or spores contain precisely one member of each homologous pair of chromosomes. If successfully completed, meiosis ensures genetic continuity from generation to generation.

The process of sexual reproduction also ensures genetic variety among members of a species. As you study meiosis, you will see that this process results in gametes that each contain unique combinations of maternally and paternally derived chromosomes in their haploid complement. With such a tremendous genetic variation among the gametes, a huge number of maternal-paternal chromosome combinations are possible at fertilization. Furthermore, you will see that the meiotic event referred to as **crossing over** results in genetic exchange between members of each homologous pair of chromosomes. This process creates intact chromosomes that are mosaics of the maternal and paternal homologs from which they arise, further enhancing the potential genetic variation in gametes and the offspring derived from them. Sexual reproduction therefore reshuffles the genetic material, producing offspring that often differ greatly from either parent. Thus, meiosis is the major source of genetic recombination within species.

An Overview of Meiosis

In the preceding discussion, we established what might be considered the goal of meiosis: the reduction to the haploid complement of chromosomes. Before considering the phases of this process systematically, we will briefly summarize how diploid cells give rise to haploid gametes or spores. You should refer to the right-hand side of Figure 2–9 during the following discussion.

We have established that in mitosis each paternally and maternally derived member of any given homologous pair of chromosomes behaves autonomously during division. By contrast, early in meiosis, homologous

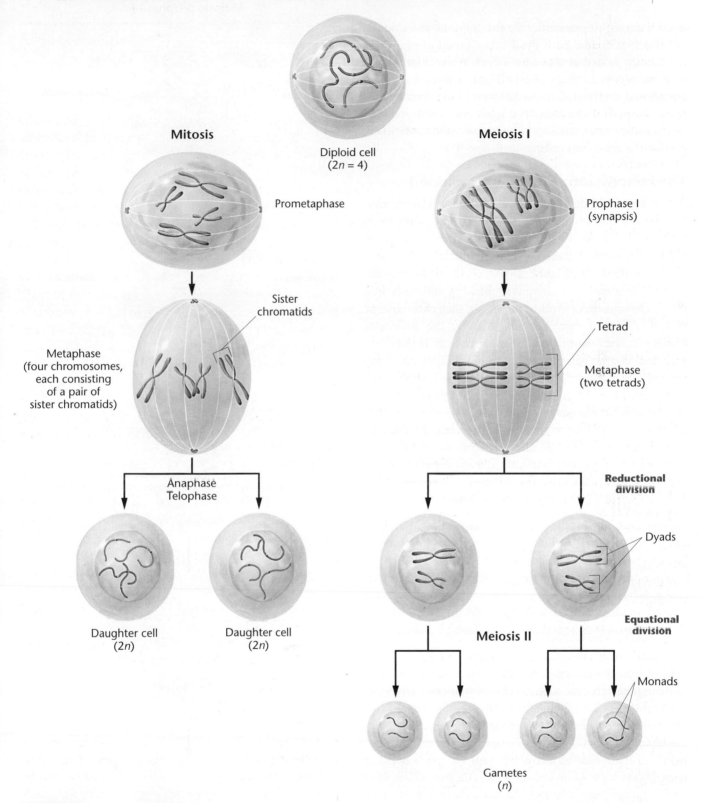

Mitosis

Diploid cell
(2n = 4)

Prometaphase

Meiosis I

Prophase I
(synapsis)

Sister
chromatids

Metaphase
(four chromosomes,
each consisting
of a pair of
sister chromatids)

Tetrad

Metaphase
(two tetrads)

Anaphase
Telophase

Reductional
division

Daughter cell
(2n)

Daughter cell
(2n)

Dyads

Equational
division

Meiosis II

Monads

Gametes
(n)

FIGURE 2–9 Overview of the major events and outcomes of mitosis and meiosis. As in Figure 2–7, two pairs of homologous chromosomes are followed.

chromosomes form pairs; that is, they *synapse* (or undergo **synapsis**). Each synapsed structure, initially called a **bivalent**, eventually gives rise to a **tetrad** consisting of four chromatids. The presence of four chromatids demonstrates that both homologs (making up the bivalent)

have, in fact, duplicated. Therefore, to achieve haploidy, two divisions are necessary. The first division occurs in meiosis I and is described as a **reductional division** (because the number of centromeres, each representing one chromosome, is *reduced* by one-half). Components of each tetrad—representing the two homologs—separate, yielding two **dyads**. Each dyad is composed of two sister chromatids joined at a common centromere. The second division occurs during meiosis II and is described as an **equational division** (because the number of centromeres remains *equal*). Here each dyad splits into two **monads** of one chromosome each. Thus, the two divisions potentially produce four haploid cells.

The First Meiotic Division: Prophase I

We turn now to a detailed account of meiosis. Like mitosis, meiosis is a continuous process. We assign names to its stages and substages only to facilitate discussion. From a genetic standpoint, three events characterize the initial stage, **prophase I** (**Figure 2–10**). First, as in mitosis, chromatin present in interphase thickens and coils into visible chromosomes. And, as in mitosis, each chromosome is a double structure, held together by the molecular complex called *cohesin*. Second, unlike mitosis, members of each homologous pair of chromosomes pair up, undergoing synapsis. Third, crossing over occurs between chromatids of synapsed homologs. Because of the complexity of these genetic events, this stage of meiosis is divided into five substages: leptonema, zygonema, pachynema, diplonema,[*] and diakinesis. As we discuss these substages, be aware that, even though it is not immediately apparent in the earliest phases of meiosis, the DNA of chromosomes has been replicated during the prior interphase.

Leptonema During the **leptotene stage**, the interphase chromatin material begins to condense, and the chromosomes, though still extended, become visible. Along each chromosome are **chromomeres**, localized condensations that resemble beads on a string. Evidence suggests that a process called **homology search**, which precedes and is essential to the initial pairing of homologs, begins during leptonema.

Zygonema The chromosomes continue to shorten and thicken during the **zygotene stage**. During the process of homology search, homologous chromosomes undergo initial alignment with one another. This so-called *rough pairing* is complete by the end of zygonema. In yeast, homologs are separated by about 300 nm, and near the end of zygonema, structures called *lateral elements* are visible between paired homologs. As meiosis proceeds, the overall length of the lateral elements along the chromosome increases, and a more extensive ultrastructural component called the **synaptonemal complex** begins to form between the homologs. This complex is believed to be the vehicle responsible for proper alignment during the pairing of homologs. In some

---

*These are the noun forms of these substages. The adjective forms (leptotene, zygotene, pachytene, and diplotene) are also used in the text.

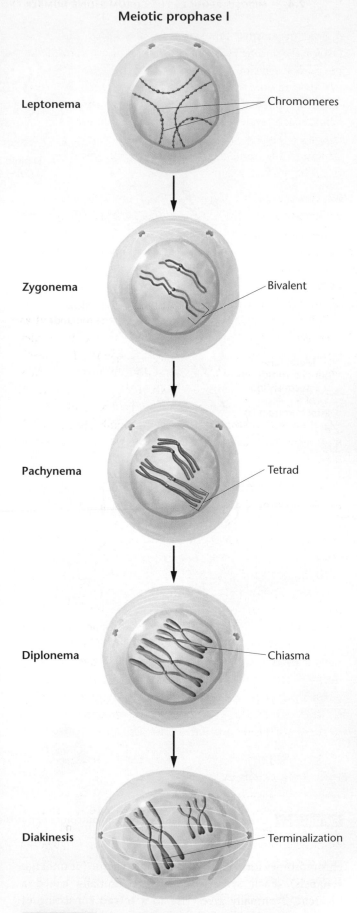

Meiotic prophase I

Leptonema — Chromomeres

Zygonema — Bivalent

Pachynema — Tetrad

Diplonema — Chiasma

Diakinesis — Terminalization

FIGURE 2–10 The substages of meiotic prophase I for the chromosomes depicted in Figure 2–9.

diploid organisms, this synapsis occurs in a zipper-like fashion, beginning at the ends of chromosomes attached to the nuclear envelope.

It is upon completion of zygonema that the paired homologs are referred to as bivalents. Although both members of each bivalent have already replicated their DNA, it is not yet visually apparent that each member is a double structure. The number of bivalents in each species is equal to the haploid (n) number.

Pachynema In the transition from the zygotene to the **pachytene stage**, the chromosomes continue to coil and shorten, and further development of the synaptonemal complex occurs between the two members of each bivalent. This leads to synapsis, a more intimate pairing. Compared to the rough-pairing characteristic of zygonema, homologs are now separated by only 100 nm.

During pachynema, each homolog is now evident as a double structure, providing visual evidence of the earlier replication of the DNA of each chromosome. Thus, each bivalent contains four chromatids. As in mitosis, replicates are called *sister chromatids*, whereas chromatids from maternal and paternal members of a homologous pair are called *nonsister chromatids*. The four-membered structure, also referred to as a *tetrad*, contains two pairs of sister chromatids.

Diplonema During the ensuing **diplotene stage**, it is even more apparent that each tetrad consists of two pairs of sister chromatids. Within each tetrad, each pair of sister chromatids begins to separate. However, one or more areas remain in contact where chromatids are intertwined. Each such area, called a **chiasma** (pl. **chiasmata**), is thought to represent a point where nonsister chromatids have undergone genetic exchange through the process referred to above as *crossing over*. Although the physical exchange between chromosome areas occurred during the previous pachytene stage, the result of crossing over is visible only when the duplicated chromosomes begin to separate. Crossing over is an important source of genetic variability, and as indicated earlier, new combinations of genetic material are formed during this process.

Diakinesis The final stage of prophase I is **diakinesis**. The chromosomes pull farther apart, but nonsister chromatids remain loosely associated at the chiasmata. As separation proceeds, the chiasmata move toward the ends of the tetrad. This process of **terminalization** begins in late diplonema and is completed during diakinesis. During this final substage, the nucleolus and nuclear envelope break down, and the two centromeres of each tetrad attach to the recently formed spindle fibers. By the completion of prophase I, the centromeres of each tetrad structure are present on the metaphase plate of the cell.

Metaphase, Anaphase, and Telophase I

The remainder of the meiotic process is depicted in **Figure 2–11**. After meiotic prophase I, stages similar to those of mitosis occur. In the first division, **metaphase I**, the chromosomes have maximally shortened and thickened. The terminal chiasmata of each tetrad are visible and appear to be the major factor holding the nonsister chromatids together. Each tetrad interacts with spindle fibers, facilitating its movement to the metaphase plate. The alignment of each tetrad prior to the first anaphase is random: Half of the tetrad (one of the dyads) will subsequently be pulled to one or the other pole, and the other half moves to the opposite pole.

During the stages of meiosis I, a single centromeric region holds each pair of sister chromatids together. It appears as a single unit, and a kinetechore forms around each one. As in our discussion of mitosis (see Figure 2–8), cohesin plays the major role in keeping sister chromatids together. At **anaphase I**, cohesin is degraded between sister chromatids, except at the centromere region, which, as in mitosis, is protected by a shugoshin complex. Then, one-half of each tetrad (a dyad) is pulled toward each pole of the dividing cell. This separation process is the physical basis of disjunction, the separation of homologous chromosomes from one another. Occasionally, errors in meiosis occur and separation is not achieved. The term **nondisjunction** describes such an error. At the completion of the normal anaphase I, a series of dyads equal to the haploid number is present at each pole.

If crossing over had not occurred in the first meiotic prophase, each dyad at each pole would consist solely of either paternal or maternal chromatids. However, the exchanges produced by crossing over create mosaic chromatids of paternal and maternal origin.

In many organisms, **telophase I** reveals a nuclear membrane forming around the dyads. In this case, the nucleus next enters into a short interphase period. If interphase occurs, the chromosomes do not replicate because they already consist of two chromatids. In other organisms, the cells go directly from anaphase I to meiosis II. In general, meiotic telophase is much shorter than the corresponding stage in mitosis.

The Second Meiotic Division

A second division, referred to as **meiosis II**, is essential if each gamete or spore is to receive only one chromatid from each original tetrad. The stages characterizing meiosis II are shown on the right side of Figure 2–11. During **prophase II**, each dyad is composed of one pair of sister chromatids attached by the common centromeric region. During **metaphase II**, the centromeres are positioned

Metaphase I   Anaphase I   Telophase I   Prophase II

Prophase II

FIGURE 2–11 The major events in meiosis in an animal cell with a diploid number of 4, beginning with metaphase I. Note that the combination of chromosomes in the cells following telophase II is dependent on the random orientation of each tetrad and dyad when they align on the equatorial plate during metaphase I and metaphase II. Several other combinations, which are not shown, can also be produced. The events depicted here are described in the text.

NOW SOLVE THIS

2–2 An organism has a diploid number of 16 in a primary oocyte. (a) How many tetrads are present in the first meiotic prophase? (b) How many dyads are present in the second meiotic prophase? (c) How many monads migrate to each pole during the second meiotic anaphase?

■ **HINT:** *This problem involves an understanding of what happens to the maternal and paternal members of each pair of homologous chromosomes during meiosis, asking you to apply your understanding of chromosome behavior in an organism with a diploid number of 16. The key to its solution is your awareness that maternal and paternal homologs synapse during meiosis. Once each chromatid has duplicated, creating a tetrad in the early phases of meiosis, each original pair behaves as a unit and leads to two dyads during anaphase I.*

For more practice, see Problems 33, 34, and 35.

on the equatorial plate. When the shugoshin complex is degraded, the centromeres separate, **anaphase II** is initiated, and the sister chromatids of each dyad are pulled to opposite poles. Because the number of dyads is equal to the haploid number, **telophase II** reveals one member of each pair of homologous chromosomes present at each pole. Each chromosome is now a monad. Following cytokinesis in telophase II, four haploid gametes may result from a single meiotic event. At the conclusion of meiosis II, not only has the haploid state been achieved, but if crossing over has occurred, each monad contains a combination of maternal and paternal genetic information. As a result, the offspring produced by any gamete will receive a mixture of genetic information originally present in his or her grandparents. Meiosis thus significantly increases the level of genetic variation in each ensuing generation.

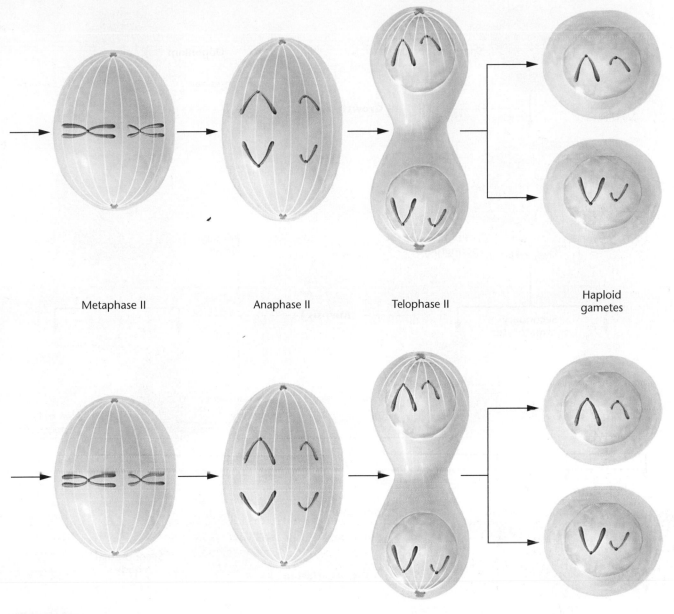

| Metaphase II | Anaphase II | Telophase II | Haploid gametes |

FIGURE 2–11   *(Continued)*

2.5 The Development of Gametes Varies in Spermatogenesis Compared to Oogenesis

Although events that occur during the meiotic divisions are similar in all cells participating in gametogenesis in most animal species, there are certain differences between the production of a male gamete (spermatogenesis) and a female gamete (oogenesis). **Figure 2–12** summarizes these processes.

Spermatogenesis takes place in the testes, the male reproductive organs. The process begins with the enlargement of an undifferentiated diploid germ cell called a spermatogonium. This cell grows to become a **primary spermatocyte**, which undergoes the first meiotic division. The products of this division, called **secondary spermatocytes**, contain a haploid number of dyads. The secondary spermatocytes then undergo meiosis II, and each of these cells produces two haploid **spermatids**. Spermatids go through a series of developmental changes, **spermiogenesis**, to become highly specialized, motile **spermatozoa**, or **sperm**. All sperm cells produced during spermatogenesis contain the haploid number of chromosomes and equal amounts of cytoplasm.

Spermatogenesis may be continuous or may occur periodically in mature male animals; its onset is determined by the species' reproductive cycles. Animals that reproduce

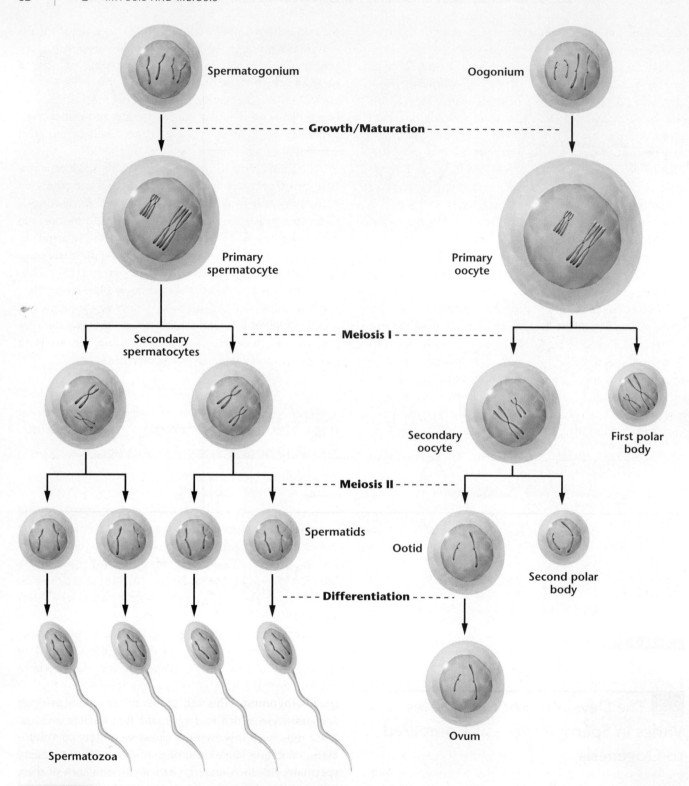

Spermatogonium

Oogonium

Growth/Maturation

Primary spermatocyte

Primary oocyte

Secondary spermatocytes

Meiosis I

Secondary oocyte

First polar body

Spermatids

Meiosis II

Ootid

Second polar body

Differentiation

Spermatozoa

Ovum

FIGURE 2–12 Spermatogenesis and oogenesis in animal cells.

year-round produce sperm continuously, whereas those whose breeding period is confined to a particular season produce sperm only during that time.

In animal **oogenesis**, the formation of **ova** (sing. **ovum**), or eggs, occurs in the ovaries, the female reproductive organs. The daughter cells resulting from the two

meiotic divisions of this process receive equal amounts of genetic material, but they do *not* receive equal amounts of cytoplasm. Instead, during each division, almost all the cytoplasm of the **primary oocyte**, itself derived from the **oogonium**, is concentrated in one of the two daughter cells. The concentration of cytoplasm is necessary because a major function of the mature ovum is to nourish the developing embryo following fertilization.

During anaphase I in oogenesis, the tetrads of the primary oocyte separate, and the dyads move toward opposite poles. During telophase I, the dyads at one pole are pinched off with very little surrounding cytoplasm to form the **first polar body**. The first polar body may or may not divide again to produce two small haploid cells. The other daughter cell produced by this first meiotic division contains most of the cytoplasm and is called the **secondary oocyte**. The mature ovum will be produced from the secondary oocyte during the second meiotic division. During this division, the cytoplasm of the secondary oocyte again divides unequally, producing an **ootid** and a **second polar body**. The ootid then differentiates into the mature ovum.

Unlike the divisions of spermatogenesis, the two meiotic divisions of oogenesis may not be continuous. In some animal species, the second division may directly follow the first. In others, including humans, the first division of all oocytes begins in the embryonic ovary but arrests in prophase I. Many years later, meiosis resumes in each oocyte just prior to its ovulation. The second division is completed only after fertilization.

NOW SOLVE THIS

2.3 Examine Figure 2–12, which shows oogenesis in animal cells. Will the genotype of the second polar body (derived from meiosis II) always be identical to that of the ootid? Why or why not?

■ **HINT:** *This problem involves an understanding of meiosis during oogenesis, asking you to demonstrate your knowledge of polar bodies. The key to its solution is to take into account that crossing over occurred between each pair of homologs during meiosis I.*

2.6 Meiosis Is Critical to Sexual Reproduction in All Diploid Organisms

The process of meiosis is critical to the successful sexual reproduction of all diploid organisms. It is the mechanism by which the diploid amount of genetic information is reduced to the haploid amount. In animals, meiosis leads to the formation of gametes, whereas in plants haploid spores are produced, which in turn lead to the formation of haploid gametes.

Each diploid organism stores its genetic information in the form of homologous pairs of chromosomes. Each pair consists of one member derived from the maternal parent and one from the paternal parent. Following meiosis,

haploid cells potentially contain either the paternal or the maternal representative of every homologous pair of chromosomes. However, the process of crossing over, which occurs in the first meiotic prophase, further reshuffles the alleles between the maternal and paternal members of each homologous pair, which then segregate and assort independently into gametes. These events result in the great amount of genetic variation present in gametes.

It is important to touch briefly on the significant role that meiosis plays in the life cycles of fungi and plants. In many fungi, the predominant stage of the life cycle consists of haploid vegetative cells. They arise through meiosis and proliferate by mitotic cell division. In multicellular plants, the life cycle alternates between the diploid **sporophyte stage** and the haploid **gametophyte stage** (**Figure 2–13**). While one or the other predominates in different plant groups during this "alternation of generations," the processes of meiosis and fertilization constitute the "bridges" between the sporophyte and gametophyte stages. Therefore, meiosis is an essential component of the life cycle of plants.

2.7 Electron Microscopy Has Revealed the Physical Structure of Mitotic and Meiotic Chromosomes

Thus far in this chapter, we have focused on mitotic and meiotic chromosomes, emphasizing their behavior during cell division and gamete formation. An interesting question is why chromosomes are invisible during interphase but visible during the various stages of mitosis and meiosis. Studies using electron microscopy clearly show why this is the case.

Recall that, during interphase, only dispersed chromatin fibers are present in the nucleus [**Figure 2–14(a)**]. Once mitosis begins, however, the fibers coil and fold, condensing into typical mitotic chromosomes [**Figure 2–14(b)**]. If the fibers comprising a mitotic chromosome are loosened, the areas of greatest spreading reveal individual fibers similar to those seen in interphase chromatin [**Figure 2–14(c)**]. Very few fiber ends seem to be present, and in some cases, none can be seen. Instead, individual fibers always seem to loop back into the interior. Such fibers are obviously twisted and coiled around one another, forming the regular pattern of folding in the mitotic chromosome. Starting in late telophase of mitosis and continuing during G1 of interphase, chromosomes unwind to form the long fibers characteristic of chromatin, which consist of DNA and associated proteins, particularly proteins called *histones*. It is in this physical arrangement that DNA can most efficiently function during transcription and replication.

Microsporangium
(produces
microspores)

Megasporangium
(produces
megaspores)

Zygote

Sporophyte

Diploid (2*n*)

Fertilization ━━━━━━━━━━━━━━━━━━━━ Meiosis

Haploid (*n*)

Megaspore (*n*)

Egg

Sperm

Female
gametophyte
(embryo sac)

Microspore (*n*)

Male
gametophyte
(pollen grain)

FIGURE 2–13 Alternation of generations between the diploid sporophyte (2*n*) and the haploid gametophyte (*n*) in a multicellular plant. The processes of meiosis and fertilization bridge the two phases of the life cycle. In angiosperms (flowering plants), like the one shown here, the sporophyte stage is the predominant phase.

Electron microscopic observations of metaphase chromosomes in varying degrees of coiling led Ernest DuPraw to postulate the **folded-fiber model**, shown in Figure 2–14(c). During metaphase, each chromosome consists of two sister chromatids joined at the centromeric region. Each arm of the chromatid appears to be a single fiber wound much like a skein of yarn. The fiber is composed of tightly coiled double-stranded DNA and protein. An orderly coiling–twisting–condensing process appears to facilitate the transition of the interphase chromatin into the more condensed mitotic chromosomes. Geneticists believe that during the transition from interphase to prophase, a 5000-fold compaction occurs in the length of DNA within the chromatin fiber! This process must be extremely precise given the highly ordered and consistent appearance of mitotic chromosomes in all eukaryotes. Note particularly in the micrographs the clear distinction between the sister chromatids constituting each chromosome. They are joined only by the common centromere that they share prior to anaphase. We will return to this general topic later in the text when we consider chromosome structure in further detail (see Chapter 12).

(a) **(b)** **(c)**

FIGURE 2–14 Comparison of (a) the chromatin fibers characteristic of the interphase nucleus with (b) metaphase chromosomes that are derived from chromatin during mitosis. Part (c) diagrams a mitotic chromosome, showing how chromatin is condensed to produce it. Part (a) is a transmission electron micrograph and part (b) is a scanning electron micrograph.

PubMed: Exploring and Retrieving Biomedical Literature

MasteringGenetics™ Visit the Study Area: Exploring Genomics

PubMed is an Internet-based search system developed by the National Center of Biotechnology Information (NCBI) at the National Library of Medicine. Using PubMed, one can access over 23 million articles in over 5600 biomedical journals. The full text of many of the journals can be obtained electronically through college or university libraries, and some journals (such as *Proceedings of the National Academy of Sciences USA; Genome Biology;* and *Science*) provide free public access to articles within certain time frames.

In this exercise, we will explore PubMed to answer questions about relationships between tubulin, human cancers, and cancer therapies.

■ **Exercise I – Tubulin, Cancer, and Mitosis**

In this chapter we were introduced to tubulin and the dynamic behavior of microtubules during the cell cycle. Cancer cells are characterized by continuous and uncontrolled mitotic divisions.

Is it possible that tubulin and microtubules contribute to the development of cancer? Could these important structures be targets for cancer therapies?

1. To begin your search for the answers, access the PubMed site at http://www.ncbi.nlm.nih.gov/pubmed/.

2. In the search box, type "tubulin cancer" and then click the "Search" button to perform the search.

3. Select several research papers and read the abstracts.

To answer the question about tubulin's association with cancer, you may want to limit your search to fewer papers, perhaps those that are review articles. To do this, click the "Review" link under the Article Types category on the left side of the page.

Explore some of the articles, as abstracts or as full text, available in your library or by free public access. Prepare a brief report or verbally share your experiences with your class. Describe two of the most important things you learned during your exploration and identify the information sources you encountered during the search.

CASE STUDY | Timing is everything

A man in his early 20s received chemotherapy and radiotherapy as treatment every 60 days for Hodgkin's disease. After unsuccessful attempts to have children, he had his sperm examined at a fertility clinic, upon which multiple chromosomal irregularities were discovered. When examined within 5 days of a treatment, extra chromosomes were often present or one or more chromosomes were completely absent. However, such irregularities were not observed at day 38 or thereafter.

1. How might a geneticist explain the time-related differences in chromosomal irregularities?

2. Do you think that exposure to chemotherapy and radiotherapy of a spermatogonium would cause more problems than exposure to a secondary spermatocyte?

3. What is the obvious advice that the man received regarding fertility while he remained under treatment?

Summary Points

MasteringGenetics™ For activities, animations, and review quizzes, go to the Study Area.

1. The structure of cells is elaborate and complex, with most components involved directly or indirectly with genetic processes.

2. In diploid organisms, chromosomes exist in homologous pairs, where each member is identical in size, centromere placement, and gene loci. One member of each pair is derived from the maternal parent, and the other from the paternal parent.

3. Mitosis and meiosis are mechanisms by which cells distribute the genetic information contained in their chromosomes to progeny cells in a precise, orderly fashion.

4. Mitosis, which is but one part of the cell cycle, is subdivided into discrete stages that initially depict the condensation of chromatin into the diploid number of chromosomes. Each chromosome first appears as a double structure, consisting of a

pair of identical sister chromatids joined at a common centromere. As mitosis proceeds, centromeres split and sister chromatids are pulled apart by spindle fibers and directed toward opposite poles of the cell. Cytoplasmic division then occurs, creating two new cells with the identical genetic information contained in the progenitor cell.

5. Meiosis converts a diploid cell into haploid gametes or spores, making sexual reproduction possible. As a result of chromosome duplication, two subsequent meiotic divisions are required to achieve haploidy, whereby each haploid cell receives one member of each homologous pair of chromosomes.

6. There is a major difference between meiosis in males and in females. Spermatogenesis partitions the cytoplasmic volume equally and produces four haploid sperm cells. Oogenesis, on the other hand, collects the bulk of cytoplasm in one egg cell and reduces the other haploid products to polar bodies. The extra cytoplasm in the egg contributes to zygote development following fertilization.

7. Meiosis results in extensive genetic variation by virtue of the exchange of chromosome segments during crossing over between maternal and paternal chromatids and by virtue of the random separation of maternal and paternal chromatids into gametes. In addition, meiosis plays an important role in the life cycles of fungi and plants, serving as the bridge between alternating generations.

8. Mitotic chromosomes are produced as a result of the coiling and condensation of chromatin fibers of interphase into the characteristic form of chromatids.

INSIGHTS AND SOLUTIONS

This appearance of "Insights and Solutions" begins a feature that will have great value to you as a student. From this point on, "Insights and Solutions" precedes the "Problems and Discussion Questions" at each chapter's end to provide sample problems and solutions that demonstrate approaches you will find useful in genetic analysis. The insights you gain by working through the sample problems will improve your ability to solve the ensuing problems in each chapter.

1. In an organism with a diploid number of $2n = 6$, how many individual chromosomal structures will align on the metaphase plate during (a) mitosis, (b) meiosis I, and (c) meiosis II? Describe each configuration.

(c) In meiosis II, the same number of structures exist (three), but in this case they are called dyads. Each dyad is a pair of sister chromatids. When crossing over has occurred, each chromatid may contain parts of one of its nonsister chromatids, obtained during exchange in prophase I.

2. Disregarding crossing over, draw all possible alignment configurations that can occur during metaphase for the chromosomes shown in Figure 2–11.

Solution: As shown in the diagram below, four configurations are possible when $n = 2$.

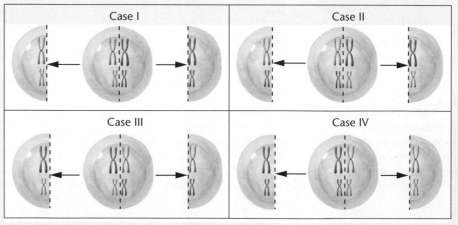

Solution for #2

Solution: (a) Remember that in mitosis, homologous chromosomes do not synapse, so there will be six double structures, each consisting of a pair of sister chromatids. In other words, the number of structures is equivalent to the diploid number.

(b) In meiosis I, the homologs have synapsed, reducing the number of structures to three. Each is called a tetrad and consists of two pairs of sister chromatids.

3. For the chromosomes in the previous problem, assume that each of the larger chromosomes has a different allele for a given gene, *A* OR *a*, as shown. Also assume that each of the smaller chromosomes has a different allele for a second gene, *B* OR *b*. Calculate the probability of generating each possible combination of these alleles (*AB, Ab, aB, ab*) following meiosis I.

Solution: As shown in the accompanying diagram:

Case I	*AB* and *ab*
Case II	*Ab* and *aB*
Case III	*aB* and *Ab*
Case IV	*ab* and *AB*

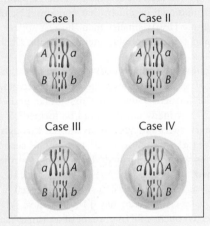

Solution for #3

Total: $AB = 2(p = 1/4)$

$Ab = 2(p = 1/4)$

$aB = 2(p = 1/4)$

$ab = 2(p = 1/4)$

4. How many different chromosome configurations can occur following meiosis I if three different pairs of chromosomes are present $(n = 3)$?

Solution: If $n = 3$, then eight different configurations would be possible. The formula 2^n, where n equals the haploid number, represents the number of potential alignment patterns. As we will see in the next chapter, these patterns are produced according to the Mendelian postulate of *segregation,* and they serve as the physical basis of another Mendelian postulate called *independent assortment.*

5. Describe the composition of a meiotic tetrad during prophase I, assuming no crossover event has occurred. What impact would a single crossover event have on this structure?

Solution: Such a tetrad contains four chromatids, existing as two pairs. Members of each pair are sister chromatids. They are held together by a common centromere. Members of one pair are maternally derived, whereas members of the other are paternally derived. Maternal and paternal members are called nonsister chromatids. A single crossover event has the effect of exchanging a portion of a maternal and a paternal chromatid, leading to a chiasma, where the two involved chromatids overlap physically in the tetrad. The process of exchange is referred to as crossing over.

Problems and Discussion Questions

HOW DO WE KNOW?

1. In this chapter, we focused on how chromosomes are distributed during cell division, both in dividing somatic cells (mitosis) and in gamete- and spore-forming cells (meiosis). We found many opportunities to consider the methods and reasoning by which much of this information was acquired. From the explanations given in the chapter, answer the following questions.
   (a) How do we know that chromosomes exist in homologous pairs?
   (b) How do we know that DNA replication occurs during interphase, not early in mitosis?
   (c) How do we know that mitotic chromosomes are derived from chromatin?

CONCEPT QUESTION

2. Review the Chapter Concepts list on page 16. All of these pertain to conceptual issues involving mitosis or meiosis. Based on these concepts, write a short essay that contrasts mitosis and meiosis, including their respective roles in organisms, the mechanisms by which they achieve their respective outcomes, and the consequences should either process fail to be executed with absolute fidelity.

3. What role do the following cellular components play in the storage, expression, or transmission of genetic information: (a) chromatin, (b) nucleolus, (c) ribosome, (d) mitochondrion, (e) centriole, (f) centromere?

4. Discuss the concepts of homologous chromosomes, diploidy, and haploidy. What characteristics do two homologous chromosomes share?

5. If two chromosomes of a species are the same length and have similar centromere placements and yet are not homologous, what is different about them?

6. Describe the events that characterize each stage of mitosis.

7. How are chromosomes named on the basis of their centromere placement?

8. Contrast telophase in plant and animal mitosis.

9. Describe the phases of the cell cycle and the events that characterize each phase.

10. Define and discuss these terms: (a) synapsis, (b) bivalents, (c) chiasmata, (d) crossing over, (e) chromomeres, (f) sister chromatids, (g) tetrads, (h) dyads, (i) monads.

11. Contrast the genetic content and the origin of sister versus nonsister chromatids during their earliest appearance in

prophase I of meiosis. How might the genetic content of these change by the time tetrads have aligned at the equatorial plate during metaphase I?

12. Given the end results of the two types of division, why is it necessary for homologs to pair during meiosis and not desirable for them to pair during mitosis?

13. Contrast spermatogenesis and oogenesis. What is the significance of the formation of polar bodies?

14. Explain why meiosis leads to significant genetic variation while mitosis does not.

15. A diploid cell contains three pairs of homologous chromosomes designated C1 and C2, M1 and M2, and S1 and S2. No crossing over occurs. What combinations of chromosomes are possible in (a) daughter cells following mitosis? (b) cells undergoing the first meiotic metaphase? (c) haploid cells following both divisions of meiosis?

16. Considering the preceding problem, predict the number of different haploid cells that could be produced by meiosis if a fourth chromosome pair (W1 and W2) were added.

17. During oogenesis in an animal species with a haploid number of 6, one dyad undergoes nondisjunction during meiosis II. Following the second meiotic division, this dyad ends up intact in the ovum. How many chromosomes are present in (a) the mature ovum and (b) the second polar body? (c) Following fertilization by a normal sperm, what chromosome condition is created?

18. What is the probability that, in an organism with a haploid number of 10, a sperm will be formed that contains all 10 chromosomes whose centromeres were derived from maternal homologs?

19. During the first meiotic prophase, (a) when does crossing over occur; (b) when does synapsis occur; (c) during which stage are the chromosomes least condensed; and (d) when are chiasmata first visible?

20. Describe the role of meiosis in the life cycle of a vascular plant.

21. Contrast the chromatin fiber with the mitotic chromosome. How are the two structures related?

22. Describe the "folded-fiber" model of the mitotic chromosome.

23. You are given a metaphase chromosome preparation (a slide) from an unknown organism that contains 12 chromosomes. Two that are clearly smaller than the rest appear identical in length and centromere placement. Describe all that you can about these chromosomes.

24. If one follows 50 primary oocytes in an animal through their various stages of oogenesis, how many secondary oocytes would be formed? How many first polar bodies would be formed? How many ootids would be formed? If one follows 50 primary spermatocytes in an animal through their various stages of spermatogenesis, how many secondary spermatocytes would be formed? How many spermatids would be formed?

25. The nuclear DNA content of a single sperm cell in *Drosophila melanogaster* is approximately 0.18 picogram. What would be the expected nuclear DNA content of a primary spermatocyte in *Drosophila*? What would be the expected nuclear DNA content of a somatic cell (non-sex cell) in the G1 phase? What would be the expected nuclear DNA content of a somatic cell at metaphase?

Extra-Spicy Problems

MasteringGenetics™ Visit for instructor-assigned tutorials and problems.

As part of the "Problems and Discussion Questions" section in this and each subsequent chapter, we shall present a number of "Extra-Spicy" genetics problems. We have chosen to set these apart in order to identify problems that are particularly challenging. You may be asked to examine and assess actual data, to design genetics experiments, or to engage in cooperative learning. Like genetic varieties of peppers, some of these experiences are just spicy and some are very hot. We hope that you will enjoy the challenges that they pose.

For Problems **26–31**, consider a diploid cell that contains three pairs of chromosomes designated AA, BB, and CC. Each pair contains a maternal and a paternal member (e.g., A^m and A^p). Using these designations, demonstrate your understanding of mitosis and meiosis by drawing chromatid combinations as requested. Be sure to indicate when chromatids are paired as a result of replication and/or synapsis. You may wish to use a large piece of brown manila wrapping paper or a cut-up paper grocery bag for this project and to work in partnership with another student. We recommend cooperative learning as an efficacious way to develop the skills you will need for solving the problems presented throughout this text.

26. In mitosis, what chromatid combination(s) will be present during metaphase? What combination(s) will be present at each pole at the completion of anaphase?

27. During meiosis I, assuming no crossing over, what chromatid combination(s) will be present at the completion of prophase? Draw all possible alignments of chromatids as migration begins during early anaphase.

28. Are there any possible combinations present during prophase of meiosis II other than those that you drew in Problem 27? If so, draw them.

29. Draw all possible combinations of chromatids during the early phases of anaphase in meiosis II.

30. Assume that during meiosis I none of the C chromosomes disjoin at metaphase, but they separate into dyads (instead of monads) during meiosis II. How would this change the alignments that you constructed during the anaphase stages in meiosis I and II? Draw them.

31. Assume that each gamete resulting from Problem 30 fuses, in fertilization, with a normal haploid gamete. What combinations will result? What percentage of zygotes will be diploid, containing one paternal and one maternal member of each chromosome pair?

32. A species of cereal rye (*Secale cereale*) has a chromosome number of 14, while a species of Canadian wild rye (*Elymus canadensis*) has a chromosome number of 28. Sterile hybrids can be produced by crossing *Secale* with *Elymus*.
(a) What would be the expected chromosome number in the somatic cells of the hybrids?
(b) Given that none of the chromosomes pair at meiosis I in the sterile hybrid (Hang and Franckowlak, 1984), speculate on the anaphase I separation patterns of these chromosomes.

33. An interesting procedure has been applied for assessing the chromosomal balance of potential secondary oocytes for use in human *in vitro* fertilization. Using fluorescence *in situ* hybridization (FISH), Kuliev and Verlinsky (2004) were able

to identify individual chromosomes in first polar bodies and thereby infer the chromosomal makeup of "sister" oocytes. Assume that when examining a first polar body you saw that it had one copy (dyad) of each chromosome but two dyads of chromosome 21. What would you expect to be the chromosomal 21 complement in the secondary oocyte? What consequences are likely in the resulting zygote, if the secondary oocyte was fertilized?

34. Assume that you were examining a first polar body and noted that it had one copy (dyad) of each chromosome except chromosome 21. Chromosome 21 was completely absent. What would you expect to be the chromosome 21 complement (only with respect to chromosome 21) in the secondary oocyte? What consequences are likely in the resulting zygote if the secondary oocyte was fertilized?

35. Kuliev and Verlinsky (2004) state that there was a relatively high number of separation errors at meiosis I. In these cases the centromere underwent a premature division, occurring at meiosis I rather than meiosis II. Regarding chromosome 21, what would you expect to be the chromosome 21 complement in the secondary oocyte in which you saw a single chromatid (monad) for chromosome 21 in the first polar body? If this secondary oocyte was involved in fertilization, what would be the expected consequences?

Gregor Johann Mendel, who in 1866 put forward the major postulates of transmission genetics as a result of experiments with the garden pea.

3 Mendelian Genetics

CHAPTER CONCEPTS

- Inheritance is governed by information stored in discrete factors called genes.

- Genes are transmitted from generation to generation on vehicles called chromosomes.

- Chromosomes, which exist in pairs in diploid organisms, provide the basis of biparental inheritance.

- During gamete formation, chromosomes are distributed according to postulates first described by Gregor Mendel, based on his nineteenth-century research with the garden pea.

- Mendelian postulates prescribe that homologous chromosomes segregate from one another and assort independently with other segregating homologs during gamete formation.

- Genetic ratios, expressed as probabilities, are subject to chance deviation and may be evaluated statistically.

- The analysis of pedigrees allows predictions concerning the genetic nature of human traits.

Although inheritance of biological traits has been recognized for thousands of years, the first significant insights into how it takes place only occurred about 150 years ago. In 1866, Gregor Johann Mendel published the results of a series of experiments that would lay the foundation for the formal discipline of genetics. Mendel's work went largely unnoticed until the turn of the twentieth century, but eventually, the concept of the gene as a distinct hereditary unit was established. Since then, the ways in which genes, as segments of chromosomes, are transmitted to offspring and control traits have been clarified. Research continued unabated throughout the twentieth century and into the present—indeed, studies in genetics, most recently at the molecular level, have remained at the forefront of biological research since the early 1900s.

When Mendel began his studies of inheritance using *Pisum sativum*, the garden pea, chromosomes and the role and mechanism of meiosis were totally unknown. Nevertheless, he determined that discrete *units of inheritance* exist and predicted their behavior in the formation of gametes. Subsequent investigators, with access to cytological data, were able to relate their own observations of chromosome behavior during meiosis and Mendel's principles of inheritance. Once this correlation was recognized, Mendel's postulates were accepted as the basis for the study of what is known as **transmission genetics**—how genes are transmitted from parents to offspring. These principles were derived directly from Mendel's experimentation.

3.1 Mendel Used a Model Experimental Approach to Study Patterns of Inheritance

Johann Mendel was born in 1822 to a peasant family in the Central European village of Heinzendorf. An excellent student in high school, he studied philosophy for several years afterward and in 1843, taking the name Gregor, was admitted to the Augustinian Monastery of St. Thomas in Brno, now part of the Czech Republic. In 1849, he was relieved of pastoral duties, and from 1851 to 1853, he attended the University of Vienna, where he studied physics and botany. He returned to Brno in 1854, where he taught physics and natural science for the next 16 years. Mendel received support from the monastery for his studies and research throughout his life.

In 1856, Mendel performed his first set of hybridization experiments with the garden pea, launching the research phase of his career. His experiments continued until 1868, when he was elected abbot of the monastery. Although he retained his interest in genetics, his new responsibilities demanded most of his time. In 1884, Mendel died of a kidney disorder. The local newspaper paid him the following tribute:

> "His death deprives the poor of a benefactor, and mankind at large of a man of the noblest character, one who was a warm friend, a promoter of the natural sciences, and an exemplary priest."

Mendel first reported the results of some simple genetic crosses between certain strains of the garden pea in 1865. Although his was not the first attempt to provide experimental evidence pertaining to inheritance, Mendel's success where others had failed can be attributed, at least in part, to his elegant experimental design and analysis.

Mendel showed remarkable insight into the methodology necessary for good experimental biology. First, he chose an organism that was easy to grow and to hybridize artificially. The pea plant is self-fertilizing in nature, but it is easy to cross-breed experimentally. It reproduces well and grows to maturity in a single season. Mendel followed seven visible features (we refer to them as characters, or characteristics), each represented by two contrasting forms, or **traits** (**Figure 3–1**). For the character stem height, for

Character	Contrasting traits		F₁ results	F₂ results	F₂ ratio
Seed shape	round/wrinkled		all round	5474 round 1850 wrinkled	2.96:1
Seed color	yellow/green		all yellow	6022 yellow 2001 green	3.01:1
Pod shape	full/constricted		all full	882 full 299 constricted	2.95:1
Pod color	green/yellow		all green	428 green 152 yellow	2.82:1
Flower color	violet/white		all violet	705 violet 224 white	3.15:1
Flower position	axial/terminal		all axial	651 axial 207 terminal	3.14:1
Stem height	tall/dwarf		all tall	787 tall 277 dwarf	2.84:1

FIGURE 3–1   Seven pairs of contrasting traits and the results of Mendel's seven monohybrid crosses of the garden pea (*Pisum sativum*). In each case, pollen derived from plants exhibiting one trait was used to fertilize the ova of plants exhibiting the other trait. In the F₁ generation, one of the two traits was exhibited by all plants. The contrasting trait reappeared in approximately 1/4 of the F₂ plants.

example, he experimented with the traits *tall* and *dwarf*. He selected six other visibly contrasting pairs of traits involving seed shape and color, pod shape and color, and flower color and position. From local seed merchants, Mendel obtained true-breeding strains, those in which each trait appeared unchanged generation after generation in self-fertilizing plants.

There were several other reasons for Mendel's success. In addition to his choice of a suitable organism, he restricted his examination to one or very few pairs of contrasting traits in each experiment. He also kept accurate quantitative records, a necessity in genetic experiments. From the analysis of his data, Mendel derived certain postulates that have become the principles of transmission genetics.

The results of Mendel's experiments went unappreciated until the turn of the century, well after his death. However, once Mendel's publications were rediscovered by geneticists investigating the function and behavior of chromosomes, the implications of his postulates were immediately apparent. He had discovered the basis for the transmission of hereditary traits!

3.2 The Monohybrid Cross Reveals How One Trait Is Transmitted from Generation to Generation

Mendel's simplest crosses involved only one pair of contrasting traits. Each such experiment is called a **monohybrid cross**. A monohybrid cross is made by mating true-breeding individuals from two parent strains, each exhibiting one of the two contrasting forms of the character under study. Initially, we examine the first generation of offspring of such a cross, and then we consider the offspring of **selfing**, that is, of self-fertilization of individuals from this first generation. The original parents constitute the P_1, or **parental generation**; their offspring are the F_1, or **first filial generation**; the individuals resulting from the selfed F_1 generation are the F_2, or **second filial generation**; and so on.

The cross between true-breeding pea plants with tall stems and dwarf stems is representative of Mendel's monohybrid crosses. *Tall* and *dwarf* are contrasting traits of the character of stem height. Unless tall or dwarf plants are crossed together or with another strain, they will undergo self-fertilization and breed true, producing their respective traits generation after generation. However, when Mendel crossed tall plants with dwarf plants,

the resulting F_1 generation consisted of only tall plants. When members of the F_1 generation were selfed, Mendel observed that 787 of 1064 F_2 plants were tall, while 277 of 1064 were dwarf. Note that in this cross (Figure 3–1), the dwarf trait disappeared in the F_1 generation, only to reappear in the F_2 generation.

Genetic data are usually expressed and analyzed as ratios. In this particular example, many identical P_1 crosses were made and many F_1 plants—all tall—were produced. As noted, of the 1064 F_2 offspring, 787 were tall and 277 were dwarf—a ratio of approximately 2.8:1.0, or about 3:1.

Mendel made similar crosses between pea plants exhibiting each of the other pairs of contrasting traits; the results of these crosses are shown in Figure 3–1. In every case, the outcome was similar to the tall/dwarf cross just described. For the character of interest, all F_1 offspring had the same trait exhibited by one of the parents, but in the F_2 offspring, an approximate ratio of 3:1 was obtained. That is, three-fourths looked like the F_1 plants, while one-fourth exhibited the contrasting trait, which had disappeared in the F_1 generation.

We note one further aspect of Mendel's monohybrid crosses. In each cross, the F_1 and F_2 patterns of inheritance were similar regardless of which P_1 plant served as the source of pollen (sperm) and which served as the source of the ovum (egg). The crosses could be made either way—pollination of dwarf plants by tall plants, or vice versa. Crosses made in both these ways are called **reciprocal crosses**. Therefore, the results of Mendel's monohybrid crosses were not sex-dependent.

To explain these results, Mendel proposed the existence of particulate *unit factors* for each trait. He suggested that these factors serve as the basic units of heredity and are passed unchanged from generation to generation, determining various traits expressed by each individual plant. Using these general ideas, Mendel proceeded to hypothesize precisely how such factors could account for the results of the monohybrid crosses.

Mendel's First Three Postulates

Using the consistent pattern of results in the monohybrid crosses, Mendel derived the following three postulates, or principles, of inheritance.

1. UNIT FACTORS IN PAIRS
Genetic characters are controlled by unit factors existing in pairs in individual organisms.

In the monohybrid cross involving tall and dwarf stems, a specific **unit factor** exists for each trait. Each diploid individual receives one factor from each parent. Because the factors occur in pairs, three combinations are possible: two factors for tall stems, two factors for dwarf stems, or one of each factor. Every individual possesses one of these three combinations, which determines stem height.

2. DOMINANCE/RECESSIVENESS

When two unlike unit factors responsible for a single character are present in a single individual, one unit factor is dominant to the other, which is said to be recessive.

In each monohybrid cross, the trait expressed in the F₁ generation is controlled by the dominant unit factor. The trait not expressed is controlled by the recessive unit factor. The terms dominant and recessive are also used to designate traits. In this case, tall stems are said to be dominant over recessive dwarf stems.

3. SEGREGATION

During the formation of gametes, the paired unit factors separate, or segregate, randomly so that each gamete receives one or the other with equal likelihood.

If an individual contains a pair of like unit factors (e.g., both specific for tall), then all its gametes receive one of that same kind of unit factor (in this case, tall). If an individual contains unlike unit factors (e.g., one for tall and one for dwarf), then each gamete has a 50 percent probability of receiving either the tall or the dwarf unit factor.

These postulates provide a suitable explanation for the results of the monohybrid crosses. Let's use the tall/dwarf cross to illustrate. Mendel reasoned that P₁ tall plants contained identical paired unit factors, as did the P₁ dwarf plants. The gametes of tall plants all receive one tall unit factor as a result of **segregation**. Similarly, the gametes of dwarf plants all receive one dwarf unit factor. Following fertilization, all F₁ plants receive one unit factor from each parent—a tall factor from one and a dwarf factor from the other—reestablishing the paired relationship, but because tall is dominant to dwarf, all F₁ plants are tall.

When F₁ plants form gametes, the postulate of segregation demands that each gamete randomly receives either the tall *or* dwarf unit factor. Following random fertilization events during F₁ selfing, four F₂ combinations will result with equal frequency:

1. tall/tall
2. tall/dwarf
3. dwarf/tall
4. dwarf/dwarf

Combinations (1) and (4) will clearly result in tall and dwarf plants, respectively. According to the postulate of dominance/recessiveness, combinations (2) and (3) will both yield tall plants. Therefore, the F₂ is predicted to consist of 3/4 tall and 1/4 dwarf, or a ratio of 3:1. This is approximately what Mendel observed in his cross between tall and dwarf plants. A similar pattern was observed in each of the other monohybrid crosses (Figure 3–1).

Modern Genetic Terminology

To analyze the monohybrid cross and Mendel's first three postulates, we must first introduce several new terms as well as a symbol convention for the unit factors. Traits such as tall or dwarf are physical expressions of the information contained in unit factors. The physical expression of a trait is the **phenotype** of the individual. Mendel's unit factors represent units of inheritance called **genes** by modern geneticists. For any given character, such as plant height, the phenotype is determined by alternative forms of a single gene, called **alleles**. For example, the unit factors representing tall and dwarf are alleles determining the height of the pea plant.

Geneticists have several different systems for using symbols to represent genes. Later in the text (see Chapter 4), we will review a number of these conventions, but for now, we will adopt one to use consistently throughout this chapter. According to this convention, the first letter of the recessive trait symbolizes the character in question; in lowercase italic, it designates the allele for the recessive trait, and in uppercase italic, it designates the allele for the dominant trait. Thus for Mendel's pea plants, we use *d* for the *dwarf* allele and *D* for the tall allele. When alleles are written in pairs to represent the two unit factors present in any individual (*DD*, *Dd*, or *dd*), the resulting symbol is called the **genotype**. The genotype designates the genetic makeup of an individual for the trait or traits it describes, whether the individual is haploid or diploid. By reading the genotype, we know the phenotype of the individual: *DD* and *Dd* are tall, and *dd* is dwarf. When both alleles are the same (*DD* or *dd*), the individual is **homozygous** for the trait, or a **homozygote**; when the alleles are different (*Dd*), we use the terms **heterozygous** and **heterozygote**. These symbols and terms are used in **Figure 3–2** to describe the monohybrid cross.

Mendel's Analytical Approach

What led Mendel to deduce that unit factors exist in pairs? Because there were two contrasting traits for each of the characters he chose, it seemed logical that two distinct factors must exist. However, why does one of the two traits or phenotypes disappear in the F_1 generation? Observation of the F_2 generation helps to answer this question. The recessive trait and its unit factor do not actually disappear in the F_1; they are merely hidden or masked, only to reappear in one-fourth of the F_2 offspring. Therefore, Mendel concluded that one unit factor for tall and one for dwarf were transmitted to each F_1 individual, but that because the tall factor or allele is dominant to the dwarf factor or allele, all F_1 plants are tall. Given this information, we can ask how Mendel explained the 3:1 F_2 ratio. As shown in Figure 3–2, Mendel deduced that the tall and dwarf alleles of the F_1 heterozygote segregate randomly into gametes. If fertilization is random, this ratio is predicted. If a large population of offspring is generated, the outcome of such a cross should reflect the 3:1 ratio.

Because he operated without the hindsight that modern geneticists enjoy, Mendel's analytical reasoning must be considered a truly outstanding scientific achievement. On the basis of rather simple but precisely executed breeding experiments, he not only proposed that discrete particulate units of heredity exist, but he also explained how they are transmitted from one generation to the next.

Punnett Squares

The genotypes and phenotypes resulting from combining gametes during fertilization can be easily visualized by constructing a diagram called a **Punnett square**, named after the person who first devised this approach, Reginald C. Punnett. **Figure 3–3** illustrates this method of analysis for our $F_1 \times F_1$ monohybrid cross. Each of the possible gametes is assigned a column or a row; the vertical columns represent those of the female parent, and the horizontal rows represent those of the male parent. After assigning the gametes to the rows and columns, we predict the new generation by entering the male and female gametic information into each box and thus producing

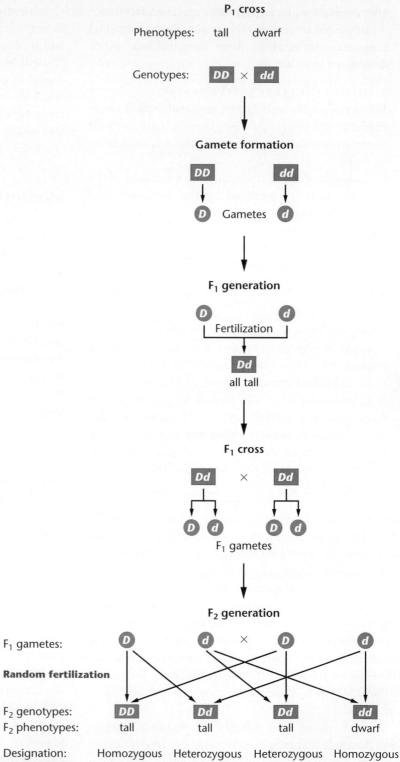

FIGURE 3–2 The monohybrid cross between tall (*D*) and dwarf (*d*) pea plants. Individuals are shown in rectangles, and gametes are shown in circles.

every possible resulting genotype. By filling out the Punnett square, we are listing all possible random fertilization events. The genotypes and phenotypes of all potential offspring are ascertained by reading the combinations in the boxes.

The Punnett square method is particularly useful when you are first learning about genetics and how to solve genetics problems. Note the ease with which the 3:1 phenotypic ratio and the 1:2:1 genotypic ratio may be derived for the F_2 generation in Figure 3–3.

NOW SOLVE THIS

3–1 Pigeons may exhibit a checkered or plain color pattern. In a series of controlled matings, the following data were obtained.

P₁ Cross	F₁ Progeny Checkered	Plain
(a) checkered × checkered	36	0
(b) checkered × plain	38	0
(c) plain × plain	0	35

Then F_1 offspring were selectively mated with the following results. (The P_1 cross giving rise to each F_1 pigeon is indicated in parentheses.)

F₁ × F₁ Crosses	F₂ Progeny Checkered	Plain
(d) checkered (a) × plain (c)	34	0
(e) checkered (b) × plain (c)	17	14
(f) checkered (b) × checkered (b)	28	9
(g) checkered (a) × checkered (b)	39	0

How are the checkered and plain patterns inherited? Select and assign symbols for the genes involved, and determine the genotypes of the parents and offspring in each cross.

■ **HINT:** *This problem asks you to analyze the data produced from several crosses involving pigeons and to determine the mode of inheritance and the genotypes of the parents and offspring in a number of instances. The key to its solution is to first determine whether or not this is a monohybrid cross. To do so, convert the data to ratios that are characteristic of Mendelian crosses. In the case of this problem, ask first whether any of the F_2 ratios match Mendel's 3:1 monohybrid ratio. If so, the second step is to determine which trait is dominant and which is recessive.*

The Testcross: One Character

Tall plants produced in the F_2 generation are predicted to have either the *DD* or the *Dd* genotype. You might ask if there is a way to distinguish the genotype. Mendel devised a rather simple method that is still used today to discover the genotype of plants and animals: the **testcross.** The organism expressing the dominant phenotype but

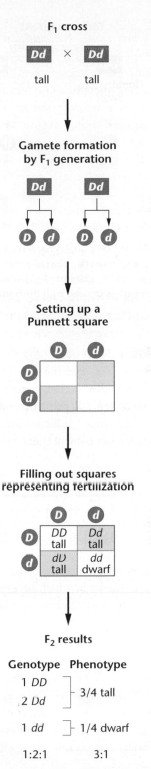

FIGURE 3–3 A Punnett square generating the F_2 ratio of the $F_1 \times F_1$ cross shown in Figure 3–2.

having an unknown genotype is crossed with a known *homozygous recessive individual.* For example, as shown in **Figure 3–4(a)**, if a tall plant of genotype *DD* is testcrossed with a dwarf plant, which must have the *dd* genotype, all offspring will be tall phenotypically and *Dd* genotypically. However, as shown in **Figure 3–4(b)**, if a tall plant is *Dd*

Testcross results

(a)

DD	×	dd
Homozygous tall		Homozygous dwarf

D   d

Dd

all tall

(b)

Dd	×	dd
Heterozygous tall		Homozygous dwarf

D d   d

Dd   dd

1/2 tall   1/2 dwarf

FIGURE 3–4 Testcross of a single character. In (a), the tall parent is homozygous, but in (b), the tall parent is heterozygous. The genotype of each tall P_1 plant can be determined by examining the offspring when each is crossed with the homozygous recessive dwarf plant.

and is crossed with a dwarf plant (*dd*), then one-half of the offspring will be tall (*Dd*) and the other half will be dwarf (*dd*). Therefore, a 1:1 tall/dwarf ratio demonstrates the heterozygous nature of the tall plant of unknown genotype. The results of the testcross reinforced Mendel's conclusion that separate unit factors control traits.

3.3 Mendel's Dihybrid Cross Generated a Unique F_2 Ratio

As a natural extension of the monohybrid cross, Mendel also designed experiments in which he examined two characters simultaneously. Such a cross, involving two pairs of

contrasting traits, is a **dihybrid cross**, or a *two-factor cross*. For example, if pea plants having yellow seeds that are round were bred with those having green seeds that are wrinkled, the results shown in **Figure 3–5** would occur: the F_1 offspring would all be yellow and round. It is therefore apparent that yellow is dominant to green and that round is dominant to wrinkled. When the F_1 individuals are selfed, approximately 9/16 of the F_2 plants express the yellow and round traits, 3/16 express yellow and wrinkled, 3/16 express green and round, and 1/16 express green and wrinkled.

A variation of this cross is also shown in Figure 3–5. Instead of crossing one P_1 parent with both dominant traits (yellow, round) to one with both recessive traits (green, wrinkled), plants with yellow, wrinkled seeds are crossed with those with green, round seeds. In spite of the change in the P_1 phenotypes, both the F_1 and F_2 results remain unchanged. Why this is so will become clear in the next section.

Mendel's Fourth Postulate: Independent Assortment

We can most easily understand the results of a dihybrid cross if we consider it theoretically as consisting of two monohybrid crosses conducted separately. Think of the two sets of traits as being inherited independently of each other; that is, the chance of any plant having yellow or green seeds is not at all influenced by the chance that this plant will have round or wrinkled seeds. Thus, because yellow is dominant to green, all F_1 plants in the first theoretical cross would have yellow seeds. In the second theoretical cross, all F_1 plants would have round seeds because round is dominant to wrinkled. When Mendel examined the F_1 plants of the dihybrid cross, all were yellow and round, as our theoretical crosses predict.

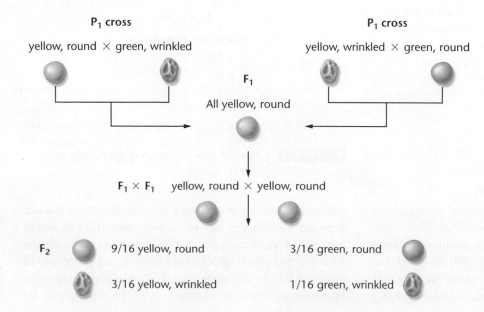

P_1 cross

yellow, round × green, wrinkled

P_1 cross

yellow, wrinkled × green, round

F_1

All yellow, round

F_1 × F_1   yellow, round × yellow, round

F_2   9/16 yellow, round   3/16 green, round

3/16 yellow, wrinkled   1/16 green, wrinkled

FIGURE 3–5 F_1 and F_2 results of Mendel's dihybrid crosses in which the plants on the top left with yellow, round seeds are crossed with plants having green, wrinkled seeds, and the plants on the top right with yellow, wrinkled seeds are crossed with plants having green, round seeds.

FIGURE 3–6 Computation of the combined probabilities of each F_2 phenotype for two independently inherited characters. The probability of each plant being yellow or green is independent of the probability of it bearing round or wrinkled seeds.

The predicted F_2 results of the first cross are 3/4 yellow and 1/4 green. Similarly, the second cross would yield 3/4 round and 1/4 wrinkled. Figure 3–5 shows that in the dihybrid cross, 12/16 F_2 plants are yellow, while 4/16 are green, exhibiting the expected 3:1 (3/4:1/4) ratio. Similarly, 12/16 of all F_2 plants have round seeds, while 4/16 have wrinkled seeds, again revealing the 3:1 ratio.

These numbers demonstrate that the two pairs of contrasting traits are inherited independently, so we can predict the frequencies of all possible F_2 phenotypes by applying the **product law** of probabilities: *When two independent events occur simultaneously, the probability of the two outcomes occurring in combination is equal to the product of their individual probabilities of occurrence.* For example, the probability of an F_2 plant having yellow and round seeds is (3/4)(3/4), or 9/16, because 3/4 of all F_2 plants should be yellow and 3/4 of all F_2 plants should be round.

In a like manner, the probabilities of the other three F_2 phenotypes can be calculated: yellow (3/4) and wrinkled (1/4) are predicted to be present together 3/16 of the time; green (1/4) and round (3/4) are predicted 3/16 of the time; and green (1/4) and wrinkled (1/4) are predicted 1/16 of the time. These calculations are shown in **Figure 3–6**.

It is now apparent why the F_1 and F_2 results are identical whether the initial cross is yellow, round plants bred with green, wrinkled plants, or whether yellow, wrinkled plants are bred with green, round plants. In both crosses, the F_1 genotype of all offspring is identical. As a result, the F_2 generation is also identical in both crosses.

On the basis of similar results in numerous dihybrid crosses, Mendel proposed a fourth postulate:

4. INDEPENDENT ASSORTMENT
During gamete formation, segregating pairs of unit factors assort independently of each other.
This postulate stipulates that segregation of any pair of unit factors occurs independently of all others. As a result of random segregation, each gamete receives one member of every pair of unit factors. For one pair, whichever unit factor is received does not influence the outcome of segregation of any other pair. Thus, according to the postulate of independent assortment, all possible combinations of gametes should be formed in equal frequency.

The Punnett square in **Figure 3–7** shows how independent assortment works in the formation of the F_2 generation. Examine the formation of gametes by the F_1 plants; segregation prescribes that every gamete receives either a G or g allele and a W or w allele. Independent assortment stipulates that all four combinations (GW, Gw, gW, and gw) will be formed with equal probabilities.

In every $F_1 \times F_1$ fertilization event, each zygote has an equal probability of receiving one of the four combinations from each parent. If many offspring are produced, 9/16 have yellow, round seeds, 3/16 have yellow, wrinkled seeds, 3/16 have green, round seeds, and 1/16 have green, wrinkled seeds, yielding what is designated as **Mendel's 9:3:3:1 dihybrid ratio**. This is an ideal ratio based on probability events involving segregation, independent assortment, and random fertilization. Because of deviation due strictly to chance, particularly if small numbers of offspring are produced, actual results are highly unlikely to match the ideal ratio.

The Testcross: Two Characters

The testcross may also be applied to individuals that express two dominant traits but whose genotypes are unknown. For example, the expression of the yellow, round seed phenotype in the F_2 generation just described may result from the *GGWW*, *GGWw*, *GgWW*, or *GgWw* genotypes. If an F_2 yellow, round plant is crossed with the homozygous recessive green, wrinkled plant (*ggww*), analysis of the offspring will indicate the exact genotype of that yellow, round plant. Each of the above genotypes results in a different set of gametes and, in a testcross, a different set of phenotypes in the resulting offspring. You should work out the results of each of these four crosses to be sure that you understand this concept.

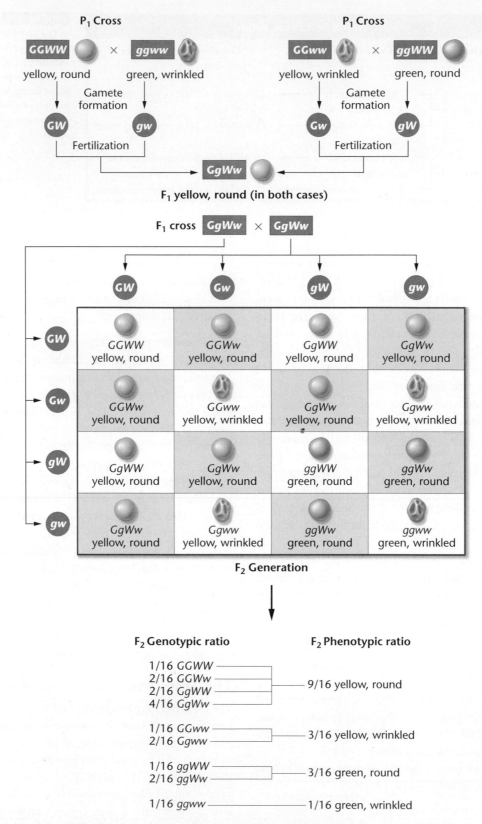

FIGURE 3-7 Analysis of the dihybrid crosses shown in Figure 3–5. The F_1 heterozygous plants are self-fertilized to produce an F_2 generation, which is computed using a Punnett square. Both the phenotypic and genotypic F_2 ratios are shown.

MODERN APPROACHES TO UNDERSTANDING GENE FUNCTION

Identifying Mendel's Gene for Regulating White Flower Color in Peas

In 2010, 150 years after Gregor Mendel studied pea flower color, an international team of researchers identified the gene responsible for regulating flower color in peas. The potential gene they focused on was called pea gene A. This gene was also found in other plants, including petunias and barrel clovers. Gene A encodes a protein that functions as a **transcription factor**—a protein that binds to DNA and regulates expression of other genes. Cells in purple flowers of pea plants accumulate anthocyanin pigment molecules that are responsible for their color. Pea plants with white flowers do not accumulate anthocyanin, even though they contain the gene that encodes the enzyme involved in anthocyanin synthesis. Researchers hypothesized that the transcription factor produced by pea gene A might regulate expression of the anthocyanin biosynthetic gene.

To test this hypothesis and confirm gene A function, they delivered normal copies of gene A into white flower petals by using a gene gun, a device that shoots metal particles coated with a gene of interest into cells. In this approach, gold particles coated with gene A enter a small percentage of cells and gene A is expressed in those cells.

Results:

Cells of white petals where gene A is expressed (left photo) accumulate anthocyanin pigment and turn purple. The inset square shows a higher magnification image enlarging spots of gene A expression. A control experiment where white petals were treated with DNA

without gene A (right photo) did not restore pigmentation. This is an example of what geneticists call a **rescue experiment** because in cells that received gene A the white flower mutant phenotype was rescued or restored to the purple, wild-type phenotype.

Conclusion:

Pea gene A encodes a transcription factor responsible for regulating expression of the anthocyanin gene in peas. Further examination of the gene A sequence from peas with white flowers revealed a single-nucleotide change in gene A that renders this transcription factor inactive. Cells with a normal copy of gene A express anthocyanin and turn purple. Cells with a mutant form of gene A do not accumulate anthocyanin and are white. The genetic mystery of Mendel's white flowers had been solved.

Reference:

Hellens, R. P., et al. (2010). Identification of Mendel's White Flower Character. *PLoS One* 5(10): e13230. doi:10.1371/journal. pone.0013230. Take a look at the YouTube video "Finding the molecular answer to Mendel's pea colour experiments" to hear Dr. Heller describe the approach his group used to identify the function of this gene. http://www .youtube.com /watch?v=BEhtyX CdcTg

Questions to Consider:

1. Why do you think that expression of gene A appears as spots in the leaves shown in the photo on the left? What does this signify?
2. If you did the same experiment with a pea plant that had a mutation in the gene for anthocyanin accumulation, would you expect that introduction of gene A would rescue the phenotype of the mutant? Why or why not?

Gene gun used to blast gold particles containing pea gene A into cells of white petals

+ Gene A   − Gene A

A-BAC   GFP alone

3.4 The Trihybrid Cross Demonstrates That Mendel's Principles Apply to Inheritance of Multiple Traits

Thus far, we have considered inheritance of up to two pairs of contrasting traits. Mendel demonstrated that the processes of segregation and independent assortment also

apply to three pairs of contrasting traits, in what is called a **trihybrid cross**, or *three-factor cross.*

Although a trihybrid cross is somewhat more complex than a dihybrid cross, its results are easily calculated if the principles of segregation and independent assortment are followed. For example, consider the cross shown in **Figure 3–8** where the gene pairs of theoretical contrasting traits are represented by the symbols *A, a, B, b, C,* and *c.* In the cross between *AABBCC* and *aabbcc* individuals, all F₁ individuals are heterozygous for all three gene pairs. Their genotype, *AaBbCc*, results in the phenotypic expression of the dominant *A*, *B*, and *C* traits. When F₁ individuals serve as parents, each produces eight different gametes in equal frequencies. At this point, we could construct a Punnett square with 64 separate boxes and read out the phenotypes—but such a method is cumbersome in a cross involving so many factors. Therefore, another method has been devised to calculate the predicted ratio.

The Forked-Line Method, or Branch Diagram

It is much less difficult to consider each contrasting pair of traits separately and then to combine these results by using the **forked-line method**, first shown in Figure 3–6. This method, also called a **branch diagram**, relies on the simple application of the laws of probability established for the dihybrid cross. Each gene pair is assumed to behave independently during gamete formation.

NOW SOLVE THIS

3–2 Considering the Mendelian traits round versus wrinkled and yellow versus green, consider the crosses below and determine the genotypes of the parental plants by analyzing the phenotypes of their offspring.

Parental Plants	Offspring
(a) round, yellow × round, yellow	3/4 round, yellow 1/4 wrinkled, yellow
(b) wrinkled, yellow ×round, yellow	6/16 wrinkled, yellow 2/16 wrinkled, green 6/16 round, yellow 2/16 round, green
(c) round, yellow × round, yellow	9/16 round, yellow 3/16 round, green 3/16 wrinkled, yellow 1/16 wrinkled, green
(d) round, yellow × wrinkled, green	1/4 round, yellow 1/4 round, green 1/4 wrinkled, yellow 1/4 wrinkled, green

■ **HINT:** *This problem involves a series of Mendelian dihybrid crosses where you are asked to determine the genotypes of the parents in a number of instances. The key to its solution is to write down everything that you know for certain. This reduces the problem to its bare essentials, clarifying what you need to determine. For example, the wrinkled, yellow plant in case (b) must be homozygous for the recessive wrinkled alleles and bear at least one dominant allele for the yellow trait. Having established this, you need only determine the remaining allele for cotyledon color.*

FIGURE 3–8 Formation of P₁ and F₁ gametes in a trihybrid cross.

When the monohybrid cross *AA* × *aa* is made, we know that:

1. All F₁ individuals have the genotype *Aa* and express the phenotype represented by the *A* allele, which is called the *A* phenotype in the discussion that follows.

2. The F₂ generation consists of individuals with either the *A* phenotype or the *a* phenotype in the ratio of 3:1.

The same generalizations can be made for the *BB* × *bb* and *CC* × *cc* crosses. Thus, in the F₂ generation, 3/4 of all organisms will express phenotype *A*, 3/4 will express *B*, and 3/4 will express *C*. Similarly, 1/4 of all organisms will express *a*, 1/4 will express *b*, and 1/4 will express *c*. The proportions of organisms that express each phenotypic combination can be predicted by assuming that fertilization, following the independent assortment of these three gene pairs during gamete formation, is a random process. We apply the product law of probabilities once again. **Figure 3–9** uses the forked-line method to calculate the phenotypic proportions of the F₂ generation. They fall into the trihybrid ratio of 27:9:9:9:3:3:3:1. The same method can be used to solve crosses involving any number of gene pairs, *provided that all gene pairs assort independently from each other.* We shall see later that gene pairs do not always assort with complete independence. However, it appeared to be true for all of Mendel's characters.

Note that in Figure 3–9, only phenotypic ratios of the F₂ generation have been derived. It is possible to generate genotypic ratios as well. To do so, we again consider the *A/a*, *B/b*, and *C/c* gene pairs separately. For example, for the *A/a* pair, the F₁ cross is *Aa* × *Aa*. Phenotypically, an F₂ ratio of 3/4 *A*:1/4 *a* is produced. Genotypically, however, the F₂ ratio is different—1/4 *AA*:1/2 *Aa*:1/4 *aa* will result. Using Figure 3–9 as a model, we would enter these

Generation of F₂ trihybrid phenotypes

FIGURE 3–9 Generation of the F_2 trihybrid phenotypic ratio using the forked-line method. This method is based on the expected probability of occurrence of each phenotype.

genotypic frequencies in the leftmost column of the diagram. Each would be connected by three lines to 1/4 *BB*, 1/2 *Bb*, and 1/4 *bb*, respectively. From each of these nine designations, three more lines would extend to the 1/4 *CC*, 1/2 *Cc*, and 1/4 *cc* genotypes. On the right side of the completed diagram, 27 genotypes and their frequencies of occurrence would appear.

In crosses involving two or more gene pairs, the calculation of gametes and genotypic and phenotypic results is quite complex. Several simple mathematical rules will enable you to check the accuracy of various steps required in working these problems. First, you must determine the number of different *heterozygous* gene pairs (n) involved in the cross—for example, where $AaBb \times AaBb$ represents the cross, $n = 2$; for $AaBbCc \times AaBcCc$, $n = 3$; for $AaBBCcDd \times AaBBCcDd$, $n = 3$ (because the B genes are not heterozygous). Once n is determined, 2^n is the number of different gametes that can be formed by each parent; 3^n is the number of different genotypes that result following fertilization; and 2^n is the number of different phenotypes that are produced from these genotypes. Table 3.1 summarizes these rules, which may be applied to crosses involving any number of genes, *provided that they assort independently from one another.*

NOW SOLVE THIS

3–3 Using the forked line, or branch diagram, method, determine the genotypic and phenotypic ratios of these trihybrid crosses: (a) $AaBbCc \times AaBBCC$, (b) $AaBBCc \times aaBBCc$, and (c) $AaBbCc \times AaBbCc$.

■ **HINT:** *This problem asks you to use the forked-line method to determine the outcome of a number of trihybrid crosses. The key to its solution is to realize that in using the forked-line method, you must consider each gene pair separately. For example, in this problem, first predict the outcome of each cross for the A/a genes, then for the B/b genes, and finally, for the C/c genes. Then you are prepared to pursue the outcome of each cross using the forked-line method.*

3.5 Mendel's Work Was Rediscovered in the Early Twentieth Century

Mendel initiated his work in 1856, presented it to the Brünn Society of Natural Science in 1865, and published it the following year. While his findings were often cited and discussed, their significance went unappreciated for about 35 years. Many explanations have been proposed for this delay.

First, Mendel's adherence to mathematical analysis of probability events was quite unusual for biological studies in those days. Perhaps it seemed foreign to his contemporaries. More important, his conclusions did not fit well with existing hypotheses concerning the cause of variation among organisms. The topic of natural variation intrigued students of evolutionary theory. This group, stimulated by the proposal developed by Charles Darwin and Alfred Russel Wallace, subscribed to the theory of **continuous variation**, which held that offspring were a blend of their parents' phenotypes. As we mentioned earlier, Mendel theorized that variation was due to a dominance–recessive relationship between discrete or particulate units, resulting

TABLE 3.1 Simple Mathematical Rules Useful in Working Genetics Problems

Crosses between Organisms Heterozygous for Genes Exhibiting Independent Assortment			
Number of Heterozygous Gene Pairs	Number of Different Types of Gametes Formed	Number of Different Genotypes Produced	Number of Different Phenotypes Produced[*]
n	2^n	3^n	2^n
1	2	3	2
2	4	9	4
3	8	27	8
4	16	81	16

*The fourth column assumes a simple dominant–recessive relationship in each gene pair.

in **discontinuous variation**. For example, note that the F$_2$ flowers in Figure 3–1 are either white or violet, never something intermediate. Mendel proposed that the F$_2$ offspring of a dihybrid cross are expressing traits produced by new combinations of previously existing unit factors. As a result, Mendel's hypotheses did not fit well with the evolutionists' preconceptions about causes of variation.

It is also likely that Mendel's contemporaries failed to realize that Mendel's postulates explained *how* variation was transmitted to offspring. Instead, they may have attempted to interpret his work in a way that addressed the issue of *why* certain phenotypes survive preferentially. It was this latter question that had been addressed in the theory of natural selection, but it was not addressed by Mendel. The collective vision of Mendel's scientific colleagues may have been obscured by the impact of Darwin's extraordinary theory of organic evolution.

The Chromosomal Theory of Inheritance

In the latter part of the nineteenth century, a remarkable observation set the scene for the recognition of Mendel's work: Walter Flemming's discovery of chromosomes in the nuclei of salamander cells. In 1879, Flemming described the behavior of these thread-like structures during cell division. As a result of his findings and the work of many other cytologists, the presence of discrete units within the nucleus soon became an integral part of scientists' ideas about inheritance.

In the early twentieth century, hybridization experiments similar to Mendel's were performed independently by three botanists, Hugo de Vries, Carl Correns, and Erich Tschermak. De Vries's work demonstrated the principle of segregation in several plant species. Apparently, he searched the existing literature and found that Mendel's work had anticipated his own conclusions! Correns and Tschermak also reached conclusions similar to those of Mendel.

About the same time, two cytologists, Walter Sutton and Theodor Boveri, independently published papers linking their discoveries of the behavior of chromosomes during meiosis to the Mendelian principles of segregation and independent assortment. They pointed out that the separation of chromosomes during meiosis could serve as the cytological basis of these two postulates. Although they thought that Mendel's unit factors were probably chromosomes rather than genes on chromosomes, their findings reestablished the importance of Mendel's work and led to many ensuing genetic investigations. Sutton and Boveri are credited with initiating the **chromosomal theory of inheritance**, the idea that the genetic material in living organisms is contained in chromosomes, which was developed during the next two decades. As we will see in subsequent chapters, work by Thomas H. Morgan, Alfred H. Sturtevant, Calvin Bridges, and others established beyond a reasonable doubt that Sutton's and Boveri's hypothesis was correct.

Unit Factors, Genes, and Homologous Chromosomes

Because the correlation between Sutton's and Boveri's observations and Mendelian postulates serves as the foundation for the modern description of transmission genetics, we will examine this correlation in some depth before moving on to other topics.

As we know, each species possesses a specific number of chromosomes in each somatic cell nucleus. For diploid organisms, this number is called the **diploid number (2n)** and is characteristic of that species. During the formation of gametes (meiosis), the number is precisely halved (n), and when two gametes combine during fertilization, the diploid number is reestablished. During meiosis, however, the chromosome number is not reduced in a random manner. It was apparent to early cytologists that the diploid number of chromosomes is composed of homologous pairs identifiable by their morphological appearance and behavior. The gametes contain one member of each pair—thus the chromosome complement of a gamete is quite specific, and the number of chromosomes in each gamete is equal to the haploid number.

With this basic information, we can see the correlation between the behavior of unit factors and chromosomes and genes. **Figure 3–10** shows three of Mendel's postulates and the chromosomal explanation of each. Unit factors are really genes located on homologous pairs of chromosomes [Figure 3–10(a)]. Members of each pair of homologs separate, or segregate, during gamete formation [Figure 3–10(b)]. In the figure, two different alignments are possible, both of which are shown.

To illustrate the principle of independent assortment, it is important to distinguish between members of any given homologous pair of chromosomes. One member of each pair is derived from the **maternal parent**, whereas the other comes from the **paternal parent**. (We represent the different parental origins with different colors.) As shown in Figure 3–10(c), following independent segregation of each pair of homologs, each gamete receives one member from each pair of chromosomes. All possible combinations are formed with equal probability. If we add the symbols used in Mendel's dihybrid cross (*G*, *g* and *W*, *w*) to the diagram, we can see why equal numbers of the four types of gametes are formed. The independent behavior of Mendel's pairs of unit factors (*G* and *W* in this example) is due to their presence on separate pairs of homologous chromosomes.

Observations of the phenotypic diversity of living organisms make it logical to assume that there are many more genes than chromosomes. Therefore, each homolog must carry genetic information for more than one trait. The currently accepted concept is that a chromosome is composed of a large number of linearly ordered, information-containing genes. Mendel's paired unit factors (which determine

(a) Unit factors in pairs (first meiotic prophase)

Homologous chromosomes in pairs

Genes are part of chromosomes

(b) Segregation of unit factors during gamete formation (first meiotic anaphase)

Homologs segregate during meiosis

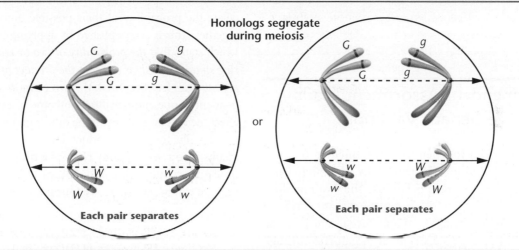

or

Each pair separates   Each pair separates

(c) Independent assortment of segregating unit factors (following many meiotic events)

Nonhomologous chromosomes assort independently

1/4   1/4   1/4   1/4

All possible gametic combinations are formed with equal probability

FIGURE 3–10 Illustrated correlation between the Mendelian postulates of (a) unit factors in pairs, (b) segregation, and (c) independent assortment, showing the presence of genes located on homologous chromosomes and their behavior during meiosis.

tall or dwarf stems, for example) actually constitute a pair of genes located on one pair of homologous chromosomes. The location on a given chromosome where any particular gene occurs is called its **locus** (pl. loci). The different alleles of a given gene (for example, *G* and *g*) contain slightly different genetic information (green or yellow) that determines the same character (seed color in this case). Although we have examined only genes with two alternative alleles, most genes

have more than two allelic forms. We conclude this section by reviewing the criteria necessary to classify two chromosomes as a homologous pair:

1. During mitosis and meiosis, when chromosomes are visible in their characteristic shapes, both members of a homologous pair are the same size and exhibit identical centromere locations. The sex chromosomes (e.g.,

the X and the Y chromosomes in mammals) are an exception.

2. During early stages of meiosis, homologous chromosomes form pairs, or synapse.

3. Although it is not generally visible under the microscope, homologs contain the identical linear order of gene loci.

EVOLVING CONCEPT OF THE GENE

Based on the pioneering work of Gregor Mendel, we can view the gene as a heritable unit factor that determines the expression of an observable trait, or phenotype. ∎

3.6 Independent Assortment Leads to Extensive Genetic Variation

One consequence of independent assortment is the production by an individual of genetically dissimilar gametes. Genetic variation results because the two members of any homologous pair of chromosomes are rarely, if ever, genetically identical. As the maternal and paternal members of all pairs are distributed to gametes through independent assortment, all possible chromosome combinations are produced, leading to extensive genetic diversity.

We have seen that the number of possible gametes, each with different chromosome compositions, is 2^n, where n equals the haploid number. Thus, if a species has a haploid number of 4, then 2^4, or 16, different gamete combinations can be formed as a result of independent assortment. Although this number is not high, consider the human species, where $n = 23$. When 2^{23} is calculated, we find that in excess of 8×10^6, or over 8 million, different types of gametes are possible through independent assortment. Because fertilization represents an event involving only one of approximately 8×10^6 possible gametes from each of two parents, each offspring represents only one of $(8 \times 10^6)^2$ or one of only 64×10^{12} potential genetic combinations. Given that this probability is less than one in one trillion, it is no wonder that, except for identical twins, each member of the human species exhibits a distinctive set of traits—this number of combinations of chromosomes is far greater than the number of humans who have ever lived on Earth! Genetic variation resulting from independent assortment has been extremely important to the process of evolution in all sexually reproducing organisms.

3.7 Laws of Probability Help to Explain Genetic Events

Recall that genetic ratios—for example, 3/4 tall:1/4 dwarf—are most properly thought of as probabilities. These values predict the outcome of each fertilization event, such that the probability of each zygote having the genetic potential for becoming tall is 3/4, whereas the potential for its being a dwarf is 1/4. Probabilities range from 0.0, where an event *is certain not to occur,* to 1.0, where an event *is certain to occur.* In this section, we consider the relation of probability to genetics. When two or more events with known probabilities occur independently but at the same time, we can calculate the probability of their possible outcomes occurring together. This is accomplished by applying the **product law,** which states that *the probability of two or more events occurring simultaneously is equal to the product of their individual probabilities* (see Section 3.3). Two or more events are independent of one another if the outcome of each one does not affect the outcome of any of the others under consideration.

To illustrate the product law, consider the possible results if you toss a penny (P) and a nickel (N) at the same time and examine all combinations of heads (H) and tails (T) that can occur. There are four possible outcomes:

$$(P_H:N_H) = (1/2)(1/2) = 1/4$$
$$(P_T:N_H) = (1/2)(1/2) = 1/4$$
$$(P_H:N_T) = (1/2)(1/2) = 1/4$$
$$(P_T:N_T) = (1/2)(1/2) = 1/4$$

The probability of obtaining a head or a tail in the toss of either coin is 1/2 and is unrelated to the outcome for the other coin. Thus, all four possible combinations are predicted to occur with equal probability.

If we want to calculate the probability when the possible outcomes of two events are independent of one another but can be accomplished in more than one way, we can apply the **sum law.** For example, what is the probability of tossing our penny and nickel and obtaining one head and one tail? In such a case, we do not care whether it is the penny or the nickel that comes up heads, provided that the other coin has the alternative outcome. As we saw above, there are two ways in which the desired outcome can be accomplished, each with a probability of 1/4. The sum law states that *the probability of obtaining any single outcome, where that outcome can be achieved by two or more events, is equal to the sum of the individual probabilities of all such events.* Thus, according to the sum law, the overall probability in our example is equal to

$$(1/4) + (1/4) = 1/2$$

One-half of all two-coin tosses are predicted to yield the desired outcome.

These simple probability laws will be useful throughout our discussions of transmission genetics and for solving genetics problems. In fact, we already applied the product law when we used the forked-line method to calculate the phenotypic results of Mendel's dihybrid and trihybrid crosses. When we wish to know the results of a cross, we need only calculate the probability of each possible outcome. The results of this calculation then allow us to predict the proportion of offspring expressing each phenotype or each genotype.

An important point to remember when you deal with probability is that predictions of possible outcomes are based on large sample sizes. If we predict that 9/16 of the offspring of a dihybrid cross will express both dominant traits, it is very unlikely that, in a small sample, exactly 9 of every 16 will express this phenotype. Instead, our prediction is that, of a large number of offspring, approximately 9/16 will do so. The deviation from the predicted ratio in smaller sample sizes is attributed to chance, a subject we examine in our discussion of statistics in the next section. As you shall see, the impact of deviation due strictly to chance diminishes as the sample size increases.

The Binomial Theorem

Probability calculations using the **binomial theorem** can be used to analyze cases where there are alternative ways to achieve a combination of events. For families of any size, we can calculate the probability of any combination of male and female children. For example, what is the probability that in a family with four children two will be male and two will be female? This question is complex because each birth is an independent event, and multiple birth orders can achieve the same overall outcome.

The expression of the binomial theorem is

$$(a + b)^n = 1$$

where a and b are the respective probabilities of the two alternative outcomes and n equals the number of trials.

n	Binomial	Expanded Binomial
1	$(a + b)^1$	$a + b$
2	$(a + b)^2$	$a^2 + 2ab + b^2$
3	$(a + b)^3$	$a^3 + 3a^2b + 3ab^2 + b^3$
4	$(a + b)^4$	$a^4 + 4a^3b + 6a^2b^2 + 4ab^3 + b^4$
5	$(a + b)^5$	$a^5 + 5a^4b + 10a^3b^2 + 10a^2b^3 + 5ab^4 + b^5$
etc.		etc.

As the value of n increases and the expanded binomial becomes more complex, Pascal's triangle, shown in **Table 3.2**, is a useful way to determine the numerical coefficient of each term in the expanded equation. Starting with the third line from the top of this triangle, each number is the sum of the two numbers immediately above it.

TABLE 3.2 Pascal's Triangle

n	Numerical Coefficients*
	1
1	1 1
2	1 2 1
3	1 3 3 1
4	1 4 6 4 1
5	1 5 10 10 5 1
6	1 6 15 20 15 6 1
7	1 7 21 35 35 21 7 1
etc.	etc.

*Notice that all numbers other than the 1's are equal to the sum of the two numbers directly above them.

To expand any binomial, the various exponents of a and b (e.g., a^3b^2) are determined using the pattern

$$(a + b)^n = a^n, a^{n-1}b, a^{n-2}b^2, a^{n-3}b^3, \ldots, b^n$$

Using these methods for setting up the expression, we find that the expansion of $(a + b)^7$ is

$$a^7 + 7a^6b + 21a^5b^2 + 35a^4b^3 + \cdots + b^7$$

Let's now return to our original question: *What is the probability that in a family with four children two will be male and two will be female?*

First, assign initial probabilities to each outcome:

$$a = \text{male} = 1/2$$
$$b = \text{female} = 1/2$$

Then write out the expanded binomial for the value of $n = 4$,

$$(a + b)^4 = a^4 + 4a^3b + 6a^2b^2 + 4ab^3 + b^4$$

Each term represents a possible outcome, with the exponent of a representing the number of males and the exponent of b representing the number of females. Therefore, the term describing the outcome of two males and two females—the expression of the probability (p) we are looking for—is

$$p = 6a^2b^2$$
$$= 6(1/2)^2(1/2)^2$$
$$= 6(1/2)^4$$
$$= 6(1/16)$$
$$= 6/16$$
$$p = 3/8$$

Thus, the probability of families of four children having two boys and two girls is 3/8. Of all families with four children, 3 out of 8 are predicted to have two boys and two girls.

Before examining one other example, we should note that if you prefer not to use Pascal's triangle, a formula can be used to determine the numerical coefficient for any set of exponents,

$$n! / (s!t!)$$

where

n = the total number of events
s = the number of times outcome a occurs
t = the number of times outcome b occurs

Therefore, $n = s + t$

The symbol ! denotes a factorial, which is the product of all the positive integers from 1 through some positive integer. For example,

$$5! = (5)(4)(3)(2)(1) = 120$$

Note that in factorials, $0! = 1$.

Using the formula, let's determine the probability that in a family with seven children, five will be males and two females. In this case, $n = 7$, $s = 5$, and $t = 2$. We begin by setting up our equation to find the term for five events having outcome a and two events having outcome b:

$$p = \frac{n!}{s!t!}a^s b^t$$

$$= \frac{7!}{5!2!}(1/2)^5(1/2)^2$$

$$= \frac{(7)\cdot(6)\cdot(5)\cdot(4)\cdot(3)\cdot(2)\cdot(1)}{(5)\cdot(4)\cdot(3)\cdot(2)\cdot(1)\cdot(2)\cdot(1)}(1/2)^7$$

$$= \frac{(7)\cdot(6)}{(2)\cdot(1)}(1/2)^7$$

$$= \frac{42}{2}(1/2)^7$$

$$= 21(1/2)^7$$

$$= 21(1/128)$$

$$p = 21/128$$

Of families with seven children, on the average, 21/128 are predicted to have five males and two females.

Calculations using the binomial theorem have various applications in genetics, including the analysis of polygenic traits (Chapter 23) and studies of population equilibrium (Chapter 25).

3.8 Chi-Square Analysis Evaluates the Influence of Chance on Genetic Data

Mendel's 3:1 monohybrid and 9:3:3:1 dihybrid ratios are hypothetical predictions based on the following assumptions: (1) each allele is dominant or recessive, (2) segregation is unimpeded, (3) independent assortment occurs, and (4) fertilization is random. The final two assumptions are influenced by chance events and therefore are subject to random fluctuation. This concept of **chance deviation** is most easily illustrated by tossing a single coin

numerous times and recording the number of heads and tails observed. In each toss, there is a probability of 1/2 that a head will occur and a probability of 1/2 that a tail will occur. Therefore, the expected ratio of many tosses is 1/2:1/2, or 1:1. If a coin is tossed 1000 times, usually *about* 500 heads and 500 tails will be observed. Any reasonable fluctuation from this hypothetical ratio (e.g., 486 heads and 514 tails) is attributed to chance.

As the total number of tosses is reduced, the impact of chance deviation increases. For example, if a coin is tossed only four times, you would not be too surprised if all four tosses resulted in only heads or only tails. For 1000 tosses, however, 1000 heads or 1000 tails would be most unexpected. In fact, you might believe that such a result would be impossible. Actually, all heads or all tails in 1000 tosses can be predicted to occur with a probability of $(1/2)^{1000}$. Since $(1/2)^{20}$ is less than one in a million times, an event occurring with a probability as small as $(1/2)^{1000}$ is virtually impossible. Two major points to keep in mind when predicting or analyzing genetic outcomes are:

1. The outcomes of independent assortment and fertilization, like coin tossing, are subject to random fluctuations from their predicted occurrences as a result of chance deviation.

2. As the sample size increases, the average deviation from the expected results decreases. Therefore, a larger sample size diminishes the impact of chance deviation on the final outcome.

Chi-Square Calculations and the Null Hypothesis

In genetics, being able to evaluate observed deviation is a crucial skill. When we assume that data will fit a given ratio such as 1:1, 3:1, or 9:3:3:1, we establish what is called the **null hypothesis** (H_0). It is so named because the hypothesis assumes that there is *no real difference* between the *measured values* (or ratio) and the *predicted values* (or ratio). Any apparent difference can be attributed purely to chance. The validity of the null hypothesis for a given set of data is measured using statistical analysis. Depending on the results of this analysis, the null hypothesis may either (1) *be rejected* or (2) *fail to be rejected*. If it is rejected, the observed deviation from the expected result is judged not to be attributable to chance alone. In this case, the null hypothesis and the underlying assumptions leading to it must be reexamined. If the null hypothesis fails to be rejected, any observed deviations are attributed to chance.

One of the simplest statistical tests for assessing the goodness of fit of the null hypothesis is **chi-square** (χ^2) **analysis**. This test takes into account the observed deviation in each component of a ratio (from what was expected)

TABLE 3.3 Chi-Square Analysis

(a) Monohybrid

Cross Expected Ratio	Observed (o)	Expected (e)	Deviation (o − e)	Deviation (d²)	d²/e
3/4	740	3/4(1000) = 750	740−750 = −10	(−10)² = 100	100/750 = 0.13
1/4	260	1/4(1000) = 250	260−250 = +10	(+10)² = 100	100/250 = 0.40
	Total = 1000				$\chi^2 = 0.53$
					$p = 0.48$

(b) Dihybrid

Cross Expected Ratio	Observed (o)	Expected (e)	Deviation (o − e)	Deviation (d²)	d²/e
9/16	587	567	+20	400	0.71
3/16	197	189	+8	64	0.34
3/16	168	189	−21	441	2.33
1/16	56	63	−7	49	0.78
	Total = 1008				$\chi^2 = 4.16$
					$p - 0.26$

as well as the sample size and reduces them to a single numerical value. The value for χ^2 is then used to estimate how frequently the observed deviation can be expected to occur strictly as a result of chance. The formula used in chi-square analysis is

$$\chi^2 = \Sigma \frac{(o - e)^2}{e}$$

where o is the observed value for a given category, e is the expected value for that category, and Σ (the Greek letter sigma) represents the sum of the calculated values for each category in the ratio. Because $(o - e)$ is the deviation (d) in each case, the equation reduces to

$$\chi^2 = \Sigma \frac{d^2}{e}$$

Table 3.3(a) shows the steps in the χ^2 calculation for the F_2 results of a hypothetical monohybrid cross. To analyze the data obtained from this cross, work from left to right across the table, verifying the calculations as appropriate. Note that regardless of whether the deviation d is positive or negative, d^2 always becomes positive after the number is squared. In Table 3.3(b) F_2 results of a hypothetical dihybrid cross are analyzed. Make sure that you understand how each number was calculated in this example.

The final step in chi-square analysis is to interpret the χ^2 value. To do so, you must initially determine a value called the **degrees of freedom (df)**, which is equal to $n - 1$, where n is the number of different categories into which the data are divided, in other words, the number of possible outcomes. For the 3:1 ratio, $n = 2$, so $df = 1$. For the 9:3:3:1 ratio, $n = 4$ and $df = 3$. Degrees of freedom must be taken into account because the greater the number of categories, the more deviation is expected as a result of chance.

Once you have determined the degrees of freedom, you can interpret the χ^2 value in terms of a corresponding **probability value (p)**. Since this calculation is complex, we usually take the p value from a standard table or graph. **Figure 3–11** shows a wide range of χ^2 values and the corresponding p values for various degrees of freedom in both a graph and a table. Let's use the graph to explain how to determine the p value. The caption for Figure 3–11(b) explains how to use the table.

To determine p using the graph, execute the following steps:

1. Locate the χ^2 value on the abscissa (the horizontal axis, or x-axis).

2. Draw a vertical line from this point up to the line on the graph representing the appropriate df.

3. From there, extend a horizontal line to the left until it intersects the ordinate (the vertical axis, or y-axis).

4. Estimate, by interpolation, the corresponding p value.

We used these steps for the monohybrid cross in Table 3.3(a) to estimate the p value of 0.48, as shown in Figure 3–11(a). Now try this method to see if you can determine the p value for the dihybrid cross [Table 3.3(b)]. Since the χ^2 value is 4.16 and $df = 3$, an approximate p value is 0.26. Checking this result in the table confirms that p values for both the monohybrid and dihybrid crosses are between 0.20 and 0.50.

Interpreting Probability Values

So far, we have been concerned with calculating χ^2 values and determining the corresponding p values. These steps bring us to the most important aspect of chi-square analysis:

(a)

Degrees of freedom (df)

(b)

	Probability (p)					
	0.90	**0.50**	**0.20**	**0.05**	**0.01**	**0.001**
1	0.02	0.46	1.64	3.84	6.64	10.83
2	0.21	1.39	3.22	5.99	9.21	13.82
3	0.58	2.37	4.64	7.82	11.35	16.27
4	1.06	3.36	5.99	9.49	13.28	18.47
5	1.61	4.35	7.29	11.07	15.09	20.52
6	2.20	5.35	8.56	12.59	16.81	22.46
df 7	2.83	6.35	9.80	14.07	18.48	24.32
8	3.49	7.34	11.03	15.51	20.09	26.13
9	4.17	8.34	12.24	16.92	21.67	27.88
10	4.87	9.34	13.44	18.31	23.21	29.59
15	8.55	14.34	19.31	25.00	30.58	37.30
25	16.47	24.34	30.68	37.65	44.31	52.62
50	37.69	49.34	58.16	67.51	76.15	86.60

χ^2 values

Fails to reject the null hypothesis
Rejects the null hypothesis

FIGURE 3–11 (a) Graph for converting χ^2 values to p values. (b) Table of χ^2 values for selected values of df and p. χ^2 values that lead to a p value of 0.05 or greater (darker blue areas) justify failure to reject the null hypothesis. Values leading to a p value of less than 0.05 (lighter blue areas) justify rejecting the null hypothesis. For example, the table in part (b) shows that for $\chi^2 = 0.53$ with 1 degree of freedom, the corresponding p value is between 0.20 and 0.50. The graph in (a) gives a more precise p value of 0.48 by interpolation. Thus, we fail to reject the null hypothesis.

understanding the meaning of the p value. It is simplest to think of the p value as a percentage. Let's use the example of the dihybrid cross in Table 3.3(b) where $p = 0.26$, which can be thought of as 26 percent. In our example, the p value indicates that if we repeat the same experiment many times, 26 percent of the trials would be expected to exhibit chance deviation as great as or greater than that seen in the initial trial. Conversely, 74 percent of the repeats would show less deviation than initially observed as a result of chance. Thus, the p value reveals that a null hypothesis (concerning the 9:3:3:1 ratio, in this case) is never proved or disproved absolutely. Instead, a relative standard is set that we use to either *reject* or *fail to reject* the null hypothesis. This standard is most often a p value of 0.05. When applied to chi-square analysis, a p value less than 0.05 means that the observed deviation in the set of results will be obtained by chance alone less than 5 percent of the time. Such a p value indicates that the difference between the observed and predicted results is substantial and requires us to reject the null hypothesis.

On the other hand, p values of 0.05 or greater (0.05 to 1.0) indicate that the observed deviation will be obtained by chance alone 5 percent or more of the time. This conclusion allows us not to reject the null hypothesis (when we are using $p = 0.05$ as our standard). Thus, with its p value of 0.26, the null hypothesis that independent assortment accounts for the results fails to be rejected. Therefore, the observed deviation can be reasonably attributed to chance.

A final note is relevant here concerning the case where the null hypothesis is rejected, that is, where $p \leq 0.05$. Suppose we had tested a dataset to assess a possible 9:3:3:1 ratio, as in Table 3.3(b), but we rejected the null hypothesis based on our calculation. What are alternative interpretations of the data? Researchers will reassess the assumptions that underlie the null hypothesis. In our dyhibrid cross, we assumed that segregation operates faithfully for both gene pairs. We also assumed that fertilization is random and that the viability of all gametes is equal regardless of genotype—that is, all gametes are equally likely to participate in fertilization. Finally, we assumed that, following fertilization, all preadult stages and adult offspring are equally viable, regardless of their genotype. If any of these assumptions is incorrect, then the original hypothesis is not necessarily invalid.

An example will clarify this point. Suppose our null hypothesis is that a dihybrid cross between fruit flies will result in 3/16 mutant wingless flies. However, perhaps fewer of the mutant embryos are able to survive their preadult development or young adulthood compared to flies whose genotype gives rise to wings. As a result, when the data are gathered, there will be fewer than 3/16 wingless flies. Rejection of the null hypothesis is not in itself cause for us to reject the validity of the postulates of segregation and independent assortment, because other factors we are unaware of may also be affecting the outcome.

NOW SOLVE THIS

3–4 In one of Mendel's dihybrid crosses, he observed 315 round, yellow, 108 round, green, 101 wrinkled, yellow, and 32 wrinkled, green F_2 plants. Analyze these data using the χ^2 test to see if
   (a) they fit a 9:3:3:1 ratio.
   (b) the round:wrinkled data fit a 3:1 ratio.
   (c) the yellow:green data fit a 3:1 ratio.

■ **HINT:** *This problem asks you to apply χ^2 analysis to a set of data and to determine whether those data fit any of several ratios. The key to its solution is to first calculate χ^2 by initially determining the expected outcomes using the predicted ratios. Then follow a stepwise approach, determining the deviation in each case, and calculating d^2/e for each category. Once you have determined the χ^2 value, you must then determine and interpret the p value for each ratio.*

For more practice, see Problems 18, 19, and 20.

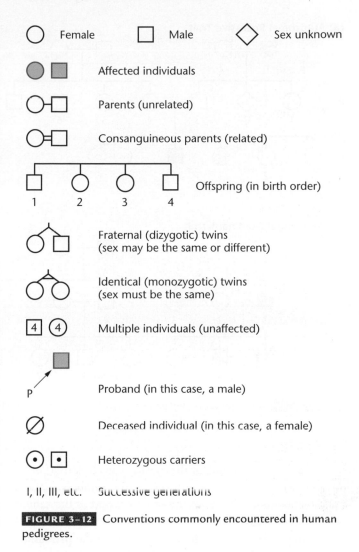

FIGURE 3–12 Conventions commonly encountered in human pedigrees.

3.9 Pedigrees Reveal Patterns of Inheritance of Human Traits

We now explore how to determine the mode of inheritance of phenotypes in humans, where experimental matings are not made and where relatively few offspring are available for study. The traditional way to study inheritance has been to construct a family tree, indicating the presence or absence of the trait in question for each member of each generation. Such a family tree is called a **pedigree**. By analyzing a pedigree, we may be able to predict how the trait under study is inherited—for example, is it due to a dominant or recessive allele? When many pedigrees for the same trait are studied, we can often ascertain the mode of inheritance.

Pedigree Conventions

Figure 3–12 illustrates some of the conventions geneticists follow in constructing pedigrees. Circles represent females and squares designate males. If the sex of an individual is unknown, a diamond is used. Parents are generally connected to each other by a single horizontal line, and vertical lines lead to their offspring. If the parents are related—that is, **consanguineous**—such as first cousins, they are connected by a double line. Offspring are called **sibs** (short for **siblings**) and are connected by a horizontal **sibship line**. Sibs are placed in birth order from left to right and are labeled with Arabic numerals. Parents also receive an Arabic number designation. Each generation is indicated by a Roman numeral. When a pedigree traces only a single trait, the circles, squares, and diamonds are shaded if the phenotype being considered is expressed and unshaded if not. In some pedigrees, those individuals that fail to express a recessive trait but are known with certainty to be heterozygous carriers have a shaded dot within their unshaded circle or square. If an individual is deceased and the phenotype is unknown, a diagonal line is placed over the circle or square.

Twins are indicated by diagonal lines stemming from a vertical line connected to the sibship line. For identical, or **monozygotic**, twins, the diagonal lines are linked by a

(a) Autosomal Recessive Trait

Either I-3 or I-4 must be heterozygous

Recessive traits typically skip generations

Recessive autosomal traits appear equally in both sexes

(b) Autosomal Dominant Trait

I-1 is heterozygous for a dominant allele

Dominant traits almost always appear in each generation

Affected individuals all have an affected parent. Dominant autosomal traits appear equally in both sexes

FIGURE 3–13 Representative pedigrees for two characteristics, each followed through three generations.

horizontal line. Fraternal, or **dizygotic**, twins lack this connecting line. A number within one of the symbols represents that number of sibs of the same sex and of the same or unknown phenotypes. The individual whose phenotype first brought attention to the family is called the **proband** and is indicated by an arrow connected to the designation **p**. This term applies to either a male or a female.

Pedigree Analysis

In **Figure 3–13**, two pedigrees are shown. The first is a representative pedigree for a trait that demonstrates autosomal recessive inheritance, such as **albinism**, where synthesis of the pigment melanin in obstructed. The male parent of the first generation (I-1) is affected. Characteristic of a situation in which a parent has a rare recessive trait, the trait "disappears" in the offspring of the next generation. Assuming recessiveness, we might predict that the unaffected female parent (I-2) is a homozygous normal individual because none of the offspring show the disorder. Had she been heterozygous, one-half of the offspring would be expected to exhibit albinism, but none do. However, such a small sample (three offspring) prevents our knowing for certain.

Further evidence supports the prediction of a recessive trait. If albinism were inherited as a dominant trait, individual II-3 would have to express the disorder in order to pass it to his offspring (III-3 and III-4), but he does not. Inspection of the offspring constituting the third generation

(row III) provides still further support for the hypothesis that albinism is a recessive trait. If it is, parents II-3 and II-4 are both heterozygous, and approximately one-fourth of their offspring should be affected. Two of the six offspring do show albinism. This deviation from the expected ratio is not unexpected in crosses with few offspring. Once we are confident that albinism is inherited as an autosomal recessive trait, we could portray the II-3 and II-4 individuals with a shaded dot within their larger square and circle. Finally, we can note that, characteristic of pedigrees for autosomal traits, both males and females are affected with equal probability. Later in the text (see Chapter 4), we will examine a pedigree representing a gene located on the sex-determining X chromosome. We will see certain patterns characteristic of the transmission of X-linked traits, such as that these traits are more prevalent in male offspring and are never passed from affected fathers to their sons.

The second pedigree illustrates the pattern of inheritance for a trait such as Huntington disease, which is caused by an autosomal dominant allele. The key to identifying a pedigree that reflects a dominant trait is that all affected offspring will have a parent that also expresses the trait. It is also possible, by chance, that none of the offspring will inherit the dominant allele. If so, the trait will cease to exist in future generations. Like recessive traits, provided that the gene is autosomal, both males and females are equally affected.

When a given autosomal dominant disease is rare within the population, and most are, then it is highly unlikely that affected individuals will inherit a copy of the mutant gene from both parents. Therefore, in most cases, affected individuals are heterozygous for the dominant allele. As a result, approximately one-half of the offspring inherit it. This is borne out in the second pedigree in Figure 3–13. Furthermore, if a mutation is dominant, and a single copy is sufficient to produce a mutant phenotype, homozygotes are likely to be even more severely affected, perhaps even failing to survive. An illustration of this is the dominant gene for **familial hypercholesterolemia**. Heterozygotes display a defect in their receptors for low-density lipoproteins, the so-called LDLs (known popularly as "bad cholesterol"). As a result, too little cholesterol is taken up by cells from the blood, and elevated plasma levels of LDLs result. Without intervention, such heterozygous individuals usually have heart attacks during the fourth decade of their life, or before. While heterozygotes have LDL levels about double that of a normal individual, rare homozygotes have been detected. They lack LDL receptors altogether, and their LDL levels are nearly ten times above the normal range. They are likely to have a heart attack very early in life, even before age 5, and almost inevitably before they reach the age of 20.

Pedigree analysis of many traits has historically been an extremely valuable research technique in human genetic studies. However, the approach does not usually provide the certainty of the conclusions obtained through experimental crosses yielding large numbers of offspring. Nevertheless, when many independent pedigrees of the same trait or disorder are analyzed, consistent conclusions can often be drawn. Table 3.4 lists numerous human traits and classifies them according to their recessive or dominant expression.

TABLE 3.4 Representative Recessive and Dominant Human Traits

Recessive Traits	Dominant Traits
Albinism	Achondroplasia
Alkaptonuria	Brachydactyly
Ataxia telangiectasia	Congenital stationary night blindness
Color blindness	Ehler–Danlos syndrome
Cystic fibrosis	Hypotrichosis
Duchenne muscular dystrophy	Huntington disease
Galactosemia	Hypercholesterolemia
Hemophilia	Marfan syndrome
Lesch–Nyhan syndrome	Myotonic dystrophy
Phenylketonuria	Neurofibromatosis
Sickle-cell anemia	Phenylthiocarbamide tasting
Tay–Sachs disease	Porphyria (some forms)

NOW SOLVE THIS

3–5 The following pedigree is for myopia (nearsightedness) in humans.

Predict whether the disorder is inherited as the result of a dominant or recessive trait. Determine the most probable genotype for each individual based on your prediction.

■ **HINT:** *This problem asks you to analyze a pedigree and determine the mode of inheritance of myopia. The key to its solution is to identify whether or not there are individuals who express the trait but neither of whose parents also express the trait. Such an observation is a powerful clue and allows you to rule out one mode of inheritance.*

3.10 Mutant Phenotypes Have Been Examined at the Molecular Level

We conclude this chapter by examining two of countless cases where the molecular basis of normal and mutant genes and their resultant phenotypes has now been revealed. Although these explanations were not forthcoming until well over 100 years after Mendel's original work, our discussion of them expands your understanding of how genes control phenotypes. First, we will discuss the molecular basis of one of Mendel's traits, and then we will turn to consideration of a human disorder.

How Mendel's Peas Become Wrinkled: A Molecular Explanation

Only recently, well over a hundred years after Mendel used wrinkled peas in his groundbreaking hybridization experiments, have we come to find out how the *wrinkled* gene makes peas wrinkled. The wild-type allele of the gene encodes a protein called *starch-branching enzyme (SBEI)*. This enzyme catalyzes the formation of highly branched starch molecules as the seed matures.

Wrinkled peas (**Figure 3–14**), which result from the homozygous presence of a mutant form of the gene, lack the activity of this enzyme. As a consequence, the production of branch points is inhibited during the synthesis of starch within the seed, which in turn leads to the accumulation of more sucrose and a higher water content while the seed develops. Osmotic pressure inside the seed rises,

FIGURE 3–14 A wrinkled and round garden pea, the phenotypic traits in one of Mendel's monohybrid crosses.

causing the seed to lose water, ultimately resulting in a wrinkled appearance at maturity. In contrast, developing seeds that bear at least one copy of the normal gene (being either homozygous or heterozygous for the dominant allele) synthesize starch and achieve an osmotic balance that minimizes the loss of water. The end result for them is a smooth-textured outer coat.

Cloning and analysis of the *SBEI* gene have provided new insight into the relationships between genotypes and phenotypes. Interestingly, the mutant gene contains a foreign sequence of some 800 base pairs that disrupts the normal coding sequence. This foreign segment closely resembles sequences called **transposable elements** that have been discovered to have the ability to move from place to place in the genome of certain organisms. Transposable elements have been found in maize (corn), parsley, snapdragons, and fruit flies, among many other organisms.

Tay—Sachs Disease: The Molecular Basis of a Recessive Disorder in Humans

Of particular interest are cases where a single mutant gene causes multiple effects associated with a severe disorder in humans. Let's consider the modern explanation of the gene that causes **Tay–Sachs disease (TSD)**, a devastating recessive disorder involving unalterable destruction of the central nervous system. Infants with TSD are unaffected at birth and appear to develop normally until they are about 6 months old. Then, a progressive loss of mental and physical abilities occurs. Afflicted infants eventually become blind, deaf, mentally retarded, and paralyzed, often within only a year or two, seldom living beyond age 5. Typical of rare autosomal recessive disorders, two unaffected heterozygous parents, who most often have no family history of the disorder, have a probability of one in four of having a Tay–Sachs child.

We know that proteins are the end products of the expression of most all genes. The protein product involved in TSD has been identified, and we now have a clear understanding of the underlying molecular basis of the disorder. TSD results from the loss of activity of a single enzyme **hexosaminidase A (Hex-A)**. Hex-A, normally found in lysosomes within cells, is needed to break down the ganglioside GM2, a lipid component of nerve cell membranes. Without functional Hex-A, gangliosides accumulate within neurons in the brain and cause deterioration of the nervous system. Heterozygous carriers of TSD with one normal copy of the gene produce only about 50 percent of the normal amount of Hex-A, but they show no symptoms of the disorder. The observation that the activity of only one gene (one wild-type allele) is sufficient for the normal development and function of the nervous system explains and illustrates the molecular basis of recessive mutations. Only when both genes are disrupted by mutation is the mutant phenotype evident. The responsible gene is located on chromosome 15 and codes for the alpha subunit of the Hex-A enzyme. More than 50 different mutations within the gene have been identified that lead to TSD phenotypes.

ANACTGACNCAC TA TAGGGCGAA TTCGAGCTCGGTACCCGGNGGATCCTCTAGAG
10   20   30   40   50

EXPLORING GENOMICS

Online Mendelian Inheritance in Man

The Online Mendelian Inheritance in Man (OMIM) database is a catalog of human genes and human disorders that are inherited in a Mendelian manner. Genetic disorders that arise from major chromosomal aberrations, such as monosomy or trisomy (the loss of a chromosome or the presence of a superfluous chromosome, respectively), are not included. The OMIM database, updated daily, is a version of the book *Mendelian Inheritance in Man*, conceived and edited by Dr. Victor McKusick of Johns Hopkins University, until he passed in 2008.

The OMIM entries provide links to a wealth of information, including DNA and protein sequences, chromosomal maps, disease descriptions, and relevant scientific publications. In this exercise, you will explore OMIM to answer questions about the recessive human disease sickle-cell anemia and other Mendelian inherited disorders.

■ **Exercise I – Sickle-cell Anemia**

In this chapter, you were introduced to recessive and dominant human traits. You will now discover more about sickle-cell anemia as an autosomal recessive disease by exploring the OMIM database.

1. To begin the search, access the OMIM site at: www.omim.org.

2. In the "SEARCH" box, type "sickle-cell anemia" and click on the "Search" button to perform the search.

3. Click on the link for the entry #603903.

4. Review the text that appears to learn about sickle-cell anemia. Examine the

list of subject headings in the right-hand column and explore these links for more information about sickle-cell anemia.

5. Select one or two references at the bottom of the page and follow them to their abstracts in PubMed.

6. Using the information in this entry, answer the following questions:

a. Which gene is mutated in individuals with sickle-cell anemia?

b. What are the major symptoms of this disorder?

c. What was the first published scientific description of sickle-cell anemia?

d. Describe two other features of this disorder that you learned from the OMIM database and state where in the database you found this information.

■ **Exercise II – Other Recessive or Dominant Disorders**

Select another human disorder that is inherited as either a dominant or recessive trait and investigate its features, following the general procedure presented above. Follow links from OMIM to other databases if you choose.

Describe several interesting pieces of information you acquired during your exploration and cite the information sources you encountered during the search.

CASE STUDY | To test or not to test

Thomas first discovered a potentially devastating piece of family history when he learned the medical diagnosis for his brother's increasing dementia, muscular rigidity, and frequency of seizures. His brother, at age 49, was diagnosed with Huntington disease (HD), a dominantly inherited condition that typically begins with such symptoms around the age of 45 and leads to death in one's early 60s. As depressing as the news was to Thomas, it helped explain his father's suicide. Thomas, 38, now wonders what his chances are of carrying the gene for HD, leading him and his wife to discuss the pros and cons of him undergoing genetic testing. Thomas and his wife have two teenage children, a boy and a girl.

1. What role might a genetic counselor play in this real-life scenario?

2. How might the preparation and analysis of a pedigree help explain the dilemma facing Thomas and his family?

3. If Thomas decides to go ahead with the genetic test, what should be the role of the health insurance industry in such cases?

4. If Thomas tests positive for HD, and you were one of his children, would you want to be tested?

Summary Points

1. Mendel's postulates help describe the basis for the inheritance of phenotypic traits. Based on the analysis of numerous monohybrid crosses, he hypothesized that unit factors exist in pairs and exhibit a dominant/recessive relationship in determining the expression of traits. He further postulated that unit factors segregate during gamete formation, such that each gamete receives one or the other factor, with equal probability.

2. Mendel's postulate of independent assortment, based initially on his analysis of dihybrid crosses, states that each pair of unit factors segregates independently of other such pairs. As a result, all possible combinations of gametes are formed with equal probability.

3. Both the Punnett square and the forked-line method are used to predict the probabilities of phenotypes or genotypes from crosses involving two or more gene pairs. The forked-line method is less complex, but just as accurate as the Punnett square.

4. The discovery of chromosomes in the late 1800s, along with subsequent studies of their behavior during meiosis, led to the rebirth of Mendel's work, linking his unit factors to chromosomes.

5. Since genetic ratios are expressed as probabilities, deriving outcomes of genetic crosses requires an understanding of the laws of probability.

6. Chi-square analysis allows us to assess the null hypothesis, which states that there is no real difference between the expected and observed values. As such, it tests the probability of whether observed variations can be attributed to chance deviation.

7. Pedigree analysis is a method for studying the inheritance pattern of human traits over several generations, providing the basis for predicting the mode of inheritance of characteristics and disorders in the absence of extensive genetic crossing and large numbers of offspring.

INSIGHTS AND SOLUTIONS

As a student, you will be asked to demonstrate your knowledge of transmission genetics by solving various problems. Success at this task requires not only comprehension of theory but also its application to more practical genetic situations. Most students find problem solving in genetics to be both challenging and rewarding. This section is designed to provide basic insights into the reasoning essential to this process.

Genetics problems are in many ways similar to word problems in algebra. The approach to solving them is identical: (1) analyze the problem carefully; (2) translate words into symbols and define each symbol precisely; and (3) choose and apply a specific technique to solve the problem. The first two steps are the most critical. The third step is largely mechanical.

The simplest problems state all necessary information about a P_1 generation and ask you to find the expected ratios of the F_1 and F_2 genotypes and/or phenotypes. Always follow these steps when you encounter this type of problem:

(a) Determine insofar as possible the genotypes of the individuals in the P_1 generation.

(b) Determine what gametes may be formed by the P_1 parents.

(c) Recombine the gametes by the Punnett square or the forked-line method, or if the situation is very simple, by inspection. From the genotypes of the F_1 generation, determine the phenotypes. Read the F_1 phenotypes.

(d) Repeat the process to obtain information about the F_2 generation.

Determining the genotypes from the given information requires that you understand the basic theory of transmission genetics. Consider this problem: *A recessive mutant allele, black, causes a very dark body in Drosophila when homozygous. The normal wild-type color is described as gray. What F_1 phenotypic ratio is predicted when a black female is crossed to a gray male whose father was black?*

To work out this problem, you must understand dominance and recessiveness, as well as the principle of segregation. Furthermore, you must use the information about the male parent's father. Here is one logical approach to solving this problem:

The female parent is black, so she must be homozygous for the mutant allele (*bb*). The male parent is gray and must therefore have at least one dominant allele (*B*). His father was black (*bb*), and he received one of the chromosomes bearing these alleles, so the male parent must be heterozygous (*Bb*).

From this point, solving the problem is simple:

Apply the approach we just studied to the following problems.

1. Mendel found that full pea pods are dominant over constricted pods, while round seeds are dominant over wrinkled seeds. One of his crosses was between full, round plants and constricted, wrinkled plants. From this cross, he obtained an F_1 generation that was all full and round. In the F_2 generation, Mendel obtained his classic 9:3:3:1 ratio. Using this information, determine the expected F_1 and F_2 results of a cross between homozygous constricted, round and full, wrinkled plants.

Solution: First, assign gene symbols to each pair of contrasting traits. Use the lowercase first letter of each recessive trait to designate that trait, and use the same letter in uppercase to designate the dominant trait. Thus, *C* and *c* indicate full and constricted pods, respectively, and *W* and *w* indicate the round and wrinkled phenotypes, respectively.

Determine the genotypes of the P_1 generation, form the gametes, combine them in the F_1 generation, and read off the phenotype(s):

P_1:	*ccWW*		*CCww*
	constricted, round	$\times$	full, wrinkled
	$\downarrow$		$\downarrow$
Gametes:	*cW*		*Cw*
F_1:		*CcWw*	
		full, round	

You can immediately see that the F_1 generation expresses both dominant phenotypes and is heterozygous for both gene pairs. Thus, you expect that the F_2 generation will yield the classic Mendelian ratio of 9:3:3:1. Let's work it out anyway, just to confirm this expectation, using the forked-line method. Both gene pairs are heterozygous and can be expected to assort independently, so we can predict the F_2 outcomes from each gene pair separately and then proceed with the forked-line method.

The F_2 offspring should exhibit the individual traits in the following proportions:

$Cc \times Cc$		$Ww \times Ww$	
$\downarrow$		$\downarrow$	
CC	}	*WW*	}
Cc	} full	*Ww*	} round
cC	}	*wW*	}
cc	constricted	*ww*	wrinkled

1. Using these proportions to complete a forked-line diagram confirms the 9:3:3:1 phenotypic ratio. (Remember that this ratio represents proportions of 9/16:3/16:3/16:1/16.) Note that we are applying the product law as we compute the final probabilities:

3/4 full
- 3/4 round $\xrightarrow{(3/4)(3/4)}$ 9/16 full, round
- 1/4 wrinkled $\xrightarrow{(3/4)(1/4)}$ 3/16 full, wrinkled

1/4 constricted
- 3/4 round $\xrightarrow{(1/4)(3/4)}$ 3/16 constricted, round
- 1/4 wrinkled $\xrightarrow{(1/4)(1/4)}$ 1/16 constricted, wrinkled

2. In another cross, involving parent plants of unknown geno-type and phenotype, the following offspring were obtained.

3/8 full, round
3/8 full, wrinkled
1/8 constricted, round
1/8 constricted, wrinkled

Determine the genotypes and phenotypes of the parents.

Solution: This problem is more difficult and requires keener insight because you must work backward to arrive at the answer. The best approach is to consider the outcomes of pod shape separately from those of seed texture.

Of all the plants, $3/8 + 3/8 = 3/4$ are full and $1/8 + 1/8 = 1/4$ are constricted. Of the various geno-typic combinations that can serve as parents, which will give rise to a ratio of 3/4:1/4? This ratio is identical to Mendel's monohybrid F_2 results, and we can propose that both unknown parents share the same genetic char-acteristic as the monohybrid F_1 parents: they must both be heterozygous for the genes controlling pod shape and thus are Cc.

Before we accept this hypothesis, let's consider the pos-sible genotypic combinations that control seed texture. If we consider this characteristic alone, we can see that the traits are expressed in a ratio of $3/8 + 1/8 = 1/2$ round: $3/8 + 1/8 = 1/2$ wrinkled. To generate such a ratio, the parents cannot both be heterozygous or their offspring would yield a 3/4:1/4 phenotypic ratio. They cannot both be homozygous or all offspring would express a single phenotype. Thus, we are left with testing the hypothesis that one parent is homozygous and one is heterozygous for the alleles controlling texture. The potential case of $WW \times Ww$ does not work because it would also yield only a single phenotype. This leaves us with the potential case of $ww \times Ww$. Offspring in such a mating will yield 1/2 Ww (round): 1/2 ww (wrinkled), exactly the outcome we are seeking.

Now, let's combine our hypotheses and predict the outcome of the cross. In our solution, we use a dash (–) to indicate that the second allele may be dominant or recessive, since we are only predicting phenotypes.

3/4 C–
- 1/2 $Ww \rightarrow$ 3/8 $C–Ww$ full, round
- 1/2 $Ww \rightarrow$ 3/8 $C–ww$ full, wrinkled

1/4 cc
- 1/2 $Ww \rightarrow$ 1/8 $ccWw$ constricted, round
- 1/2 $Ww \rightarrow$ 1/8 $ccww$ constricted, wrinkled

As you can see, this cross produces offspring in proportions that match our initial information, and we have solved the problem. Note that, in the solution, we have used genotypes in the forked-line method, in contrast to the use of pheno-types in Solution 1.

3. In the laboratory, a genetics student crossed flies with nor-mal long wings with flies expressing the *dumpy* mutation (truncated wings), which she believed was a recessive trait. In the F_1 generation, all flies had long wings. The following results were obtained in the F_2 generation:

792 long-winged flies

208 dumpy-winged flies

The student tested the hypothesis that the dumpy wing is inherited as a recessive trait using χ^2 analysis of the F_2 data.

(a) What ratio was hypothesized?

(b) Did the analysis support the hypothesis?

(c) What do the data suggest about the *dumpy* mutation?

Solution:

(a) The student hypothesized that the F_2 data (792:208) fit Mendel's 3:1 monohybrid ratio for recessive genes.

(b) The initial step in χ^2 analysis is to calculate the expected results (e) for a ratio of 3:1. Then we can compute deviation $o - e$ (d) and the remaining numbers.

Ratio	o	e	d	d^2	d^2/e
3/4	792	750	42	1764	2.35
1/4	208	250	–42	1764	7.06
Total = 1000					

$$\chi^2 = \Sigma \frac{d^2}{e}$$
$$= 2.35 + 7.06$$
$$= 9.41$$

We consult Figure 3–11 to determine the probability (p) and to decide whether the deviations can be attributed to chance. There are two possible outcomes ($n = 2$), so the degrees of freedom (df) $= n - 1$, or 1. The table in Figure 3–11(b) shows that p is a value between 0.01 and 0.001; the graph in Figure 3–11(a) gives an estimate of about 0.001. Since $p < 0.05$, we reject the null hypothesis. The data do not fit a 3:1 ratio.

(c) When the student hypothesized that Mendel's 3:1 ratio was a valid expression of the monohybrid cross, she was tac-itly making numerous assumptions. Examining these under-lying assumptions may explain why the null hypothesis was rejected. For one thing, she assumed that all the genotypes resulting from the cross were equally viable—that genotypes yielding long wings are equally likely to survive from fertil-ization through adulthood as the genotype yielding dumpy wings. Further study would reveal that dumpy-winged flies are somewhat less viable than normal flies. As a result, we would expect *less* than 1/4 of the total offspring to express dumpy wings. This observation is borne out in the data, although we have not proven that this is true.

(continued)

Insights and Solutions—continued

4. If two parents, both heterozygous carriers of the autosomal recessive gene causing cystic fibrosis, have five children, what is the probability that exactly three will be normal?

Solution: This is an opportunity to use the binomial theorem. To do so requires two facts you already possess: the probability of having a normal child during each pregnancy is

$$p_a = \text{normal} = 3/4$$

and the probability of having an afflicted child is

$$p_b = \text{afflicted} = 1/4$$

Insert these into the formula

$$\frac{n!}{s!t!}\, a^s b^t$$

where $n = 5$, $s = 3$, and $t = 2$

$$p = \frac{(5)\cdot(4)\cdot(3)\cdot(2)\cdot(1)}{(3)\cdot(2)\cdot(1)\cdot(2)\cdot(1)}(3/4)^3(1/4)^2$$

$$= \frac{(5)\cdot(4)}{(2)\cdot(1)}(3/4)^3(1/4)^2$$

$$= 10(27/64)\cdot(1/16)$$

$$= 10(27/1024)$$

$$= 270/1024$$

$$p = \sim 0.26$$

Problems and Discussion Questions

MasteringGenetics™ Visit for instructor-assigned tutorials and problems.

When working out genetics problems in this and succeeding chapters, always assume that members of the P_1 generation are homozygous, unless the information or data you are given require you to do otherwise.

HOW DO WE KNOW?

1. In this chapter, we focused on the Mendelian postulates, probability, and pedigree analysis. We also considered some of the methods and reasoning by which these ideas, concepts, and techniques were developed. On the basis of these discussions, what answers would you propose to the following questions:
(a) How was Mendel able to derive postulates concerning the behavior of "unit factors" during gamete formation, when he could not directly observe them?
(b) How do we know whether an organism expressing a dominant trait is homozygous or heterozygous?
(c) In analyzing genetic data, how do we know whether deviation from the expected ratio is due to chance rather than to another, independent factor?
(d) Since experimental crosses are not performed in humans, how do we know how traits are inherited?

CONCEPT QUESTION

2. Review the Chapter Concepts list on p. 40. The first five concepts provide a modern interpretation of Mendelian postulates. Based on these concepts, write a short essay that correlates Mendel's four postulates with what is now known about genes, alleles, and homologous chromosomes.
3. Albinism in humans is inherited as a simple recessive trait. For the following families, determine the genotypes of the parents and offspring. (When two alternative genotypes are possible, list both.)
(a) Two normal parents have five children, four normal and one albino.
(b) A normal male and an albino female have six children, all normal.
(c) A normal male and an albino female have six children, three normal and three albino.
(d) Construct a pedigree of the families in (b) and (c). Assume that one of the normal children in (b) and one of the albino

children in (c) become the parents of eight children. Add these children to the pedigree, predicting their phenotypes (normal or albino).
4. Which of Mendel's postulates are illustrated by the pedigree that you constructed in Problem 3? List and define these postulates.
5. Discuss how Mendel's monohybrid results served as the basis for all but one of his postulates. Which postulate was not based on these results? Why?
6. What advantages were provided by Mendel's choice of the garden pea in his experiments?
7. Mendel crossed peas having round seeds and yellow cotyledons (seed leaves) with peas having wrinkled seeds and green cotyledons. All the F_1 plants had round seeds with yellow cotyledons. Diagram this cross through the F_2 generation, using both the Punnett square and forked-line, or branch diagram, methods.
8. Based on the preceding cross, what is the probability that an organism in the F_2 generation will have round seeds and green cotyledons *and* be true breeding?
9. Which of Mendel's postulates can only be demonstrated in crosses involving at least two pairs of traits? State the postulate.
10. In a cross between a black and a white guinea pig, all members of the F_1 generation are black. The F_2 generation is made up of approximately 3/4 black and 1/4 white guinea pigs.
(a) Diagram this cross, showing the genotypes and phenotypes.
(b) What will the offspring be like if two F_2 white guinea pigs are mated?
(c) Two different matings were made between black members of the F_2 generation, with the following results.

Cross	Offspring
Cross 1	All black
Cross 2	3/4 black, 1/4 white

Diagram each of the crosses.
11. What is the basis for homology among chromosomes?

12. In *Drosophila*, *gray* body color is dominant to *ebony* body color, while *long* wings are dominant to *vestigial* wings. Assuming that the P₁ individuals are homozygous, work the following crosses through the F₂ generation, and determine the genotypic and phenotypic ratios for each generation.
    (a) gray, long × ebony, vestigial
    (b) gray, vestigial × ebony, long
    (c) gray, long × gray, vestigial

13. How many different types of gametes can be formed by individuals of the following genotypes: (a) *AaBb*, (b) *AaBB*, (c) *AaBbCc*, (d) *AaBBcc*, (e) *AaBbcc*, and (f) *AaBbCcDdEe*? What are the gametes in each case?

14. Mendel crossed peas having green seeds with peas having yellow seeds. The F₁ generation produced only yellow seeds. In the F₂, the progeny consisted of 6022 plants with yellow seeds and 2001 plants with green seeds. Of the F₂ yellow-seeded plants, 519 were self-fertilized with the following results: 166 bred true for yellow and 353 produced an F₃ ratio of 3/4 yellow: 1/4 green. Explain these results by diagramming the crosses.

15. In a study of black guinea pigs and white guinea pigs, 100 black animals were crossed with 100 white animals, and each cross was carried to an F₂ generation. In 94 of the crosses, all the F₁ offspring were black and an F₂ ratio of 3 black:1 white was obtained. In the other 6 cases, half of the F₁ animals were black and the other half were white. Why? Predict the results of crossing the black and white F₁ guinea pigs from the 6 exceptional cases.

16. Mendel crossed peas having round green seeds with peas having wrinkled yellow seeds. All F₁ plants had seeds that were round and yellow. Predict the results of testcrossing these F₁ plants.

17. Thalassemia is an inherited anemic disorder in humans. Affected individuals exhibit either a minor anemia or a major anemia. Assuming that only a single gene pair and two alleles are involved in the inheritance of these conditions, is thalassemia a dominant or recessive disorder?

18. The following are F₂ results of two of Mendel's monohybrid crosses.

(a) full pods	882
constricted pods	299
(b) violet flowers	705
white flowers	224

For each cross, state a null hypothesis to be tested using χ^2 analysis. Calculate the χ^2 value and determine the p value for both. Interpret the p values. Can the deviation in each case be attributed to chance or not? Which of the two crosses shows a greater amount of deviation?

19. In assessing data that fell into two phenotypic classes, a geneticist observed values of 250:150. She decided to perform a χ^2 analysis by using the following two different null hypotheses: (a) the data fit a 3:1 ratio, and (b) the data fit a 1:1 ratio. Calculate the χ^2 values for each hypothesis. What can be concluded about each hypothesis?

20. The basis for rejecting any null hypothesis is arbitrary. The researcher can set more or less stringent standards by deciding to raise or lower the p value used to reject or not reject the hypothesis. In the case of the chi-square analysis of genetic crosses, would the use of a standard of $p = 0.10$ be more or less stringent about not rejecting the null hypothesis? Explain.

21. Consider the following pedigree.

Predict the mode of inheritance of the trait of interest and the most probable genotype of each individual. Assume that the alleles *A* and *a* control the expression.

22. Draw all possible conclusions concerning the mode of inheritance of the trait portrayed in each of the following limited pedigrees. (Each of the four cases is based on a different trait.)

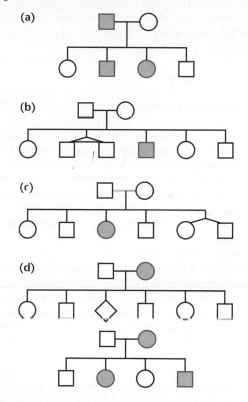

23. In a family of five children, what is the probability that
    (a) all are males?
    (b) three are males and two are females?
    (c) two are males and three are females?
    (d) all are the same sex?

    Assume that the probability of a male child is equal to the probability of a female child ($p = 1/2$).

24. In a family of eight children, where both parents are heterozygous for albinism, what mathematical expression predicts the probability that six are normal and two are albinos?

25. For decades scientists have been perplexed by different circumstances surrounding families with rare, early-onset auditory neuropathy (deafness). In some families, parents and grandparents of the proband have normal hearing, while in

other families, a number of affected (deaf) family members are scattered throughout the pedigree, appearing in every generation. Assuming a genetic cause for each case, offer a reasonable explanation for the genetic origin of such deafness in the two types of families.

26. A "wrongful birth" case was recently brought before a court in which a child with Smith–Lemli–Opitz syndrome was born to apparently healthy parents. This syndrome is characterized by a cluster of birth defects including cleft palate, and an array of problems with the reproductive and urinary organs. Originally considered by their physician as having a nongenetic basis, the parents decided to have another child, who was also born with Smith–Lemli–Opitz syndrome. In the role of a genetic counselor, instruct the court about what occurred, including the probability of the parents having two affected offspring, knowing that the disorder is inherited as a recessive trait.

Extra-Spicy Problems

MasteringGenetics™ Visit for instructor-assigned tutorials and problems.

27. Two true-breeding pea plants were crossed. One parent is round, terminal, violet, constricted, while the other expresses the respective contrasting phenotypes of wrinkled, axial, white, full. The four pairs of contrasting traits are controlled by four genes, each located on a separate chromosome. In the F_1 only round, axial, violet, and full were expressed. In the F_2, all possible combinations of these traits were expressed in ratios consistent with Mendelian inheritance.
    (a) What conclusion about the inheritance of the traits can be drawn based on the F_1 results?
    (b) In the F_2 results, which phenotype appeared most frequently? Write a mathematical expression that predicts the probability of occurrence of this phenotype.
    (c) Which F_2 phenotype is expected to occur least frequently? Write a mathematical expression that predicts this probability.
    (d) In the F_2 generation, how often is either of the P_1 phenotypes likely to occur?
    (e) If the F_1 plants were testcrossed, how many different phenotypes would be produced? How does this number compare with the number of different phenotypes in the F_2 generation just discussed?

28. Tay–Sachs disease (TSD) is an inborn error of metabolism that results in death, often by the age of 2. You are a genetic counselor interviewing a phenotypically normal couple who tell you the male had a female first cousin (on his father's side) who died from TSD and the female had a maternal uncle with TSD. There are no other known cases in either of the families, and none of the matings have been between related individuals. Assume that this trait is very rare.
    (a) Draw a pedigree of the families of this couple, showing the relevant individuals.
    (b) Calculate the probability that both the male and female are carriers for TSD.
    (c) What is the probability that neither of them is a carrier?
    (d) What is the probability that one of them is a carrier and the other is not? [*Hint:* The p values in (b), (c), and (d) should equal 1.]

29. *Datura stramonium* (the Jimsonweed) expresses flower colors of purple and white and pod textures of smooth and spiny. The results of two crosses in which the parents were not necessarily true breeding are shown at the top of the next column.

| white spiny × white spiny | → 3/4 white spiny: 1/4 white smooth |
| purple smooth × purple smooth | → 3/4 purple smooth: 1/4 white smooth |

    (a) Based on these results, put forward a hypothesis for the inheritance of the purple/white and smooth/spiny traits.
    (b) Assuming that true-breeding strains of all combinations of traits are available, what single cross could you execute and carry to an F_2 generation that will prove or disprove your hypothesis? Assuming your hypothesis is correct, what results of this cross will support it?

30. The wild-type (normal) fruit fly, *Drosophila melanogaster,* has straight wings and long bristles. Mutant strains have been isolated that have either curled wings or short bristles. The genes representing these two mutant traits are located on separate chromosomes. Carefully examine the data from the five crosses shown on the top of the following page (running across both columns).
    (a) Identify each mutation as either dominant or recessive. In each case, indicate which crosses support your answer.
    (b) Assign gene symbols and, for each cross, determine the genotypes of the parents.

31. An alternative to using the expanded binomial equation and Pascal's triangle in determining probabilities of phenotypes in a subsequent generation when the parents' genotypes are known is to use the following equation:

$$\frac{n!}{s!t!}a^s b^t$$

    where *n* is the total number of offspring, *s* is the number of offspring in one phenotypic category, *t* is the number of offspring in the other phenotypic category, *a* is the probability of occurrence of the first phenotype, and *b* is the probability of the second phenotype. Using this equation, determine the probability of a family of 5 offspring having exactly 2 children afflicted with sickle-cell anemia (an autosomal recessive disease) when both parents are heterozygous for the sickle-cell allele.

Cross	Progeny			
	straight wings, long bristles	straight wings, short bristles	curled wings, long bristles	curled wings, short bristles
1. straight, short × straight, short	30	90	10	30
2. straight, long × straight, long	120	0	40	0
3. curled, long × straight, short	40	40	40	40
4. straight, short × straight, short	40	120	0	0
5. curled, short straight, short	20	60	20	60

32. To assess Mendel's law of segregation using tomatoes, a true-breeding tall variety (SS) is crossed with a true-breeding short variety (ss). The heterozygous F_1 tall plants (Ss) were crossed to produce two sets of F_2 data, as follows.

Set I	Set II
30 tall	300 tall
5 short	50 short

(a) Using the χ^2 test, analyze the results for both datasets. Calculate χ^2 values and estimate the p values in both cases.
(b) From the above analysis, what can you conclude about the importance of generating large datasets in experimental conditions?

33. Albinism, caused by a mutational disruption in melanin (skin pigment) production, has been observed in many species, including humans. In 1991, the only documented observation of an albino humpback whale (named "Migaloo") was observed near New South Wales. Recently, Polanowski and coworkers (Polanowski, A., S. Robinson-Laverick, and D. Paton. 2012. *Journal of Heredity* 103: 130–133) studied the genetics of humpback whales from the east coast of Australia, including Migaloo.
(a) Do you think that Migaloo's albinism is more likely caused by a dominant or recessive mutation? Explain your reasoning.
(b) What data would be helpful in determining the answer to part (a)?

34. (a) Assuming that Migaloo's albinism is caused by a rare recessive gene, what would be the likelihood of the establishment of a natural robust subpopulation of albino white humpback whales in this population?
(b) Assuming that Migaloo's albinism is caused by a rare dominant gene, what would be the likelihood of the establishment of a natural robust subpopulation of albino white humpback whales in this population?

35. Assume that Migaloo's albinism is caused by a rare recessive gene.
(a) In a mating of two heterozygous, normally pigmented whales, what is the probability that the first three offspring will all have normal pigmentation?
(b) What is the probability that the first female offspring is normally pigmented?
(c) What is the probability that the first offspring is a normally pigmented female?

36. *Dentinogenesis imperfecta* is a tooth disorder involving the production of dentin sialophosphoprotein, a bone-like component of the protective middle layer of teeth. The trait is inherited as an autosomal dominant allele located on chromosome 4 in humans and occurs in about 1 in 6000 to 8000 people. Assume that a man with *dentinogenesis imperfecta*, whose father had the disease but whose mother had normal teeth, married a woman with normal teeth. They have six children. What is the probability that their first child will be a male with *dentinogenesis imperfecta*? What is the probability that three of their six children will have the disease?

Labrador retriever puppies expressing brown (chocolate), golden (yellow), and black coat colors, traits controlled by two gene pairs.

4 Extensions of Mendelian Genetics

CHAPTER CONCEPTS

- While alleles are transmitted from parent to offspring according to Mendelian principles, they often do not display the clear-cut dominant/recessive relationship observed by Mendel.

- In many cases, in a departure from Mendelian genetics, two or more genes are known to influence the phenotype of a single characteristic.

- Still another exception to Mendelian inheritance occurs when genes are located on the X chromosome, because one of the sexes receives only one copy of that chromosome, eliminating the possibility of heterozygosity.

- The result of the various exceptions to Mendelian principles is the occurrence of phenotypic ratios that differ from those produced by standard monohybrid, dihybrid, and trihybrid crosses.

- Phenotypes are often the combined result of genetics and the environment within which genes are expressed.

We discussed the fundamental principles of transmission genetics. We saw that genes are present on homologous chromosomes and that these chromosomes segregate from each other and assort independently from other segregating chromosomes during gamete formation. These two postulates are the basic principles of gene transmission from parent to offspring. Once an offspring has received the total set of genes, it is the expression of genes that determines the organism's phenotype. When gene expression does not adhere to a simple dominant/recessive mode, or when more than one pair of genes influences the expression of a single character, the classic 3:1 and 9:3:3:1 F_2 ratios are usually modified. In this and the next several chapters, we consider more complex modes of inheritance. In spite of the greater complexity of these situations, the fundamental principles set down by Mendel still hold.

In this chapter, we restrict our initial discussion to the inheritance of traits controlled by only one set of genes. In diploid organisms, which have homologous pairs of chromosomes, two copies of each gene influence such traits. The copies need not be identical since alternative forms of genes, *alleles*, occur within populations. How alleles influence phenotypes will be our primary focus. We will then consider **gene interaction**, a situation in which a single phenotype is affected by more than one set of genes. Numerous examples will be presented to illustrate a variety of heritable patterns observed in such situations.

Thus far, we have restricted our discussion to chromosomes other than the X and Y pair. By examining cases where genes are present on the X chromosome, illustrating **X-linkage**, we will see yet another modification of Mendelian ratios. Our discussion of modified ratios also includes the consideration of sex-limited and sex-influenced inheritance, where the sex of the individual, but not necessarily the genes on the X chromosome, influences the phenotype. We conclude the chapter by showing how a given phenotype often varies depending on the overall environment in which a gene, a cell, or an organism finds itself. This discussion points out that phenotypic expression depends on more than just the genotype of an organism. Please note that some of the topics disussed in this chapter are explored in greater depth later in the text (see Special Topic Chapter 1—Epigenetics).

4.1 Alleles Alter Phenotypes in Different Ways

Following the rediscovery of Mendel's work in the early 1900s, research focused on the many ways in which genes influence an individual's phenotype. This course of investigation, stemming from Mendel's findings, is called neo-Mendelian genetics (*neo* from the Greek word meaning *since* or *new*).

Each type of inheritance described in this chapter was investigated when observations of genetic data did not conform precisely to the expected Mendelian ratios. Hypotheses that modified and extended the Mendelian principles were proposed and tested with specifically designed crosses. The explanations proffered to account for these observations were constructed in accordance with the principle that a phenotype is under the influence of one or more genes located at specific loci on one or more pairs of homologous chromosomes.

To understand the various modes of inheritance, we must first consider the potential function of an **allele**. An allele is an alternative form of a gene. The allele that occurs most frequently in a population, the one that we arbitrarily designate as normal, is called the *wild-type allele*. This is often, but not always, dominant. Wild-type alleles are responsible for the corresponding wild-type phenotype and are the standards against which all other mutations occurring at a particular locus are compared.

A mutant allele contains modified genetic information and often specifies an altered gene product. For example, in human populations, there are many known alleles of the gene encoding the β chain of human hemoglobin. All such alleles store information necessary for the synthesis of the β chain polypeptide, but each allele specifies a slightly different form of the same molecule. Once the allele's product has been manufactured, the product's function may or may not be altered.

The process of mutation is the source of alleles. For a new allele to be recognized by observation of an organism, the allele must cause a change in the phenotype. A new phenotype results from a change in functional activity of the cellular product specified by that gene. Often, the mutation causes the diminution or the loss of the specific wild-type function. For example, if a gene is responsible for the synthesis of a specific enzyme, a mutation in that gene may ultimately change the conformation of this enzyme and reduce or eliminate its affinity for the substrate. Such a mutation is designated as a **loss-of-function mutation**. If the loss is complete, the mutation has resulted in what is called a **null allele**.

Conversely, other mutations may enhance the function of the wild-type product. Most often when this occurs, it is the result of increasing the quantity of the gene product. For example, the mutation may be affecting the regulation of transcription of the gene under consideration. Such mutations, designated **gain-of-function mutations**, most often result in dominant alleles, since one copy of the mutation in a diploid organism is sufficient to alter the normal phenotype. Examples of gain-of-function mutations include the genetic conversion of *proto-oncogenes*, which regulate the cell cycle, to *oncogenes*, where regulation is overridden by excess gene product. The result is the creation of a cancerous cell. Another example is a mutation that alters the sensitivity of a receptor, whereby an inhibitory signal molecule is unable to quell a particular biochemical response. In a sense, the function of the gene product is always turned on.

Having introduced the concepts of gain- and loss-of-function mutations, we should note the possibility that a mutation will create an allele that produces no detectable change in function. In this case, the mutation would not be immediately apparent since no phenotypic variation would be evident. However, such a mutation could be detected if the DNA sequence of the gene was examined directly. These are sometimes referred to as **neutral mutations** since the gene product presents no change to either the phenotype or the evolutionary fitness of the organism.

Finally, we note that while a phenotypic trait may be affected by a single mutation in one gene, traits are often influenced by many gene products. For example, enzymatic reactions are most often part of complex metabolic pathways leading to the synthesis of an end product, such as an amino acid. Mutations in any of a pathway's reactions can have a common effect—the failure to synthesize the end product. Therefore, phenotypic traits related to the end product are often influenced by more than one gene. Such is the case in *Drosophila* eye color mutations. Eye color results from the synthesis and deposition of a brown and a bright red pigment in the facets of the compound eye. This causes the wild-type eye color to appear brick red. There are a series of recessive loss-of-function mutations that interrupt the multistep pathway leading to the synthesis of the brown pigment. While these mutations represent genes located on different chromosomes, they all result in the same phenotype: a bright red eye whose color is due to the absence of the brown pigment. Examples are the mutations *vermilion*, *cinnabar*, and *scarlet*, which are indistinguishable phenotypically.

In each of the many crosses discussed in the next few chapters, only one or a few gene pairs are involved. Keep in mind that in each cross, all genes that are not under consideration are assumed to have no effect on the inheritance patterns described.

4.2 Geneticists Use a Variety of Symbols for Alleles

Earlier in the text, we learned a standard convention used to symbolize alleles for very simple Mendelian traits (see Chapter 3). The initial letter of the name of a recessive trait, lowercased and italicized, denotes the recessive allele, and the same letter in uppercase refers to the dominant allele. Thus, in the case of tall and dwarf, where dwarf is recessive, *D* and *d* represent the alleles responsible for these respective traits. Mendel used upper- and lowercase letters such as these to symbolize his unit factors.

Another useful system was developed in genetic studies of the fruit fly *Drosophila melanogaster* to discriminate between wild-type and mutant traits. This system uses the initial letter, or a combination of several letters, from the name of the mutant trait. If the trait is recessive, lowercase is used; if it is dominant, uppercase is used. The contrasting wild-type trait is denoted by the same letters, but with a superscript +. For example, *ebony* is a recessive body color mutation in *Drosophila*. The normal wild-type body color is gray. Using this system, we denote *ebony* by the symbol e, while gray is denoted by e^+. The responsible locus may be occupied by either the wild-type allele (e^+) or the mutant allele (e). A diploid fly may thus exhibit one of three possible genotypes (the two phenotypes are indicated parenthetically):

e^+/e^+	**gray homozygote (wild type)**
e^+/e	**gray heterozygote (wild type)**
e /e	**ebony homozygote (mutant)**

The slash between the letters indicates that the two allele designations represent the same locus on two homologous chromosomes. If we instead consider a mutant allele that is dominant to the normal wild-type allele, such as *Wrinkled* wing in *Drosophila*, the three possible genotypes are Wr/Wr, Wr/Wr^+, and Wr^+/Wr^+. The initial two genotypes express the mutant wrinkled-wing phenotype.

One advantage of this system is that further abbreviation can be used when convenient: The wild-type allele may simply be denoted by the + symbol. With *ebony* as an example, the designations of the three possible genotypes become the following:

$+/+$	**gray homozygote (wild type)**
$+/e$	**gray heterozygote (wild type)**
e/e	**ebony homozygote (mutant)**

Another variation is utilized when no dominance exists between alleles (a situation we will explore in Section 4.3). We simply use uppercase letters and superscripts to denote alternative alleles (e.g., R^1 and R^2, L^M and L^N, and I^A and I^B).

Many diverse systems of genetic nomenclature are used to identify genes in various organisms. Usually, the symbol selected reflects the function of the gene or even a disorder caused by a mutant gene. For example, in yeast, *cdk* is the abbreviation for the *c*yclin-*d*ependent *k*inase gene, whose product is involved in the cell-cycle regulation mechanism (discussed in Chapter 2). In bacteria, *leu*⁻ refers to a mutation that interrupts the biosynthesis of the amino acid leucine, and the wild-type gene is designated *leu*⁺. The symbol *dnaA* represents a bacterial gene involved in DNA replication (and DnaA, without italics, is the protein made by that gene). In humans, italicized capital letters are used to name genes: *BRCA1* represents one of the genes associated with susceptibility to *br*east *ca*ncer. Although these different systems may seem complex, they are useful ways to symbolize genes.

4.3 Neither Allele Is Dominant in Incomplete, or Partial, Dominance

Unlike the Mendelian crosses (reported in Chapter 3), a cross between parents with contrasting traits may sometimes generate offspring with an intermediate phenotype. For example, if a four-o'clock or a snapdragon plant with red flowers is crossed with a white-flowered plant, the offspring have pink flowers. Because some red pigment is produced in the F_1 intermediate-colored plant, neither the red nor white flower color is dominant. Such a situation is known as **incomplete**, or **partial, dominance**.

If the phenotype is under the control of a single gene and two alleles, where neither is dominant, the results of the F_1 (pink) × F_1 (pink) cross can be predicted. The resulting F_2 generation shown in **Figure 4–1** confirms the hypothesis that only one pair of alleles determines these phenotypes. The genotypic ratio (1:2:1) of the F_2 generation is identical to that of Mendel's monohybrid cross. However, because neither allele is dominant, the phenotypic ratio is identical to the genotypic ratio (in contrast to the 3:1 phenotypic

$R^1 R^1$ × $R^2 R^2$ P_1
red   white

$R^1 R^2$ F_1
pink

$R^1 R^2 \times R^1 R^2$ $F_1 \times F_1$

1/4 $R^1 R^1$ red
1/2 $R^1 R^2$ pink F_2
1/4 $R^2 R^2$ white

FIGURE 4–1   Incomplete dominance shown in the flower color of snapdragons.

ratio of a Mendelian monohybrid cross). Note that because neither allele is recessive, we have chosen not to use upper- and lowercase letters as symbols. Instead, we denote the red and white alleles as R^1 and R^2. We could have chosen W^1 and W^2 or still other designations such as C^W and C^R, where C indicates "color" and the W and R superscripts indicate white and red, respectively.

How are we to interpret lack of dominance whereby an intermediate phenotype characterizes heterozygotes? The most accurate way is to consider gene expression in a quantitative way. In the case of flower color above, the mutation causing white flowers is most likely one where complete "loss of function" occurs. In this case, it is likely that the gene product of the wild-type allele (R^1) is an enzyme that participates in a reaction leading to the synthesis of a red pigment. The mutant allele (R^2) produces an enzyme that cannot catalyze the reaction leading to pigment. The end result is that the heterozygote produces only about half the pigment of the red-flowered plant and the phenotype is pink.

Clear-cut cases of incomplete dominance are relatively rare. However, even when one allele seems to have complete dominance over the other, careful examination of the gene product and its activity, rather than the phenotype, often reveals an intermediate level of gene expression. An example is the human biochemical disorder **Tay–Sachs disease**, in which homozygous recessive individuals are severely affected with a fatal lipid-storage disorder and neonates die during their first one to three years of life. In afflicted individuals, there is almost no activity of **hexosaminidase A**, an enzyme normally involved in lipid metabolism. Heterozygotes, with only a single copy of the mutant gene, are phenotypically normal, but with only about 50 percent of the enzyme activity found in homozygous normal individuals. Fortunately, this level of enzyme activity is adequate to achieve normal biochemical function. This situation is not uncommon in enzyme disorders and illustrates the concept of the **threshold effect**, whereby normal phenotypic expression occurs anytime a certain level of gene product is attained. Most often, and in particular in Tay–Sachs disease, the threshold is less than 50 percent.

4.4 In Codominance, the Influence of Both Alleles in a Heterozygote Is Clearly Evident

If two alleles of a single gene are responsible for producing two distinct, detectable gene products, a situation different from incomplete dominance or dominance/recessiveness arises. In this case, *the joint expression of both alleles in a heterozygote* is called **codominance**. The **MN blood group** in humans illustrates this phenomenon. Karl Landsteiner and Philip Levine discovered a glycoprotein molecule found on the surface of red blood cells that acts as a native antigen, providing biochemical and immunological identity to individuals. In the human population, two forms of this glycoprotein exist, designated M and N; an individual may exhibit either one or both of them.

The MN system is under the control of a locus found on chromosome 4, with two alleles designated L^M and L^N. Because humans are diploid, three combinations are possible, each resulting in a distinct blood type:

Genotype	Phenotype
$L^M L^M$	M
$L^M L^N$	MN
$L^N L^N$	N

As predicted, a mating between two heterozygous MN parents may produce children of all three blood types, as follows:

$$L^M L^N \times L^M L^N$$
$$\downarrow$$
$$1/4\ L^M L^M$$
$$1/2\ L^M L^N$$
$$1/4\ L^N L^N$$

Once again, the genotypic ratio 1:2:1 is upheld.

Codominant inheritance is characterized by *distinct expression of the gene products of both alleles*. This characteristic distinguishes codominance from incomplete dominance, where heterozygotes express an intermediate, blended phenotype. For codominance to be studied, both products must be phenotypically detectable. We shall see another example of codominance when we examine the ABO blood-type system.

4.5 Multiple Alleles of a Gene May Exist in a Population

The information stored in any gene is extensive, and mutations can modify this information in many ways. Each change produces a different allele. Therefore, for any gene, the number of alleles within members of a population need not be restricted to two. When three or more alleles of the same gene—which we designate as **multiple alleles**—are present in a population, the resulting mode of inheritance may be unique. It is important to realize that *multiple alleles can be studied only in populations*. Any individual diploid organism has, at most, two homologous gene loci that may be occupied by different alleles of the same gene. However, among members of a species, numerous alternative forms of the same gene can exist.

The ABO Blood Groups

The simplest case of multiple alleles occurs when three alternative alleles of one gene exist. This situation is illustrated in the inheritance of the **ABO blood groups** in humans, discovered by Karl Landsteiner in the early 1900s. The ABO system, like the MN blood types, is characterized by the presence of antigens on the surface of red blood cells. The A and B antigens are distinct from the MN antigens and are under the control of a different gene, located on chromosome 9. As in the MN system, one combination of alleles in the ABO system exhibits a codominant mode of inheritance.

The ABO phenotype of any individual is ascertained by mixing a blood sample with an antiserum containing type A or type B antibodies. If an antigen is present on the surface of the person's red blood cells, it will react with the corresponding antibody and cause clumping, or agglutination, of the red blood cells. When an individual is tested in this way, one of four phenotypes may be revealed. Each individual has the A antigen (A phenotype), the B antigen (B phenotype), the A and B antigens (AB phenotype), or neither antigen (O phenotype).

In 1924, it was hypothesized that these phenotypes were inherited as the result of three alleles of a single gene. This hypothesis was based on studies of the blood types of many different families. Although different designations can be used, we will use the symbols I^A, I^B, and i to distinguish these three alleles. The I designation stands for *isoagglutinogen*, another term for antigen. If we assume that the I^A and I^B alleles are responsible for the production of their respective A and B antigens and that i is an allele that does not produce any detectable A or B antigens, we can list the various genotypic possibilities and assign the appropriate phenotype to each:

Genotype	Antigen	Phenotype
$I^A I^A$	A	A
$I^A i$	A	
$I^B I^B$	B	B
$I^B i$	B	
$I^A I^B$	A, B	AB
$i\ i$	Neither	O

In these assignments, the I^A and I^B alleles are dominant to the i allele, but codominant to each other.

Our knowledge of human blood types has several practical applications, including compatible blood transfusions and successful organ transplants.

The A and B Antigens

The biochemical basis of the ABO blood type system has now been carefully worked out. The A and B antigens are actually carbohydrate groups (sugars) that are bound to lipid molecules (fatty acids) protruding from the membrane of the red blood cell. The specificity of the A and B antigens is based on the terminal sugar of the carbohydrate group.

Almost all individuals possess what is called the **H substance**, to which one or two terminal sugars are added. As shown in **Figure 4–2**, the H substance itself contains three sugar molecules—galactose (Gal), *N*-acetylglucosamine (AcGluNH), and fucose—chemically linked together. The I^A allele is responsible for an enzyme that can add the terminal sugar *N*-acetylgalactosamine (AcGalNH) to the H substance. The I^B allele is responsible for a modified enzyme that

FIGURE 4–2 The biochemical basis of the ABO blood groups. The wild-type *FUT1* allele, present in almost all humans, directs the conversion of a precursor molecule to the H substance by adding a molecule of fucose to it. The *I^A* and *I^B* alleles are then able to direct the addition of terminal sugar residues to the H substance. The *i* allele is unable to direct either of these terminal additions. Failure to produce the H substance results in the Bombay phenotype, in which individuals are type O regardless of the presence of an *I^A* or *I^B* allele. Gal: galactose; AcGluNH: *N*-acetylglucosamine; AcGalNH: *N*-acetylgalactosamine.

cannot add *N*-acetylgalactosamine, but instead can add a terminal galactose. Heterozygotes ($I^A I^B$) add either one or the other sugar at the many sites (substrates) available on the surface of the red blood cell, illustrating the biochemical basis of codominance in individuals of the AB blood type. Finally, persons of type O (*ii*) cannot add either terminal sugar; these persons have only the H substance protruding from the surface of their red blood cells.

The Bombay Phenotype

In 1952, a very unusual situation provided information concerning the genetic basis of the H substance. A woman in Bombay displayed a unique genetic history inconsistent with her blood type. In need of a transfusion, she was found to lack both the A and B antigens and was thus typed as O. However, as shown in the partial pedigree in **Figure 4–3**, one of her parents was type AB, and she herself was the

FIGURE 4–3 A partial pedigree of a woman with the Bombay phenotype. Functionally, her ABO blood group behaves as type O. Genetically, she is type B.

TABLE 4.1 Some of the Alleles Present at the *white* Locus of *Drosophila*

Allele	Name	Eye Color
w	*white*	pure white
w^a	*white-apricot*	yellowish orange
w^{bf}	*white-buff*	light buff
w^{bl}	*white-blood*	yellowish ruby
w^{cf}	*white-coffee*	deep ruby
w^e	*white-eosin*	yellowish pink
w^{mo}	*white-mottled orange*	light mottled orange
w^{sat}	*white-satsuma*	deep ruby
w^{sp}	*white-spotted*	fine grain, yellow mottling
w^t	*white-tinged*	light pink

obvious donor of an I^B allele to two of her offspring. Thus, she was genetically type B but functionally type O!

This woman was subsequently shown to be homozygous for a rare recessive mutation in a gene designated *FUT1* (encoding an enzyme, fucosyl transferase), which prevented her from synthesizing the complete H substance. In this mutation, the terminal portion of the carbohydrate chain protruding from the red cell membrane lacks fucose, normally added by the enzyme. In the absence of fucose, the enzymes specified by the I^A and I^B alleles apparently are unable to recognize the incomplete H substance as a proper substrate. Thus, neither the terminal galactose nor *N*-acetylgalactosamine can be added, even though the appropriate enzymes capable of doing so are present and functional. As a result, the ABO system genotype cannot be expressed in individuals homozygous for the mutant form of the *FUT1* gene; even though they may have the I^A and/or the I^B alleles, neither antigen is added to the cell surface, and they are functionally type O. To distinguish them from the rest of the population, they are said to demonstrate the **Bombay phenotype**. The frequency of the mutant *FUT1* allele is exceedingly low. Hence, the vast majority of the human population can synthesize the H substance.

The *white* Locus in *Drosophila*

Many other phenotypes in plants and animals are influenced by multiple allelic inheritance. In *Drosophila*, many alleles are present at practically every locus. The recessive mutation that causes white eyes, discovered by Thomas H. Morgan and Calvin Bridges in 1912, is one of over 100 alleles that can occupy this locus. In this allelic series, eye colors range from complete absence of pigment in the *white* allele to deep ruby in the *white-satsuma* allele, orange in the *white-apricot* allele, and a buff color in the *white-buff* allele. These alleles are designated w, w^{sat}, w^a, and w^{bf}, respectively. In each case, the total amount of pigment in these mutant eyes is reduced to

less than 20 percent of that found in the brick-red wild-type eye. Table 4.1 lists these and other *white* alleles and their color phenotypes.

It is interesting to note the biological basis of the original *white* mutation in *Drosophila*. Given what we know about eye color in this organism, it might be logical to presume that the mutant allele somehow interrupts the biochemical synthesis of pigments making up the brick-red eye of the wild-type fly. However, it is now clear that the product of the *white* locus is a protein that is involved in transporting pigments into the ommatidia (the individual units) comprising the compound eye. While flies expressing the *white* mutation can synthesize eye pigments normally, they cannot transport them into these structural units of the eye, thus rendering the white phenotype.

4.6 Lethal Alleles Represent Essential Genes

Many gene products are essential to an organism's survival. Mutations resulting in the synthesis of a gene product that is nonfunctional can often be tolerated in the heterozygous state; that is, one wild-type allele may be sufficient to produce enough of the essential product to allow survival. However, such a mutation behaves as a **recessive lethal allele**, and homozygous recessive individuals will not survive. The time of death will depend on when the product is essential. In mammals, for example, this might occur during development, early childhood, or even adulthood.

In some cases, the allele responsible for a lethal effect when homozygous may also result in a distinctive mutant

4–1 In the guinea pig, one locus involved in the control of coat color may be occupied by any of four alleles: C (full color), c^k (sepia), c^d (cream), or c^a (albino), with an order of dominance of: $C > c^k > c^d > c^a$. (C is dominant to all others, c^k is dominant to c^d and c^a, but not C, etc.) In the following crosses, determine the parental genotypes and predict the phenotypic ratios that would result:

(a) sepia × cream, where both guinea pigs had an albino parent

(b) sepia × cream, where the sepia guinea pig had an albino parent and the cream guinea pig had two sepia parents

(c) sepia × cream, where the sepia guinea pig had two full-color parents and the cream guinea pig had two sepia parents

(d) sepia × cream, where the sepia guinea pig had a full-color parent and an albino parent and the cream guinea pig had two full-color parents

■ **HINT:** *This problem involves an understanding of multiple alleles. The key to its solution is to note particularly the hierarchy of dominance of the various alleles. Remember also that even though there can be more than two alleles in a population, an individual can have at most two of these. Thus, the allelic distribution into gametes adheres to the principle of segregation.*

phenotype when present heterozygously. *It is behaving as a recessive lethal allele but is dominant with respect to the phenotype.* For example, a mutation that causes a yellow coat in mice was discovered in the early part of this century. The yellow coat varies from the normal agouti (wild-type) coat phenotype, as shown in **Figure 4–4**. Crosses between the various combinations of the two strains yield unusual results:

	Crosses			
(A) agouti	×	agouti	⟶	all agouti
(B) yellow	×	yellow	⟶	2/3 yellow: 1/3 agouti
(C) agouti	×	yellow	⟶	1/2 yellow: 1/2 agouti

These results are explained on the basis of a single pair of alleles. With regard to coat color, the mutant *yellow* allele (A^Y) is dominant to the wild-type *agouti* allele (A), so heterozygous mice will have yellow coats. However, the *yellow* allele is also a homozygous recessive lethal. When present in two copies, the mice die before birth. Thus, there are no homozygous yellow mice. The genetic basis for these three crosses is shown in Figure 4–4.

In other cases, a mutation may behave as a **dominant lethal allele**. In such cases, the presence of just one copy of the allele results in the death of the individual. In humans, a disorder called **Huntington disease** is due to a dominant autosomal allele H, where the onset of the disease in heterozygotes (Hh) is delayed, usually well into adulthood. Affected individuals then undergo gradual nervous and motor degeneration until they die. This lethal disorder is particularly tragic because it has such a late onset, typically at about age 40. By that time, the affected individual may have produced a family, and each of their children has a 50 percent probability of inheriting the lethal allele, transmitting the allele to his or her offspring, and eventually developing the disorder. The American folk singer and composer Woody Guthrie (father of modern-day folk singer Arlo Guthrie) died from this disease at age 39.

Dominant lethal alleles are rarely observed. For these alleles to exist in a population, the affected individuals must reproduce before the lethal allele is expressed, as can occur in Huntington disease. If all affected individuals die before reaching reproductive age, the mutant gene will not be passed to future generations, and the mutation will disappear from the population unless it arises again as a result of a new mutation.

The Molecular Basis of Dominance, Recessiveness, and Lethality: The *agouti* Gene

Molecular analysis of the gene resulting in the agouti and yellow mice has provided insight into how a mutation can be both dominant for one phenotypic effect (hair color) and recessive for another (embryonic development). The A^Y allele is a classic example of a gain-of-function mutation. Animals homozygous for the wild-type A allele have yellow pigment deposited as a band on the otherwise black hair shaft, resulting in the agouti phenotype (see Figure 4–4). Heterozygotes deposit yellow pigment along the entire length of hair shafts as a result of the deletion of the regulatory region preceding the DNA coding region of the A^Y allele. Without any means to regulate its expression, one copy of the A^Y allele is always turned on in heterozygotes, resulting in the gain of function leading to the dominant effect.

The homozygous lethal effect has also been explained by molecular analysis of the mutant gene. The extensive deletion of genetic material that produced the A^Y allele actually extends into the coding region of an adjacent gene (*Merc*), rendering it nonfunctional. It is this gene that is critical to embryonic development, and the loss of its function in A^Y/A^Y homozygotes is what causes lethality. Heterozygotes exceed the threshold level of the wild-type Merc gene product and thus survive.

FIGURE 4–4 Inheritance patterns in three crosses involving the *agouti* allele (A) and the mutant *yellow* allele (A^Y) in the mouse. Note that the mutant allele behaves dominantly to the normal allele in controlling coat color, but it also behaves as a homozygous recessive lethal allele. Mice with the genotype $A^Y A^Y$ do not survive.

4.7 Combinations of Two Gene Pairs with Two Modes of Inheritance Modify the 9:3:3:1 Ratio

Each example discussed so far modifies Mendel's 3:1 F_2 monohybrid ratio. Therefore, combining any two of these modes of inheritance in a dihybrid cross will also modify the classical 9:3:3:1 dihybrid ratio. Having established the foundation of the modes of inheritance of incomplete dominance, codominance, multiple alleles, and lethal alleles, we can now deal with the situation of two modes of inheritance occurring simultaneously. Mendel's principle of independent assortment applies to these situations, provided that the genes controlling each character are not located on the same chromosome—in other words, that they do not demonstrate what is called *genetic linkage*.

Consider, for example, a mating between two humans who are both heterozygous for the autosomal recessive gene that causes albinism and who are both of blood type AB. What is the probability of a particular phenotypic combination occurring in each of their children? Albinism is inherited in the simple Mendelian fashion, and the blood types are determined by the series of three multiple alleles, I^A, I^B, and i. The solution to this problem is diagrammed in **Figure 4–5** using the forked-line method. This dihybrid cross does not yield four phenotypes in the classical 9:3:3:1 ratio. Instead, six phenotypes occur in a 3:6:3:1:2:1 ratio, establishing the expected probability for each phenotype. This is just one of the many variants of modified ratios that are possible when different modes of inheritance are combined.

EVOLVING CONCEPT OF A GENE

Based on the work of many geneticists following the rediscovery of Mendel's work in the very early part of the twentieth century, the chromosome theory of inheritance was put forward, which hypothesized that chromosomes are the carriers of genes and that meiosis is the physical basis of Mendel's postulates. In the ensuing 40 years, the concept of a gene evolved to reflect that

FIGURE 4–5 Calculation of the probabilities in a mating involving the ABO blood type and albinism in humans, using the forked-line method.

this hereditary unit can exist in multiple forms, or alleles, each of which can impact on the phenotype in different ways, leading to incomplete dominance, codominance, and even lethality. It became clear that the process of mutation was the source of new alleles. ∎

4.8 Phenotypes Are Often Affected by More Than One Gene

Soon after Mendel's work was rediscovered, experimentation revealed that in many cases a given phenotype is affected by more than one gene. This was a significant discovery because it revealed that genetic influence on the phenotype is often much more complex than the situations Mendel encountered in his crosses with the garden pea. Instead of single genes controlling

the development of individual parts of a plant or animal body, it soon became clear that phenotypic characters such as eye color, hair color, or fruit shape can be influenced by many different genes and their products.

The term **gene interaction** is often used to express the idea that several genes influence a particular characteristic. This does not mean, however, that two or more genes or their products necessarily interact directly with one another to influence a particular phenotype. Rather, the term means that the cellular function of numerous gene products contributes to the development of a common phenotype. For example, the development of an organ such as the eye of an insect is exceedingly complex and leads to a structure with multiple phenotypic manifestations, for example, to an eye having a specific size, shape, texture, and color. The development of the eye is a complex cascade of developmental events leading to that organ's formation. This process illustrates the developmental concept of **epigenesis**, whereby each step of development increases the complexity of the organ or feature of interest and is under the control and influence of many genes.

An enlightening example of epigenesis and multiple gene interaction involves the formation of the inner ear in mammals, allowing organisms to detect and interpret sound. The structure and function of the inner ear are exceedingly complex. Its formation includes distinctive anatomical features not only to capture, funnel, and transmit external sound toward and through the middle ear, but also to convert sound waves into nerve impulses within the inner ear. Thus, the ear forms as a result of a cascade of intricate developmental events influenced by many genes. Mutations that interrupt many of the steps of ear development lead to a common phenotype: **hereditary deafness**. In a sense, these many genes "interact" to produce a common phenotype. In such situations, the mutant phenotype is described as a **heterogeneous trait**, reflecting the many genes involved. In humans, while a few common alleles are responsible for the vast majority of cases of hereditary deafness, over 50 genes are involved in the development of the ability to discern sound.

Epistasis

Some of the best examples of gene interaction are those showing the phenomenon of **epistasis**, where the expression of one gene pair masks or modifies the effect of another gene pair. Sometimes the genes involved influence the same general phenotypic characteristic in an antagonistic manner, which leads to masking. In other cases, however, the genes involved exert their influence on one another in a complementary, or cooperative, fashion.

For example, the homozygous presence of a recessive allele may prevent or override the expression of other alleles at a second locus (or several other loci). In this case, the alleles at the first locus are said to be *epistatic* to those at the second locus, and the alleles at the second locus are *hypostatic* to those at the first locus. As we will see, there are several variations on this theme. In another example, a single dominant allele at the first locus may be epistatic to the expression of the alleles at a second gene locus. In a third example, two gene pairs may *complement* one another such that at least one dominant allele in each pair is required to express a particular phenotype.

The Bombay phenotype discussed earlier is an example of the homozygous recessive condition at one locus masking the expression of a second locus. There we established that the homozygous presence of the mutant form of the *FUT1* gene masks the expression of the I^A and I^B alleles. Only individuals containing at least one wild-type *FUT1* allele can form the A or B antigen. As a result, individuals whose genotypes include the I^A or I^B allele and who have no wild-type *FUT1* allele are of the type O phenotype, regardless of their potential to make either antigen. An example of the outcome of matings between individuals heterozygous at both loci is illustrated in **Figure 4–6**. If many such

FIGURE 4–6 The outcome of a mating between individuals heterozygous at two genes determining their ABO blood type. Final phenotypes are calculated by considering each gene separately and then combining the results using the forked-line method.

individuals have children, the phenotypic ratio of 3 A: 6 AB: 3 B: 4 O is expected in their offspring.

It is important to note two things when examining this cross and the predicted phenotypic ratio:

1. A key distinction exists between this cross and the modified dihybrid cross shown in Figure 4–5: *only one characteristic—blood type—is being followed*. In the modified dihybrid cross in Figure 4–5, blood type *and* skin pigmentation are followed as separate phenotypic characteristics.

2. Even though only a single character was followed, the phenotypic ratio comes out in sixteenths. If we knew nothing about the H substance and the gene controlling it, we could still be confident (because the proportions are in sixteenths) that a second gene pair, other than that controlling the A and B antigens, was involved in the phenotypic expression. *When a single character is being studied, a ratio that is expressed in 16 parts (e.g., 3:6:3:4) suggests that two gene pairs are "interacting" in the expression of the phenotype under consideration.*

The study of gene interaction reveals a number of inheritance patterns that are modifications of the Mendelian dihybrid F_2 ratio (9:3:3:1). In several of the subsequent examples, epistasis has the effect of combining one or more of the four phenotypic categories in various ways. The generation of these four groups is reviewed in **Figure 4–7**, along with several modified ratios.

As we discuss these and other examples (see **Figure 4–8**), we will make several assumptions and adopt certain conventions:

1. In each case, distinct phenotypic classes are produced, each clearly discernible from all others. Such traits illustrate discontinuous variation, where phenotypic categories are discrete and qualitatively different from one another.

2. The genes considered in each cross are on different chromosomes and therefore assort independently of one another during gamete formation. To allow you to easily compare the results of different crosses, we designated alleles as *A, a* and *B, b* in each case.

3. When we assume that complete dominance exists within a gene pair, such that *AA* and *Aa* or *BB* and *Bb* are equivalent in their genetic effects, we use the designations *A–* or *B–* for both combinations, where the dash (–) indicates that either allele may be present without consequence to the phenotype.

4. All P_1 crosses involve homozygous individuals (e.g., $AABB \times aabb, AAbb \times aaBB \times aaBB \times AAbb$). Therefore, each F_1 generation consists of only heterozygotes of genotype *AaBb*.

5. In each example, the F_2 generation produced from these heterozygous parents is our main focus of analysis. When two genes are involved (Figure 4–7), the F_2

FIGURE 4–7 Generation of various modified dihybrid ratios from the nine unique genotypes produced in a cross between individuals heterozygous at two genes.

genotypes fall into four categories: 9/16 $A-B-$, 3/16 $A-bb$, 3/16 $aaB-$, and 1/16 $aabb$. Because of dominance, all genotypes in each category are equivalent in their effect on the phenotype.

Case 1 is the inheritance of coat color in mice (Figure 4–8). Normal wild-type coat color is agouti, a grayish pattern formed by alternating bands of pigment on each hair (see Figure 4–4). Agouti is dominant to black (nonagouti) hair, which results from the homozygous expression of a recessive mutation that we designate a. Thus, $A-$ results in agouti, whereas aa yields black coat color. When a recessive mutation, b, at a separate locus is homozygous, it eliminates pigmentation altogether, yielding albino mice (bb), regardless of the genotype at the a locus. Thus, in a cross between agouti ($AABB$) and albino ($aabb$) parents, members of the F_1 are all $AaBb$ and have agouti coat color. In the F_2 progeny of a cross between two F_1 double heterozygotes, the following genotypes and phenotypes are observed:

$$F_1: AaBb \times AaBb$$
$$\downarrow$$

F_2 Ratio	Genotype	Phenotype	Final Phenotypic Ratio
9/16	$A-B-$	agouti	9/16 agouti
3/16	$A-bb$	albino	3/16 black
3/16	$aaB-$	black	4/16 albino
1/16	$aabb$	albino	

We can envision gene interaction yielding the observed 9:3:4 F_2 ratio as a two-step process:

In the presence of a B allele, black pigment can be made from a colorless substance. In the presence of an A allele, the black pigment is deposited during the development of hair in a pattern that produces the agouti phenotype. If the aa genotype occurs, all of the hair remains black. If the bb genotype occurs, no black pigment is produced, regardless of the presence of the A or a alleles, and the mouse is albino. Therefore, the bb genotype masks or suppresses the expression of the A allele. As a result, this is referred to as *recessive epistasis*.

A second type of epistasis, called *dominant epistasis*, occurs when a dominant allele at one genetic locus masks the expression of the alleles of a second locus. For instance, Case 2 of Figure 4–8 deals with the inheritance of fruit color in summer squash. Here, the dominant allele A results in white fruit color regardless of the genotype at a second locus, B. In the absence of a dominant A allele (the aa genotype), BB or Bb results in yellow color, while bb results in

Case	Organism	Character	F₂ Phenotypes 9/16	3/16	3/16	1/16	Modified ratio
1	Mouse	Coat color	agouti	albino	black	albino	9:3:4
2	Squash	Color	white		yellow	green	12:3:1
3	Pea	Flower color	purple	white			9:7
4	Squash	Fruit shape	disc	sphere		long	9:6:1
5	Chicken	Color	white		colored	white	13:3
6	Mouse	Color	white-spotted	white	colored	white-spotted	10:3:3
7	Shepherd's purse	Seed capsule	triangular			ovoid	15:1
8	Flour beetle	Color	6/16 sooty and 3/16 red	black	jet	black	6:3:3:4

FIGURE 4–8 The basis of modified dihybrid F_2 phenotypic ratios resulting from crosses between doubly heterozygous F_1 individuals. The four groupings of the F_2 genotypes shown in Figure 4–7 and across the top of this figure are combined in various ways to produce these ratios.

green color. Therefore, if two white-colored double heterozygotes (*AaBb*) are crossed, this type of epistasis generates an interesting phenotypic ratio:

$$F_1: AaBb \times AaBb$$

F₂ Ratio	Genotype	Phenotype	Final Phenotypic Ratio
9/16	A–B–	white	12/16 white
3/16	A–bb	white	
3/16	aaB–	yellow	3/16 yellow
1/16	aabb	green	1/16 green

Of the offspring, 9/16 are *A–B–* and are thus white. The 3/16 bearing the genotypes *A–bb* are also white. Of the remaining squash, 3/16 are yellow (*aaB–*), while 1/16 are green (*aabb*). Thus, the modified phenotypic ratio of 12:3:1 occurs.

Our third example (Case 3 of Figure 4–8), first discovered by William Bateson and Reginald Punnett (of Punnett square fame), is demonstrated in a cross between two true-breeding strains of white-flowered sweet peas. Unexpectedly, the results of this cross yield all purple F₁ plants, and the F₂ plants occur in a ratio of 9/16 purple to 7/16 white. The proposed explanation suggests that the presence of at least one dominant allele of each of two gene pairs is essential in order for flowers to be purple. Thus, this cross represents a case of *complementary gene interaction*. All other genotype combinations yield white flowers because the homozygous condition of either recessive allele masks the expression of the dominant allele at the other locus.

The cross is shown as follows:

$$P_1: AAbb \times aaBB$$
$$\text{white} \quad \text{white}$$
$$\downarrow$$
$$F_1: \text{All } AaBb \text{ (purple)}$$

F₂ Ratio	Genotype	Phenotype	Final Phenotypic Ratio
9/16	A–B–	purple	9/16 purple
3/16	A–bb	white	
3/16	aaB–	white	7/16 white
1/16	aabb	white	

We can now envision how two gene pairs might yield such results:

	Gene A			Gene B	
Precursor substance (colorless)	↓ ⟶ A–	Intermediate product (colorless)	↓ ⟶ B–	Final product (purple)	

At least one dominant allele from each pair of genes is necessary to ensure both biochemical conversions to the final product, yielding purple flowers. In the preceding cross, this will occur in 9/16 of the F₂ offspring. All other plants (7/16) have flowers that remain white.

These three examples illustrate in a simple way how the products of two genes interact to influence the development of a common phenotype. In other instances, more than two genes and their products are involved in controlling phenotypic expression.

Novel Phenotypes

Other cases of gene interaction yield novel, or new, phenotypes in the F₂ generation, in addition to producing modified dihybrid ratios. Case 4 in Figure 4–8 depicts the inheritance of fruit shape in the summer squash *Cucurbita pepo*. When plants with disc-shaped fruit (*AABB*) are crossed with plants with long fruit (*aabb*), the F₁ generation all have disc fruit. However, in the F₂ progeny, fruit with a novel shape—sphere—appear, as well as fruit exhibiting the parental phenotypes. A variety of fruit shapes are shown in **Figure 4–9**.

The F₂ generation, with a modified 9:6:1 ratio, is generated as follows:

$$F_1: AaBb \times AaBb$$
$$\text{disc} \quad \text{disc}$$
$$\downarrow$$

F₂ Ratio	Genotype	Phenotype	Final Phenotypic Ratio
9/16	A–B–	disc	9/16 disc
3/16	A–bb	sphere	6/16 sphere
3/16	aaB–	sphere	
1/16	aabb	long	1/16 long

In this example of gene interaction, both gene pairs influence fruit shape equally. A dominant allele at either locus ensures a sphere-shaped fruit. In the absence of dominant alleles, the fruit is long. However, if both dominant alleles (*A* and *B*) are present, the fruit displays a flattened, disc shape.

FIGURE 4–9 Summer squash exhibiting various fruit-shape phenotypes, including disc, long, and sphere.

NOW SOLVE THIS

4–2 In some plants a red flower pigment, cyanidin, is synthesized from a colorless precursor. The addition of a hydroxyl group (OH⁻) to the cyanidin molecule causes it to become purple. In a cross between two randomly selected purple varieties, the following results were obtained:

94 purple

31 red

43 white

How many genes are involved in the determination of these flower colors? Which genotypic combinations produce which phenotypes? Diagram the purple × purple cross.

■ **HINT:** *This problem describes a plant in which flower color, a single characteristic, can take on one of three variations. The key to its solution is to first analyze the raw data and convert the numbers to a meaningful ratio. This will guide you in determining how many gene pairs are involved. Then you can group the genotypes in a way that corresponds to the phenotypic ratio.*

For more practice, see Problems 15, 16, 17, and 18.

Another interesting example of an unexpected phenotype arising in the F₂ generation is the inheritance of eye color in *Drosophila melanogaster*. As mentioned earlier, the wild-type eye color is brick red. When two autosomal recessive mutants, *brown* and *scarlet*, are crossed, the F₁ generation consists of flies with wild-type eye color. In the F₂ generation, wild, scarlet, brown, and white-eyed flies are found in a 9:3:3:1 ratio. While this ratio is numerically the same as Mendel's dihybrid ratio, the *Drosophila* cross involves only one character: eye color. This is an important distinction to make when modified dihybrid ratios resulting from gene interaction are studied.

The *Drosophila* cross is an excellent example of gene interaction because the biochemical basis of eye color in this organism has been determined (**Figure 4–10**). *Drosophila*, as a typical arthropod, has compound eyes made up of hundreds of individual visual units called ommatidia. The wild-type eye color is due to the deposition and mixing of two separate pigment groups in each ommatidium—the bright-red **drosopterins** and the brown **xanthommatins**. Each type

FIGURE 4–10 A theoretical explanation of the biochemical basis of the four eye color phenotypes produced in a cross between *Drosophila* with brown eyes and scarlet eyes. In the presence of at least one wild-type *bw⁺* allele, an enzyme is produced that converts substance b to c, and the pigment drosopterin is synthesized. In the presence of at least one wild-type *st⁺* allele, substance e is converted to f, and the pigment xanthommatin is synthesized. The homozygous presence of the recessive *st* or *bw* mutant allele blocks the synthesis of the respective pigment molecule. Either one, both, or neither of these pathways can be blocked, depending on the genotype.

Wild type: *bw⁺bw⁺; st⁺st⁺*

Brown mutant: *bwbw; st⁺st⁺*

Scarlet mutant: *bw⁺bw⁺; stst*

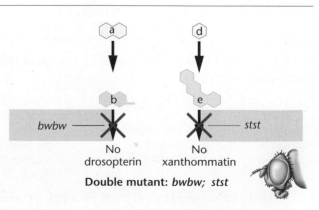

Double mutant: *bwbw; stst*

of pigment is produced by a separate biosynthetic pathway. Each step of each pathway is catalyzed by a separate enzyme and is thus under the control of a separate gene. As shown in Figure 4–10, the *brown* mutation, when homozygous, interrupts the pathway leading to the synthesis of the bright-red pigments. Because only xanthommatin pigments are present, the eye is brown. The *scarlet* mutation, affecting a gene located on a separate autosome, interrupts the pathway leading to the synthesis of the brown xanthommatins and renders the eye color bright red in homozygous mutant flies. Each mutation apparently causes the production of a nonfunctional enzyme. Flies that are double mutants and thus homozygous for both *brown* and *scarlet* lack both functional enzymes and can make neither of the pigments; they represent the novel white-eyed flies appearing in 1/16 of the F_2 generation. Note that the absence of pigment in these flies is not due to the X-linked *white* mutation, in which pigments can be synthesized but the necessary precursors cannot be transported into the cells making up the ommatidia.

Other Modified Dihybrid Ratios

The remaining cases (5–8) in Figure 4–8 illustrate additional modifications of the dihybrid ratio and provide still other examples of gene interactions. As you will note, ratios of 13:3, 10:3:3; 15:1, and 6:3:3:4 are illustrated. These cases, like the four preceding them, have two things in common. First, we need not violate the principles of segregation and independent assortment to explain the inheritance pattern of each case. Therefore, the added complexity of inheritance in these examples does not detract from the validity of Mendel's conclusions. Second, the F_2 phenotypic ratio in each example has been expressed in sixteenths. When sixteenths are seen in the ratios of crosses where the inheritance pattern is unknown, they suggest to geneticists that two gene pairs are controlling the observed phenotypes. You should make the same inference in your analysis of genetics problems. Other insights into solving genetics problems are provided in "Insights and Solutions" at the conclusion of this chapter.

4.9 Complementation Analysis Can Determine if Two Mutations Causing a Similar Phenotype Are Alleles of the Same Gene

An interesting situation arises when two mutations that both produce a similar phenotype are isolated independently. Suppose that two investigators independently isolate and establish a true-breeding strain of wingless *Drosophila* and demonstrate that each mutant phenotype is due to a recessive

mutation. We might assume that both strains contain mutations in the same gene. However, since we know that many genes are involved in the formation of wings, we must consider the possibility that mutations in any one of them might inhibit wing formation during development. This is the case with any *heterogeneous trait*, a concept introduced earlier in this chapter in our discussion of hereditary deafness. An analytical procedure called **complementation analysis** allows us to determine whether two independently isolated mutations are in the same gene—that is, whether they are alleles—or whether they represent mutations in separate genes.

To repeat, our analysis seeks to answer this simple question: *Are two mutations that yield similar phenotypes present in the same gene or in two different genes?* To find the answer, we cross the two mutant strains and analyze the F_1 generation. The two possible alternative outcomes and their interpretations are shown in **Figure 4–11**. To discuss these possibilities (Case 1 and Case 2), we designate one of the mutations m^a and the other m^b.

Case 1. *All offspring develop normal wings.*
Interpretation: The two recessive mutations are in separate genes and are not alleles of one another. Following the cross, all F_1 flies are heterozygous for both genes. Since each mutation is in a separate gene and each F_1 fly is heterozygous at both loci, the normal products of both genes are produced (by the one normal copy of each gene), and wings develop. Under such circumstances, the genes complement one another in restoration of the wild-type phenotype, and complementation is said to occur because the two mutations are in different genes.

Case 2. *All offspring fail to develop wings.*
Interpretation: The two mutations affect the same gene and are alleles of one another. Complementation does not occur. Since the two mutations affect the same gene, the F_1 flies are homozygous for the two mutant alleles (the m^a allele and the m^b allele). No normal product of the gene is produced, and in the absence of this essential product, wings do not form.

Complementation analysis, as originally devised by the *Drosophila* geneticist Edward B. Lewis, may be used to screen any number of individual mutations that result in the same phenotype. Such an analysis may reveal that only a single gene is involved or that two or more genes are involved. All mutations determined to be present in any single gene are said to fall into the same **complementation group**, and they will complement mutations in all other groups. When large numbers of mutations affecting the same trait are available and studied using complementation analysis, it is possible to predict the total number of genes involved in the determination of that trait.

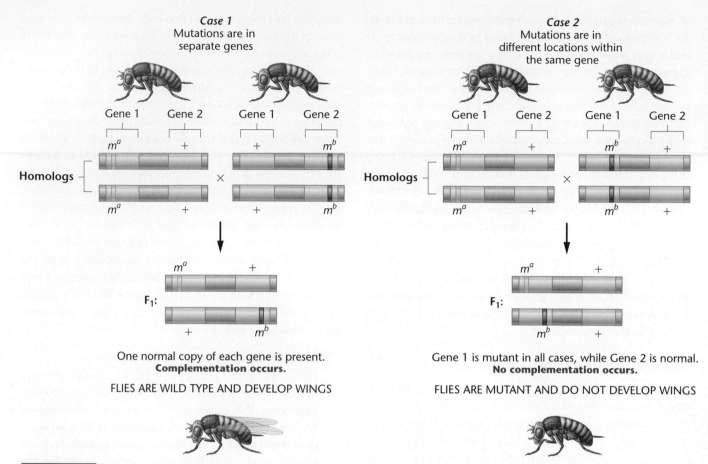

FIGURE 4–11 Complementation analysis of alternative outcomes of two wingless mutations in *Drosophila* (m^a and m^b). In Case 1, the mutations are not alleles of the same gene, while in Case 2, the mutations are alleles of the same gene.

4.10 Expression of a Single Gene May Have Multiple Effects

While the previous sections have focused on the effects of two or more genes on a single characteristic, the converse situation, where expression of a single gene has multiple phenotypic effects, is also quite common. This phenomenon, which often becomes apparent when phenotypes are examined carefully, is referred to as **pleiotropy**. Many excellent examples can be drawn from human disorders, and we will review two such cases to illustrate this point.

The first disorder is **Marfan syndrome**, a human malady resulting from an autosomal dominant mutation in the gene encoding the connective tissue protein *fibrillin*. Because this protein is widespread in many tissues in the body, one would expect multiple effects of such a defect. In fact, fibrillin is important to the structural integrity of the lens of the eye, to the lining of vessels such as the aorta, and to bones, among other tissues. As a result, the phenotype associated with Marfan syndrome includes lens dislocation, increased risk of aortic aneurysm, and lengthened long

bones in limbs. This disorder is of historical interest in that speculation abounds that Abraham Lincoln was afflicted.

A second example involves another human autosomal dominant disorder, **porphyria variegata**. Afflicted individuals cannot adequately metabolize the porphyrin component of hemoglobin when this respiratory pigment is broken down as red blood cells are replaced. The accumulation of excess porphyrins is immediately evident in the urine, which takes on a deep red color. However, this phenotypic characteristic is merely diagnostic. The severe features of the disorder are due to the toxicity of the buildup of porphyrins in the body, particularly in the brain. Complete phenotypic characterization includes abdominal pain, muscular weakness, fever, a racing pulse, insomnia, headaches, vision problems (that can lead to blindness), delirium, and ultimately convulsions. As you can see, deciding which phenotypic trait best characterizes the disorder is impossible.

Like Marfan syndrome, porphyria variegata is also of historical significance. George III, King of England during the American Revolution, is believed to have suffered from episodes involving all of the above symptoms. He ultimately became blind and senile prior to his death.

We could cite many other examples to illustrate pleiotropy, but suffice it to say that if one looks carefully, most mutations display more than a single manifestation when expressed.

4.11 X-Linkage Describes Genes on the X Chromosome

In many animals and some plant species, one of the sexes contains a pair of unlike chromosomes that are involved in sex determination. In many cases, these are designated as X and Y. For example, in both *Drosophila* and humans, males contain an X and a Y chromosome, whereas females contain two X chromosomes. The Y chromosome must contain a region of pairing homology with the X chromosome if the two are to synapse and segregate during meiosis, but a major portion of the Y chromosome in humans as well as other species is considered to be relatively inert genetically. While we now recognize a number of male-specific genes on the human Y chromosome, it lacks copies of most genes present on the X chromosome. As a result, genes present on the X chromosome exhibit patterns of inheritance that are very different from those seen with autosomal genes. The term **X-linkage** is used to describe these situations.

In the following discussion, we will focus on inheritance patterns resulting from genes present on the X but absent from the Y chromosome. This situation results in a modification of Mendelian ratios, the central theme of this chapter.

X-Linkage in *Drosophila*

One of the first cases of X-linkage was documented in 1910 by Thomas H. Morgan during his studies of the *white* eye mutation in *Drosophila* (**Figure 4–12**). The normal wild-type red eye color is dominant to white eye color.

Morgan's work established that the inheritance pattern of the white-eye trait was clearly related to the sex of the parent carrying the mutant allele. Unlike the outcome of the typical Mendelian monohybrid cross where F_1 and F_2 data were similar regardless of which P_1 parent exhibited the recessive mutant trait, reciprocal crosses between white-eyed and red-eyed flies did not yield identical results. Morgan's analysis led to the conclusion that the *white* locus is present on the X chromosome rather than on one of the autosomes. Both the gene and the trait are said to be X-linked.

Results of reciprocal crosses between white-eyed and red-eyed flies are shown in Figure 4–12. The obvious differences in phenotypic ratios in both the F_1 and F_2 generations are dependent on whether or not the P_1 white-eyed parent was male or female.

FIGURE 4–12 The F_1 and F_2 results of T. H. Morgan's reciprocal crosses involving the X-linked *white* mutation in *Drosophila melanogaster*. The actual data are shown in parentheses. The photographs show white eye and the brick-red wild-type eye color.

Morgan was able to correlate these observations with the difference found in the sex-chromosome composition of male and female *Drosophila*. He hypothesized that the recessive allele for white eye is found on the X chromosome, but its corresponding locus is absent from the Y chromosome. Females thus have two available gene loci, one on each X chromosome, whereas males have only one available locus, on their single X chromosome.

Morgan's interpretation of X-linked inheritance, shown in **Figure 4–13**, provides a suitable theoretical explanation for his results. Since the Y chromosome lacks homology with almost all genes on the X chromosome, these alleles present on the X chromosome of the males will be directly expressed in the phenotype. Males cannot be either homozygous or heterozygous for X-linked genes; instead, their condition—possession of only one copy of a gene in an otherwise diploid cell—is referred to as **hemizygosity**. The individual is said to

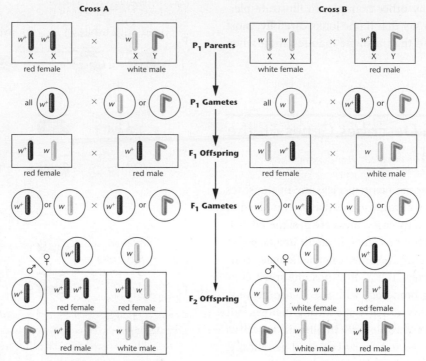

FIGURE 4–13 The chromosomal explanation of the results of the X-linked crosses shown in Figure 4–12.

be **hemizygous**. One result of X-linkage is the *crisscross pattern of inheritance*, in which phenotypic traits controlled by recessive X-linked genes are passed from homozygous mothers to all sons. This pattern occurs because females exhibiting a recessive trait must contain the mutant allele on both X chromosomes. Because male offspring receive one of their mother's two X chromosomes and are hemizygous for all alleles present on that X, all sons will express the same recessive X-linked traits as their mother.

Morgan's work has taken on great historical significance. By 1910, the correlation between Mendel's work and the behavior of chromosomes during meiosis had provided the basis for the **chromosome theory of inheritance**. Morgan's work, and subsequently that of his student, Calvin Bridges, around 1920, provided direct

evidence that genes are transmitted on specific chromosomes, and is considered the first solid experimental evidence in support of this theory.

X-Linkage in Humans

In humans, many genes and the respective traits controlled by them are recognized as being linked to the X chromosome (see **Table 4.2**). These X-linked traits can be easily identified in a pedigree because of the crisscross pattern of inheritance. A pedigree for one form of human **color blindness** is shown in **Figure 4–14**. The mother in generation I passes the trait to all her sons but to none of her daughters. If the offspring in generation II marry normal individuals, the color-blind sons will produce all normal male and female offspring (III-1, 2, and 3); the normal-visioned daughters will produce normal-visioned

FIGURE 4–14 A human pedigree of the X-linked color-blindness trait. The photograph is of an Ishihara color-blindness chart, which tests for red–green color blindness. Those with normal vision will see the number 15, while those with red–green color blindness will see the number 17.

Condition	Characteristics
Color blindness, deutan type	Insensitivity to green light
Color blindness, protan type	Insensitivity to red light
Fabry's disease	Deficiency of galactosidase A; heart and kidney defects, early death
G-6-PD deficiency	Deficiency of glucose-6-phosphate dehydrogenase; severe anemic reaction following intake of primaquines in drugs and certain foods, including fava beans
Hemophilia A	Classic form of clotting deficiency; deficiency of clotting factor VIII
Hemophilia B	Christmas disease; deficiency of clotting factor IX
Hunter syndrome	Mucopolysaccharide storage disease resulting from iduronate sulfatase enzyme deficiency; short stature, claw-like fingers, coarse facial features, slow mental deterioration, and deafness
Ichthyosis	Deficiency of steroid sulfatase enzyme; scaly dry skin, particularly on extremities
Lesch–Nyhan syndrome	Deficiency of hypoxanthine-guanine phosphoribosyltransferase enzyme (HPRT) leading to motor and mental retardation, self-mutilation, and early death
Duchenne muscular dystrophy	Progressive, life-shortening disorder characterized by muscle degeneration and weakness; sometimes associated with mental retardation; deficiency of the protein dystrophin

TABLE 4.2 Human X-Linked Traits

NOW SOLVE THIS

1–3 Below are three pedigrees. For each trait, consider whether it is or is not consistent with X-linked recessive inheritance. In a sentence or two, indicate why or why not.

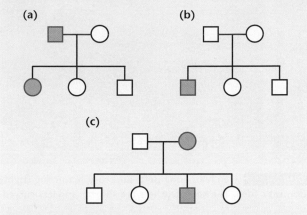

■ HINT: *This problem involves potential X-linked recessive traits as analyzed in pedigrees. The key to its solution is to focus on hemizygosity, where an X-linked recessive allele is always expressed in males, but never passed from a father to his sons. Homozygous females, on the other hand, pass the trait to all sons, but not to their daughters unless the father is also affected.*

4.12 In Sex-Limited and Sex-Influenced Inheritance, an Individual's Sex Influences the Phenotype

In contrast to X-linked inheritance, patterns of gene expression may be affected by the sex of an individual even when the genes are not on the X chromosome. In numerous examples in different organisms, the sex of the individual plays a determining role in the expression of a phenotype. In some cases, the expression of a specific phenotype is absolutely limited to one sex; in others, the sex of an individual influences the expression of a phenotype that is not limited to one sex or the other. This distinction differentiates **sex-limited inheritance** from **sex-influenced inheritance**.

In both types of inheritance, autosomal genes are responsible for the existence of contrasting phenotypes, but the expression of these genes is dependent on the hormone constitution of the individual. Thus, the heterozygous genotype may exhibit one phenotype in males and the contrasting one in females. In domestic fowl, for example, tail and neck plumage is often distinctly different in males and females (**Figure 4–15**), demonstrating *sex-limited inheritance*. Cock feathering is longer, more curved, and pointed, whereas hen feathering is shorter and less curved. Inheritance of these feather phenotypes is controlled by a single

female offspring (III-4, 6, and 7), as well as color-blind (III-8) and normal-visioned (III-5) male offspring.

The way in which X-linked genes are transmitted causes unusual circumstances associated with recessive X-linked disorders, in comparison to recessive autosomal disorders. For example, if an X-linked disorder debilitates or is lethal to the affected individual prior to reproductive maturation, the disorder occurs exclusively in males. This is so because the only sources of the lethal allele in the population are in heterozygous females who are "carriers" and do not express the disorder. They pass the allele to one-half of their sons, who develop the disorder because they are hemizygous but rarely, if ever, reproduce. Heterozygous females also pass the allele to one-half of their daughters, who become carriers but do not develop the disorder. An example of such an X-linked disorder is *Duchenne muscular dystrophy*. The disease has an onset prior to age 6 and is often lethal around age 20. It normally occurs only in males.

FIGURE 4–15 Hen feathering (left) and cock feathering (right) in domestic fowl. The hen's feathers are shorter and less curved.

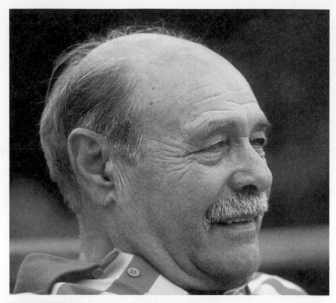

FIGURE 4–16 Pattern baldness, a sex-influenced autosomal trait in humans.

pair of autosomal alleles whose expression is modified by the individual's sex hormones. As shown in the following chart, hen feathering is due to a dominant allele, *H*, but regardless of the homozygous presence of the recessive *h* allele, all females remain hen-feathered. Only in males does the *hh* genotype result in cock feathering.

Genotype	Phenotype	
	♀	♂
HH	Hen-feathered	Hen-feathered
Hh	Hen-feathered	Hen-feathered
hh	Hen-feathered	Cock-feathered

In certain breeds of fowl, the hen feathering or cock feathering allele has become fixed in the population. In the Leghorn breed, all individuals are of the *hh* genotype; as a result, males always differ from females in their plumage. Seabright bantams are all *HH*, showing no sexual distinction in feathering phenotypes.

Another example of sex-limited inheritance involves the autosomal genes responsible for milk yield in dairy cattle. Regardless of the overall genotype that influences the quantity of milk production, those genes are obviously expressed only in females.

Cases of *sex-influenced inheritance* include pattern baldness in humans, horn formation in certain breeds of sheep (e.g., Dorsett Horn sheep), and certain coat patterns in cattle. In such cases, autosomal genes are responsible for the contrasting phenotypes, and while the trait may be displayed by both males and females, the expression of these genes is dependent on the hormone constitution of the individual. Thus, the heterozygous genotype exhibits one phenotype in one sex and the contrasting one in the other. For example, pattern baldness in humans, where the hair is very thin or absent on the top of the head (**Figure 4–16**), is inherited in the following way:

Genotype	Phenotype	
	♀	♂
BB	Bald	Bald
Bb	Not bald	Bald
bb	Not bald	Not bald

Females can display pattern baldness, but this phenotype is much more prevalent in males. When females do inherit the *BB* genotype, the phenotype is less pronounced than in males and is expressed later in life.

4.13 Genetic Background and the Environment May Alter Phenotypic Expression

In the final section of this chapter we consider *phenotypic expression*. We assumed that the genotype of an organism is always directly expressed in its phenotype (Chapters 2 and 3). For example, pea plants homozygous for the recessive *d* allele (*dd*) will always be dwarf. We discussed gene expression as though the genes operate in a closed system in which the presence or absence of functional products directly determines the collective phenotype of an individual. The situation is actually much more complex. Most gene products function within the internal milieu of the cell, and cells interact with one another in various ways. Furthermore, the organism exists under diverse environmental influences. Thus, gene expression and the resultant phenotype are often modified through the interaction between an individual's particular genotype and the external environment. In this final section of this chapter, we will deal with some of the variables that are known to modify gene expression.

Penetrance and Expressivity

Some mutant genotypes are always expressed as a distinct phenotype, whereas others produce a proportion of individuals whose phenotypes cannot be distinguished from normal (wild type). The degree of expression of a particular trait can be studied quantitatively by determining the *penetrance* and *expressivity* of the genotype under investigation.

The percentage of individuals that show at least some degree of expression of a mutant genotype defines the **penetrance** of the mutation. For example, the phenotypic expression of many of the mutant alleles found in *Drosophila* can overlap with wild-type expression. If 15 percent of flies with a given mutant genotype show the wild-type appearance, the mutant gene is said to have a penetrance of 85 percent.

By contrast, **expressivity** reflects the *range of expression* of the mutant genotype. Flies homozygous for the recessive mutant gene *eyeless* exhibit phenotypes that range from the presence of normal eyes to a partial reduction in size to the complete absence of one or both eyes (**Figure 4–17**). Although the average reduction of eye size is one-fourth to one-half, expressivity ranges from complete loss of both eyes to completely normal eyes.

FIGURE 4–17   Variable expressivity as shown in flies homozygous for the *eyeless* mutation in *Drosophila*. Gradations in phenotype range from wild type to partial reduction to eyeless.

Examples such as the expression of the *eyeless* gene have provided the basis for experiments to determine the causes of phenotypic variation. If the laboratory environment is held constant and extensive variation is still observed, other genes may be influencing or modifying the phenotype. On the other hand, if the genetic background is not the cause of the phenotypic variation, environmental factors such as temperature, humidity, and nutrition may be involved. In the case of the *eyeless* phenotype, experiments have shown that both genetic background and environmental factors influence its expression.

Genetic Background: Position Effects

Although it is difficult to assess the specific effect of the **genetic background** and the expression of a gene responsible for determining a potential phenotype, one effect of genetic background has been well characterized, called the **position effect**. In such instances, the physical location of a gene in relation to other genetic material may influence its expression. For example, if a region of a chromosome is relocated or rearranged (called a translocation or inversion event), normal expression of genes in that chromosomal region may be modified. This is particularly true if the gene is relocated to or near certain areas of the chromosome that are condensed and genetically inert, referred to as **heterochromatin**.

An example of a position effect involves female *Drosophila* heterozygous for the X-linked recessive eye color mutant *white* (*w*). The w^+/w genotype normally results in a wild-type brick-red eye color. However, if the region of the X chromosome containing the wild-type w^+ allele is translocated so that it is close to a heterochromatic region, expression of the w^+ allele is modified. Instead of having a red color, the eyes are variegated, or mottled with red and white patches (**Figure 4–18**). Therefore, following translocation, the dominant effect of the normal w^+ allele is intermittent. A similar position effect is produced if a heterochromatic region is relocated next to the *white* locus on the X chromosome. Apparently, heterochromatic regions inhibit the expression of adjacent genes. Loci in many other organisms also exhibit position effects, providing proof that alteration of the normal arrangement of genetic information can modify its expression.

Temperature Effects—An Introduction to Conditional Mutations

Chemical activity depends on the kinetic energy of the reacting substances, which in turn depends on the surrounding temperature. We can thus expect temperature to influence phenotypes. An example is seen in the evening primrose, which produces red flowers when grown at 23°C and white flowers when grown at 18°C. An even more striking example is seen in Siamese cats and Himalayan rabbits,

(a)

(b)

FIGURE 4–18 Position effect, as illustrated in the eye phenotype in two female *Drosophila* heterozygous for the gene *white*. (a) Normal dominant phenotype showing brick-red eye color. (b) Variegated color of an eye caused by translocation of the *white* gene to another location in the genome.

which exhibit dark fur in certain regions where their body temperature is slightly cooler, particularly the nose, ears, and paws (**Figure 4–19**). In these cases, it appears that the enzyme normally responsible for pigment production is functional only at the lower temperatures present in the extremities, but it loses its catalytic function at the slightly higher temperatures found throughout the rest of the body.

Mutations whose expression is affected by temperature, called **temperature-sensitive mutations**, are examples of **conditional mutations**, whereby phenotypic expression is determined by environmental conditions. Examples of temperature-sensitive mutations are known in viruses and a variety of organisms, including bacteria, fungi, and *Drosophila*. In extreme cases, an organism carrying a mutant allele may express a mutant phenotype when grown at one temperature but express the wild-type phenotype when reared at another temperature. This type of temperature effect is useful in studying mutations that interrupt essential processes during development and are thus normally detrimental or lethal. For example, if bacterial viruses are cultured under *permissive conditions* of 25°C, the mutant gene product is functional, infection proceeds normally, and new viruses are produced and can be studied. However, if bacterial viruses carrying temperature-sensitive mutations infect bacteria cultured at 42°C—the *restrictive condition*—infection progresses up to the point where the essential gene product is required (e.g., for viral assembly) and then arrests. Temperature-sensitive mutations are easily induced and isolated in viruses, and have added immensely to the study of viral genetics.

Nutritional Effects

Another category of phenotypes that are not always a direct reflection of the organism's genotype consists of **nutritional mutations**. In microorganisms, mutations that prevent synthesis of nutrient molecules are quite common, such as when an enzyme essential to a biosynthetic pathway becomes inactive. A microorganism bearing such a mutation is called an **auxotroph**. If the end product of a biochemical pathway can no longer be synthesized, and if that molecule is essential to normal growth and development, the mutation prevents growth and may be lethal. For example, if the bread mold *Neurospora* can no longer synthesize the amino acid leucine, proteins cannot be synthesized. If leucine is present in the growth medium, the detrimental effect is overcome. Nutritional mutants have been crucial to genetic studies in bacteria and also served as the basis for George Beadle and Edward Tatum's proposal, in the early 1940s, that one gene functions to produce one enzyme. (See Chapter 14.)

A slightly different set of circumstances exists in humans. The ingestion of certain dietary substances that normal individuals may consume without harm can adversely affect individuals with abnormal genetic constitutions. Often, a mutation may prevent an individual from metabolizing some substance commonly found in normal diets. For example, those afflicted with the genetic disorder **phenylketonuria** cannot metabolize the amino acid phenylalanine. Those with **galactosemia** cannot metabolize galactose.

(a)

(b)

FIGURE 4–19 (a) A Himalayan rabbit. (b) A Siamese cat. Both show dark fur color on the snout, ears, and paws. These patches are due to the effect of a temperature-sensitive allele responsible for pigment production.

Those with **lactose intolerance** cannot metabolize lactose. However, if the dietary intake of the involved molecule is drastically reduced or eliminated, the associated phenotype may be ameliorated.

Onset of Genetic Expression

Not all genetic traits become apparent at the same time during an organism's life span. In most cases, the age at which a mutant gene exerts a noticeable phenotype depends on events during the normal sequence of growth and development. In humans, the prenatal, infant, preadult, and adult phases require different genetic information. As a result, many severe inherited disorders are not manifested until after birth. **Tay–Sachs disease**, inherited as an autosomal recessive, is a lethal lipid-metabolism disease involving an abnormal enzyme, hexosaminidase A. Newborns appear to be phenotypically normal for the first few months. Then, developmental retardation, paralysis, and blindness ensue, and most affected children die around the age of 3.

The **Lesch–Nyhan syndrome**, inherited as an X-linked recessive disease, is characterized by abnormal nucleic acid metabolism (inability to salvage nitrogenous purine bases), leading to the accumulation of uric acid in blood and tissues, mental retardation, palsy, and self-mutilation of the lips and fingers. The disorder is due to a mutation in the gene encoding hypoxanthine-guanine phosphoribosyl transferase (HPRT). Newborns are normal for six to eight months prior to the onset of the first symptoms.

Still another example is **Duchenne muscular dystrophy (DMD)**, an X-linked recessive disorder associated with progressive muscular wasting. It is not usually diagnosed until a child is 3 to 5 years old. Even with modern medical intervention, the disease is often fatal in the early 20s.

Perhaps the most delayed and highly variable age of onset for a genetic disorder in humans is seen in **Huntington disease**. Inherited as an autosomal dominant disorder, Huntington disease affects the frontal lobes of the cerebral cortex, where progressive cell death occurs over a period of more than a decade. Brain deterioration is accompanied by spastic uncontrolled movements, intellectual deterioration, and ultimately death. While onset of these symptoms has been reported at all ages, they are most often initially observed between ages 30 and 50, with a mean onset age of 38 years.

These examples support the concept that gene products may play more essential roles at certain times during the life cycle of an organism. One may be able to tolerate the impact of a mutant gene for a considerable period of time without noticeable effect. At some point, however, a mutant phenotype is manifested. Perhaps this is the result of the internal physiological environment of an organism changing during development and with age.

Genetic Anticipation

Interest in studying the genetic onset of phenotypic expression has intensified with the discovery of heritable disorders that *exhibit a progressively earlier age of onset and an increased severity of the disorder in each successive generation.* This phenomenon is referred to as **genetic anticipation**.

Myotonic dystrophy (DM1), the most common type of adult muscular dystrophy, clearly illustrates genetic anticipation. Individuals afflicted with this autosomal dominant disorder exhibit extreme variation in the severity of symptoms. Mildly affected individuals develop cataracts as adults, but have little or no muscular weakness. Severely affected individuals demonstrate more extensive weakness, as well as myotonia (muscle hyperexcitability) and in some cases mental retardation. In its most extreme form, the disease is fatal just after birth. A great deal of excitement was generated in 1989, when C. J. Howeler and colleagues confirmed the correlation of increased severity and earlier onset with successive generations of inheritance. The researchers studied 61 parent–child pairs, and in 60 of the cases, age of onset was earlier and more severe in the child than in his or her affected parent.

In 1992, an explanation was put forward to explain both the molecular cause of the mutation responsible for DM1 and the basis of genetic anticipation in the disorder. As we will see later in the text, a three nucleotide sequence of DNA within the *DMPK* gene is repeated a variable number of times and is unstable (see Chapter 17). Normal individuals have about 5 to 35 copies of this sequence; affected individuals have between 150 and 2000 copies. Those with a greater number of repeats are more severely affected. The most remarkable observation was that, in successive generations of DM1 individuals, the size of the repeated segment increases. We now know that the RNA transcribed from mutant genes is the culprit in the disorder and alters the expression of still other genes. Several other inherited human disorders, including a second form of myotonic dystrophy (DM2), fragile-X syndrome, Kennedy disease, and Huntington disease, also reveal an association between the number of copies of a repeated DNA sequence and disease severity.

Genomic (Parental) Imprinting and Gene Silencing

A final example involving genetic background involves what is called **genomic**, or **parental, imprinting**, whereby the process of selective *gene silencing* occurs during early development, impacting on subsequent phenotypic expression. Examples involve cases where genes or regions of a chromosome are imprinted on one homolog but not the other. The impact of silencing depends on the parental origin of the genes or regions that are involved. Such silencing leads to the direct phenotypic expression of the allele(s) on the homolog that is not silenced. Thus, the imprinting step, the critical issue in understanding this phenomenon, is thought to occur before or during gamete formation, leading to differentially marked genes (or chromosome regions) in sperm-forming versus egg-forming tissues.

The first example of genomic imprinting was discovered in 1991, in three specific mouse genes. One is the gene encoding insulin-like growth factor II (*Igf2*). A mouse that carries two normal alleles of this gene is normal in size, whereas a mouse that carries two mutant alleles lacks the growth factor and is dwarf. The size of a heterozygous mouse—one allele normal and one mutant—depends on the parental origin of the wild-type allele. The mouse is normal in size if the normal allele comes from the father, but it is dwarf if the normal allele came from the mother. From this, we can deduce that the normal *Igf2* gene is imprinted and thus silenced during egg production, but it functions normally when it has passed through sperm-producing tissue in males. The imprint is inherited in the sense that the *Igf2* gene in all progeny cells formed during development remain silenced. Imprinting in the next generation then depends on whether the gene passes through sperm-producing or egg-forming tissue.

An example in humans involves two distinct genetic disorders thought to be caused by differential imprinting of the same region of the long arm of chromosome 15 (15q1). In both cases, the disorders are due to an identical deletion of this region in one member of the chromosome 15 pair. The first disorder, **Prader–Willi syndrome (PWS)**, results when the paternal segment is deleted and an undeleted maternal chromosome remains. If the maternal segment is deleted and an undeleted paternal chromosome remains, an entirely different disorder, **Angelman syndrome (AS)**, results.

These two conditions exhibit different phenotypes. PWS entails mental retardation, a severe eating disorder marked by an uncontrollable appetite, obesity, diabetes,

and growth retardation. Angelman syndrome also involves mental retardation, but involuntary muscle contractions (chorea) and seizures characterize the disorder. We can conclude that the involved region of chromosome 15 is imprinted differently in male and female gametes and that both an undeleted maternal and a paternal region are required for normal development.

Although numerous questions remain unanswered regarding genomic imprinting, it is now clear that many genes are subject to this process. More than 50 have been identified in mammals thus far. It appears that regions of chromosomes rather than specific genes are imprinted. This phenomenon is an example of the more general topic of **epigenetics**, where genetic expression is *not* the direct result of the information stored in the nucleotide sequence of DNA. Instead, the DNA is altered in a way that affects its expression. These changes are stable in the sense that they are transmitted during cell division to progeny cells, and often through gametes to future generations.

The precise molecular mechanism of imprinting and other epigenetic events is still a matter for conjecture, but it seems certain that **DNA methylation** is involved. In most eukaryotes, methyl groups can be added to the carbon atom at position 5 in cytosine (see Chapter 10) as a result of the activity of the enzyme DNA methyltransferase. Methyl groups are added when the dinucleotide CpG or groups of CpG units (called CpG islands) are present along a DNA chain.

DNA methylation is a reasonable mechanism for establishing a molecular imprint, since there is evidence that a high level of methylation can inhibit gene activity and that active genes (or their regulatory sequences) are often undermethylated. This phenomenon is a fascinating topic. We will discuss the most recent findings involving the above topics later in the text (see Special Topic Chapter 1—Epigenetics).

GENETICS, TECHNOLOGY, AND SOCIETY

Improving the Genetic Fate of Purebred Dogs

For dog lovers, nothing is quite so heartbreaking as watching a dog slowly go blind, struggling to adapt to a life of perpetual darkness. That's what happens in progressive retinal atrophy (PRA), a group of inherited disorders first described in Gordon setters in 1909. Since then, PRA has been

detected in more than 100 other breeds of dogs, including Irish setters, border collies, Norwegian elkhounds, toy poodles, miniature schnauzers, cocker spaniels, and Siberian huskies.

The products of many genes are required for the development and maintenance of healthy retinas, and a defect

in any one of these genes may cause retinal dysfunction. Decades of research have led to the identification of five such genes (*PDE6A*, *PDE6B*, *PRCD*, *rhodopsin*, and *PRGR*), and more may be discovered. Different mutant alleles are present in different breeds, and each allele is associated with a different form of PRA

(continued)

that varies slightly in its clinical symptoms and rate of progression. Mutations of *PDE6A, PDE6B,* and *PRCD* genes are inherited in a recessive pattern, mutations of the *rhodopsin* gene (such as those found in Mastiffs) are dominant, and *PRGR* mutations (in Siberian huskies and Samoyeds) are X-linked.

PRA is almost ten times more common in certain purebred dogs than in mixed breeds. The development of distinct breeds of dogs has involved intensive selection for desirable attributes, such as a particular size, shape, color, or behavior. Many desired characteristics are determined by recessive alleles. The fastest way to increase the homozygosity of these alleles is to mate close relatives, which are likely to carry the same alleles. For example, dogs may be mated to a cousin or a grandparent. Some breeders, in an attempt to profit from impressive pedigrees, also produce hundreds of offspring from individual dogs that have won major prizes at dog shows. This "popular sire effect," as it has been termed, further increases the homozygosity of alleles in purebred dogs.

Unfortunately, the generations of inbreeding that have established favorable characteristics in purebreeds have also increased the homozygosity of certain harmful recessive alleles, resulting in a high incidence of inherited diseases. More than 300 genetic diseases have been characterized in purebred dogs, and many breeds have a predisposition to more than 20 of them. According to researchers at Cornell University, purebred dogs suffer the highest incidence of inherited disease of any animal: 25 percent of the 20 million purebred dogs in America are affected with one genetic ailment or another.

Fortunately, advances in canine genetics are beginning to provide new tools to increase the health of purebred dogs. As of 2007, genetic tests are available to detect 30 different retinal diseases in dogs. Tests for PRA are now being used to identify heterozygous carriers of *PRCD* mutations. These carriers show no symptoms of PRA but, if mated with other carriers, pass the trait on to about 25 percent of their offspring. Eliminating PRA carriers from breeding programs has almost eradicated this condition from Portuguese water dogs and has greatly reduced its prevalence in other breeds.

Scientists will be able to identify more genes underlying canine inherited diseases thanks to the completion of the Dog Genome Project in 2005. In addition, new therapies that correct gene-based defects will emerge.

The Dog Genome Project may have benefits for humans beyond the reduction of disease in their canine companions. Eighty-five percent of the genes in the dog genome have equivalents in humans, and over 300 diseases affecting dogs also affect humans, including heart disease, epilepsy, allergies, and some cancers. The identification of a disease-causing gene in dogs can be a shortcut to the isolation of the corresponding gene in humans. By contributing to the cure of human diseases, dogs may prove to be "man's best friend" in an entirely new way.

Your Turn

Take time, individually or in groups, to answer the following questions. Investigate the references and links, to help you understand some of the issues surrounding the genetics of purebred dogs.

1. What are some of the limitations of genetic tests, especially as they apply to purebred dog genetic diseases?
This topic is discussed on the OptiGen website (http://www.optigen.com). OptiGen is a company that offers gene tests for all known forms of PRA in dogs and is developing tests for other inherited disorders. From their TESTS list, select prcd-PRA, and visit the link "Benefits and Limits to All Genetic Testing."

2. Which human disease is similar to PRA in the Siberian husky?
To learn more about these genes and diseases, visit the "Inherited Diseases in Dogs" database (http://www.vet.cam.ac.uk/idid/) and search the database for Progressive Retinal Atrophy in the Siberian husky. Once there, follow the OMIM reference link to learn about the human version of PRA in the Siberian husky.

3. Chinese Shar-Pei dogs have been selected for their unique wrinkled skin. Unfortunately, these purebred dogs are also predisposed to hereditary fevers. Recently, a gene called *HAS2* was identified in these dogs. It encodes the enzyme hyaluronic acid synthase 2, and a mutation associated with the gene is responsible for both skin appearance and fever. Describe how the *HAS2* gene can have these pleiotropic effects and why this finding is important to human health.

Read about the HAS2 gene discovery in Olsson, M. et al. 2011. A novel unstable duplication upstream of HAS2 predisposes to a breed-defining skin phenotype and a periodic fever syndrome in Chinese Shar-Pei dogs. PLoS Genetics 7(3):e1001332.

CASE STUDY | But he isn't deaf

Researching their family histories, a deaf couple learns that each of them has relatives through several generations who are deaf. With a rudimentary understanding of genetics, they also learn that one of many forms of deafness can be inherited as an autosomal recessive trait. They plan to have children, and based on the above information, they are concerned that some or all of their children may be deaf. To their delight, their first child has normal hearing. The couple turns to you as a geneticist to help explain this situation.

1. Is it likely that these parents inherited their deafness as an autosomal recessive trait?

2. What is the likelihood that each future child will be deaf?

3. What conclusions could be drawn if their first child had been deaf?

Summary Points

MasteringGenetics™ For activities, animations, and review quizzes, go to the Study Area.

1. Since Mendel's work was rediscovered, transmission genetics has been expanded to include many alternative modes of inheritance, including the study of incomplete dominance, codominance, multiple alleles, and lethal alleles.

2. Mendel's classic F_2 ratio is often modified in instances when gene interaction controls phenotypic variation. Many such instances involve epistasis, whereby the expression of one gene influences or inhibits the expression of another gene.

3. Complementation analysis determines whether independently isolated mutations that produce similar phenotypes are alleles of one another, or whether they represent separate genes.

4. Pleiotropy refers to multiple phenotypic effects caused by a single mutation.

5. Genes located on the X chromosome result in a characteristic mode of genetic transmission referred to as X-linkage, displaying so-called criss-cross inheritance, whereby affected mothers pass X-linked traits to all of their sons.

6. Sex-limited and sex-influenced inheritance occurs when the sex of the organism affects the phenotype controlled by a gene located on an autosome.

7. Phenotypic expression is not always the direct reflection of the genotype. Variable expressivity may be observed, or a percentage of organisms may not express the expected phenotype at all, the basis of the penetrance of a mutant allele. In addition, the phenotype can be modified by genetic background, temperature, and nutrition. Finally, the onset of expression of a gene may vary during the lifetime of an organism, and even depend on whether the mutant allele is transmitted by the male or female parent, the basis of genomic imprinting.

INSIGHTS AND SOLUTIONS

Genetic problems take on added complexity if they involve two independent characters and multiple alleles, incomplete dominance, or epistasis. The most difficult types of problems are those that pioneering geneticists faced during laboratory or field studies. They had to determine the mode of inheritance by working backward from the observations of offspring to parents of unknown genotype.

1. Consider the problem of comb-shape inheritance in chickens, where walnut, rose, pea, and single are observed as distinct phenotypes. These variations are shown in the accompanying photographs. Considering the following data, determine how comb shape is inherited and what genotypes are present in the P1 generation of each cross.

Cross 1:	single × single	⟶	all single
Cross 2:	walnut × walnut	⟶	all walnut
Cross 3:	rose × pea	⟶	all walnut
Cross 4:	F_1 × F_1 of Cross 3		
	walnut × walnut	⟶	93 walnut
			28 rose
			32 pea
			10 single

Solution: At first glance, this problem appears quite difficult. However, working systematically and breaking the analysis into steps simplify it. To start, look at the data carefully for any useful information. Once you identify something that is clearly helpful, follow an empirical approach; that is, formulate a hypothesis and test it against the given data. Look for a pattern of inheritance that is consistent with all cases.

This problem gives two immediately useful facts. First, in cross 1, P_1 singles breed true. Second, while P_1 walnut breeds true in cross 2, a walnut phenotype is also produced in cross 3 between rose and pea. When these F_1 walnuts are mated in cross 4, all four comb shapes are produced in a ratio that approximates 9:3:3:1. This observation immediately suggests a cross involving two gene pairs, because the resulting data display the same ratio as in Mendel's dihybrid crosses. Since only one character is involved (comb shape), epistasis may be occurring. This could serve as your working hypothesis, and you must now propose how the two gene pairs "interact" to produce each phenotype.

If you call the allele pairs *A*, *a* and *B*, *b*, you might predict that because walnut represents 9/16 of the offspring in cross 4, *A–B–* will produce walnut. (Recall that *A–* and *B–* mean *AA* or *Aa* and *BB* or *Bb*, respectively.) You might also hypothesize that in cross 2, the genotypes are *AABB* × *AABB* where walnut bred true.

The phenotype representing 1/16 of the offspring of cross 4 is single; therefore you could predict that the single phenotype is the result of the *aabb* genotype. This is consistent with cross 1.

Now you have only to determine the genotypes for rose and pea. The most logical prediction is that at least one dominant *A* or *B* allele combined with the double recessive condition of the other allele pair accounts for these phenotypes. For example,

$$A\text{–}bb \longrightarrow \text{rose}$$
$$aaB\text{–} \longrightarrow \text{pea}$$

If *AAbb* (rose) is crossed with *aaBB* (pea) in cross 3, all offspring would be *AaBb* (walnut). This is consistent with the data, and you need now look at only cross 4. We predict these walnut genotypes to be *AaBb* (as above), and from the cross

$$AaBb \text{ (walnut)} \times AaBb \text{ (walnut)}$$

(continued)

Insights and Solutions—continued

we expect

9/16	A–B–	(walnut)
3/16	A–bb	(rose)
3/16	aaB–	(pea)
1/16	aabb	(single)

Our prediction is consistent with the data given. The initial hypothesis of the interaction of two gene pairs proves consistent throughout, and the problem is solved.

This problem demonstrates the usefulness of a basic theoretical knowledge of transmission genetics. With such knowledge, you can search for clues that will enable you to proceed in a stepwise fashion toward a solution. Mastering problem-solving requires practice, but can give you a great deal of satisfaction. Apply the same general approach to the following problems.

Walnut

Pea

Rose

Single

2. In radishes, flower color may be red, purple, or white. The edible portion of the radish may be long or oval. When only flower color is studied, no dominance is evident, and red × white crosses yield all purple. If these F_1 purples are interbred, the F_2 generation consists of 1/4 red: 1/2 purple: 1/4 white. Regarding radish shape, long is dominant to oval in a normal Mendelian fashion.

(a) Determine the F_1 and F_2 phenotypes from a cross between a true-breeding red, long radish and a radish that is white and oval. Be sure to define all gene symbols at the start.

(b) A red oval plant was crossed with a plant of unknown genotype and phenotype, yielding the following offspring:

103 red long: 101 red oval
98 purple long: 100 purple oval

Determine the genotype and phenotype of the unknown plant.

Solution: First, establish gene symbols:

RR = red	$O–$ = long
Rr = purple	oo = oval
rr = white	

(a) This is a modified dihybrid cross where the gene pair controlling color exhibits incomplete dominance. Shape is controlled conventionally.

P_1: RROO   ×   rroo
       (red long)   (white oval)
F_1: all RrOo (purple long)
$F_1 \times F_1$: $RrOo \times RrOo$

F_2:
1/4 RR → 3/4 O–	3/16 RRO–	red long
1/4 RR → 1/4 oo	1/16 RRoo	red oval
2/4 Rr → 3/4 O–	6/16 RrO–	purple long
2/4 Rr → 1/4 oo	2/16 Rroo	purple oval
1/4 rr → 3/4 O–	3/16 rrO–	white long
1/4 rr → 1/4 oo	1/16 rroo	white oval

Note that to generate the F_2 results, we have used the forked-line method. First, we consider the outcome of crossing F_1 parents for the color genes ($Rr \times Rr$). Then the outcome of shape is considered ($Oo \times Oo$).

(b) The two characters appear to be inherited independently, so consider them separately. The data indicate a 1/4:1/4:1/ 4:1/4 proportion. First, consider color:

P_1:   red × ???   (unknown)
F_1:   204 red   (1/2)
        198 purple   (1/2)

Because the red parent must be RR, the unknown must have a genotype of Rr to produce these results. Thus it is purple. Now, consider shape:

P_1:   oval × ???   (unknown)
F_1:   201 long   (1/2)
        201 oval   (1/2)

Since the oval plant must be oo, the unknown plant must have a genotype of Oo to produce these results. Thus it is long. The unknown plant is

RrOo purple long

3. In humans, red–green color blindness is inherited as an X-linked recessive trait. A woman with normal vision whose father is color-blind marries a male who has normal vision. Predict the color vision of their male and female offspring.

Solution: The female is heterozygous, since she inherited an X chromosome with the mutant allele from her father. Her husband is normal. Therefore, the parental genotypes are

$Cc \times C\Upsilon$ (Υ represents the Y chromosome)

All female offspring are normal (CC or Cc). One-half of the male children will be color-blind ($c\Upsilon$), and the other half will have normal vision ($C\Upsilon$).

(continued)

Insights and Solutions—continued

4. Consider the two very limited unrelated pedigrees shown here. Of the four combinations of X-linked recessive, X-linked dominant, autosomal recessive, and autosomal

(a)

(b)

dominant, which modes of inheritance can be absolutely ruled out in each case?

Solution: For both pedigrees, X-linked recessive and autosomal recessive remain possible, provided that the maternal parent is heterozygous in pedigree (b). Autosomal dominance seems at first glance unlikely in pedigree (a), since at least half of the offspring should express a dominant trait expressed by one of their parents. However, while it is true that if the affected parent carries an autosomal dominant gene heterozygously, each offspring has a 50 percent chance of inheriting and expressing the mutant gene, the sample size of four offspring is too small to rule this possibility out. In pedigree (b), autosomal dominance is clearly possible. In both cases, one can rule out X-linked dominance because the female offspring would inherit and express the dominant allele, and they do not express the trait in either pedigree.

Problems and Discussion Questions

MasteringGenetics™ Visit for instructor-assigned tutorials and problems.

HOW DO WE KNOW?

1. In this chapter, we focused on extensions and modifications of Mendelian principles and ratios. In the process, we encountered many opportunities to consider how this information was acquired. On the basis of these discussions, what answers would you propose to the following fundamental questions?
   (a) How were early geneticists able to ascertain inheritance patterns that did not fit typical Mendelian ratios?
   (b) How did geneticists determine that inheritance of some phenotypic characteristics involves the interactions of two or more gene pairs? How were they able to determine how many gene pairs were involved?
   (c) How do we know that specific genes are located on the sex-determining chromosomes rather than on autosomes?
   (d) For genes whose expression seems to be tied to the sex of individuals, how do we know whether a gene is X-linked in contrast to exhibiting sex-limited or sex-influenced inheritance?

CONCEPT QUESTION

2. Review the Chapter Concepts list on page 70. These all relate to exceptions to the inheritance patterns encountered by Mendel. Write a short essay that explains why multiple and lethal alleles often result in a modification of the classic Mendelian monohybrid and dihybrid ratios.

3. In shorthorn cattle, coat color may be red, white, or roan. Roan is an intermediate phenotype expressed as a mixture of red and white hairs. The following data were obtained from various crosses:

red	×	red	⟶ all red
white	×	white	⟶ all white
red	×	white	⟶ all roan
roan	×	roan	⟶ 1/4 red:1/2 roan: 1/4 white

How is coat color inherited? What are the genotypes of parents and offspring for each cross?

4. In foxes, two alleles of a single gene, *P* and *p*, may result in lethality (*PP*), platinum coat (*Pp*), or silver coat (*pp*). What ratio is obtained when platinum foxes are interbred? Is the *P* allele behaving dominantly or recessively in causing (a) lethality; (b) platinum coat color?

5. In mice, a short-tailed mutant was discovered. When it was crossed to a normal long-tailed mouse, 4 offspring were short-tailed and 3 were long-tailed. Two short-tailed mice from the F₁ generation were selected and crossed. They produced 6 short-tailed and 3 long-tailed mice. These genetic experiments were repeated three times with approximately the same results. What genetic ratios are illustrated? Hypothesize the mode of inheritance and diagram the crosses.

6. List all possible genotypes for the A, B, AB, and O phenotypes. Is the mode of inheritance of the ABO blood types representative of dominance? of recessiveness? of codominance?

7. With regard to the ABO blood types in humans, determine the genotype of the male parent and female parent shown here:

   Male parent: Blood type B; mother type O
   Female parent: Blood type A; father type B

   Predict the blood types of the offspring that this couple may have and the expected proportion of each.

8. In a disputed parentage case, the child is blood type O, while the mother is blood type A. What blood type would exclude a male from being the father? Would the other blood types prove that a particular male was the father?

9. The A and B antigens in humans may be found in water-soluble form in secretions, including saliva, of some individuals (*Se/Se* and *Se/se*) but not in others (*se/se*). The population thus contains "secretors" and "nonsecretors."

(a) Determine the proportion of various phenotypes (blood type and ability to secrete) in matings between individuals that are blood type AB and type O, both of whom are *Se/se*.

(b) How will the results of such matings change if both parents are heterozygous for the gene controlling the synthesis of the H substance (*Hh*)?

10. In chickens, a condition referred to as "creeper" exists whereby the bird has very short legs and wings, and appears to be creeping when it walks. If creepers are bred to normal chickens, one-half of the offspring are normal and one-half are creepers. Creepers never breed true. If bred together, they yield two-thirds creepers and one-third normal. Propose an explanation for the inheritance of this condition.

11. In rabbits, a series of multiple alleles controls coat color in the following way: *C* is dominant to all other alleles and causes full color. The chinchilla phenotype is due to the *c^{ch}* allele, which is dominant to all alleles other than *C*. The *c^h* allele, dominant only to *c^a* (albino), results in the Himalayan coat color. Thus, the order of dominance is $C > c^{ch} > c^h > c^a$. For each of the following three cases, the phenotypes of the P$_1$ generations of two crosses are shown, as well as the phenotype of *one member* of the F$_1$ generation.

	P$_1$ Phenotypes		F$_1$ Phenotypes
(a)	Himalayan × Himalayan	⟶	albino
	×	⟶ ??	
	full color × albino	⟶	chinchilla
(b)	albino × chinchilla	⟶	albino
	×	⟶ ??	
	full color × albino	⟶	full color
(c)	chinchilla × albino	⟶	Himalayan
	×	⟶ ??	
	full color × albino	⟶	Himalayan

For each case, determine the genotypes of the P$_1$ generation and the F$_1$ offspring, and predict the results of making each indicated cross between F$_1$ individuals.

12. Three gene pairs located on separate autosomes determine flower color and shape as well as plant height. The first pair exhibits incomplete dominance, where the color can be red, pink (the heterozygote), or white. The second pair leads to personate (dominant) or peloric (recessive) flower shape, while the third gene pair produces either the dominant tall trait or the recessive dwarf trait. Homozygous plants that are red, personate, and tall are crossed to those that are white, peloric, and dwarf. Determine the F$_1$ genotype(s) and phenotype(s). If the F$_1$ plants are interbred, what proportion of the offspring will exhibit the same phenotype as the F$_1$ plants?

personate   peloric

13. As in Problem 12, flower color may be red, white, or pink, and flower shape may be personate or peloric. For the following crosses, determine the P$_1$ and F$_1$ genotypes:

(a) red, peloric × white, personate
↓
F$_1$: all pink, personate

(b) red, personate × white, peloric
↓
F$_1$: all pink, personate

(c) pink, personate × red, peloric → F$_1$
{ 1/4 red, personate
1/4 red, peloric
1/4 pink, peloric
1/4 pink, personate

(d) pink, personate × white, peloric → F$_1$
{ 1/4 white, personate
1/4 white, peloric
1/4 pink, personate
1/4 pink, peloric

(e) What phenotypic ratios would result from crossing the F$_1$ of (a) to the F$_1$ of (b)?

14. Horses can be cremello (a light cream color), chestnut (a brownish color), or palomino (a golden color with white in the horse's tail and mane). Of these phenotypes, only palominos never breed true.

cremello × palomino	⟶	1/2 cremello 1/2 palomino
chestnut × palomino	⟶	1/2 chestnut 1/2 palomino
palomino × palomino	⟶	1/4 chestnut 1/2 palomino 1/4 cremello

(a) From the results given above, determine the mode of inheritance by assigning gene symbols and indicating which genotypes yield which phenotypes.

(b) Predict the F$_1$ and F$_2$ results of many initial matings between cremello and chestnut horses.

Chestnut   Palomino

Cremello

15. With reference to the eye color phenotypes produced by the recessive, autosomal, unlinked *brown* and *scarlet* loci in *Drosophila* (see Figure 4–10), predict the F_1 and F_2 results of the following P_1 crosses. (Recall that when both the *brown* and *scarlet* alleles are homozygous, no pigment is produced, and the eyes are white.)
    (a) wild type × white
    (b) wild type × scarlet
    (c) brown × white

16. Pigment in mouse fur is only produced when the *C* allele is present. Individuals of the *cc* genotype are white. If color is present, it may be determined by the *A, a* alleles. *AA* or *Aa* results in agouti color, while *aa* results in black coats.
    (a) What F_1 and F_2 genotypic and phenotypic ratios are obtained from a cross between *AACC* and *aacc* mice?
    (b) In three crosses between agouti females whose genotypes were unknown and males of the *aacc* genotype, the following phenotypic ratios were obtained:

(1)	8 agouti	(2)	9 agouti	(3)	4 agouti
	8 white		10 black		5 black
					10 white

What are the genotypes of these female parents?

17. In rats, the following genotypes of two independently assorting autosomal genes determine coat color:

A–B–	(gray)
A–bb	(yellow)
aaB–	(black)
aabb	(cream)

A third gene pair on a separate autosome determines whether or not any color will be produced. The *CC* and *Cc* genotypes allow color according to the expression of the *A* and *B* alleles. However, the *cc* genotype results in albino rats regardless of the *A* and *B* alleles present. Determine the F_1 phenotypic ratio of the following crosses:
    (a) *AAbbCC* × *aaBBcc*
    (b) *AaBBCC* × *AABbcc*
    (c) *AaBbCc* × *AaBbcc*
    (d) *AaBBCc* × *AaBBCc*
    (e) *AABbCc* × *AABbcc*

18. Given the inheritance pattern of coat color in rats described in Problem 17, predict the genotype and phenotype of the parents who produced the following offspring:
    (a) 9/16 gray: 3/16 yellow: 3/16 black: 1/16 cream
    (b) 9/16 gray: 3/16 yellow: 4/16 albino
    (c) 27/64 gray: 16/64 albino: 9/64 yellow: 9/64 black: 3/64 cream
    (d) 3/8 black: 3/8 cream: 2/8 albino
    (e) 3/8 black: 4/8 albino: 1/8 cream

19. In a species of the cat family, eye color can be gray, blue, green, or brown, and each trait is true breeding. In separate crosses involving homozygous parents, the following data were obtained:

Cross	P_1	F_1	F_2
A	green × gray	all green	3/4 green: 1/4 gray
B	green × brown	all green	3/4 green: 1/4 brown
C	gray × brown	all green	9/16 green: 3/16 brown
			3/16 gray: 1/16 blue

(a) Analyze the data. How many genes are involved? Define gene symbols and indicate which genotypes yield each phenotype.
(b) In a cross between a gray-eyed cat and one of unknown genotype and phenotype, the F_1 generation was not observed. However, the F_2 resulted in the same F_2 ratio as in cross C. Determine the genotypes and phenotypes of the unknown P_1 and F_1 cats.

20. In a plant, a tall variety was crossed with a dwarf variety. All F_1 plants were tall. When F_1 × F_1 plants were interbred, 9/16 of the F_2 were tall and 7/16 were dwarf.
    (a) Explain the inheritance of height by indicating the number of gene pairs involved and by designating which genotypes yield tall and which yield dwarf. (Use dashes where appropriate.)
    (b) What proportion of the F_2 plants will be true breeding if self-fertilized? List these genotypes.

21. In a unique species of plants, flowers may be yellow, blue, red, or mauve. All colors may be true breeding. If plants with blue flowers are crossed to red-flowered plants, all F_1 plants have yellow flowers. When these produced an F_2 generation, the following ratio was observed:

    9/16 yellow: 3/16 blue: 3/16 red: 1/16 mauve

In still another cross using true-breeding parents, yellow-flowered plants are crossed with mauve-flowered plants. Again, all F_1 plants had yellow flowers and the F_2 showed a 9:3:3:1 ratio, as just shown.
    (a) Describe the inheritance of flower color by defining gene symbols and designating which genotypes give rise to each of the four phenotypes.
    (b) Determine the F_1 and F_2 results of a cross between true-breeding red and true-breeding mauve-flowered plants.

22. Five human matings (1–5), identified by both maternal and paternal phenotypes for ABO and MN blood-group antigen status, are shown on the left side of the following table:

	Parental Phenotypes		Offspring	
(1)	A, M	× A, N	(a)	A, N
(2)	B, M	× B, M	(b)	O, N
(3)	O, N	× B, N	(c)	O, MN
(4)	AB, M	× O, N	(d)	B, M
(5)	AB, MN	× AB, MN	(e)	B, MN

Each mating resulted in one of the five offspring shown in the right-hand column (a–e). Match each offspring with one correct set of parents, using each parental set only once. Is there more than one set of correct answers?

23. A husband and wife have normal vision, although both of their fathers are red–green color-blind, an inherited X-linked

recessive condition. What is the probability that their first child will be (a) a normal son? (b) a normal daughter? (c) a color-blind son? (d) a color-blind daughter?

24. In humans, the ABO blood type is under the control of autosomal multiple alleles. Color blindness is a recessive X-linked trait. If two parents who are both type A and have normal vision produce a son who is color-blind and is type O, what is the probability that their next child will be a female who has normal vision and is type O?

25. In *Drosophila*, an X-linked recessive mutation, *scalloped* (*sd*), causes irregular wing margins. Diagram the F_1 and F_2 results if (a) a scalloped female is crossed with a normal male; (b) a scalloped male is crossed with a normal female. Compare these results with those that would be obtained if the *scalloped* gene were autosomal.

26. Another recessive mutation in *Drosophila*, *ebony* (*e*), is on an autosome (chromosome 3) and causes darkening of the body compared with wild-type flies. What phenotypic F_1 and F_2 male and female ratios will result if a scalloped-winged female with normal body color is crossed with a normal-winged ebony male? Work out this problem by both the Punnett square method and the forked-line method.

27. In *Drosophila*, the X-linked recessive mutation *vermilion* (*v*) causes bright red eyes, in contrast to the brick-red eyes of wild type. A separate autosomal recessive mutation, *suppressor of vermilion* (*su-v*), causes flies homozygous or hemizygous for *v* to have wild-type eyes. In the absence of *vermilion* alleles, *su-v* has no effect on eye color. Determine the F_1 and F_2 phenotypic ratios from a cross between a female with wild-type alleles at the *vermilion* locus, but who is homozygous for *su-v*, with a *vermilion* male who has wild-type alleles at the *su-v* locus.

28. While *vermilion* is X-linked in *Drosophila* and causes the eye color to be bright red, *brown* is an autosomal recessive mutation that causes the eye to be brown. Flies carrying both mutations lose all pigmentation and are white-eyed. Predict the F_1 and F_2 results of the following crosses:
    (a) vermilion females × brown males
    (b) brown females × vermilion males
    (c) white females × wild-type males

29. In a cross in *Drosophila* involving the X-linked recessive eye mutation *white* and the autosomally linked recessive eye mutation *sepia* (resulting in a dark eye), predict the F_1 and F_2 results of crossing true-breeding parents of the following phenotypes:
    (a) white females × sepia males
    (b) sepia females × white males
    Note that white is epistatic to the expression of sepia.

30. Consider the three pedigrees at the top of the right column, all involving a single human trait.
    (a) Which combination of conditions, if any, can be excluded?
       dominant and X-linked
       dominant and autosomal
       recessive and X-linked
       recessive and autosomal
    (b) For each combination that you excluded, indicate the single individual in generation II (e.g., II-1, II-2) that was most instrumental in your decision to exclude it. If none were excluded, answer "none apply."

(c) Given your conclusions in part (a), indicate the genotype of the following individuals:

II-1, II-6, II-9

If more than one possibility applies, list all possibilities. Use the symbols *A* and *a* for the genotypes.

31. In goats, the development of the beard is due to a recessive gene. The following cross involving true-breeding goats was made and carried to the F_2 generation:

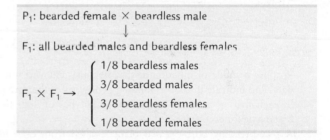

P$_1$: bearded female × beardless male
↓
F$_1$: all bearded males and beardless females

F$_1$ × F$_1$ →
  1/8 beardless males
  3/8 bearded males
  3/8 beardless females
  1/8 bearded females

Offer an explanation for the inheritance and expression of this trait, diagramming the cross. Propose one or more crosses to test your hypothesis.

32. Predict the F_1 and F_2 results of crossing a male fowl that is cock-feathered with a true-breeding hen-feathered female fowl. Recall that these traits are sex limited.

33. Two mothers give birth to sons at the same time at a busy urban hospital. The son of mother 1 is afflicted with hemophilia, a disease caused by an X-linked recessive allele. Neither parent has the disease. Mother 2 has a normal son, despite the fact that the father has hemophilia. Several years later, couple 1 sues the hospital, claiming that these two newborns were swapped in the nursery following their birth. As a genetic counselor, you are called to testify. What information can you provide the jury concerning the allegation?

34. Discuss the topic of phenotypic expression and the many factors that impinge on it.

35. Contrast penetrance and expressivity as the terms relate to phenotypic expression.

Extra-Spicy Problems

MasteringGenetics™ Visit for instructor-assigned tutorials and problems.

36. Labrador retrievers may be black, brown (chocolate), or golden (yellow) in color (see chapter-opening photo on p. 70). While each color may breed true, many different outcomes are seen when numerous litters are examined from a variety of matings where the parents are not necessarily true breeding. Following are just some of the many possibilities.

(a)	black	×	brown	⟶	all black
(b)	black	×	brown	⟶	1/2 black
					1/2 brown
(c)	black	×	brown	⟶	3/4 black
					1/4 golden
(d)	black	×	golden	⟶	all black
(e)	black	×	golden	⟶	4/8 golden
					3/8 black
					1/8 brown
(f)	black	×	golden	⟶	2/4 golden
					1/4 black
					1/4 brown
(g)	brown	×	brown	⟶	3/4 brown
					1/4 golden
(h)	black	×	black	⟶	9/16 black
					4/16 golden
					3/16 brown

Propose a mode of inheritance that is consistent with these data, and indicate the corresponding genotypes of the parents in each mating. Indicate as well the genotypes of dogs that breed true for each color.

37. A true-breeding purple-leafed plant isolated from one side of El Yunque, the rain forest in Puerto Rico, was crossed to a true-breeding white variety found on the other side. The F_1 offspring were all purple. A large number of $F_1 \times F_1$ crosses produced the following results:

purple: 4219   white: 5781   (Total = 10,000)

Propose an explanation for the inheritance of leaf color. As a geneticist, how might you go about testing your hypothesis? Describe the genetic experiments that you would conduct.

38. In Dexter and Kerry cattle, animals may be polled (hornless) or horned. The Dexter animals have short legs, whereas the Kerry animals have long legs. When many offspring were obtained from matings between polled Kerrys and horned Dexters, half were found to be polled Dexters and half polled Kerrys. When these two types of F_1 cattle were mated to one another, the following F_2 data were obtained:

3/8 polled Dexters
3/8 polled Kerrys
1/8 horned Dexters
1/8 horned Kerrys

A geneticist was puzzled by these data and interviewed farmers who had bred these cattle for decades. She learned that Kerrys were true breeding. Dexters, on the other hand, were not true breeding and never produced as many offspring as Kerrys. Provide a genetic explanation for these observations.

39. A geneticist from an alien planet that prohibits genetic research brought with him to Earth two pure-breeding lines of frogs. One line croaks by *uttering* "rib-it rib-it" and has purple eyes. The other line croaks more softly by *muttering* "knee-deep knee-deep" and has green eyes. With a new-found freedom of inquiry, the geneticist mated the two types of frogs, producing F_1 frogs that were all utterers and had blue eyes. A large F_2 generation then yielded the following ratios:

27/64	blue-eyed, "rib-it" utterer
12/64	green-eyed, "rib-it" utterer
9/64	blue-eyed, "knee-deep" mutterer
9/64	purple-eyed, "rib-it" utterer
4/64	green-eyed, "knee-deep" mutterer
3/64	purple-eyed, "knee-deep" mutterer

(a) How many total gene pairs are involved in the inheritance of both traits? Support your answer.
(b) Of these, how many are controlling eye color? How can you tell? How many are controlling croaking?
(c) Assign gene symbols for all phenotypes and indicate the genotypes of the P_1 and F_1 frogs.
(d) Indicate the genotypes of the six F_2 phenotypes.
(e) After years of experiments, the geneticist isolated pure-breeding strains of all six F_2 phenotypes. Indicate the F_1 and F_2 phenotypic ratios of the following cross using these pure-breeding strains:

blue-eyed, "knee-deep" mutterer × purple-eyed, "rib-it" utterer

(f) One set of crosses with his true-breeding lines initially caused the geneticist some confusion. When he crossed true-breeding purple-eyed, "knee-deep" mutterers with true-breeding green-eyed, "knee-deep" mutterers, he often got different results. In some matings, all offspring were blue-eyed, "knee-deep" mutterers, but in other matings all offspring were purple-eyed, "knee-deep" mutterers. In still a third mating, 1/2 blue-eyed, "knee-deep" mutterers and 1/2 purple-eyed, "knee-deep" mutterers were observed. Explain why the results differed.
(g) In another experiment, the geneticist crossed two purple-eyed, "rib-it" *utterers* together with the results shown here:

9/16	purple-eyed, "rib-it" utterer
3/16	purple-eyed, "knee-deep" mutterer
3/16	green-eyed, "rib-it" utterer
1/16	green-eyed, "knee-deep" mutterer

What were the genotypes of the two parents?

40. The following pedigree is characteristic of an inherited condition known as male precocious puberty, where affected males show signs of puberty by age 4. Propose a genetic explanation of this phenotype.

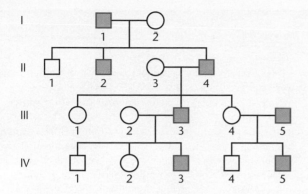

41. Students taking a genetics exam were expected to answer the following question by converting data to a "meaningful ratio" and then solving the problem. The instructor assumed that the final ratio would reflect two gene pairs, and most correct answers did. Here is the exam question:

"Flowers may be white, orange, or brown. When plants with white flowers are crossed with plants with brown flowers, all the F_1 flowers are white. For F_2 flowers, the following data were obtained:

48	white
12	orange
4	brown

Convert the F_2 data to a meaningful ratio that allows you to explain the inheritance of color. Determine the number of genes involved and the genotypes that yield each phenotype."

(a) Solve the problem for two gene pairs. What is the final F_2 ratio?

(b) A number of students failed to reduce the ratio for two gene pairs as described above and solved the problem using three gene pairs. When examined carefully, their solution was deemed a valid response by the instructor. Solve the problem using three gene pairs.

(c) We now have a dilemma. The data are consistent with two alternative mechanisms of inheritance. Propose an experiment that executes crosses involving the original parents that would distinguish between the two solutions proposed by the students. Explain how this experiment would resolve the dilemma.

42. In four o'clock plants, many flower colors are observed. In a cross involving two true-breeding strains, one crimson and the other white, all of the F_1 generation were rose color. In the F_2, four new phenotypes appeared along with the P_1 and F_1 parental colors. The following ratio was obtained:

1/16 crimson	4/16 rose
2/16 orange	2/16 pale yellow
1/16 yellow	4/16 white
2/16 magenta	

Propose an explanation for the inheritance of these flower colors.

43. Proto-oncogenes stimulate cells to progress through the cell cycle and begin mitosis. In cells that stop dividing, transcription of proto-oncogenes is inhibited by regulatory molecules. As is typical of all genes, proto-oncogenes contain a regulatory DNA region followed by a coding DNA region that specifies the amino acid sequence of the gene product. Consider two types of mutation in a proto-oncogene, one in the regulatory region that eliminates transcriptional control and the other in the coding region that renders the gene product inactive. Characterize both of these mutant alleles as either gain-of-function or loss-of-function mutations and indicate whether each would be dominant or recessive.

44. Below is a partial pedigree of hemophilia in the British Royal Family descended from Queen Victoria, who is believed to be the original "carrier" in this pedigree. Analyze the pedigree and indicate which females are also certain to be carriers. What is the probability that Princess Irene is a carrier?

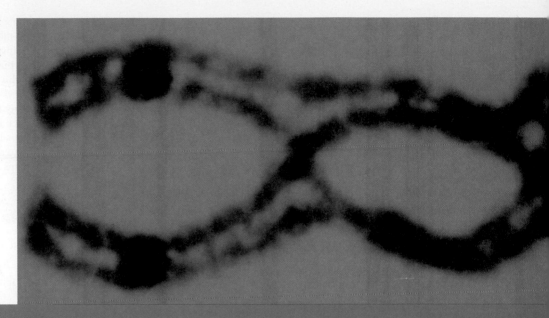

Chiasmata present
between synapsed
homologs during
the first meiotic prophase.

5 Chromosome Mapping in Eukaryotes

CHAPTER CONCEPTS

- Chromosomes in eukaryotes contain large numbers of genes, whose locations are fixed along the length of the chromosomes.

- Unless separated by crossing over, alleles on the same chromosome segregate as a unit during gamete formation.

- Crossing over between homologs during meiosis creates recombinant gametes with different combinations of alleles that enhance genetic variation.

- Crossing over between homologs serves as the basis for the construction of chromosome maps. The greater the distance between two genes on a chromosome, the higher the frequency of crossing over is between them.

- While exchanges also occur between sister chromatids during mitosis, no new recombinant chromatids are created.

Walter Sutton, along with Theodor Boveri, was instrumental in uniting the fields of cytology and genetics. As early as 1903, Sutton pointed out the likelihood that there must be many more "unit factors" than chromosomes in most organisms. Soon thereafter, genetic studies with several organisms revealed that certain genes segregate as if they were somehow joined or linked together. Further investigations showed that such genes are part of the same chromosome, and they may indeed be transmitted as a single unit. We now know that most chromosomes contain a very large number of genes. Those that are part of the same chromosome are said to be *linked* and to demonstrate **linkage** in genetic crosses.

Because the chromosome, not the gene, is the unit of transmission during meiosis, linked genes are not free to undergo independent assortment. Instead, the alleles at all loci of one chromosome should, in theory, be transmitted as a unit during gamete formation. However, in many instances this does not occur. As we saw during the first meiotic prophase, when homologs are paired, or synapsed, a reciprocal exchange of chromosome segments may take place (Chapter 2). This **crossing over** results in the reshuffling, or **recombination,** of the alleles between homologs and always occurs during the tetrad stage.

Crossing over is currently viewed as an actual physical breaking and rejoining process that occurs during meiosis. You can see an example in the micrograph that opens this chapter. The exchange of chromosome segments provides an enormous potential for genetic variation in the gametes formed by any individual. This type of variation, in combination with that resulting from independent assortment, ensures that all offspring will contain a diverse mixture of maternal and paternal alleles.

The frequency of crossing over between any two loci on a single chromosome is proportional to the distance between them. Thus, depending on which loci are being considered, the percentage of recombinant gametes varies. This correlation allows us to construct **chromosome maps,** which indicate the relative locations of genes on the chromosomes.

In this chapter, we will discuss linkage, crossing over, and chromosome mapping in more detail. We will also consider a variety of other topics involving the exchange of genetic information, concluding the chapter with the rather intriguing question of why Mendel, who studied seven genes in an organism with seven chromosomes, did not encounter linkage. Or did he?

5.1 Genes Linked on the Same Chromosome Segregate Together

A simplified overview of the major theme of this chapter is given in **Figure 5–1**, which contrasts the meiotic consequences of (a) independent assortment, (b) linkage *without* crossing over, and (c) linkage *with* crossing over. In **Figure 5–1(a)** we see the results of independent assortment of two pairs of chromosomes, each containing one heterozygous gene pair. No linkage is exhibited. When these same two chromosomes are observed in a large number of meiotic events, they are seen to form four genetically different gametes in equal proportions, each containing a different combination of alleles of the two genes.

Now let's compare these results with what occurs if the same genes are linked on the same chromosome. If no crossing over occurs between the two genes [**Figure 5–1(b)**], only two genetically different kinds of gametes are formed. Each gamete receives the alleles present on one homolog or the other, which is transmitted intact as the result of segregation. This case illustrates *complete linkage*, which produces only **parental,** or **noncrossover, gametes.** The two parental gametes are formed in equal proportions. Though complete linkage between two genes seldom occurs, it is useful to consider the theoretical consequences of this concept.

Figure 5–1(c) shows the results when crossing over occurs between two linked genes. As you can see, this

FIGURE 5–1   Results of gamete formation when two heterozygous genes are (a) on two different pairs of chromosomes; (b) on the same pair of homologs, but with no exchange occurring between them; and (c) on the same pair of homologs, but with an exchange occurring between two nonsister chromatids. Note in this and the following figures that members of homologous pairs of chromosomes are shown in two different colors. (This convention was established in Chapter 2; see, for example, Figure 2–7 and Figure 2–11.)

(a)   **Independent assortment: Two genes on two different homologous pairs of chromosomes**

(b)   **Linkage: Two genes on a single pair of homologs; no exchange occurs**

(c)   **Linkage: Two genes on a single pair of homologs; exchange occurs between two nonsister chromatids**

crossover involves only two nonsister chromatids of the four chromatids present in the tetrad. This exchange generates two new allele combinations, called **recombinant, or crossover, gametes.** The two chromatids not involved in the exchange result in noncrossover gametes, like those in Figure 5–1(b). Importantly, the frequency with which crossing over occurs between any two linked genes is proportional to the distance separating the respective loci along the chromosome. As the distance between the two genes increases, the proportion of recombinant gametes increases and that of the parental gametes decreases. In theory, two randomly selected genes can be so close to each other that crossover events are too infrequent to be easily detected. As shown in Figure 5–1(b), this complete linkage produces only parental gametes. On the other hand, if a small, but distinct, distance separates two genes, few recombinant and many parental gametes will be formed.

As we will discuss again later in this chapter, when the loci of two linked genes are far apart, the number of recombinant gametes approaches, but does not exceed, 50 percent. If 50 percent recombinants occur, the result is a 1:1:1:1 ratio of the four types (two parental and two recombinant gametes). In this case, transmission of two linked genes is indistinguishable from that of two unlinked, independently assorting genes. That is, the proportion of the four possible genotypes would be identical, as shown in Figure 5–1(a) and Figure 5–1(c).

The Linkage Ratio

If complete linkage exists between two genes because of their close proximity, and organisms heterozygous at both loci are mated, a unique F_2 phenotypic ratio results, which we designate the **linkage ratio.** To illustrate this ratio, let's consider a cross involving the closely linked, recessive, mutant genes *heavy* wing vein (*hv*) and *brown* eye (*bw*) in *Drosophila melanogaster* (**Figure 5–2**). The normal, wild-type alleles hv^+ and bw^+ are both dominant and result in thin wing veins and red eyes, respectively.

In this cross, flies with normal thin wing veins and mutant brown eyes are mated to flies with mutant heavy wing veins and normal red eyes. In more concise terms, heavy-veined flies are crossed with brown-eyed flies. Linked genes are represented by placing their allele designations (the genetic symbols established in Chapter 4) above and below a single or double horizontal line. Those above the line are located at loci on one homolog, and those below the line are located at the homologous loci on the other homolog. Thus, we represent the P_1 generation as follows:

$$P_1: \frac{hv^+ \, bw}{hv^+ \, bw} \times \frac{hv \, bw^+}{hv \, bw^+}$$

thin, brown   heavy, red

Because these genes are located on an autosome, no designation of male or female is necessary.

In the F_1 generation, each fly receives one chromosome of each pair from each parent. All flies are heterozygous for both gene pairs and exhibit the dominant traits of thin veins and red eyes:

$$F_1 = \frac{hv^+ \, bw}{hv \, bw^+}$$

thin, red

As shown in Figure 5–2(a), when the F_1 generation is interbred, each F_1 individual forms only parental gametes because of complete linkage. Following fertilization, the F_2 generation is produced in a 1:2:1 phenotypic and genotypic ratio. One-fourth of this generation shows thin wing veins and brown eyes; one-half shows both wild-type traits, namely, thin veins and red eyes; and one-fourth will show heavy wing veins and red eyes. Therefore, the ratio is 1 heavy: 2 wild: 1 brown. Such a 1:2:1 ratio is characteristic of complete linkage. Complete linkage is usually observed only when genes are very close together and the number of progeny is relatively small.

Figure 5–2(b) demonstrates the results of a testcross with the F_1 flies. Such a cross produces a 1:1 ratio of thin, brown and heavy, red flies. Had the genes controlling these traits been incompletely linked or located on separate autosomes, the testcross would have produced four phenotypes rather than two.

When large numbers of mutant genes in any given species are investigated, genes located on the same chromosome show evidence of linkage to one another. As a result, **linkage groups** can be identified, one for each chromosome. In theory, the number of linkage groups should correspond to the haploid number of chromosomes. In diploid organisms in which large numbers of mutant genes are available for genetic study, this correlation has been confirmed.

NOW SOLVE THIS

5–1 Consider two hypothetical recessive autosomal genes *a* and *b*, where a heterozygote is testcrossed to a double-homozygous mutant. Predict the phenotypic ratios under the following conditions:

(a) *a* and *b* are located on separate autosomes.

(b) *a* and *b* are linked on the same autosome but are so far apart that a crossover always occurs between them.

(c) *a* and *b* are linked on the same autosome but are so close together that a crossover almost never occurs.

■ **HINT:** *This problem involves an understanding of linkage, crossing over, and independent assortment. The key to its solution is to be aware that results are indistinguishable when two genes are unlinked compared to the case where they are linked but so far apart that crossing over always intervenes between them during meiosis.*

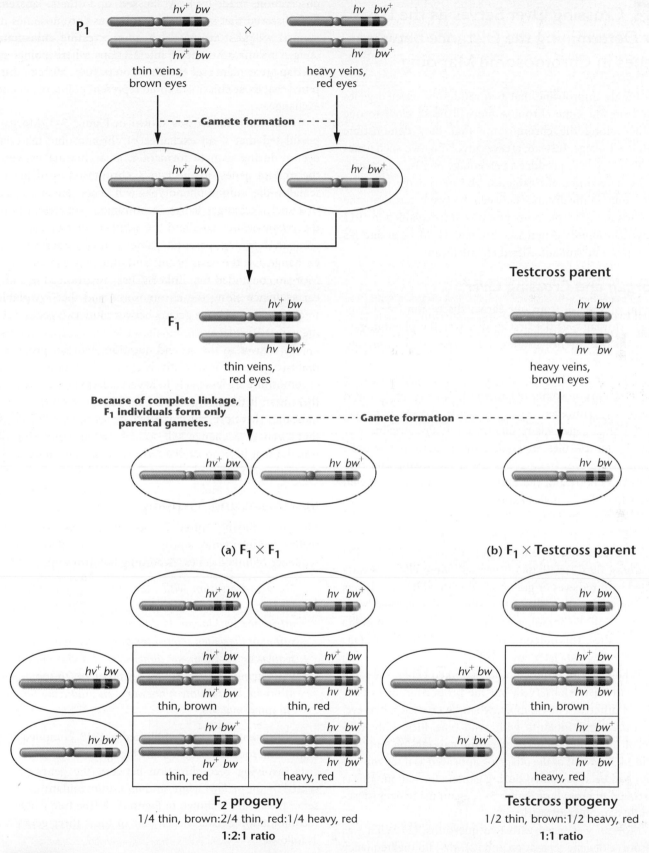

(a) F₁ × F₁

(b) F₁ × Testcross parent

F₂ progeny
1/4 thin, brown:2/4 thin, red:1/4 heavy, red
1:2:1 ratio

Testcross progeny
1/2 thin, brown:1/2 heavy, red
1:1 ratio

FIGURE 5-2 Results of a cross involving two genes located on the same chromosome and demonstrating complete linkage. (a) The F₂ results of the cross. (b) The results of a testcross involving the F₁ progeny.

5.2 Crossing Over Serves as the Basis for Determining the Distance between Genes in Chromosome Mapping

It is highly improbable that two randomly selected genes linked on the same chromosome will be so close to one another along the chromosome that they demonstrate complete linkage. Instead, crosses involving two such genes will almost always produce a percentage of offspring resulting from recombinant gametes. The percentage will vary depending on the distance between the two genes along the chromosome. This phenomenon was first explained in 1911 by two *Drosophila* geneticists, Thomas H. Morgan and his undergraduate student, Alfred H. Sturtevant.

Morgan and Crossing Over

As you may recall from our earlier discussion (see Chapter 4), Morgan was the first to discover the phenomenon of X-linkage. In his studies, he investigated numerous *Drosophila* mutations located on the X chromosome. His original analysis, based on crosses involving only one gene on the X chromosome, led to the discovery of X-linked inheritance. However, when he made crosses involving two X-linked genes, his results were initially puzzling. For example, female flies expressing the mutant *yellow* body (*y*) and *white* eyes (*w*) alleles were crossed with wild-type males (gray body and red eyes). The F_1 females were wild type, while the F_1 males expressed both mutant traits. In the F_2 the vast majority of the total offspring showed the expected parental phenotypes—yellow-bodied, white-eyed flies and wild-type flies (gray-bodied, red-eyed). The remaining flies, less than 1.0 percent, were either yellow-bodied with red eyes or gray-bodied with white eyes. It was as if the two mutant alleles had somehow separated from each other on the homolog during gamete formation in the F_1 female flies. This outcome is illustrated in cross A of **Figure 5–3**, using data later compiled by Sturtevant.

When Morgan studied other X-linked genes, the same basic pattern was observed, but the proportion of F_2 phenotypes differed. For example, when he crossed *white*-eye, *miniature*-wing mutants with wild-type flies, only 65.5 percent of all the F_2 flies showed the parental phenotypes, while 34.5 percent of the offspring appeared as if the mutant genes had been separated during gamete formation. This is illustrated in cross B of Figure 5–3, again using data subsequently compiled by Sturtevant.

Morgan was faced with two questions: (1) What was the source of gene separation and (2) why did the frequency of the apparent separation vary depending on the genes being studied? The answer Morgan proposed for the first question was based on his knowledge of earlier cytological

observations made by F. A. Janssens and others. Janssens had observed that synapsed homologous chromosomes in meiosis wrapped around each other, creating **chiasmata** (sing. chiasma), X-shaped intersections where points of overlap are evident (see the photo on p. 104). Morgan proposed that these chiasmata could represent points of genetic exchange.

Regarding the crosses shown in Figure 5–3, Morgan postulated that if an exchange of chromosome material occurs during gamete formation, at a chiasma between the mutant genes on the two X chromosomes of the F_1 females, the unique phenotypes will occur. He suggested that such exchanges led to recombinant gametes in both the *yellow–white* cross and the *white–miniature* cross, as compared to the parental gametes that underwent no exchange. On the basis of this and other experimentation, Morgan concluded that linked genes are arranged in a linear sequence along the chromosome and that a variable frequency of exchange occurs between any two genes during gamete formation.

In answer to the second question, Morgan proposed that two genes located relatively close to each other along a chromosome are less likely to have a chiasma form between them than if the two genes are farther apart on the chromosome. Therefore, the closer two genes are, the less likely that a genetic exchange will occur between them. Morgan was the first to propose the term *crossing over* to describe the physical exchange leading to recombination.

Sturtevant and Mapping

Morgan's student, Alfred H. Sturtevant, was the first to realize that his mentor's proposal could be used to map the sequence of linked genes. According to Sturtevant,

> *"In a conversation with Morgan . . . I suddenly realized that the variations in strength of linkage, already attributed by Morgan to differences in the spatial separation of the genes, offered the possibility of determining sequences in the linear dimension of a chromosome. I went home and spent most of the night (to the neglect of my undergraduate homework) in producing the first chromosomal map."*

Sturtevant, in a paper published in 1913, compiled data from numerous crosses made by Morgan and other geneticists involving recombination between the genes represented by the *yellow*, *white*, and *miniature* mutants. A subset of these data is shown in Figure 5–3. The frequencies of recombination between each pair of these three genes are as follows:

(1)	*yellow, white*	0.5%
(2)	*white, miniature*	34.5%
(3)	*yellow, miniature*	35.4%

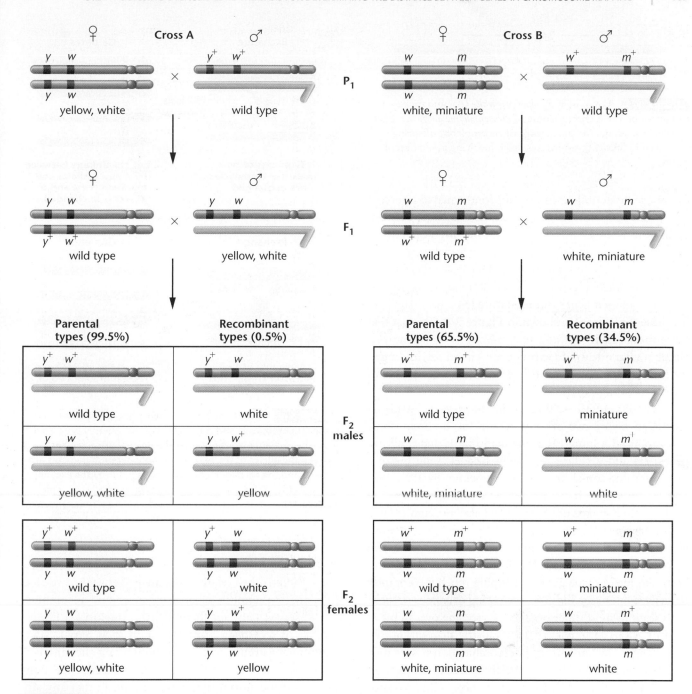

FIGURE 5–3   The F_1 and F_2 results of crosses involving the *yellow* (*y*), *white* (*w*) mutations (cross A), and the *white*, *miniature* (*m*) mutations (cross B), as compiled by Sturtevant. In cross A, 0.5 percent of the F_2 flies (males and females) demonstrate recombinant phenotypes, which express either *white* or *yellow*. In cross B, 34.5 percent of the F_2 flies (males and females) demonstrate recombinant phenotypes, which are either *miniature* or *white* mutants.

Because the sum of (1) and (2) approximately equals (3), Sturtevant suggested that the recombination frequencies between linked genes are additive. On this basis, he predicted that the order of the genes on the X chromosome is *yellow–white–miniature*. In arriving at this conclusion, he reasoned as follows: The *yellow* and *white* genes are apparently close to each other because the recombination frequency is low. However, both of these genes are quite far from the *miniature* gene because the *white–miniature* and

yellow–miniature combinations show larger recombination frequencies. Because *miniature* shows more recombination with *yellow* than with *white* (35.4 percent vs. 34.5 percent), it follows that *white* is located between the other two genes, not outside of them.

Sturtevant knew from Morgan's work that the frequency of exchange could be used as an estimate of the distance between two genes or loci along the chromosome. He constructed a chromosome map of the three genes on the X

FIGURE 5-4 A map of the *yellow* (*y*), *white* (*w*), and *miniature* (*m*) genes on the X chromosome of *Drosophila melanogaster*. Each number represents the percentage of recombinant offspring produced in one of three crosses, each involving two different genes.

chromosome, setting one map unit (mu) equal to 1 percent recombination between two genes.* The distance between *yellow* and *white* is thus 0.5 mu, and the distance between *yellow* and *miniature* is 35.4 mu. It follows that the distance between *white* and *miniature* should be 35.4 − 0.5 = 34.9 mu. This estimate is close to the actual frequency of recombination between *white* and *miniature* (34.5 mu). The map for these three genes is shown in **Figure 5-4**. The fact that these numbers do not add up perfectly is due to normal variation that one would expect between crosses, leading to the minor imprecisions encountered in independently conducted mapping experiments.

In addition to these three genes, Sturtevant considered crosses involving two other genes on the X chromosome and produced a more extensive map that included all five genes. He and a colleague, Calvin Bridges, soon began a search for autosomal linkage in *Drosophila*. By 1923, they had clearly shown that linkage and crossing over are not restricted to X-linked genes but could also be demonstrated with autosomes. During this work, they made another interesting observation. In *Drosophila*, crossing over was shown to occur only in females. The fact that no crossing over occurs in males made genetic mapping much less complex to analyze in *Drosophila*. While crossing over does occur in both sexes in most other organisms, crossing over in males is often observed to occur less frequently than in females. For example, in humans, such recombination occurs only about 60 percent as often in males compared to females.

Although many refinements have been added to chromosome mapping since Sturtevant's initial work, his basic principles are accepted as correct. These principles are used to produce detailed chromosome maps of organisms for which large numbers of linked mutant genes are known. Sturtevant's findings are also historically significant to the broader field of genetics. In 1910, the chromosomal theory of inheritance was still widely disputed—even Morgan was skeptical of this theory before he conducted his experiments. Research has now firmly established that chromosomes contain genes in a linear order and that these genes are the equivalent of Mendel's unit factors.

---

*In honor of Morgan's work, map units are often referred to as centi-Morgans (cM).

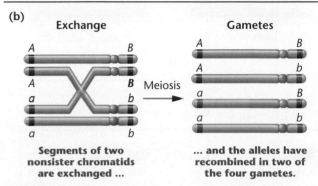

FIGURE 5-5 Two examples of a single crossover between two nonsister chromatids and the gametes subsequently produced. In (a) the exchange does not alter the linkage arrangement between the alleles of the two genes, only parental gametes are formed, and the exchange goes undetected. In (b) the exchange separates the alleles, resulting in recombinant gametes, which are detectable.

Single Crossovers

Why should the relative distance between two loci influence the amount of crossing over and recombination observed between them? During meiosis, a limited number of crossover events occur in each tetrad. These recombinant events occur randomly along the length of the tetrad. Therefore, the closer that two loci reside along the axis of the chromosome, the less likely that any **single crossover** event will occur between them. The same reasoning suggests that the farther apart two linked loci, the more likely a random crossover event will occur in between them.

In **Figure 5–5(a)**, a single crossover occurs between two nonsister chromatids, but not between the two loci being studied; therefore, the crossover is undetected because no recombinant gametes are produced for the two traits of interest. In Figure 5–5(b), where the two loci under study are quite far apart, the crossover does occur between them, yielding gametes in which the traits of interest are recombined.

When a single crossover occurs between two nonsister chromatids, the other two chromatids of the tetrad are not

FIGURE 5–6 The consequences of a single exchange between two nonsister chromatids occurring in the tetrad stage. Two noncrossover (parental) and two crossover (recombinant) gametes are produced.

involved in the exchange and enter the gamete unchanged. Even if a single crossover occurs 100 percent of the time between two linked genes, recombination is subsequently observed in only 50 percent of the potential gametes formed. This concept is diagrammed in **Figure 5–6**. Theoretically, if we assume only single exchanges between a given pair of loci and observe 20 percent recombinant gametes, we will conclude that crossing over actually occurs between these two loci in 40 percent of the tetrads. The general rule is that, under these conditions, the percentage of tetrads involved in an exchange between two genes is twice as great as the percentage of recombinant gametes produced. Therefore, the theoretical limit of observed recombination due to crossing over is 50 percent.

When two linked genes are more than 50 map units apart, a crossover can theoretically be expected to occur between them in 100 percent of the tetrads. If this prediction were achieved, each tetrad would yield equal proportions of the four gametes shown in Figure 5–6, just as if the genes were on different chromosomes and assorting independently. For a variety of reasons, this theoretical limit is seldom achieved.

5.3 Determining the Gene Sequence during Mapping Requires the Analysis of Multiple Crossovers

The study of single crossovers between two linked genes provides a basis for determining the *distance* between them. However, when many linked genes are studied, their *sequence* along the chromosome is more difficult to determine. Fortunately, the discovery that multiple crossovers occur between the chromatids of a tetrad has facilitated the process of producing more extensive chromosome maps. As we shall see next, when three or more linked genes are

investigated simultaneously, it is possible to determine first the sequence of genes and then the distances between them.

NOW SOLVE THIS

5–2 With two pairs of genes involved (*P/p* and *Z/z*), a testcross (*ppzz*) with an organism of unknown genotype indicated that the gametes produced were in the following proportions:

PZ, 42.4%; *Pz*, 6.9%; *pZ*, 7.1%; *pz*, 43.6%

Draw all possible conclusions from these data.

■ **HINT:** *This problem involves an understanding of the proportionality between crossover frequency and distance between genes. The key to its solution is to be aware that noncrossover and crossover gametes occur in reciprocal pairs of approximately equal proportions.*

Multiple Exchanges

It is possible that in a single tetrad, two, three, or more exchanges will occur between nonsister chromatids as a result of several crossing over events. Double exchanges of genetic material result from **double crossovers (DCOs),** as shown in **Figure 5–7**. To study a double exchange, three gene pairs must be investigated, each heterozygous for two alleles. Before we determine the frequency of recombination among all three loci, let's review some simple probability calculations.

As we have seen, the probability of a single exchange occurring in between the *A* and *B* or the *B* and *C* genes is related directly to the distance between the respective loci. The closer *A* is to *B* and *B* is to *C*, the less likely it is that a single exchange will occur in between either of the two sets of loci. In the case of a double crossover, two separate and independent events or exchanges must occur simultaneously. The mathematical probability of two independent events occurring simultaneously is equal to the product of

Double-crossover gametes

Noncrossover gametes

FIGURE 5–7 Consequences of a double exchange occurring between two nonsister chromatids. Because the exchanges involve only two chromatids, two noncrossover gametes and two double-crossover gametes are produced. The chapter-opening photograph on p. 104 illustrates two chiasmata present in a tetrad isolated during the first meiotic prophase stage.

the individual probabilities. (This is the *product law* introduced in Chapter 3.)

Suppose that crossover gametes resulting from single exchanges are recovered 20 percent of the time ($p = 0.20$) between A and B, and 30 percent of the time ($p = 0.30$) between B and C. The probability of recovering a double-crossover gamete arising from two exchanges (between A and B and between B and C) is predicted to be $(0.20)(0.30) = 0.06$, or 6 percent. It is apparent from this calculation that the expected frequency of double-crossover gametes is always expected to be much lower than that of either single-crossover class of gametes.

If three genes are relatively close together along one chromosome, the expected frequency of double-crossover gametes is extremely low. For example, suppose that the A–B distance in Figure 5–7 is 3 mu and the B–C distance is 2 mu. The expected double-crossover frequency is $(0.03)(0.02) = 0.0006$, or 0.06 percent. This translates to only six events in 10,000. Thus in a mapping experiment where closely linked genes are involved, very large numbers of offspring are required to detect double-crossover events. In this example, it is unlikely that a double crossover will be observed even if 1000 offspring are examined. Thus, it is evident that if four or five genes are being mapped, even fewer triple and quadruple crossovers can be expected to occur.

Three-Point Mapping in *Drosophila*

The information presented in the previous section enables us to map three or more linked genes in a single cross. To illustrate the mapping process in its entirety, we examine two situations involving three linked genes in two quite different organisms.

To execute a successful mapping cross, three criteria must be met:

1. The genotype of the organism producing the crossover gametes must be heterozygous at all loci under consideration. If homozygosity occurred at any locus, all gametes produced would contain the same allele, precluding mapping analysis.

2. The cross must be constructed so that the genotypes of all gametes can be accurately determined by observing the phenotypes of the resulting offspring. This is necessary because the gametes and their genotypes can never be observed directly. To overcome this problem, each phenotypic class must reflect the genotype of the gametes of the parents producing it.

3. A sufficient number of offspring must be produced in the mapping experiment to recover a representative sample of all crossover classes.

These criteria are met in the three-point mapping cross of *Drosophila melanogaster* shown in **Figure 5–8**. In this cross three X-linked recessive mutant genes—*yellow* body color, *white* eye color, and *echinus* eye shape—are considered. To diagram the cross, *we must assume some theoretical sequence, even though we do not yet know if it is correct.* In Figure 5–8, we initially assume the sequence of the three genes to be *y–w–ec*. If this is incorrect, our analysis shall demonstrate it and reveal the correct sequence.

In the P_1 generation, males hemizygous for all three wild-type alleles are crossed to females that are homozygous for all three recessive mutant alleles. Therefore, the P_1 males are wild type with respect to body color, eye color, and eye shape. They are said to have a *wild-type phenotype*. The females, on the other hand, exhibit the three mutant traits: yellow body color, white eyes, and echinus eye shape.

This cross produces an F_1 generation consisting of females that are heterozygous at all three loci and males that, because of the Y chromosome, are hemizygous for the three mutant alleles. Phenotypically, all F_1 females are wild type, while all F_1 males are yellow, white, and echinus. The genotype of the F_1 females fulfills the first criterion for constructing a map of the three linked genes; that is, it is heterozygous at the three loci and may serve as the source of recombinant gametes generated by crossing over. Note that, because of the genotypes of the P_1 parents, all three of the mutant alleles are on one homolog and all three wild-type alleles are on the other homolog. With other parents, *other arrangements would be possible that could produce a heterozygous genotype.* For example, a heterozygous female could have the *y* and *ec* mutant alleles on one homolog and the *w* allele on the other. This would occur if one of her parents was yellow, echinus and the other parent was white.

Origin of female gametes	Gametes			F₂ phenotype	Observed number	Category, total, and percentage
NCO	① *y w ec*	*y w ec* / *y w ec*	*y w cc*	*y w ec*	4685	Non-crossover
	② *y⁺ w⁺ ec⁺*	*y⁺ w⁺ ec⁺* / *y w ec*	*y⁺ w⁺ ec⁺*	*y⁺ w⁺ ec⁺*	4759	9444 94.44%
SCO	③ *y w⁺ ec⁺*	*y w⁺ ec⁺* / *y w ec*	*y w⁺ ec⁺*	*y w⁺ ec⁺*	80	Single crossover between *y* and *w*
	④ *y⁺ w ec*	*y⁺ w ec* / *y w ec*	*y⁺ w ec*	*y⁺ w ec*	70	150 1.50%
SCO	⑤ *y w ec⁺*	*y w ec⁺* / *y w ec*	*y w ec⁺*	*y w ec⁺*	193	Single crossover between *w* and *ec*
	⑥ *y⁺ w⁺ ec*	*y⁺ w⁺ ec* / *y w ec*	*y⁺ w⁺ ec*	*y⁺ w⁺ ec*	207	400 4.00%
DCO	⑦ *y w⁺ ec*	*y w⁺ ec* / *y w ec*	*y w⁺ ec*	*y w⁺ ec*	3	Double crossover between *y* and *w* and between *w* and *ec*
	⑧ *y⁺ w ec⁺*	*y⁺ w ec⁺* / *y w ec*	*y⁺ w ec⁺*	*y⁺ w ec⁺*	3	6 0.06%

Map of *y*, *w*, and *ec* loci

├─1.56─┼───4.06───┤

FIGURE 5–8 A three-point mapping cross involving the *yellow* (*y* or *y⁺*), *white* (*w* or *w⁺*), and *echinus* (*ec* or *ec⁺*) genes in *Drosophila melanogaster*. NCO, SCO, and DCO refer to noncrossover, single-crossover, and double-crossover groups, respectively. Centromeres are not drawn on the chromosomes, and only two nonsister chromatids are initially shown in the left-hand column.

In our cross, the second criterion is met as a result of the gametes formed by the F₁ males. Every gamete contains either an X chromosome bearing the three mutant alleles or a Y chromosome, which does not contain any of the three loci being considered. Whichever type participates in fertilization, the genotype of the gamete produced by the F₁ female will be expressed phenotypically in the F₂ female and male offspring derived from it. As a result, all noncrossover and crossover gametes produced by the F₁ female parent can be determined by observing the F₂ phenotypes.

With these two criteria met, we can construct a chromosome map from the crosses illustrated in Figure 5–8. First, we must determine which F₂ phenotypes correspond to the various noncrossover and crossover categories. To determine the **noncrossover** F₂ phenotypes, we must identify individuals derived from the parental gametes formed by the F₁ female. Each such gamete contains *an X chromosome unaffected by crossing over*. As a result of segregation, approximately equal proportions of the two types of gametes, and subsequently their F₂ phenotypes, are produced. Because they derive from a heterozygote, the genotypes of the two parental gametes and the F₂ phenotypes complement one another. For example, if one is wild type, the other is mutant for all three genes. This is the case in the cross being considered. In other situations, if one chromosome shows one mutant allele, the second chromosome shows the other two mutant alleles, and so on. These are therefore called **reciprocal classes** of gametes and phenotypes.

The two noncrossover phenotypes are most easily recognized because *they occur in the greatest proportion of offspring.* Figure 5–8 shows that gametes (1) and (2) are present in the greatest numbers. Therefore, flies that are yellow, white, and echinus and those that are normal, or wild type, for all three characters constitute the noncrossover category and represent 94.44 percent of the F₂ offspring.

The second category that can be easily detected is represented by the double-crossover phenotypes. Because of their low probability of occurrence, *they must be present in the least numbers.* Remember that this group represents two independent but simultaneous single-crossover events. Two reciprocal phenotypes can be identified: gamete 7, which shows the mutant traits yellow and echinus, but normal eye color; and gamete 8, which shows the mutant trait white, but normal body color and eye shape. Together these double-crossover phenotypes constitute only 0.06 percent of the F₂ offspring.

The remaining four phenotypic classes fall into two categories resulting from single crossovers. Gametes 3 and 4, reciprocal phenotypes produced by single-crossover events occurring between the *yellow* and *white* loci, are equal to 1.50 percent of the F₂ offspring. Gametes 5 and 6, constituting 4.00 percent of the F₂ offspring, represent the reciprocal phenotypes resulting from single-crossover events occurring between the *white* and *echinus* loci.

We can now calculate the map distances between the three loci. The distance between y and w, or between w and ec, is equal to the percentage of all detectable exchanges occurring between them. For any two genes under consideration, this includes all related single crossovers as well as all double crossovers. *The latter are included because they represent two simultaneous single crossovers.* For the y and w genes, this includes gametes 3, 4, 7, and 8, totaling 1.50% + 0.06%, or 1.56 mu. Similarly, the distance between w and ec is equal to the percentage of offspring resulting from an exchange between these two loci: gametes 5, 6, 7, and 8, totaling 4.00% + 0.06%, or 4.06 mu. The map of these three loci on the X chromosome is shown at the bottom of Figure 5–8.

Determining the Gene Sequence

In the preceding example, we assumed that the sequence (or order) of the three genes along the chromosome was y–w–ec. Our analysis established that the sequence is consistent with the data. However, in most mapping experiments, the gene sequence is not known, and this constitutes another variable in the analysis. In our example, had the gene order been unknown, we could have used one of two methods (which we will study next) to determine it. In your own work, you should select one of these methods and use it consistently.

Method I This method is based on the fact that there are only three possible arrangements, each containing a different one of the three genes between the other two:

(I)   w–y–ec   (y is in the middle)

(II) y–ec–w   (ec is in the middle)

(III) y–w–ec   (w is in the middle)

Use the following steps during your analysis to determine the gene order:

1. Assuming any of the three orders, first determine the *arrangement of alleles* along each homolog of the heterozygous parent giving rise to noncrossover and crossover gametes (the F₁ female in our example).

2. Determine whether a double-crossover event occurring within that arrangement will produce the *observed double-crossover phenotypes.* Remember that these phenotypes occur least frequently and are easily identified.

3. If this order does not produce the correct phenotypes, try each of the other two orders. One must work!

These steps are shown in **Figure 5–9**, using our y–w–ec cross. The three possible arrangements are labeled I, II, and III, as shown above.

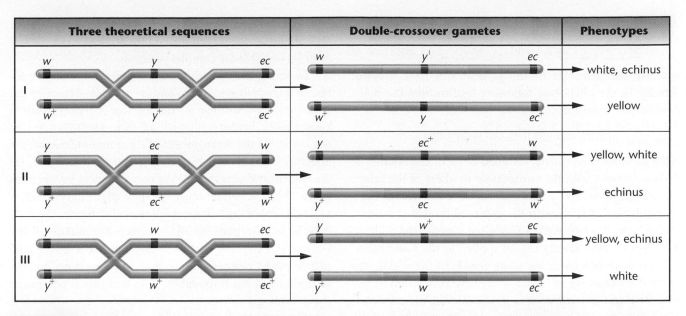

FIGURE 5–9 The three possible sequences of the *white, yellow,* and *echinus* genes, the results of a double crossover in each case, and the resulting phenotypes produced in a testcross. For simplicity, the two noncrossover chromatids of each tetrad are omitted.

1. Assuming that y is between w and ec (arrangement I), the distribution of alleles between the homologs of the F_1 heterozygote is:

$$\frac{w \qquad y \qquad ec}{w^+ \qquad y^+ \qquad ec^+}$$

We know this because of the way in which the P_1 generation was crossed: The P_1 female contributes an X chromosome bearing the w, y, and ec alleles, while the P_1 male contributed an X chromosome bearing the w^+, y^+, and ec^+ alleles.

2. A double crossover within that arrangement yields the following gametes:

$$\frac{w \qquad y^+ \qquad ec}{\quad} \quad \text{and} \quad \frac{w^+ \qquad y \qquad ec^+}{\quad}$$

Following fertilization, if y is in the middle, the F_2 double-crossover phenotypes will correspond to these gametic genotypes, yielding offspring that express the white, echinus phenotype and offspring that express the yellow phenotype. Instead, determination of the actual double crossovers reveals them to be yellow, echinus flies and white flies. *Therefore, our assumed order is incorrect.*

3. If we consider arrangement II, with the ec/ec^+ alleles in the middle, or arrangement III, with the w/w^+ alleles in the middle:

$$\text{(II)} \; \frac{y \qquad ec \qquad w}{y^+ \qquad ec^+ \qquad w^+} \quad \text{or} \quad \text{(III)} \; \frac{y \qquad w \qquad ec}{y^+ \qquad w^+ \qquad ec^+}$$

we see that arrangement II again provides predicted double-crossover phenotypes that do not correspond to the actual (observed) double-crossover phenotypes. The predicted phenotypes are yellow, white flies and echinus flies in the F_2 generation. *Therefore, this order is also incorrect.* However, arrangement III produces the observed phenotypes—yellow, echinus flies and white flies. *Therefore, this arrangement, with the w gene in the middle, is correct.*

To summarize Method I: First, determine the arrangement of alleles on the homologs of the heterozygote yielding the crossover gametes by identifying the reciprocal non-crossover phenotypes. Then, test each of the three possible orders to determine which one yields the observed double-crossover phenotypes—*the one that does so represents the correct order.* This method is summarized in Figure 5–9.

Method II Method II also begins by determining the arrangement of alleles along each homolog of the heterozygous parent. In addition, it requires one further assumption: *Following a double-crossover event, the allele in the middle position will fall between the outside, or flanking, alleles that were present on the opposite parental homolog.*

To illustrate, assume order I, w–y–ec, in the following arrangement:

$$\frac{w \qquad y \qquad ec}{w^+ \qquad y^+ \qquad ec^+}$$

Following a double-crossover event, the y and y^+ alleles would be switched to this arrangement:

$$\frac{w \qquad y^+ \qquad ec}{w^+ \qquad y \qquad ec^+}$$

After segregation, two gametes would be formed:

$$\underline{w \quad y^+ \quad ec} \quad \text{and} \quad \underline{w^+ \quad y \quad ec^+}$$

Because the genotype of the gamete will be expressed directly in the phenotype following fertilization, the double-crossover phenotypes will be:

white, echinus flies and yellow flies

Note that the *yellow* allele, assumed to be in the middle, is now associated with the two outside markers of the other homolog, w^+ and ec^+. However, these predicted phenotypes do not coincide with the observed double-crossover phenotypes. Therefore, the *yellow* gene is not in the middle.

This same reasoning can be applied to the assumption that the *echinus* gene or the *white* gene is in the middle. In the former case, we will reach a negative conclusion. If we assume that the *white* gene is in the middle, the *predicted* and *actual* double crossovers coincide. Therefore, we conclude that the *white* gene is located between the *yellow* and *echinus* genes.

To summarize Method II, determine the arrangement of alleles on the homologs of the heterozygote yielding crossover gametes. Then examine the actual double-crossover phenotypes and identify the single allele that has been switched so that it is now no longer associated with its original neighboring alleles. That allele will be the one located between the other two in the sequence.

In our example *y*, *ec*, and *w* are on one homolog in the F_1 heterozygote, and y^+, ec^+, and w^+ are on the other. In the F_2 double-crossover classes, it is *w* and w^+ that have been switched. The *w* allele is now associated with y^+ and ec^+, while the w^+ allele is now associated with the *y* and *ec* alleles. Therefore, the *white* gene is in the middle, and the *yellow* and *echinus* genes are the flanking markers.

A Mapping Problem in Maize

Having established the basic principles of chromosome mapping, we will now consider a related problem in maize (corn). This analysis differs from the preceding example in two ways. First, the previous mapping cross involved X-linked genes. Here, we consider autosomal genes. Second, in the discussion of this cross, we will change our use of symbols (as first suggested in Chapter 4). Instead of using the gene symbols and superscripts (e.g., bm^+, v^+, and pr^+), we simply use + to denote each wild-type allele. This system is easier to manipulate but requires a better understanding of mapping procedures.

When we look at three autosomally linked genes in maize, our experimental cross must still meet the same three criteria we established for the X-linked genes in *Drosophila*: (1) One parent must be heterozygous for all traits under consideration; (2) the gametic genotypes produced by the heterozygote must be apparent from observing the phenotypes of the offspring; and (3) a sufficient sample size must be available for complete analysis.

In maize, the recessive mutant genes *bm* (*brown* midrib), *v* (*virescent* seedling), and *pr* (*purple* aleurone) are linked on chromosome 5. Assume that a female plant is known to be heterozygous for all three traits, but we do not know: (1) the arrangement of the mutant alleles on the maternal and paternal homologs of this heterozygote; (2) the sequence of genes; or (3) the map distances between the genes. What genotype must the male plant have to allow successful mapping? To meet the second criterion, the male must be homozygous for all three recessive mutant alleles. Otherwise, offspring of this cross showing a given phenotype might represent more than one genotype, making accurate mapping impossible. Note that this is equivalent to performing a testcross.

Figure 5–10 diagrams this cross. As shown, we know neither the *arrangement of alleles* nor the *sequence of loci* in the heterozygous female. Several possibilities are shown, but we have yet to determine which is correct. We don't know the sequence in the testcross male parent either, so we must designate it randomly. Note that we initially placed *v* in the middle. *This may or may not be correct.*

The offspring have been arranged in groups of two, representing each pair of reciprocal phenotypic classes. The four reciprocal classes are derived from no crossing over (NCO), each of two possible single-crossover events (SCO), and a double-crossover event (DCO).

To solve this problem, refer to Figures 5–10 and 5–11 as you consider the following questions:

1. *What is the correct heterozygous arrangement of alleles in the female parent?*

   Determine the two noncrossover classes, those that occur with the highest frequency. In this case, they are $\underline{+ \; v \; bm}$ and $\underline{pr \; + \; +}$. Therefore, the alleles on the homologs of the female parent must be distributed as shown in **Figure 5–11(a)**. These homologs segregate into gametes, unaffected by any recombination event. Any other arrangement of alleles will not yield the observed noncrossover classes. (Remember that $\underline{+ \; v \; bm}$ is equivalent to $\underline{pr^+ \; v \; bm}$ and that $\underline{pr \; + \; +}$ is equivalent to $\underline{pr \; v^+ \; bm^+}$.)

2. *What is the correct sequence of genes?*

   To answer this question, we will first use the approach described in Method I. We know, based on the answer to question 1, that the correct arrangement of alleles is

   $$\frac{+ \qquad v \qquad bm}{pr \qquad + \qquad +}$$

   But is the gene sequence correct? That is, will a double-crossover event yield the observed double-crossover

(a) Some possible allele arrangements and gene sequences in a heterozygous female

Which of the above is correct?

Heterozygous female   ×   Testcross male

(b) Actual results of mapping cross*

Phenotypes of offspring	Number	Total and percentage	Exchange classification
+ v bm	230	467 42.1%	Noncrossover (NCO)
pr + +	237		
+ + bm	82	161 14.5%	Single crossover (SCO)
pr v +	79		
+ v +	200	395 35.6%	Single crossover (SCO)
pr + bm	195		
pr v bm	44	86 7.8%	Double crossover (DCO)
+ + +	42		

*The sequence *pr* – *v* – *bm* may or may not be correct.

FIGURE 5–10 (a) Some possible allele arrangements and gene sequences in a heterozygous female. The data from a three-point mapping cross, depicted in (b), where the female is testcrossed, provide the basis for determining which combination of arrangement and sequence is correct. [See Figure 5–11(d).]

phenotypes following fertilization? *Observation shows that it will not* [**Figure 5–11(b)**]. Now try the other two orders [**Figure 5–11(c)** and **Figure 5–11(d)**], *keeping the same allelic arrangement:*

$$\frac{+ \quad bm \quad v}{pr \quad + \quad +} \quad \text{or} \quad \frac{v \quad + \quad bm}{+ \quad pr \quad +}$$

Only the order on the right yields the observed double-crossover gametes [Figure 5–11(d)]. Therefore, the *pr* gene is in the middle.

The same conclusion is reached if we use Method II to analyze the problem. In this case, no assumption of gene sequence is necessary. The arrangement of alleles along homologs in the heterozygous parent is

$$\frac{+ \quad v \quad bm}{pr \quad + \quad +}$$

The double-crossover gametes are also known:

$$\underline{pr \quad v \quad bm} \quad \text{and} \quad \underline{+ \quad + \quad +}$$

Possible allele arrangements and sequences	Testcross phenotypes	Explanation
(a) ![chromosome: + v bm / pr + +]	+ v bm and pr + +	Noncrossover phenotypes provide the basis for determining the correct arrangement of alleles on homologs
(b) ![+ v bm / pr + +]	+ + bm and pr v +	Expected double-crossover phenotypes if *v* is in the middle
(c) ![+ bm v / pr + +]	+ + v and pr bm +	Expected double-crossover phenotypes if *bm* is in the middle
(d) ![v + bm / + pr +]	v pr bm and + + +	Expected double-crossover phenotypes if *pr* is in the middle **(This is the *actual situation*.)**
(e) ![v + bm / + pr +]	v pr + and + + bm	Given that (a) and (d) are correct, single-crossover phenotypes when exchange occurs between *v* and *pr*
(f) ![v + bm / + pr +]	v + + and + pr bm	Given that (a) and (d) are correct, single-crossover phenotypes when exchange occurs between *pr* and *bm*
(g) Final map — v — pr — bm; 22.3, 43.4		

FIGURE 5–11 Producing a map of the three genes in the cross in Figure 5–10, where neither the arrangement of alleles nor the sequence of genes in the heterozygous female parent is known.

We can see that it is the *pr* allele that has shifted relative to its noncrossover arrangement, so as to be associated with *v* and *bm* following a double crossover. The latter two alleles (*v* and *bm*) were present together on one homolog, and they stayed together. Therefore, *pr* is the odd gene, so to speak, and is located in the middle. Thus, we arrive at the same arrangement and sequence as we did with Method I:

$$\frac{v \quad + \quad bm}{+ \quad pr \quad +}$$

3. *What is the distance between each pair of genes?*
Having established the correct sequence of loci as *v–pr–bm*, we can now determine the distance between

v and *pr* and between *pr* and *bm*. Remember that the map distance between two genes is calculated on the basis of all detectable recombinational events occurring between them. This includes both the single and double-crossover events.

Figure 5–11(e) shows that the phenotypes *v pr +* and *+ + bm* result from single crossovers between *v* and *pr*, and Figure 5–10 shows that those single crossovers account for 14.5 percent of the offspring. By adding the percentage of double crossovers (7.8 percent) to the number obtained for those single crossovers, we calculate the total distance between *v* and *pr* to be 22.3 mu.

Figure 5–11(f) shows that the phenotypes *v + +* and *+ pr bm* result from single crossovers between the *pr* and *bm* loci, totaling 35.6 percent, according to Figure 5–10. Adding the double-crossover classes (7.8 percent), we compute the distance between *pr* and *bm* as 43.4 mu. The final map for all three genes in this example is shown in **Figure 5–11(g)**.

N O W   S O L V E   T H I S

5–3 In *Drosophila*, a heterozygous female for the X-linked recessive traits *a*, *b*, and *c* was crossed to a male that phenotypically expressed *a*, *b*, and *c*. The offspring occurred in the following phenotypic ratios.

+	*b*	*c*	460
a	+	+	450
a	*b*	*c*	32
+	+	+	38
a	+	*c*	11
+	*b*	+	9

No other phenotypes were observed.
  (a) What is the genotypic arrangement of the alleles of these genes on the X chromosome of the female?
  (b) Determine the correct sequence and construct a map of these genes on the X chromosome.
  (c) What progeny phenotypes are missing? Why?

■ **HINT:** *This problem involves a three-point mapping experiment where only six phenotypic categories are observed, even though eight categories are typical of such a cross. The key to its solution is to be aware that if the distances between the loci are relatively small, the sample size may be too small for the predicted number of double crossovers to be recovered, even though reciprocal pairs of single crossovers are seen. You should write the missing gametes down as double crossovers and record zeros for their frequency of appearance.*

For more practice, see Problems 15, 16, and 17.

5.4   As the Distance between Two Genes Increases, Mapping Estimates Become More Inaccurate

So far, we have assumed that crossover frequencies are directly proportional to the distance between any two loci along the chromosome. However, it is not always possible to detect all crossover events. A case in point is a double exchange that occurs between the two loci

in question. As shown in **Figure 5–12(a)**, if a double exchange occurs, the original arrangement of alleles on each nonsister homolog is recovered. Therefore, even though crossing over has occurred, it is impossible to detect. This phenomenon is true for all even-numbered exchanges between two loci.

Furthermore, as a result of complications posed by multiple-strand exchanges, mapping determinations usually underestimate the actual distance between two genes. The farther apart two genes are, the greater the probability that undetected crossovers will occur. While the discrepancy is minimal for two genes relatively close together, the degree of inaccuracy increases as the distance increases, as shown in the graph of recombination frequency versus map distance in **Figure 5–12(b)**. There, the theoretical frequency where a direct correlation between recombination and map distance exists is contrasted with the actual frequency observed as the distance between two genes increases. The most accurate maps are constructed from experiments in which genes are relatively close together.

Interference and the Coefficient of Coincidence

As review of the product law in Section 5.3 would indicate, the expected frequency of multiple exchanges, such as double crossovers, can be predicted once the distance between genes is established. For example, in the maize cross of the previous section, the distance between *v* and *pr* is 22.3 mu, and the distance between *pr* and *bm* is 43.4 mu. If the two single crossovers that make up a double crossover occur independently of one another, we can calculate the expected frequency of double crossovers (DCO_{exp}) as follows:

$$DCO_{exp} = (0.223) \times (0.434) = 0.097 = 9.7\%$$

Often in mapping experiments, the observed DCO frequency is less than the expected number of DCOs. In the maize cross, for example, only 7.8 percent of the DCOs are observed when 9.7 percent are expected. **Interference (*I*)**, the inhibition of further crossover events by a crossover event in a nearby region of the chromosome, causes this reduction.

To quantify the disparities that result from interference, we calculate the **coefficient of coincidence (*C*)**:

$$C = \frac{\text{Observed DCO}}{\text{Expected DCO}}$$

In the maize cross, we have

$$C = \frac{0.078}{0.097} = 0.804$$

(a) Two-strand double exchange

No detectable recombinants

(b)

(a) A double crossover is undetected because no rearrangement of alleles occurs. (b) The theoretical and actual percentage of recombinant chromatids versus map distance. The straight line shows the theoretical relationship if a direct correlation between recombination and map distance exists. The curved line is the actual relationship derived from studies of *Drosophila*, *Neurospora*, and *Zea mays*.

Once we have found *C*, we can quantify interference (*I*) by using this simple equation

$$I = 1 - C$$

In the maize cross, we have

$$I = 1.000 - 0.804 = 0.196$$

If interference is complete and no double crossovers occur, then $I = 1.0$. If fewer DCOs than expected occur, *I* is a positive number and **positive interference** has occurred. If more DCOs than expected occur, *I* is a negative number and **negative interference** has occurred. In this example, *I* is a positive number (0.196), indicating that 19.6 percent fewer double crossovers occurred than expected.

Positive interference is most often observed in eukaryotic systems. In *C. elegans*, for example, only one crossover event per chromosome is observed, and interference along each chromosome is complete ($C = 1.0$). In other organisms, the closer genes are to one another along the chromosome, the more positive interference occurs. Interference in *Drosophila* is often complete within a distance of 10 map units. This observation suggests that physical constraints preventing the formation of closely spaced chiasmata contribute to interference. The interpretation is consistent with the finding that interference decreases as the genes in question are located farther apart. In the maize cross illustrated in Figures 5–10 and 5–11, the three genes are relatively far apart, and 80 percent of the expected double crossovers are observed.

5.5 *Drosophila* Genes Have Been Extensively Mapped

In organisms such as fruit flies, maize, and the mouse, where large numbers of mutants have been discovered and where mapping crosses are possible, extensive maps of each chromosome have been constructed. **Figure 5–13** presents partial maps of the four chromosomes of *Drosophila melanogaster*. Virtually every morphological feature of the fruit fly has been subjected to mutation. Each locus affected by mutation is first localized to one of the four chromosomes, or linkage groups, and then mapped in relation to other genes present on that chromosome. As you can see, the genetic map of the X chromosome is somewhat shorter than that of autosome II or III. In comparison to these three, autosome IV is miniscule. Cytological evidence has shown that the relative lengths of the genetic maps correlate roughly with the relative physical lengths of these chromosomes.

EVOLVING CONCEPT OF THE GENE

Based on the gene-mapping studies in *Drosophila* and many other organisms from the 1920s through the mid-1950s, geneticists regarded genes as hereditary units organized in a specific sequence along chromosomes, between which recombination could occur. Genes were thus viewed as indivisible "beads on a string." ■

FIGURE 5–13 A partial genetic map of the four chromosomes of *Drosophila melanogaster*. The circle on each chromosome represents the position of the centromere. Chromosome I is the X chromosome. Chromosome IV is not drawn to scale; that is, it is relatively smaller than indicated.

5.6 Lod Score Analysis and Somatic Cell Hybridization Were Historically Important in Creating Human Chromosome Maps

In humans, genetic experiments involving carefully planned crosses and large numbers of offspring are neither ethical nor feasible, so the earliest linkage studies were based on pedigree analysis. These studies attempted to establish whether certain traits were X-linked or autosomal. As we showed earlier in the text (see Chapter 4), traits determined by genes located on the X chromosome result in characteristic pedigrees; thus, such genes were easier to identify. For autosomal traits, geneticists tried to distinguish clearly whether pairs of traits demonstrated linkage or independent assortment. When extensive pedigrees are available, it is possible to conclude that two genes under consideration are closely linked (i.e., rarely separated by crossing over) from the fact that the two traits segregate together. This approach established linkage between the genes encoding the **Rh antigens** and the gene responsible for the phenotype referred to as **elliptocytosis,** where the shape of erythrocytes is oval. It was hoped that from these kinds of observations a human gene map could be created.

A difficulty arises, however, when two genes of interest are separated on a chromosome to the degree that recombinant gametes are formed, obscuring linkage in a pedigree. In these cases, an approach relying on probability calculations, called the **lod score method,** helps to demonstrate linkage. First devised by J. B. S. Haldane and C. A. Smith in 1947 and refined by Newton Morton in 1955, the lod score (standing for *log* of the *odds* favoring linkage) assesses the probability that a particular pedigree (or several pedigrees for the same traits of interest) involving two traits reflects genetic linkage between them. First, the probability is calculated that the family (pedigree) data concerning two traits conform to transmission without linkage—that is, the traits appear to be independently assorting. Then the probability is calculated that the identical family data for these same traits result from linkage with a specified recombination frequency. These probability calculations factor in the statistical significance at the $p = 0.05$ level. The ratio of these probability values is then calculated and converted to the logarithm of this value, which reflects the "odds" for, and against, linkage. Traditionally, a value of 3.0 or higher strongly indicates linkage, whereas a value of -2.0 or less argues strongly against linkage. Values between -2.0 and 3.0 are considered to be inconclusive.

The lod score method represented an important advance in assigning human genes to specific chromosomes and in constructing preliminary human chromosome maps. However, its accuracy is limited by the extent of the pedigree, and the initial results were discouraging—both because of this limitation and because of the relatively high haploid number of human chromosomes (23). By 1960, very little autosomal linkage information had become available. Today, however, in contrast to its restricted impact when originally developed, this elegant technique has become important in human linkage analysis, owing to the discovery of countless molecular *DNA markers* along every human chromosome. The discovery of these markers, which behave just as genes do in occupying a particular locus along a chromosome, was a result of recombinant DNA techniques (Chapter 20) and genomic analysis (Chapter 21). Any human trait may now be tested for linkage with such markers. We will return to a consideration of DNA markers in Section 5.7.

In the 1960s, a new technique, **somatic cell hybridization,** proved to be an immense aid in assigning human genes to their respective chromosomes. This technique, first discovered by Georges Barski, relies on the fact that two cells in culture can be induced to fuse into a single hybrid cell. Barski used two mouse-cell lines, but it soon became evident that cells from different organisms could also be fused. When fusion occurs, an initial cell type called a **heterokaryon** is produced. The hybrid cell contains two nuclei in a common cytoplasm. Using the proper techniques, we can fuse human and mouse cells, for example, and isolate the hybrids from the parental cells.

As the heterokaryons are cultured *in vitro,* two interesting changes occur. Eventually, the nuclei fuse together, creating a **synkaryon.** Then, as culturing is continued for many generations, chromosomes from one of the two parental species are gradually lost. In the case of the human–mouse hybrid, human chromosomes are lost randomly until eventually the synkaryon has a full complement of mouse chromosomes and only a few human chromosomes. It is the preferential loss of human chromosomes (rather than mouse chromosomes) that makes possible the assignment of human genes to the chromosomes on which they reside.

The experimental rationale is straightforward. If a specific human gene product is synthesized in a synkaryon containing three human chromosomes, for example, then the gene responsible for that product must reside on one of the three human chromosomes remaining in the hybrid cell. On the other hand, if the human gene product is not synthesized in the synkaryon, the responsible gene cannot be present on any of the remaining three human chromosomes. Ideally, one would have a panel of 23 hybrid cell lines, each with a different human chromosome, allowing the immediate assignment to a particular chromosome of any human gene for which the product could be characterized.

In practice, a panel of cell lines each of which contains several remaining human chromosomes is most often used. The correlation of the presence or absence of each chromosome with the presence or absence of each gene product is called **synteny testing.** Consider, for example, the hypothetical data provided in **Figure 5–14,** where four gene products (A, B, C, and D) are tested in relationship to eight human chromosomes. Let us carefully analyze the results to locate the gene that produces product A.

1. Product A is not produced by cell line 23, but chromosomes 1, 2, 3, and 4 are present in cell line 23. Therefore, we can rule out the presence of gene *A* on those four chromosomes and conclude that it might be on chromosome 5, 6, 7, or 8.

2. Product A is produced by cell line 34, which contains chromosomes 5 and 6, but not 7 and 8. Therefore, gene *A* is on chromosome 5 or 6, but cannot be on 7 or 8 because they are absent, even though product A is produced.

3. Product A is also produced by cell line 41, which contains chromosome 5 but not chromosome 6. Therefore, gene *A* is on chromosome 5, according to this analysis.

Using a similar approach, we can assign gene *B* to chromosome 3. Perform the analysis for yourself to demonstrate that this is correct.

Hybrid cell lines	Human chromosomes present								Gene products expressed			
	1	2	3	4	5	6	7	8	A	B	C	D
23	●	●	●	●					−	+	−	+
34	●	●			●	●			+	−	−	+
41	●		●		●		●		+	+	−	+

FIGURE 5–14 A hypothetical grid of data used in synteny testing to assign genes to their appropriate human chromosomes. Three somatic hybrid cell lines, designated 23, 34, and 41, have each been scored for the presence, or absence, of human chromosomes 1 through 8, as well as for their ability to produce the hypothetical human gene products A, B, C, and D.

Gene *C* presents a unique situation. The data indicate that it is not present on chromosomes 1–7. While it might be on chromosome 8, no direct evidence supports this conclusion. Other panels are needed. We leave gene *D* for you to analyze. Upon what chromosome does it reside?

By using the approach just described, researchers were able to assign literally hundreds of human genes to one chromosome or another. To map genes for which the products have yet to be discovered, researchers have had to rely on other approaches. For example, by combining recombinant DNA technology with pedigree analysis, it was possible to assign the genes responsible for Huntington disease, cystic fibrosis, and neurofibromatosis to their respective chromosomes 4, 7, and 17. Modern genomic analysis has expanded our knowledge of the mapping location of countless other human traits, as described in the next section.

5.7 Chromosome Mapping Is Now Possible Using DNA Markers and Annotated Computer Databases

Although traditional methods based on recombination analysis have produced detailed chromosomal maps in several organisms, maps in other organisms (including humans) that do not lend themselves to such studies are greatly limited. Fortunately, the development of technology allowing direct analysis of DNA has greatly enhanced mapping in those organisms. We will address this topic using humans as an example.

Progress has initially relied on the discovery of **DNA markers** (mentioned earlier) that have been identified during recombinant DNA and genomic studies. These markers are short segments of DNA whose sequence and location are known, making them useful landmarks for mapping purposes. The analysis of human genes in relation to these markers has extended our knowledge of the location within the genome of countless genes, which is the ultimate goal of mapping (see Figure 21–11).

The earliest examples are the DNA markers referred to as **restriction fragment length polymorphisms (RFLPs)** (see Chapter 22) and **microsatellites** or **short tandem repeats** (see Chapter 12). RFLPS are polymorphic sites generated when specific DNA sequences are recognized and cut by restriction enzymes. Microsatellites are short repetitive sequences that are found throughout the genome, and they vary in the number of repeats at any given site. For example, the two-nucleotide sequence CA is repeated 5–50 times per site [$(CA)_n$] and appears throughout the genome approximately every 10,000 bases, on average. Microsatellites may be identified not only by the number of repeats but by the DNA sequences that flank them. More recently, variation in single nucleotides, called **single-nucleotide polymorphisms** (**SNPs**, also called "snips"), has been utilized. Found throughout the genome, up to several million of these variations may be screened for an association with a disease or trait of interest, thus providing geneticists with a means to identify and locate related genes.

Cystic fibrosis offers an early example of a gene located by using DNA markers. It is a life-shortening autosomal recessive exocrine disorder resulting in excessive, thick mucus that impedes the function of organs such as the lung and pancreas. After scientists established that the gene causing this disorder is located on chromosome 7, they were then able to pinpoint its exact location on the long arm (the q arm) of that chromosome.

Several years ago (June 2007), using SNPs as DNA markers, associations between 24 genomic locations were established with seven common human diseases: *Type 1* (insulin dependent) and *Type 2 diabetes*, *Crohn's disease* (inflammatory bowel disease), *hypertension*, *coronary artery disease*, *bipolar* (manic-depressive) *disorder*, and *rheumatoid arthritis*. In each case, an inherited susceptibility effect was mapped to a specific location on a specific chromosome within the genome. In some cases, this either confirmed or led to the identification of a specific gene involved in the cause of the disease.

During the past 15 years or so, dramatic improvements in DNA sequencing technology have resulted in a proliferation of **sequence maps** for humans and many other species. Sequence maps provide the finest level of mapping detail because they pinpoint the nucleotide sequence of genes (and noncoding sequences) on a chromosome. The Human Genome Project resulted in sequence maps for all human chromosomes, providing an incredible level of detail about human gene sequences, the specific location of genes on a chromosome, and the proximity of genes and noncoding sequences to each other, among other details. For instance, when human chromosome sequences were analyzed by software programs, an approach called **bioinformatics**, to be discussed later in the text (see Chapter 22), geneticists could utilize such data to map possible protein-coding sequences in the genome. This led to the identification of thousands of potential genes that were previously unknown.

The many Human Genome Project databases that are now available make it possible to map genes along a human chromosome in base-pair distances rather than recombination frequency. This distinguishes what is referred to as a *physical map* of the genome from the *genetic maps* described above. When the genome sequence of a species is available, mapping by linkage or other genetic mapping approaches becomes obsolete.

(For an example of a physical map developed by DNA sequencing refer to Figure 21–12.) Also, try the Exploring Genomics feature at the end of this chapter to visit Human Genome Project databases that detail sequence maps of human chromosomes. From these sites you can pinpoint the nucleotide sequence of all known or potential genes revealed by the Human Genome Project to date! We will return to this topic in much greater detail later in the text (see Chapters 21 and 22).

5.8 Crossing Over Involves a Physical Exchange between Chromatids

Once genetic mapping techniques had been developed, they were used to study the relationship between the chiasmata observed in meiotic prophase I and crossing over. For example, are chiasmata visible manifestations of crossover events? If so, then crossing over in higher organisms appears to be the result of an actual physical exchange between homologous chromosomes. That this is the case was demonstrated independently in the 1930s by Harriet Creighton and Barbara McClintock in *Zea mays* (maize) and by Curt Stern in *Drosophila*.

Because the experiments are similar, we will consider only one of them, the work with maize. Creighton and McClintock studied two linked genes on chromosome 9 of the maize plant. At one locus, the alleles *colorless* (*c*) and *colored* (*C*) control endosperm coloration (the endosperm is the nutritive tissue inside the corn kernel). At the other locus, the alleles *starchy* (*Wx*) and *waxy* (*wx*) control the carbohydrate characteristics of the endosperm. The maize plant studied was heterozygous at both loci. The key to this experiment is that one of the homologs contained two unique cytological markers. The markers consisted of a densely stained knob at one end of the chromosome and a translocated piece of another chromosome (8) at the other end. The arrangements of these alleles and markers could be detected cytologically and are shown in **Figure 5–15**.

Creighton and McClintock crossed this plant to one homozygous for the *colorless* allele (*c*) and heterozygous for the *waxy/starchy* alleles. They obtained a variety of different phenotypes in the offspring, but they were most interested in one that occurred as a result of a crossover involving the chromosome with the unique cytological markers. They examined the chromosomes of this plant,

FIGURE 5–15 The phenotypes and chromosome compositions of parents and recombinant offspring in Creighton and McClintock's experiment in maize. The knob and translocated segment served as cytological markers, which established that crossing over involves an actual exchange of chromosome arms.

having a colorless, waxy phenotype (Case I in Figure 5–15), for the presence of the cytological markers. If genetic crossing over was accompanied by a physical exchange between homologs, the translocated chromosome would still be present, but the knob would not. This was the case! In a second plant (Case II), the phenotype colored, starchy should result from either nonrecombinant gametes or crossing over. Some of the cases then ought to contain chromosomes with the dense knob but not the translocated chromosome. This condition was also found, and the conclusion that a physical exchange had taken place was again supported. Along with Curt Stern's findings in *Drosophila*, this work clearly established that crossing over has a cytological basis.

Once we have discussed DNA in more detail (see Chapter 10), we will return to the topic of crossing over to examine how breakage and reunion occur between strands of DNA in chromatids. This discussion (see Chapter 11) will provide a better understanding of genetic recombination.

5.9   Exchanges Also Occur between Sister Chromatids during Mitosis

Considering that crossing over occurs between synapsed homologs in meiosis, we might ask whether such a physical exchange occurs between sister chromatids that are aligned together during mitosis. Each individual chromosome in prophase and metaphase of mitosis consists of two identical sister chromatids, joined at a common centromere. A number of experiments have demonstrated that reciprocal exchanges similar to crossing over do occur between sister chromatids. While these **sister chromatid exchanges (SCEs)** do not produce new allelic combinations, evidence is accumulating that attaches significance to these events.

Identification and study of SCEs are facilitated by several unique staining techniques. In one approach, cells are allowed to replicate for two generations in the presence of the thymidine analog bromodeoxyuridine (BrdU). Following two rounds of replication, each pair of sister chromatids has one member with one strand of DNA "labeled" with BrdU and the other member with both strands labeled with BrdU. Using a differential stain, chromatids with the analog in both strands stain *less brightly* than chromatids with BrdU in only one strand. As a result, any SCEs are readily detectable. In **Figure 5–16**, numerous instances of SCE events are clearly evident. Because of their patterns of alternating patches, these sister chromatids are sometimes referred to as **harlequin chromosomes.**

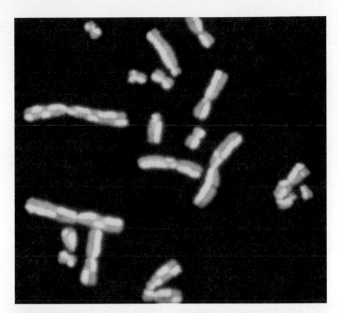

FIGURE 5–16   Demonstration of sister chromatid exchanges (SCEs) in mitotic chromosomes. Sometimes called harlequin chromosomes because of the alternating patterns they exhibit, sister chromatids containing the thymidine analog BrdU are seen to fluoresce *less* brightly where they contain the analog in both DNA strands than when they contain the analog in only one strand. These chromosomes were stained with 33258-Hoechst reagent and acridine orange and then viewed under fluorescence microscopy.

The significance of SCEs is still uncertain, but several observations have led to great interest in this phenomenon. We know, for example, that agents that induce chromosome damage (e.g., viruses, X rays, ultraviolet light, and certain chemical mutagens) also increase the frequency of SCEs. Further, the frequency of SCEs is elevated in **Bloom syndrome,** a human disorder caused by a mutation in the *BLM* gene on chromosome 15. This rare, recessively inherited disease is characterized by prenatal and postnatal retardation of growth, a great sensitivity of the facial skin to the sun, immune deficiency, a predisposition to malignant and benign tumors, and abnormal behavior patterns. The chromosomes from cultured leukocytes, bone marrow cells, and fibroblasts derived from homozygotes are very fragile and unstable when compared with those derived from homozygous and heterozygous normal individuals. Increased breaks and rearrangements between nonhomologous chromosomes are observed in addition to excessive amounts of sister chromatid exchanges. Work by James German and colleagues suggests that the *BLM* gene encodes an enzyme called **DNA helicase,** which is best known for its role in DNA replication (see Chapter 11).

The mechanisms of exchange between nonhomologous chromosomes and between sister chromatids may prove to share common features because the frequency of both events increases substantially in individuals with certain genetic disorders. These findings suggest that further study of sister chromatid exchange may contribute to the understanding of recombination mechanisms and to the relative stability of normal and genetically abnormal chromosomes. We shall encounter still another demonstration of SCEs when we consider replication of DNA (see Chapter 11).

5.10 Did Mendel Encounter Linkage?

We conclude this chapter by examining a modern-day interpretation of the experiments that form the cornerstone of transmission genetics—Mendel's crosses with garden peas.

Some observers believe that Mendel had extremely good fortune in his classic experiments with the garden pea. In their view, he did not encounter any linkage relationships between the seven mutant characters in his crosses. Had Mendel obtained highly variable data characteristic of linkage and crossing over, these observers say, he might not have succeeded in recognizing the basic patterns of inheritance and interpreting them correctly.

The article by Stig Blixt, reprinted in its entirety in the box that follows, demonstrates the inadequacy of this hypothesis. As we shall see, some of Mendel's genes were indeed linked. We shall leave it to Stig Blixt to enlighten you as to why Mendel did not detect linkage.

Why Didn't Gregor Mendel Find Linkage?

It is quite often said that Mendel was very fortunate not to run into the complication of linkage during his experiments. He used seven genes, and the pea has only seven chromosomes. Some have said that had he taken just one more, he would have had problems. This, however, is a gross oversimplification. The actual situation, most probably, is that Mendel worked with three genes in chromosome 4, two genes in chromosome 1, and one gene in each of chromosomes 5 and 7. (See Table 1.)

It seems at first glance that, out of the 21 dihybrid combinations Mendel theoretically could have studied, no less than four (that is, a–i, v–fa, v–le, fa–le) ought to have resulted in linkages. As found, however, in hundreds of crosses and shown by the genetic map of the pea, a and i in chromosome 1 are so distantly located on the chromosome that no linkage is normally detected. The same is true for v and le on the one hand, and fa on the other, in chromosome 4. This leaves v–le, which ought to have shown linkage.

Mendel, however, does not seem to have published this particular combination and thus, presumably, never made the appropriate cross to obtain both genes segregating simultaneously.

It is therefore not so astonishing that Mendel did not run into the complication of linkage, although he did not avoid it by choosing one gene from each chromosome.

Stig Blixt

Weibullsholm Plant Breeding Institute, Landskrona, Sweden, and Centro de Energia Nuclear na Agricultura, Piracicaba, SP, Brazil

Source: Reprinted by permission from Macmillan Publishers Ltd: Nature, "Molecular Structure of Nucleic Acids: A Structure for Deoxyribose Nucleic Acid" by F.H.C. Crick and J.D. Watson, *Nature*, Vol. 171, No. 4356, pp. 737–38. Copyright 1953. www.nature.com

TABLE 1 Relationship between Modern Genetic Terminology and Character Pairs Used by Mendel

Character Pair Used by Mendel	Alleles in Modern Terminology	Located in Chromosome
Seed color, yellow–green	I–i	1
Seed coat and flowers, colored–white	A–a	1
Mature pods, smooth expanded–wrinkled indented	V–v	4
Inflorescences, from leaf axis–umbellate in top of plant	Fa–fa	4
Plant height, 0.5–1 m	Le–le	4
Unripe pods, green–yellow	Gp–gp	5
Mature seeds, smooth–wrinkled	R–r	7

Human Chromosome Maps on the Internet

MasteringGenetics™ Visit the
Study Area: Exploring Genomics

In this chapter we discussed how recombination data can be analyzed to develop chromosome maps based on linkage. Although linkage analysis and chromosome mapping continue to be important approaches in genetics, chromosome maps are increasingly being developed for many species using genomics techniques to sequence entire chromosomes. As a result of the Human Genome Project, maps of human chromosomes are now freely available on the Internet. With the click of a mouse you can have immediate access to an incredible wealth of information. In this exercise we will explore the **National Center for Biotechnology Information (NCBI) Genes and Disease** Web site to learn more about human chromosome maps.

■ **NCBI Genes and Disease**

The NCBI Web site is an outstanding resource for genome data. Here we explore the Genes and Disease site, which presents human chromosome maps that show the locations of specific disease genes.

1. Access the Genes and Disease site at http://www.ncbi.nlm.nih.gov/books/ NBK22183/

2. Under contents, click on "Chromosome Map" to see a page with an image of a karyotype of human chromosomes. Click on a chromosome in the chromosome map image, scroll down the page to view a chromosome or click on a chromosome listed on the right side of the page. For example, click on chromosome 7. Notice that the number of genes on the chromosomes and the number of base pairs the chromosome contains are displayed above the image.

3. Look again at chromosome 7. At first you might think there are only five disease genes on this chromosome because the initial view shows only selected disease genes. However, if you click the "MapViewer" link for the chromosome (just above the drawing), you will see detailed information about the chromosome, including a complete "Master Map" of the genes it contains, including the symbols used in naming genes.

    Links: The items in the "Links" column provide access to OMIM (Online Mendelian Inheritance in Man, discussed in the "Exploring Genomics" feature for Chapter 3) data for a particular gene, as well as to protein information (*pr*) and lists of homologous genes (*hm;* these are other genes that have similar sequences).

4. Click on the links in MapViewer to learn more about a gene of interest.

5. Scan the chromosome maps in Map Viewer until you see one of the genes listed as a "hypothetical gene or protein."

    a. What does it mean if a gene or protein is referred to as hypothetical?

    b. What information do you think genome scientists use to assign a gene locus for a gene encoding a hypothetical protein?

Visit the **NCBI Map Viewer** homepage (http://www.ncbi.nlm.nih.gov/projects/ mapview/) for an excellent database containing chromosome maps for a wide variety of different organisms. Search this database to learn more about chromosome maps for an organism you are interested in.

CASE STUDY | Links to autism

As parents of an autistic child, a couple decided that entering a research study would not only educate them about their son's condition, but also help further research into this complex, behaviorally defined disorder. In an interview, researchers explained to the parents that autism results from the action of hundreds of genes and that no single gene accounts for more than a small percentage of cases. Recent studies have identified 18 genes that have a higher likelihood of involvement, referred to as candidate genes; three of these, on chromosomes 2, 7, and 14, are regarded as very strong candidate genes. Generally unaware of the principles of basic genetics, the couple asked a number of interesting questions. If you were the interviewer, how would you respond to them?

1. How might identification of a "candidate" gene be helpful in treating autism?

2. Because there are hundreds of genes involved, is it possible that our children might inherit several or even many mutant versions of these genes?

3. With such a complex genetic condition that may also depend on environmental factors, is there a way to calculate the risk that our next child will be autistic?

4. Is prenatal diagnosis for autism possible?

Summary Points

1. Genes located on the same chromosome are said to be linked. Alleles of linked genes located close together on the same homolog are usually transmitted together during gamete formation.
2. Crossover frequency between linked genes during gamete formation is proportional to the distance between genes, providing the experimental basis for mapping the location of genes relative to one another along the chromosome.
3. Determining the sequence of genes in a three-point mapping experiment requires analysis of double-crossover gametes, as reflected in the phenotype of the offspring receiving those gametes.
4. Interference describes the extent to which a crossover in one region of a chromosome influences the occurrence of a cross-

over in an adjacent region of the chromosome and is quantified by calculating the coefficient of coincidence (*C*).
5. Human linkage studies, initially relying on pedigree and lod score analysis, and subsequently on somatic cell hybridization techniques, are now enhanced by the use of newly discovered molecular DNA markers.
6. Cytological investigations of both maize and *Drosophila* reveal that crossing over involves a physical exchange of segments between nonsister chromatids.
7. Recombination events are known to occur between sister chromatids in mitosis and are referred to as sister chromatid exchanges (SCEs).

INSIGHTS AND SOLUTIONS

1. In a series of two-point mapping crosses involving three genes linked on chromosome III in *Drosophila*, the following distances were calculated:

$$cd-sr \text{ 13 mu}$$
$$cd-ro \text{ 16 mu}$$

(a) Why can't we determine the sequence and construct a map of these three genes?

(b) What mapping data will resolve the issue?

(c) Can we tell which of the sequences shown here is correct?

$$ro \xrightarrow{\quad 16 \quad} cd \xrightarrow{\quad 13 \quad} sr$$

or

$$sr \xrightarrow{\quad 13 \quad} cd \xrightarrow{\quad 16 \quad} ro$$

Solution:

(a) It is impossible to do so because there are two possibilities based on these limited data:

Case 1: $$cd \xrightarrow{\quad 13 \quad} sr \xrightarrow{\ 3\ } ro$$

or

Case 2: $$ro \xrightarrow{\quad 16 \quad} cd \xrightarrow{\quad 13 \quad} sr$$

(b) The map distance is determined by crossing over between *ro* and *sr*. If case 1 is correct, it should be 3 mu, and if case 2 is correct, it should be 29 mu. In fact, this distance is 29 mu, demonstrating that case 2 is correct.

(c) No; based on the mapping data, they are equivalent.

2. In *Drosophila*, *Lyra (Ly)* and *Stubble (Sb)* are dominant mutations located at loci 40 and 58, respectively, on chromosome III. A recessive mutation with bright red eyes was discovered and shown also to be on chromosome III. A map is obtained by crossing a female who is heterozygous for all three mutations to a male homozygous for the *bright red* mutation (which we refer to here as *br*). The data in the table are generated. Determine the location of the *br* mutation on

chromosome III. By referring to Figure 5–13, predict what mutation has been discovered. How could you be sure?

Phenotype			Number
(1) *Ly*	*Sb*	*br*	404
(2) +	+	+	422
(3) *Ly*	+	+	18
(4) +	*Sb*	*br*	16
(5) *Ly*	+	*br*	75
(6) +	*Sb*	+	59
(7) *Ly*	*Sb*	+	4
(8) +	+	*br*	2
Total			=1000

Solution: First determine the distribution of the alleles between the homologs of the heterozygous crossover parent (the female in this case). To do this, locate the most frequent reciprocal phenotypes, which arise from the noncrossover gametes. These are phenotypes 1 and 2. Each phenotype represents the alleles on one of the homologs. Therefore, the distribution of alleles is

Second, determine the correct *sequence* of the three loci along the chromosome. This is done by determining which sequence yields the observed double-crossover phenotypes that are the least frequent reciprocal phenotypes (7 and 8). If the sequence is correct as written, then a double crossover, depicted here, would yield *Ly* + *br* and + *Sb* + as phenotypes. Inspection shows that these categories (5 and 6) are actually single crossovers, not double crossovers. Therefore, the sequence, as written, is incorrect. There are only two other possible sequences. Either the *Ly* gene (Case A below) or the *br* gene (Case B below) is in the middle between the other two genes.

Comparison with the actual data shows that case B is correct. The double-crossover gametes 7 and 8 yield flies that express *Ly* and *Sb* but not *br*, or express *br* but not *Ly* and *Sb*. Therefore, the correct *arrangement* and *sequence* are as follows:

Once the sequence is found, determine the location of *br* relative to *Ly* and *Sb*. A single crossover between *Ly* and *br*, as shown here,

yields flies that are *Ly* + + and + *br Sb* (phenotypes 3 and 4). Therefore, the distance between the *Ly* and *br* loci is equal to

$$\frac{18 + 16 + 4 + 2}{1000} = \frac{40}{1000} = 0.04 = 4 \text{ mu}$$

Remember that, because we need to know the frequency of all crossovers between *Ly* and *br*, we must add in the double crossovers, since they represent two single crossovers occurring simultaneously. Similarly, the distance between the *br* and *Sb* loci is derived mainly from single crossovers between them.

This event yields *Ly br* + and + + *Sb* phenotypes (phenotypes 5 and 6). Therefore, the distance equals

$$\frac{75 + 59 + 4 + 2}{1000} = \frac{140}{1000} = 0.14 = 14 \text{ mu}$$

The final map shows that *br* is located at locus 44, since *Lyra* and *Stubble* are known:

Inspection of Figure 5–13 reveals that the mutation *scarlet*, which produces bright red eyes, is known to sit at locus 44, so it is reasonable to hypothesize that the *bright red* eye mutation is an allele of *scarlet*. To test this hypothesis, we could cross females of our *bright red* mutant with known *scarlet* males. If the two mutations are alleles, no complementation will occur, and all progeny will reveal a bright red mutant eye phenotype. If complementation occurs, all progeny will show normal brick-red (wild-type) eyes, since the *bright red* mutation and *scarlet* are at different loci. (They are probably very close together.) In such a case, all progeny will be heterozygous at both the *bright red* and the *scarlet* loci and will not express either mutation because they are both recessive. This cross represents what is called an *allelism test.*

3. In rabbits, black color (*B*) is dominant to brown (*b*), while full color (*C*) is dominant to chinchilla (*c^{ch}*). The genes controlling these traits are linked. Rabbits that are heterozygous for both traits and express black, full color were crossed with rabbits that express brown, chinchilla, with the following results:

31 brown, chinchilla

34 black, full color

16 brown, full color

19 black, chinchilla

Determine the arrangement of alleles in the heterozygous parents and the map distance between the two genes.

Solution: This is a two-point mapping problem. The two most prevalent reciprocal phenotypes are the noncrossovers, and the less frequent reciprocal phenotypes arise from a single crossover. The distribution of alleles is derived from the noncrossover phenotypes because they enter gametes intact.

The single crossovers give rise to 35/100 offspring (35 percent). Therefore, the distance between the two genes is 35 mu.

Problems and Discussion Questions

HOW DO WE KNOW?

1. In this chapter, we focused on linkage, chromosomal mapping, and many associated phenomena. In the process, we found many opportunities to consider the methods and reasoning by which much of this information was acquired. From the explanations given in the chapter, what answers would you propose to the following fundamental questions?
(a) How was it established experimentally that the frequency of recombination (crossing over) between two genes is related to the distance between them along the chromosome?
(b) How do we know that specific genes are linked on a single chromosome, in contrast to being located on separate chromosomes?
(c) How do we know that crossing over results from a physical exchange between chromatids?
(d) How do we know that sister chromatids undergo recombination during mitosis?
(e) When designed matings cannot be conducted in an organism (for example, in humans), how do we learn that genes are linked, and how do we map them?

CONCEPT QUESTION

2. Review the Chapter Concepts list on page 104. Most of these center around the process of crossing over between linked genes. Write a short essay that discusses how crossing over can be detected and how the resultant data provide the basis of chromosome mapping.

3. Describe the cytological observation that suggests that crossing over occurs during the first meiotic prophase.

4. Why does more crossing over occur between two distantly linked genes than between two genes that are very close together on the same chromosome?

5. Explain why a 50 percent recovery of single-crossover products is the upper limit, even when crossing over *always* occurs between two linked genes?

6. Why are double-crossover events expected less frequently than single-crossover events?

7. What is the proposed basis for positive interference?

8. What two essential criteria must be met in order to execute a successful mapping cross?

9. The genes *dumpy* (*dp*), *clot* (*cl*), and *apterous* (*ap*) are linked on chromosome II of *Drosophila*. In a series of two-point mapping crosses, the following genetic distances were determined. What is the sequence of the three genes?

dp–ap	42
dp–cl	3
ap–cl	39

10. Colored aleurone in the kernels of corn is due to the dominant allele *R*. The recessive allele *r*, when homozygous, produces colorless aleurone. The plant color (not the kernel color) is controlled by another gene with two alleles, *Y* and *y*. The dominant *Y* allele results in green color, whereas the homozygous presence of the recessive *y* allele causes the plant to appear yellow. In a testcross between a plant of unknown genotype and a plant that is homozygous recessive for both traits, the following progeny were obtained:

colored, green	88
colored, yellow	12
colorless, green	8
colorless, yellow	92

Explain how these results were obtained by determining the exact genotype and phenotype of the unknown plant, including the precise arrangement of the alleles on the homologs.

11. In the cross shown here, involving two linked genes, *ebony* (*e*) and *claret* (*ca*), in *Drosophila*, where crossing over does not occur in males, offspring were produced in a 2 + : 1 *ca* : 1 *e* phenotypic ratio:

♀		♂
$\dfrac{e \quad ca^+}{e^+ \quad ca}$	×	$\dfrac{e \quad ca^+}{e^+ \quad ca}$

These genes are 30 units apart on chromosome III. What did crossing over in the female contribute to these phenotypes?

12. In a series of two-point mapping crosses involving five genes located on chromosome II in *Drosophila*, the following recombinant (single-crossover) frequencies were observed:

pr–adp	29%
pr–vg	13
pr–c	21
pr–b	6
adp–b	35
adp–c	8
adp–vg	16
vg–b	19
vg–c	8
c–b	27

(a) Given that the *adp* gene is near the end of chromosome II (locus 83), construct a map of these genes.
(b) In another set of experiments, a sixth gene, *d*, was tested against *b* and *pr*:

d–b	17%
d–pr	23%

Predict the results of two-point mapping between *d* and *c*, *d* and *vg*, and *d* and *adp*.

13. Two different female *Drosophila* were isolated, each heterozygous for the autosomally linked genes *b* (*black body*), *d* (*dachs tarsus*), and *c* (*curved wings*). These genes are in the order *d–b–c*, with *b* being closer to *d* than to *c*. Shown here is the

genotypic arrangement for each female along with the various gametes formed by both:

Female A		Female B	
$\dfrac{d\ b\ +}{+\ +\ c}$		$\dfrac{d\ +\ +}{+\ b\ c}$	
↓	Gamete formation	↓	
(1) $d\ b\ c$	(5) $d\ +\ +$	(1) $d\ b\ +$	(5) $d\ b\ c$
(2) $+\ +\ +$	(6) $+\ b\ c$	(2) $+\ +\ c$	(6) $+\ +\ +$
(3) $+\ +\ c$	(7) $d\ +\ c$	(3) $d\ +\ c$	(7) $d\ +\ +$
(4) $d\ b\ +$	(8) $+\ b\ +$	(4) $+\ b\ +$	(8) $+\ b\ C$

Identify which categories are noncrossovers (NCOs), single crossovers (SCOs), and double crossovers (DCOs) in each case. Then, indicate the relative frequency in which each will be produced.

14. In *Drosophila*, a cross was made between females—all expressing the three X-linked recessive traits *scute* bristles (*sc*), *sable* body (*s*), and *vermilion* eyes (*v*)—and wild-type males. In the F_1, all females were wild type, while all males expressed all three mutant traits. The cross was carried to the F_2 generation, and 1000 offspring were counted, with the results shown in the following table.

Phenotype			Offspring
sc	*s*	*v*	314
+	+	+	280
+	*s*	*v*	150
sc	+	+	156
sc	+	*v*	46
+	*s*	+	30
sc	*s*	+	10
+	+	*v*	14

No determination of sex was made in the data.

(a) Using proper nomenclature, determine the genotypes of the P_1 and F_1 parents.
(b) Determine the sequence of the three genes and the map distances between them.
(c) Are there more or fewer double crossovers than expected?
(d) Calculate the coefficient of coincidence. Does it represent positive or negative interference?

15. Another cross in *Drosophila* involved the recessive, X-linked genes *yellow* (*y*), *white* (*w*), and *cut* (*ct*). A yellow-bodied, white-eyed female with normal wings was crossed to a male whose eyes and body were normal but whose wings were cut. The F_1 females were wild type for all three traits, while the F_1 males expressed the yellow-body and white-eye traits. The cross was carried to an F_2 progeny, and only male offspring were tallied. On the basis of the data shown here, a genetic map was constructed.

Phenotype			Male Offspring
y	+	*ct*	9
+	*w*	+	6
y	*w*	*ct*	90
+	+	+	95
+	+	*ct*	424
y	*w*	+	376
y	+	+	0
+	*w*	*ct*	0

(a) Diagram the genotypes of the F_1 parents.
(b) Construct a map, assuming that *white* is at locus 1.5 on the X chromosome.
(c) Were any double-crossover offspring expected?
(d) Could the F_2 female offspring be used to construct the map? Why or why not?

16. In *Drosophila*, Dichaete (*D*) is a mutation on chromosome III with a dominant effect on wing shape. It is lethal when homozygous. The genes *ebony* body (*e*) and *pink* eye (*p*) are recessive mutations on chromosome III. Flies from a *Dichaete* stock were crossed to homozygous ebony, pink flies, and the F_1 progeny, with a Dichaete phenotype, were backcrossed to the ebony, pink homozygotes. Using the results of this backcross shown in the table,

(a) Diagram this cross, showing the genotypes of the parents and offspring of both crosses.
(b) What is the sequence and interlocus distance between these three genes?

Phenotype	Number
Dichaete	401
ebony, pink	389
Dichaete, ebony	84
pink	96
Dichaete, pink	2
ebony	3
Dichaete, ebony, pink	12
wild type	13

17. *Drosophila* females homozygous for the third chromosomal genes *pink* and *ebony* (the same genes from Problem 16) were crossed with males homozygous for the second chromosomal gene *dumpy*. Because these genes are recessive, all offspring were wild type (normal). F_1 females were testcrossed to triply recessive males. If we assume that the two linked genes, *pink* and *ebony*, are 20 mu apart, predict the results of this cross. If the reciprocal cross were made (F_1 males—where no crossing over occurs—with triply recessive females), how would the results vary, if at all?

18. In *Drosophila*, two mutations, Stubble (*Sb*) and *curled* (*cu*), are linked on chromosome III. *Stubble* is a dominant gene that is lethal in a homozygous state, and *curled* is a recessive gene. If a female of the genotype

$$\dfrac{Sb \qquad cu}{+ \qquad +}$$

is to be mated to detect recombinants among her offspring, what male genotype would you choose as a mate?

19. If the cross described in Problem 18 were made, and if *Sb* and *cu* are 8.2 map units apart on chromosome III, and if 1000 offspring were recovered, what would be the outcome of the cross, assuming that equal numbers of males and females were observed?

20. Are mitotic recombinations and sister chromatid exchanges effective in producing genetic variability in an individual? in the offspring of individuals?

21. What possible conclusions can be drawn from the observations that in male *Drosophila*, no crossing over occurs, and that during meiosis, synaptonemal complexes are not seen in males but are observed in females where crossing over occurs?

22. An organism of the genotype *AaBbCc* was testcrossed to a triply recessive organism (*aabbcc*). The genotypes of the progeny are presented in the following table.

20	*AaBbCc*	20	*AaBbcc*
20	*aabbCc*	20	*aabbcc*
5	*AabbCc*	5	*Aabbcc*
5	*aaBbCc*	5	*aaBbcc*

(a) If these three genes were all assorting independently, how many genotypic and phenotypic classes would result in the offspring, and in what proportion, assuming simple dominance and recessiveness in each gene pair?

(b) Answer part (a) again, assuming the three genes are so tightly linked on a single chromosome that no crossover gametes were recovered in the sample of offspring.

(c) What can you conclude from the *actual* data about the location of the three genes in relation to one another?

23. Based on our discussion of the potential inaccuracy of mapping (see Figure 5–12), would you revise your answer to Problem 22? If so, how?

24. Traditional gene mapping has been applied successfully to a variety of organisms including yeast, fungi, maize, and *Drosophila*. However, human gene mapping has only recently shared a similar spotlight. What factors have delayed the application of traditional gene-mapping techniques in humans?

25. DNA markers have greatly enhanced the mapping of genes in humans. What are DNA markers, and what advantage do they confer?

26. In a certain plant, fruit is either red or yellow, and fruit shape is either oval or long. Red and oval are the dominant traits. Two plants, both heterozygous for these traits, were testcrossed, with the following results.

	Progeny	
Phenotype	Plant A	Plant B
red, long	46	4
yellow, oval	44	6
red, oval	5	43
yellow, long	5	47
	100	100

Determine the location of the genes relative to one another and the genotypes of the two parental plants.

27. Two plants in a cross were each heterozygous for two gene pairs (*Ab/aB*) whose loci are linked and 25 mu apart. Assuming that crossing over occurs during the formation of both male and female gametes and that the *A* and *B* alleles are dominant, determine the phenotypic ratio of their offspring.

Extra-Spicy Problems

MasteringGenetics™ Visit for instructor-assigned tutorials and problems.

28. A number of human–mouse somatic cell hybrid clones were examined for the expression of specific human genes and the presence of human chromosomes. The results are summarized in the following table. Assign each gene to the chromosome on which it is located.

	Hybrid Cell Clone					
	A	B	C	D	E	F
Genes expressed						
ENO1 (enolase-1)	−	+	−	+	+	−
MDH1 (malate dehydrogenase-1)	+	+	−	+	−	+
PEPS (peptidase S)	+	−	+	−	−	−
PGM1 (phosphoglucomutase-1)	−	+	−	+	+	−
Chromosomes (present or absent)						
1	−	+	−	+	+	−
2	+	+	−	+	−	+
3	+	+	−	−	+	−
4	+	−	+	−	−	−
5	−	+	+	+	+	+

29. A female of genotype

$$\frac{a \quad b \quad c}{+ \quad + \quad +}$$

produces 100 meiotic tetrads. Of these, 68 show no crossover events. Of the remaining 32, 20 show a crossover between *a* and *b*, 10 show a crossover between *b* and *c*, and 2 show a double crossover between *a* and *b* and between *b* and *c*. Of the 400 gametes produced, how many of each of the 8 different genotypes will be produced? Assuming the order *a–b–c* and the allele arrangement previously shown, what is the map distance between these loci?

30. In laboratory class, a genetics student was assigned to study an unknown mutation in *Drosophila* that had a whitish eye. He crossed females from his true-breeding mutant stock to wild-type (brick-red-eyed) males, recovering all wild-type F_1 flies. In the F_2 generation, the following offspring were recovered in the following proportions:

wild type	5/8
bright red	1/8
brown eye	1/8
white eye	1/8

The student was stumped until the instructor suggested that perhaps the whitish eye in the original stock was the result of homozygosity for a mutation causing brown eyes *and* a mutation causing bright red eyes, illustrating gene interaction (see Chapter 4). After much thought, the student was able to analyze the data, explain the results, and learn several things about the location of the two genes relative to one another. One key to his understanding was that crossing over occurs in *Drosophila* females but not in males. Based on his analysis, what did the student learn about the two genes?

31. *Drosophila melanogaster* has one pair of sex chromosomes (XX or XY) and three pairs of autosomes, referred to as chromosomes II, III, and IV. A genetics student discovered a male fly with very short (*sh*) legs. Using this male, the student was able to establish a pure breeding stock of this mutant and found that it was recessive. She then incorporated the mutant into a stock containing the recessive gene *black* (*b*, body color located on chromosome II) and the recessive gene *pink* (*p*, eye color located on chromosome III). A female from the homozygous black, pink, short stock was then mated to a wild-type male. The F_1 males of this cross were all wild type and were then backcrossed to the homozygous *b, p, sh* females. The F_2 results appeared as shown in the following table. No other phenotypes were observed.

	Wild	Pink*	Black, Short*	Black, Pink, Short
Females	63	58	55	69
Males	59	65	51	60

*Other trait or traits are wild type.

(a) Based on these results, the student was able to assign *short* to a linkage group (a chromosome). Which one was it? Include your step-by-step reasoning.

(b) The student repeated the experiment, making the reciprocal cross, F_1 females backcrossed to homozygous *b, p, sh* males. She observed that 85 percent of the offspring fell into the given classes, but that 15 percent of the offspring were equally divided among *b + p, b + +, + sh p,* and *+ sh +* phenotypic males and females. How can these results be explained, and what information can be derived from the data?

32. In *Drosophila*, a female fly is heterozygous for three mutations, *Bar* eyes (*B*), *miniature* wings (*m*), and *ebony* body (*e*). Note that *Bar* is a dominant mutation. The fly is crossed to a male with normal eyes, miniature wings, and ebony body. The results of the cross are as follows.

111 miniature	101 Bar, ebony
29 wild type	31 Bar, miniature, ebony
117 Bar	35 ebony
26 Bar, miniature	115 miniature, ebony

Interpret the results of this cross. If you conclude that linkage is involved between any of the genes, determine the map distance(s) between them.

33. The gene controlling the Xg blood group alleles (Xg^+ and Xg^-) and the gene controlling a newly described form of inherited recessive muscle weakness called *episodic muscle weakness* (*EMWX*) (Ryan et al., 1999) are closely linked on the X chromosome in humans at position Xp22.3 (the tip of the short arm). A male with EMWX who is Xg^- marries a woman who is Xg^+, and they have eight daughters and one son, all of whom are normal for muscle function, the male being Xg^+ and all the daughters being heterozygous at both the *EMWX* and *Xg* loci. Following is a table that lists three of the daughters with the phenotypes of their husbands and children.

	Husband's Phenotype	Offspring's Sex	Offspring's Phenotype
Daughter 1:	Xg^+	female	Xg^+
		male	EMWX, Xg^+
Daughter 2:	Xg^-	male	Xg^-
		female	Xg^+
		male	EMWX, Xg^-
Daughter 3:	Xg^-	male	EMWX, Xg^-
		male	Xg^+
		male	Xg^-
		male	EMWX, Xg^+
		male	Xg^-
		male	EMWX, Xg^-
		female	Xg^+
		female	Xg^-
		female	Xg^+

(a) Create a pedigree that represents all data stated above and in the following table.

(b) For each of the offspring, indicate whether or not a crossover was required to produce the phenotypes that are given.

34. Because of the relatively high frequency of meiotic errors that lead to developmental abnormalities in humans, many research efforts have focused on identifying correlations between error frequency and chromosome morphology and behavior. Tease et al. (2002) studied human fetal oocytes of chromosomes 21, 18, and 13 using an immunocytological approach that allowed a direct estimate of the frequency and position of meiotic recombination. Below is a summary of information (modified from Tease et al., 2002) that compares recombination frequency with the frequency of trisomy for chromosomes 21, 18, and 13. (*Note:* You may want to read appropriate portions of Chapter 8 for descriptions of these trisomic conditions.)

Trisomic	Mean Recombination Frequency	Live-born Frequency
Chromosome 21	1.23	1/700
Chromosome 18	2.36	1/3000–1/8000
Chromosome 13	2.50	1/5000–1/19,000

(a) What conclusions can be drawn from these data in terms of recombination and nondisjunction frequencies? How might recombination frequencies influence trisomic frequencies?

(b) Other studies indicate that the number of crossovers per oocyte is somewhat constant, and it has been suggested that positive chromosomal interference acts to spread out a limited number of crossovers among as many chromosomes as possible. Considering information in part (a), speculate on the selective advantage positive chromosomal interference might confer.

Transmission electron micrograph of conjugating *Escherichia coli.*

6

Genetic Analysis and Mapping in Bacteria and Bacteriophages

CHAPTER CONCEPTS

- Bacterial genomes are most often contained in a single circular chromosome.

- Bacteria have developed numerous ways of exchanging and recombining genetic information between individual cells, including conjugation, transformation, and transduction.

- The ability to undergo conjugation and to transfer the bacterial chromosome from one cell to another is governed by genetic information contained in the DNA of a "fertility," or F, factor.

- The F factor can exist autonomously in the bacterial cytoplasm as a plasmid, or it can integrate into the bacterial chromosome, where it facilitates the transfer of the host chromosome to the recipient cell, leading to genetic recombination.

- Genetic recombination during conjugation provides the basis for mapping bacterial genes.

- Bacteriophages are viruses that have bacteria as their hosts. Viral DNA is injected into the host cell, where it replicates and directs the reproduction of the bacteriophage and the lysis of the bacterium.

- Rarely, following infection, bacteriophage DNA integrates into the host chromosome, becoming a prophage, where it is replicated along with the bacterial DNA.

- Bacteriophages undergo both intergenic and intragenic recombination.

In this chapter, we shift from consideration of transmission genetics and mapping in eukaryotes to discussion of the analysis of genetic recombination and mapping in bacteria and bacteriophages, viruses that have bacteria as their host. As we focus on these topics, it will become clear that complex processes have evolved in bacteria and bacteriophages that transfer genetic information between individual cells within populations. These processes provide geneticists with the basis for chromosome mapping.

The study of bacteria and bacteriophages has been essential to the accumulation of knowledge in many areas of genetic study. For example, much of what we know about the expression and regulation of genetic information was initially derived from experimental work with them. Furthermore, as we shall see (Chapter 20), our extensive knowledge of bacteria and their resident plasmids has served as the basis for their widespread use in DNA cloning and other recombinant DNA procedures.

The value of bacteria and their viruses as research organisms in genetics is based on two important characteristics that they display. First, they have extremely short reproductive cycles. Literally hundreds of generations, amounting to billions of genetically identical bacteria or phages, can be produced in short periods of time. Second, they can also be studied in pure culture. That is, a single species or mutant strain of bacteria or one type of virus can with ease be isolated and investigated independently of other similar organisms. As a result, they have been indispensable to the progress made in genetics over the past half century.

6.1 Bacteria Mutate Spontaneously and Grow at an Exponential Rate

Genetic studies using bacteria depend on our ability to study mutations in these organisms. It has long been known that genetically homogeneous cultures of bacteria occasionally give rise to cells exhibiting heritable variation, particularly with respect to growth under unique environmental conditions. Prior to 1943, the source of this variation was hotly debated. The majority of bacteriologists believed that environmental factors induced changes in certain bacteria, leading to their survival or adaptation to the new conditions. For example, strains of *E. coli* are known to be sensitive to infection by the bacteriophage T1. Infection by the bacteriophage T1 leads to reproduction of the virus at the expense of the bacterial host, from which new phages are released as the host cell is disrupted, or lysed. If a plate of *E. coli* is uniformly sprayed with T1, almost all cells are lysed. Rare *E. coli* cells, however, survive infection and are not lysed. If these cells are isolated and established in pure culture, all their descendants are resistant to T1 infection. The **adaptation hypothesis,** put forth to explain this type of observation, implies that the interaction of the phage and bacterium is essential to the acquisition of immunity. In other words, exposure to the phage "induces" resistance in the bacteria.

On the other hand, the occurrence of **spontaneous mutations,** which occur regardless of the presence or absence of bacteriophage T1, suggested an alternative model to explain the origin of resistance in *E. coli*. In 1943, Salvador Luria and Max Delbrück presented the first convincing evidence that bacteria, like eukaryotic organisms, are capable of spontaneous mutation. Their experiment, referred to as the **fluctuation test,** marks the initiation of modern bacterial genetic study. (We will explore this discovery in Chapter 16.) Mutant cells that arise spontaneously in otherwise pure cultures can be isolated and established independently from the parent strain by the use of selection techniques. *Selection* refers to culturing the organism under conditions where only the desired mutant grows well, while the wild type does not grow. With carefully designed selection, mutations for almost any desired characteristic can now be isolated. Because bacteria and viruses usually contain only one copy of a single chromosome, and are therefore haploid, all mutations are expressed directly in the descendants of mutant cells, adding to the ease with which these microorganisms can be studied.

Bacteria are grown either in a liquid culture medium or in a petri dish on a semisolid agar surface. If the nutrient components of the growth medium are very simple and consist only of an organic carbon source (such as glucose or lactose) and various inorganic ions, including Na^+, K^+, Mg^{2+}, Ca^{2+}, and NH_4^+ present as inorganic salts, it is called **minimal medium.** To grow on such a medium, a bacterium must be able to synthesize all essential organic compounds (e.g., amino acids, purines, pyrimidines, sugars, vitamins, and fatty acids). A bacterium that can accomplish this remarkable biosynthetic feat—one that the human body cannot duplicate—is a **prototroph.** It is said to be wild type for all growth requirements. On the other hand, if a bacterium loses, through mutation, the ability to synthesize one or more organic components, it is an **auxotroph.** For example, a bacterium that loses the ability to make histidine is designated as a *his⁻* auxotroph, in contrast to its prototrophic *his⁺* counterpart. For the *his⁻* bacterium to grow, this amino acid must be added as a supplement to the minimal medium. Medium that has been extensively supplemented is called *complete medium.*

To study bacterial growth quantitatively, an inoculum of bacteria—a small amount of a bacteria-containing solution, for example, 0.1 or 1.0 mL—is placed in liquid culture medium. A graph of the characteristic growth pattern for a bacteria culture is shown in **Figure 6–1.** Initially, during the **lag phase,** growth is slow. Then, a period of rapid growth, called the **logarithmic (log) phase,** ensues. During this phase, cells divide continually with a fixed time interval between cell divisions, resulting in exponential growth. When a cell density of about 10^9 cells/mL of culture medium is reached, nutrients become limiting and cells cease dividing; at this point, the cells enter the **stationary phase.** The doubling time during the log phase can be as short as 20 minutes. Thus, an initial inoculum of a few

FIGURE 6–1 Typical bacterial population growth curve showing the initial lag phase, the subsequent log phase where exponential growth occurs, and the stationary phase that occurs when nutrients are exhausted. Eventually, all cells will die.

FIGURE 6–2 Results of the serial dilution technique and subsequent culture of bacteria. Each dilution varies by a factor of 10. Each colony was derived from a single bacterial cell.

thousand cells added to the culture easily achieves maximum cell density during an overnight incubation.

Cells grown in liquid medium can be quantified by transferring them to the semisolid medium of a petri dish. Following incubation and many divisions, each cell gives rise to a colony visible on the surface of the medium. By counting colonies, it is possible to estimate the number of bacteria present in the original culture. If the number of colonies is too great to count, then successive dilutions (in a technique called *serial dilution*) of the original liquid culture are made and plated, until the colony number is reduced to the point where it can be counted (**Figure 6–2**). This technique allows the number of bacteria present in the original culture to be calculated.

For example, let's assume that the three petri dishes in Figure 6–2 represent dilutions of the liquid culture by 10^{-3}, 10^{-4}, and 10^{-5} (from left to right).[*] We need only select the dish in which the number of colonies can be counted accurately. Because each colony presumably arose from a single bacterium, the number of colonies times the dilution factor represents the number of bacteria in each milliliter (mL) of the initial inoculum before it was diluted. In Figure 6–2, the rightmost dish contains 12 colonies. The dilution factor for a 10^{-5} dilution is 10^{5}. Therefore, the initial number of bacteria was 12×10^{5} per mL.

6.2 Genetic Recombination Occurs in Bacteria

Development of techniques that allowed the identification and study of bacterial mutations led to detailed investigations of the transfer of genetic information between individual organisms. As we shall see, as with meiotic crossing over in eukaryotes, the process of **genetic recombination** in bacteria provided the basis for the development of

chromosome mapping methodology. It is important to note at the outset of our discussion that the term *genetic recombination*, as applied to bacteria, refers to the *replacement* of one or more genes present in the chromosome of one cell with those from the chromosome of a genetically distinct cell. While this is somewhat different from our use of the term in eukaryotes—where it describes crossing over *resulting in a reciprocal exchange*—the overall effect is the same: Genetic information is transferred and results in an altered genotype.

We will discuss three processes that result in the transfer of genetic information from one bacterium to another: *conjugation, transformation,* and *transduction.* Collectively, knowledge of these processes has helped us understand the origin of genetic variation between members of the same bacterial species, and in some cases, between members of different species. When transfer of genetic information occurs between members of the same species, the term **vertical gene transfer** applies. When transfer occurs between members of related but distinct bacterial species, the term **horizontal gene transfer** is used. The horizontal gene transfer process has played a significant role in the evolution of bacteria. Often, the genes discovered to be involved in horizontal transfer are those that also confer survival advantages to the recipient species. For example, one species may transfer antibiotic resistance genes to another species. Or genes conferring enhanced pathogenicity may be transferred. Thus, the potential for such transfer is a major concern in the medical community. In addition, horizontal gene transfer has been a major factor in the process of speciation in bacteria. Many, if not most, bacterial species have been the recipient of genes from other species.

Conjugation in Bacteria: The Discovery of F⁺ and F⁻ Strains

Studies of bacterial recombination began in 1946, when Joshua Lederberg and Edward Tatum showed that bacteria undergo **conjugation,** a process by which genetic information from one bacterium is transferred to and recombined

---
[*]10^{-5} represents a 1:100,000 dilution.

Auxotrophic strains grown separately
in complete medium

Strain A
(*met⁻ bio⁻ thr⁺ leu⁺ thi⁺*)

Strain B
(*met⁺ bio⁺ thr⁻ leu⁻ thi⁻*)

Mix A and B in complete
medium; incubate overnight

Control

Strains A + B
met⁻ bio⁻ thr⁺ leu⁺ thi⁺
and
met⁺ bio⁺ thr⁻ leu⁻ thi⁻

Control

Plate on minimal
medium and incubate

Plate on minimal
medium and incubate

Plate on minimal
medium and incubate

Colonies of
prototrophs

**No growth
(no prototrophs)**

**Only *met⁺ bio⁺ thr⁺ leu⁺ thi⁺* cells
grow, occurring at a frequency
of 1/10⁷ of total cells**

**No growth
(no prototrophs)**

FIGURE 6–3 Production of prototrophs as a result of genetic recombination between two auxotrophic strains. Neither auxotrophic strain will grow on minimal medium, but prototrophs do, suggesting that genetic recombination has occurred.

simultaneously at two or three independent locations to become wild-type cells. Therefore, the researchers assumed that any prototrophs recovered must have arisen as a result of some form of genetic exchange and recombination between the two mutant strains.

In this experiment, prototrophs were recovered at a rate of $1/10^7$ (or 10^{-7}) cells plated. The controls for this experiment consisted of separate plating of cells from strains A and B on minimal medium. No prototrophs were recovered. On the basis of these observations, Lederberg and Tatum proposed that, while the events were indeed rare, genetic recombination had occurred.

Lederberg and Tatum's findings were soon followed by numerous experiments that elucidated the physical nature and the genetic basis of conjugation. It quickly became evident that different strains of bacteria were capable of effecting a unidirectional transfer of genetic material. When cells serve as donors of parts of their chromosomes, they are designated as **F⁺ cells** (F for "fertility"). Recipient bacteria, designated as **F⁻ cells**, receive the donor chromosome material (now known to be DNA) and recombine it with part of their own chromosome.

Experimentation subsequently established that cell-to-cell contact is essential for chromosome transfer. Support for this concept was provided by Bernard Davis, who designed the Davis U-tube for growing F⁺ and F⁻ cells (**Figure 6–4**). At the base of the tube is a sintered glass filter with a pore size that allows passage of the liquid medium but is too small to allow passage of bacteria. The F⁺ cells are placed on one side of the filter and F⁻ cells on the other side. The medium passes back and forth across the filter so that it is shared by both sets of bacterial cells during incubation. When Davis plated samples from both sides of the tube on minimal medium, no prototrophs were found, and he logically concluded that *physical contact between cells of the two strains is essential to genetic recombination.* We now know that this physical interaction is the initial stage of the process of conjugation and is mediated by a structure called the **F pilus** (or **sex pilus;** pl. pili), a 6- to 9-nm tubular extension of the cell (see the chapter-opening photograph on p. 134). Bacteria often have many

with that of another bacterium. Their initial experiments were performed with two multiple auxotrophs (nutritional mutants) of *E. coli* strain K12. As shown in **Figure 6–3**, strain A required methionine (met) and biotin (bio) in order to grow, whereas strain B required threonine (thr), leucine (leu), and thiamine (thi). Neither strain would grow on minimal medium. The two strains were first grown separately in supplemented media, and then cells from both were mixed and grown together for several more generations. They were then plated on minimal medium. Any cells that grew on minimal medium were prototrophs. It is highly improbable that any of the cells containing two or three mutant genes would undergo spontaneous mutation

FIGURE 6–4 When strain A and strain B auxotrophs are grown in a common medium but separated by a filter, as in this Davis U-tube apparatus, no genetic recombination occurs and no prototrophs are produced.

pili of different types performing different cellular functions, but all pili are involved in some way with adhesion (the binding together of cells). After contact has been initiated between mating pairs, chromosome transfer is possible.

Later evidence established that F$^+$ cells contain a **fertility factor (F factor)** that confers the ability to donate part of their chromosome during conjugation. Experiments by Joshua and Esther Lederberg and by William Hayes and Luca Cavalli-Sforza showed that certain environmental conditions eliminate the F factor from otherwise fertile cells. However, if these "infertile" cells are then grown with fertile donor cells, the F factor is regained. These findings led to the hypothesis that the F factor is a mobile element, a conclusion further supported by the observation that, after conjugation, recipient F$^-$ cells always become F$^+$. Thus, in addition to the rare cases of gene transfer (genetic recombination) that result from conjugation, the F factor itself is passed to *all* recipient cells. Accordingly, the initial cross of Lederberg and Tatum (Figure 6–3) can be described as follows:

Strain A		Strain B
F$^+$		F$^-$
(DONOR)	×	(RECIPIENT)

Characterization of the F factor confirmed these conclusions. Like the bacterial chromosome, though distinct from it, the F factor has been shown to consist of a circular, double-stranded DNA molecule; it is equivalent in size to about 2 percent of the bacterial chromosome (about 100,000 nucleotide pairs) and contains as many as 40 genes. Many are *tra* genes, whose products are involved in the *tra*nsfer of genetic information, including the genes essential to the formation of the sex pilus.

Geneticists believe that transfer of the F factor during conjugation involves separation of the two strands of its double helix and movement of one of the two strands into the recipient cell. The other strand remains in the donor cell. Both strands, one moving across the conjugation tube and one remaining in the donor cell, are replicated. The result is that both the donor and the recipient cells become F$^+$. This process is diagrammed in **Figure 6–5**.

To summarize, an *E. coli* cell may or may not contain the F factor. When it is present, the cell is able to form a sex pilus and potentially serve as a donor of genetic information. During conjugation, a copy of the F factor is almost always transferred from the F$^+$ cell to the F$^-$ recipient, converting the recipient to the F$^+$ state. The question remained as to exactly why such a low proportion of these matings (10^{-7}) also results in genetic recombination. Also, it was unclear what the transfer of the F factor had to do with the transfer and recombination of particular genes. The answers to these questions awaited further experimentation.

As you soon shall see, the F factor is in reality an autonomous genetic unit referred to as a *plasmid*. However, in covering the history of its discovery, in this chapter we will continue to refer to it as a "factor."

Hfr Bacteria and Chromosome Mapping

Subsequent discoveries not only clarified how genetic recombination occurs but also defined a mechanism by which the *E. coli* chromosome could be mapped. Let's address chromosome mapping first.

In 1950, Cavalli-Sforza treated an F$^+$ strain of *E. coli* K12 with nitrogen mustard, a potent chemical known to induce mutations. From these treated cells, he recovered a genetically altered strain of donor bacteria that underwent recombination at a rate of 1/10^4 (or 10^{-4}), 1000 times more frequently than the original F$^+$ strains. In 1953, William Hayes isolated another strain that demonstrated a similarly elevated frequency of recombination. Both strains were designated **Hfr,** for **high-frequency recombination.** Hfr cells constitute a special class of F$^+$ cells.

In addition to the higher frequency of recombination, another important difference was noted between Hfr

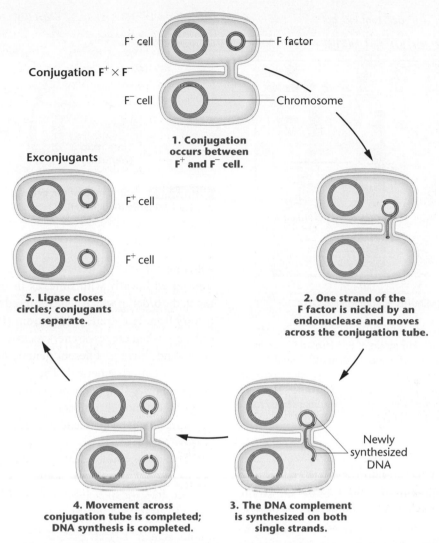

FIGURE 6–5 An $F^+ \times F^-$ mating, demonstrating how the recipient F^- cell is converted to F^+. During conjugation, the DNA of the F factor is replicated, with one new copy entering the recipient cell, converting it to F^+. The bars drawn on the F factors indicate their clockwise rotation during replication. Newly replicated DNA is depicted by a lighter shade of blue as the F factor is transferred.

strains and the original F^+ strains. If a donor cell is from an Hfr strain, recipient cells, though sometimes displaying genetic recombination, *never become Hfr*; thus they remain F^-. In comparison, then,

$F^+ \times F^- \rightarrow$ recipient becomes F^+ (low rate of recombination)

Hfr $\times F^- \rightarrow$ recipient remains F^- (high rate of recombination)

Perhaps the most significant characteristic of Hfr strains is the *specific nature of recombination*. In a given Hfr strain, certain genes are more frequently recombined than others, and some do not recombine at all. This *nonrandom* pattern of gene transfer was shown to vary among Hfr strains. Although these results were puzzling, Hayes interpreted them to mean that some physiological alteration of the F factor had occurred to produce Hfr strains of *E. coli*.

In the mid-1950s, experimentation by Ellie Wollman and François Jacob explained the differences between Hfr cells and F^+ cells and showed how Hfr strains would allow genetic mapping of the *E. coli* chromosome. In Wollman and Jacob's experiments, Hfr and antibiotic-resistant F^- strains with suitable marker genes were mixed, and recombination of these genes was assayed at different times. Specifically, a culture containing a mixture of an Hfr and an F^- strain was incubated, and samples were removed at intervals and placed in a blender. The shear forces created in the blender separated conjugating bacteria so that the transfer of the chromosome was terminated. Then the sampled cells were grown on medium containing the antibiotic, so that only recipient cells would be recovered. These cells were subsequently tested for the transfer of specific genes.

Hfr H *(thr⁺ leu⁺ aziᴿ tonˢ lac⁺ gal⁺)*
×
F⁻ *(thr⁻ leu⁻ aziˢ tonᴿ lac⁻ gal⁻)*

FIGURE 6–6 The progressive transfer during conjugation of various genes from a specific Hfr strain of *E. coli* to an F⁻ strain. Certain genes (*azi* and *ton*) transfer sooner than others and recombine more frequently. Others (*lac* and *gal*) transfer later, and recombinants are found at a lower frequency. Still others (*thr* and *leu*) are always transferred and were used in the initial screen for recombinants but are not shown here.

FIGURE 6–7 A time map of the genes studied in the experiment depicted in Figure 6–6.

This process, called the **interrupted mating technique,** demonstrated that, depending on the specific Hfr strain, certain genes are transferred and recombined sooner than others. The graph in **Figure 6–6** illustrates this point. During the first 8 minutes after the two strains were mixed, no genetic recombination was detected. At about 10 minutes, recombination of the *azi*ᴿ gene could be detected, but no transfer of the *ton*ˢ, *lac*⁺, or *gal*⁺ genes was noted. By 15 minutes, 50 percent of the recombinants were *azi*ᴿ and 15 percent were also *ton*ˢ; but none was *lac*⁺ or *gal*⁺. Within 20 minutes, the *lac*⁺ gene was found among the recombinants; and within 25 minutes, *gal*⁺ was also beginning to be transferred. Wollman and Jacob had demonstrated an *ordered transfer of genes* that correlated with the length of time conjugation proceeded.

It appeared that the chromosome of the Hfr bacterium was transferred linearly, so that the gene order and distance between genes, as measured in minutes, could be predicted from experiments such as Wollman and Jacob's (**Figure 6–7**). This information, sometimes referred to as **time mapping,** served as the basis for the first genetic map of the *E. coli* chromosome. Minutes in bacterial mapping provide a measure similar to map units in eukaryotes.

Wollman and Jacob repeated the same type of experiment with other Hfr strains, obtaining similar results but

with one important difference. Although genes were always transferred linearly with time, as in their original experiment, the order in which genes entered the recipient seemed to vary from Hfr strain to Hfr strain [**Figure 6–8(a)**]. Nevertheless, when the researchers reexamined the entry rate of genes, and thus the different genetic maps for each strain, a distinct pattern emerged. The major difference between each strain was simply the point of the origin (*O*)—the first part of the donor chromosome to enter the recipient—and the direction in which entry proceeded from that point [**Figure 6–8(b)**].

To explain these results, Wollman and Jacob postulated that the *E. coli* chromosome is circular (a closed circle, with no free ends). If the point of origin (*O*) varies from strain to strain, a different sequence of genes will be transferred in each case. But what determines *O*? They proposed that, in various Hfr strains, the F factor integrates into the chromosome at different points, and its position determines the *O* site. One such case of integration is shown in step 1 of **Figure 6–9**. During conjugation between an Hfr and an F⁻ cell, the position of the F factor determines the initial point of transfer (steps 2 and 3). Those genes adjacent to *O* are transferred first, and the F factor becomes the last part that can be transferred (step 4). However, conjugation rarely, if ever, lasts long enough to allow the entire chromosome to pass across the conjugation tube (step 5). *This proposal explains why recipient cells, when mated with Hfr cells, remain F⁻.*

Figure 6–9 also depicts the way in which the two strands making up a donor's DNA molecule behave during transfer, allowing for the entry of one strand of DNA into the recipient (step 3). Following its replication in the recipient, the entering DNA has the potential to recombine with the region homologous to it on the host chromosome. The DNA strand that remains in the donor also undergoes replication.

Use of the interrupted mating technique with different Hfr strains allowed researchers to map the entire *E. coli*

(a)

Hfr strain	(earliest)			Order of transfer				(latest)
H	thr –	leu –	azi –	ton –	pro –	lac –	gal –	thi
1	leu –	thr –	thi –	gal –	lac –	pro –	ton –	azi
2	pro –	ton –	azi –	leu –	thr –	thi –	gal –	lac
7	ton –	azi –	leu –	thr –	thi –	gal –	lac –	pro

(b)

FIGURE 6–8 (a) The order of gene transfer in four Hfr strains, suggesting that the *E. coli* chromosome is circular. (b) The point where transfer originates (O) is identified in each strain. The origin is the point of integration of the F factor into the chromosome; the direction of transfer is determined by the orientation of the F factor as it integrates. The arrowheads indicate the points of initial transfer.

chromosome. Mapped in time units, strain K12 (or *E. coli* K12) was shown to be 100 minutes long. While modern genome analysis of the *E. coli* chromosome has now established the presence of just over 4000 protein-coding sequences, this original mapping procedure established the location of approximately 1000 genes.

NOW SOLVE THIS

6–1 When the interrupted mating technique was used with five different strains of Hfr bacteria, the following orders of gene entry and recombination were observed. On the basis of these data, draw a map of the bacterial chromosome. Do the data support the concept of circularity?

Hfr Strain			Order		
1	T	C	H	R	O
2	H	R	O	M	B
3	M	O	R	H	C
4	M	B	A	K	T
5	C	T	K	A	B

■ **HINT:** *This problem involves an understanding of how the bacterial chromosome is transferred during conjugation, leading to recombination and providing data for mapping. The key to its solution is to understand that chromosome transfer is strain-specific and depends on where in the chromosome, and in which orientation, the F factor has integrated.*

Recombination in F⁺ × F⁻ Matings: A Reexamination

The preceding model helped geneticists better understand how genetic recombination occurs during the $F^+ \times F^-$ matings. Recall that recombination occurs much less frequently in them than in Hfr $\times$ F⁻ matings and that random gene transfer is involved. The current belief is that when F⁺ and F⁻ cells are mixed, conjugation occurs readily, and each F⁻ cell involved in conjugation with an F⁺ cell receives a copy of the F factor, *but no genetic recombination occurs.* However, at an extremely low frequency in a population of F⁺ cells, the F factor integrates spontaneously into a random point in the bacterial chromosome, converting that F⁺ cell to the Hfr state as shown in Figure 6–9. Therefore, in F⁺ × F⁻ matings, the extremely low frequency of genetic recombination (10^{-7}) is attributed to the rare, newly formed Hfr cells, which then undergo conjugation with F⁻ cells. Because the point of integration of the F factor is random, the genes transferred by any newly formed Hfr donor *will also appear to be random within the larger* F⁺/F⁻ *population.* The recipient bacterium will appear as a recombinant but will, in fact, remain F⁻. If it subsequently undergoes conjugation with an F⁺ cell, it will be converted to F⁺.

The F′ State and Merozygotes

In 1959, during experiments with Hfr strains of *E. coli,* Edward Adelberg discovered that the F factor could lose its integrated status, causing the cell to revert to the F⁺ state

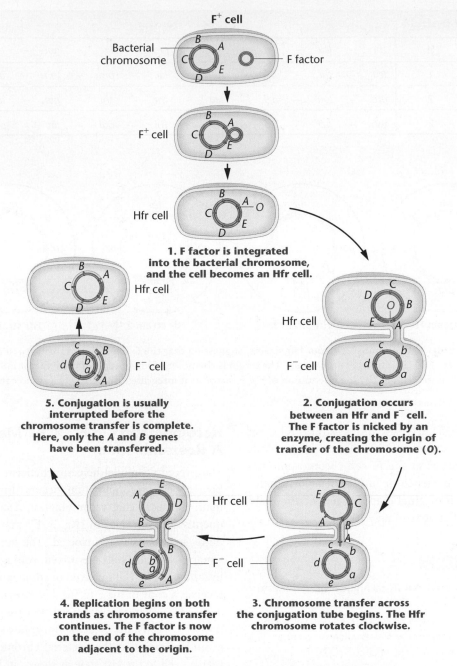

FIGURE 6–9 Conversion of F⁺ to an Hfr state occurs by integration of the F factor into the bacterial chromosome. The point of integration determines the origin (O) of transfer. During conjugation, an enzyme nicks the F factor, now integrated into the host chromosome, initiating the transfer of the chromosome at that point. Conjugation is usually interrupted prior to complete transfer. Here, only the A and B genes are transferred to the F⁻ cell; they may recombine with the host chromosome. Newly replicated DNA of the chromosome is depicted by a lighter shade of orange.

(**Figure 6–10**, step 1). When this occurs, the F factor frequently carries several adjacent bacterial genes along with it (step 2). Adelberg designated this condition F′ to distinguish it from F⁺ and Hfr. F′, like Hfr, is thus another special case of F⁺.

The presence of bacterial genes within a cytoplasmic F factor creates an interesting situation. An F′ bacterium behaves like an F⁺ cell by initiating conjugation with F⁻ cells (Figure 6–10, step 3). When this occurs, the F factor,

containing chromosomal genes, is transferred to the F⁻ cell (step 4). As a result, whatever chromosomal genes are part of the F factor are now present as duplicates in the recipient cell (step 5) because the recipient still has a complete chromosome. This creates a partially diploid cell called a **merozygote**. Pure cultures of F′ merozygotes can be established. They have been extremely useful in the study of genetic regulation in bacteria, as we will discuss later in the text (see Chapter 16).

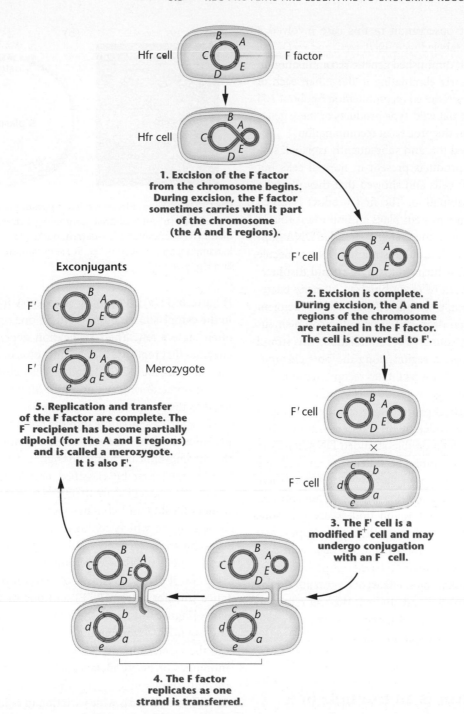

FIGURE 6–10 Conversion of an Hfr bacterium to F′ and its subsequent mating with an F⁻ cell. The conversion occurs when the F factor loses its integrated status. During excision from the chromosome, the F factor may carry with it one or more chromosomal genes (in this case, *A* and *E*). Following conjugation, the recipient cell becomes partially diploid and is called a merozygote. It also behaves as an F⁺ donor cell.

6.3 Rec Proteins Are Essential to Bacterial Recombination

Once researchers established that a unidirectional transfer of DNA occurs between bacteria, they became interested in determining how the actual recombination event occurs in the recipient cell. Just how does the donor DNA replace the homologous region in the recipient chromosome? As with many systems, the biochemical mechanism by which recombination occurs was deciphered through genetic studies. Major insights were gained as a result of the isolation of a group of mutations that impaired the process of recombination and led to the discovery of *rec* (for recombination) genes.

The first relevant observation in this case involved a series of mutant genes labeled *recA*, *recB*, *recC*, and *recD*. The first mutant gene, *recA*, diminished genetic recombination in bacteria 1000-fold, nearly eliminating it altogether; each of the other *rec* mutations reduced recombination by about 100 times. Clearly, the normal wild-type products of these genes play an essential role in the process of recombination.

Researchers looked for, and subsequently isolated, several functional gene products present in normal cells but missing in *rec* mutant cells and showed that they played a role in genetic recombination. The first product is called the **RecA protein.** [*] This protein plays an important role in recombination involving either a single-stranded DNA molecule or the linear end of a double-stranded DNA molecule that has unwound. As it turns out, **single-strand displacement** is a common form of recombination in many bacterial species. When double-stranded DNA enters a recipient cell, one strand is often degraded, leaving the complementary strand as the only source of recombination. This strand must find its homologous region along the host chromosome, and once it does, RecA facilitates recombination.

The second related gene product is a more complex protein called the **RecBCD protein,** an enzyme consisting of polypeptide subunits encoded by three other *rec* genes. This protein is important when double-stranded DNA serves as the source of genetic recombination. RecBCD unwinds the helix, facilitating recombination that involves RecA. These discoveries have extended our knowledge of the process of recombination considerably and underscore the value of isolating mutations, establishing their phenotypes, and determining the biological role of the normal, wild-type genes. The model of recombination based on the *rec* discoveries also applies to eukaryotes: eukaryotic proteins similar to RecA have been isolated and studied. We will return to this topic later in the text (see Chapter 11) where we will discuss two models of DNA recombination.

6.4 The F Factor Is an Example of a Plasmid

The preceding sections introduced the extrachromosomal heredity unit called the F factor that bacteria require for conjugation. When it exists autonomously in the bacterial cytoplasm, it is composed of a double-stranded closed circle of DNA. These characteristics place the F factor in the more general category of genetic structures called **plasmids**

---

[*] Note that the names of bacterial genes use lowercase letters and are italicized, while the names of the corresponding gene products begin with capital letters and are not italicized. For example, the *recA* gene encodes the RecA protein.

(a) **(b)**

FIGURE 6–11 (a) Electron micrograph of plasmids isolated from *E. coli*. (b) An R plasmid containing a resistance transfer factor (RTF) and multiple r-determinants (Tc, tetracycline; Kan, kanamycin; Sm, streptomycin; Su, sulfonamide; Amp, ampicillin; and Hg, mercury).

[Figure 6–11(a)]. Plasmids often exist in multiple copies in the cytoplasm; each may contain one or more genes and often quite a few. Their replication depends on the same enzymes that replicate the chromosome of the host cell, and they are distributed to daughter cells along with the host chromosome during cell division. Many plasmids are confined to the cytoplasm of the bacterial cell. Others, such as the F factor, can integrate into the host chromosome. Those plasmids that can exist autonomously or can integrate into the chromosome are further designated as **episomes**.

Plasmids can be classified according to the genetic information specified by their DNA. The F factor plasmid confers fertility and contains genes essential for sex pilus formation, on which conjugation and subsequent genetic recombination depend. Other examples of plasmids include the R and the Col plasmids.

Most **R plasmids** consist of two components: the **resistance transfer factor (RTF)** and one or more **r-determinants** [Figure 6–11(b)]. The RTF encodes genetic information essential to transferring the plasmid between bacteria, and the r-determinants are genes conferring resistance to antibiotics or heavy metals such as mercury. While RTFs are quite similar in a variety of plasmids from different bacterial species, there is wide variation in r-determinants, each of which is specific for resistance to one class of antibiotic. Determinants with resistance to tetracycline, streptomycin, ampicillin, sulfanilamide, kanamycin, or chloramphenicol are the most frequently encountered. Sometimes plasmids contain many r-determinants, conferring resistance to several antibiotics [Figure 6–11(b)]. Bacteria bearing such plasmids are of great medical significance, not only because of their multiple resistance but also because of the ease with which the plasmids may be transferred to other pathogenic bacteria, rendering those bacteria resistant to a wide range of antibiotics.

The first known case of such a plasmid occurred in Japan in the 1950s in the bacterium *Shigella*, which causes dysentery. In hospitals, bacteria were isolated that were resistant to as many as five of the above antibiotics. Obviously, this phenomenon represents a major health threat. Fortunately, a bacterial cell sometimes contains r-determinant plasmids but no RTF. Although such a cell is resistant, it cannot transfer the genetic information for resistance to recipient cells. The most commonly studied plasmids, however, contain the RTF as well as one or more r-determinants.

The **Col plasmid,** ColE1 (derived from *E. coli*), is clearly distinct from R plasmids. It encodes one or more proteins that are highly toxic to bacterial strains that do not harbor the same plasmid. These proteins, called **colicins,** can kill neighboring bacteria, and bacteria that carry the plasmid are said to be *colicinogenic*. Present in 10 to 20 copies per cell, the Col plasmid also contains a gene encoding an immunity protein that protects the host cell from the toxin. Unlike an R plasmid, the Col plasmid is not usually transmissible to other cells.

Interest in plasmids has increased dramatically because of their role in recombinant DNA research. As we will see (in Chapter 20), specific genes from any source can be inserted into a plasmid, which may then be inserted into a bacterial cell. As the altered cell replicates its DNA and undergoes division, the foreign gene is also replicated, thus being cloned.

6.5 Transformation Is a Second Process Leading to Genetic Recombination in Bacteria

Transformation provides another mechanism for recombining genetic information in some bacteria. Small pieces of extracellular (exogenous) DNA are taken up by a living bacterium, potentially leading to a stable genetic change in the recipient cell. We discuss transformation in this chapter because in those bacterial species in which it occurs, the process can be used to map bacterial genes, though in a more limited way than conjugation. As we will see later in the text (see Chapter 10), the process of transformation was also instrumental in proving that DNA is the genetic material. Further, in recombinant DNA

studies (Chapter 20), transformation, albeit an artificial version enhanced by *electroporation* (electric current), is instrumental in gene cloning.

The Transformation Process

The process of transformation (**Figure 6–12**) consists of numerous steps that achieve two basic outcomes: (1) entry of foreign DNA into a recipient cell; and (2) recombination between the foreign DNA and its homologous region in the recipient chromosome. While completion of both outcomes is required for genetic recombination, the first step of transformation can occur without the second step, resulting in the addition of foreign DNA to the bacterial cytoplasm but not to its chromosome.

In a population of bacterial cells, only those in a particular physiological state of **competence** take up DNA.

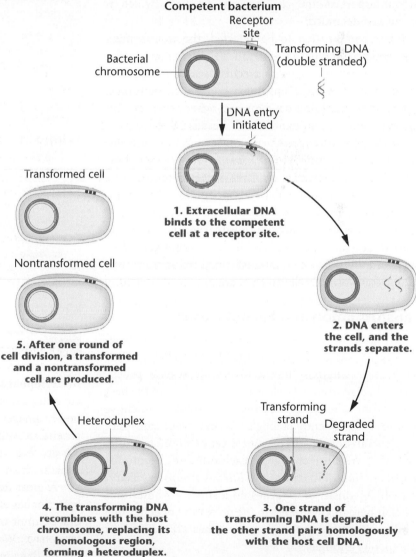

FIGURE 6–12 Proposed steps for transformation of a bacterial cell by exogenous DNA. Only one of the two strands of the entering DNA is involved in the transformation event, which is completed following cell division.

Studies have shown that various kinds of bacteria readily undergo transformation naturally (e.g., *Haemophilus influenzae, Bacillus subtilis, Shigella paradysenteriae, Streptococcus pneumoniae,* and *E. coli*). Others can be induced in the laboratory to become competent. Entry of DNA is thought to occur at a limited number of receptor sites on the surface of a competent bacterial cell (Figure 6–12, step 1). Passage into the cell is thought to be an active process that requires energy and specific transport molecules. This model is supported by the fact that substances that inhibit energy production or protein synthesis also inhibit transformation.

Soon after entry, one of the two strands of the double helix is digested by nucleases, leaving only a single strand to participate in transformation (Figure 6–12, steps 2 and 3). The surviving DNA strand aligns with the complementary region of the bacterial chromosome. In a process involving several enzymes, this segment of DNA replaces its counterpart in the chromosome (step 4), which is excised and degraded.

For recombination to be detected, the transforming DNA must be derived from a different strain of bacteria that bears some distinguishing genetic variation, such as a mutation. Once this is integrated into the chromosome, the recombinant region contains one host strand (present originally) and one mutant strand. Because these strands are from different sources, the region is referred to as a **heteroduplex,** which usually contains some mismatch of base sequence. This mismatch activates a repair process (see Chapter 15). Following repair and one round of DNA replication, one chromosome is restored to its original DNA sequence, identical to that of the original recipient cell, and the other contains the properly aligned mutant gene. Following cell division, one nontransformed cell (nonmutant) and one transformed cell (mutant) are produced (step 5).

Transformation and Linked Genes

In early transformation studies, the most effective exogenous DNA was a size containing 10,000–20,000 nucleotide pairs, a length sufficient to encode several genes.* Genes adjacent to or very close to one another on the bacterial chromosome can be carried on a single segment of this size. Consequently, a single transfer event can result in the **cotransformation** of several genes simultaneously. Genes that are close enough to each other to be cotransformed are *linked*. In contrast to *linkage groups* in eukaryotes, which consist of all genes on a single chromosome, note that here *linkage* refers to the proximity of genes that permits cotransformation (i.e., the genes are next to, or close to, one another).

---

*Today, we know that a 2000 nucleotide pair length of DNA is highly effective in gene cloning experiments.

If two genes are not linked, simultaneous transformation occurs only as a result of two independent events involving two distinct segments of DNA. As with double crossovers in eukaryotes, the probability of two independent events occurring simultaneously is equal to the product of the individual probabilities. Thus, the frequency of two unlinked genes being transformed simultaneously is much lower than if they are linked. Under certain conditions, relative distances between linked genes can be determined from transformation data in a manner analogous to chromosome mapping in eukaryotes, though somewhat more complex.

NOW SOLVE THIS

6–2 In a transformation experiment involving a recipient bacterial strain of genotype $a^- b^-$, the following results were obtained. What can you conclude about the location of the *a* and *b* genes relative to each other?

Transforming DNA	Transformants (%)		
	$a^+ b^-$	$a^- b^+$	$a^+ b^+$
$a^+ b^+$	3.1	1.2	0.04
$a^+ b^-$ and $a^- b^+$	2.4	1.4	0.03

■ **HINT:** *This problem involves an understanding of how transformation can be used to determine if bacterial genes are closely "linked." You are asked to predict the location of two genes relative to one another. The key to its solution is to understand that cotransformation (of two genes) occurs according to the laws of probability. Two "unlinked" genes are transformed only as a result of two independent events. In such a case, the probability of that occurrence is equal to the product of the individual probabilities.*

6.6 Bacteriophages Are Bacterial Viruses

Bacteriophages, or **phages** as they are commonly known, are viruses that have bacteria as their hosts. The reproduction of phages can lead to still another mode of bacterial genetic recombination, called transduction. To understand this process, we first must consider the genetics of bacteriophages, which themselves can undergo recombination.

A great deal of genetic research has been done using bacteriophages as a model system. In this section, we will first examine the structure and life cycle of one type of bacteriophage. We then discuss how these phages are studied during their infection of bacteria. Finally, we contrast two possible modes of behavior once initial phage infection occurs. This information is background for our discussion of *transduction* and *bacteriophage recombination*.

Head with packaged DNA

Tube

Collar

Sheath

Tail

Tail fibers

Base plate

Mature T4 phage

FIGURE 6–13 The structure of bacteriophage T4, which includes an icosahedral head filled with DNA; a tail consisting of a collar, tube, and sheath; and a base plate with tail fibers. During assembly, the tail components are added to the head and then tail fibers are added.

Phage T4: Structure and Life Cycle

Bacteriophage T4 is one of a group of related bacterial viruses referred to as T-even phages. It exhibits the intricate structure shown in **Figure 6–13**. Its genetic material, DNA, is contained within an icosahedral (referring to a polyhedron with 20 faces) protein coat, making up the head of the virus. The DNA is sufficient in quantity to encode more than 150 average-sized genes. The head is connected to a tail that contains a collar and a contractile sheath surrounding a central core. Tail fibers, which protrude from the tail, contain binding sites in their tips that specifically recognize unique areas of the outer surface of the cell wall of the bacterial host, *E. coli*.

The life cycle of phage T4 (**Figure 6–14**) is initiated when the virus binds by adsorption to the bacterial host cell. Then, it has been proposed that an ATP-driven contraction of the tail sheath causes the central core to penetrate the cell wall. The DNA in the head is extruded, and it moves across the cell membrane into the bacterial cytoplasm. Within minutes, all bacterial DNA, RNA, and protein synthesis is inhibited, and synthesis of viral molecules begins. At the same time, degradation of the host DNA is initiated.

A period of intensive viral gene activity characterizes infection. Initially, phage DNA replication occurs, leading to a pool of viral DNA molecules. Then, the components of the head, tail, and tail fibers are synthesized. The assembly of mature viruses is a complex process that has been well studied by William Wood, Robert Edgar, and others. Three sequential pathways take part: (1) DNA packaging as the viral heads are assembled, (2) tail assembly, and (3) tail-fiber assembly. Once DNA is packaged into the head, that structure combines with the tail components, to which tail fibers are added. Total construction is a combination of self-assembly and enzyme-directed processes.

When approximately 200 new viruses are constructed, the bacterial cell is ruptured by the action of lysozyme (a phage gene product), and the mature phages are released from the host cell. This step during infection is referred to as **lysis**, and it completes what is referred to as the **lytic cycle**. The 200 new phages infect other available bacterial cells, and the process repeats itself over and over again.

The Plaque Assay

Bacteriophages and other viruses have played a critical role in our understanding of molecular genetics.

Host chromosome

1. Phage is adsorbed to bacterial host cell.

Host chromosome

5. Host cell is lysed; phages are released.

2. Phage DNA is injected; host DNA is degraded.

4. Mature phages are assembled.

3. Phage DNA is replicated; phage protein components are synthesized.

FIGURE 6–14 Life cycle of bacteriophage T4.

Serial dilutions of a bacteriophage culture

Total volume	10 mL	10 mL	10 mL	10 mL	10 mL
Dilution	0	10^{-1}	10^{-3}	10^{-5}	10^{-7}
Dilution factor	0	10	10^3	10^5	10^7

10^{-3} dilution
All bacteria lysed
(plaques fused)

10^{-5} dilution
23 plaques

10^{-7} dilution
Lawn of bacteria
(no plaques)

Layer of nutrient agar
plus bacteria

Plaque

Uninfected
bacterial growth

Base of
agar

FIGURE 6–15 A plaque assay for bacteriophage analysis. First, serial dilutions are made of a bacterial culture infected with bacteriophages. Then, three of the dilutions (10^{-3}, 10^{-5}, and 10^{-7}) are analyzed using the plaque assay technique. Each plaque represents the initial infection of one bacterial cell by one bacteriophage. In the 10^{-3} dilution, so many phages are present that all bacteria are lysed. In the 10^{-5} dilution, 23 plaques are produced. In the 10^{-7} dilution, the dilution factor is so great that no phages are present in the 0.1-mL sample, and thus no plaques form. From the 0.1-mL sample of the 10^{-5} dilution, the original bacteriophage density is calculated to be $23 \times 10 \times 10^5$ phages/mL (230×10^5). The photograph shows phage T2 plaques on lawns of *E. coli*.

During infection of bacteria, enormous quantities of bacteriophages may be obtained for investigation. Often, more than 10^{10} viruses are produced per milliliter of culture medium. Many genetic studies have relied on our ability to determine the number of phages produced following infection under specific culture conditions. The **plaque assay**, routinely used for such determinations, is invaluable in quantitative analysis during mutational and recombinational studies of bacteriophages.

This assay is illustrated in **Figure 6–15**, where actual plaque morphology is also shown. A serial dilution of the original virally infected bacterial culture is performed.

Then, a 0.1-mL sample (an aliquot, meaning a fractional portion) from a dilution is added to a small volume of melted nutrient agar (about 3 mL) into which a few drops of a healthy bacterial culture have been added. The solution is then poured evenly over a base of solid nutrient agar in a petri dish and allowed to solidify before incubation. A clear area called a **plaque** occurs wherever a single virus initially infected one bacterium in the culture (the lawn) that has grown up during incubation. The plaque represents clones of the single infecting bacteriophage, created as reproduction cycles are repeated. If the dilution factor is too low, the plaques will be plentiful, and they may fuse, lysing the entire lawn of bacteria. This has occurred in the 10^{-3} dilution in Figure 6–15. However, if the dilution factor is increased appropriately, plaques can be counted, and the density of viruses in the initial culture can be estimated:

initial phage density = (plaque number/mL) × (dilution factor)

Figure 6–15 shows that 23 phage plaques were derived from the 0.1-mL aliquot of the 10^{-5} dilution. Therefore, we estimate a density of 230 phages/mL *at this dilution* (since the initial aliquot was 0.1 mL). The initial phage density in the undiluted sample, given that 23 plaques were observed from 0.1 mL of the 10^{-5} dilution, is calculated as

initial phage density = (230/mL) × (10^5) = $(230 × 10^5)$/mL

Because this figure is derived from the 10^{-5} dilution, we can also estimate that there would be only 0.23 phage/0.1 mL in the 10^{-7} dilution. Thus, if 0.1 mL from this tube were assayed, we would predict that no phage particles would be present. This prediction is borne out in Figure 6–15, where an intact lawn of bacteria lacking any plaques is depicted. The dilution factor is simply too great.

Use of the plaque assay has been invaluable in mutational and recombinational studies of bacteriophages. We will apply this technique more directly later in this chapter when we discuss Seymour Benzer's elegant genetic analysis of a single gene in phage T4.

Lysogeny

Infection of a bacterium by a virus does not always result in viral reproduction and lysis. As early as the 1920s, it was known that a virus can enter a bacterial cell and coexist with it. The precise molecular basis of this relationship is now well understood. Upon entry, the viral DNA is integrated into the bacterial chromosome instead of replicating in the bacterial cytoplasm; this integration characterizes the developmental stage referred to as **lysogeny**. Subsequently, each time the bacterial chromosome is replicated, the viral DNA is also replicated and passed to daughter bacterial cells following division. No new viruses are produced, and no lysis of the bacterial cell occurs. However, under certain stimuli, such as chemical or ultraviolet-light treatment, the viral DNA loses its integrated status and initiates replication, phage reproduction, and lysis of the bacterium.

Several terms are used in describing this relationship. The viral DNA integrated into the bacterial chromosome is called a **prophage.** Viruses that can either lyse the cell or behave as a prophage are called **temperate phages.** Those that can only lyse the cell are referred to as **virulent phages.** A bacterium harboring a prophage has been **lysogenized** and is said to be **lysogenic;** that is, it is capable of being lysed as a result of induced viral reproduction. The viral DNA (like the F factor discussed earlier) is classified as an *episome*, meaning a genetic molecule that can replicate either in the cytoplasm of a cell or as part of its chromosome.

6.7 Transduction Is Virus-Mediated Bacterial DNA Transfer

In 1952, Norton Zinder and Joshua Lederberg were investigating possible recombination in the bacterium *Salmonella typhimurium*. Although they recovered prototrophs from mixed cultures of two different auxotrophic strains, subsequent investigations showed that recombination was not due to the presence of an F factor and conjugation, as in *E. coli*. What they discovered was a process of bacterial recombination mediated by bacteriophages and now called **transduction.**

The Lederberg–Zinder Experiment

Lederberg and Zinder mixed the *Salmonella* auxotrophic strains LA-22 and LA-2 together, and when the mixture was plated on minimal medium, they recovered prototrophic cells. The LA-22 strain was unable to synthesize the amino acids phenylalanine and tryptophan ($phe^- trp^-$), and LA-2 could not synthesize the amino acids methionine and histidine ($met^- his^-$). Prototrophs ($phe^+ trp^+$ $met^+ his^+$) were recovered at a rate of about $1/10^5$ (or 10^{-5}) cells.

Although these observations at first suggested that the recombination was the type observed earlier in conjugative strains of *E. coli*, experiments using the Davis U-tube soon showed otherwise (**Figure 6–16**). The two auxotrophic strains were separated by a sintered glass filter, thus preventing contact between the strains while allowing them to grow in a common medium. Surprisingly, when samples were removed from both sides of the filter and plated

FIGURE 6–16 The Lederberg–Zinder experiment using *Salmonella*. After placing two auxotrophic strains on opposite sides of a Davis U-tube, Lederberg and Zinder recovered prototrophs from the side with the LA-22 strain but not from the side containing the LA-2 strain.

independently on minimal medium, prototrophs *were* recovered, but only from the side of the tube containing LA-22 bacteria. Recall that if conjugation were responsible, the Davis U-tube should have *prevented* recombination altogether (see Figure 6–4).

Since LA-2 cells appeared to be the source of the new genetic information (*phe*⁺ and *trp*⁺), how that information crossed the filter from the LA-2 cells to the LA-22 cells, allowing recombination to occur, was a mystery. The unknown source was designated simply as a **filterable agent (FA)**.

Three observations were used to identify the FA:

1. The FA was produced by the LA-2 cells only when they were grown in association with LA-22 cells. If LA-2 cells were grown independently in a culture medium that was later added to LA-22 cells, recombination did not occur. Therefore, the LA-22 cells played some role in the production of FA by LA-2 cells but did so only when the two strains were sharing a common growth medium.

2. The addition of DNase, which enzymatically digests DNA, did not render the FA ineffective. Therefore, the FA is not exogenous DNA, ruling out transformation.

3. The FA could not pass across the filter of the Davis U-tube when the pore size was reduced below the size of bacteriophages.

Aided by these observations and aware that temperate phages could lysogenize *Salmonella*, researchers proposed that the genetic recombination event was mediated by bacteriophage P22, present initially as a prophage in the chromosome of the LA-22 *Salmonella* cells. They hypothesized that P22 prophages sometimes enter the vegetative, or lytic, phase, reproduce, and are released by the LA-22 cells. Such P22 phages, being much smaller than a bacterium, then cross the filter of the U-tube and subsequently infect and lyse some of the LA-2 cells. In the process of lysis of LA-2, the P22 phages occasionally package a region of the LA-2 chromosome in their heads. If this region contains the *phe*⁺ and *trp*⁺ genes, and if the phages subsequently pass back across the filter and infect LA-22 cells, these newly lysogenized cells will behave as prototrophs. This process of transduction, whereby bacterial recombination is mediated by bacteriophage P22, is diagrammed in **Figure 6–17**.

The Nature of Transduction

Further studies have revealed the existence of transducing phages in other species of bacteria. For example, *E. coli* can be transduced by phage P1, and *B. subtilis* and *Pseudomonas aeruginosa* can be transduced by phages SPO1 and F116, respectively. The details of several different modes of transduction have also been established. Even though the initial discovery of transduction involved a temperate phage and a lysogenized bacterium, the same process can occur during the normal lytic cycle. Sometimes a small piece of bacterial DNA is packaged *along with* the viral chromosome, *or instead of it*, so that the transducing phage either contains both viral and bacterial DNA, or just bacterial DNA. In either case, only a few bacterial genes are present in the transducing phage, although the phage head is capable of enclosing up to 1 percent of the bacterial chromosome. In either case, the ability to infect a host cell is unrelated to the type of DNA in the phage head, making transduction possible.

When bacterial rather than viral DNA is injected into the host cell, it either remains in the cytoplasm or recombines with the homologous region of the bacterial chromosome. If the bacterial DNA remains in the cytoplasm, it does not replicate but is transmitted to one progeny cell following each division. When this happens, only a single cell, partially diploid for the transduced genes, is produced—a phenomenon called *abortive transduction*. If the bacterial DNA recombines with its homologous region of the bacterial chromosome, *complete transduction* occurs, whereby the transduced genes

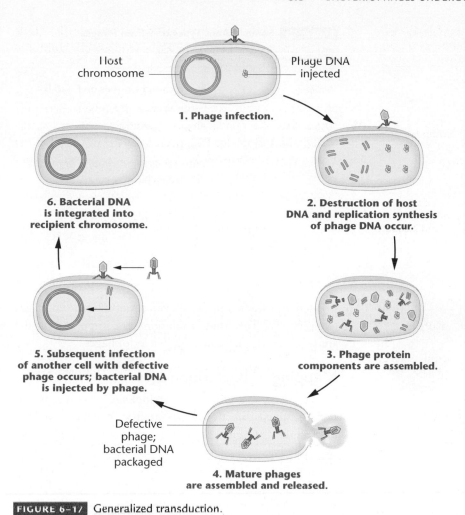

1. Phage infection.

Host chromosome

Phage DNA injected

2. Destruction of host DNA and replication synthesis of phage DNA occur.

3. Phage protein components are assembled.

4. Mature phages are assembled and released.

Defective phage; bacterial DNA packaged

5. Subsequent infection of another cell with defective phage occurs; bacterial DNA is injected by phage.

6. Bacterial DNA is integrated into recipient chromosome.

FIGURE 6–17 Generalized transduction.

become a permanent part of the chromosome, which is passed to all daughter cells.

Both abortive and complete transduction are subclasses of the broader category of *generalized transduction*, which is characterized by the random nature of DNA fragments and genes that are transduced. Each fragment of the bacterial chromosome has a finite but small chance of being packaged in the phage head and subsequently recombined during transduction. Most cases of generalized transduction are of the abortive type; some data suggest that complete transduction occurs 10 to 20 times less frequently. In contrast to generalized transduction, *specialized transduction* occurs when transfer of bacterial DNA is not random, but instead, only strain-specific genes are transduced. This occurs when the DNA representing a temperate bacteriophage breaks out of the host chromosome, bringing with it bacterial DNA on either of its ends.

Transduction and Mapping

Like transformation, transduction has been used in linkage and mapping studies of the bacterial chromosome. The fragment of bacterial DNA involved in a transduction event may be large enough to include several genes. As a result, two genes that are close to one another along the bacterial chromosome (i.e., are linked) can be transduced simultaneously, a process called **cotransduction**. If two genes are not close enough to one another along the chromosome to be included on a single DNA fragment, two independent transduction events must occur to carry them into a single cell. Since this occurs with a much lower probability than cotransduction, linkage can be determined by comparing the frequency of specific simultaneous recombinations.

By concentrating on two or three linked genes, transduction studies can also determine the precise order of these genes. The closer linked genes are to each other, the greater the frequency of cotransduction. Mapping studies can be done on three closely aligned genes, predicated on the same rationale that underlies other mapping techniques.

6.8 Bacteriophages Undergo Intergenic Recombination

Around 1947, several research teams demonstrated that genetic recombination can be detected in bacteriophages. This led to the discovery that gene mapping can be performed in these viruses. Such studies relied on finding numerous phage mutations that could be visualized or assayed. As in bacteria and eukaryotes, these mutations allow genes to be identified and followed in mapping experiments. Before considering recombination and mapping in these bacterial viruses, we briefly introduce several of the mutations that were studied.

Bacteriophage Mutations

Phage mutations often affect the morphology of the plaques formed following lysis of bacterial cells. For example, in 1946, Alfred Hershey observed unusual T2 plaques on plates of *E. coli* strain B. Normal T2 plaques are small and have a clear center surrounded by a diffuse (nearly invisible) halo. In contrast, the unusual plaques were larger

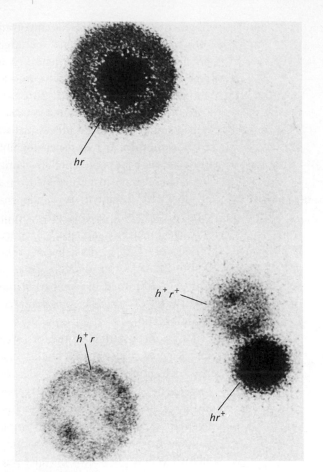

FIGURE 6–18 Plaque morphology phenotypes observed following simultaneous infection of *E. coli* by two strains of phage T2, h^+r and hr^+. In addition to the parental genotypes, recombinant plaques hr and h^+r^+ are shown.

TABLE 6.1	Some Mutant Types of T-Even Phages
Name	**Description**
minute	Forms small plaques
turbid	Forms turbid plaques on *E. coli* B
star	Forms irregular plaques
UV-sensitive	Alters UV sensitivity
acriflavin-resistant	Forms plaques on acriflavin agar
osmotic shock	Withstands rapid dilution into distilled water
lysozyme	Does not produce lysozyme
amber	Grows in *E. coli* K12 but not B
temperature-sensitive	Grows at 25°C but not at 42°C

Table 6.1 lists other types of mutations that have been isolated and studied in the T-even series of bacteriophages (e.g., T2, T4, T6). These mutations are important to the study of genetic phenomena in bacteriophages.

Mapping in Bacteriophages

Genetic recombination in bacteriophages was discovered during **mixed infection experiments**, in which two distinct mutant strains were allowed to *simultaneously* infect the same bacterial culture. These studies were designed so that the number of viral particles sufficiently exceeded the number of bacterial cells to ensure simultaneous infection of most cells by both viral strains. If two loci are involved, recombination is referred to as **intergenic**.

For example, in one study using the T2/*E. coli* system, the parental viruses were of either the h^+r (wild-type host range, rapid lysis) or the hr^+ (extended host range, normal lysis) genotype. If no recombination occurred, these two parental genotypes would be the only expected phage progeny. However, the recombinants h^+r^+ and hr were detected in addition to the parental genotypes (see Figure 6–18). As with eukaryotes, the percentage of recombinant plaques divided by the total number of plaques reflects the relative distance between the genes:

recombinational frequency = $(h^+r^+ + hr)$/total plaques × 100

Sample data for the h and r loci are shown in **Table 6.2**.

and possessed a distinctive outer perimeter (compare the lighter plaques in **Figure 6–18**). When the viruses were isolated from these plaques and replated on *E. coli* B cells, the resulting plaque appearance was identical. Thus, the plaque phenotype was an inherited trait resulting from the reproduction of mutant phages. Hershey named the mutant *rapid lysis* (*r*) because the plaques' larger size was thought to be due to a more rapid or more efficient life cycle of the phage. We now know that, in wild-type phages, reproduction is inhibited once a particular-sized plaque has been formed. The *r* mutant T2 phages overcome this inhibition, producing larger plaques.

Salvador Luria discovered another bacteriophage mutation, *host range* (*h*). This mutation extends the range of bacterial hosts that the phage can infect. Although wild-type T2 phages can infect *E. coli* B (a unique strain), they normally cannot attach or be adsorbed to the surface of *E. coli* B-2 (a different strain). The *h* mutation, however, confers the ability to adsorb to and subsequently infect *E. coli* B-2. When grown on a mixture of *E. coli* B and B-2, the *h* plaque has a center that appears much darker than that of the h^+ plaque (Figure 6–18).

TABLE 6.2	Results of a Cross Involving the *h* and *r* Genes in Phage T2 ($hr^+ \times h^+r$)		
Genotype	**Plaques**	**Designation**	
$h\,r^+$	42	Parental progeny	
h^+r	34	76%	
h^+r^+	12	Recombinants	
$h\,r$	12	24%	

Source: Data derived from Hershey and Rotman (1949).

Similar recombinational studies have been conducted with numerous mutant genes in a variety of bacteriophages. Data are analyzed in much the same way as in eukaryotic mapping experiments. Two- and three-point mapping crosses are possible, and the percentage of recombinants in the total number of phage progeny is calculated. This value is proportional to the relative distance between two genes along the DNA molecule constituting the chromosome.

Investigations into phage recombination support a model similar to that of eukaryotic crossing over—a breakage and reunion process between the viral chromosomes. A fairly clear picture of the dynamics of viral recombination has emerged. Following the early phase of infection, the chromosomes of the phages begin replication. As this stage progresses, a pool of chromosomes accumulates in the bacterial cytoplasm. If double infection by phages of two genotypes has occurred, then the pool of chromosomes initially consists of the two parental types. Genetic exchange between these two types will occur before, during, and after replication, producing recombinant chromosomes.

In the case of the h^+r and hr^+ example discussed here, recombinant h^+r^+ and hr chromosomes are produced. Each of these chromosomes can undergo replication, with new replicates undergoing exchange with each other and with parental chromosomes. Furthermore, recombination is not restricted to exchange between two chromosomes—three or more may be involved simultaneously. As phage development progresses, chromosomes are randomly removed from the pool and packed into the phage head, forming mature phage particles. Thus, a variety of parental and recombinant genotypes are represented in progeny phages.

As we will see in the next section, powerful selection systems have made it possible to detect *intragenic* recombination in viruses, where exchanges occur at points within a single gene, as opposed to intergenic recombination, where exchanges occur at points located between genes. Such studies have led to what has been called the fine-structure analysis of the gene.

6.9 Intragenic Recombination Occurs in Phage T4

We conclude this chapter with an account of an ingenious example of genetic analysis. In the early 1950s, Seymour Benzer undertook a detailed examination of a single locus, *rII*, in phage T4. Benzer successfully designed experiments to recover the extremely rare genetic recombinants arising as a result of intragenic exchange. Such recombination is equivalent to eukaryotic crossing over, but in this case, within a gene rather than at a point between two genes.

Benzer demonstrated that such recombination occurs between the DNA of individual bacteriophages during simultaneous infection of the host bacterium *E. coli*.

The end result of Benzer's work was the production of a detailed map of the *rII* locus. Because of the extremely detailed information provided by his analysis, and because these experiments occurred decades before DNA-sequencing techniques were developed, the insights concerning the internal structure of the gene were particularly noteworthy.

The *rII* Locus of Phage T4

The primary requirement in genetic analysis is the isolation of a large number of mutations in the gene being investigated. Mutants at the *rII* locus produce distinctive plaques when plated on *E. coli* strain B, allowing their easy identification. Figure 6–18 illustrates mutant *r* plaques compared to their wild-type r^+ counterparts in the related T2 phage. Benzer's approach was to isolate many independent *rII* mutants—he eventually obtained about 20,000—and to perform recombinational studies so as to produce a genetic map of this locus. Benzer assumed that most of these mutations, because they were randomly isolated, would represent different locations within the *rII* locus and would thus provide an ample basis for mapping studies.

The key to Benzer's analysis was that *rII* mutant phages, though capable of infecting and lysing *E. coli* B, could not successfully lyse a second related strain, *E. coli* K12(λ).* Wild-type phages, by contrast, could lyse both the B and the K12 strains. Benzer reasoned that these conditions provided the potential for a highly sensitive screening system. If phages from any two different mutant strains were allowed to simultaneously infect *E. coli* B, exchanges between the two mutant sites within the locus would produce rare wild-type recombinants (**Figure 6–19**). If the progeny phage population, which contained more than 99.9 percent *rII* phages and less than 0.1 percent wild-type phages, were then allowed to infect strain K12, the wild-type recombinants would successfully reproduce and produce wild-type plaques. *This is the critical step in recovering and quantifying rare recombinants.*

By using serial dilution techniques, Benzer was able to determine the total number of mutant *rII* phages produced on *E. coli* B and the total number of recombinant wild-type phages that would lyse *E. coli* K12. These data provided the basis for calculating the frequency of recombination, a value proportional to the distance within the gene between the two mutations being studied. As we will see, this experimental design was extraordinarily sensitive. Remarkably, it was possible for Benzer to detect as few as one recombinant

*The inclusion of "(λ)" in the designation of K12 indicates that this bacterial strain is lysogenized by phage λ. This, in fact, is the reason that *rII* mutants cannot lyse such bacteria. In future discussions, this strain will simply be abbreviated as *E. coli* K12.

FIGURE 6–19 Illustration of intragenic recombination between two mutations in the *rII* locus of phage T4. The result is the production of a wild-type phage, which will grow on both *E. coli* B and K12, and of a phage that has incorporated both mutations into the *rII* locus. The latter will grow on *E. coli* B but not on *E. coli* K12.

wild-type phage among 100 million mutant phages. When information from many such experiments is combined, a detailed map of the locus is possible.

Before we discuss this mapping, we need to describe an important discovery Benzer made during the early development of his screen—a discovery that led to the development of a technique used widely in genetics labs today, the **complementation assay** you learned about earlier (see Chapter 4).

Complementation by *rII* Mutations

Before Benzer was able to initiate these intragenic recombination studies, he had to resolve a problem encountered during the early stages of his experimentation. While doing a control study in which K12 bacteria were simultaneously infected with pairs of different *rII* mutant strains, Benzer sometimes found that certain pairs of the *rII* mutant strains lysed the K12 bacteria. This was initially quite puzzling, since only the wild-type *rII* was supposed to be capable of lysing K12 bacteria. How could two mutant strains of *rII*, each of which was thought to contain a defect in the same gene, show a wild-type function?

Benzer reasoned that, during simultaneous infection, each mutant strain provided something that the other lacked, thus restoring wild-type function. This phenomenon, which he called **complementation**, is illustrated in **Figure 6–20(a)**. When many pairs of mutations were tested, each mutation fell into one of two possible **complementation groups,** A or B. Those that failed to complement one another were placed in the same complementation group, while those that did

complement one another were each assigned to a different complementation group. Benzer coined the term **cistron,** which he defined as the smallest functional genetic unit, to describe a complementation group. In modern terminology, we know that a cistron represents a gene.

We now know that Benzer's A and B cistrons represent two separate genes in what we originally referred to as the *rII* locus (because of the initial assumption that it was a single gene). Complementation occurs when K12 bacteria are infected with two *rII* mutants, one with a mutation in the A gene and one with a mutation in the B gene. Therefore, there is a source of both wild-type gene products, since the A mutant provides wild-type B and the B mutant provides wild-type A. We can also explain why two strains that fail to complement, say two A-cistron mutants, are actually mutations in the same gene. In this case, if two A-cistron mutants are combined, there will be an immediate source of the wild-type B product, but no immediate source of the wild-type A product [**Figure 6–20(b)**].

Once Benzer was able to place all *rII* mutations in either the A or the B cistron, he was set to return to his intragenic recombination studies, testing mutations in the A cistron against each other and testing mutations in the B cistron against each other.

NOW SOLVE THIS

6–3 In complementation studies of the *rII* locus of phage T4, three groups of three different mutations were tested. For each group, only two combinations were tested. On the basis of each set of data (shown here), predict the results of the third experiment for each group.

Group A	Group B	Group C
d × *e*–lysis	*g* × *b*–no lysis	*j* × *k*–lysis
d × *f*–no lysis	*g* × *i*–no lysis	*j* × *l*–lysis
e × *f*–?	*b* × *i*–?	*k* × *l*–?

■ **HINT:** *This problem involves an understanding of why complementation occurs during simultaneous infection of a bacterial cell by two bacteriophage strains, each with a different mutation within the rII locus. The key to its solution is to be aware that if each mutation alters a different genetic product, then each strain will provide the product that the other is missing, thus leading to complementation.*

For more practice, see Problems 19, 20, and 22.

Recombinational Analysis

Of the approximately 20,000 *rII* mutations, roughly half fell into each cistron. Benzer set about mapping the mutations within each one. For example, if two *rII* A mutants (i.e., two phage strains with different mutations in the A cistron) were first allowed to infect *E. coli* B in a liquid culture, and if a recombination event occurred between the mutational sites in the A cistron, then wild-type progeny viruses would be produced at low frequency. If samples of the progeny viruses from such an experiment were then plated on *E. coli* K12, only the wild-type recombinants would lyse the bacteria and produce plaques. The total number of nonrecombinant progeny viruses would be determined by plating samples on *E. coli* B.

This experimental protocol is illustrated in **Figure 6–21**. The percentage of recombinants can be determined by counting the plaques at the appropriate dilution in each case. As in eukaryotic mapping experiments, the frequency of recombination is an estimate of the distance between the two mutations within the cistron. For example, if the number of recombinants is equal to 4×10^3/mL, and the total number of progeny is 8×10^9/mL, then the frequency of recombination between the two mutants is

$$2\left(\frac{4 \times 10^3}{8 \times 10^9}\right) = 2(0.5 \times 10^{-6})$$
$$= 10^{-6}$$
$$= 0.000001$$

Multiplying by 2 is necessary because each recombinant event yields two reciprocal products, only one of which—the wild type—is detected.

Deletion Testing of the *rII* Locus

Although the system for assessing recombination frequencies described earlier allowed for mapping mutations within each cistron, testing 1000 mutants two at a time in all combinations would have required millions of experiments. Fortunately,

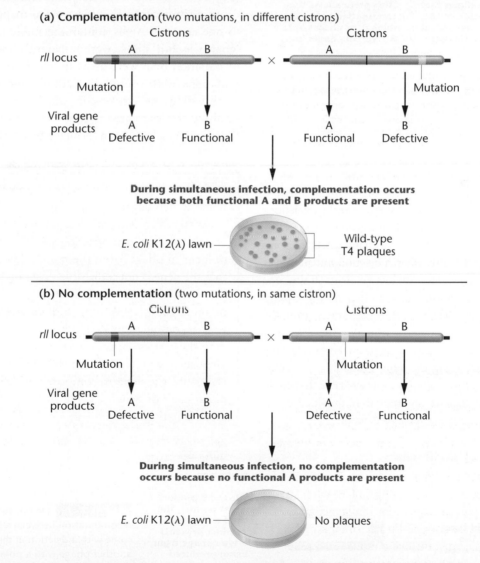

(a) Complementation (two mutations, in different cistrons)

During simultaneous infection, complementation occurs because both functional A and B products are present

(b) No complementation (two mutations, in same cistron)

During simultaneous infection, no complementation occurs because no functional A products are present

FIGURE 6–20 Comparison of two pairs of *rII* mutations. (a) In one case, they complement one another. (b) In the other case, they do not complement one another. Complementation occurs when each mutation is in a separate cistron. Failure to complement occurs when the two mutations are in the same cistron.

Recombinant (wild-type) phages infect *E. coli* K12(λ)

Nonrecombinant (*rII* mutants) phages infect *E. coli* B

Simultaneous infection with two *rIIA* or two *rIIB* mutations

E. coli B

10^{-3} | Serial dilutions and plaque assay | 10^{-9}

plaques

E. coli K12(λ)

E. coli B

This plate allows the determination of the number of recombinants: 4×10^3 recombinant phages/mL

This plate allows the determination of the total number of phages/mL: 8×10^9 *rII* phages/mL

FIGURE 6–21 The experimental protocol for recombination studies between pairs of mutations in the same cistron. In this figure, all phage infecting *E. coli* B (in the flask) contain one of two mutations in the A cistron, as shown in the depiction of their chromosomes to the left of the flask.

Benzer was able to overcome this obstacle when he devised an analytical approach referred to as **deletion testing**. He discovered that some of the *rII* mutations were, in reality, deletions of small parts of both cistrons. That is, the genetic changes giving rise to the *rII* properties were not a characteristic of point mutations. Most importantly, when a deletion mutation was tested using simultaneous infection by two phage strains, one having the deletion mutation and the other having a point mutation located in the deleted part of the same cistron, the test never yielded wild-type recombinants. The reason is illustrated in **Figure 6–22**. Because the deleted area is lacking the area of DNA containing the point mutation, no recombination is possible. Thus, a method was available that could roughly, but quickly, localize any mutation, provided it was contained within a region covered by a deletion.

Deletion testing could thus provide data for the initial localization of each mutation. For example, as shown in **Figure 6–23**, seven overlapping deletions spanning various regions of the A cistron were used for the initial screening of point mutations in that cistron. Depending on whether the viral chromosome bearing a point mutation does or does not undergo recombination with the chromosome bearing a deletion, each point mutation can be assigned to a specific area of the cistron. Further deletions within each of the seven areas can be used to localize, or map, each *rII* point mutation more precisely. Remember that, in each case, a point mutation is localized in the area of a deletion when it fails to give rise to any wild-type recombinants.

The *rII* Gene Map

After several years of work, Benzer produced a genetic map of the two cistrons composing the *rII* locus of phage T4 (**Figure 6–24**). From the 20,000 mutations analyzed, 307 distinct sites within this locus were mapped in relation to one another. Areas containing many mutations, designated as **hot spots**, were apparently more susceptible to mutation than were areas in which only one or a few mutations were found. In addition, Benzer discovered areas within the cistrons in which no mutations were localized. He estimated that as many as 200 recombinational units had not been localized by his studies.

EVOLVING CONCEPT OF A GENE

In the early 1950s, genes were regarded as indivisible units of heredity that could undergo mutation and between which *intergenic* recombination could occur. Seymour Benzer's pioneering genetic analysis of the *rII* locus in phage T4 in the mid-1950s demonstrated that the gene is not indivisible. Instead, he established that multiple sites exist within a gene, each capable of undergoing mutation, and between which *intragenic* recombination can occur. Benzer was able to map these sites within the *rII* locus. As we will see in an ensuing chapter, around the same time, it became clear that the gene is composed of DNA nucleotide pairs, each of which can be the site of mutation or recombination. ∎

Area of deletion — Deletion mutation × Point mutation

Since recombination cannot occur in the area of the deletion, no wild-type recombinants of the A cistron can be produced

While the B product remains normal, the lack of a functional A product prevents wild-type phage from being produced

FIGURE 6–22 Demonstration that recombination between a phage chromosome with a deletion in the A cistron and another phage with a point mutation overlapped by that deletion cannot yield a chromosome with wild-type A and B cistrons.

FIGURE 6–23 Three series of overlapping deletions in the A cistron of the *rII* locus used to localize the position of an unknown *rII* mutation. For example, if a mutant strain tested against each deletion (dashed areas) in Series I for the production of recombinant wild-type progeny shows the results at the right (− or +), the mutation must be in segment *A5*. In Series II, the mutation is further narrowed to segment *A5c*, and in Series III to segment *A5c3*.

FIGURE 6–24 A partial map of mutations in the A and B cistrons of the *rII* locus of phage T4. Each square represents an independently isolated mutation. Note the two areas in which the largest number of mutations are present, referred to as "hot spots" (*A6cd* and *B5*).

GENETICS, TECHNOLOGY, AND SOCIETY

From Cholera Genes to Edible Vaccines

Using an expanding toolbox of molecular genetic tools, scientists are tackling some of the most serious bacterial diseases affecting our species. Our ability to clone bacterial genes and transfer them into other organisms is leading directly to exciting new treatments. The story of edible vaccines for the treatment of cholera illustrates how genetic engineering is being applied to control a serious human disease.

Cholera is caused by *Vibrio cholerae*, a curved, rod-shaped bacterium found in rivers and oceans. Most genetic strains of *V. cholerae* are harmless; only a few are pathogenic. Infection occurs when a person drinks water or eats food contaminated with pathogenic *V. cholerae*. Once in the digestive system, these bacteria colonize the small intestine and produce proteins called enterotoxins that invade the mucosal cells lining the intestine. This triggers a massive secretion of water and dissolved salts, resulting in violent diarrhea, severe dehydration, muscle cramps, lethargy, and often death. The enterotoxin consists of two polypeptides, called the A and B subunits, encoded by two separate genes.

Cholera remains a leading cause of human deaths throughout the Third World, where basic sanitation is lacking and water supplies are often contaminated. For example, in July 1994, 70,000 cases of cholera leading to 12,000 fatalities were reported among the Rwandans crowded into refugee camps in Goma, Zaire. And after an absence of over 100 years, cholera reappeared in Latin America in 1991, spreading from Peru to Mexico and claiming more than 10,000 lives. Following the 2010 earthquakes in Haiti, a severe cholera outbreak spread through the country, claiming more than 4000 lives.

A new gene-based technology is emerging to attack cholera. This technology centers on genetically engineered plants that act as vaccines. Scientists introduce a cloned gene—such as a gene encoding a bacterial protein—into the plant genome. The transgenic plant produces the new gene product, and immunity is acquired when an animal eats the plant. The gene product in the plant acts as an antigen, stimulating the production of antibodies

to protect against bacterial infection or the effects of their toxins. Since the B subunit of the cholera enterotoxin binds to intestinal cells, research has focused on using this polypeptide as the antigen, with the hope that antibodies against it will prevent toxin binding and render the bacteria harmless.

Leading the efforts to develop an edible vaccine are Charles Arntzen and associates at Cornell University. To test the system, they are using the B subunit of an *E. coli* enterotoxin, which is similar in structure and immunological properties to the cholera protein. Their first step was to obtain the DNA clone of the gene encoding the B subunit and to attach it to a promoter that would induce transcription in all tissues of the plant. Second, the researchers introduced the hybrid gene into potato plants by means of *Agrobacterium*-mediated transformation. The engineered plants expressed their new gene and produced the enterotoxin B subunit. Third, they fed mice a few grams of the genetically engineered tubers. Arntzen's group found that the mice produced specific antibodies against the B subunit and secreted them into the small intestine. When they fed purified enterotoxin to the mice, the mice were protected from its effects and did not develop the symptoms of cholera. In clinical trials conducted using humans in 1998, almost all of the volunteers developed an immune response, and none experienced adverse side effects.

Arntzen's experiments have served as models for other research efforts involving edible vaccines. Currently, scientists are developing edible vaccines against bacterial diseases such as anthrax and tetanus, as well as viral diseases such as rabies, AIDS, and measles.

Your Turn

Take time, individually or in groups, to answer the following questions. Investigate the references and links to help you understand some of the issues that surround the development and uses of edible vaccines.

1. What are the latest research developments on edible vaccines for cholera?

A source of information is the PubMed Web site (http://www.ncbi.nlm.nih.gov/pubmed), as described in an "Exploring Genomics" feature (see Chapter 2).

2. Several oral vaccines against cholera are currently available. Given the availability of these vaccines, why do you think that scientists are also developing edible vaccines for cholera? Which vaccine type would you choose for vaccinating populations at risk for cholera?

Read about these cholera vaccines on the World Health Organization Web site at http://www.who.int/cholera/vaccines/en

3. Cholera is spread through ingestion of contaminated water and food. Despite its severity, cholera patients can be effectively treated by oral rehydration. Cholera becomes a major health problem only when proper sanitation and medical treatment are lacking. Given these facts, how much research funding do you think we should spend to develop cholera vaccines, relative to funds spent on improved sanitation, water treatment, and education about treatments?

A discussion of sanitation versus cholera vaccination can be found on the Web site of the Integrated Regional Information Network at http://www.irinnews.org/Report/84386/

4. In a recent study, scientists from UC San Diego used the *Vibrio cholerae* gene that encodes the enterotoxin B subunit in a unique way. They fused the gene to another gene that encodes a malaria protein, expressed the recombinant fusion gene in algae, and used the freeze-dried algae as an edible vaccine. Describe the significance of this study, for control of both cholera and other food and water-borne diseases.

For details, see Quest for edible malarial vaccine leads to other potential medical uses for algae, *at* http://phys.org/news/2013-04-quest-edible-malarial-vaccine-potential.html
Also see Gregory, J.A., et al. 2013. Algae-produced cholera toxin-Pfs25 fusion proteins as oral vaccines. *Appl. Environ. Microbiol.* 79: 3917–3925.

CASE STUDY | To treat or not to treat

A 4-month-old infant had been running a moderate fever for 36 hours, and a nervous mother made a call to her pediatrician. Examination and testing revealed no outward signs of infection or cause of the fever. The anxious mother asked the pediatrician about antibiotics, but the pediatrician recommended watching the infant carefully for two days before making a decision. He explained that decades of rampant use of antibiotics in medicine and agriculture had caused a worldwide surge in bacteria that are now resistant to such drugs. He also said that the reproductive behavior of bacteria allows them to exchange antibiotic resistance traits with a wide range of other disease-causing bacteria, and that many strains are now resistant to multiple antibiotics. The physician's information raises several interesting questions.

1. Was the physician correct in saying that bacteria can share resistance?

2. Where do bacteria carry antibiotic resistance genes, and how are they exchanged?

3. If the infant was given an antibiotic as a precaution, how might it contribute to the production of resistant bacteria?

4. Aside from hospitals, where else would infants and children come in contact with antibiotic-resistant strains of bacteria? Does the presence of such bacteria in the body always mean an infection?

Summary Points

MasteringGenetics™ For activities, animations, and review quizzes, go to the Study Area.

1. Genetic recombination in bacteria takes place in three ways: conjugation, transformation, and transduction.

2. Conjugation may be initiated by a bacterium housing a plasmid called the F factor in its cytoplasm, making it a donor cell. Following conjugation, the recipient cell receives a copy of the F factor and is converted to the F^+ status.

3. When the F factor is integrated from the cytoplasm into the chromosome, the cell remains as a donor and is referred to as an Hfr cell. Upon mating, the donor chromosome moves unidirectionally into the recipient, initiating recombination and providing the basis for time mapping of the bacterial chromosome.

4. Plasmids, such as the F factor, are autonomously replicating DNA molecules found in the bacterial cytoplasm, sometimes containing unique genes conferring antibiotic resistance as well as the genes necessary for plasmid transfer during conjugation.

5. Transformation in bacteria, which does not require cell-to-cell contact, involves exogenous DNA that enters a recipient bacterium and recombines with the host's chromosome. Linkage mapping of closely aligned genes is possible during the analysis of transformation.

6. Bacteriophages, viruses that infect bacteria, demonstrate a well-defined life cycle where they reproduce within the host cell and can be studied using the plaque assay.

7. Bacteriophages can be lytic, meaning they infect the host cell, reproduce, and then lyse it, or in contrast, they can lysogenize the host cell, where they infect it and integrate their DNA into the host chromosome, but do not reproduce.

8. Transduction is virus-mediated bacterial DNA recombination. When a lysogenized bacterium subsequently reenters the lytic cycle, the new bacteriophages serve as vehicles for the transfer of host (bacterial) DNA.

9. Various mutant phenotypes, including mutations in plaque morphology and host range, have been studied in bacteriophages and have served as the basis for mapping in these viruses.

10. Transduction is also used for bacterial linkage and mapping studies.

11. Various mutant phenotypes, including mutations in plaque morphology and host range, have been studied in bacteriophages. These have served as the basis for investigating genetic exchange and mapping in these viruses.

12. Genetic analysis of the *rII* locus in bacteriophage T4 allowed Seymour Benzer to study intragenic recombination. By isolating *rII* mutants and performing complementation analysis, recombinational studies, and deletion mapping, Benzer was able to locate and map more than 300 distinct sites within the two cistrons of the *rII* locus.

INSIGHTS AND SOLUTIONS

1. Time mapping is performed in a cross involving the genes *his*, *leu*, *mal*, and *xyl*. The recipient cells were auxotrophic for all four genes. After 25 minutes, mating was interrupted with the following results in recipient cells. Diagram the positions of these genes relative to the origin (*O*) of the F factor and to one another.

   (a) 90% were *xyl*$^+$
   (b) 80% were *mal*$^+$
   (c) 20% were *his*$^+$
   (d) none were *leu*$^+$

   Solution: The *xyl* gene was transferred most frequently, which shows it is closest to *O* (very close). The *mal* gene is

next closest and reasonably near *xyl*, followed by the more distant *his* gene. The *leu* gene is far beyond these three, since no recombinants are recovered that include it. The diagram shows these relative locations along a piece of the circular chromosome.

2. Three strains of bacteria, each bearing a ser... *a*$^-$, *b*$^-$, or *c*$^-$, are the sources of donor ... mation experiment. Recipient cells are ... genes but express the mutation *d*$^-$.

Insights and Solutions—continued

(a) Based on the following data, and assuming that the location of the *d* gene precedes the *a*, *b*, and *c* genes, propose a linkage map for the four genes.

DNA Donor	Recipient	Transformants	Frequency of Transformants
a^-d^+	a^+d^-	a^+d^+	0.21
b^-d^+	b^+d^-	b^+d^+	0.18
c^-d^+	c^+d^-	c^+d^+	0.63

(b) If the donor DNA were wild type and the recipient cells were either a^-b^-, a^-c^-, or b^-c^-, which of the crosses would be expected to produce the greatest number of wild-type transformants?

Solution: (a) These data reflect the relative distances between the *a*, *b*, and *c* genes, individually, and the *d* gene. The *a* and *b* genes are about the same distance from the *d* gene and are thus tightly linked to one another. The *c* gene is more distant. Assuming that the *d* gene precedes the others, the map looks like this:

(b) Because the *a* and *b* genes are closely linked, they most likely cotransform in a single event. Thus, recipient cells a^-b^- are most likely to convert to wild type.

3. For his fine-structure analysis of the *rII* locus in phage T4, Benzer was able to perform complementation testing of any pair of mutations once it was clear that the locus contained two cistrons. Complementation was assayed by simultaneously infecting *E. coli* K12 with two phage strains, each with an independent mutation, neither of which could alone lyse K12. From the data that follow, determine which mutations are in which cistron, assuming that mutation *1* (*M-1*) is in the A cistron and mutation *2* (*M-2*) is in the B cistron. Are there any cases where the mutation cannot be properly assigned?

Test Pair	Results*
1, 2	+
1, 3	–
1, 4	–
1, 5	+
2, 3	–
2, 4	+
2, 5	–

*+ or – indicates complementation or the failure of complementation, respectively.

Solution: *M-1* and *M-5* complement one another and, therefore, are not in the same cistron. Thus, *M-5* must be in the B cistron. *M-2* and *M-4* complement one another. By the same reasoning, *M-4* is not with *M-2* and, therefore, is in the A cistron. *M-3* fails to complement either *M-1* or *M-2*, and so it would seem to be in both cistrons. One explanation is that the physical cause of *M-3* somehow overlaps both the A and the B cistrons. It might be a double mutation with one sequence change in each cistron. It might also be a deletion that overlaps both cistrons and thus could not complement either *M-1* or *M-2*.

4. Another mutation, *M-6*, was tested with the results shown here:

Test Pair	Results
1, 6	+
2, 6	–
3, 6	–
4, 6	+
5, 6	–

Draw all possible conclusions about *M-6*.

Solution: These results are consistent with assigning *M-6* to the B cistron.

5. Recombination testing was then performed for *M-2*, *M-5*, and *M-6* so as to map the B cistron. Recombination analysis using both *E. coli* B and K12 showed that recombination occurred between *M-2* and *M-5* and between *M-5* and *M-6*, but not between *M-2* and *M-6*. Why not?

Solution: Either *M-2* and *M-6* represent identical mutations, or one of them may be a deletion that overlaps the other but does not overlap *M-5*. Furthermore, the data cannot rule out the possibility that both are deletions.

6. In recombination studies of the *rII* locus in phage T4, what is the significance of the value determined by calculating phage growth in the K12 versus the B strains of *E. coli* following simultaneous infection in *E. coli* B? Which value is always greater?

Solution: When plaque analysis is performed on *E. coli* B, in which the wild-type and mutant phages are both lytic, the total number of phages per milliliter can be determined. Because almost all cells are *rII* mutants of one type or another, this value is much larger than the value obtained with K12. To avoid total lysis of the plate, extensive dilution is necessary. In K12, *rII* mutations will not grow, but wild-type phages will. Because wild-type phages are the rare recombinants, there are relatively few of them and extensive dilution is not required.

Problems and Discussion Questions

HOW DO WE KNOW?

1. In this chapter, we have focused on genetic systems present in bacteria and on the viruses that use bacteria as hosts (bacteriophages). In particular, we discussed mechanisms by which bacteria and their phages undergo genetic recombination, which allows geneticists to map bacterial and bacteriophage chromosomes. In the process, we found many opportunities to consider how this information was acquired. From the explanations given in the chapter, what answers would you propose to the following questions?
(a) How do we know that genes exist in bacteria and bacteriophages?
(b) How do we know that bacteria undergo genetic recombination, allowing the transfer of genes from one organism to another?
(c) How do we know whether or not genetic recombination between bacteria involves cell-to-cell contact?
(d) How do we know that bacteriophages recombine genetic material through transduction and that cell-to-cell contact is not essential for transduction to occur?
(e) How do we know that intergenic exchange occurs in bacteriophages?
(f) How do we know that in bacteriophage T4 the *rII* locus is subdivided into two regions, or cistrons?

CONCEPT QUESTION

2. Review the Chapter Concepts list on p. 134. Many of these center around the findings that genetic recombination occurs in bacteria and in bacteriophages. Write a short summary that contrasts how recombination occurs in bacteria and bacteriophages.
3. With respect to F^+ and F^- bacterial matings, answer the following questions:
(a) How was it established that physical contact between cells was necessary?
(b) How was it established that chromosome transfer was unidirectional?
(c) What is the genetic basis for a bacterium's being F^+?
4. List all major differences between (a) the $F^+ \times F^-$ and the Hfr $\times F^-$ bacterial crosses; and (b) the F^+, F^- Hfr, and F' bacteria.
5. Describe the basis for chromosome mapping in the Hfr $\times F^-$ crosses.
6. In general, when recombination experiments are conducted with bacteria, participating bacteria are mixed in complete medium, then transferred to a minimal growth medium. Why isn't the protocol reversed: minimal medium first, complete medium second?
7. Why are the recombinants produced from an Hfr $\times F^-$ cross rarely, if ever, F^+?
8. Describe the origin of F' bacteria and merozygotes.
9. In a transformation experiment, donor DNA was obtained from a prototroph bacterial strain ($a^+b^+c^+$), and the recipient was a triple auxotroph ($a^-b^-c^-$). What general conclusions can you draw about the linkage relationships among the three genes from the following transformant classes that were recovered?

$a^+\,b^-\,c^-$	180
$a^-\,b^+\,c^-$	150
$a^+\,b^+\,c^-$	210
$a^-\,b^-\,c^+$	179
$a^+\,b^-\,c^+$	2
$a^-\,b^+\,c^+$	1
$a^+\,b^+\,c^+$	3

10. Describe the role of heteroduplex formation during transformation.
11. Explain the observations that led Zinder and Lederberg to conclude that the prototrophs recovered in their transduction experiments were not the result of F^+ mediated conjugation.
12. Define plaque, lysogeny, and prophage.
13. Differentiate between generalized and specialized transduction.
14. Two theoretical genetic strains of a virus ($a^-b^-c^-$ and $a^+b^+c^+$) were used to simultaneously infect a culture of host bacteria. Of 10,000 plaques scored, the following genotypes were observed. Determine the genetic map of these three genes on the viral chromosome. Decide whether interference was positive or negative.

$a^+\,b^+\,c^+$	4100	$a^-\,b^+\,c^-$	160
$a^-\,b^-\,c^-$	3990	$a^+\,b^-\,c^+$	140
$a^+\,b^-\,c^-$	740	$a^-\,b^-\,c^+$	90
$a^-\,b^+\,c^+$	670	$a^+\,b^+\,c^-$	110

15. The bacteriophage genome consists of many genes encoding proteins that make up the head, collar, tail, and tail fibers. When these genes are transcribed following phage infection, how are these proteins synthesized, since the phage genome lacks genes essential to ribosome structure?
16. If a single bacteriophage infects one *E. coli* cell present on a lawn of bacteria and, upon lysis, yields 200 viable viruses, how many phages will exist in a single plaque if three more lytic cycles occur?
17. A phage-infected bacterial culture was subjected to a series of dilutions, and a plaque assay was performed in each case, with the results shown in the following table. What conclusion can be drawn in the case of each dilution, assuming that 0.1 mL was used in each plaque assay?

	Dilution Factor	Assay Results
(a)	10^4	All bacteria lysed
(b)	10^5	14 plaques
(c)	10^6	0 plaques

18. In recombination studies of the *rII* locus in phage T4, what is the significance of the value determined by calculating phage growth in the K12 versus the B strains of *E. coli* following simultaneous infection in *E. coli* B? Which value is always greater?

19. In an analysis of *rII* mutants, complementation testing yielded the following results:

Mutants	Results (+/− lysis)
1, 2	+
1, 3	+
1, 4	−
1, 5	−

Predict the results of testing 2 and 3, 2 and 4, and 3 and 4 together.

20. If further testing of the mutations in Problem 19 yielded the following results, what would you conclude about mutant 5?

Mutants	Results
2, 5	−
3, 5	−
4, 5	−

21. Using mutants 2 and 3 from the previous problem, following mixed infection on *E. coli* B, progeny viruses were plated in a series of dilutions on both *E. coli* B and K12 with the following results. (a) What is the recombination frequency between the two mutants?

Strain Plated	Dilution	Plaques
E. coli B	10^{-5}	2
E. coli K12	10^{-1}	5

(b) Another mutation, 6, was tested in relation to mutations 1 through 5 from the previous problems. In initial testing, mutant 6 complemented mutants 2 and 3. In recombination testing with 1, 4, and 5, mutant 6 yielded recombinants with 1 and 5, but not with 4. What can you conclude about mutation 6?

Extra-Spicy Problems

22. During the analysis of seven *rII* mutations in phage T4, mutants 1, 2, and 6 were in cistron A, while mutants 3, 4, and 5 were in cistron B. Of these, mutant 4 was a deletion overlapping mutant 5. The remainder were point mutations. Nothing was known about mutant 7. Predict the results of complementation (+ or −) between 1 and 2; 1 and 3; 2 and 4; and 4 and 5.

23. In studies of recombination between mutants 1 and 2 from the previous problem, the results shown in the following table were obtained.

Strain	Dilution	Plaques	Phenotypes
E. coli B	10^{-7}	4	*r*
E. coli K12	10^{-2}	8	1

(a) Calculate the recombination frequency.
(b) When mutant 6 was tested for recombination with mutant 1, the data were the same as those shown above for strain B, but not for K12. The researcher lost the K12 data, but remembered that recombination was ten times more frequent than when mutants 1 and 2 were tested. What were the lost values (dilution and colony numbers)?
(c) Mutant 7 (Problem 22) failed to complement any of the other mutants (1–6). Define the nature of mutant 7.

24. In *Bacillus subtilis*, linkage analysis of two mutant genes affecting the synthesis of two amino acids, tryptophan (trp_2^-) and tyrosine (tyr_1^-), was performed using transformation. Examine the following data and draw all possible conclusions regarding linkage. What is the purpose of Part B of the experiment? [Reference: E. Nester, M. Schafer, and J. Lederberg (1963).]

Donor DNA	Recipient Cell	Transformants	No.
A. $trp_2^+\ tyr_1^+$	$trp_2^-\ tyr_1^-$	$trp^+\ tyr^-$	196
		$trp^-\ tyr^+$	328
		$trp^+\ tyr^+$	367
B. $trp_2^+\ tyr_1^-$ and $trp_2^-\ tyr_1^+$	$trp_2^-\ tyr_1^-$	$trp^+\ tyr^-$	190
		$trp^-\ tyr^+$	256
		$trp^+\ tyr^+$	2

25. An Hfr strain is used to map three genes in an interrupted mating experiment. The cross is $Hfr/a^+b^+c^+rif \times F^-/a^-b^-c^-rif^{\,r}$. (No map order is implied in the listing of the alleles; $rif^{\,r}$ is resistance to the antibiotic rifampicin.) The a^+ gene is required for the biosynthesis of nutrient A, the b^+ gene for nutrient B, and c^+ for nutrient C. The minus alleles are auxotrophs for these nutrients. The cross is initiated at time = 0, and at various times, the mating mixture is plated on three types of medium. Each plate contains minimal medium (MM) plus rifampicin plus specific supplements that are indicated in the following table. (The results for each time interval are shown as the number of colonies growing on each plate.)

	Time of Interruption			
	5 min	10 min	15 min	20 min
Nutrients A and B	0	0	4	21
Nutrients B and C	0	5	23	40
Nutrients A and C	4	25	60	82

(a) What is the purpose of rifampicin in the experiment?
(b) Based on these data, determine the approximate location on the chromosome of the *a*, *b*, and *c* genes relative to one another and to the F factor.
(c) Can the location of the *rif* gene be determined in this experiment? If not, design an experiment to determine the location of *rif* relative to the F factor and to gene *b*.

26. A plaque assay is performed beginning with 1 mL of a solution containing bacteriophages. This solution is serially diluted three times by combining 0.1 mL of each sequential dilution with 9.9 mL of liquid medium. Then 0.1 mL of the final dilution is plated in the plaque assay and yields 17 plaques. What is the initial density of bacteriophages in the original 1 mL?

27. In a cotransformation experiment, using various combinations of genes two at a time, the following data were produced. Determine which genes are "linked" to which others.

Successful Cotransformation	Unsuccessful Cotransformation
a and d; b and c; b and f	a and b; a and c; a and f; d and b; d and c; d and f; a and e; b and e; c and e; d and e; f and e

28. For the experiment in Problem 27, another gene, g, was studied. It demonstrated positive cotransformation when tested with gene f. Predict the results of testing gene g with genes a, b, c, d, and e.

29. Bacterial conjugation, mediated mainly by conjugative plasmids such as F, represents a potential health threat through the sharing of genes for pathogenicity or antibiotic resistance. Given that more than 400 different species of bacteria coinhabit a healthy human gut and more than 200 coinhabit human skin, Francisco Dionisio [*Genetics* (2002) 162:1525–1532] investigated the ability of plasmids to undergo between-species conjugal transfer. The following data are presented for various species of the enterobacterial genus *Escherichia*. The data are presented as "log base 10" values; for example, −2.0 would be equivalent to 10^{-2} as a rate of transfer. Assume that all differences between values presented are statistically significant.
(a) What general conclusion(s) can be drawn from these data?
(b) In what species is within-species transfer most likely? In what species pair is between-species transfer most likely?
(c) What is the significance of these findings in terms of human health?

	Donor			
Recipient	E. chrysanthemi	E. blattae	E. fergusonii	E. coli
E. chrysanthemi	−2.4	−4.7	−5.8	−3.7
E. blattae	−2.0	−3.4	−5.2	−3.4
E. fergusonii	−3.4	−5.0	−5.8	−4.2
E. coli	−1.7	−3.7	−5.3	−3.5

30. A study was conducted in an attempt to determine which functional regions of a particular conjugative transfer gene (*tra1*) are involved in the transfer of plasmid R27 in *Salmonella enterica*. The R27 plasmid is of significant clinical interest because it is capable of encoding multiple-antibiotic resistance to typhoid fever. To identify functional regions responsible for conjugal transfer, an analysis by Lawley et al. (2002. *J. Bacteriol.* 184:2173–2180) was conducted in which particular regions of the *tra1* gene were mutated and tested for their impact on conjugation. Shown here is a map of the regions tested and believed to be involved in conjugative transfer of the plasmid. Similar coloring indicates related function. Numbers correspond to each functional region subjected to mutation analysis.

Accompanying the map is a table showing the effects of these mutations on R27 conjugation.

Effects of Mutations in Functional Regions of Transfer Region 1 (*tra1*) on R27 Conjugation

R27 Mutation in Region	Conjugative Transfer	Relative Conjugation Frequency (%)
1	+	100
2	+	100
3	−	0
4	+	100
5	−	0
6	−	0
7	+	12
8	−	0
9	−	0
10	−	0
11	+	13
12	−	0
13	−	0
14		0

(a) Given the data, do all functional regions appear to influence conjugative transfer?
(b) Which regions appear to have the most impact on conjugation?
(c) Which regions appear to have a limited impact on conjugation?
(d) What general conclusions might one draw from these data?

31. Influenza (the flu) is responsible for approximately 250,000 to 500,000 deaths annually, but periodically its toll has been much higher. For example, the 1918 flu pandemic killed approximately 30 million people worldwide and is considered the worst spread of a deadly illness in recorded history. With highly virulent flu strains emerging periodically, it is little wonder that the scientific community is actively studying influenza biology. In 2007, the National Institute of Allergy and Infectious Diseases completed sequencing of 2035 human and avian influenza virus strains. Influenza strains undergo recombination as described in this chapter, and they have a high mutation rate owing to the error-prone replication of their genome (which consists of RNA rather than DNA). In addition, they are capable of chromosome reassortment in which various combinations of their eight chromosomes (or portions thereof) can be packaged into progeny viruses when two or more strains infect the same cell. The end result is that we can make vaccines, but they must change annually, and even then, we can only guess at what specific viral strains will be prevalent in any given year. Based on the above information, consider the following questions:
(a) Of what evolutionary value to influenza viruses are high mutation and recombination rates coupled with chromosome reassortment?
(b) Why can't humans combat influenza just as they do mumps, measles, or chicken pox?
(c) Why are vaccines available for many viral diseases but not influenza?

A human X chromosome highlighted using fluorescence *in situ* hybridization (FISH), a method in which specific probes bind to specific sequences of DNA. The probe producing green fluorescence binds to the DNA of the X chromosome centromeres. The probe producing red fluorescence binds to the DNA sequence of the X-linked Duchenne muscular dystrophy (DMD) gene.

7

Sex Determination and Sex Chromosomes

CHAPTER CONCEPTS

- A variety of mechanisms have evolved that result in sexual differentiation, leading to sexual dimorphism and greatly enhancing the production of genetic variation within species.

- Often, specific genes, usually on a single chromosome, cause maleness or femaleness during development.

- In humans, the presence of extra X or Y chromosomes beyond the diploid number may be tolerated but often leads to syndromes demonstrating distinctive phenotypes.

- While segregation of sex-determining chromosomes should theoretically lead to a one-to-one sex ratio of males to females, in humans the actual ratio greatly favors males at conception.

- In mammals, females inherit two X chromosomes compared to one in males, but the extra genetic information in females is compensated for by random inactivation of one of the X chromosomes early in development.

- In some reptilian species, temperature during incubation of eggs determines the sex of offspring.

In the biological world, a wide range of reproductive modes and life cycles are observed. Some organisms are entirely asexual, displaying no evidence of sexual reproduction. Some organisms alternate between short periods of sexual reproduction and prolonged periods of asexual reproduction. In most diploid eukaryotes, however, sexual reproduction is the only natural mechanism for producing new members of the species. Orderly transmission of genetic material from parents to offspring, and the resultant phenotypic variability, relies on the processes of segregation and independent assortment that occur during meiosis. Meiosis produces haploid gametes so that, following fertilization, the resulting offspring maintain the diploid number of chromosomes characteristic of their kind. Thus, meiosis ensures genetic constancy within members of the same species.

These events, seen in the perpetuation of all sexually reproducing organisms, depend ultimately on an efficient union of gametes during fertilization. In turn, successful fertilization depends on some form of sexual differentiation in the reproductive organisms. Even though it is not overtly evident, this differentiation occurs in such diverse organisms as bacteria, archaea, and unicellular eukaryotes such as algae. In many animal species, including humans, the differentiation of the sexes is more evident as phenotypic dimorphism of males and females. The ancient symbol for iron and for Mars, depicting a shield and spear (♂), and the ancient symbol for copper and for Venus, depicting a mirror (♀), have also come to symbolize maleness and femaleness, respectively.

Dissimilar, or **heteromorphic chromosomes**, such as the XY pair in mammals, characterize one sex or the other in a wide range of species, resulting in their label as **sex chromosomes**. Nevertheless, in many species, genes rather than chromosomes ultimately serve as the underlying basis of **sex determination**. As we will see, some of these genes are present on sex chromosomes, but others are autosomal. Extensive investigation has revealed variation in sex-chromosome systems—even in closely related organisms—suggesting that mechanisms controlling sex determination have undergone rapid evolution many times in the history of life.

In this chapter, we review some representative modes of sexual differentiation by examining the life cycles of three model organisms often studied in genetics: the green alga *Chlamydomonas*; the maize plant, *Zea mays*; and the nematode (roundworm), *Caenorhabditis elegans*. These organisms contrast the different roles that sexual differentiation plays in the lives of diverse organisms. Then, we delve more deeply into what is known about the genetic basis for the determination of sexual differences, with a particular emphasis on two organisms: our own species, representative of mammals; and *Drosophila*, on which pioneering sex-determining studies were performed.

Please note that some of the topics discussed in this chapter are explored in greater depth later in the text (see Special Topic Chapter 1—Epigenetics).

7.1 Life Cycles Depend on Sexual Differentiation

In describing sexual dimorphism (differences between males and females) in multicellular animals, biologists distinguish between **primary sexual differentiation**, which involves only the gonads, where gametes are produced, and **secondary sexual differentiation**, which involves the overall appearance of the organism, including clear differences in such organs as mammary glands and external genitalia as well as in nonreproductive organs. In plants and animals, the terms **unisexual, dioecious**, and **gonochoric** are equivalent; they all refer to an individual containing only male *or* only female reproductive organs. Conversely, the terms **bisexual, monoecious**, and **hermaphroditic** refer to individuals containing both male *and* female reproductive organs, a common occurrence in both the plant and animal kingdoms. These organisms can produce both eggs and sperm. The term **intersex** is usually reserved for individuals of an intermediate sexual condition, most of whom are sterile.

Chlamydomonas

The life cycle of the green alga *Chlamydomonas* (Cla-may-da-moan-us), shown in **Figure 7–1**, is representative of organisms exhibiting only infrequent periods of sexual reproduction. Such organisms spend most of their life cycle in a haploid phase, asexually producing daughter cells by mitotic divisions. However, under unfavorable nutrient conditions, such as nitrogen depletion, certain daughter cells function as gametes, joining together in fertilization. Following fertilization, a diploid zygote, which may withstand the unfavorable environment, is formed. When conditions change for the better, meiosis ensues and haploid vegetative cells are again produced.

In such species, there is little visible difference between the haploid vegetative cells that reproduce asexually and the haploid gametes that are involved in sexual reproduction. Moreover, the two gametes that fuse during mating are not usually morphologically distinguishable from one another, which is why they are called **isogametes** (*iso-* means equal, or uniform). Species producing them are said to be **isogamous**.

Over half a century ago, it was demonstrated that gametes in *Chlamydomonas* could be subdivided into two mating types. Working with clones derived from single haploid cells, they showed that cells from a given clone mate with cells from some but not all other clones. When they tested the mating abilities of large numbers of clones, all could be placed into one of two mating categories, either mt^+ or mt^- cells. "Plus" cells mate only with "minus" cells, and vice versa. Following fertilization, which involves fusion of entire cells, and subsequently, meiosis, the four haploid cells, or **zoospores**, produced (see the top of Figure 7–1) were found to consist of two plus types and two minus types.

Further experimentation established that plus and minus cells differ chemically. When extracts are prepared from cloned *Chlamydomonas* cells (or their flagella) of one type and then added to cells of the opposite mating type, clumping, or agglutination, occurs. No such agglutination occurs if the extracts are added to cells of the mating type from which they were derived. These observations suggest that despite the morphological similarities between isogametes, they are differentiated biochemically. Therefore, in this alga, a primitive means of sex differentiation exists, even though there is no morphological indication that such differentiation has occurred. Further research has pinpointed the *mt* locus to *Chlamydomonas* chromosome VI and has identified the gene that mediates the expression of the mt^- mating type, which is essential for cell fusion in response to nitrogen depletion.

Zea mays

The life cycles of many plants alternate between the *haploid gametophyte stage* and the *diploid sporophyte stage* (see Figure 2–13). The processes of meiosis and fertilization link the two phases during the life cycle. The relative amount of time

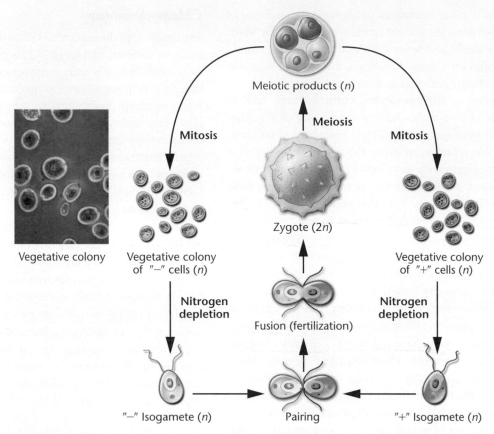

FIGURE 7–1 The life cycle of *Chlamydomonas*. Unfavorable conditions stimulate the formation of isogametes of opposite mating types that may fuse in fertilization. The resulting zygote undergoes meiosis, producing two haploid cells of each mating type. The photograph shows vegetative cells of this green alga.

spent in the two phases varies between the major plant groups. In some nonseed plants, such as mosses, the haploid gametophyte phase and the morphological structures representing this stage predominate. The reverse is true in seed plants.

Maize (*Zea mays*), familiar to you as corn, exemplifies a *monoecious* seed plant, meaning a plant in which the sporophyte phase and the morphological structures representing that phase predominate during the life cycle. Both male and female structures are present on the adult plant. Thus, sex determination occurs differently in different tissues of the same organism, as shown in the life cycle of this plant (**Figure 7–2**). The stamens, which collectively constitute the tassel, produce diploid microspore mother cells, each of which undergoes meiosis and gives rise to four haploid microspores. Each haploid microspore in turn develops into a mature male microgametophyte—the pollen grain—which contains two haploid sperm nuclei.

Equivalent female diploid cells, known as megaspore mother cells, are produced in the pistil of the sporophyte. Following meiosis, only one of the four haploid megaspores survives. It usually divides mitotically three times, producing a total of eight haploid nuclei enclosed in the embryo sac. Two of these nuclei unite near the center of the embryo sac, becoming the endosperm nuclei. At the micropyle end of the

sac, where the sperm enters, sit three other nuclei: the oocyte nucleus and two synergids. The remaining three, antipodal nuclei, cluster at the opposite end of the embryo sac.

Pollination occurs when pollen grains make contact with the silks (or stigma) of the pistil and develop long pollen tubes that grow toward the embryo sac. When contact is made at the micropyle, the two sperm nuclei enter the embryo sac. One sperm nucleus unites with the haploid oocyte nucleus, and the other sperm nucleus unites with two endosperm nuclei. This process, known as *double fertilization*, creates the diploid zygote nucleus and the triploid endosperm nucleus, respectively. Each ear of corn can contain as many as 1000 of these structures, each of which develops into a single kernel. Each kernel, if allowed to germinate, gives rise to a new plant, the *sporophyte*.

The mechanism of sex determination and differentiation in a monoecious plant such as *Zea mays*, where the tissues that form the male and female gametes have the same genetic constitution, was difficult to unravel at first. However, the discovery of a number of mutant genes that disrupt normal tassel and pistil formation supports the concept that normal products of these genes play an important role in sex determination by affecting the differentiation of male or female tissue in several ways.

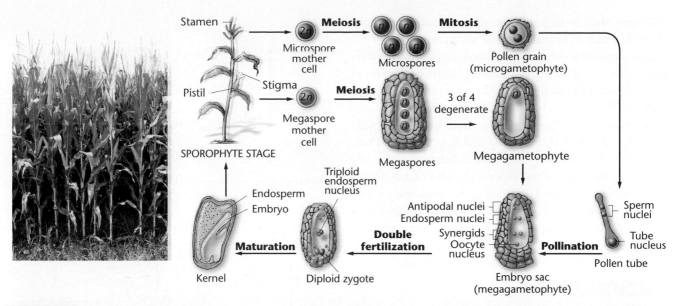

FIGURE 7–2 The life cycle of maize (*Zea mays*). The diploid sporophyte bears stamens and pistils that give rise to haploid microspores and megaspores, which develop into the pollen grain and the embryo sac that ultimately house the sperm and oocyte, respectively. Following fertilization, the embryo develops within the kernel and is nourished by the endosperm. Germination of the kernel gives rise to a new sporophyte (the mature corn plant), and the cycle repeats itself.

For example, mutant genes altering the sexual development of florets provide valuable information. When homozygous, mutations classified as *tassel seed* (*ts1* and *ts2*) convert male tassels to female pistils. The wild-type form of these genes normally eliminates the cells forming pistils by inducing their cell death. Thus, a single gene can cause a normally monoecious plant to become exclusively female. On the other hand, the recessive mutations *silkless* (*sk*) and *barren stalk* (*ba*) interfere with the development of the pistil, resulting in plants with only male-functioning reproductive organs, provided that the plant has wild-type *ts* genes.

Data gathered from studies of these and other mutants suggest that the products of many wild-type alleles of these genes interact in controlling sex determination. Following sexual differentiation of florets into either male or female structures, male or female gametes are produced.

Caenorhabditis elegans

The nematode worm *Caenorhabditis elegans* [*C. elegans*, for short; **Figure 7–3(a)**] is a popular organism in genetic studies, particularly for investigating the genetic control of development. Its usefulness is based on the fact that adults consist of 959 somatic cells, the precise lineage of which can be traced back to specific embryonic origins.

There are two sexual phenotypes in these worms: males, which have only testes, and hermaphrodites, which during larval development form two gonads, which subsequently produce both sperm and eggs. The eggs that are produced are fertilized by the stored sperm in a process of self-fertilization.

The outcome of this process is quite interesting [**Figure 7–3(b)**]. The vast majority of organisms that result are hermaphrodites, like the parental worm; less than 1 percent of the offspring are males. As adults,

(a)

(b)

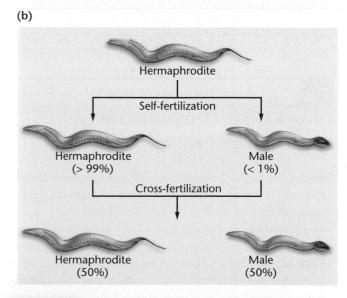

FIGURE 7–3 (a) Photomicrograph of a hermaphroditic nematode, *C. elegans*; (b) the outcomes of self-fertilization in a hermaphrodite, and a mating of a hermaphrodite and a male worm.

males can mate with hermaphrodites, producing about half male and half hermaphrodite offspring.

The signal that determines maleness in contrast to hermaphroditic development is provided by the expression of genes located on both the X chromosome and autosomes. *C. elegans* lacks a Y chromosome altogether—hermaphrodites have two X chromosomes, while males have only one X chromosome. It is believed that the ratio of X chromosomes to the number of sets of autosomes ultimately determines the sex of these worms. A ratio of 1.0 (two X chromosomes and two copies of each autosome) results in hermaphrodites, and a ratio of 0.5 results in males. The absence of a heteromorphic Y chromosome is not uncommon in organisms.

NOW SOLVE THIS

7–1 The marine echiurid worm *Bonellia viridis* is an extreme example of environmental influence on sex determination. Undifferentiated larvae either remain free-swimming and differentiate into females, or they settle on the proboscis of an adult female and become males. If larvae that have been on a female proboscis for a short period are removed and placed in seawater, they develop as intersexes. If larvae are forced to develop in an aquarium where pieces of proboscises have been placed, they develop into males. Contrast this mode of sexual differentiation with that of mammals. Suggest further experimentation to elucidate the mechanism of sex determination in *B. viridis*.

■ **HINT:** *This problem asks you to analyze experimental findings related to sex determination. The key to its solution is to devise further testing with the goal of isolating the unknown factor affecting sex determination and testing it experimentally.*

For more practice, see Problems 30, 31, and 32.

7.2 X and Y Chromosomes Were First Linked to Sex Determination Early in the Twentieth Century

How sex is determined has long intrigued geneticists. In 1891, H. Henking identified a nuclear structure in the sperm of certain insects, which he labeled the X-body. Several years later, Clarence McClung showed that some of the sperm in grasshoppers contain an unusual genetic structure, which he called a *heterochromosome*, but the remainder of the sperm lack this structure. He mistakenly associated the presence of the heterochromosome with the production of male progeny. In 1906, Edmund B. Wilson clarified Henking and McClung's findings when

(a)

(b)

FIGURE 7–4 (a) Sex determination where the heterogametic sex (the male in this example) is X0 and produces gametes with or without the X chromosome; (b) sex determination, where the heterogametic sex (again, the male in this example) is XY and produces gametes with either an X or a Y chromosome. In both cases, the chromosome composition of the offspring determines its sex.

he demonstrated that female somatic cells in the butterfly *Protenor* contain 14 chromosomes, including two X chromosomes. During oogenesis, an even reduction occurs, producing gametes with seven chromosomes, including one X chromosome. Male somatic cells, on the other hand, contain only 13 chromosomes, including one X chromosome. During spermatogenesis, gametes are produced containing either six chromosomes, without an X, or seven chromosomes, one of which is an X. Fertilization by X-bearing sperm results in female offspring, and fertilization by X-deficient sperm results in male offspring [**Figure 7–4(a)**].

The presence or absence of the X chromosome in male gametes provides an efficient mechanism for sex determination in this species and also produces a 1:1 sex ratio in the resulting offspring. As we saw earlier, *C. elegans* exhibits this system of sex determination.

Wilson also experimented with the milkweed bug *Lygaeus turcicus*, in which both sexes have 14 chromosomes. Twelve of these are autosomes (A). In addition, the females have two X chromosomes, while the males have only a single X and a smaller heterochromosome labeled the **Y chromosome**. Females in this species produce only gametes of the (6A + X) constitution, but males produce two types of gametes in equal proportions, (6A + X) and (6A + Y). Therefore, following random fertilization, equal numbers of male and female progeny will be produced with distinct chromosome complements [**Figure 7–4(b)**].

In *Protenor* and *Lygaeus* insects, males produce unlike gametes. As a result, they are described as the **heterogametic sex**, and in effect, their gametes ultimately determine the sex of the progeny in those species. In such cases, the female, which has like sex chromosomes, is the **homogametic sex**, producing uniform gametes with regard to chromosome numbers and types.

The male is not always the heterogametic sex. In some organisms, the female produces unlike gametes, exhibiting either the *Protenor* XX/XO or *Lygaeus* XX/XY mode of sex determination. Examples include certain moths and butterflies, some fish, reptiles, amphibians, at least one species of plants (*Fragaria orientalis*), and most birds. To immediately distinguish situations in which the female is the heterogametic sex, some geneticists use the notation **ZZ/ZW**, where ZZ is the homogametic male and ZW is the heterogametic female, instead of the XX/XY notation. For example, chickens are so denoted.

7.3 The Y Chromosome Determines Maleness in Humans

The first attempt to understand sex determination in our own species occurred almost 100 years ago and involved the visual examination of chromosomes in dividing cells. Efforts were made to accurately determine the diploid chromosome number of humans, but because of the relatively large number of chromosomes, this proved to be quite difficult. In 1912, H. von Winiwarter counted 47 chromosomes in a spermatogonial metaphase preparation. It was believed that the sex-determining mechanism in humans was based on the presence of an extra chromosome in females, who were thought to have 48 chromosomes. However, in the 1920s, Theophilus Painter counted between 45 and 48 chromosomes in cells of testicular tissue and also discovered the small Y chromosome, which is now known to occur only in males. In his original paper, Painter favored 46 as the diploid number in humans, but he later concluded incorrectly that 48 was the chromosome number in both males and females.

For 30 years, this number was accepted. Then, in 1956, Joe Hin Tjio and Albert Levan discovered a better way to prepare chromosomes for viewing. This improved technique led to a strikingly clear demonstration of metaphase stages showing that 46 was indeed the human diploid number. Later that same year, C. E. Ford and John L. Hamerton, also working with testicular tissue, confirmed this finding. The familiar karyotypes of humans are shown in **Figure 7–5**.

Of the normal 23 pairs of human chromosomes, one pair was shown to vary in configuration in males and females. These two chromosomes were designated the X and Y sex chromosomes. The human female has two X chromosomes, and the human male has one X and one Y chromosome.

We might believe that this observation is sufficient to conclude that the Y chromosome determines maleness. However, several other interpretations are possible. The Y could play no role in sex determination; the presence of two X chromosomes could cause femaleness; or maleness could result from the lack of a second X chromosome. The evidence that clarified which explanation was correct came from study of the effects of human sex-chromosome variations, described below. As such investigations revealed, the Y chromosome does indeed determine maleness in humans.

(a)

(b)

FIGURE 7–5 The traditional human karyotypes derived from a normal female and a normal male. Each contains 22 pairs of autosomes and two sex chromosomes. The female (a) contains two X chromosomes, while the male (b) contains one X and one Y chromosome.

Klinefelter and Turner Syndromes

In about 1940, scientists identified two human abnormalities characterized by aberrant sexual development, **Klinefelter syndrome (47,XXY)** and **Turner syndrome (45,X)**.* Individuals with Klinefelter syndrome are generally tall and have long arms and legs and large hands and feet. They usually have genitalia and internal ducts that are male, but their testes are rudimentary and fail to produce sperm. At the same time, feminine sexual development is not entirely suppressed. Slight enlargement of the breasts (gynecomastia) is common, and the hips are often rounded. This ambiguous sexual development, referred to as intersexuality, can lead to abnormal social development. Intelligence is often below the normal range as well.

In Turner syndrome, the affected individual has female external genitalia and internal ducts, but the ovaries are rudimentary. Other characteristic abnormalities include short stature (usually under 5 feet), cognitive impairment, skin folds on the back of the neck, and underdeveloped breasts. A broad, shieldlike chest is sometimes noted. In 1959, the karyotypes of individuals with these syndromes were determined to be abnormal with respect to the sex chromosomes. Individuals with Klinefelter syndrome have more than one X chromosome. Most often they have an XXY complement in addition to 44 autosomes [**Figure 7–6(a)**], which is why people with this karyotype are designated 47,XXY. Individuals with Turner syndrome most often have only 45 chromosomes, including just a single X chromosome; thus, they are designated 45,X [**Figure 7–6(b)**]. Note the convention used in designating these chromosome compositions: the number states the total number of chromosomes present, and the symbols after the comma indicate the deviation from the normal diploid content. Both conditions result from **nondisjunction**, the failure of the X chromosomes to segregate properly during meiosis (nondisjunction is described in Chapter 8 and illustrated in Figure 8–1).

These Klinefelter and Turner karyotypes and their corresponding sexual phenotypes led scientists to conclude that the Y chromosome determines maleness and thus is the basis for phenotypic sex determination in humans. In its absence, the person's sex is female, even if only a single X chromosome is present. The presence of the Y chromosome in the presence of two X chromosomes characteristic of Klinefelter syndrome is sufficient to determine maleness, even though male development is not complete. Similarly, in the absence of a Y chromosome, as in the case of individuals with Turner syndrome, no masculinization occurs. Note that we cannot conclude anything regarding sex determination under circumstances where a Y chromosome is present without an X because Y-containing human embryos lacking an X chromosome (designated 45,Y) do not survive.

Klinefelter syndrome occurs in about 1 of every 660 male births. The karyotypes **48,XXXY, 48,XXYY, 49,XXXXY**, and **49,XXXYY** are similar phenotypically to 47,XXY, but manifestations are often more severe in individuals with a greater number of X chromosomes.

Turner syndrome can also result from karyotypes other than 45,X, including individuals called **mosaics**, whose somatic cells display two different genetic cell lines, each exhibiting a different karyotype. Such cell lines result from a mitotic error during early development, the most common chromosome combinations being **45,X/46,XY** and **45,X/46,XX**. Thus, an embryo that began life with a normal karyotype can give rise to an individual whose cells show a mixture of karyotypes and who exhibits varying aspects of this syndrome.

---

*Although the possessive form of the names of eponymous syndromes is sometimes used (e.g., Klinefelter's syndrome), the current preference is to use the nonpossessive form.

(a)

(b)

FIGURE 7–6 The karyotypes of individuals with (a) Klinefelter syndrome (47,XXY) and (b) Turner syndrome (45,X).

Setting	Restriction	Number Studied	Number XYY	Frequency XYY
Control population	Newborns	28,366	29	0.10%
Mental-penal	No height restriction	4,239	82	1.93
Penal	No height restriction	5,805	26	0.44
Mental	No height restriction	2,562	8	0.31
Mental-penal	Height restriction	1,048	48	4.61
Penal	Height restriction	1,683	31	1.84
Mental	Height restriction	649	9	1.38

TABLE 7.1 Frequency of XYY Individuals in Various Settings

Source: Compiled from data presented in Hook, 1973, Tables 1–8. Copyright 1973 by the American Association for the Advancement of Science.

Turner syndrome is observed in about 1 in 2000 female births, a frequency much lower than that for Klinefelter syndrome. One explanation for this difference is the observation that the majority of 45,X fetuses die *in utero* and are aborted spontaneously. Thus, a similar frequency of the two syndromes may occur at conception.

47,XXX Syndrome

The abnormal presence of three X chromosomes along with a normal set of autosomes (**47,XXX**) results in female differentiation. The highly variable syndrome that accompanies this genotype, often called **triplo-X**, occurs in about 1 of 1000 female births. Frequently, 47,XXX women are perfectly normal and may remain unaware of their abnormality in chromosome number unless a karyotype is done. In other cases, underdeveloped secondary sex characteristics, sterility, delayed development of language and motor skills, and mental retardation may occur. In rare instances, **48,XXXX** (tetra-X) and **49,XXXXX** (penta-X) karyotypes have been reported. The syndromes associated with these karyotypes are similar to but more pronounced than the 47,XXX syndrome. Thus, in many cases, the presence of additional X chromosomes appears to disrupt the delicate balance of genetic information essential to normal female development.

47,XYY Condition

Another human condition involving the sex chromosomes is **47,XYY**. Studies of this condition, where the only deviation from diploidy is the presence of an additional Y chromosome in an otherwise normal male karyotype, were initiated in 1965 by Patricia Jacobs. She discovered that 9 of 315 males in a Scottish maximum security prison had the 47,XYY karyotype. These males were significantly above average in height and had been incarcerated as a result of antisocial (nonviolent) criminal acts. Of the nine males studied, seven were of subnormal intelligence, and all suffered personality disorders. Several other studies produced similar findings.

The possible correlation between this chromosome composition and criminal behavior piqued considerable interest, and extensive investigation of the phenotype and frequency of the 47,XYY condition in both criminal and noncriminal populations ensued. Above-average height (usually over 6 feet) and subnormal intelligence have been generally substantiated, and the frequency of males displaying this karyotype is indeed higher among people in penal and mental institutions than among unincarcerated populations (see Table 7.1). A particularly relevant question involves the characteristics displayed by XYY males who are not incarcerated. The only nearly constant association is that such individuals are over 6 feet tall.

A study addressing this issue was initiated to identify 47,XYY individuals at birth and to follow their behavioral patterns during preadult and adult development. By 1974, the two investigators, Stanley Walzer and Park Gerald, had identified about 20 XYY newborns in 15,000 births at Boston Hospital for Women. However, they soon came under great pressure to abandon their research. Those opposed to the study argued that the investigation could not be justified and might cause great harm to individuals who displayed this karyotype. The opponents argued that (1) no association between the additional Y chromosome and abnormal behavior had been previously established in the population at large, and (2) "labeling" the individuals in the study might create a self-fulfilling prophecy. That is, as a result of participation in the study, parents, relatives, and friends might treat individuals identified as 47,XYY differently, ultimately producing the expected antisocial behavior. Despite the support of a government funding agency and the faculty at Harvard Medical School, Walzer and Gerald abandoned the investigation in 1975.

Since Walzer and Gerald's work, it has become clear that many XYY males are present in the population who do not exhibit antisocial behavior and who lead normal lives. Therefore, we must conclude that there is a high, but not constant, correlation between the extra Y chromosome and the predisposition of these males to exhibit behavioral problems.

Sexual Differentiation in Humans

Once researchers had established that, in humans, it is the Y chromosome that houses genetic information necessary for maleness, they attempted to pinpoint a specific gene or genes capable of providing the "signal" responsible for sex determination. Before we delve into this topic, it is useful to consider how sexual differentiation occurs in order to better comprehend how humans develop into sexually dimorphic males and females. During early development, every human embryo undergoes a period when it is potentially hermaphroditic. By the fifth week of gestation, gonadal primordia (the tissues that will form the gonad) arise as a pair of **gonadal (genital) ridges** associated with each embryonic kidney. The embryo is potentially hermaphroditic because at this stage its gonadal phenotype is sexually indifferent—male or female reproductive structures cannot be distinguished, and the gonadal ridge tissue can develop to form male or female gonads. As development progresses, primordial germ cells migrate to these ridges, where an outer cortex and inner medulla form (*cortex* and *medulla* are the outer and inner tissues of an organ, respectively). The cortex is capable of developing into an ovary, while the medulla may develop into a testis. In addition, two sets of undifferentiated ducts called the Wolffian and Müllerian ducts exist in each embryo. Wolffian ducts differentiate into other organs of the male reproductive tract, while Müllerian ducts differentiate into structures of the female reproductive tract.

Because gonadal ridges can form either ovaries or testes, they are commonly referred to as **bipotential gonads**. What is the switch that triggers gonadal ridge development into testes or ovaries? The presence or absence of a Y chromosome is the key. If cells of the ridge have an XY constitution, development of the medulla into a testis is initiated around the seventh week. However, in the absence of the Y chromosome, no male development occurs, the cortex of the ridge subsequently forms ovarian tissue, and the Müllerian duct forms oviducts (Fallopian tubes), uterus, cervix, and portions of the vagina. Depending on which pathway is initiated, parallel development of the appropriate male or female duct system then occurs, and the other duct system degenerates. If testes differentiation is initiated, the embryonic testicular tissue secretes hormones that are essential for continued male sexual differentiation. As we will discuss in the next section, presence of a Y chromosome and development of the testes also inhibit formation of female reproductive organs.

In females, as the 12th week of fetal development approaches, oogonia within the ovaries begin meiosis, and primary oocytes can be detected. By the 25th week of gestation, all oocytes become arrested in meiosis and remain dormant until puberty is reached some 10 to 15 years later.

In males, on the other hand, primary spermatocytes are not produced until puberty is reached (refer to Figure 2–12).

The Y Chromosome and Male Development

The human Y chromosome, unlike the X, was long thought to be mostly blank genetically. It is now known that this is not true, even though the Y chromosome contains far fewer genes than does the X. Data from the Human Genome Project indicate that the Y chromosome has about 50 genes, compared to about 1000 genes on the X. The human X and Y chromosomes are believed to have originated from a homologous pair of autosomes about 200 million years ago. Yet they now share a relatively small degree of sequence similarity. Current analysis of these genes and regions with potential genetic function reveals that some have homologous counterparts on the X chromosome and others do not. For example, present on both ends of the Y chromosome are so-called **pseudoautosomal regions (PARs)** that share homology with regions on the X chromosome and synapse and recombine with it during meiosis. The presence of such a pairing region is critical to segregation of the X and Y chromosomes during male gametogenesis. The remainder of the chromosome, about 95 percent of it, does not synapse or recombine with the X chromosome. As a result, it was originally referred to as the *nonrecombining region of the Y (NRY)*. More recently, researchers have designated this region as the **male-specific region of the Y (MSY)**. As you will see, some portions of the MSY share homology with genes on the X chromosome, and others do not.

The human Y chromosome is diagrammed in **Figure 7–7**. The MSY is divided about equally between *euchromatic* regions, containing functional genes, and *heterochromatic* regions, lacking genes. Within euchromatin, adjacent to the PAR of the short arm of the Y chromosome, is a critical gene that controls male sexual development, called the *sex-determining region Y (SRY)*. In humans, the absence of a Y chromosome almost always leads to female development; thus, this gene is absent from the X chromosome. At 6 to 8 weeks of development, the

FIGURE 7–7 The regions of the human Y chromosome.

SRY gene becomes active in XY embryos. *SRY* encodes a protein that causes the undifferentiated gonadal tissue of the embryo to form testes. This protein is called the **testis-determining factor (TDF)**.

SRY (or a closely related version) is present in all mammals thus far examined, indicative of its essential function throughout this diverse group of animals. It is interesting to note that in chickens, a similar gene has recently been identified. Called *DMRT1*, it is located on the Z chromosome. Our ability to identify the presence or absence of DNA sequences in rare individuals whose sex-chromosome composition does not correspond to their sexual phenotype has provided evidence that *SRY* is the gene responsible for male sex determination. For example, there are human males who have two X and no Y chromosomes. Often, attached to one of their X chromosomes is the region of the Y that contains *SRY*. There are also females who have one X and one Y chromosome. Their Y is almost always missing the *SRY* gene.

Further support of this conclusion involves experiments using **transgenic mice**. These animals are produced from fertilized eggs injected with foreign DNA that is subsequently incorporated into the genetic composition of the developing embryo. In normal mice, a chromosome region designated *Sry* has been identified that is comparable to *SRY* in humans. When mouse DNA containing *Sry* is injected into normal XX mouse eggs, most of the offspring develop into males.

The question of how the product of this gene triggers development of embryonic gonadal tissue into testes rather than ovaries has been under investigation for a number of years. TDF functions as a *transcription factor*, a DNA-binding protein that interacts directly with regulatory sequences of other genes to stimulate their expression. Thus, while TDF behaves as a master switch that controls other genes downstream in the process of sexual differentiation, identifying TDF target genes has been difficult. To date, *Sox9* in mice is one such gene. Another potential target for activation by TDF that has been extensively studied is the gene for **Müllerian inhibiting substance (MIS**, also called Müllerian inhibiting hormone, MIH, or anti-Müllerian hormone). Cells of the developing testes secrete MIS. As its name suggests, MIS protein causes regression (atrophy) of cells in the Müllerian duct. Degeneration of the duct prevents formation of the female reproductive tract.

Other *autosomal genes* are part of a cascade of genetic expression initiated by *SRY*. Examples include the human *SOX9* gene, which when activated by *SRY*, leads to the differentiation of cells that form the seminiferous tubules that contain male germ cells. In the mouse, fibroblast growth factor 9 (*Fgf9*) is upregulated in XY gonads. Testis development is completely blocked in gonads lacking *Fgf9*, and

signs of ovarian development occur. Another gene, *SF1*, is involved in the regulation of enzymes affecting steroid metabolism. In mice, this gene is initially active in both the male and female bisexual genital ridge, persisting until the point in development when testis formation is apparent. At that time, its expression persists in males but is extinguished in females. Recent work using mice has suggested that testicular development may be actively repressed throughout the life of females by downregulating expression of specific genes. This is based on experiments showing that, in adult female mice, deletion of a gene *Foxl2*, which encodes a transcription factor, leads to transdifferentiation of the ovary into the testis. Establishment of the link between these various genes and sex determination has brought us closer to a complete understanding of how males and females arise in humans, but much work remains to be done.

Findings by David Page and his many colleagues have now provided a reasonably complete picture of the MSY region of the human Y chromosome. Page has spearheaded the detailed study of the Y chromosome for the past several decades. The MSY consists of about 23 million base pairs (23 Mb) and can be divided into three regions. The first region is the *X-transposed region*. It comprises about 15 percent of the MSY and was originally derived from the X chromosome in the course of human evolution (about 3 to 4 million years ago). The X-transposed region is 99 percent identical to region Xq21 of the modern human X chromosome. Two genes, both with X chromosome homologs, are present in this region.

Research by Page and others has also revealed that sequences called **palindromes**—sequences of base pairs that read the same but in the opposite direction on complementary strands—are present throughout the MSY. Recombination between palindromes on sister chromatids of the Y during replication is a mechanism used to repair mutations in the Y. This discovery has fascinating implications concerning how the Y chromosome may maintain its size and structure.

In early 2010, Page and colleagues demonstrated the first comprehensive comparison of the Y chromosome structure from two species. One interesting finding was that the MSY of the human Y chromosome is very different in sequence structure than the MSY from chimpanzees. The study indicates that rapid evolution has occurred since separation of these species over 6 million years ago—a surprise given that primate sex chromosomes have been in existence for hundreds of millions of years. Over 30 percent of the chimpanzee MSY sequence has no homologous sequence in the human MSY. The chimpanzee MSY has lost many protein-coding genes compared to common ancestors but contains twice the number of palindromic sequences as the human MSY.

The second area of the MSY is designated the *X-degenerative region*. Comprising about 20 percent of the MSY, this region contains DNA sequences that are even more distantly related to those present on the X chromosome. The X-degenerative region contains 27 single-copy genes and a number of *pseudogenes* (genes whose sequences have degenerated sufficiently during evolution to render them nonfunctional). As with the genes present in the X-transposed region, all share some homology with counterparts on the X chromosome. One of these is the *SRY* gene, discussed earlier. Other X-degenerative genes that encode protein products are expressed ubiquitously in all tissues in the body, but *SRY* is expressed only in the testes.

The third area, the *ampliconic region*, contains about 30 percent of the MSY, including most of the genes closely associated with the development of testes. These genes lack counterparts on the X chromosome, and their expression is limited to the testes. There are 60 transcription units (genes that yield a product) divided among nine gene families in this region, most represented by multiple copies. Members of each family have nearly identical (>98 percent) DNA sequences. Each repeat unit is an **amplicon** and is contained within seven segments scattered across the euchromatic regions of both the short and long arms of the Y chromosome. Genes in the ampliconic region encode proteins specific to the development and function of the testes, and the products of many of these genes are directly related to fertility in males. It is currently believed that a great deal of male sterility in our population can be linked to mutations in these genes.

A more recent area of investigation has involved the Y chromosome and paternal aging. For many years, it has been known that maternal age is correlated with an elevated rate of offspring with chromosomal defects, including Down syndrome (see Chapter 8). Advanced paternal age has now been associated with an increased risk in offspring of congenital disorders with a genetic basis, including certain cancers, schizophrenia, autism, and other conditions, collectively known as *paternal age effects (PAE)*. Studies in which the genomes of sperm have been sequenced have demonstrated the presence of specific PAE mutations including numerous ones on the Y chromosome. Evidence suggests that PAE mutations are positively selected for and result in an enrichment of mutant sperm over time.

This recent work has greatly expanded our picture of the genetic information carried by this unique chromosome. It clearly refutes the so-called *wasteland theory*, prevalent some 25 years ago, that depicted the human Y chromosome as almost devoid of genetic information other than a few genes that cause maleness. The knowledge we have gained provides the basis for a much clearer picture of how maleness is determined.

NOW SOLVE THIS

7–2 Campomelic dysplasia (CMD1) is a congenital human syndrome featuring malformation of bone and cartilage. It is caused by an autosomal dominant mutation of a gene located on chromosome 17. Consider the following observations in sequence, and in each case, draw whatever appropriate conclusions are warranted.

  (a) Of those with the syndrome who are karyotypically 46,XY, approximately 75 percent are sex reversed, exhibiting a wide range of female characteristics.

  (b) The nonmutant form of the gene, called *SOX9*, is expressed in the developing gonad of the XY male, but not the XX female.

  (c) The *SOX9* gene shares 71 percent amino acid coding sequence homology with the Y-linked *SRY* gene.

  (d) CMD1 patients who exhibit a 46,XX karyotype develop as females, with no gonadal abnormalities.

■ **HINT:** *This problem asks you to apply the information presented in this chapter to a real-life example. The key to its solution is knowing that some genes are activated and produce their normal product as a result of expression of products of other genes found on different chromosomes—in this case, perhaps one that is on the Y chromosome.*

7.4 The Ratio of Males to Females in Humans Is Not 1.0

The presence of heteromorphic sex chromosomes in one sex of a species but not the other provides a potential mechanism for producing equal proportions of male and female offspring. This potential depends on the segregation of the X and Y (or Z and W) chromosomes during meiosis, such that half of the gametes of the heterogametic sex receive one of the chromosomes and half receive the other one. As we learned in the previous section, small pseudoautosomal regions of pairing homology do exist at both ends of the human X and Y chromosomes, suggesting that the X and Y chromosomes do synapse and then segregate into different gametes. Provided that both types of gametes are equally successful in fertilization and that the two sexes are equally viable during fetal and embryonic development, a 1:1 ratio of male and female offspring should result.

The actual proportion of male to female offspring, referred to as the **sex ratio**, has been assessed in two ways.

The **primary sex ratio** reflects the proportion of males to females conceived in a population. The **secondary sex ratio** reflects the proportion of each sex that is born. The secondary sex ratio is much easier to determine but has the disadvantage of not accounting for any disproportionate embryonic or fetal mortality.

When the secondary sex ratio in the human population was determined in 1969 by using worldwide census data, it was found not to equal 1.0. For example, in the Caucasian population in the United States, the secondary ratio was a little less than 1.06, indicating that about 106 males were born for each 100 females. (In 1995, this ratio dropped to slightly less than 1.05.) In the African-American population in the United States, the ratio was 1.025. In other countries the excess of male births is even greater than is reflected in these values. For example, in Korea, the secondary sex ratio was 1.15.

Despite these ratios, it is possible that the primary sex ratio is 1.0 and is later altered between conception and birth. For the secondary ratio to exceed 1.0, then, prenatal female mortality would have to be greater than prenatal male mortality. However, this hypothesis has been examined and shown to be false. In fact, just the opposite occurs. In a Carnegie Institute study, reported in 1948, the sex of approximately 6000 embryos and fetuses recovered from miscarriages and abortions was determined, and fetal mortality was actually higher in males. On the basis of the data derived from that study, the primary sex ratio in U.S. Caucasians was estimated to be 1.079. It is now believed that the figure may be much higher, perhaps above 1.20, suggesting that many more males than females are conceived in the human population.

It is not clear why such a radical departure from the expected primary sex ratio of 1.0 occurs. To come up with a suitable explanation, researchers must examine the assumptions on which the theoretical ratio is based:

1. Because of segregation, males produce equal numbers of X- and Y-bearing sperm.

2. Each type of sperm has equivalent viability and motility in the female reproductive tract.

3. The egg surface is equally receptive to both X- and Y-bearing sperm.

No direct experimental evidence contradicts any of these assumptions; however, the human Y chromosome is smaller than the X chromosome and therefore of less mass. Thus, it has been speculated that Y-bearing sperm are more motile than X-bearing sperm. If this is true, then the probability of a fertilization event leading to a male zygote is increased, providing one possible explanation for the observed primary ratio.

7.5 Dosage Compensation Prevents Excessive Expression of X-Linked Genes in Mammals

The presence of two X chromosomes in normal human females and only one X in normal human males is unique compared with the equal numbers of autosomes present in the cells of both sexes. This disparity creates a "genetic dosage" difference between males and females, with attendant problems, for all X-linked genes. There is the potential for females to produce twice as much of each product of all X-linked genes. The additional X chromosomes in both males and females exhibiting the various syndromes discussed earlier in this chapter are thought to compound this dosage problem. Embryonic development depends on proper timing and precisely regulated levels of gene expression. Otherwise, disease phenotypes or embryonic lethality can occur. In this section, we will highlight examples of research findings regarding X-linked gene expression that demonstrate a genetic mechanism of **dosage compensation** that balances the dose of X chromosome gene expression in females and males.

Barr Bodies

Murray L. Barr and Ewart G. Bertram's experiments with female cats, as well as Keith Moore and Barr's subsequent study in humans, demonstrate a genetic mechanism in mammals that compensates for X chromosome dosage disparities. Barr and Bertram observed a darkly staining body in interphase nerve cells of female cats that was absent in similar cells of males. In humans, this body can be easily demonstrated in female cells derived from the buccal mucosa (cheek cells) or in fibroblasts (undifferentiated connective tissue cells), but not in similar male cells (**Figure 7–8**). This highly condensed structure, about 1 μm in diameter, lies against the nuclear envelope of interphase cells. It stains positively in the Feulgen reaction, a cytochemical test for DNA.

This structure, called a **sex chromatin body**, or simply a **Barr body**, is an inactivated X chromosome. Susumu Ohno was the first to suggest that the Barr body arises from one of the two X chromosomes. Ohno's hypothesis was attractive because it provided a possible mechanism for dosage compensation. If one of the two X chromosomes is inactive in the cells of females, the dosage of genetic information that can be expressed in males and females will be equivalent. Convincing, though indirect, evidence for this hypothesis comes from the study of the sex-chromosome syndromes described earlier in this chapter. Regardless of how many X chromosomes a somatic cell possesses, all but one of them

FIGURE 7-8 Photomicrographs comparing cheek epithelial cell nuclei from a male that fails to reveal Barr bodies (right) with a nucleus from a female that demonstrates a Barr body (indicated by the arrow in the left image). This structure, also called a sex chromatin body, represents an inactivated X chromosome.

appear to be inactivated and can be seen as Barr bodies. For example, no Barr body is seen in the somatic cells of Turner 45,X females; one is seen in Klinefelter 47,XXY males; two in 47,XXX females; three in 48,XXXX females; and so on (**Figure 7–9**). Therefore, the number of Barr bodies follows an $N - 1$ rule, where N is the total number of X chromosomes present.

Although this apparent inactivation of all but one X chromosome increases our understanding of dosage compensation, it further complicates our perception of other matters. For example, because one of the two X chromosomes is inactivated in normal human females, why then is the Turner 45,X individual not entirely normal? Why aren't females with the triplo-X and tetra-X karyotypes (47,XXX and 48,XXXX) completely

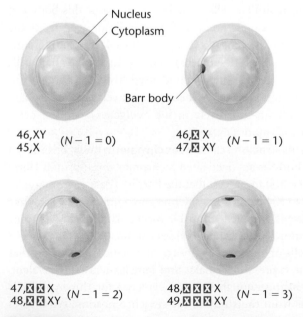

46,XY
45,X $(N - 1 = 0)$

46,⊠ X
47,⊠ XY $(N - 1 = 1)$

47,⊠ ⊠ X
48,⊠ ⊠ XY $(N - 1 = 2)$

48,⊠ ⊠ ⊠ X
49,⊠ ⊠ ⊠ XY $(N - 1 = 3)$

FIGURE 7-9 Occurrence of Barr bodies in various human karyotypes, where all X chromosomes except one ($N - 1$) are inactivated.

unaffected by the additional X chromosomes? Furthermore, in Klinefelter syndrome (47,XXY), X chromosome inactivation effectively renders the person 46,XY. Why aren't these males unaffected by the extra X chromosome in their nuclei?

One possible explanation is that chromosome inactivation does not normally occur in the very early stages of development of those cells destined to form gonadal tissues. Another possible explanation is that not all of each X chromosome forming a Barr body is inactivated. Recent studies have indeed demonstrated that as many as 15 percent of the human X-chromosomal genes actually escape inactivation. Clearly, then, not every gene on the X requires inactivation. In either case, excessive expression of certain X-linked genes might still occur at critical times during development despite apparent inactivation of superfluous X chromosomes.

The Lyon Hypothesis

In mammalian females, one X chromosome is of maternal origin, and the other is of paternal origin. Which one is inactivated? Is the inactivation random? Is the same chromosome inactive in all somatic cells? In 1961, Mary Lyon and Liane Russell independently proposed a hypothesis that answers these questions. They postulated that the inactivation of X chromosomes occurs randomly in somatic cells at a point early in embryonic development, most likely sometime during the blastocyst stage of development. Once inactivation has occurred, all descendant cells have the same X chromosome inactivated as their initial progenitor cell.

This explanation, which has come to be called the **Lyon hypothesis**, was initially based on observations of female mice heterozygous for X-linked coat color genes. The pigmentation of these heterozygous females was mottled, with large patches expressing the color allele on one X and other patches expressing the allele on the other X. This is the phenotypic pattern that would be expected if different X chromosomes were inactive in adjacent patches of cells. Similar mosaic patterns occur in the black and yellow-orange patches of female tortoiseshell and calico cats (**Figure 7–10**). Such X-linked coat color patterns do not occur in male cats because all their cells contain the single maternal X chromosome and are therefore hemizygous for only one X-linked coat color allele.

Evidence in support of the Lyon hypothesis came from studies of gene expression in clones of human fibroblast cells. Individual cells are isolated following biopsy and cultured *in vitro*. A culture of cells derived from a single cell is called a **clone**. The synthesis of the enzyme glucose-6-phosphate dehydrogenase (G6PD) is controlled by an

(a)

(b)

FIGURE 7–10 (a) The random distribution of orange and black patches in a calico cat illustrates the Lyon hypothesis. The white patches are due to another gene, distinguishing calico cats from tortoiseshell cats (b), which lack the white patches.

X-linked gene. Numerous mutant alleles of this gene have been detected, and their gene products can be differentiated from the wild-type enzyme by their migration pattern in an electrophoretic field.

Fibroblasts have been taken from females heterozygous for different allelic forms of *G6PD* and studied. The Lyon hypothesis predicts that if inactivation of an X chromosome occurs randomly early in development, and thereafter all progeny cells have the same X chromosome inactivated as their progenitor, such a female should show two types of clones, each containing only one electrophoretic form of *G6PD*, in approximately equal proportions.

In 1963, Ronald Davidson and colleagues performed an experiment involving 14 clones from a single heterozygous female. Seven showed only one form of the enzyme, and 7 showed only the other form. Most important was the finding that none of the 14 clones showed both forms of the enzyme. Studies of *G6PD* mutants thus provide strong support for the random permanent inactivation of either the maternal or paternal X chromosome.

Another consequence of X-inactivation is that mammalian females are mosaics for all heterozygous X-linked alleles—some areas of the body express only the maternally derived alleles, and others express only the paternally derived alleles. An especially interesting example involves **red-green color blindness**, an X-linked recessive disorder. In humans, hemizygous males are fully color-blind in all retinal cells. However, heterozygous females display mosaic retinas, with patches of defective color perception and surrounding areas with normal color perception. In this example, random inactivation of one or the other X chromosome early in the development of heterozygous females has led to these phenotypes.

NOW SOLVE THIS

7–3 CC (Carbon Copy), the first cat produced from a clone, was created from an ovarian cell taken from her genetic donor, Rainbow, a calico cat. The diploid nucleus from the cell was extracted and then injected into an enucleated egg. The resulting zygote was then allowed to develop in a petri dish, and the cloned embryo was implanted in the uterus of a surrogate mother cat, who gave birth to CC. CC's surrogate mother was a tabby (see the photo on page 187 at the end of this chapter). Geneticists were very interested in the outcome of cloning a calico cat, because they were not certain if the cat would have patches of orange and black, just orange, or just black. Taking into account the Lyon hypothesis, explain the basis of the uncertainty. Would you expect CC to appear identical to Rainbow? Explain why or why not.

■ **HINT:** *This problem involves an understanding of the Lyon hypothesis. The key to its solution is to realize that the donor nucleus was from a differentiated ovarian cell of an adult female cat, which itself had inactivated one of its X chromosomes.*

The Mechanism of Inactivation

Understanding the mechanism of X chromosome inactivation is an active area of research. Somehow, either DNA, the attached histone proteins, or both DNA and histone proteins, are chemically modified, silencing most genes that are part of that chromosome. Once silenced, a memory is created that keeps the same homolog inactivated following chromosome replications and cell divisions. Such a process, whereby expression of genes on one homolog, but not the other, is affected, is referred to as **imprinting**. This term also applies to a number of other examples in which genetic information is modified and gene expression is repressed. Collectively, such events are part of the growing field of **epigenetics**. Please note that other topics involving this field are explored later in the text (see Special Topic Chapter 1—Epigenetics).

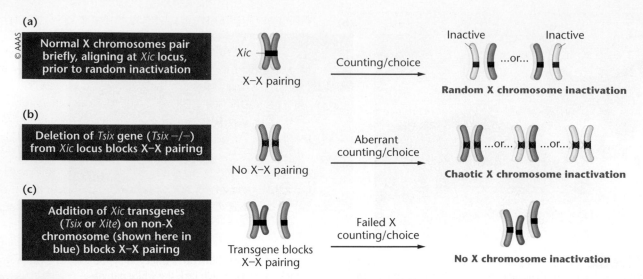

(a)

Normal X chromosomes pair briefly, aligning at *Xic* locus, prior to random inactivation

Xic

X–X pairing

Counting/choice

Inactive   Inactive

...or...

Random X chromosome inactivation

(b)

Deletion of *Tsix* gene (*Tsix –/–*) from *Xic* locus blocks X–X pairing

No X–X pairing

Aberrant counting/choice

...or...   ...or...

Chaotic X chromosome inactivation

(c)

Addition of *Xic* transgenes (*Tsix* or *Xite*) on non-X chromosome (shown here in blue) blocks X–X pairing

Transgene blocks X–X pairing

Failed X counting/choice

No X chromosome inactivation

FIGURE 7–11 (a) Transient pairing of X chromosomes may be required for initiating X-inactivation. (b) Deleting the *Tsix* gene of the *Xic* locus prevents X–X pairing and leads to chaotic X-inactivation. (c) Blocking X–X pairing by addition of *Xic*-containing transgenes blocks X–X pairing and prevents X-inactivation.

Ongoing investigations are beginning to clarify the mechanism of inactivation. A region of the mammalian X chromosome is the major control unit. This region, located on the proximal end of the p arm in humans, is called the **X inactivation center** (**Xic**), and its genetic expression *occurs only on the X chromosome that is inactivated*. The *Xic* is about 1 Mb (10^6 base pairs) in length and is known to contain several putative regulatory units and four genes. One of these, *X-inactive specific transcript (XIST)*, is now known to be a critical gene for X-inactivation.

Several interesting observations have been made regarding the RNA that is transcribed from the *XIST* gene, many coming from experiments that used the equivalent gene in the mouse (*Xist*). First, the RNA product is quite large and does not encode a protein, and thus is not translated. The RNA products of *Xist* spread over and coat the X chromosome *bearing the gene that produced them*. Two other noncoding genes at the *Xic* locus, *Tsix* (an antisense partner of *Xist*) and *Xite*, are also believed to play important roles in X-inactivation.

A second observation is that transcription of *Xist* initially occurs at low levels on all X chromosomes. As the inactivation process begins, however, transcription continues, and is enhanced, only on the X chromosome that becomes inactivated. In 1996, a research group led by Neil Brockdorff and Graeme Penny provided convincing evidence that transcription of *Xist* is the critical event in chromosome inactivation. These researchers introduced a targeted deletion (7 kb) into this gene, disrupting its sequence. As a result, the chromosome bearing the deletion lost its ability to become inactivated. Interesting questions remain regarding imprinting and inactivation. For example, in cells with more than two X chromosomes, what sort of

"counting" mechanism exists that designates all but one X chromosome to be inactivated? Studies by Jeannie T. Lee and colleagues suggest that maternal and paternal X chromosomes must first pair briefly and align at their *Xic* loci as a mechanism for counting the number of X chromosomes prior to X-inactivation [**Figure 7–11(a)**]. Using mouse embryonic stem cells, Lee's group deleted the *Tsix* gene contained in the *Xic* locus. This deletion blocked X–X pairing and resulted in chaotic inactivation of 0, 1, or 2 X chromosomes [**Figure 7–11(b)**]. Lee and colleagues provided further evidence for the role of *Xic* locus in chromosome counting by adding copies of genetically engineered non-X chromosomes containing multiple copies of *Tsix* or *Xite*. (These are referred to as **transgenes** because they are artificially introduced into the organism.) This experimental procedure effectively blocked X–X pairing and prevented X chromosome inactivation [**Figure 7–11(c)**].

Other genes and protein products are being examined for their role in X chromosome pairing and counting. Recent studies by Lee and colleagues have provided evidence that the inactivated X must associate with regions at the periphery of the nucleus to maintain a state of silenced gene expression. Indeed, in a majority of human female somatic cells the inactivated X, present as a Barr body, is observed attached to the nuclear envelope.

Many questions remain. What "blocks" the *Xic* locus of the active chromosome, preventing further transcription of *Xist*? How does imprinting impart a memory such that inactivation of the same X chromosome or chromosomes is subsequently maintained in progeny cells, as the Lyon hypothesis calls for? Whatever the answers to these questions, scientists have taken exciting steps toward understanding how dosage compensation is accomplished in mammals.

7.6 The Ratio of X Chromosomes to Sets of Autosomes Determines Sex in *Drosophila*

Because males and females in *Drosophila melanogaster* (and other *Drosophila* species) have the same general sex-chromosome composition as humans (males are XY and females are XX), we might assume that the Y chromosome also causes maleness in these flies. However, the elegant work of Calvin Bridges in 1916 showed this not to be true. His studies of flies with quite varied chromosome compositions led him to the conclusion that the Y chromosome is not involved in sex determination in this organism. Instead, Bridges proposed that the X chromosomes and autosomes together play a critical role in sex determination. Recall that in the nematode *C. elegans*, which lacks a Y chromosome, both the sex chromosomes and autosomes are critical to sex determination.

Bridges' work can be divided into two phases: (1) A study of offspring resulting from nondisjunction of the X chromosomes during meiosis in females and (2) subsequent work with progeny of females containing three copies of each chromosome, called triploid ($3n$) females. As we have seen previously in this chapter (and as you will see in Figure 8–1), nondisjunction is the failure of paired chromosomes to segregate or separate during the anaphase stage of the first or second meiotic divisions. The result is the production of two types of abnormal gametes, one of which contains an extra chromosome ($n + 1$) and the other of which lacks a chromosome ($n − 1$). Fertilization of such aberrant gametes with a haploid gamete produces $2n + 1$ or $2n − 1$ zygotes. As in humans, if nondisjunction involves the X chromosome, in addition to the normal complement of autosomes, both an XXY and an X0 sex-chromosome composition may result. (The "0" signifies that neither a second

X nor a Y chromosome is present, as occurs in X0 genotypes of individuals with Turner syndrome.)

Contrary to what was later discovered in humans, Bridges found that the XXY flies were normal females and the X0 flies were sterile males. The presence of the Y chromosome in the XXY flies did not cause maleness, and its absence in the X0 flies did not produce femaleness. From these data, he concluded that the Y chromosome in *Drosophila* lacks male-determining factors, but since the X0 males were sterile, it does contain genetic information essential to male fertility. Recent work has shown that the Y chromosome in *Drosophila* contains only about 20 protein-coding genes but mutation of these genes has significant impacts on regulating expression of hundreds of genes on other chromosomes, including genes on the X chromosome.

Bridges was able to clarify the mode of sex determination in *Drosophila* by studying the progeny of triploid females ($3n$), which have three copies each of the haploid complement of chromosomes. *Drosophila* has a haploid number of 4, thereby possessing three pairs of autosomes in addition to its pair of sex chromosomes. Triploid females apparently originate from rare diploid eggs fertilized by normal haploid sperm. Triploid females have heavy-set bodies, coarse bristles, and coarse eyes, and they may be fertile. Because of the odd number of each chromosome (3), during meiosis, a variety of different chromosome complements are distributed into gametes that give rise to offspring with a variety of abnormal chromosome constitutions. Correlations between the sexual morphology and chromosome composition, along with Bridges' interpretation, are shown in **Figure 7–12**.

Bridges realized that the critical factor in determining sex is *the ratio of X chromosomes to the number of haploid sets of autosomes (A) present*. Normal (2X:2A) and triploid (3X:3A) females each have a ratio equal to 1.0, and both

Normal diploid male

2 sets of autosomes
+
X   Y

Chromosome formulation	Ratio of X chromosomes to autosome sets	Sexual morphology
3X:2A	1.5	Metafemale
3X:3A	1.0	Female
2X:2A	1.0	Female
3X:4A	0.75	Intersex
2X:3A	0.67	Intersex
X:2A	0.50	Male
XY:2A	0.50	Male
XY:3A	0.33	Metamale

FIGURE 7–12 Chromosome compositions, the corresponding ratios of X chromosomes to sets of autosomes, and the resultant sexual morphology seen in *Drosophila melanogaster*. The normal diploid male chromosome composition is shown as a reference on the left (XY:2A). The rows representing normally occurring females and males are lightly shaded.

are fertile. As the ratio exceeds unity (3X:2A, or 1.5, for example), what was once called a *superfemale* is produced. Because such females are most often inviable, they are now more appropriately called **metafemales**.

Normal (XY:2A) and sterile (X0:2A) males each have a ratio of 1:2, or 0.5. When the ratio decreases to 1:3, or 0.33, as in the case of an XY:3A male, infertile **metamales** result. Other flies recovered by Bridges in these studies had an X:A ratio intermediate between 0.5 and 1.0. These flies were generally larger, and they exhibited a variety of morphological abnormalities and rudimentary bisexual gonads and genitalia. They were invariably sterile and expressed both male and female morphology, thus being designated as **intersexes**.

Bridges' results indicate that, in *Drosophila*, factors that cause a fly to develop into a male are not located on the sex chromosomes but are instead found on the autosomes. Some female-determining factors, however, are located on the X chromosomes. Thus, with respect to primary sex determination, male gametes containing one of each autosome plus a Y chromosome result in male offspring not because of the presence of the Y but because they fail to contribute an X chromosome. This mode of sex determination is explained by the **genic balance theory**. Bridges proposed that a threshold for maleness is reached when the X:A ratio is 1:2 (X:2A), but that the presence of an additional X (XX:2A) alters the balance and results in female differentiation.

Numerous mutant genes have been identified that are involved in sex determination in *Drosophila*. Recessive mutations in the autosomal gene, *transformer* (*tra*), discovered over 75 years ago by Alfred H. Sturtevant, clearly demonstrated that a single autosomal gene could have a profound impact on sex determination. Females homozygous for *tra* are transformed into sterile males, but homozygous males are unaffected.

More recently, another gene, *Sex-lethal* (*Sxl*), has been shown to play a critical role, serving as a "master switch" in sex determination. Activation of the X-linked *Sxl* gene, which relies on a ratio of X chromosomes to sets of autosomes that equals 1.0, is essential to female development. In the absence of activation—as when, for example, the X:A ratio is 0.5—male development occurs. It is interesting to note that mutations that inactivate the *Sxl* gene, as originally studied in 1960 by Hermann J. Muller, kill female embryos but have no effect on male embryos, consistent with the role of the gene. Although it is not yet exactly clear how this ratio influences the *Sxl* locus, we do have some insights into the question. The *Sxl* locus is part of a hierarchy of gene expression and exerts control over other genes, including *tra* (discussed in the previous paragraph) and *dsx* (*doublesex*). The wild-type allele of *tra* is activated by the product of *Sxl* only in females and in turn influences the expression of *dsx*.

Depending on how the initial RNA transcript of *dsx* is processed (spliced, as explained below), the resultant dsx protein activates either male- or female-specific genes required for sexual differentiation. Each step in this regulatory cascade requires a form of processing called **RNA splicing**, in which portions of the RNA are removed and the remaining fragments are "spliced" back together prior to translation into a protein. In the case of the *Sxl* gene, the RNA transcript may be spliced in different ways, a phenomenon called **alternative splicing**. A different RNA transcript is produced in females than in males. In potential females, the transcript encodes a functional protein and initiates a cascade of regulatory gene expression, ultimately leading to female differentiation. In potential males, the transcript encodes a nonfunctional protein, leading to a different pattern of gene activity, whereby male differentiation occurs. Later in the text (see Chapter 17), alternative splicing is again addressed as one of the mechanisms involved in the regulation of genetic expression in eukaryotes.)

Dosage Compensation in *Drosophila*

Since *Drosophila* females contain two copies of X-linked genes, whereas males contain only one copy, a dosage problem exists as it does in mammals such as humans and mice. However, the mechanism of dosage compensation in *Drosophila* differs considerably from that in mammals, since X chromosome inactivation is not observed. Instead, male X-linked genes are transcribed at twice the level of the comparable genes in females. Interestingly, if groups of X-linked genes are moved (translocated) to autosomes, dosage compensation still affects them, even though they are no longer part of the X chromosome.

As in mammals, considerable gains have been made recently in understanding the process of dosage compensation in *Drosophila*. At least four autosomal genes are known to be involved, under the same master-switch gene, *Sxl*, that induces female differentiation during sex determination. Mutations in any of these genes severely reduce the increased expression of X-linked genes in males, causing lethality.

Evidence supporting a mechanism of increased genetic activity in males is now available. The well-accepted model proposes that one of the autosomal genes, *mle* (*maleless*), encodes a protein that binds to numerous sites along the X chromosome, causing enhancement of genetic expression. The products of three other autosomal genes also participate in and are required for *mle* binding. In addition, proteins called male-specific lethals (MSLs) have been shown to bind to gene-rich regions of the X to increase gene expression in male flies. Collectively, this cluster of gene-activating proteins is called the **dosage**

MODERN APPROACHES TO UNDERSTANDING GENE FUNCTION

Drosophila Sxl Gene Induces Female Development

Recently, scientists have investigated a critical step involved in determining how germ-cell development, the ability to form either sperm or egg cells, is regulated in fruit flies. As discussed in this chapter, in *Drosophila* the *Sxl* gene encodes a protein that binds to RNA and regulates RNA splicing events. While the molecular mechanism that initiates female germ-cell fate is not known, researchers have hypothesized that the *Sxl* gene product might provide the critical switch that regulates this process. To test this hypothesis, they expressed *Sxl* in **primordial germ cells** (**PGCs**), undifferentiated diploid germ cells from XY male flies that would normally become sperm. *Sxl*-containing PGCs were then implanted into the ovaries of female flies and induced to enter oogenesis.

Donor PGCs	Number of Female Adults with Transplanted Germ-line Cells	Number of Female Adults with Transplanted Germ-line Cells Executing Oogenesis	Number of Female Adults with Transplanted Germ-line Cells Producing Progeny
XY	13	0 (0%)	0
XY + *Sxl*	18	13 (72%)	8
XY-nullo *Sxl*	15	0 (0%)	0
XX	25	25 (100%)	25

(Table modified from Hashiyama et al., Table 1.)

Results:

The following table summarizes *Sxl* implantation results. Implanted cells were tracked to determine whether or not they produced oocytes and whether such oocytes were capable of being fertilized and producing progeny. As shown in the table, XY donor PGCs lacking *Sxl* did not produce oocytes when transplanted into ovaries. When XY PGCs containing the *Sxl* gene were transplanted, 72 percent produced eggs, and these eggs were capable of being fertilized and producing progeny! Thus, the addition of a single gene to Y chromosome containing cells destined to become sperm is sufficient to change the fate of these cells to induce female germ-cell development. Various control experiments were conducted, including XY donor cells with a mutant, nonfunction version of *Sxl* (XY-nullo *Sxl*).

Conclusion:

Sxl functions to initiate development of female germ cells in *Drosophila*. Many questions remain, such as how *Sxl* is activated in female germ cells and which RNA molecules are affected by the *Sxl* gene product in female germ cells. Nonetheless, this result is very exciting because germ-line sexual development is thought to be highly conserved between animal species. Understanding how genes such as *Sxl* regulate germ-cell development in *Drosophila* is expected to help scientists understand key aspects of gamete development in mammals, including humans.

References:

Van Doren, M. 2011. Determining sexual identity. *Science* 333:829–830.
Hashiyama, K., et al. 2011. *Drosophila* sex lethal gene initiates female development in germline progenitors. *Science* 333:885–888.

Questions to Consider:

1. Which of the four experiments shown in the above table are controls?
2. Discuss the role of each control experiment. Are the results what you would predict?

compensation complex (DCC). **Figure 7–13** illustrates the presence of these proteins bound to the X chromosome in *Drosophila* in contrast to their failure to bind to the autosomes. The location of DCC proteins may be identified when fluorescent antibodies against these proteins are added to preparations of the large polytene chromosomes characteristic of salivary gland cells in fly larvae (see Chapter 12).

This model predicts that the master-switch *Sxl* gene plays an important role during dosage compensation. In XY flies, *Sxl* is inactive; therefore, the autosomal genes are activated, causing enhanced X chromosome activity. On the other hand, *Sxl* is active in XX females and functions to inactivate one or more of the male-specific autosomal genes, perhaps *mle*. By dampening the activity of these autosomal genes, it ensures that they will not serve to double the expression of X-linked genes in females, which would further compound the dosage problem.

Tom Cline has proposed that, before the aforementioned dosage compensation mechanism is activated, *Sxl* acts as a sensor for the expression of several other X-linked genes. In a way, *Sxl* counts X chromosomes. When it registers the dose of their expression as being high—for example, as the result of the presence of two X chromosomes—the *Sxl* gene product is modified to

FIGURE 7–13 Fluorescent antibodies against proteins in the dosage compensation complex (DCC) bind only to the X chromosome in *Drosophila* polytene chromosome preparations, providing evidence concerning the role of the DCC in increasing the expression of X-linked genes.

FIGURE 7–14 A bilateral gynandromorph of *Drosophila melanogaster* formed following the loss of one X chromosome in one of the two cells during the first mitotic division. The left side of the fly, composed of male cells containing a single X, expresses the mutant *white*-eye and *miniature*-wing alleles. The right side is composed of female cells containing two X chromosomes heterozygous for the two recessive alleles.

dampen the expression of the autosomal genes. Although this model may yet be revised or refined, it is useful for guiding future research.

Clearly, an entirely different mechanism of dosage compensation exists in *Drosophila* (and probably many related organisms) than that seen in mammals. The development of elaborate mechanisms to equalize the expression of X-linked genes demonstrates the critical importance of level of gene expression. A delicate balance of gene products is necessary to maintain normal development of both males and females.

Drosophila Mosaics

Our knowledge of sex determination and our discussion of X-linkage in *Drosophila* (Chapter 4) helps us to understand the unusual appearance of a unique fruit fly, shown in **Figure 7–14**. This fly was recovered from a stock in which all other females were heterozygous for the X-linked genes *white* eye (*w*) and *miniature* wing (*m*). It is a **bilateral gynandromorph**, which means that one-half of its body (the left half) has developed as a male and the other half (the right half) as a female.

We can account for the presence of both sexes in a single fly in the following way. If a female zygote (heterozygous for *white* eye and *miniature* wing) were to lose one of its X chromosomes during the first mitotic division, the two cells would be of the XX and X0 constitution, respectively. Thus, one cell would be female and the other would be male. Each of these cells is responsible for producing all progeny cells that make up either the right half or the left half of the body during embryogenesis.

In the case of the bilateral gynandromorph, the original cell of X0 constitution apparently produced only identical progeny cells and gave rise to the left half of the fly, which, because of its chromosomal constitution, was male. Since the male half demonstrated the *white*, *miniature* phenotype, the X chromosome bearing the w^+, m^+ alleles was lost, while the *w*, *m*-bearing homolog was retained. All cells on the right side of the body were derived from the original XX cell, leading to female development. These cells, which remained heterozygous for both mutant genes, expressed the wild-type eye–wing phenotypes.

Depending on the orientation of the spindle during the first mitotic division, gynandromorphs can be produced that have the "line" demarcating male versus female development along or across any axis of the fly's body.

7.7 Temperature Variation Controls Sex Determination in Reptiles

We conclude this chapter by discussing several cases involving reptiles, in which the environment—specifically temperature—has a profound influence on sex determination. In contrast to **genotypic sex determination (GSD)**, in which sex is determined genetically (as is true of all examples thus far presented in the chapter), the cases that we will now discuss are categorized as **temperature-dependent sex determination (TSD)**. As we shall see, the investigations leading to this information may well have come closer to revealing the true nature of the underlying basis of sex determination than any findings previously discussed.

In many species of reptiles, GSD is involved at conception based on sex-chromosome composition, as is the case in most organisms already considered in this chapter. For example, in many snakes, including vipers, a ZZ/ZW mode is in effect, in which the female is the heterogamous sex (ZW). However, in boas and pythons, it is impossible to distinguish one sex chromosome from the other in either sex. In many lizards, both the XX/XY and ZZ/ZW systems are found, depending on the species.

In still other reptilian species, however, TSD is the norm, including all crocodiles, most turtles, and some lizards, where sex determination is achieved according to the incubation temperature of eggs during a critical period of embryonic development. Three distinct patterns of TSD emerge (cases I–III in **Figure 7–15**). In case I, low temperatures yield 100 percent females, and high temperatures yield 100 percent males. Just the opposite occurs in case II. In case III, low *and* high temperatures yield 100 percent females, while intermediate temperatures yield various proportions of males. The third pattern is seen in various species of crocodiles, turtles, and lizards, although other members of these groups are known to exhibit the other patterns.

Noteworthy is the observation that in all three patterns one or more temperatures result in both males and females. A temperature at which approximately equal numbers of males and females result is called the pivotal temperature (T_p). The central question raised by this observation is this: What are the metabolic or physiological parameters affected by temperature that lead to the differentiation of one sex or the other?

The answer is thought to involve steroids (mainly estrogens) and the enzymes involved in their synthesis. Studies clearly demonstrate that the effects of temperature on estrogens, androgens, and inhibitors of the enzymes controlling their synthesis are involved in the sexual differentiation of ovaries and testes. One enzyme in particular, **aromatase**, converts androgens (male hormones such as testosterone) to estrogens (female hormones such as estradiol). The activity of this enzyme is correlated with the pathway of reactions that occurs during gonadal differentiation activity and is high in developing ovaries and low in developing testes. Researchers in this field, including Claude Pieau and colleagues, have proposed that a thermosensitive factor mediates the transcription of the reptilian aromatase gene, leading to temperature-dependent sex determination. Several other genes are likely to be involved in this mediation.

The involvement of sex steroids in gonadal differentiation has also been documented in birds, fishes, and amphibians. Thus, sex-determining mechanisms involving estrogens seem to be characteristic of nonmammalian vertebrates. The regulation of such systems, while temperature dependent in many reptiles, appears to be controlled by sex chromosomes (XX/XY or ZZ/ZW) in many of these other organisms. A final intriguing thought on this matter is that the product of *SRY*, a key component in mammalian sex determination, has been shown to bind *in vitro* to a regulatory portion of the aromatase gene, suggesting a mechanism whereby it could act as a repressor of ovarian development.

FIGURE 7–15 Three different patterns of temperature-dependent sex determination (TSD) in reptiles, as described in the text. The pivotal temperature T_p is crucial to sex determination during a critical point during embryonic development. FT = Female-determining temperature; MT = male-determining temperature.

GENETICS, TECHNOLOGY, AND SOCIETY

A Question of Gender: Sex Selection in Humans

Throughout history, people have attempted to influence the gender of their unborn offspring by following varied and sometimes bizarre procedures. In medieval Europe, prospective parents would place a hammer under the bed to help them conceive a boy, or a pair of scissors to conceive a girl. Other practices were based on the ancient belief that semen from the right testicle created male offspring and that from the left testicle created females. As late as the eighteenth century, European men might tie off or remove their left testicle to increase the chances of getting a male heir. In some cultures, efforts to control the sex of offspring has had a darker side—female infanticide. In ancient Greece, the murder of female infants was so common that the male:female ratio in some areas approached 4:1. In some parts of rural India, hundreds of families admitted to female infanticide as late as the 1990s. In 1997, the World Health Organization reported population data showing that about 50 million women were "missing" in China, likely because of selective abortion of female fetuses and institutionalized neglect of female children.

In recent times, amniocentesis and ultrasound testing, followed by sex-specific abortion, have replaced much of the traditional female infanticide. Studies in India estimate that approximately 10 million female fetuses were aborted from 1986 to 2006, resulting in a childhood female:male sex ratio of 927:1000. In some northern states, the ratio was as low as 600:1000. In 2010, the sex ratio at birth in China was 120 males to 100 females.

New genetic and reproductive technologies offer parents ways to select their children's gender prior to implantation of the embryo in the uterus—called *preimplantation gender selection (PGS)*. Following *in vitro* fertilization, embryos are biopsied and assessed for gender. Only sex-selected embryos are then implanted. The simplest method involves separating X and Y chromosome-bearing spermatozoa based on their DNA content. Because of the difference in size of the X and Y chromosomes, X-bearing sperm contain 2.8 to 3.0 percent more DNA than Y-bearing sperm. Sperm samples are treated with a fluorescent DNA stain, and then passed through a laser beam in a Fluorescence-Activated Cell Sorter machine that separates the sperm into two fractions based on the intensity of their DNA-fluorescence. The sorted sperm are then used for standard intrauterine insemination.

The emerging PGS methods raise a number of legal and ethical issues. Some people feel that prospective parents have the legal right to use sex-selection techniques as part of their fundamental procreative liberty. Proponents state that PGS will reduce the suffering of many families. For example, people at risk for transmitting X-linked diseases such as hemophilia or Duchenne muscular dystrophy would be able to enhance their chance of conceiving a female child, who will not express the disease.

The majority of people who undertake PGS, however, do so for nonmedical reasons—to "balance" their families. A possible argument in favor of this use is that the ability to intentionally select the sex of an offspring may reduce overpopulation and economic burdens for families who would repeatedly reproduce to get the desired gender. By the same token, PGS may reduce the number of abortions. It is also possible that PGS may increase the happiness of both parents and children, as the children would be more "wanted."

On the other hand, some argue that PGS serves neither the individual nor the common good. They argue that PGS is inherently sexist, having its basis in the idea that one sex is superior to the other, and leads to an increase in linking a child's worth to gender. Other critics fear that social approval of PGS will open the door to other genetic manipulations of children's characteristics. It is difficult to predict the full effects that PGS will bring to the world. But the gender-selection genie is now out of the bottle and is unwilling to return.

Your Turn

Take time, individually or in groups, to answer the following questions. Investigate the references and links to help you understand some of the issues that surround the topic of gender selection.

1. What do you think are valid arguments for and against the use of PGS?

2. A generally accepted moral and legal concept is that of reproductive autonomy—the freedom to make individual reproductive decisions without external interference. Are there circumstances under which reproductive autonomy should be restricted?

   The above questions, and others, are explored in a series of articles in the American Journal of Bioethics, Volume 1 (2001). See the article by J. A. Robertson on pages 2–9 for a summary of the moral and legal issues surrounding PGS.

3. What do you think are the reasons that some societies practice female infanticide and prefer the birth of male children?

   For a discussion of this topic, visit the "Gendercide Watch" Web site http://www.gendercide.org.

4. If safe and efficient methods of PGS were available to you, do you think that you would use them to help you with family planning? Under what circumstances might you use them?

   Studies in 2009 and 2012 suggest that information about preimplantation genetic testing available on fertility clinic Web sites may be of poor quality and may minimize the risks. Investigate this topic in: Klitzman, R. et al. 2009. Preimplantation genetic diagnosis (PDG) on in-vitro fertilization (IVF) websites: presentations of risks, benefits and other information. Fertil. Steril. 92(4):1276–1283.

CASE STUDY | Doggone it!

A dog breeder discovers one of her male puppies has abnormal genitalia. After a visit to the veterinary clinic at a nearby university, the breeder learns that the dog's karyotype lacks a Y chromosome, and instead has an XX chromosome pair, with one of the X chromosomes slightly larger than usual (being mammals, male dogs are normally XY and females are XX). The veterinarian tells her that in other breeds, some females display an XY chromosome pair, with the Y chromosome being slightly shorter than normal. These observations raise several interesting questions:

1. Can you speculate as to how the chromosomal composition of the breeder's dog led to its ambiguous sexuality?

2. How could such a case be used to locate the gene(s) responsible for maleness?

3. Suppose you discover a female dog with a normal-sized XY chromosome pair. What kind of mutation might be involved in this case?

4. Suppose you discover a female dog with only a single X chromosome. What predictions might you make about the sex organs and reproductive capacity of this dog?

Summary Points

1. Sexual reproduction depends on the differentiation of male and female structures responsible for the production of male and female gametes, which in turn is controlled by specific genes, most often housed on specific sex chromosomes.

2. Specific sex chromosomes contain genetic information that controls sex determination and sexual differentiation.

3. The presence or absence of a Y chromosome that contains an intact *SRY* gene is responsible for causing maleness in humans and other mammals.

4. In humans, while many more males than females are conceived, and although fewer male than female embryos and fetuses survive *in utero*, there are nevertheless more males than females born.

5. In mammals, female somatic cells randomly inactivate one of two X chromosomes during early embryonic development, a process important for balancing the expression of X chromosome linked genes in males and females.

6. The Lyon hypothesis states that early in development, inactivation of either the maternal or paternal X chromosome occurs in each cell, and that all progeny cells subsequently inactivate the same chromosome. Mammalian females thus develop as mosaics for the expression of heterozygous X-linked alleles.

7. Many reptiles show temperature-dependent effects on sex determination. Although specific sex chromosomes determine genotypic sex in many reptiles, temperature effects on genes involved in sexual determination affect whether an embryo develops a male or female phenotype.

INSIGHTS AND SOLUTIONS

1. In *Drosophila*, the X chromosomes may become attached to one another $(\widehat{XX})$ such that they always segregate together. Some flies thus contain a set of attached X chromosomes plus a Y chromosome.

(a) What sex would such a fly be? Explain why this is so.

(b) Given the answer to part (a), predict the sex of the offspring that would occur in a cross between this fly and a normal one of the opposite sex.

(c) If the offspring described in part (b) are allowed to interbreed, what will be the outcome?

Solution:

(a) The fly will be a female. The ratio of X chromosomes to sets of autosomes—which determines sex in *Drosophila*—will be 1.0, leading to normal female development. The Y chromosome has no influence on sex determination in *Drosophila*.

(b) All progeny flies will have two sets of autosomes along with one of the following sex-chromosome compositions:

(1) $\widehat{XX}X \rightarrow$ a metafemale with 3 X's (called a trisomic)

(2) $\widehat{XX}Y \rightarrow$ a female like her mother

(3) XY $\rightarrow$ a normal male

(4) YY $\rightarrow$ no development occurs

(c) A stock will be created that maintains attached-X females generation after generation.

2. The Xg cell-surface antigen is coded for by a gene located on the X chromosome. No equivalent gene exists on the Y chromosome. Two codominant alleles of this gene have been identified: *Xg1* and *Xg2*. A woman of genotype *Xg2/Xg2* bears children with a man of genotype *Xg1/Y*, and they produce a son with Klinefelter syndrome of genotype *Xg1/Xg2/Y*. Using proper genetic terminology, briefly explain how this individual was generated. In which parent and in which meiotic division did the mistake occur?

Solution: Because the son with Klinefelter syndrome is *Xg1/Xg2/Y*, he must have received both the *Xg1* allele and the Y chromosome from his father. Therefore, nondisjunction must have occurred during meiosis I in the father.

Problems and Discussion Questions

HOW DO WE KNOW?

1. In this chapter, we focused on sex differentiation, sex chromosomes, and genetic mechanisms involved in sex determination. At the same time, we found many opportunities to consider the methods and reasoning by which much of this information was acquired. From the explanations given in the chapter, what answers would you propose to the following fundamental questions?

   (a) How do we know that specific genes in maize play a role in sexual differentiation?

   (b) How do we know whether or not a heteromorphic chromosome such as the Y chromosome plays a crucial role in the determination of sex?

   (c) How do we know that in humans the X chromosomes play no role in human sex determination, while the Y chromosome causes maleness and its absence causes femaleness?

   (d) How did we learn that, although the sex ratio at birth in humans favors males slightly, the sex ratio at conception favors them much more?

   (e) How do we know that *Drosophila* utilizes a different sex-determination mechanism than mammals, even though it has the same sex-chromosome compositions in males and females?

   (f) How do we know that X chromosomal inactivation of either the paternal or maternal homolog is a random event during early development in mammalian females?

CONCEPT QUESTION

2. Review the Chapter Concepts list on p. 164. These all center around sex determination or the expression of genes encoded on sex chromosomes. Write a short essay that discusses sex chromosomes as they contrast with autosomes.

3. Contrast the life cycle of a plant such as *Zea mays* with an animal such as *C. elegans*.

4. Distinguish between the terms *homomorphic* and *heteromorphic chromosomes*, and between *isogamous* and *heterogamous* organisms.

5. Distinguish between the concepts of sexual differentiation and sex determination.

6. Contrast the XX/XY and XX/X0 modes of sex determination.

7. Describe the major difference between sex determination in *Drosophila* and in humans.

8. How do mammals, including humans, solve the "dosage problem" caused by the presence of an X and Y chromosome in one sex and two X chromosomes in the other sex?

9. The phenotype of an early-stage human embryo is considered sexually indifferent. Explain why this is so even though the embryo's genotypic sex is already fixed.

10. What specific observations (evidence) support the conclusions about sex determination in *Drosophila* and humans?

11. Describe how nondisjunction in human female gametes can give rise to Klinefelter and Turner syndrome offspring following fertilization by a normal male gamete.

12. An insect species is discovered in which the heterogametic sex is unknown. An X-linked recessive mutation for *reduced wing* (*rw*) is discovered. Contrast the F_1 and F_2 generations from a cross between a female with reduced wings and a male with normal-sized wings when

    (a) the female is the heterogametic sex.

    (b) the male is the heterogametic sex.

13. When cows have twin calves of unlike sex (fraternal twins), the female twin is usually sterile and has masculinized reproductive organs. This calf is referred to as a freemartin. In cows, twins may share a common placenta and thus fetal circulation. Predict why a freemartin develops.

14. An attached-X female fly, $\widehat{XX}Y$ (see the "Insights and Solutions" box), expresses the recessive X-linked *white*-eye mutation. It is crossed to a male fly that expresses the X-linked recessive *miniature*-wing mutation. Determine the outcome of this cross in terms of sex, eye color, and wing size of the offspring.

15. Assume that on rare occasions the attached X chromosomes in female gametes become unattached. Based on the parental phenotypes in Problem 14, what outcomes in the F_1 generation would indicate that this has occurred during female meiosis?

16. It has been suggested that any male-determining genes contained on the Y chromosome in humans cannot be located in the limited region that synapses with the X chromosome during meiosis. What might be the outcome if such genes were located in this region?

17. What is a Barr body, and where is it found in a cell?

18. Indicate the expected number of Barr bodies in interphase cells of individuals with Klinefelter syndrome; Turner syndrome; and karyotypes 47,XYY, 47,XXX, and 48,XXXX.

19. Define the Lyon hypothesis.

20. Can the Lyon hypothesis be tested in a human female who is homozygous for one allele of the X-linked *G6PD* gene? Why, or why not?

21. Predict the potential effect of the Lyon hypothesis on the retina of a human female heterozygous for the X-linked red-green color blindness trait.

22. Cat breeders are aware that kittens expressing the X-linked calico coat pattern and tortoiseshell pattern are almost invariably females. Why are they certain of this?

23. What does the apparent need for dosage compensation mechanisms suggest about the expression of genetic information in normal diploid individuals?

24. How does X chromosome dosage compensation in *Drosophila* differ from that process in humans?

25. What type of evidence supports the conclusion that the primary sex ratio in humans is much higher than the secondary sex ratio?

26. Devise as many hypotheses as you can that might explain why so many more human male conceptions than human female conceptions occur.

27. In mice, the *Sry* gene (see Section 7.3) is located on the Y chromosome very close to one of the pseudoautosomal regions that pairs with the X chromosome during male meiosis. Given this information, propose a model to explain the generation of unusual males who have two X chromosomes (with an *Sry*-containing piece of the Y chromosome attached to one X chromosome).

28. The genes encoding the red- and green-color-detecting proteins of the human eye are located next to one another on the X chromosome and probably evolved from a common ancestral pigment gene. The two proteins demonstrate 76 percent homology in their amino acid sequences. A normal-visioned woman (with both genes present on each of her two X chromosomes) has a red-color-blind son who was shown to have one copy of the green-detecting gene and no copies of the red-detecting gene. Devise an explanation for these observations at the chromosomal level (involving meiosis).

29. What is the role of the enzyme aromatase in sexual differentiation in reptiles?

Extra-Spicy Problems

MasteringGenetics™ Visit for instructor assigned tutorials and problems.

30. In the wasp *Bracon hebetor*, a form of parthenogenesis (the development of unfertilized eggs into progeny) resulting in haploid organisms is not uncommon. All haploids are males. When offspring arise from fertilization, females almost invariably result. P. W. Whiting has shown that an X-linked gene with nine multiple alleles (X_a, X_b, etc.) controls sex determination. Any homozygous or hemizygous condition results in males, and any heterozygous condition results in females. If an X_a/X_b female mates with an X_a male and lays 50 percent fertilized and 50 percent unfertilized eggs, what proportion of male and female offspring will result?

31. Since the mid-1800s, sex in honeybees (*Apis mellifera*) was thought to be determined by the fertilization (for females) or nonfertilization (for males) of eggs. These conclusions were later supported by cytological observations. However, male honeybees can also be derived from inbred diploid, fertilized eggs, leading to the finding that fertilization also occurs in nature to produce diploid males. Such males are eaten by female worker bees right after hatching from the egg. Based on the method of sex determination in *Bracon hebetor*, described in Problem 30, suggest a model for sex determination in honeybees that includes the production of diploid male embryos.

32. In mice, the X-linked dominant mutation *Testicular feminization* (*Tfm*) eliminates the normal response to the testicular hormone testosterone during sexual differentiation. An XY mouse bearing the *Tfm* allele on the X chromosome develops testes, but no further male differentiation occurs—the external genitalia of such an animal are female. From this information, what might you conclude about the role of the *Tfm* gene product and the X and Y chromosomes in sex determination and sexual differentiation in mammals? Can you devise an experiment, assuming you can "genetically engineer" the chromosomes of mice, to test and confirm your explanation?

33. When the cloned cat Carbon Copy (CC) was born (see the Now Solve This question on p. 177), she had black patches and white patches, but completely lacked any orange patches. The knowledgeable students of genetics were not surprised at this outcome. Starting with the somatic ovarian cell used as the source of the nucleus in the cloning process, explain how this outcome occurred.

Carbon Copy with her surrogate mother.

34. In a number of organisms, including *Drosophila* and butterflies, genes that alter the sex ratio have been described. In the pest species *Musca domesticus* (the house fly), *Aedes aegypti* (the mosquito that is the vector for yellow fever), and *Culex pipiens* (the mosquito vector for filariasis and some viral diseases), scientists are especially interested in such genes. Sex in *Culex* is determined by a single gene pair, *Mm* being male and *mm* being female. Males homozygous for the recessive gene *dd* never produce many female offspring. The *dd* combination in males causes fragmentation of the *m*-bearing dyad during the first meiotic division, hence its failure to complete spermatogenesis.

    (a) Account for this sex-ratio distortion by drawing labeled chromosome arrangements in primary and secondary spermatocytes for each of the following genotypes: *Mm Dd* and *Mm dd*. How do meiotic products differ between *Dd* and *dd* genotypes? Note that the diploid chromosome number is 6 in *Culex pipiens* and both *D* and *M* loci are linked on the same chromosome.

    (b) How might a sex-ratio distorter such as *dd* be used to control pest population numbers?

35. In chickens, a key gene involved in sex determination has recently been identified. Called *DMRT1*, it is located on the Z chromosome and is absent on the W chromosome. Like *SRY* in humans, it is male determining. Unlike *SRY* in humans, however, female chickens (ZW) have a single copy while males (ZZ) have two copies of the gene. Nevertheless, it is transcribed only in the developing testis. Working in the laboratory of Andrew Sinclair (a co-discoverer of the human *SRY* gene), Craig Smith and colleagues were able to "knock down" expression of *DMRT1* in ZZ embryos using RNA interference techniques (see Chapter 17). In such cases, the developing gonads look more like ovaries than testes [*Nature* 461: 267 (2009)]. What conclusions can you draw about the role that the *DMRT1* gene plays in chickens in contrast to the role the *SRY* gene plays in humans?

36. The paradigm in vertebrates is that, once sex determination occurs and testes or ovaries are formed, secondary sexual differentiation (male vs. female characteristics) is dependent on male or female hormones that are produced. Recently, D. Zhao and colleagues studied three chickens that were bilateral gynandromorphs, with the right side of the body being clearly female and the left side of the body clearly male [*Nature* 464: 237 (2010)]. Propose experimental questions that can be investigated using these chickens to test this paradigm. What alternative interpretation contrasts with the paradigm?

Spectral karyotyping of human chromosomes, utilizing differentially labeled "painting" probes.

8 Chromosome Mutations: Variation in Number and Arrangement

CHAPTER CONCEPTS

- The failure of chromosomes to properly separate during meiosis results in variation in the chromosome content of gametes and subsequently in offspring arising from such gametes.

- Plants often tolerate an abnormal genetic content, but, as a result, they often manifest unique phenotypes. Such genetic variation has been an important factor in the evolution of plants.

- In animals, genetic information is in a delicate equilibrium whereby the gain or loss of a chromosome, or part of a chromosome, in an otherwise diploid organism often leads to lethality or to an abnormal phenotype.

- The rearrangement of genetic information within the genome of a diploid organism may be tolerated by that organism but may affect the viability of gametes and the phenotypes of organisms arising from those gametes.

- Chromosomes in humans contain fragile sites—regions susceptible to breakage, which lead to abnormal phenotypes.

I n previous chapters, we have emphasized how mutations and the resulting alleles affect an organism's phenotype and how traits are passed from parents to offspring according to Mendelian principles. In this chapter,

we look at phenotypic variation that results from more substantial changes than alterations of individual genes—modifications at the level of the chromosome.

Although most members of diploid species normally contain precisely two haploid chromosome sets, many known cases vary from this pattern. Modifications include a change in the total number of chromosomes, the deletion or duplication of genes or segments of a chromosome, and rearrangements of the genetic material either within or among chromosomes. Taken together, such changes are called **chromosome mutations** or **chromosome aberrations**, to distinguish them from gene mutations. Because the chromosome is the unit of genetic transmission, according to Mendelian laws, chromosome aberrations are passed to offspring in a predictable manner, resulting in many unique genetic outcomes.

Because the genetic component of an organism is delicately balanced, even minor alterations of either content or location of genetic information within the genome can result in some form of phenotypic variation. More substantial changes may be lethal, particularly in animals. Throughout this chapter, we consider many types of chromosomal aberrations, the phenotypic consequences for the organism that harbors an aberration, and the impact of the aberration on the offspring of an affected individual. We will also discuss the role of chromosome aberrations in the evolutionary process.

8.1 Variation in Chromosome Number: Terminology and Origin

Variation in chromosome number ranges from the addition or loss of one or more chromosomes to the addition of one or more haploid sets of chromosomes. Before we embark on our discussion, it is useful to clarify the terminology that describes such changes. In the general condition known as **aneuploidy**, an organism gains or loses one or more chromosomes but not a complete set. The loss of a single chromosome from an otherwise diploid genome is called *monosomy*. The gain of one chromosome results in *trisomy*. These changes are contrasted with the condition of **euploidy**, where complete haploid sets of chromosomes are present. If more than two sets are present, the term **polyploidy** applies. Organisms with three sets are specifically *triploid*, those with four sets are *tetraploid*, and so on. Table 8.1 provides an organizational framework for you to follow as we discuss each of these categories of aneuploid and euploid variation and the subsets within them.

As we consider cases that include the gain or loss of chromosomes, it is useful to examine how such aberrations originate. For instance, how do the syndromes arise where the number of sex-determining chromosomes in humans is altered, (Chapter 7)? As you may recall, the gain (47,XXY) or loss (45,X) of an X chromosome from an otherwise diploid genome affects the phenotype, resulting in **Klinefelter syndrome** or **Turner syndrome**, respectively (see Figure 7–6). Human females may contain extra X chromosomes (e.g., 47,XXX, 48,XXXX), and some males contain an extra Y chromosome (47,XYY).

Such chromosomal variation originates as a random error during the production of gametes, a phenomenon

NOW SOLVE THIS

8–1 A human female with Turner syndrome (47,X) also expresses the X-linked trait hemophilia, as did her father. Which of her parents underwent nondisjunction during meiosis, giving rise to the gamete responsible for the syndrome?

■ **HINT:** *This problem involves an understanding of how nondisjunction leads to aneuploidy. The key to its solution is first to review Turner syndrome, discussed above and in more detail later in the text (see Chapter 7), then to factor in that she expresses hemophilia, and finally, to consider which parent contributed a gamete with an X chromosome that underwent normal meiosis.*

For more practice, see Problems 27, 28, and 29.

referred to as **nondisjunction**, whereby paired homologs fail to disjoin during segregation. This process disrupts the normal distribution of chromosomes into gametes. The results of nondisjunction during meiosis I and meiosis II for a single chromosome of a diploid organism are shown in **Figure 8–1**. As you can see, abnormal gametes can form containing either two members of the affected chromosome or none at all. Fertilizing these with a normal haploid gamete produces a zygote with either three members (trisomy) or only one member (monosomy) of this chromosome. Nondisjunction leads to a variety of aneuploid conditions in humans and other organisms.

8.2 Monosomy and Trisomy Result in a Variety of Phenotypic Effects

We turn now to a consideration of variations in the number of autosomes and the genetic consequence of such changes. The most common examples of *aneuploidy,* where an organism has a chromosome number other than an exact multiple of the haploid set, are cases in which a single chromosome is either added to, or lost from, a normal diploid set.

Monosomy

The loss of one chromosome produces a $2n - 1$ complement called **monosomy**. Although monosomy for the X chromosome occurs in humans, as we have seen in 45,X Turner syndrome, monosomy for any of the autosomes is not usually tolerated in humans or other animals. In *Drosophila,* flies that are monosomic for the very small chromosome IV (containing less than 5 percent of the organism's genes) develop more slowly, exhibit reduced body size, and have impaired viability. Monosomy for the larger autosomal

TABLE 8.1   Terminology for Variation in Chromosome Numbers

Term	Explanation
Aneuploidy	$2n \pm x$ chromosomes
Monosomy	$2n - 1$
Disomy	$2n$
Trisomy	$2n + 1$
Tetrasomy, pentasomy, etc.	$2n + 2, 2n + 3$, etc.
Euploidy	Multiples of n
Diploidy	$2n$
Polyploidy	$3n, 4n, 5n, \ldots$
Triploidy	$3n$
Tetraploidy, pentaploidy, etc.	$4n, 5n$, etc.
Autopolyploidy	Multiples of the same genome
Allopolyploidy (amphidiploidy)	Multiples of closely related genomes

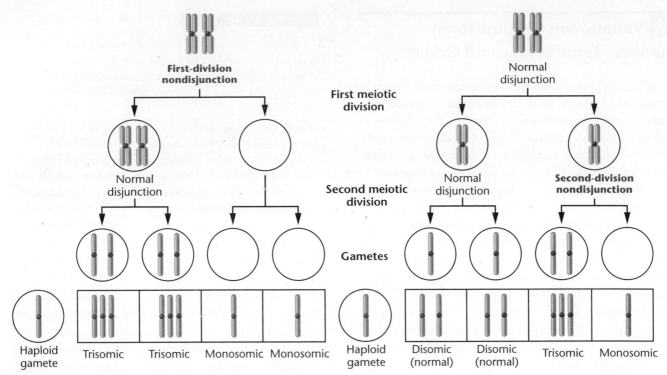

FIGURE 8-1 Nondisjunction during the first and second meiotic divisions. In both cases, some of the gametes that are formed either contain two members of a specific chromosome or lack that chromosome. After fertilization by a gamete with a normal haploid content, monosomic, disomic (normal), or trisomic zygotes are produced.

chromosomes II and III is apparently lethal because such flies have never been recovered.

The failure of monosomic individuals to survive is at first quite puzzling, since at least a single copy of every gene is present in the remaining homolog. However, if just one of those genes is represented by a lethal allele, the unpaired chromosome condition will result in the death of the organism. This will occur because monosomy unmasks recessive lethals that are otherwise tolerated in heterozygotes carrying the corresponding wild-type alleles. Another possible cause of lethality of aneuploidy is that a single copy of a recessive gene may be insufficient to provide adequate function for sustaining the organism, a phenomenon called **haploinsufficiency**.

Aneuploidy is better tolerated in the plant kingdom. Monosomy for autosomal chromosomes has been observed in maize, tobacco, the evening primrose (*Oenothera*), and the jimson weed (*Datura*), among many other plants. Nevertheless, such monosomic plants are usually less viable than their diploid derivatives. Haploid pollen grains, which undergo extensive development before participating in fertilization, are particularly sensitive to the lack of one chromosome and are seldom viable.

Trisomy

In general, the effects of **trisomy** (2n + 1) parallel those of monosomy. However, the addition of an extra chromosome produces somewhat more viable individuals in both animal and plant species than does the loss of a chromosome. In animals, this is often true, provided that the chromosome involved is relatively small. However, the addition of a large autosome to the diploid complement in both *Drosophila* and humans has severe effects and is usually lethal during development.

In plants, trisomic individuals are viable, but their phenotype may be altered. A classical example involves the jimson weed, *Datura,* whose diploid number is 24. Twelve primary trisomic conditions are possible, and examples of each one have been recovered. Each trisomy alters the phenotype of the plant's capsule (**Figure 8–2**) sufficiently to produce a unique phenotype. These capsule phenotypes were first thought to be caused by mutations in one or more genes.

Still another example is seen in the rice plant (*Oryza sativa*), which has a haploid number of 12. Trisomic strains for each chromosome have been isolated and studied—the plants of 11 strains can be distinguished from one another and from wild-type plants. Trisomics for the longer chromosomes are the most distinctive, and the plants grow more slowly. This is in keeping with the belief that larger chromosomes cause greater genetic imbalance than smaller ones. Leaf structure, foliage, stems, grain morphology, and plant height also vary among the various trisomies.

FIGURE 8-2 The capsule of the fruit of the jimson weed, *Datura stramonium,* the phenotype of which is uniquely altered by each of the possible 12 trisomic conditions.

Down Syndrome: Trisomy 21

The only human autosomal trisomy in which a significant number of individuals survive longer than a year past birth was discovered in 1866 by Langdon Down. The condition is now known to result from trisomy of chromosome 21, one of the G group*(**Figure 8–3**), and is called **Down syndrome** or simply **trisomy 21** (designated 47,21+). This trisomy is found in approximately 1 infant in every 800 live births. While this might seem to be a rare, improbable event, there

are approximately 4000–5000 such births annually in the United States, and there are currently over 250,000 individuals with Down syndrome.

Typical of other conditions classified as syndromes, many phenotypic characteristics *may* be present in trisomy 21, but any single affected individual usually exhibits only a subset of these. In the case of Down syndrome, there are 12 to 14 such characteristics, with each individual, on average, expressing 6 to 8 of them. Nevertheless, the outward appearance of these individuals is very similar, and they bear a striking resemblance to one another. This is largely due to a prominent epicanthic fold in each eye** and the typically flat face and round head. Those with Down syndrome are also characteristically short and may have a protruding, furrowed tongue (which causes the mouth to remain partially open) and short, broad hands with characteristic palm and fingerprint patterns. Physical, psychomotor, and mental development is retarded, and poor muscle tone is characteristic. While life expectancy is shortened to an average of about 50 years, individuals are known to survive into their 60s.

Children afflicted with Down syndrome are also prone to respiratory disease and heart malformations, and they show an incidence of leukemia approximately 20 times higher than that of the normal population. In addition, death in older Down syndrome adults is frequently due to Alzheimer disease, the onset of which occurs at a much earlier age than in the normal population.

*On the basis of size and centromere placement, human autosomal chromosomes are divided into seven groups: A (1–3), B (4–5), C (6–12), D (13–15), E (16–18), F (19–20), and G (21–22).

**The epicanthic fold, or epicanthus, is a skin fold of the upper eyelid, extending from the nose to the inner side of the eyebrow. It covers and appears to lower the inner corner of the eye, giving the eye a slanted, or almond-shaped, appearance. The epicanthus is a prominent normal component of the eyes in many Asian groups.

© Design Pics/Alamy

FIGURE 8-3 The karyotype and a photograph of a child with Down syndrome (hugging her unaffected sister on the right). In the karyotype, three members of the G-group chromosome 21 are present, creating the 47,21+ condition.

The Down Syndrome Critical Region (DSCR)

Because Down syndrome is common in our population, a comprehensive understanding of the underlying genetic basis has long been a research goal. Investigations have given rise to the idea that a critical region of chromosome 21 contains the genes that are dosage sensitive in this trisomy and responsible for the many phenotypes associated with the syndrome. This hypothetical portion of the chromosome has been called the **Down syndrome critical region (DSCR)**. A mouse model was created in 2004 that is trisomic for the DSCR, although some mice do not exhibit the characteristics of the syndrome. Nevertheless, this remains an important investigative approach, which is explored in the box below.

MODERN APPROACHES TO UNDERSTANDING GENE FUNCTION

Mouse Models of Down Syndrome

The underlying hypothesis concerning the genetic basis of Down syndrome is that the presence of three copies of chromosome 21 leads to the overexpression of some portion of the genes on that chromosome and that the resulting gene products are responsible for the multiple characteristics associated with the complete phenotype. It is possible that, even though Down syndrome is not caused by a single gene, individual genes may be responsible for specific characteristics making up the syndrome. Elucidation of which genes are involved has long been the goal of numerous research investigations.

In many of the "Modern Approaches to Understanding Gene Function" features, we focus on experimental approaches that involve the study of one or a few genes. However, geneticists can create model organisms with trisomy, making possible the simultaneous analysis of the function of many genes. Relevant to this discussion, trisomy (Ts) mouse models for Down syndrome have been created and for over two decades have been available to investigators. We focus here on several Ts mouse models that may prove invaluable to our future understanding of the genetic basis of the syndrome and to our developing potential treatments for affected humans.

Human chromosome 21 (Hsa21) and mouse chromosome 16 contain *syntenic* regions—chromosomal regions in different species that contain much of the same content and arrangement of *orthologs*, genes with similar sequences that are present in different species. One of the earliest models created (Ts16) has an extra copy of mouse chromosome 16, and indeed it displays some, but not all, human Down syndrome characteristics. Therefore Ts16 mice are missing some of the critical orthologs present on Hsa21. Ts16 mice also have extra copies of other genes not present on Hsa21.

Further investigation has established that mouse chromosomes 10 and 17 also contain orthologs for genes on Hsa21. Thus, an important goal of this research effort was to create an extended mouse model that contains most, if not all, of the genes on Hsa21, and in particular, the 33 genes that are part of the Down syndrome critical region (DSCR) discussed earlier in this chapter. This goal was achieved in 2010 when scientists at the Roswell Park Cancer Institute in Buffalo, New York, developed a mouse model of Down syndrome that is trisomic for all syntenic regions of Hsa21 by combining regions of mouse chromosome 10, 16, and 17 (Mmu 10, 16, 17).

Results:

Mmu 10, 16, 17 trisomic mice display the learning and memory deficits characteristic of Down syndrome that were determined through various behavioral tests and electrophysiological recordings of the brain. These mice also show anatomical abnormalities associated with human Down syndrome such as hydrocephalus, accumulation of cerebrospinal fluid in the brain, and a resulting rounded and enlarged cranium. There are no known genes on Hsa21 that are directly associated with hydrocephalus in humans, so this condition is likely caused by expressing multiple copies of several orthologs.

Conclusion:

Research with mouse models has demonstrated that no single gene is responsible for all phenotypes associated with Down syndrome, but instead that overexpression of many genes is necessary to produce the full human syndrome. The creation of new models such as the Mmu 10, 16, 17 animals demonstrates their potential value for understanding the genetics of Down syndrome and for developing treatments for Down syndrome patients. Clearly, adding an entire chromosome to an organism's genome has extended our ability to investigate complex human disorders such as Down syndrome.

Reference:

Yu, T. et al. 2010. A mouse model of Down syndrome trisomic for all human chromosome 21 syntenic regions. *Human Mol. Genet.* 19:2780–2791.

Questions to Consider:

1. What are two limitations in creating a mouse model for Down syndrome that is an exact genetic replica of human trisomy 21?

2. How might mouse model animals that are trisomic only for certain syntenic regions of Mmu 10, 16, and 17 be valuable for identifying human orthologs responsible for particular phenotypes observed in Down syndrome?

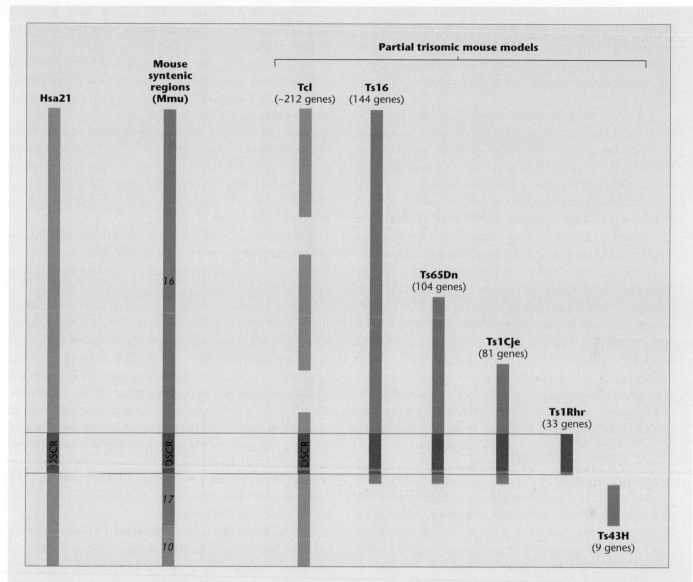

Schematic representation focusing on the q-arm of human chromosome 21 (Hsa1) where the DSCR is located, compared with syntenic regions of mouse chromosomes (Mmu) 10, 16, and 17, and chromosomal configurations of partial trisomic mouse models.
© American Society of Hematology

Current studies of the DSCR in both humans and mice have led to several interesting findings. Research investigations have now led us to believe that the presence of three copies of the genes present in this region is necessary, but not sufficient for the cognitive deficiencies characteristic of the syndrome. Another finding involves an important observation about Down syndrome—that such individuals have a decreased risk of developing a number of cancers involving solid tumors, including lung cancer and melanoma. This health benefit has been correlated with the presence of an extra copy of the *DSCR1* gene, which encodes a protein that suppresses *vascular endothelial growth factor* (*VEGF*). This suppression, in turn, blocks the

process of angiogenesis. As a result, the overexpression of this gene inhibits tumors from forming proper vascularization, diminishing their growth. A 14-year study published in 2002 involving 17,800 Down syndrome individuals revealed an approximate 10 percent reduction in cancer mortality in contrast to a control population. No doubt, further information will be forthcoming from the study of the DSCR.

The Origin of the Extra 21st Chromosome in Down Syndrome

Most frequently, this trisomic condition occurs through nondisjunction of chromosome 21 during meiosis. Failure of paired homologs to disjoin during either anaphase I or II may lead to gametes with the *n* + 1 chromosome composition. About 75 percent of these errors leading to Down syndrome are attributed to nondisjunction during meiosis I. Subsequent fertilization with a normal gamete creates the trisomic condition.

Chromosome analysis has shown that, while the additional chromosome may be derived from either the mother or father, the ovum is the source in about 95 percent of 47,21+ trisomy cases. Before the development of techniques using polymorphic markers to distinguish paternal from maternal homologs, this conclusion was supported by the more indirect evidence derived from studies of the age of mothers giving birth to infants afflicted with Down syndrome. **Figure 8–4** shows the relationship between the incidence of Down syndrome births and maternal age, illustrating the dramatic increase as the age of the mother increases. While the frequency is about 1 in 1000 at maternal age 30, a tenfold increase to a frequency of 1 in 100 is noted at age 40. The frequency increases still further to about 1 in 30 at age 45. A very alarming statistic is that as the age of childbearing women exceeds 45, the probability of a Down syndrome birth continues to increase substantially. In spite of these statistics, substantially more than half of Down syndrome births occur to women younger than 35 years, because the overwhelming proportion of pregnancies in the general population involve women under that age.

Although the nondisjunctional event clearly increases with age, we do not know with certainty why this is so. However, one observation may be relevant. Meiosis is initiated in all the eggs of a human female when she is still a fetus, until the point where the homologs synapse and recombination has begun. Then oocyte development is arrested in meiosis I. Thus, all primary oocytes have been formed by birth. When ovulation begins at puberty, meiosis is reinitiated in one egg during each ovulatory cycle and continues into meiosis II. The process is once again arrested after ovulation and is not completed unless fertilization occurs.

The end result of this progression is that each ovum that is released has been arrested in meiosis I for about a month longer than the one released during the preceding cycle. As a consequence, women 30 or 40 years old produce ova that are significantly older and that have been arrested longer than those they ovulated 10 or 20 years previously. In spite of the logic underlying this hypothesis explaining the cause of the increased incidence of Down syndrome as women age, it remains difficult to prove directly.

These statistics obviously pose a serious problem for the woman who becomes pregnant late in her reproductive years. Genetic counseling early in such pregnancies is highly recommended. Counseling informs prospective parents about the probability that their child will be affected and educates them about Down syndrome. Although some individuals with Down syndrome must be institutionalized, others benefit greatly from special education programs and may be cared for at home. (Down syndrome children in general are noted for their affectionate, loving nature.) A genetic counselor may also recommend a prenatal diagnostic technique in which fetal cells are isolated and cultured.

In **amniocentesis** and **chorionic villus sampling (CVS)**, the two most familiar approaches, fetal cells are obtained from the amniotic fluid or the chorion of the placenta, respectively. In a newer approach, fetal cells and DNA are derived directly from the maternal circulation, a technique referred to as **noninvasive prenatal genetic diagnosis (NIPGD)**. Requiring only a 10-mL maternal blood sample, this procedure will become increasingly more common because it poses no risk to the fetus. After fetal cells are obtained and cultured, the karyotype can be determined by cytogenetic analysis. If the fetus is diagnosed as being affected, a therapeutic abortion is one option currently available to parents. Obviously, this is a difficult decision involving a number of religious and ethical issues.

Since Down syndrome is caused by a random error—nondisjunction of chromosome 21 during maternal or paternal meiosis—the occurrence of the disorder is *not* expected to be inherited. Nevertheless, Down syndrome occasionally runs in families. These instances, referred to as *familial Down syndrome*, involve a translocation of chromosome 21, another type of chromosomal aberration, which we will discuss later in the chapter.

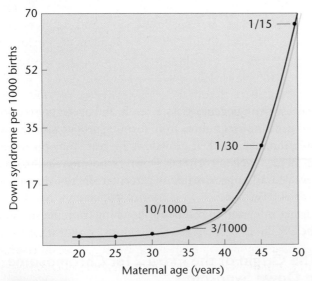

FIGURE 8–4 Incidence of Down syndrome births related to maternal age.

Human Aneuploidy

Besides Down syndrome, only two human trisomies, and no monosomies, survive to term: **Patau** and **Edwards syndromes** (47,13+ and 47,18+, respectively). Even so, these individuals manifest severe malformations and early lethality. **Figure 8–5** illustrates the abnormal karyotype and the many defects characterizing Patau infants.

The above observation leads us to ask whether many other aneuploid conditions arise but that the affected fetuses do not survive to term. That this is the case has been confirmed by karyotypic analysis of spontaneously aborted fetuses. These studies reveal two striking statistics: (1) Approximately 20 percent of all conceptions terminate in spontaneous abortion (some estimates are considerably higher); and (2) about 30 percent of all spontaneously aborted fetuses demonstrate some form of chromosomal imbalance. This suggests that at least 6 percent (0.20×0.30) of conceptions contain an abnormal chromosome complement. A large percentage of fetuses demonstrating chromosomal abnormalities are aneuploids.

An extensive review of this subject by David H. Carr has revealed that a significant percentage of aborted fetuses are trisomic for one of the chromosome groups. Trisomies for every human chromosome have been recovered. Interestingly, the monosomy with the highest incidence among abortuses is the 45,X condition, which produces an infant with Turner syndrome, if the fetus survives to term. Autosomal monosomies are seldom found, however, even though nondisjunction should produce $n - 1$ gametes with a frequency equal to $n + 1$ gametes. This finding suggests that gametes lacking a single chromosome are functionally impaired to a serious degree or that the embryo dies so early in its development that recovery occurs infrequently. We discussed the potential causes of monosomic lethality earlier in this chapter. Carr's study also found various forms of polyploidy and other miscellaneous chromosomal anomalies.

These observations support the hypothesis that normal embryonic development requires a precise diploid complement of chromosomes to maintain the delicate equilibrium in the expression of genetic information. The prenatal mortality of most aneuploids provides a barrier against the introduction of these genetic anomalies into the human population.

Mental retardation	Microcephaly
Growth failure	Cleft lip and palate
Low-set, deformed ears	Polydactyly
Deafness	Deformed finger nails
Atrial septal defect	Kidney cysts
Ventricular septal defect	Double ureter
Abnormal polymorphonuclear granulocytes	Umbilical hernia
	Developmental uterine abnormalities
	Cryptorchidism

FIGURE 8–5 The karyotype and phenotypic description of an infant with Patau syndrome, where three members of the D-group chromosome 13 are present, creating the 47,13+ condition.

8.3 Polyploidy, in Which More Than Two Haploid Sets of Chromosomes Are Present, Is Prevalent in Plants

The term *polyploidy* describes instances in which more than two multiples of the haploid chromosome set are found. The naming of polyploids is based on the number of sets of chromosomes found: A triploid has $3n$ chromosomes; a tetraploid has $4n$; a pentaploid, $5n$; and so forth (Table 8.1). Several general statements can be made about polyploidy. This condition is relatively infrequent in many animal species but is well known in lizards, amphibians, and fish, and is much more common in plant species. Usually, odd numbers of chromosome sets are not reliably maintained from generation to generation because a polyploid organism with an uneven number of homologs often does not produce genetically balanced gametes. For this reason, triploids, pentaploids, and so on, are not usually found in plant species that depend solely on sexual reproduction for propagation.

Polyploidy originates in two ways: (1) the addition of one or more extra sets of chromosomes, identical to the normal haploid complement of the same species, resulting in **autopolyploidy**; or (2) the combination of chromosome sets from different species occurring as a consequence of hybridization, resulting in **allopolyploidy** (from the Greek

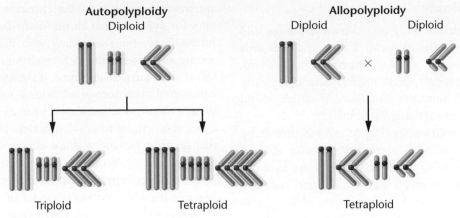

FIGURE 8–6 Contrasting chromosome origins of an autopolyploid versus an allopolyploid karyotype.

word *allo*, meaning "other" or "different"). The distinction between auto- and allopolyploidy is based on the genetic origin of the extra chromosome sets, as shown in **Figure 8–6**.

In our discussion of polyploidy, we use the following symbols to clarify the origin of additional chromosome sets. For example, if *A* represents the haploid set of chromosomes of any organism, then

$$A = a_1 + a_2 + a_3 + a_4 + \cdots + a_n$$

where a_1, a_2, and so on, are individual chromosomes and *n* is the haploid number. A normal diploid organism is represented simply as *AA*.

Autopolyploidy

In autopolyploidy, each additional set of chromosomes is identical to the parent species. Therefore, triploids are represented as *AAA*, tetraploids are *AAAA*, and so forth.

Autotriploids arise in several ways. A failure of all chromosomes to segregate during meiotic divisions can produce a diploid gamete. If such a gamete is fertilized by a haploid gamete, a zygote with three sets of chromosomes is produced. Or, rarely, two sperm may fertilize an ovum, resulting in a triploid zygote. Triploids are also produced under experimental conditions by crossing diploids with tetraploids. Diploid organisms produce gametes with *n* chromosomes, while tetraploids produce 2*n* gametes. Upon fertilization, the desired triploid is produced.

Because they have an even number of chromosomes, **autotetraploids** (4*n*) are theoretically more likely to be found in nature than are autotriploids. Unlike triploids, which often produce genetically unbalanced gametes with odd numbers of

chromosomes, tetraploids are more likely to produce balanced gametes when involved in sexual reproduction.

How polyploidy arises naturally is of great interest to geneticists. In theory, if chromosomes have replicated, but the parent cell never divides and instead reenters interphase, the chromosome number will be doubled. That this very likely occurs is supported by the observation that tetraploid cells can be produced experimentally from diploid cells. This process is accomplished by applying cold or heat shock to meiotic cells or by applying colchicine to somatic cells undergoing mitosis. **Colchicine**, an alkaloid derived from the autumn crocus, interferes with spindle formation, and thus replicated chromosomes cannot separate at anaphase and do not migrate to the poles. When colchicine is removed, the cell can reenter interphase. When the paired sister chromatids separate and uncoil, the nucleus contains twice the diploid number of chromosomes and is therefore 4*n*. This process is shown in **Figure 8–7**.

In general, autopolyploids are larger than their diploid relatives. This increase seems to be due to larger cell size

FIGURE 8–7 The potential involvement of colchicine in doubling the chromosome number. Two pairs of homologous chromosomes are shown. While each chromosome had replicated its DNA earlier during interphase, the chromosomes do not appear as double structures until late prophase. When anaphase fails to occur normally, the chromosome number doubles if the cell reenters interphase.

rather than greater cell number. Although autopolyploids do not contain new or unique information compared with their diploid relatives, the flower and fruit of plants are often increased in size, making such varieties of greater horticultural or commercial value. Economically important triploid plants include several potato species of the genus *Solanum*, Winesap apples, commercial bananas, seedless watermelons, and the cultivated tiger lily *Lilium tigrinum*. These plants are propagated asexually. Diploid bananas contain hard seeds, but the commercial triploid "seedless" variety has edible seeds. Tetraploid alfalfa, coffee, peanuts, and McIntosh apples are also of economic value because they are either larger or grow more vigorously than do their diploid or triploid counterparts. Many of the most popular varieties of hosta plant are tetraploid. In each case, leaves are thicker and larger, the foliage is more vivid, and the plant grows more vigorously. The commercial strawberry is an octoploid.

We have long been curious about how cells with increased ploidy values, where no new genes are present, express different phenotypes from their diploid counterparts. Our current ability to examine gene expression using modern biotechnology has provided some interesting insights. For example, Gerald Fink and his colleagues have been able to create strains of the yeast *Saccharomyces cerevisiae* with one, two, three, or four copies of the genome. Thus, each strain contains identical genes (they are said to be isogenic) but different ploidy values. These scientists then examined the expression levels of all genes during the entire cell cycle of the organism. Using the rather stringent standards of a tenfold increase or decrease of gene expression, Fink and coworkers proceeded to identify ten cases where, as ploidy increased, gene expression was increased at least tenfold and seven cases where it was reduced by a similar level.

One of these genes provides insights into how polyploid cells become larger than their haploid or diploid counterparts. In polyploid yeast, two **G1 cyclins**, Cln1, and Pcl1, are repressed when ploidy increases, while the size of the yeast cells increases. This is explained by the observation that G1 cyclins facilitate the cell's movement through G1, which is delayed when expression of these genes is repressed. The polyploid cell stays in the G1 phase longer and, on average, grows to a larger size before it moves beyond the G1 stage of the cell cycle. Yeast cells also show different morphology as ploidy increases. Several of the other genes, repressed as ploidy increases, have been linked to cytoskeletal dynamics that account for the morphological changes.

Allopolyploidy

Polyploidy can also result from hybridizing two closely related species. If a haploid ovum from a species with chromosome sets AA is fertilized by sperm from a species with sets BB, the resulting hybrid is AB, where $A = a_1, a_2, a_3, \ldots a_n$

and $B = b_1, b_2, b_3, \ldots b_n$. The hybrid plant may be sterile because of its inability to produce viable gametes. Most often, this occurs when some or all of the a and b chromosomes are not homologous and therefore cannot synapse in meiosis. As a result, unbalanced genetic conditions result. If, however, the new AB genetic combination undergoes a natural or an induced chromosomal doubling, two copies of all a chromosomes and two copies of all b chromosomes will be present, and they will pair during meiosis. As a result, a fertile $AABB$ tetraploid is produced. These events are shown in **Figure 8–8**. Since this polyploid contains the equivalent of four haploid genomes derived from separate species, such an organism is called an **allotetraploid**. When both original species are known, an equivalent term, **amphidiploid**, is preferred in describing the allotetraploid.

Amphidiploid plants are often found in nature. Their reproductive success is based on their potential for forming balanced gametes. Since two homologs of each specific chromosome are present, meiosis occurs normally (Figure 8–8) and fertilization successfully propagates the plant sexually.

FIGURE 8–8 The origin and propagation of an amphidiploid. Species 1 contains genome A consisting of three distinct chromosomes, a_1, a_2, and a_3. Species 2 contains genome B consisting of two distinct chromosomes, b_1 and b_2. Following fertilization between members of the two species and chromosome doubling, a fertile amphidiploid containing two complete diploid genomes ($AABB$) is formed.

FIGURE 8–9 The pods of the amphidiploid form of *Gossypium,* the cultivated American cotton plant.

This discussion assumes the simplest situation, where none of the chromosomes in set *A* are homologous to those in set *B.* In amphidiploids, formed from closely related species, some homology between *a* and *b* chromosomes is likely. Allopolyploids are rare in most animals because mating behavior is most often species-specific, and thus the initial step in hybridization is unlikely to occur.

A classical example of amphidiploidy in plants is the cultivated species of American cotton, *Gossypium* (**Figure 8–9**). This species has 26 pairs of chromosomes: 13 are large and 13 are much smaller. When it was discovered that Old World cotton had only 13 pairs of large chromosomes, allopolyploidy was suspected. After an examination of wild American cotton revealed 13 pairs of small chromosomes, this speculation was strengthened. J. O. Beasley reconstructed the origin of cultivated cotton experimentally by crossing the Old World strain with the wild American strain and then treating the hybrid with colchicine to double the chromosome number. The result of these treatments was a fertile amphidiploid variety of cotton. It contained 26 pairs of chromosomes as well as characteristics similar to the cultivated variety.

Amphidiploids often exhibit traits of both parental species. An interesting example, but one with no practical economic importance, is that of the hybrid formed between the radish *Raphanus sativus* and the cabbage *Brassica oleracea.* Both species have a haploid number *n* = 9. The initial hybrid consists of nine *Raphanus* and nine *Brassica* chromosomes (9R + 9B). Although hybrids are almost always sterile, some fertile amphidiploids (18R + 18B) have been produced. Unfortunately, the root of this plant is more like the cabbage and its shoot is more like the radish; had the converse occurred, the hybrid might have been of economic importance.

A much more successful commercial hybridization uses the grasses wheat and rye. Wheat (genus *Triticum*) has a basic haploid genome of seven chromosomes. In addition to normal diploids (2n = 14), cultivated autopolyploids exist, including tetraploid (4n = 28) and hexaploid (6n = 42) species. Rye (genus *Secale*) also has a genome consisting of seven chromosomes. The only cultivated species is the diploid plant (2n = 14).

Using the technique outlined in Figure 8–8, geneticists have produced various hybrids. When tetraploid wheat is crossed with diploid rye and the F_1 plants are treated with colchicine, a hexaploid variety (6n = 42) is obtained; the hybrid, designated *Triticale,* represents a new genus. Fertile hybrid varieties derived from various wheat and rye species can be crossed or backcrossed. These crosses have created many variations of the genus *Triticale.* The hybrid plants demonstrate characteristics of both wheat and rye. For example, certain hybrids combine the high-protein content of wheat with rye's high content of the amino acid lysine. (The lysine content is low in wheat and thus is a limiting nutritional factor.) Wheat is considered to be a high-yielding grain, whereas rye is noted for its versatility of growth in unfavorable environments. *Triticale* species, which combine both traits, have the potential of significantly increasing grain production. Programs designed to improve crops through hybridization have long been underway in several developing countries.

Endopolyploidy

Endopolyploidy is the condition in which only certain cells in an otherwise diploid organism are polyploid. In such cells, the set of chromosomes replicates repeatedly without nuclear division. Numerous examples of naturally occurring endopolyploidy have been observed. For example, vertebrate liver cell nuclei, including human ones, often contain 4n, 8n, or 16n chromosome sets. The stem and parenchymal tissue of apical regions of flowering plants are also often endopolyploid. Cells lining the gut of mosquito larvae attain a 16n ploidy, but during the pupal stages, such cells undergo very quick reduction divisions, giving rise to smaller diploid cells. In the water strider *Gerris,* wide variations in chromosome numbers are found in different tissues, with as many as 1024 to 2048 copies of each chromosome in the salivary gland cells. Since the diploid number in this organism is 22, the nuclei of these cells may contain more than 40,000 chromosomes.

Although the role of endopolyploidy is not clear, the proliferation of chromosome copies often occurs in cells where high levels of certain gene products are required. In fact, it is well established that certain genes whose product is in high demand in *every* cell exist naturally in multiple copies in the genome. Ribosomal and transfer RNA genes are examples of multiple-copy genes. In certain cells of organisms, where even this condition may not allow for a sufficient amount of a particular gene product, it may be necessary to replicate the entire genome, allowing an even greater rate of expression of that gene.

NOW SOLVE THIS

8–2 When two plants belonging to the same genus but different species are crossed, the F$_1$ hybrid is more viable and has more ornate flowers. Unfortunately, this hybrid is sterile and can only be propagated by vegetative cuttings. Explain the sterility of the hybrid and what would have to occur for the sterility of this hybrid to be reversed.

■ **HINT:** *This problem involves an understanding of allopolyploid plants. The key to its solution is to focus on the origin and composition of the chromosomes in the F$_1$ and how they might be manipulated.*

8.4 Variation Occurs in the Composition and Arrangement of Chromosomes

The second general class of chromosome aberrations includes changes that delete, add, or rearrange substantial portions of one or more chromosomes. Included in this broad category are deletions and duplications of genes or part of a chromosome and rearrangements of genetic material in which a chromosome segment is inverted, exchanged with a segment of a nonhomologous chromosome, or merely transferred to another chromosome. Exchanges and transfers are called *translocations*, in which the locations of genes are altered within the genome. These types of chromosome alterations are illustrated in **Figure 8–10**.

In most instances, these structural changes are due to one or more breaks along the axis of a chromosome, followed by either the loss or rearrangement of genetic material. Chromosomes can break spontaneously, but the rate of breakage may increase in cells exposed to chemicals or radiation. Although the actual ends of chromosomes, known as telomeres, do not readily fuse with newly created ends of "broken" chromosomes or with other telomeres, the ends produced at points of breakage are "sticky" and can rejoin other broken ends. If breakage and rejoining do not reestablish the original relationship and if the alteration occurs in germ cells, the gametes will contain the structural rearrangement, which is heritable.

If the aberration is found in one homolog, but not the other, the individual is said to be *heterozygous for the aberration*. In such cases, unusual but characteristic pairing

FIGURE 8–10 An overview of the five different types of gain, loss, or rearrangement of chromosome segments.

configurations are formed during meiotic synapsis. These patterns are useful in identifying the type of change that has occurred. If no loss or gain of genetic material occurs, individuals bearing the aberration "heterozygously" are likely to be unaffected phenotypically. However, the unusual pairing arrangements often lead to gametes that are duplicated or deficient for some chromosomal regions. When this occurs, the offspring of "carriers" of certain aberrations have an increased probability of demonstrating phenotypic changes.

8.5 A Deletion Is a Missing Region of a Chromosome

When a chromosome breaks in one or more places and a portion of it is lost, the missing piece is called a **deletion** (or a **deficiency**). The deletion can occur either near one end or within the interior of the chromosome. These are **terminal** and **intercalary deletions**, respectively [**Figure 8–11(a)** and **8–11(b)**]. The portion of the chromosome that retains the centromere region is usually maintained when the cell divides, whereas the segment without the centromere is eventually

(a) Origin of terminal deletion

A B C D E F → B C D E F
Break
A + (Lost)

(b) Origin of intercalary deletion

Break D C Break
A B E F
→ D C
A B E F

A B E F
Deleted chromosome
+ D C
(Lost)

(c) Formation of deletion loop

Area missing in deleted chromosome
A B [C D] E F
Normal chromosome
A B E F
Homolog with deleted region C and D

Synapsis →

C D
A B E F
A B E F
Formation of deletion loop

FIGURE 8–11 Origins of (a) a terminal and (b) an intercalary deletion. In (c), pairing occurs between a normal chromosome and one with an intercalary deletion by looping out the undeleted portion to form a deletion (or compensation) loop.

lost in progeny cells following mitosis or meiosis. For synapsis to occur between a chromosome with a large intercalary deletion and a normal homolog, the unpaired region of the normal homolog must "buckle out" into a **deletion**, or **compensation, loop** [**Figure 8–11(c)**].

If only a small part of a chromosome is deleted, the organism might survive. However, a deletion of a portion of a chromosome need not be very great before the effects become severe. We see an example of these effects in the following discussion of the cri du chat syndrome in humans. If even more genetic information is lost as a result of a deletion, the aberration is often lethal, in which case the chromosome mutation never becomes available for study.

Cri du Chat Syndrome in Humans

In humans, the **cri du chat syndrome** results from the deletion of a small terminal portion of chromosome 5. It might be considered a case of *partial monosomy,* but since the region that is missing is so small, it is better referred to as a **segmental deletion**. This syndrome was first reported by Jérôme LeJeune in 1963, when he described the clinical symptoms, including an eerie cry similar to the meowing of a cat, after which the syndrome is named. This syndrome is associated with the loss of a small, variable part of the short arm of chromosome 5 (**Figure 8–12**). Thus, the genetic constitution may be designated as 46,5p–, meaning that the individual has all 46 chromosomes but that some or all of the p arm (the petite, or short, arm) of one member of the chromosome 5 pair is missing.

Infants with this syndrome may exhibit anatomic malformations, including gastrointestinal and cardiac complications, and they are often mentally retarded. Abnormal development of the glottis and larynx (leading to the characteristic cry) is typical of this syndrome.

Since 1963, hundreds of cases of cri du chat syndrome have been reported worldwide. An incidence of 1 in 25,000–50,000 live births has been estimated. Most often, the condition is not inherited but instead results from the sporadic loss of chromosomal material in gametes. The length of the short arm that is deleted varies somewhat; longer deletions appear to have a greater impact on the physical, psychomotor, and mental skill levels of those children who survive. Although the effects of the syndrome are severe, most individuals achieve motor and language skills and may be home-cared. In 2004, it was reported that the portion of the chromosome that is missing contains the *TERT* gene, which encodes *telomerase reverse transcriptase,* an enzyme essential for the maintenance of telomeres during DNA replication (see Chapter 11). Whether the absence of this gene on one homolog is related to the multiple phenotypes of cri du chat infants is still unknown.

FIGURE 8–12 A representative karyotype and a photograph of a child exhibiting cri du chat syndrome (46,5p–). In the karyotype, the arrow identifies the absence of a small piece of the short arm of one member of the chromosome 5 homologs.

8.6 A Duplication Is a Repeated Segment of a Chromosome

When any part of the genetic material—a single locus or a large piece of a chromosome—is present more than once in the genome, it is called a **duplication**. As in deletions, pairing in heterozygotes can produce a compensation loop. Duplications may arise as the result of unequal crossing over between synapsed chromosomes during meiosis (**Figure 8–13**) or through a replication error prior to meiosis. In the former case, both a duplication and a deletion are produced.

We consider three interesting aspects of duplications. First, they may result in gene redundancy. Second, as with deletions, duplications may produce phenotypic variation. Third, according to one convincing theory, duplications have also been an important source of genetic variability during evolution.

Gene Redundancy and Amplification—Ribosomal RNA Genes

Duplication of chromosomal segments has the potential to amplify the number of copies of individual genes. This has clearly been the case with the gene encoding ribosomal RNA, which is needed in abundance in the ribosomes of all cells to support protein synthesis. We might hypothesize that a single copy of the gene encoding rRNA is inadequate in many cells that demonstrate intense metabolic activity. Studies using the technique of molecular hybridization, which enables us to determine the percentage of the genome that codes for specific RNA sequences, show that our hypothesis is correct. Indeed, multiple copies of genes code for rRNA. Such DNA is called **rDNA**, and the general phenomenon is referred to as **gene redundancy**. For example, in the common intestinal bacterium *Escherichia coli* (*E. coli*), about 0.7 percent of the haploid genome consists of rDNA—the equivalent of seven copies of the gene. In *Drosophila melanogaster*, 0.3 percent of the haploid genome, equivalent to 130 gene copies, consists of rDNA. Although the presence of multiple copies of the same gene is not restricted to those coding for rRNA, we will focus on those genes in this section.

Interestingly, in some cells, particularly oocytes, even the normal redundancy of rDNA is insufficient to provide adequate amounts of rRNA needed to construct ribosomes. Oocytes store abundant nutrients, including huge quantities of ribosomes, for use by the embryo during early development. More ribosomes are included in oocytes than in any other cell type. By considering how the amphibian *Xenopus laevis* acquires this abundance of ribosomes, we shall see a second way in which the amount of rRNA is increased. This phenomenon is called **gene amplification**.

The genes that code for rRNA are located in an area of the chromosome known as the **nucleolar organizer region (NOR)**. The NOR is intimately associated with the nucleolus, which is a processing center for ribosome production. Molecular hybridization analysis has shown that each NOR in the frog *Xenopus* contains the equivalent of 400 redundant gene copies coding for rRNA. Even this number of genes is apparently inadequate to synthesize the vast

FIGURE 8–13 The origin of duplicated and deficient regions of chromosomes as a result of unequal crossing over. The tetrad on the left is mispaired during synapsis. A single crossover between chromatids 2 and 3 results in the deficient (chromosome 2) and duplicated (chromosome 3) chromosomal regions shown on the right. The two chromosomes uninvolved in the crossover event remain normal in gene sequence and content.

amount of ribosomes that must accumulate in the amphibian oocyte to support development following fertilization.

To further amplify the number of rRNA genes, the rDNA is selectively replicated, and each new set of genes is released from its template. Because each new copy is equivalent to one NOR, multiple small nucleoli are formed in the oocyte. As many as 1500 of these "micronucleoli" have been observed in a single *Xenopus* oocyte. If we multiply the number of micronucleoli (1500) by the number of gene copies in each NOR (400), we see that amplification in *Xenopus* oocytes can result in over half a million gene copies! If each copy is transcribed only 20 times during the maturation of the oocyte, in theory, sufficient copies of rRNA are produced to result in well over 12 million ribosomes.

The *Bar* Mutation in *Drosophila*

Duplications can cause phenotypic variation that might at first appear to be caused by a simple gene mutation. The *Bar*-eye phenotype in *Drosophila* (**Figure 8–14**) is a classic example. Instead of the normal oval-eye shape, *Bar*-eyed flies have narrow, slitlike eyes. This phenotype is inherited in the same way as a dominant X-linked mutation.

In the early 1920s, Alfred H. Sturtevant and Thomas H. Morgan discovered and investigated this "mutation." Normal wild-type females (B^+/B^+) have about 800 facets in each eye. Heterozygous females (B/B^+) have about 350 facets, while homozygous females (B/B) average only about 70 facets. Females were occasionally recovered with even fewer facets and were designated as *double Bar* (B^D/B^+).

About 10 years later, Calvin Bridges and Herman J. Muller compared the polytene X chromosome banding pattern of the *Bar* fly with that of the wild-type fly. These chromosomes contain specific banding patterns that have been well categorized into regions. Their studies revealed that one copy of the region designated as 16A is present on both X chromosomes of wild-type flies but that this region was duplicated in *Bar* flies and triplicated in *double Bar* flies. These observations provided evidence that the *Bar* phenotype is not the result of a simple chemical change in the gene but is instead a duplication.

The Role of Gene Duplication in Evolution

During the study of evolution, it is intriguing to speculate on the possible mechanisms of genetic variation. The origin of unique gene products present in more recently evolved organisms but absent in ancestral forms is a topic of particular interest. In other words, how do "new" genes arise? As we will see below, the process of gene duplication is hypothesized to be the major source of new genes, as proposed in 1970 by Susumu Ohno in his provocative monograph, *Evolution by Gene Duplication*. Ohno's thesis is based on the supposition that the products of many genes, present as only a single copy in the genome, are indispensable to the survival of members of any species during evolution. Therefore, unique genes are not free to accumulate mutations sufficient to alter their primary function and give rise to new genes.

However, if an essential gene is duplicated in the germ line, major mutational changes in this extra copy will be tolerated in future generations because the original gene provides the genetic information for its essential function. The duplicated copy will be free to acquire many mutational changes over extended periods of time. Over short intervals, the new genetic information may be of no practical advantage. However, over long evolutionary periods, the duplicated gene may change sufficiently so that its product assumes a divergent role in the cell. The new function may impart an "adaptive" advantage to organisms, enhancing their fitness. Ohno has outlined a mechanism through which sustained genetic variability may have originated.

Ohno's thesis is supported by the discovery of genes that have a substantial amount of their DNA sequence in common, but whose gene products are distinct. The genes encoding the digestive enzymes *trypsin* and *chymotrypsin* are examples, as are those that encode the respiratory molecules *myoglobin* and the various forms of *hemoglobin*. We conclude that the genes arose from a common ancestral gene through duplication. During evolution, the related genes diverged sufficiently that their products became unique.

Other support includes the presence of **gene families**—groups of contiguous genes whose products perform the same, or very similar functions. Again, members of a family show DNA sequence homology sufficient to conclude that they share a common origin and arose through the process of gene duplication. One of the most interesting supporting examples is the case of the *SRGAP2* gene in primates. This gene is known to be involved in the development of the brain. Humans have at least four similar copies of

B^+/B^+

B/B^+

B/B

FIGURE 8–14 *Bar*-eye phenotypes in contrast to the wild-type eye in *Drosophila*.

the gene, while all nonhuman primates have only a single copy. Several duplication events can be traced back to 3.4 million years ago, to 2.4 million years ago, and finally to 1 million years ago, resulting in distinct forms of *SRGAP2* labeled A–D. These evolutionary periods coincide with the emergence of the human lineage in primates. The function of these genes has now been related to the regulation and formation of dendritic spines in the brain, which is believed to contribute to the evolution of expanded brain function in humans, including the development of language and social cognition.

Other examples of gene families arising from duplication during evolution include the various types of human hemoglobin polypeptide chains, as well as the immunologically important T-cell receptors and antigens encoded by the major histocompatibility complex.

Duplications at the Molecular Level: Copy Number Variants (CNVs)

As we entered the era of genomics and became capable of sequencing entire genomes (see Chapters 20, 21, and 22), we quickly realized that duplications of *portions of genes*, most often involving thousands of base pairs, occur on a regular basis. When individuals in the same species are compared, the number of copies of any given duplicated sequence is found to vary—sometimes there are larger and sometimes smaller numbers of copies. These variations, because they represent *quantitative differences in the number of large DNA sequences,* are termed **copy number variants (CNVs)** and are found in both coding and noncoding regions of the genome.

CNVs are of major interest in genetics because they are now believed to play crucial roles in the expression of many of our individual traits. In 2004, two research groups independently described the presence of CNVs in the genomes of healthy individuals with no known genetic disorders. CNVs were initially defined as regions of DNA at least 1 kb in length (1000 base pairs) that display at least 90 percent sequence identity. This initial study revealed 50 CNV loci, and in 2005, 300 additional sites were identified. In 2010 the number of CNV sites, when scaled down to sequences of DNA of at least 500 base pairs, was estimated at over 10,000 regions, representing a substantial proportion of the total genetic variability within humans. Future studies will no doubt uncover many more unique CNVs in the human genome.

Current studies have focused on finding associations with human diseases. CNVs appear to have both positive and negative associations with many diseases in which the genetic basis is not yet fully understood. For example, an association has been reported between CNVs and autism, the well-known neurodevelopmental disorder that impairs communication, behavior, and social interaction. Interestingly, a mutant CNV site has been found to appear *de novo* (anew) in 10 percent of so-called sporadic cases of autism, where unaffected parents lack the CNV mutation. This is in contrast to only 2 percent of affected individuals where the disease appears to be familial (that is, to run in the family).

Often, entire gene sequences are duplicated and impact individuals. For example, a higher than average copy number of the gene *CCL3L1* imparts an HIV-suppressive effect during viral infection, diminishing the progression to AIDS. Another finding has associated specific mutant CNV sites with certain subset populations of individuals with lung cancer—the greater number of copies of the *EGFR* (*Epidermal Growth Factor Receptor*) gene, the more responsive are patients with non–small-cell lung cancer to treatment. Finally, the greater the reduction in the copy number of the gene designated *DEFB*, the greater the risk of developing Crohn's disease, a condition affecting the colon. Relevant to this chapter, these findings reveal that duplications and deletions are no longer restricted to textbook examples of these chromosomal mutations. We will return to this interesting topic later in the text (see Chapter 21), when genomics is discussed in detail.

8.7   Inversions Rearrange the Linear Gene Sequence

The **inversion**, another class of structural variation, is a type of chromosomal aberration in which a segment of a chromosome is turned around 180 degrees within a chromosome. An inversion does not involve a loss of genetic information but simply rearranges the linear gene sequence. An inversion requires breaks at two points along the length of the chromosome and subsequent reinsertion of the inverted segment. **Figure 8–15** illustrates how an inversion might arise. By forming a chromosomal loop prior to breakage, the newly created "sticky ends" are brought close together and rejoined.

The inverted segment may be short or quite long and may or may not include the centromere. If the centromere is not part of the rearranged chromosome segment, it is a **paracentric inversion**. If the centromere is part of the inverted segment, it is described as a **pericentric inversion**, which is the type shown in Figure 8–15.

Although inversions appear to have a minimal impact on the individuals bearing them, their consequences are of great interest to geneticists. Organisms that are heterozygous for inversions may produce aberrant gametes that have a major impact on their offspring.

FIGURE 8–15 One possible origin of a pericentric inversion.

Consequences of Inversions during Gamete Formation

If only one member of a homologous pair of chromosomes has an inverted segment, normal linear synapsis during meiosis is not possible. Organisms with one inverted chromosome and one noninverted homolog are called **inversion heterozygotes.** Two such chromosomes in meiosis can be paired only if they form an **inversion loop (Figure 8–16).**

If crossing over does not occur within the inverted segment of the inversion loop, the homologs will segregate, which results in two normal and two inverted chromatids that are distributed into gametes. However, if crossing over does occur within the inversion loop, abnormal chromatids are produced. The effect of a single crossover (SCO) event within a paracentric inversion is diagrammed in **Figure 8–16(a).**

In any meiotic tetrad, a single crossover between nonsister chromatids produces two parental chromatids and two recombinant chromatids. When the crossover occurs within a paracentric inversion, however, one recombinant **dicentric chromatid** (two centromeres) and one recombinant **acentric chromatid** (lacking a centromere) are produced. Both contain duplications and deletions of chromosome segments as well. During anaphase, an acentric chromatid moves randomly to one pole or the other or may be lost, while a dicentric chromatid is pulled in two directions. This polarized movement produces *dicentric bridges* that are cytologically recognizable. A dicentric chromatid usually breaks at some point so that part of the chromatid goes into one gamete and part into another gamete during the reduction divisions. Therefore, gametes containing either recombinant chromatid

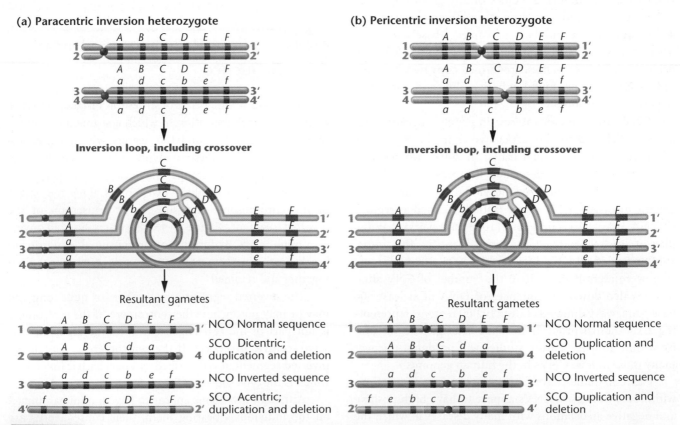

FIGURE 8–16 (a) The effects of a single crossover (SCO) within an inversion loop in a paracentric inversion heterozygote, where two altered chromosomes are produced, one acentric and one dicentric. Both chromosomes also contain duplicated and deficient regions. (b) The effects of a crossover in a pericentric inversion heterozygote, where two altered chromosomes are produced, both with duplicated and deficient regions.

are deficient in genetic material. When such a gamete participates in fertilization, the zygote most often develops abnormally, if at all.

A similar chromosomal imbalance is produced as a result of a crossover event between a chromatid bearing a pericentric inversion and its noninverted homolog, as shown in **Figure 8–16(b)**. The recombinant chromatids that are directly involved in the exchange have duplications and deletions. In plants, gametes receiving such aberrant chromatids fail to develop normally, leading to aborted pollen or ovules. Thus, lethality occurs prior to fertilization, and inviable seeds result. In animals, the gametes have developed prior to the meiotic error, so fertilization is more likely to occur in spite of the chromosome error. However, the end result is the production of inviable embryos following fertilization. In both cases, viability is reduced.

Because offspring bearing crossover gametes are inviable and not recovered, it *appears* as if the inversion suppresses crossing over. Actually, in inversion heterozygotes, the inversion has the effect of *suppressing the recovery of crossover products* when chromosome exchange occurs within the inverted region. If crossing over always occurred within a paracentric or pericentric inversion, 50 percent of the gametes would be ineffective. The viability of the resulting zygotes is therefore greatly diminished. Furthermore, up to one-half of the viable gametes have the inverted chromosome, and the inversion will be perpetuated within the species. The cycle will be repeated continuously during meiosis in future generations.

Evolutionary Advantages of Inversions

Because recovery of crossover products is suppressed in inversion heterozygotes, groups of specific alleles at adjacent loci within inversions may be preserved from generation to generation. If the alleles of the involved genes confer a survival advantage on organisms maintaining them, the inversion is beneficial to the evolutionary survival of the species. For example, if a set of alleles *ABcDef* is more adaptive than sets *AbCdeF* or *abcdEF*, effective gametes will contain this favorable set of genes, undisrupted by crossing over.

In laboratory studies, the same principle is applied using **balancer chromosomes**, which contain inversions. When an organism is heterozygous for a balancer chromosome, desired sequences of alleles are preserved during experimental work.

8.8 Translocations Alter the Location of Chromosomal Segments in the Genome

Translocation, as the name implies, is the movement of a chromosomal segment to a new location in the genome. Reciprocal translocation, for example, involves the exchange of segments between two nonhomologous chromosomes. The least complex way for this event to occur is for two nonhomologous chromosome arms to come close to each other so that an exchange is facilitated. **Figure 8–17(a)** shows a simple reciprocal translocation in which only two breaks are required. If the exchange includes internal chromosome segments, four breaks are required, two on each chromosome.

The genetic consequences of reciprocal translocations are, in several instances, similar to those of inversions. For example, genetic information is not lost or gained. Rather, there is only a rearrangement of genetic material. The presence of a translocation does not, therefore, directly alter the viability of individuals bearing it.

Homologs that are heterozygous for a reciprocal translocation undergo unorthodox synapsis during meiosis. As shown in **Figure 8–17(b)**, pairing results in a cruciform, or crosslike, configuration. As with inversions, some of the gametes produced are genetically unbalanced as a result of an unusual alignment during meiosis. In the case of translocations, however, aberrant gametes are not necessarily the result of crossing over. To see how unbalanced gametes are produced, focus on the homologous centromeres in Figure 8–17(b) and 8–17(c). According to the principle of independent assortment, the chromosome containing centromere 1 migrates randomly toward one pole of the spindle during the first meiotic anaphase; it travels along with *either* the chromosome having centromere 3 *or* the chromosome having centromere 4. The chromosome with centromere 2 moves to the other pole, along with the chromosome containing *either* centromere 3 *or* centromere 4. This results in four potential meiotic products. The 1,4 combination contains chromosomes that are not involved in the translocation and are normal. The 2,3 combination, however, contains the translocated chromosomes, but these contain a complete complement of genetic information and are balanced. When this result is achieved [the top configuration in Figure 8–17(c)], the segregation pattern at the first meiotic division is referred to as **alternate segregation**. A second pattern [the bottom configuration in **Figure 8–17(c)**] produces the other two potential products, the 1,3 and 2,4 combinations, which contain chromosomes displaying duplicated and deleted (deficient) segments. This pattern is called **adjacent**

NOW SOLVE THIS

8–3 What is the effect of a rare double crossover (a) within a chromosome segment that is heterozygous for a pericentric inversion; and (b) within a segment that is heterozygous for a paracentric inversion?

■ **HINT:** *This problem involves an understanding of how homologs synapse in the presence of a heterozygous inversion, as well as the distinction between pericentric and paracentric inversions. The key to its solution is to draw out the tetrad and follow the chromatids undergoing a double crossover.*

(a) Possible origin of a reciprocal translocation between two nonhomologous chromosomes

(b) Synapsis of translocation heterozygote

(c) Two possible segregation patterns leading to gamete formation

Normal   Balanced translocation

Meiosis I and II   Meiosis I and II

Duplicated and deficient   Duplicated and deficient

FIGURE 8–17 (a) Possible origin of a reciprocal translocation. (b) Synaptic configuration formed during meiosis in an individual that is heterozygous for the translocation. (c) Two possible segregation patterns, one of which leads to a normal and a balanced gamete (called alternate segregation) and one that leads to gametes containing duplications and deficiencies (called adjacent segregation-1).

segregation-1. Note that a third type of arrangement, where homologous centromeres segregate to the same pole during meiosis (called *adjacent segregation-2*), has not been included in this figure. This type of segregation has an outcome similar to adjacent segregation-1, with meiotic products containing genetically unbalanced duplicated and deleted chromosomal material.

When genetically unbalanced gametes participate in fertilization in animals, the resultant offspring do not usually survive. Fewer than 50 percent of the progeny of parents heterozygous for a reciprocal translocation survive. This condition in a parent is called **semisterility**, and its impact on the

reproductive fitness of organisms plays a role in evolution. In humans, such an unbalanced condition results in partial monosomy or trisomy, leading to a variety of birth defects.

Translocations in Humans: Familial Down Syndrome

Research conducted since 1959 has revealed numerous translocations in members of the human population. One common type of translocation involves breaks at the extreme ends of the short arms of two nonhomologous acrocentric chromosomes. These small segments are lost, and the larger segments fuse at their centromeric region. This type of translocation produces a new, large submetacentric or metacentric chromosome, often called a **Robertsonian translocation**.

One such translocation accounts for cases in which Down syndrome is familial (inherited). Earlier in this chapter, we pointed out that most instances of Down syndrome are due to trisomy 21. This chromosome composition results from nondisjunction during meiosis in one parent. Trisomy accounts for over 95 percent of all cases of Down syndrome. In such instances, the chance of the same parents producing a second affected child is extremely low. However, in the remaining families with a Down child, the syndrome occurs with much greater frequency over several generations—it "runs in families."

Cytogenetic studies of the parents and their offspring from these unusual cases explain the cause of **familial Down syndrome**. Analysis reveals that one of the parents contains a **14/21, D/G translocation** (**Figure 8–18**). That is, one parent has the majority of the G-group chromosome 21 translocated to one end of the D-group chromosome 14. This individual is phenotypically normal, even though he or she has only 45 chromosomes and is referred to as a *balanced translocation carrier*. During meiosis in such an individual, one of the gametes contains two copies of chromosome 21—a normal chromosome and a second copy translocated to chromosome 14. When such a gamete is fertilized by a standard haploid gamete, the resulting zygote has 46 chromosomes but three copies of chromosome 21. These individuals exhibit Down syndrome. Other potential surviving offspring contain either the standard diploid genome (without a translocation) or the balanced translocation like the parent. Both cases result in normal individuals. In the fourth case, a monosomic individual is produced, which is lethal. Although not illustrated, adjacent-2 segregation is also thought to occur, but rarely. Such gametes are unbalanced, and upon fertilization, lethality occurs.

The above findings have allowed geneticists to resolve the seeming paradox of an inherited trisomic phenotype in an individual with an apparent diploid number of chromosomes. Interestingly, the "carrier," who has 45 chromosomes and exhibits a normal phenotype, does not contain the complete diploid amount of genetic material. A small

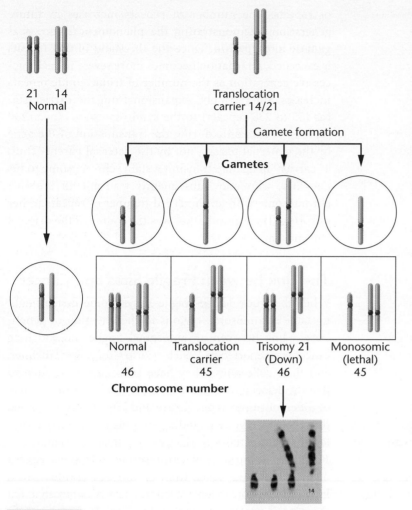

21 14
Normal

Translocation
carrier 14/21

Gamete formation

Gametes

Normal
46

Translocation
carrier
45

Trisomy 21
(Down)
46

Monosomic
(lethal)
45

Chromosome number

FIGURE 8–18 Chromosomal involvement and translocation in familial Down syndrome. The photograph shows the relevant chromosomes from a trisomy 21 offspring produced by a translocation carrier parent.

region is lost from both chromosomes 14 and 21 during the translocation event. This occurs because the ends of both chromosomes have broken off prior to their fusion. These specific regions are known to be two of many chromosomal locations housing multiple copies of the genes encoding rRNA, the major component of ribosomes. Despite the loss of up to 20 percent of these genes, the carrier is unaffected.

8.9 Fragile Sites in Human Chromosomes Are Susceptible to Breakage

We conclude this chapter with a brief discussion of the results of an intriguing discovery made around 1970 during observations of metaphase chromosomes prepared following human cell culture. In cells derived from certain individuals, a specific area along one of the chromosomes failed to stain, giving the appearance of a gap. In other individuals whose chromosomes displayed such morphology, the gaps appeared at other positions within the set of chromosomes. Such areas eventually became known as **fragile sites**, since they appeared to be susceptible to chromosome breakage when cultured in the absence of certain chemicals such as folic acid, which is normally present in the culture medium.

The cause of the fragility at these sites is unknown. However, since they represent points along the chromosome that are susceptible to breakage, these sites may indicate regions where the chromatin is not tightly coiled. Note that even though almost all studies of fragile sites have been carried out *in vitro* using mitotically dividing cells, interest in them increased when clear associations were established between several of these sites and a corresponding altered phenotype, including mental retardation and cancer.

Fragile-X Syndrome

While most fragile sites do not appear to be associated with any clinical syndrome, individuals bearing a folate-sensitive site on the X chromosome (**Figure 8–19**) exhibit the **fragile-X syndrome** (FXS), the most common form of inherited mental retardation. This syndrome affects about 1 in 4000 males and 1 in 8000 females. Since affected females usually carry only one fragile X chromosome the disorder is considered a dominant trait. Fortunately, penetrance is not complete, and the trait is fully expressed in only about 30 percent of fragile X-bearing females and 80 percent of fragile X-bearing males. In addition to mental retardation, affected males have characteristic long, narrow faces with protruding chins, enlarged ears, and increased testicular size. Female carriers also express premature ovarian insufficiency.

A gene that spans the fragile site is now known to be responsible for this syndrome. This gene, *FMR1*, is one of a growing number in which a sequence of three nucleotides is repeated many times, expanding the size of the gene. Such **trinucleotide repeats** are also characteristic of other human disorders, including Huntington disease and myotonic dystrophy. In *FMR1*, the trinucleotide sequence CGG is repeated in an untranslated area adjacent to the coding sequence of the gene (called the "upstream" region). The number of repeats varies within the human population, and a high number correlates directly with

FIGURE 8–19   A human fragile X chromosome. The "gap" region (near the bottom of the chromosome) is associated with the fragile-X syndrome.

expression of fragile-X syndrome. Normal individuals have between 6 and 54 repeats, whereas those with 55 to 230 repeats are unaffected but are considered "carriers" of the disorder. More than 230 repeats lead to expression of the syndrome. The primary impact of the increased number of repeats in FXS is the loss of expression of *FMR1*. A particularly interesting aspect of the study of FXS is the finding that the product of the *FMR1* gene, named FMRP, is an RNA-binding protein. Thus, the neurological expression of FXS is the result of disruption of the regulation of neuron-specific RNA function.

It is thought that, once the gene contains this increased number of repeats, it becomes chemically modified so that the bases within and around the repeats are methylated, which inactivates the gene. The normal product of the gene is an RNA-binding protein, FMRP, known to be expressed in the brain. Evidence is now accumulating that directly links the absence of the protein in the brain with the cognitive defects associated with the syndrome.

From a genetic standpoint, an interesting aspect of fragile-X syndrome is the instability of the CGG repeats. An individual with 6 to 54 repeats transmits a gene containing the same number of copies to his or her offspring. However, carrier individuals with 55 to 230 repeats, though not at risk to develop the syndrome, may transmit to their offspring a gene with an increased number of repeats. The number of repeats increases in future generations, demonstrating the phenomenon known as **genetic anticipation**. Once the threshold of 230 repeats is exceeded, retardation becomes more severe in each successive generation as the number of trinucleotide repeats increases. Interestingly, expansion from the carrier status (55 to 230 repeats) to the syndrome status (over 230 repeats) occurs only during the transmission of the gene by the maternal parent, not by the paternal parent. Thus, a "carrier" male may transmit a stable chromosome to his daughter, who may subsequently transmit an unstable chromosome with an increased number of repeats to her offspring. Their grandfather was the source of the original chromosome.

The Link between Fragile Sites and Cancer

While the study of the fragile-X syndrome first brought unstable chromosome regions to the attention of geneticists, a link between an autosomal fragile site and lung cancer was reported in 1996 by Carlo Croce, Kay Huebner, and their colleagues. They have subsequently postulated that the defect is associated with the formation of a variety of different tumor types. Croce and Huebner first showed that the *FHIT* gene (standing for *f*ragile *hi*stidine *t*riad), located within the well-defined fragile site designated as *FRA3B* on the p arm of chromosome 3, is often altered or missing in cells taken from tumors of individuals with lung cancer. More extensive studies have now revealed that the normal protein product of this gene is absent in cells of many other cancers, including those of the esophagus, breast, cervix, liver, kidney, pancreas, colon, and stomach. Genes such as *FHIT* that are located within fragile regions undoubtedly have an increased susceptibility to mutations and deletions.

More recently, Muller Fabbri and Kay Huebner, working with others in Croce's lab, have identified and studied another fragile site, with most interesting results. Found within the *FRA16D* site on chromosome 16 is the *WWOX* gene. Like the *FHIT* gene, it has been implicated in a range of human cancers. In particular, like *FHIT*, it has been found to be either lost or genetically silenced in the large majority of lung tumors, as well as in cancer tissue of the breast, ovary, prostate, bladder, esophagus, and pancreas. When the gene is present but silent, its DNA is thought to be heavily methylated, rendering it inactive. Furthermore, the active gene is also thought to behave as a *tumor suppressor*, providing a surveillance function by recognizing cancer cells and inducing apoptosis, effectively eliminating them before malignant tumors can be initiated.

GENETICS, TECHNOLOGY, AND SOCIETY

Down Syndrome and Prenatal Testing—The New Eugenics?

Down syndrome is the most common chromosomal abnormality seen in newborn babies. Each year, about 4000–5000 babies are born with Down syndrome in the United States. Prenatal diagnostic tests for Down syndrome have been available for decades, especially to older pregnant women who have an increased risk of bearing a Down syndrome child. Scientists estimate that there is an abortion rate of about 30 percent for fetuses that test positive for Down syndrome in the United States, and rates of up to 85 percent in other parts of the world, such as Taiwan and France.

In addition to Down syndrome testing, prenatal genetic tests for other chromosomal and gene-specific defects are entering medical practice. As new genomic methods gain prevalence, we will soon see inexpensive genetic screens for hundreds of genetic defects and gene variants.

Many people agree that it is morally acceptable to prevent the birth of a genetically abnormal fetus. However, many others argue that prenatal genetic testing and the elimination of congenital disorders are both unethical. These arguments often center around their views about abortion and self-determination. In addition, some people argue that prenatal genetic tests followed by selective abortion is eugenic.

These eugenics arguments are highly emotionally charged, and some people contend they are inappropriate arguments to use when discussing screening for genetic diseases. It is safe to say that most people on both sides of the eugenics debate are unclear about the definition of eugenics and even less clear about how it may relate to prenatal genetic testing.

So, what is eugenics? And how does eugenics apply, if at all, to screening for Down syndrome and other human genetic defects? The term *eugenics* was first defined by Francis Galton in 1883 as "the science which deals with all influences that improve the inborn qualities of a race; also with those that develop them to the utmost advantage." Galton believed that human traits such as intelligence and personality were hereditary and that humans could selectively mate with each other to create gifted groups of people—analogous to the creation of purebred dogs with specific traits. Galton did not propose coercion but thought that people would voluntarily enter matings for beneficial outcomes.

In the early to mid-twentieth century, countries throughout the world adopted eugenic policies with the aim of enhancing desirable human traits and eliminating undesirable ones. Two distinct approaches to eugenics developed: *positive eugenics*, in which those with desirable mental and physical traits were encouraged to reproduce, and *negative eugenics*, in which those with undesirable traits were discouraged or prevented from reproducing. Many countries, including Britain, Canada, and the United States, enacted compulsory sterilization programs for the "feeble-minded," mentally ill, and criminals. The eugenic policies of Nazi Germany were particularly infamous, resulting in forced human genetic experimentation and the killing of tens of thousands of disabled people. The eugenics movement was discredited after World War II, and the evils perpetuated in its name have tainted the term *eugenics* ever since.

Given the history of the eugenics movement, is it fair to use the term *eugenics* when we speak about genetic testing for Down syndrome and other genetic disorders? Some people argue that it is not eugenic to select for healthy children because there is no coercion, the state is not involved, and the goal is the elimination of suffering. Others point out that such voluntary actions still constitute eugenics, since they involve a form of bioengineering for better human beings.

Now that we are entering an era of unprecedented knowledge about our genomes and our predisposition to genetic disorders, we must make decisions about whether our attempts to control or improve human genomes is ethical, and what limits we should place on these efforts. The story of the eugenics movement provides us with a powerful cautionary tale about the potential misuses of genetic information.

Your Turn

Take time, individually or in groups, to answer the following questions. Investigate the references and links to help you discuss some of the issues surrounding genetic testing and eugenics.

1. Do you think that modern prenatal and preimplantation genetic testing followed by selective abortion is eugenic? Why or why not?

For background on these questions, see McCabe, L. and McCabe, E., 2011. Down syndrome: Coercion and eugenics. *Genet. Med.* 13: 708–710. *Another useful discussion can be found in* Scully, J. L., 2008. Disability and genetics in the era of genomic medicine. *Nature Reviews Genetics* 9: 797–802.

2. Is it desirable, or even possible, for genetic counseling to be nondirective?

One of the arguments that genetic tests followed by selective abortion are eugenic is that there are strong pressures on pregnant women to produce "normal" children. Some of these pressures may come from genetic counselors. For a discussion of this topic, see King, D. S., 1999. Preimplantation genetic diagnosis and the "new" eugenics. *J. Med. Ethics* 25: 176–182.

3. If genetic technologies were more advanced than today, and you could choose the traits of your children, would you take advantage of that option? Which traits would you choose—height, weight, intellectual abilities, athleticism, artistic talents? If so, would this be eugenic?

To read about similar questions answered by groups of Swiss law and medical students, read Elger, B. and Harding, T., 2003. Huntington's disease: Do future physicians and lawyers think eugenically? *Clin. Genet.* 64: 327–338.

CASE STUDY | Fish tales

Aquatic vegetation overgrowth, usually controlled by dredging or herbicides, represents a significant issue in maintaining private and public waterways. In 1963, diploid grass carp were introduced in Arkansas to consume vegetation, but they reproduced prodigiously and spread to eventually become a hazard to aquatic ecosystems in 35 states. In the 1980s, many states adopted triploid grass carp as an alternative because of their high, but not absolute, sterility level and their longevity of seven to ten years. Today, most states require permits for vegetation control by triploid carp, requiring their containment in the body of water to which they are introduced. Genetic modifications of organisms to achieve specific outcomes will certainly become more common in the future and raise several interesting questions.

1. Taking triploid carp as an example, what controversies may emerge as similar modified species become available for widespread use?

2. If you were a state employee in charge of a specific waterway, what questions would you ask before you approved the introduction of a laboratory-produced, polyploid species into your waterway?

3. Why would the creation and use of a tetraploid carp species be less desirable in the above situation?

Summary Points

MasteringGenetics™ For activities, animations, and review quizzes, go to the Study Area.

1. Alterations of the precise diploid content of chromosomes are referred to as chromosomal aberrations or chromosomal mutations.
2. Studies of monosomic and trisomic disorders are increasing our understanding of the delicate genetic balance that is essential for normal development.
3. When more than two haploid sets of chromosomes are present, these may be derived from the same or different species, the basis of autopolyploidy and allotetraploidy, respectively.
4. Deletions or duplications of segments of a gene or a chromosome may be the source of mutant phenotypes, such as cri du chat syndrome in humans and Bar eyes in *Drosophila*, while

duplications can be particularly important as a source of amplified or new genes.
5. Inversions and translocations may initially cause little or no loss of genetic information or deleterious effects. However, heterozygous combinations of the involved chromosome segments may result in genetically abnormal gametes following meiosis, with lethality or inviability often ensuing.
6. Fragile sites in human mitotic chromosomes have sparked research interest because one such site on the X chromosome is associated with the most common form of inherited mental retardation, while other autosomal sites have been linked to various forms of cancer.

INSIGHTS AND SOLUTIONS

1. In a cross using maize that involves three genes, *a*, *b*, and *c*, a heterozygote (*abc*/+++) is testcrossed to *abc*/*abc*. Even though the three genes are separated along the chromosome, thus predicting that crossover gametes and the resultant phenotypes should be observed, only two phenotypes are recovered: *abc* and +++. In addition, the cross produced significantly fewer viable plants than expected. Can you propose why no other phenotypes were recovered and why the viability was reduced?

   Solution: One of the two chromosomes may contain an inversion that overlaps all three genes, effectively precluding the recovery of any "crossover" offspring. If this is a paracentric inversion and the genes are clearly separated (assuring that a significant number of crossovers occurs between them), then numerous acentric and dicentric chromosomes will form, resulting in the observed reduction in viability.

2. A male *Drosophila* from a wild-type stock is discovered to have only seven chromosomes, whereas normally 2*n* = 8. Close examination reveals that one member of chromosome

IV (the smallest chromosome) is attached to (translocated to) the distal end of chromosome II and is missing its centromere, thus accounting for the reduction in chromosome number.

(a) Diagram all members of chromosomes II and IV during synapsis in meiosis I.

Solution:

(b) If this male mates with a female with a normal chromosome composition who is homozygous for the recessive chromosome IV mutation *eyeless* (*ey*), what chromosome compositions will occur in the offspring regarding chromosomes II and IV?

Solution:

Normal female   Translocation male

(1) (2) (3) (4)

(c) Referring to the diagram in the solution to part (b), what phenotypic ratio will result regarding the presence of eyes, assuming all abnormal chromosome compositions survive?

Solution:

1. normal (heterozygous)

2. eyeless (monosomic, contains chromosome IV from mother)

3. normal (heterozygous; trisomic and may die)

4. normal (heterozygous; balanced translocation)

The final ratio is 3/4 normal: 1/4 eyeless.

Problems and Discussion Questions

MasteringGenetics™ Visit for instructor-assigned tutorials and problems.

HOW DO WE KNOW?

1. In this chapter, we have focused on chromosomal mutations resulting from a change in number or arrangement of chromosomes. In our discussions, we found many opportunities to consider the methods and reasoning by which much of this information was acquired. From the explanations given in the chapter, what answers would you propose to the following fundamental questions?
   (a) How do we know that the extra chromosome causing Down syndrome is usually maternal in origin?
   (b) How do we know that human aneuploidy for each of the 22 autosomes occurs at conception, even though most often human aneuploids do not survive embryonic or fetal development and thus are never observed at birth?
   (c) How do we know that specific mutant phenotypes are due to changes in chromosome number or structure?
   (d) How do we know that the mutant Bar-eye phenotype in *Drosophila* is due to a duplicated gene region rather than to a change in the nucleotide sequence of a gene?

CONCEPT QUESTION

2. Review the Chapter Concepts list on page 188. These all center around chromosome aberrations that create variations from the "normal" diploid genome. Write a short essay that discusses five altered phenotypes that result from specific chromosomal aberrations.

3. Define these pairs of terms, and distinguish between them.
   aneuploidy/euploidy
   monosomy/trisomy
   Patau syndrome/Edwards syndrome
   autopolyploidy/allopolyploidy
   autotetraploid/amphidiploid
   paracentric inversion/pericentric inversion

4. For a species with a diploid number of 18, indicate how many chromosomes will be present in the somatic nuclei of individuals that are haploid, tetraploid, trisomic, and monosomic.

5. What evidence suggests that Down syndrome is more often the result of nondisjunction during oogenesis rather than during spermatogenesis?

6. What evidence indicates that humans with aneuploid karyotypes occur at conception but are usually inviable?

7. Contrast the fertility of an allotetraploid with an autotriploid and an autotetraploid.

8. Describe the origin of cultivated American cotton.

9. Predict how the synaptic configurations of homologous pairs of chromosomes might appear when one member is normal and the other member has sustained a deletion or duplication.

10. Inversions are said to "suppress crossing over." Is this terminology technically correct? If not, restate the description accurately.

11. Contrast the genetic composition of gametes derived from tetrads of inversion heterozygotes where crossing over occurs within a paracentric versus a pericentric inversion.

12. Human adult hemoglobin is a tetramer containing two alpha (α) and two beta (β) polypeptide chains. The α gene cluster on chromosome 16 and the β gene cluster on chromosome 11 share amino acid similarities such that 61 of the amino acids of the α-globin polypeptide (141 amino acids long) are shared in identical sequence with the β-globin polypeptide (146 amino acids long). How might one explain the existence of two polypeptides with partially shared function and structure on two different chromosomes?

13. Discuss Ohno's hypothesis on the role of gene duplication in the process of evolution. What evidence supports this hypothesis?

14. What roles have inversions and translocations played in the evolutionary process?

15. The primrose, *Primula kewensis,* has 36 chromosomes that are similar in appearance to the chromosomes in two related species, *P. floribunda* ($2n = 18$) and *P. verticillata* ($2n = 18$). How could *P. kewensis* arise from these species? How would you describe *P. kewensis* in genetic terms?

16. Certain varieties of chrysanthemums contain 18, 36, 54, 72, and 90 chromosomes; all are multiples of a basic set of nine chromosomes. How would you describe these varieties genetically? What feature do the karyotypes of each variety share? A variety with 27 chromosomes has been discovered, but it is sterile. Why?

17. *Drosophila* may be monosomic for chromosome 4, yet remain fertile. Contrast the F_1 and F_2 results of the following crosses involving the recessive chromosome 4 trait, bent bristles: (a) monosomic IV, bent bristles × diploid, normal bristles; (b) monosomic IV, normal bristles × diploid, bent bristles.

18. Mendelian ratios are modified in crosses involving auto-tetraploids. Assume that one plant expresses the dominant trait green seeds and is homozygous (*WWWW*). This plant is crossed to one with white seeds that is also homozygous (*wwww*). If only one dominant allele is sufficient to produce green seeds, predict the F_1 and F_2 results of such a cross. Assume that synapsis between chromosome pairs is random during meiosis.

19. Having correctly established the F_2 ratio in Problem 18, predict the F_2 ratio of a "dihybrid" cross involving two independently assorting characteristics (e.g., $P_1 = WWWWAAAA \times wwwwaaaa$).

20. The mutations called *bobbed* in *Drosophila* result from variable reductions (deletions) in the number of amplified genes coding for rRNA. Researchers trying to maintain *bobbed* stocks have often documented their tendency to revert to wild type in successive generations. Propose a mechanism based on meiotic recombination which could account for this reversion phenomenon. Why would wild-type flies become more prevalent in *Drosophila* cultures?

21. The outcome of a single crossover between nonsister chromatids in the inversion loop of an inversion heterozygote varies depending on whether the inversion is of the paracentric or pericentric type. What differences are expected?

22. A couple planning their family are aware that through the past three generations on the husband's side a substantial number of stillbirths have occurred and several malformed babies were born who died early in childhood. The wife has studied genetics and urges her husband to visit a genetic counseling clinic, where a complete karyotype-banding analysis is performed. Although the tests show that he has a normal complement of 46 chromosomes, banding analysis reveals that one member of the chromosome 1 pair (in group A) contains an inversion covering 70 percent of its length. The homolog of chromosome 1 and all other chromosomes show the normal banding sequence.
(a) How would you explain the high incidence of past still-births?
(b) What can you predict about the probability of abnormality/normality of their future children?
(c) Would you advise the woman that she will have to bring each pregnancy to term to determine whether the fetus is normal? If not, what else can you suggest?

Extra-Spicy Problems

MasteringGenetics™ Visit for instructor-assigned tutorials and problems.

23. In a cross in *Drosophila*, a female heterozygous for the autosomally linked genes *a*, *b*, *c*, *d*, and *e* (*abcde*/+++++) was testcrossed with a male homozygous for all recessive alleles. Even though the distance between each of the loci was at least 3 map units, only four phenotypes were recovered, yielding the following data:

Phenotype	No. of Flies
+ + + + +	440
a b c d e	460
+ + + + e	48
a b c d +	52
	Total = 1000

Why are many expected crossover phenotypes missing? Can any of these loci be mapped from the data given here? If so, determine map distances.

24. A woman who sought genetic counseling is found to be heterozygous for a chromosomal rearrangement between the second and third chromosomes. Her chromosomes, compared to those in a normal karyotype, are diagrammed to the right.
(a) What kind of chromosomal aberration is shown?
(b) Using a drawing, demonstrate how these chromosomes would pair during meiosis. Be sure to label the different segments of the chromosomes.

(c) This woman is phenotypically normal. Does this surprise you? Why or why not? Under what circumstances might you expect a phenotypic effect of such a rearrangement?

25. The woman in Problem 24 has had two miscarriages. She has come to you, an established genetic counselor, with these questions: Is there a genetic explanation of her frequent miscarriages? Should she abandon her attempts to have a child of her own? If not, what is the chance that she could have a normal child? Provide an informed response to her concerns.

26. In a recent cytogenetic study on 1021 cases of Down syndrome, 46 were the result of translocations, the most frequent of which was symbolized as t(14;21). What does this symbol represent, and how many chromosomes would you expect to be present in t(14;21) Down syndrome individuals?

27. A boy with Klinefelter syndrome (47,XXY) is born to a mother who is phenotypically normal and a father who has the

X-linked skin condition called anhidrotic ectodermal dysplasia. The mother's skin is completely normal with no signs of the skin abnormality. In contrast, her son has patches of normal skin and patches of abnormal skin.

(a) Which parent contributed the abnormal gamete?

(b) Using the appropriate genetic terminology, describe the meiotic mistake that occurred. Be sure to indicate in which division the mistake occurred.

(c) Using the appropriate genetic terminology, explain the son's skin phenotype.

28. Most cases of Turner syndrome are attributed to nondisjunction of one or more of the sex chromosomes during gametogenesis, from either the male or female parent. However, some females possess a rare form of Turner syndrome in which some of the cells of the body (somatic cells) lack an X chromosome, while other cells have the normal two X chromosomes. Often detected in blood and/or skin cells, such individuals with mosaic Turner syndrome may exhibit relatively mild symptoms. An individual may be specified as 45,X(20)/46,XX(80) if, for example, 20 percent of the cells examined were X monosomic. How might mitotic events cause such mosaicism, and what parameter(s) would likely determine the percentages and distributions of X0 cells?

29. To investigate the origin of nondisjunction, 200 human oocytes that had failed to be fertilized during *in vitro* fertilization procedures were subsequently examined (Angel, R. 1997. *Am. J. Hum. Genet.* 61: 23–32). These oocytes had completed meiosis I and were arrested in metaphase II (MII). The majority (67 percent) had a normal MII-metaphase complement, showing 23 chromosomes, each consisting of two sister chromatids joined at a common centromere. The remaining oocytes all had abnormal chromosome compositions. Surprisingly, when trisomy was considered, none of the abnormal oocytes had 24 chromosomes.

(a) Interpret these results in regard to the origin of trisomy, as it relates to nondisjunction, and when it occurs. Why are the results surprising?

(b) A large number of the abnormal oocytes contained 22 1/2 chromosomes; that is, 22 chromosomes plus a single chromatid representing the 1/2 chromosome. What chromosome compositions will result in the zygote if such oocytes proceed through meiosis and are fertilized by normal sperm?

(c) How could the complement of 22 1/2 chromosomes arise? Provide a drawing that includes several pairs of MII chromosomes.

(d) Do your answers support or dispute the generally accepted theory regarding nondisjunction and trisomy, as outlined in Figure 8–1?

30. A 3-year-old child exhibited some early indication of Turner syndrome, which results from a 45,X chromosome composition. Karyotypic analysis demonstrated two cell types: 46,XX (normal) and 45,X. Propose a mechanism for the origin of this mosaicism.

31. A normal female is discovered with 45 chromosomes, one of which exhibits a Robertsonian translocation containing most of chromosomes 15 and 21. Discuss the possible outcomes in her offspring when her husband contains a normal karyotype.

32. Prader-Willi and Angelman syndromes (see Chapter 4) are human conditions that result in part through the process of genomic imprinting, where a particular gene is "marked" during gamete formation in the parent of origin. In the case of these two syndromes, a portion of the long arm of chromosome 15 (15q11 to 15q13) is imprinted. Another condition, Beckwith-Wiedemann syndrome (accelerated growth and increased risk of cancer), is associated with abnormalities of imprinted genes on the short arm of chromosome 11. All three of the above syndromes occur when imprinted sequences become abnormally exposed by some genetic or chromosomal event. One such event is uniparental disomy (UPD), in which a person receives two homologs of one chromosome (or part of a chromosome) from one parent and no homolog from the other. In many cases, UPD is without consequence; however, if chromosome 11 or 15 is involved, then, coupled with genomic imprinting, complications can arise. Listed below are possible origins of UPD. Provide a diagram and explanation for each.

1. *Trisomic rescue*: loss of a chromosome in a trisomic zygote

2. *Monosomic rescue*: gain of a chromosome in a monosomic zygote

3. *Gamete complementation*: fertilization of a gamete with two copies of a chromosome by a gamete with no copies of that chromosome

4. *Isochromosome formation*: a chromosome that contains two copies of an arm (15q-15q, for example) rather than one

A mammalian cell demonstrating the presence of mtDNA (stained green), which is located in the nucleoids in the tubular mitochondrial network (stained red). The nucleus of the cell is stained in blue.

9 Extranuclear Inheritance

CHAPTER CONCEPTS

- Extranuclear inheritance occurs when phenotypes result from genetic influence other than the biparental transmission of genes located on chromosomes housed within the nucleus.

- Organelle heredity, an example of extranuclear inheritance, is due to the transmission of genetic information contained in mitochondria or chloroplasts, most often from only one parent.

- Traits determined by mitochondrial DNA are most often transmitted uniparentally through the maternal gamete, while traits determined by chloroplast DNA may be transmitted uniparentally or biparentally.

- Mitochondrial mutations have been linked to many human disease conditions as well as to the aging process.

- Maternal effect, the expression of the maternal nuclear genotype during gametogenesis and during early development, may have a strong influence on the phenotype of an organism.

Throughout the history of genetics, occasional reports have challenged the basic tenet of Mendelian transmission genetics—that the phenotype is transmitted by nuclear genes located on the chromosomes of both parents. Observations have revealed inheritance patterns that fail to reflect Mendelian principles, and some indicate an apparent extranuclear influence on the phenotype. Before the role of DNA in genetics was firmly established, such observations were commonly regarded with skepticism. However, with the increasing knowledge of molecular genetics and the discovery of DNA in mitochondria and chloroplasts, extranuclear inheritance is now recognized as an important aspect of genetics.

There are several varieties of extranuclear inheritance. One major type, referred to above, is also described as **organelle heredity**. In this type of inheritance, DNA contained in mitochondria or chloroplasts determines certain phenotypic characteristics of the offspring. Examples are often recognized on the basis of the uniparental transmission of these organelles, usually from the female parent through the egg to progeny. A second type, called **infectious heredity**, results from a symbiotic or parasitic association with a microorganism. In such cases, an inherited phenotype is affected by the presence of the microorganism in the cytoplasm of the host cells. A third variety involves the **maternal effect** on the phenotype, whereby nuclear gene products are stored in the egg and then transmitted through the ooplasm to offspring. These gene products are distributed to cells of the developing embryo and influence its phenotype.

The common element in all of these examples is the transmission of genetic information to offspring through the cytoplasm rather than through the nucleus, most often from only one of the parents. This shall constitute our definition of **extranuclear inheritance**.

9.1 Organelle Heredity Involves DNA in Chloroplasts and Mitochondria

In this section and the next, we will examine examples of inheritance patterns arising from chloroplast and mitochondrial function. Such patterns are now appropriately called **organelle heredity**. Before DNA was discovered in these organelles, the exact mechanism of transmission of the traits we are about to discuss was not clear, except that their inheritance appeared to be linked to something in the cytoplasm rather than to genes in the nucleus. Most often (but not in all cases), the traits appeared to be transmitted from the maternal parent through the ooplasm, causing the results of reciprocal crosses to vary.

Analysis of the inheritance patterns resulting from mutant alleles in chloroplasts and mitochondria has been difficult for two major reasons. First, the function of these organelles is dependent on gene products from both nuclear and organelle DNA, making the discovery of the genetic origin of mutations affecting organelle function difficult. Second, large numbers of these organelles are contributed to each progeny cell following cell division. If only one or a few of the organelles acquire a new mutation or contain an existing one in a cell with a population of mostly normal organelles, the corresponding mutant phenotype may not be revealed, since the organelles lacking the mutation perform the wild-type function for the cell. Such variation in the genetic content of organelles is called **heteroplasmy**. Analysis is thus much more complex for traits controlled by genes encoded by organelle DNA than for Mendelian characters controlled by nuclear genes.

We will begin our discussion with several of the classical examples that ultimately called attention to organelle heredity. After that, we will discuss information concerning the DNA and the resultant genetic function in each organelle.

Chloroplasts: Variegation in Four O'Clock Plants

In 1908, Carl Correns (one of the rediscoverers of Mendel's work) provided the earliest example of inheritance linked to chloroplast transmission. Correns discovered a variant of the four o'clock plant, *Mirabilis jalapa*, in which some branches had white leaves, some had green, and some had variegated leaves. The completely white leaves and the white areas in variegated leaves lack chlorophyll that otherwise provides green color. Chlorophyll is the light-absorbing pigment made within chloroplasts.

Correns was curious about how inheritance of this phenotypic trait occurred. Inheritance in all possible combinations of crosses is strictly determined by the phenotype of the ovule source (**Figure 9–1**). For example, if the seeds (representing the progeny) were derived from ovules on branches with green leaves, all progeny plants bore only green leaves, regardless of the phenotype of the source of pollen. Correns concluded that inheritance was transmitted through the cytoplasm of the maternal parent because the pollen, which contributes little or no cytoplasm to the zygote, had no apparent influence on the progeny phenotypes.

Since leaf coloration is a function of the chloroplast, genetic information either contained in that organelle or somehow present in the cytoplasm and influencing the chloroplast must be responsible for the inheritance pattern. It now seems certain that the genetic "defect" that eliminates the green chlorophyll in the white patches on leaves is a mutation in the DNA housed in the chloroplast.

Chloroplast Mutations in *Chlamydomonas*

The unicellular green alga *Chlamydomonas reinhardtii* has provided an excellent system for the investigation of plastid inheritance. This haploid eukaryotic organism has a single large chloroplast containing about 75 copies of a circular double-stranded DNA molecule. Matings that reestablish diploidy are immediately followed by meiosis, and the various stages of the life cycle are easily studied in culture in the laboratory. The first known cytoplasmic mutation, streptomycin resistance (str^R) in *Chlamydomonas*, was reported in 1954 by Ruth Sager. Although *Chlamydomonas*'s two mating types, mt^+ and mt^-, appear to make equal cytoplasmic contributions to the zygote, Sager determined that the str^R phenotype is transmitted only through the mt^+ parent (**Figure 9–2**). Reciprocal crosses between sensitive and resistant strains yield different results depending on the genotype of the mt^+ parent, which is expressed in all offspring. As shown in the figure, one-half of the offspring are mt^+ and one-half of them are mt^-, indicating that mating type is controlled by a nuclear gene that segregates in a Mendelian fashion.

Since Sager's discovery, a number of other *Chlamydomonas* mutations (including resistance to, or dependence on, a variety of bacterial antibiotics) that show a similar uniparental inheritance pattern have been discovered. These mutations have all been linked to the transmission of the chloroplast, and their study has extended our knowledge of chloroplast inheritance.

Following fertilization, which involves the fusion of two cells of opposite mating type, the single chloroplasts of the two mating types fuse. After the resulting zygote has undergone meiosis and haploid cells are produced, it is apparent that the genetic information in the chloroplast of progeny cells is derived only from the mt^+ parent. The

	Location of Ovule		
Source of Pollen	White branch	Green branch	Variegated branch
White branch	White	Green	White, green, or variegated
Green branch	White	Green	White, green, or variegated
Variegated branch	White	Green	White, green, or variegated

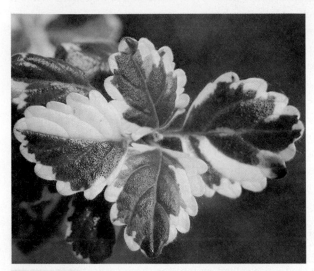

FIGURE 9–1 Offspring of crosses involving leaves from various branches of variegated four o'clock plants. The photograph illustrates variegation in the leaves of the madagascar spur.

$$str^R \; mt^+ \; \times \; str^S \; mt^-$$

$$\downarrow$$

1/2 mt^+	1/2 mt^-
all str^R	

$$str^S \; mt^+ \; \times \; str^R \; mt^-$$

$$\downarrow$$

1/2 mt^+	1/2 mt^-
all str^S	

FIGURE 9–2 The results of reciprocal crosses between streptomycin-resistant (str^R) and streptomycin-sensitive (str^S) strains in the green alga *Chlamydomonas* (shown in the photograph).

genetic information originally present within the mt^- chloroplast has degenerated.

NOW SOLVE THIS

9–1 *Chlamydomonas*, a eukaryotic green alga, may be sensitive to the antibiotic erythromycin, which inhibits protein synthesis in prokaryotes. There are two mating types in this alga, mt^+ and mt^-. If an mt^+ cell sensitive to the antibiotic is crossed with an mt^- cell that is resistant, all progeny cells are sensitive. The reciprocal cross (mt^+ resistant and mt^- sensitive) yields all resistant progeny cells. Assuming that the mutation for resistance is in the chloroplast DNA, what can you conclude from the results of these crosses?

■ **HINT:** *This problem involves an understanding of the cytoplasmic transmission of organelles in unicellular algae. The key to its solution is to consider the results you would expect from two possibilities: that inheritance of the trait is uniparental or that inheritance is biparental.*

The inheritance of phenotypes influenced by mitochondria is also uniparental in *Chlamydomonas*. However, studies of the transmission of several cases of antibiotic resistance governed by mitochondria have shown that it is the mt^- parent that transmits the mitochondrial genetic information to progeny cells. This is just the opposite of what occurs with chloroplast-derived phenotypes, such as str^R. The significance of inheriting one organelle from one parent and the other organelle from the other parent is not yet established.

Mitochondrial Mutations: Early Studies in *Neurospora* and Yeast

As alluded to earlier, mutations affecting mitochondrial function have also been discovered and studied, revealing that mitochondria, too, contain a distinctive genetic system. As with chloroplasts, mitochondrial mutations are transmitted through the cytoplasm during reproduction. In 1952, Mary B. Mitchell and Herschel K. Mitchell studied the pink bread mold *Neurospora crassa* (**Figure 9–3**). They discovered a slow-growing mutant strain and named it *poky*. (It is also designated *mi-1*, for *maternal inheritance*.) Slow growth is associated with impaired mitochondrial function,

FIGURE 9–3 Micrograph illustrating the bread mold *Neurospora crassa*.

Normal colonies

Petite colonies

FIGURE 9–4 A comparison of normal versus petite colonies in the yeast *Saccharomyces cerevisiae*.

specifically caused by the absence of several cytochrome proteins essential for electron transport. In the absence of cytochromes, aerobic respiration leading to ATP synthesis is curtailed. Results of genetic crosses between wild-type and *poky* strains suggest that the trait is maternally inherited. If one mating type is *poky* and the other is wild type, all progeny colonies are *poky*, yet the reciprocal cross produces normal wild-type colonies.

Another study of mitochondrial mutations has been performed with the yeast *Saccharomyces cerevisiae*. The first such mutation, described by Boris Ephrussi and his coworkers in 1956, was named *petite* because of the small size of the yeast colonies (**Figure 9–4**). Many independent *petite* mutations have since been discovered and studied, and all have a common characteristic: a deficiency in cellu-

lar respiration involving abnormal electron transport, as performed by mitochondria. This organism is a *facultative anaerobe* (an organism that can function both with and without the presence of oxygen), so in the absence of oxygen it can grow by fermenting glucose through glycolysis. Thus, it may survive the loss of mitochondrial function by generating energy anaerobically.

The complex genetics of *petite* mutations is diagrammed in **Figure 9–5**. A small proportion of these mutants are the result of nuclear mutations in genes whose products are transported to and function in mitochondria. They exhibit Mendelian inheritance and are thus called **segregational petites**. The remaining mutants demonstrate cytoplasmic transmission, indicating alterations in the DNA of the mitochondria. They produce one of two effects in matings. **Neutral petites**, when crossed to wild type, yield meiotic products (called ascospores) that give rise only to wild-type, or normal, colonies. The same pattern continues if the progeny of such crosses are backcrossed to *neutral petites*. The majority of "neutrals" lack mtDNA completely or have lost a substantial portion of it, so for their offspring to be normal, the neutrals must also be inheriting mitochondria capable of aerobic respiration from the normal parent following reproduction. This establishes that in yeast, mitochondria are inherited from

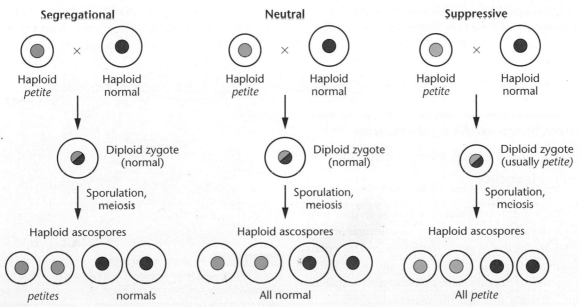

FIGURE 9–5 The outcome of crosses involving the three types of *petite* mutations affecting mitochondrial function in the yeast *Saccharomyces cerevisiae*.

both parental cells. The functional mitochondria from the normal parent are replicated in offspring and support aerobic respiration.

The third mutational type, **suppressive petites**, provides different results. Crosses between mutant and wild type give rise to diploid zygotes, which after meiosis, yield haploid cells that all express the *petite* phenotype. Assuming that the offspring have received mitochondria from both parents, the *petite* cells behave as what is called a **dominant-negative mutation**, which somehow suppresses the function of the wild-type mitochondria.

Two major hypotheses concerning the organelle DNA have been advanced to explain this suppressiveness. One explanation suggests that the mutant (or deleted) DNA in the mitochondria (mtDNA) replicates more rapidly, resulting in the mutant mitochondria "taking over" or dominating the phenotype by numbers alone. The second explanation suggests that recombination occurs between the mutant and wild-type mtDNA, introducing errors into or disrupting the normal mtDNA. It is not yet clear which one, if either, of these explanations is correct.

NOW SOLVE THIS

9–2 In aerobically cultured yeast, a *petite* mutant is isolated. To determine the type of mutation causing this phenotype, the *petite* and wild-type strains are crossed. Such a cross has three potential outcomes.

   (a) all wild type
   (b) some *petite*, some wild type
   (c) all *petite*

For each set of results, what conclusion about the type of *petite* mutation is justified?

■ **HINT:** *This problem involves the understanding that the petite phenotype is related to mitochondrial function and to how mitochondria are inherited. The key to its solution is to remember that in yeast, inheritance of mitochondria is biparental.*

9.2 Knowledge of Mitochondrial and Chloroplast DNA Helps Explain Organelle Heredity

That both mitochondria and chloroplasts contain their own DNA and a system for expressing genetic information was first suggested by the discovery of mutations and the resultant inheritance patterns in plants, yeast, and other fungi, as already discussed. Because both mitochondria and chloroplasts are inherited through the maternal cytoplasm in most organisms, and because each of the above-mentioned

examples of mutations could be linked hypothetically to the altered function of either chloroplasts or mitochondria, geneticists set out to look for more direct evidence of DNA in these organelles. Not only was unique DNA found to be a normal component of both mitochondria and chloroplasts, but careful examination of the nature of this genetic information would provide essential clues as to the evolutionary origin of these organelles.

Organelle DNA and the Endosymbiotic Theory

Electron microscopists not only documented the presence of DNA in mitochondria and chloroplasts, but they also saw that it exists there in a form quite unlike the form seen in the nucleus of the eukaryotic cells that house these organelles (**Figures 9–6** and **9–7**). The DNA in chloroplasts and mitochondria looks remarkably similar to the DNA seen in bacteria. This similarity, along with the observation of the presence of a unique genetic system capable of organelle-specific transcription and translation, led Lynn Margulis and others to the postulate known as the **endosymbiotic theory**. Basically, the theory states that mitochondria and chloroplasts arose independently about 2 billion years ago from free-living protobacteria (primitive bacteria). Progenitors possessed the abilities now attributed to these organelles—aerobic respiration and photosynthesis, respectively. This idea proposes that these ancient bacteria-like cells were engulfed by larger primitive eukaryotic cells, which originally lacked the ability to respire aerobically or to capture energy from sunlight. A beneficial, symbiotic relationship subsequently developed, whereby the bacteria eventually lost their ability to function autonomously, while the eukaryotic host cells gained the

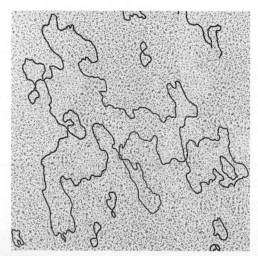

FIGURE 9–6 An electron micrograph of chloroplast DNA (cpDNA) derived from lettuce. Genes encoded by cpDNA impart photosynthetic function to the plant as well as providing the basis for transcription and translation of genetic information within the organelle.

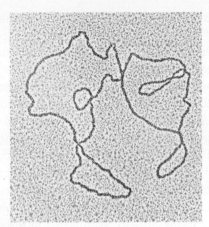

FIGURE 9–7 Electron micrograph of mitochondrial DNA derived from the frog *Xenopus laevis*.

ability to perform either oxidative respiration or photosynthesis, as the case may be. Although some questions remain unanswered, evidence continues to accumulate in support of this theory, and its basic tenets are now widely accepted.

A brief examination of modern-day mitochondria will help us better understand endosymbiotic theory. During the course of evolution subsequent to the invasion event, distinct branches of diverse eukaryotic organisms arose. As the evolution of the host cells progressed, the companion bacteria also underwent their own independent changes. The primary alteration was the transfer of many of the genes from the invading bacterium to the nucleus of the host. The *products* of these genes, though still functioning in the organelle, are nevertheless now encoded and transcribed in the nucleus and translated in the cytoplasm prior to their transport into the organelle. The amount of DNA remaining today in the typical mitochondrial genome is minuscule compared with that in the free-living bacteria from which it was derived. The most gene-rich organelles now have fewer than 10 percent of the genes present in the smallest bacterium known.

Similar changes have characterized the evolution of chloroplasts. In the subsequent sections of this chapter, we will explore in some detail what is known about modern-day chloroplasts and mitochondria.

Molecular Organization and Gene Products of Chloroplast DNA

The details of the autonomous genetic system of chloroplasts have now been worked out, providing further support of the endosymbiotic theory. The chloroplast, responsible for photosynthesis, contains both DNA (as a source of genetic information) and a complete protein-synthesizing apparatus. The molecular components of the chloroplast's translation apparatus are derived from both nuclear and organelle genetic information.

Chloroplast DNA (cpDNA), shown in Figure 9–6, is fairly uniform in size among different organisms, ranging between 100 and 225 kb in length. It shares many similarities to DNA found in prokaryotic cells. It is circular and double stranded, and it is free of the associated proteins characteristic of eukaryotic DNA. Compared with nuclear DNA from the same organism, it invariably shows a different density and base composition.

The size of cpDNA is much larger than that of mtDNA. To some extent, this can be accounted for by a larger number of genes. However, most of the difference appears to be due to the presence in cpDNA of many long noncoding nucleotide sequences both between and within genes, the latter being introns, or noncoding DNA characteristic of eukaryotic nuclear DNA (See Chapter 13). Duplications of many DNA sequences are also present. Since such noncoding sequences vary in different plants, they indicate that independent evolution occurred in chloroplasts following their initial invasion of a primitive eukaryotic-like cell.

In the green alga *Chlamydomonas*, there are about 75 copies of the chloroplast DNA molecule per organelle. In higher plants, such as the sweet pea, multiple copies of the DNA molecule are also present in each organelle, but the molecule (134 kb) is considerably smaller than that in *Chlamydomonas* (195 kb). Interestingly, genetic recombination between the multiple copies of DNA within chloroplasts has been documented in some organisms.

Numerous gene products encoded by chloroplast DNA function during translation within the organelle. Two sets each of the genes coding for the ribosomal RNAs—16S, and 23S rRNA—are present. S refers to the Svedberg coefficient (described in Chapter 10), which is related to the molecule's size and shape. In addition, cpDNA encodes numerous transfer RNAs (tRNAs), as well as many ribosomal proteins specific to the chloroplast ribosomes. In the liverwort, whose cpDNA was the first to be sequenced, there are genes encoding 30 tRNAs, RNA polymerase, multiple rRNAs, and numerous ribosomal proteins. The variations in the gene products encoded in the cpDNA of different plants again attest to the independent evolution that occurred within chloroplasts.

Chloroplast ribosomes differ significantly from those present in the cytoplasm and encoded by nuclear genes. They have a Svedberg coefficient slightly less than 70S, which characterizes bacterial ribosomes. Even though some chloroplast ribosomal proteins are encoded by chloroplast DNA and some by nuclear DNA, most, if not all, such proteins are chemically distinct from their counterparts present in cytoplasmic ribosomes. Both observations provide direct support for the endosymbiotic theory.

Still other chloroplast genes specific to the photosynthetic function, the major role normally associated with this organelle, have been identified. For example, in the moss, there are 92 chloroplast genes encoding proteins that are part of the thylakoid membrane, a cellular component integral to the light-dependent reactions of photosynthesis. Mutations in these genes may inactivate photosynthesis. A typical distribution of genes between the nucleus and the chloroplast is illustrated by one of the major photosynthetic enzymes, ribulose-1-5-bisphosphate carboxylase (known as *Rubisco*). This enzyme has its small subunit encoded by a nuclear gene, whereas the large subunit is encoded by cpDNA.

Molecular Organization and Gene Products of Mitochondrial DNA

Extensive information is also available concerning the structure and gene products of mitochondrial DNA (mtDNA). In most eukaryotes, mtDNA exists as a double-stranded, closed circle (Figure 9–7) that, like cpDNA, is free of the chromosomal proteins characteristic of eukaryotic chromosomal DNA. An exception is found in some ciliated protozoans, in which the DNA is linear.

In size, mtDNA is much smaller than cpDNA and varies greatly among organisms, as demonstrated in **Table 9.1**. In a variety of animals, including humans, mtDNA consists of about 16,000 to 18,000 bp (16 to 18 kb). However, yeast (*Saccharomyces*) mtDNA consists of 75 kb. Plants typically exceed this amount—367 kb is present in mitochondria in the mustard plant, *Arabidopsis*. Vertebrates have 5 to 10 such DNA molecules per organelle, while plants have 20 to 40 copies per organelle.

There are several other noteworthy aspects of mtDNA. With only rare exceptions, and unlike cpDNA, introns are absent from mitochondrial genes, and gene repetitions are seldom present. Nor is there usually much in the way of intergenic spacer DNA. This is particularly true in species whose mtDNA is fairly small in size, such as humans. In *Saccharomyces*, with a much larger mtDNA molecule, much of the excess DNA is accounted for by introns and intergenic spacer DNA. As will be discussed later in the text (see Chapter 13),

the expression of mitochondrial genes uses several modifications of the otherwise standard genetic code. Also of interest is the fact that replication in mitochondria is dependent on enzymes encoded by nuclear DNA.

Human mtDNA encodes two ribosomal RNAs (rRNAs), 22 transfer RNAs (tRNAs), and 13 polypeptides essential to the oxidative respiration functions of the organelle. For instance, mitochondrial-encoded gene products are present in all of the protein complexes of the electron transport chain found in the inner membrane of mitochondria. In most cases, these polypeptides are part of multichain proteins, many of which also contain subunits that are encoded in the nucleus, synthesized in the cytoplasm, and then transported into the organelle. Thus, the protein-synthesizing apparatus and the molecular components for cellular respiration are jointly derived from nuclear and mitochondrial genes.

Another interesting observation is that in vertebrate mtDNA, the two strands vary in density, as revealed by centrifugation. This provides researchers with a way to isolate the strands for study, designating one heavy (H) and the other light (L). While most of the mitochondrial genes are encoded by the H strand, several are encoded by the complementary L strand.

As might be predicted by the endosymbiotic theory, ribosomes found in the organelle differ from those present in the neighboring cytoplasm. Mitochondrial ribosomes of different species vary considerably in their Svedberg coefficients, ranging from 55*S* to 80*S*, while cytoplasmic ribosomes are uniformly 80*S*. The majority of proteins that function in mitochondria are encoded by nuclear genes. In fact, over 1100 nuclear-coded gene products are essential to biological activity in the organelle. They include, for example, DNA and RNA polymerases, initiation and elongation factors essential for translation, ribosomal proteins, aminoacyl tRNA synthetases, and several tRNA species. Notably, these imported components are distinct from their cytoplasmic counterparts, even though both sets are coded by nuclear genes, providing further support for the endosymbiotic theory. For example, the synthetase enzymes essential for charging mitochondrial tRNA molecules (a process essential to translation) show a distinct affinity for the mitochondrial tRNA species as compared with the cytoplasmic tRNAs. Similar affinity has been shown for the initiation and elongation factors. Furthermore, while bacterial and nuclear RNA polymerases are known to be composed of numerous subunits, the mitochondrial variety consists of only one polypeptide chain. This polymerase is generally sensitive to antibiotics that inhibit bacterial RNA synthesis, but not to eukaryotic inhibitors. The various contributions of some of the nuclear and mitochondrial gene products are contrasted in **Figure 9–8**.

TABLE 9.1   The Size of mtDNA in Different Organisms

Organism	Size (kb)
Homo sapiens (human)	16.6
Mus musculus (mouse)	16.2
Xenopus laevis (frog)	18.4
Drosophila melanogaster (fruit fly)	18.4
Saccharomyces cerevisiae (yeast)	75.0
Pisum sativum (pea)	110.0
Arabidopsis thaliana (mustard plant)	367.0

FIGURE 9–8 Gene products that are essential to mitochondrial function. Those shown entering the organelle are derived from the cytoplasm and encoded by nuclear genes.

NOW SOLVE THIS

9–3 DNA in human mitochondria encodes 22 different tRNA molecules. However, 32 different tRNA molecules are required for translation of proteins within mitochondria. Explain.

■ **HINT:** *This problem involves understanding the origin of mitochondria in eukaryotes. The key to its solution is to consider the endosymbiotic theory and its ramifications.*

For more practice, see Problems 16, 17, and 18.

9.3 Mutations in Mitochondrial DNA Cause Human Disorders

The DNA found in human mitochondria has been completely sequenced and contains 16,569 base pairs. As mentioned earlier, mtDNA gene products include 13 proteins required for aerobic cellular respiration. Because a cell's energy supply is largely dependent on aerobic cellular respiration to generate ATP, disruption of any mitochondrial gene by mutation may potentially have a severe impact on that organism. We have seen this in our previous discussion of the *petite* mutations in yeast, which would be lethal were it not for this organism's ability to respire anaerobically. In fact, mtDNA is particularly vulnerable to mutations, for at least three reasons. First, mtDNA does not have the structural protection from mutations provided by histone proteins present in nuclear DNA. Second, DNA repair

mechanisms for mtDNA are limited. Third, mitochondria concentrate highly mutagenic **reactive oxygen species** (**ROS**) generated by cell respiration. In such a confined space, ROS are toxic to the contents of the organelle and are known to damage proteins, lipids, and mtDNA. Ultimately, this increases the frequency of point mutations and deletions in the mitochondria. As a result, mutations in mtDNA occur at a rate that is at least tenfold higher than in nuclear DNA.

The number of copies of mtDNA in human cells can range from several hundred in somatic cells to approximately 100,000 copies of mtDNA in an oocyte. Fortunately, a zygote receives a large number of organelles through the egg, so if only one organelle or a few of them contain a mutation, its impact is greatly diluted by the many mitochondria that lack the mutation and function normally. However, during early development, cell division disperses the initial population of mitochondria present in the zygote, and in the newly formed cells, these organelles reproduce autonomously. Therefore, if a deleterious mutation arises or is present in the initial population of organelles, adults will have cells with a variable mixture of both normal and abnormal organelles. This variation in the genetic content of organelles, as indicated earlier in the chapter, is called *heteroplasmy*.

In order for a human disorder to be attributable to genetically altered mitochondria, several criteria must be met:

1. Inheritance must exhibit a maternal rather than a Mendelian pattern.

2. The disorder must reflect a deficiency in the bioenergetic function of the organelle.

3. There must be a mutation in one or more of the mitochondrial genes.

Today over 150 highly diverse human syndromes are known to demonstrate these characteristics. Some are expressed in infancy, while others are not expressed until adulthood. Some impact on multiple organ systems, and some are highly organ-specific. For example, **myoclonic epilepsy and ragged-red fiber disease** (**MERRF**) demonstrates a pattern of inheritance consistent with maternal transmission. Only the offspring of affected mothers inherit the disorder; the offspring of affected fathers are normal. Individuals with this rare disorder express ataxia (lack of muscular coordination), deafness, dementia, and epileptic seizures. The disease is so named because of the presence of "ragged-red" skeletal muscle fibers that exhibit blotchy red patches resulting from the proliferation of aberrant mitochondria (**Figure 9–9**). Brain function, which has a high energy demand, is affected in this disorder, leading to the neurological symptoms described.

(a)

(b)

FIGURE 9–9 Ragged-red fibers in skeletal muscle cells from patients with the mitochondrial disease MERRF. (a) The muscle fiber has mild proliferation of mitochondria. (See red rim and speckled cytoplasm.) (b) Marked proliferation in which mitochondria have replaced most cellular structures.

Analysis of mtDNA from patients with MERRF has revealed a mutation in one of the 22 mitochondrial genes encoding a transfer RNA. Specifically, the gene encoding tRNA^{Lys} (the tRNA that delivers lysine during translation) contains an A-to-G transition within its sequence. This genetic alteration apparently interferes with the capacity for translation within the organelle, which in turn leads to the various manifestations of the disorder.

The cells of affected individuals exhibit heteroplasmy, containing a mixture of normal and abnormal mitochondria. Different patients contain different proportions of the two, and even different cells from the same patient exhibit various levels of abnormal mitochondria. Were it not for heteroplasmy, the mutation would very likely be lethal, testifying to the essential nature of mitochondrial function and its reliance on the genes encoded by mtDNA within the organelle.

A second disorder, **Leber's hereditary optic neuropathy (LHON)**, also exhibits maternal inheritance as well as mtDNA lesions. The disorder is characterized by sudden bilateral blindness. The average age of vision loss is 27, but onset is quite variable. Four mutations have been identified, all of which disrupt normal oxidative phosphorylation, the final pathway of respiration in cells. More than 50 percent of cases are due to a mutation at a specific position in the mitochondrial gene encoding a subunit of NADH dehydrogenase. This mutation is transmitted maternally through the mitochondria to all offspring. Noteworthy is the observation that in many instances of LHON, there is no family history; a significant number of cases are "sporadic," resulting from newly arisen mutations.

Individuals severely affected by a third disorder, **Kearns–Sayre syndrome (KSS)**, lose their vision, experience hearing loss, and display heart conditions. The genetic basis of KSS involves deletions at various positions within mtDNA. Many KSS patients are symptom-free as children but display progressive symptoms as adults. The proportion of mtDNAs that reveal deletion mutations increases as the severity of symptoms increases.

Mitochondria, Human Health, and Aging

The study of hereditary mitochondrial-based disorders provides insights into the critical importance of this organelle during normal development. In fact, mitochondrial dysfunction seems to be implicated in most all major human disease conditions, including anemia, blindness, Type II (late-onset) diabetes, autism, atherosclerosis, infertility, neurodegenerative diseases such as Parkinson, Alzheimer, and Huntington disease, schizophrenia and bipolar disorders, and a variety of cancers. It is becoming evident, for example, that mutations in mtDNA are present in such human malignancies as skin, colorectal, liver, breast, pancreatic, lung, prostate, and bladder cancers.

Over 400 mtDNA mutations associated with more than 150 distinct mtDNA-based genetic syndromes have been identified. Genetic tests for detecting mutations in the mtDNA genome that may serve as early-stage disease markers have been developed. For example, mtDNA mutations in skin cells have been detected as a biomarker of cumulative exposure of ultraviolet light and development of skin cancer. However, it is still unclear whether mtDNA mutations are causative effects contributing to development of malignant tumors or whether they are the consequences of tumor formation. Nonetheless, there is an interesting link between mtDNA mutations and cancer, including data suggesting that many chemical carcinogens have significant mutation effects on mtDNA.

The study of hereditary mitochondrial-based disorders has also suggested a link between the progressive decline of mitochondrial function and the aging process. It has been hypothesized that the accumulation of sporadic mutations in mtDNA leads to an increased prevalence of defective mitochondria (and the concomitant decrease in the supply of ATP) in cells over a lifetime. This condition in turn plays a significant role in aging. It has been suggested that cells require a threshold level of ATP production resulting from oxidative phosphorylation for normal function. When the level drops below this threshold, the aging process is accelerated.

Many studies have now documented that aging tissues contain mitochondria with increased levels of DNA damage. As with cancer, the major question is whether such changes are simply biomarkers of the aging process or whether they lead to a decline in physiological function that contributes significantly to aging. In support of the latter hypothesis, one study links age-related muscle fiber atrophy in rats to deletions in mtDNA and electron transport abnormalities. Such deletions appear to be present in the fibers of atrophied muscle, but are absent from fibers in regions of normal tissue. Another study using genetically altered mice is even more convincing. Such mice have a nuclear gene altered that diminishes proofreading during the replication of mtDNA. These mice display reduced fertility and accumulate mutations over time at a much higher rate than is normal. Such mice also show many characteristics of premature aging, as observed by loss and graying of hair, reduction in bone density and muscle mass, decline in fertility, anemia, and reduced life span.

These, and other studies, continue to speak to the importance of generating adequate ATP as a result of oxidative phosphorylation under the direction of DNA in mitochondria. As cells undergo genetic damage, which appears to be a natural phenomenon, their function declines, which may be an underlying factor in aging as well as in the progression of age-related disorders.

Future Prevention of the Transmission of mtDNA-Based Disorders

Estimates suggest that 1 in 5000 humans either have a mtDNA-based disease or are at risk for developing such a genetic disorder. Many mtDNA-based genetic disorders can now be detected by genetic testing, but there are currently no cures for these disorders. However, new therapeutic approaches are being developed that can prevent *transmission of mtDNA mutations* from an affected mother to her offspring. In 2010, scientists demonstrated that the mtDNA genome can effectively be replaced in the eggs of a nonhuman primate, the rhesus monkey (*Macaca mulatta*). As illustrated in **Figure 9–10**, this was accomplished by transplanting the nuclear genome from an egg of one mother to an *enucleated* recipient egg (one with its nucleus removed) of another female with a normal content of mito-

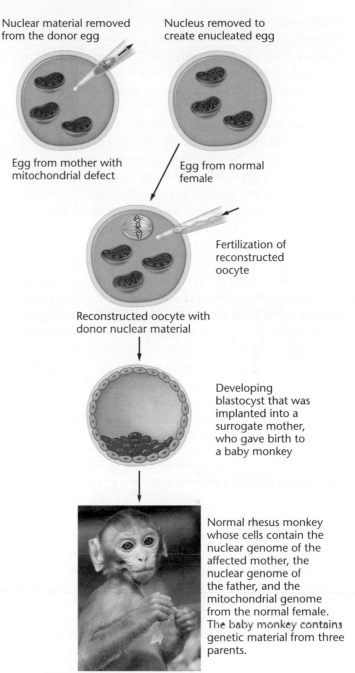

FIGURE 9–10 Illustration of mitochondrial swapping, working with oocytes from rhesus monkeys. The nuclear material (red) from one oocyte with defective mitochondria was removed and transferred to an enucleated egg containing normal mitochondria. The father's sperm was injected and following fertilization, the developing blastocyst was implanted in a surrogate mother. A healthy monkey resulted. This mtDNA swapping approach has the potential to prevent transmission of mtDNA-based mutations if used for *in vitro* fertilization.

chondria. These reconstructed eggs were fertilized and implanted in the uterus of the original mother. The result was the production of healthy offspring with nuclear DNA from the transplanted nuclear genome, and mitochondria from the recipient egg, but devoid of mitochondria from the egg that provided the nuclear genome.

Sometimes referred to as **mitochondrial swapping**, this technology has now been extended to human reproductive research. Near the end of 2012, the same technology described above was adopted using human eggs and *in vitro* fertilization. The successful zygotes developed normally to the blastocyst stage (the 100-cell stage), which was then used to develop cultured embryonic cell lines, which were tested in numerous ways. These cell lines behaved and tested similarly to those that had not undergone mitochondrial swapping. Thus, this technology may potentially offer a future treatment option for preventing mtDNA disease transmission in families with known histories of mtDNA-based disorders.

Several technical and ethical hurdles need to be overcome if this approach is to be used for humans. For instance, this technique produces offspring with genetic contributions from three parents. Is this ethically acceptable? As of 2013, the United Kingdom was on the verge of becoming the first nation to legalize *in vitro* fertilization techniques, as described above, involving nuclear DNA transplantation designed to prevent children from inheriting diseases caused by mutations in mtDNA. Thus women with mtDNA-based diseases could possibly bear healthy children derived from their own nuclear DNA and mitochondria derived from a third party.

NOW SOLVE THIS

9–4 Given the maternal origin of mitochondria, from mother to offspring through the egg, and coupled with the relatively high mutation rate of mitochondrial DNA, one would expect that a high percentage of mutated, nonfunctional mitochondria would accumulate in cells of adults. One could envision that as a result, a mitochondrial meltdown would eventually occur as generations ensue. Such is not the case, however, and data indicate that over generations, mutations in mtDNA tend to be reduced in frequency in a given lineage. How might this phenomenon be explained?

■ **HINT:** *This problem involves an understanding of heteroplasmy in mitochondria. The key to its solution is to consider factors that drive evolution, particularly natural selection, and to apply this concept to the presence of many mitochondria in each cell.*

9.4 In Maternal Effect, the Maternal Genotype Has a Strong Influence during Early Development

In **maternal effect**, also referred to as *maternal influence*, an offspring's phenotype for a particular trait is under the control of nuclear gene products present in the egg. This is in contrast to biparental inheritance, where both parents transmit information on genes in the nucleus that determines the offspring's phenotype. In cases of maternal effect, the nuclear genes of the female gamete are transcribed, and the genetic products (either proteins or untranslated RNAs) accumulate in the egg cytoplasm. After fertilization, these products are distributed among newly formed cells and influence the patterns or traits established during early development. Two examples will illustrate such an influence of the maternal genome on particular traits.

Lymnaea Coiling

Shell coiling (chirality) in the snail *Lymnaea peregra* is an excellent example of maternal effect on a permanent rather than a transitory phenotype. Some strains of this snail have left-handed, or sinistrally, coiled shells (*dd*), while others have right-handed, or dextrally, coiled shells (*DD* or *Dd*). These snails are hermaphroditic and may undergo either cross- or self-fertilization, providing a variety of types of matings.

Figure 9–10 illustrates the results of reciprocal crosses between true-breeding snails. As you can see, these crosses yield different outcomes, even though both are between sinistral and dextral organisms and produce all heterozygous offspring. Examination of the progeny reveals that their phenotypes depend on the genotype of the female parent. If we adopt that conclusion as a working hypothesis, we can test it by examining the offspring in subsequent generations of self-fertilization events. In each case, the hypothesis is upheld. Ovum donors that are *DD* or *Dd* produce only dextrally coiled progeny. Maternal parents that are *dd* produce only sinistrally coiled progeny. The coiling pattern of the progeny snails is determined by *the genotype of the parent producing the egg, regardless of the phenotype of that parent.*

Investigation of the developmental events in *Lymnaea* reveals that the orientation of the cleavage pattern following the eight-cell embryo stage determines the direction of coiling. Cell-cell interaction is influenced by a maternal gene in a way that establishes the orientation of dividing cells. The dextral allele (*D*) produces an active gene product that causes right-handed coiling. If ooplasm from dextral eggs is injected into uncleaved sinistral eggs, they cleave in a dextral pattern. However, in the converse experiment, sinistral ooplasm has no effect when injected into dextral eggs. Apparently, the sinistral allele is the result of a classic recessive mutation that encodes an inactive gene product.

We can conclude, then, that females that are either *DD* or *Dd* produce oocytes that synthesize the *D* gene product, which is stored in the ooplasm. Even if the oocyte contains only the *d* allele following meiosis and is fertilized by a *d*-bearing sperm, the resulting *dd* snail will be dextrally coiled (right handed).

FIGURE 9–11 Inheritance of coiling in the snail *Lymnaea peregra*. Coiling is either dextral (right handed) or sinistral (left handed). A maternal effect is evident in generations II and III, where the genotype of the maternal parent, rather than the offspring's own genotype, controls the phenotype of the offspring. The photograph illustrates right- versus left-handed coiled snails.

Embryonic Development in *Drosophila*

A more recently documented example of maternal effect involves various genes that control embryonic development in *Drosophila melanogaster*. The genetic control of embryonic development in *Drosophila*, discussed in greater detail later in the text (see Chapter 18), is a fascinating story. The protein products of the maternal-effect genes function to activate other genes, which may in turn activate still other genes. This cascade of gene activity leads to a normal embryo whose subsequent development yields a normal adult fly. The extensive work by Edward B. Lewis, Christiane Nüsslein-Volhard,

and Eric Wieschaus (who shared the 1995 Nobel Prize for Physiology or Medicine for their findings) has clarified how these and other genes function. Genes that illustrate maternal effect have products that are synthesized by the developing egg and stored in the oocyte prior to fertilization. Following fertilization, these products create molecular gradients that determine spatial organization as development proceeds.

For example, the gene *bicoid* (bcd^+) plays an important role in specifying the development of the anterior portion of the fly. The RNA transcribed by this gene is deposited anteriorly in the egg (**Figure 9–12**), and upon translation, forms a gradient highest at the anterior end and gradually diluted posteriorly. Embryos derived from mothers who are homozygous for the mutant allele (bcd^-/bcd^-) fail to develop anterior areas that normally give rise to the head and thorax of the adult fly. Embryos whose mothers contain at least one wild-type allele (bcd^+) develop normally, even if the genotype of the embryo is homozygous for the mutation. Consistent with the concept of *maternal effect*, the *genotype of the female parent, not the genotype of the embryo* determines the phenotype of the offspring. Nüsslein-Volhard, and Wieschaus, using large-scale mutant screens, discovered many other maternal-effect genes critical to normal *Drosophila* development, influencing not only anterior and posterior morphogenesis, but also the expression of zygotic (nuclear) genes that control segmentation in this arthropod. When we return to our discussion of this general topic later in the text (see Chapter 18), we will see examples of other genes illustrating maternal effect that influence both anterior and posterior morphogenesis. Many of these genes function to regulate the spatial expression of "zygotic" (nuclear) genes that influence other aspects of development and that behave genetically in the conventional Mendelian fashion.

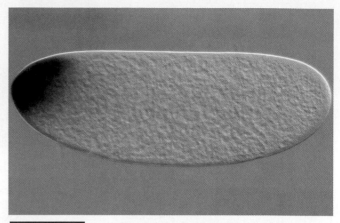

FIGURE 9-12 A gradient of *bicoid* mRNA (blue stain) as concentrated in anterior region of the *Drosophila* embryo during early development.

GENETICS, TECHNOLOGY, AND SOCIETY

Mitochondrial DNA and the Mystery of the Romanovs

In 1917, after more than 300 years of Romanov Imperial Russian rule and a violent Bolshevik revolution, the last Romanov ruler abdicated his crown. Tsar Nicholas II, his wife Tsarina Alexandra, and their five children—Olga, Tatiana, Maria, Anastasia, and Alexei—were arrested and sent into exile in the town of Ekaterinburg in western Siberia. They were accompanied by their family doctor and three loyal servants.

Just after midnight on July 17, 1918, the group was awakened and brought downstairs to a cellar room, where they were told that they would be moved to a safer location. Instead, eleven men with revolvers entered the room and shot the family and their staff. To complete the execution, the bodies were bayoneted and their faces smashed with rifle butts. The corpses were then hauled away and thrown down a mineshaft. Two days later, the bodies were removed from the mineshaft and buried in shallow graves in the woods. There they rested for more than 60 years.

An air of mystery soon developed around the demise of the Romanovs. Because the burial location was unknown and there were few eyewitness accounts of the assassination, speculation arose that some—or perhaps all—of the family may have survived. Romantic mythologies developed over the possible survival of the youngest daughter, Anastasia, and the heir to the throne, Alexei, both of whom were said to have escaped from Russia and awaited the restoration of their imperial birthrights. Since 1918, more than 200 people have claimed to be the Grand Duchess Anastasia.

The solution to the Romanov mystery began in 1979, when a Siberian geologist discovered four skulls in a shallow grave near Ekaterinburg. In the summer of 1991, after the establishment of *glasnost* in the former Soviet Union, exhumation of the site began. Altogether, almost 1000 bone fragments were recovered, which were reassembled into nine skeletons—five females and four males. Based on measurements of the bones and computer-assisted superimposition of the skulls onto photographs, the remains were tentatively identified as belonging to the murdered Romanovs and their four staff members. But there were two missing bodies—those of one daughter and the boy Alexei.

The next step in authenticating the remains involved DNA analysis. The goals were to establish family relationships among the remains, and then to determine, by comparisons with living relatives, whether the family group was in fact the Romanovs. The scientists extracted small amounts of DNA from bone fragments from each skeleton. Genomic DNA typing confirmed the familial relationships between an adult male and female (the presumed parents) and three young females. DNA typing

(continued)

Genetics, Technology, and Society, continued

from four of the adult skeletons revealed that they were not related to each other or to the family group.

After nuclear DNA typing, the scientists analyzed mitochondrial DNA (mtDNA). Since mitochondria are transmitted strictly from mother to offspring, mtDNA sequences can be used to trace maternal lineages without the complicating effects of meiotic crossing over. Scientists determined the nucleotide sequences of two highly variable regions of mtDNA from all nine bone samples. The sequences from the presumed Tsarina Alexandra were an exact match with those from Prince Philip of England, who is her grandnephew, verifying her identity. However, identification was more complicated for the Tsar.

The Tsar's mtDNA sequences were compared with those from two living relatives—the Countess Xenia Cheremeteff-Sfiri (his great-grandniece) and James George Alexander Bannerman Carnegie, third Duke of Fife (descended from a line of women stretching back to the Tsar's grandmother). These comparisons produced a surprise. At position 16,169 of the mtDNA, the Tsar seemed to have either one or another base, a C or a T. The Countess and the Duke, in contrast, had only a T at this position. The conclusion was that Tsar Nicholas had two different populations of mitochondria in his cells, each with a different base at position 16,169 of its DNA. This condition, called heteroplasmy, is now believed to

occur in 10 to 20 percent of humans. To clarify the discrepancy between the Tsar's mtDNA and that of his living relatives, the Russian government granted a request to analyze the remains of the Tsar's younger brother, Grand Duke Georgij Romanov, who died in 1899 of tuberculosis. The Grand Duke's mtDNA contained the same heteroplasmic variant at position 16,169. It was concluded that the Ekaterinburg bones were the doomed imperial family. With years of controversy finally resolved, the authenticated remains of Tsar Nicholas II, Tsarina Alexandra, and three of their daughters were buried in the Saint Peter and Paul Cathedral in Saint Petersburg on July 17, 1998, 80 years to the day after they were murdered.

Your Turn

Take time, individually or in groups, to answer the following questions. Investigate the references and links, to help you understand some of the technologies and issues surrounding the identification of the Romanov family.

1. In 2007, a second grave was discovered near the mass grave of the Romanovs. This one contained the remains of an adolescent male and female, consistent with accounts from eyewitnesses in 1918 that Alexei and one of his sisters had been

buried nearby after unsuccessful attempts to burn their bodies. Were these the remains of the last two Romanovs?

Read about the forensic DNA analyses involved in identifying these remains in Coble, M. D., et al. 2009. Mystery solved: The identification of the two missing Romanov children using DNA analysis. *PLoS ONE* 4: 1–9.

2. One of the most famous people claiming to be Grand Duchess Anastasia was Anna Anderson, who died in the United States in 1984. What types of DNA analyses were used to verify the true identity of Ms. Anderson, and what were the conclusions from these studies?

Begin your search by reading Stoneking, M., et al. 1995. Establishing the identity of Anna Anderson Manahan. *Nature Genet.* 9: 9–10.

3. Alexei Romanov suffered from hemophilia, inherited through his mother from Queen Victoria of England. Historians consider that his condition contributed to the Russian Revolution and the demise of the Romanovs. Explain how this came about and the genetic basis for his disease.

An interesting account of the "Royal Disease" and how Alexei's hemophilia contributed to history can be found in Rogaev, E. I., et al. 2009. Genotype analysis identifies the cause of the "Royal Disease." *Science* 326: 817.

CASE STUDY | A twin difference

In 2000, Rocco Baldelli was a first-round draft pick by the Tampa Bay Rays baseball team. Two years later, his early success in professional baseball was followed by disabling muscle injuries and fatigue. His mysterious illness was traced to a disorder called mitochondrial myopathy. This diagnosis brought not only personal clarification to one set of identical twin brothers, but also national awareness of an array of similar disorders that affect thousands of children and adults regardless of age, gender, race, or position in society. For 14 years the twin brothers competed on equal terms until Rocco began to suffer loss of visual acuity and muscularity. Diagnosis of a mitochondrial disorder explained the cause and forecasted supportive treatment, but also raised some important questions.

1. The parents and other relatives of the twins are apparently healthy, so how could this genetic disorder have arisen?

2. How could one identical twin have an inherited mitochondrial disorder and not the other?

3. Will the unaffected brother be guaranteed continued good health?

Summary Points

1. Patterns of inheritance sometimes vary from those expected from the biparental transmission of nuclear genes. Often, phenotypes appear to result from genetic information transmitted through the ooplasm of the egg.
2. Organelle heredity is based on the genotypes of chloroplast and mitochondrial DNA, as these organelles are transmitted to offspring. Chloroplast mutations affect the photosynthetic capabilities of plants, whereas mitochondrial mutations affect cells highly dependent on energy (ATP) generated through cellular respiration. The resulting mutants display phenotypes related to the loss of function of these organelles.
3. Both chloroplasts and mitochondria first appeared in primitive eukaryotic cells some 2 billion years ago, originating as invad-

ing protobacteria, which then coevolved with the host cell according to the endosymbiotic theory. Evidence in support of this endosymbiotic theory is extensive and centers around many observations involving the DNA and genetic machinery present in modern-day chloroplasts and mitochondria.
4. Mutations in human mtDNA are the underlying causes of a range of heritable genetic disorders in humans.
5. Maternal-effect patterns result when nuclear gene products expressed by the maternal genotype of the egg influence early development. Coiling in snails and gene expression during early development in *Drosophila* are examples.

INSIGHTS AND SOLUTIONS

1. Analyze the following hypothetical pedigree, determine the most consistent interpretation of how the trait is inherited, and point out any inconsistencies:

Solution: The trait is passed from all affected male parents to all but one offspring, but it is *never* passed maternally. Individual IV-7 (a female) is the only exception.

2. Can the explanation in Solution 1 be attributed to a gene on the Y chromosome? Defend your answer.

Solution: No, because male parents pass the trait to their daughters as well as to their sons.

3. Is the above pedigree an example of a paternal effect or of paternal inheritance?

Solution: It has all the characteristics of paternal inheritance because males pass the trait to almost all of their offspring. To assess whether the trait is due to a paternal effect (resulting from a nuclear gene in the male gamete), analysis of further matings would be needed.

Problems and Discussion Questions

HOW DO WE KNOW?

1. In this chapter, we focused on extranuclear inheritance and how traits can be determined by genetic information contained in mitochondria and chloroplasts, and we discussed how expression of maternal genotypes can affect the phenotype of an organism. At the same time, we found many opportunities to consider the methods and reasoning by which much of this information was acquired. From the explanations given in the chapter, what answers would you propose to the following fundamental questions?
(a) How was it established that particular phenotypes are inherited as a result of genetic information present in the chloroplast rather than in the nucleus?

(b) How did the discovery of three categories of *petite* mutations in yeast lead researchers to postulate extranuclear inheritance of colony size?
(c) What observations support the endosymbiotic theory?
(d) What key observations in crosses between dextrally and sinistrally coiled snails support the explanation that this phenotype is the result of maternal-effect inheritance?
(e) What findings demonstrate a maternal effect as the basis of a mode of inheritance?

CONCEPT QUESTION

2. Review the Chapter Concepts list on page 214. The first three center around extranuclear inheritance involving DNA in

organelles. The fourth involves what is called maternal effect. Write a short essay that distinguishes between organelle heredity and maternal effect.

3. Streptomycin resistance in *Chlamydomonas* may result from a mutation in either a chloroplast gene or a nuclear gene. What phenotypic results would occur in a cross between a member of an mt^+ strain resistant in both genes and a member of a strain sensitive to the antibiotic? What results would occur in the reciprocal cross?

4. A plant may have green, white, or green-and-white (variegated) leaves on its branches, owing to a mutation in the chloroplast that prevents color from developing. Predict the results of the following crosses:

Ovule Source		Pollen Source
(a) Green branch	×	White branch
(b) White branch	×	Green branch
(c) Variegated branch	×	Green branch
(d) Green branch	×	Variegated branch

5. In diploid yeast strains, sporulation and subsequent meiosis can produce haploid ascospores, which may fuse to reestablish diploid cells. When ascospores from a *segregational petite* strain fuse with those of a normal wild-type strain, the diploid zygotes are all normal. Following meiosis, ascospores are *petite* and normal. Is the *segregational petite* phenotype inherited as a dominant or a recessive trait?

6. Predict the results of a cross between ascospores from a *segregational petite* strain and a *neutral petite* strain. Indicate the phenotype of the zygote and the ascospores it may subsequently produce.

7. In *Lymnaea*, what results would you expect in a cross between a *Dd* dextrally coiled and a *Dd* sinistrally coiled snail, assuming cross-fertilization occurs as shown in Figure 9–11? What results would occur if the *Dd* dextral produced only eggs and the *Dd* sinistral produced only sperm?

8. In a cross of *Lymnaea*, the snail contributing the eggs was dextral but of unknown genotype. Both the genotype and the phenotype of the other snail are unknown. All F_1 offspring exhibited dextral coiling. Ten of the F_1 snails were allowed to undergo self-fertilization. One-half produced only dextrally coiled offspring, whereas the other half produced only sinistrally coiled offspring. What were the genotypes of the original parents?

9. In *Drosophila subobscura*, the presence of a recessive gene called *grandchildless* (*gs*) causes the offspring of homozygous females, but not those of homozygous males, to be sterile. Can you offer an explanation as to why females and not males are affected by the mutant gene?

10. A male mouse from a true-breeding strain of hyperactive animals is crossed with a female mouse from a true-breeding strain of lethargic animals. (These are both hypothetical strains.) All the progeny are lethargic. In the F_2 generation, all offspring are lethargic. What is the best genetic explanation for these observations? Propose a cross to test your explanation.

11. Consider the case where a mutation occurs that disrupts translation in a single human mitochondrion found in the oocyte participating in fertilization. What is the likely impact of this mutation on the offspring arising from this oocyte?

12. What is the endosymbiotic theory, and why is this theory relevant to the study of extranuclear DNA in eukaryotic organelles?

13. In an earlier Problems and Discussion section (see Chapter 7, Problem 33), we described CC, the cat created by nuclear transfer cloning, whereby a diploid nucleus from one cell is injected into an enucleated egg cell to create an embryo. Cattle, sheep, rats, dogs, and several other species have been cloned using nuclei from somatic cells. Embryos and adults produced by this approach often show a number of different mitochondrial defects. Explain possible reasons for the prevalence of mitochondrial defects in embryos created by nuclear transfer cloning.

Extra-Spicy Problems

14. The specification of the anterior–posterior axis in *Drosophila* embryos is initially controlled by various gene products that are synthesized and stored in the mature egg following oogenesis. Mutations in these genes result in abnormalities of the axis during embryogenesis. These mutations illustrate *maternal effect*. How do such mutations vary from those produced by organelle heredity? Devise a set of parallel crosses and expected outcomes involving mutant genes that contrast maternal effect and organelle heredity.

15. The maternal-effect mutation *bicoid* (*bcd*) is recessive. In the absence of the bicoid protein product, embryogenesis is not completed. Consider a cross between a female heterozygous for the *bicoid* alleles (bcd^+/bcd^-) and a male homozygous for the mutation (bcd^-/bcd^-).
(a) How is it possible for a male homozygous for the mutation to exist?

(b) Predict the outcome (normal vs. failed embryogenesis) in the F_1 and F_2 generations of the cross described.

16. (a) In humans the mitochondrial genome encodes a low number of proteins, rRNAs, and tRNAs but imports approximately 1100 proteins encoded by the nuclear genome. Yet, with such a small proportion from the mitochondrial genome encoding proteins and RNAs, a disproportionately high number of genetic disorders due to mtDNA mutations have been identified (Bigger, B. et al. 1999). What inheritance pattern would you expect in a three-generation pedigree in which the grandfather expresses the initial mtDNA defect? What inheritance pattern would you expect in a three-generation pedigree in which the grandmother expresses the initial mtDNA defect?
(b) Considering the description in part (a) above, how would your pedigrees change if you knew that the mutation that caused the mitochondrial defect was recessive and located in

the nuclear genome, was successfully transported into mitochondria, and negated a physiologically important mitochondrial function?

17. Mutations in mitochondrial DNA appear to be responsible for a number of neurological disorders, including myoclonic epilepsy and ragged-red fiber disease, Leber's hereditary optic neuropathy, and Kearns–Sayre syndrome. In each case, the disease phenotype is expressed when the ratio of mutant to wild-type mitochondria exceeds a threshold peculiar to each disease, but usually in the 60 to 95 percent range.

(a) Given that these are debilitating conditions, why has no cure been developed? Can you suggest a general approach that might be used to treat, or perhaps even cure, these disorders?

(b) Compared with the vast number of mitochondria in an embryo, the number of mitochondria in an ovum is relatively small. Might such an ooplasmic mitochondrial bottleneck present an opportunity for therapy or cure? Explain.

18. Researchers examined a family with an interesting distribution of Leigh syndrome symptoms. In this disorder, individuals may show a progressive loss of motor function (ataxia, A) with peripheral neuropathy (PN, meaning impairment of the peripheral nerves). A mitochondrial DNA (mtDNA) mutation that reduces ATPase activity was identified in various tissues of affected individuals. The accompanying table summarizes the presence of symptoms in an extended family.

Person	Condition	Percent Mitochondria with Mutation
Proband	A and PN	>90%
Brother	A and PN	>90%
Brother	Asymptomatic	17%
Mother	PN	86%
Maternal uncle	PN	85%
Maternal cousin	A and PN	90%
Maternal cousin	A and PN	91%
Maternal grandmother	Asymptomatic	56%

(a) Develop a pedigree that summarizes the information presented in the table.

(b) Provide an explanation for the pattern of inheritance of the disease. What term describes this pattern?

(c) How can some individuals in the same family show such variation in symptoms? What term, as related to organelle heredity, describes such variation?

(d) In what way does a condition caused by mtDNA differ in expression and transmission from a mutation that causes albinism?

19. Payne, B. A. et al. (2013) present evidence that a low level of heteroplasmic mtDNA exists in all tested healthy individuals.

(a) What are two likely sources of such heteroplasmy?

(b) What genetic conditions within a given mitochondrion are likely to contribute to such a variable pool of mitochondria?

10 DNA Structure and Analysis

CHAPTER CONCEPTS

- Except in some viruses, DNA serves as the genetic material in all living organisms on Earth.

- According to the Watson–Crick model, DNA exists in the form of a right-handed double helix.

- The strands of the double helix are antiparallel and are held together by hydrogen bonding between complementary nitrogenous bases.

- The structure of DNA provides the means of storing and expressing genetic information.

- RNA has many similarities to DNA but exists mostly as a single-stranded molecule.

- In some viruses, RNA serves as the genetic material.

- Many techniques have been developed that facilitate the analysis of nucleic acids, most based on detection of the complementarity of nitrogenous bases.

U p to this point in the text, we have described chromosomes as containing genes that control phenotypic traits transmitted through gametes to future offspring. Logically, genes must contain some sort of information that, when passed to a new generation, influences the form and characteristics of each individual. We refer to that information as the **genetic material**. Logic also suggests that this same information in some way directs the many complex processes that lead to an organism's adult form.

Until 1944, it was not clear what chemical component of the chromosome makes up genes and constitutes the genetic material. Because chromosomes were known to have both a nucleic acid and a protein component, both were candidates. In 1944, however, direct experimental evidence emerged showing that the nucleic acid DNA serves as the informational basis for the process of heredity.

Once the importance of DNA to genetic processes was realized, work was intensified with the hope of discerning not only the structure of this molecule but also the relationship of its structure to its function. Between 1944 and 1953, many scientists sought information that might answer the most significant and intriguing question in the history of biology: How does DNA serve as the genetic basis for living processes? Researchers believed the answer must depend strongly on the chemical structure of the DNA molecule, given the complex but orderly functions ascribed to it.

These efforts were rewarded in 1953, when James Watson and Francis Crick put forth their hypothesis for the double-helical nature of DNA. The assumption that the molecule's functions would be easier to clarify once its general structure was determined proved to be correct. In this chapter, we first review the evidence that DNA is the genetic material and then discuss the elucidation of its structure. We conclude the chapter with a discussion of various analytical techniques useful during the investigation of the nucleic acids, DNA and RNA.

Please note that some of the topics discussed in this chapter are explored in greater depth later in the text (see Special Topic Chapter 2—Emerging Roles of RNA).

10.1 The Genetic Material Must Exhibit Four Characteristics

For a molecule to serve as the genetic material, it must exhibit four crucial characteristics: **replication, storage of information, expression of information**, and **variation by mutation**. *Replication* of the genetic material is one facet of the cell cycle and as such is a fundamental property of all living organisms. Once the genetic material of cells replicates and is doubled in amount, it must then be partitioned equally—through mitosis—into daughter cells. The genetic material is also replicated during the formation of gametes, but is partitioned so that each cell gets only one-half of the original amount of genetic material—the process of *meiosis* (discussed in Chapter 2). Although the products of mitosis and meiosis are different, these processes are both part of the more general phenomenon of cellular reproduction.

Storage of information requires the molecule to act as a repository of genetic information that may or may not be expressed by the cell in which it resides. It is clear that while most cells contain a complete copy of the organism's genome, at any point in time they express only a part of this genetic potential. For example, in bacteria many genes "turn on" in response to specific environmental cues and "turn off" when conditions change. In vertebrates, skin cells may display active melanin genes but never activate their hemoglobin genes; in contrast, digestive cells activate many genes specific to their function but do not activate their melanin genes.

Inherent in the concept of storage is the need for the genetic material to be able to encode the vast variety of gene products found among the countless forms of life on our planet. The chemical language of the genetic material must have the capability of storing such diverse information and transmitting it to progeny cells and organisms.

Expression of the stored genetic information is a complex process that is the underlying basis for the concept of **information flow** within the cell (**Figure 10–1**). The initial event in this flow of information is the **transcription** of DNA, in which three main types of RNA molecules are synthesized: messenger RNA (mRNA), transfer RNA (tRNA), and ribosomal RNA (rRNA). Of these, mRNAs are translated into proteins, by means of a process mediated by the tRNA and rRNA. Each mRNA is the product of a specific gene and leads to the synthesis of a different protein. In

FIGURE 10–1 Simplified diagram of information flow (the central dogma) from DNA to RNA to produce the proteins within cells.

translation, the chemical information in mRNA directs the construction of a chain of amino acids, called a polypeptide, which then folds into a protein. Collectively, these processes serve as the foundation for the **central dogma of molecular genetics**: "DNA makes RNA, which makes proteins."

The genetic material is also the source of *variability* among organisms, through the process of mutation. If a mutation—a change in the chemical composition of DNA—occurs, the alteration is reflected during transcription and translation, affecting the specific protein. If a mutation is present in a gamete, it may be passed to future generations and, with time, become distributed in the population. Genetic variation, which also includes alterations of chromosome number and rearrangements within and between chromosomes (as discussed in Chapter 8), provides the raw material for the process of evolution.

10.2 Until 1944, Observations Favored Protein as the Genetic Material

The idea that genetic material is physically transmitted from parent to offspring has been accepted for as long as the concept of inheritance has existed. Beginning in the late nineteenth century, research into the structure of biomolecules progressed considerably, setting the stage for describing the genetic material in chemical terms. Although proteins and nucleic acid were both considered major candidates for the role of genetic material, until the 1940s many geneticists favored proteins.

This is not surprising, since proteins were known to be both diverse and abundant in cells, and much more was known about protein than about nucleic acid chemistry.

DNA was first studied in 1869 by a Swiss chemist, Friedrich Miescher. He isolated cell nuclei and derived an acidic substance, now known to contain DNA, that he called **nuclein.** As investigations of DNA progressed, however, showing it to be present in chromosomes, the substance seemed to lack the chemical diversity necessary to store extensive genetic information.

This conclusion was based largely on Phoebus A. Levene's observations in 1910 that DNA contained approximately equal amounts of four similar molecules called *nucleotides*. Levene postulated incorrectly that identical groups of these four components were repeated over and over, which was the basis of his **tetranucleotide hypothesis** for DNA structure. Attention was thus directed away from DNA, thereby favoring proteins. However, in the 1940s, Erwin Chargaff showed that Levene's proposal was incorrect when he demonstrated that most organisms do not contain precisely equal proportions of the four nucleotides. We shall see later that the structure of DNA accounts for Chargaff's observations.

10.3 Evidence Favoring DNA as the Genetic Material Was First Obtained during the Study of Bacteria and Bacteriophages

The 1944 publication by Oswald Avery, Colin MacLeod, and Maclyn McCarty concerning the chemical nature of a "transforming principle" in bacteria was the initial event leading to the acceptance of DNA as the genetic material. Their work, along with subsequent findings of other research teams, constituted the first direct experimental proof that DNA, and not protein, is the biomolecule responsible for heredity. It marked the beginning of the *era of molecular genetics*, a period of discovery in biology that made biotechnology feasible and has moved us closer to an understanding of the basis of life. The impact of their initial findings on future research and thinking paralleled that of the publication of Darwin's theory of evolution and the subsequent rediscovery of Mendel's postulates of transmission genetics. Together, these events constitute three great revolutions in biology.

Transformation: Early Studies

The research that provided the foundation for Avery, MacLeod, and McCarty's work was initiated in 1927 by Frederick Griffith, a medical officer in the British Ministry of Health. He performed experiments with several different strains of the bacterium *Diplococcus pneumoniae*.* Some were *virulent*, that is, infectious, strains that cause pneumonia in certain vertebrates (notably humans and mice), whereas others were *avirulent*, or noninfectious strains, which do not cause illness.

The difference in virulence depends on the presence of a polysaccharide capsule; virulent strains have this capsule, whereas avirulent strains do not. The nonencapsulated bacteria are readily engulfed and destroyed by phagocytic cells in the host animal's circulatory system. Virulent bacteria, which possess the polysaccharide coat, are not easily engulfed; they multiply and cause pneumonia.

The presence or absence of the capsule causes a visible difference between colonies of virulent and avirulent strains. Encapsulated bacteria form smooth, shiny-surfaced colonies (*S*) when grown on an agar culture plate; nonencapsulated strains produce rough colonies (*R*). Thus, virulent and avirulent strains are easily distinguished by standard microbiological culture techniques.

Each strain of *Diplococcus* may be one of dozens of different types called *serotypes* that differ in the precise chemical structure of the polysaccharide constituent of the thick, slimy capsule. Serotypes are identified by immunological techniques and are usually designated by Roman numerals. In the United States, types I and II are the most common in causing pneumonia. Griffith used types II*R* and III*S* in his critical experiments that led to new concepts about the genetic material. Table 10.1 summarizes the characteristics of Griffith's two strains, while **Figure 10–2** on p. 234 depicts his experiment.

Griffith knew from the work of others that only living virulent cells would produce pneumonia in mice. If heat-killed virulent bacteria are injected into mice, no pneumonia results, just as living avirulent bacteria fail to produce the disease. Griffith's critical experiment (Figure 10–2) involved an injection into mice of living II*R* (avirulent) cells combined with heat-killed III*S* (virulent) cells. Since neither cell type caused death in mice when injected alone, Griffith expected that the double injection would not kill the mice. But, after five days, all of the mice that received both types of cells were dead. Paradoxically, analysis of their blood revealed a large number of living type III*S* (virulent) bacteria.

As far as could be determined, these III*S* bacteria were identical to the III*S* strain from which the heat-killed cell preparation had been made. The control mice, injected

TABLE 10.1   Strains of *Diplococcus pneumonia* Used by Frederick Griffith in His Original Transformation Experiments

Serotype	Colony Morphology	Capsule	Virulence
II*R*	Rough	Absent	Avirulent
III*S*	Smooth	Present	Virulent

*This organism is now named *Streptococcus pneumoniae*.

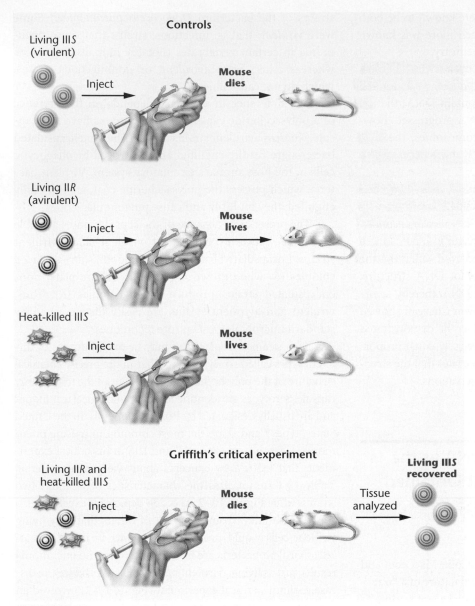

Controls

Living IIIS
(virulent)

Inject → Mouse dies →

Living IIR
(avirulent)

Inject → Mouse lives →

Heat-killed IIIS

Inject → Mouse lives →

Griffith's critical experiment

Living IIR and
heat-killed IIIS

Inject → Mouse dies → Tissue analyzed → Living IIIS recovered

FIGURE 10–2 Griffith's transformation experiment.

Griffith's work led other physicians and bacteriologists to research the phenomenon of transformation. By 1931, M. Henry Dawson at the Rockefeller Institute had confirmed Griffith's observations and extended his work one step further. Dawson and his coworkers showed that transformation could occur *in vitro* (in a test tube). When heat-killed IIIS cells were incubated with living IIR cells, living IIIS cells were recovered. Therefore, injection into mice was not necessary for transformation to occur. By 1933, J. Lionel Alloway had refined the *in vitro* experiments by using crude extracts of IIIS cells and living IIR cells. The soluble filtrate from the heat-killed IIIS cells was as effective in inducing transformation as were the intact cells. Alloway and others did not view transformation as a genetic event, but rather as a physiological modification of some sort. Nevertheless, the experimental evidence that a chemical substance was responsible for transformation was quite convincing.

Transformation: The Avery, MacLeod, and McCarty Experiment

The critical question, of course, was what molecule serves as the transforming principle? In 1944, after 10 years of work, Avery, MacLeod, and McCarty published their results in what is now regarded as a classic paper in the field of molecular genetics. They reported that they had obtained the transforming principle in a purified state and that beyond reasonable doubt it was DNA.

The details of their work, sometimes called the Avery, MacLeod, and McCarty experiment, are outlined in **Figure 10–3**. These researchers began their isolation procedure with large quantities (50–75 liters) of liquid cultures of type IIIS virulent cells. The cells were centrifuged, collected, and heat killed. Following homogenization and several extractions with the detergent deoxycholate (DOC), the researchers obtained a soluble filtrate that retained the ability to induce transformation of type IIR avirulent cells. Protein was removed from the active filtrate by several chloroform extractions, and polysaccharides were enzymatically digested and

only with living avirulent IIR bacteria for this set of experiments, did not develop pneumonia and remained healthy. This ruled out the possibility that the avirulent IIR cells simply changed (or mutated) to virulent IIIS cells in the absence of the heat-killed IIIS bacteria. Instead, some type of interaction had taken place between living IIR and heat-killed IIIS cells.

Griffith concluded that the heat-killed IIIS bacteria somehow converted live avirulent IIR cells into virulent IIIS cells. Calling the phenomenon **transformation**, he suggested that the *transforming principle* might be some part of the polysaccharide capsule or a compound required for capsule synthesis, although the capsule alone did not cause pneumonia. To use Griffith's term, the transforming principle from the dead IIIS cells served as a "pabulum"— that is, a nutrient source—for the IIR cells.

FIGURE 10-3 Summary of Avery, MacLeod, and McCarty's experiment demonstrating that DNA is the transforming principle.

removed. Finally, precipitation with ethanol yielded a fibrous mass that still retained the ability to induce transformation of type IIR avirulent cells. From the original 75-liter sample, the procedure yielded 10 to 25 mg of this "active factor."

Further testing clearly established that the transforming principle was DNA. The fibrous mass was first analyzed for its nitrogen: phosphorus ratio, which was shown to coincide with the ratio of "sodium desoxyribonucleate," the chemical name then used to describe DNA. To solidify their findings, Avery, MacLeod, and McCarty sought to eliminate, to the greatest extent possible, all probable contaminants from their final product. Thus, it was treated with the proteolytic enzymes trypsin and chymotrypsin and then with an RNA-digesting enzyme, called **ribonuclease (RNase)**. Such treatments destroyed any remaining activity of proteins and RNA. Nevertheless, transforming activity still remained. Chemical testing of the final product gave strong positive reactions for DNA.

The final confirmation came with experiments using crude samples of the DNA-digesting enzyme **deoxyribonuclease (DNase)**, which was isolated from dog and rabbit sera. Digestion with this enzyme destroyed the transforming activity of the filtrate—thus Avery and his coworkers were certain that the active transforming principle in these experiments was DNA.

The great amount of work involved in this research, the confirmation and reconfirmation of the conclusions drawn, and the unambiguous logic of the experimental design are truly impressive. Avery, MacLeod, and McCarty's conclusion in the 1944 publication was, however, very simply stated: "The evidence presented supports the belief that a nucleic acid of the desoxyribose* type is the fundamental unit of the transforming principle of *Pneumococcus* Type III."

_____

*Desoxyribose is now spelled deoxyribose.

Avery and his colleagues recognized the genetic and biochemical implications of their work. They observed that "nucleic acids of this type must be regarded not merely as structurally important but as functionally active in determining the biochemical activities and specific characteristics of pneumococcal cells." This suggested that the transforming principle interacts with the II*R* cell and gives rise to a coordinated series of enzymatic reactions culminating in the synthesis of the type III*S* capsular polysaccharide. Avery, MacLeod, and McCarty emphasized that, once transformation occurs, the capsular polysaccharide is produced in successive generations. Transformation is therefore heritable, and the process affects the genetic material.

Immediately after publication of the report, several investigators turned to, or intensified, their studies of transformation in order to clarify the role of DNA in genetic mechanisms. In particular, the work of Rollin Hotchkiss was instrumental in confirming that the critical factor in transformation was DNA and not protein. In 1949, in a separate study, Harriet Taylor isolated an **extremely rough** (*ER*) mutant strain from a rough (*R*) strain. This *ER* strain produced colonies that were more irregular than the *R* strain. The DNA from *R* accomplished the transformation of *ER* to *R*. Thus, the *R* strain, which served as the recipient in the Avery experiments, was shown also to be able to serve as the DNA donor in transformation.

Transformation has now been shown to occur in *Haemophilus influenzae, Bacillus subtilis, Shigella paradysenteriae*, and *Escherichia coli*, among many other microorganisms. Transformation of numerous genetic traits other than colony morphology has also been demonstrated, including traits involving resistance to antibiotics. These observations further strengthened the belief that transformation by DNA is primarily a genetic event rather than simply a physiological change. We will pursue this idea again in the "Insights and Solutions" section at the end of this chapter.

The Hershey–Chase Experiment

The second major piece of evidence supporting DNA as the genetic material was provided during the study of the bacterium *Escherichia coli* and one of its infecting viruses, **bacteriophage T2**. Often referred to simply as a **phage**, the virus consists of a protein coat surrounding a core of DNA. Electron micrographs reveal that the phage's external structure is composed of a hexagonal head plus a tail. **Figure 10–4** shows as much of the life cycle as was known

FIGURE 10–4 Life cycle of a T-even bacteriophage, as known in 1952. The electron micrograph shows an *E. coli* cell during infection by numerous T2 phages (shown in blue).

in 1952 for a T-even bacteriophage such as T2. Briefly, the phage adsorbs to the bacterial cell, and some genetic component of the phage enters the bacterial cell. Following infection, the viral component "commandeers" the cellular machinery of the host and causes viral reproduction. In a reasonably short time, many new phages are constructed and the bacterial cell is lysed, releasing the progeny viruses. This process is referred to as the **lytic cycle**.

In 1952, Alfred Hershey and Martha Chase published the results of experiments designed to clarify the events leading to phage reproduction. Several of the experiments clearly established the independent functions of phage protein and nucleic acid in the reproduction process associated with the bacterial cell. Hershey and Chase knew from existing data that:

1. T2 phages consist of approximately 50 percent protein and 50 percent DNA.

2. Infection is initiated by adsorption of the phage by its tail fibers to the bacterial cell.

3. The production of new viruses occurs within the bacterial cell.

It appeared that some molecular component of the phage—DNA or protein (or both)—entered the bacterial cell and directed viral reproduction. Which was it?

Hershey and Chase used the radioisotopes ^{32}P and ^{35}S to follow the molecular components of phages during infection. Because DNA contains phosphorus (P) but not sulfur, ^{32}P effectively labels DNA; because proteins contain sulfur (S) but not phosphorus, ^{35}S labels protein. *This is a key feature of the experiment.* If *E. coli* cells are first grown in the presence of ^{32}P *or* ^{35}S and then infected with T2 viruses, the progeny phages will have *either* a radioactively labeled DNA core *or* a radioactively labeled protein coat, respectively. These labeled phages can be isolated and used to infect unlabeled bacteria (**Figure 10–5**).

When labeled phages and unlabeled bacteria were mixed, an adsorption complex was formed as the phages attached their tail fibers to the bacterial wall. These complexes were isolated and subjected to a high shear force in a blender. The force stripped off the attached phages so that the phages and bacteria could be analyzed separately. Centrifugation separated the lighter phage particles from the heavier bacterial cells (Figure 10–5). By tracing the radioisotopes, Hershey and Chase were able to demonstrate that most of the ^{32}P-labeled DNA had been transferred into the bacterial cell following adsorption; on the other hand, almost all of the ^{35}S-labeled protein remained outside the bacterial cell and was recovered in the phage "ghosts" (empty phage coats) after the blender treatment.

Following this separation, the bacterial cells, which now contained viral DNA, were eventually lysed as new phages were produced. These progeny phages contained ^{32}P, but not ^{35}S.

Hershey and Chase interpreted these results as indicating that the protein of the phage coat remains outside the host cell and is not involved in directing the production of new phages. On the other hand, and most important, phage DNA enters the host cell and directs phage reproduction. Hershey and Chase had demonstrated that the genetic material in phage T2 is DNA, not protein.

These experiments, along with those of Avery and his colleagues, provided convincing evidence that DNA was the molecule responsible for heredity. This conclusion has since served as the cornerstone of the field of molecular genetics.

NOW SOLVE THIS

10–1 Would an experiment similar to that performed by Hershey and Chase work if the basic design were applied to the phenomenon of transformation? Explain why or why not.

■ **HINT:** *This problem involves an understanding of the protocol of the Hershey–Chase experiment as applied to the investigation of transformation. The key to its solution is to remember that in transformation, exogenous DNA enters the soon-to-be transformed cell and that no cell-to-cell contact is involved in the process.*

Transfection Experiments

During the eight years following publication of the Hershey–Chase experiment, additional research using bacterial viruses provided even more solid proof that DNA is the genetic material. In 1957, several reports demonstrated that if *E. coli* is treated with the enzyme lysozyme, the outer wall of the cell can be removed without destroying the bacterium. Enzymatically treated cells are naked, so to speak, and contain only the cell membrane as their outer boundary. Such structures are called **protoplasts** (or **spheroplasts**). John Spizizen and Dean Fraser independently reported that by using protoplasts, they were able to initiate phage reproduction with disrupted T2 particles. That is, provided protoplasts were used, a virus did not have to be intact for infection to occur. Thus, the outer protein coat structure may be essential to the movement of DNA through the intact cell wall, but it is not essential for infection when protoplasts are used.

Similar, but more refined, experiments were reported in 1960 by George Guthrie and Robert Sinsheimer. DNA was purified from bacteriophage ϕX174, a small phage

Phage T2 (unlabeled)

Phage added to *E. coli* in radioactive medium

(▇ ³²P or ³⁵S ▇)

³²P

³⁵S

Progeny phages become labeled

Labeled phages infect unlabeled bacteria

Separation of phage "ghosts" from bacterial cells

Phage "ghosts" are unlabeled + Infected bacteria are labeled with ³²P

Phage "ghosts" are labeled with ³⁵S + Infected bacteria are unlabeled

Viable ³²P-labeled phages are produced

Viable unlabeled phages produced

FIGURE 10–5 Summary of the Hershey–Chase experiment demonstrating that DNA, and not protein, is responsible for directing the reproduction of phage T2 during the infection of *E. coli*.

that contains a single-stranded circular DNA molecule of some 5386 nucleotides. When added to *E. coli* protoplasts, the purified DNA resulted in the production of complete φX174 bacteriophages. This process of infection by only the viral nucleic acid, called **transfection**, proves conclusively

that φX174 DNA alone contains all the necessary information for production of mature viruses. Thus, the evidence that DNA serves as the genetic material was further strengthened, even though all direct evidence to that point had been obtained from bacterial and viral studies.

10.4 Indirect and Direct Evidence Supports the Concept that DNA Is the Genetic Material in Eukaryotes

In 1950, eukaryotic organisms were not amenable to the types of experiments that used bacteria and viruses to demonstrate that DNA is the genetic material. Nevertheless, it was generally assumed that the genetic material would be a universal substance serving the same role in eukaryotes. Initially, support for this assumption relied on several circumstantial observations that, taken together, indicated that DNA does serve as the genetic material in eukaryotes. Subsequently, direct evidence established unequivocally the central role of DNA in genetic processes.

Indirect Evidence: Distribution of DNA

The genetic material should be found where it functions—in the nucleus as part of chromosomes. Both DNA and protein fit this criterion. However, protein is also abundant in the cytoplasm, whereas DNA is not. Both mitochondria and chloroplasts are known to perform genetic functions, and DNA is also present in these organelles. Thus, DNA is found only where primary genetic functions occur. Protein, on the other hand, is found everywhere in the cell. These observations are consistent with the interpretation favoring DNA over proteins as the genetic material.

Because it had earlier been established that chromosomes within the nucleus contain the genetic material, a correlation was expected to exist between the ploidy (n, $2n$, etc.) of a cell and the quantity of the substance that functions as the genetic material. Meaningful comparisons can be made between gametes (sperm and eggs) and somatic or body cells. The latter are recognized as being diploid ($2n$) and containing twice the number of chromosomes as gametes, which are haploid (n).

Table 10.2 compares, for a variety of organisms, the amount of DNA found in haploid sperm to the amount found in diploid nucleated precursors of red blood cells. The amount of DNA and the number of sets of chromosomes is closely

TABLE 10.2 DNA Content of Haploid versus Diploid Cells of Various Species*

Organism	n (pg)	2n (pg)
Human	3.25	7.30
Chicken	1.26	2.49
Trout	2.67	5.79
Carp	1.65	3.49
Shad	0.91	1.97

*Sperm (n) and nucleated precursors to red blood cells ($2n$) were used to contrast ploidy levels.

correlated. No such consistent correlation can be observed between gametes and diploid cells for proteins. These data thus provide further circumstantial evidence favoring DNA over proteins as the genetic material of eukaryotes.

Indirect Evidence: Mutagenesis

Ultraviolet (UV) light is one of a number of agents capable of inducing mutations in the genetic material. Simple organisms such as yeast and other fungi can be irradiated with various wavelengths of ultraviolet light and the effectiveness of each wavelength measured by the number of mutations it induces. When the data are plotted, an **action spectrum** of UV light as a mutagenic agent is obtained. This action spectrum can then be compared with the **absorption spectrum** of any molecule suspected to be the genetic material (**Figure 10–6**). *The molecule serving as the genetic material is expected to absorb at the wavelength(s) found to be mutagenic.*

UV light is most mutagenic at the wavelength l of 260 nanometers (nm), and both DNA and RNA absorb UV light most strongly at 260 nm. On the other hand, protein absorbs most strongly at 280 nm, yet no significant mutagenic effects are observed at that wavelength. This indirect evidence supports the idea that a nucleic acid, rather than protein, is the genetic material.

Direct Evidence: Recombinant DNA Studies

Although the circumstantial evidence just described does not constitute direct proof that DNA is the genetic material

— Nucleic acids
— Proteins

FIGURE 10–6 Comparison of the action spectrum (which determines the most effective mutagenic UV wavelength) and the absorption spectrum (which shows the range of wavelength where nucleic acids and proteins absorb UV light).

in eukaryotes, those observations spurred researchers to forge ahead using this supposition as the underlying hypothesis. Today, there is no doubt of its validity; DNA *is* the genetic material in all eukaryotes. The strongest evidence is provided by molecular analysis utilizing **recombinant DNA technology**. In this procedure, segments of eukaryotic DNA corresponding to specific genes are isolated and spliced into bacterial DNA. The resulting complex can be inserted into a bacterial cell, and then its genetic expression is monitored. If a eukaryotic gene is introduced, the subsequent production of the corresponding eukaryotic protein product demonstrates directly that the eukaryotic DNA is now present and functional in the bacterial cell. This has been shown to be the case in countless instances. For example, the products of the human genes specifying insulin and interferon are produced by bacteria after the human genes that encode these proteins are inserted. As the bacterium divides, the eukaryotic DNA replicates along with the bacterial DNA and is distributed to the daughter cells, which also express the human genes by creating the corresponding proteins.

The availability of vast amounts of DNA coding for specific genes, derived from recombinant DNA research, has led to other direct evidence that DNA serves as the genetic material. Work in the laboratory of Beatrice Mintz has demonstrated that DNA encoding the human *β-globin* gene, when microinjected into a fertilized mouse egg, is later found to be present and expressed in adult mouse tissue and transmitted to and expressed in that mouse's progeny. These mice are examples of what are called **transgenic animals**. Other work has introduced rat DNA encoding a growth hormone into fertilized mouse eggs. About one-third of the resultant mice grew to twice their normal size, indicating that foreign DNA was present and functional. Subsequent generations of mice inherited this genetic information and also grew to a large size. This clearly demonstrates that DNA meets the requirement of expression of genetic information in eukaryotes. Later, we will see exactly how DNA is stored, replicated, expressed, and mutated.

10.5 RNA Serves as the Genetic Material in Some Viruses

Some viruses contain an RNA core rather than a DNA core. In these viruses, it appears that RNA serves as the genetic material—an exception to the general rule that DNA performs this function. In 1956, it was demonstrated that when purified RNA from **tobacco mosaic virus (TMV)** was spread on tobacco leaves, the characteristic lesions caused by viral infection subsequently appeared. Thus, it was concluded that RNA is the genetic material of this virus.

In 1965 and 1966, Norman Pace and Sol Spiegelman demonstrated that RNA from the phage Qβ can be isolated and replicated *in vitro*. Replication depends on an enzyme, **RNA replicase**, which is isolated from host *E. coli* cells following normal infection. When the RNA replicated *in vitro* is added to *E. coli* protoplasts, infection and viral multiplication (*transfection*) occur. Thus, RNA synthesized in a test tube serves as the genetic material in these phages by directing the production of all the components necessary for viral reproduction. While many viruses, such the T2 virus used by Hershey and Chase, use DNA as their hereditary material, another group of RNA-containing viruses bears mention. These are the **retroviruses**, which replicate in an unusual way. Their RNA serves as a template for the synthesis of the complementary DNA molecule. The process, **reverse transcription**, occurs under the direction of an RNA-dependent DNA polymerase enzyme called **reverse transcriptase**. This DNA intermediate can be incorporated into the genome of the host cell, and when the host DNA is transcribed, copies of the original retroviral RNA chromosomes are produced. Retroviruses include the human immunodeficiency virus (HIV), which causes AIDS, as well as several RNA tumor viruses.

10.6 Knowledge of Nucleic Acid Chemistry Is Essential to the Understanding of DNA Structure

Having established the critical importance of DNA and RNA in genetic processes, we will now take a brief look at the chemical structures of these molecules. As we shall see, the structural components of DNA and RNA are very similar. This chemical similarity is important in the coordinated functions played by these molecules during gene expression. Like the other major groups of organic biomolecules (proteins, carbohydrates, and lipids), nucleic acid chemistry is based on a variety of similar building blocks that are polymerized into chains of varying lengths.

Nucleotides: Building Blocks of Nucleic Acids

DNA is a nucleic acid, and **nucleotides** are the building blocks of all nucleic acid molecules. Sometimes called mononucleotides, these structural units consist of three essential components: a **nitrogenous base**, a **pentose sugar** (a 5-carbon sugar), and a **phosphate group**. There are two kinds of nitrogenous bases: the nine-member double-ring **purines** and the six-member single-ring **pyrimidines**.

Two types of purines and three types of pyrimidines are commonly found in nucleic acids. The two purines are **adenine** and **guanine**, abbreviated **A** and **G**. The three

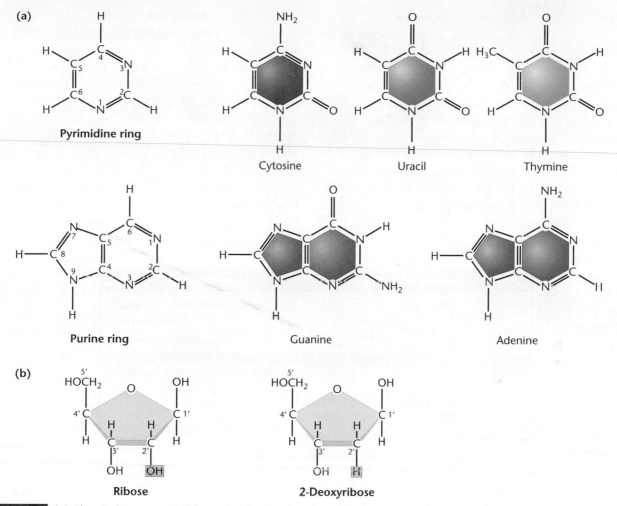

FIGURE 10-7 (a) Chemical structures of the pyrimidines and purines that serve as the nitrogenous bases in RNA and DNA. The convention for numbering carbon and nitrogen atoms making up the two categories of bases is shown within the structures that appear on the left. (b) Chemical ring structures of ribose and 2-deoxyribose, which serve as the pentose sugars in RNA and DNA, respectively.

pyrimidines are **cytosine**, **thymine**, and **uracil**, abbreviated **C, T**, and **U**, respectively. The chemical structures of A, G, C, T, and U are shown in **Figure 10–7(a)**. Both DNA and RNA contain A, C, and G, but only DNA contains the base T and only RNA contains the base U. Each nitrogen or carbon atom of the ring structures of purines and pyrimidines is designated by an unprimed number. Note that corresponding atoms in the two rings are numbered differently in most cases.

The pentose sugars found in nucleic acids give them their names. Ribonucleic acids (RNA) contain **ribose**, while deoxyribonucleic acids (DNA) contain **deoxyribose**. **Figure 10–7(b)** shows the ring structures for these two pentose sugars. Each carbon atom is distinguished by a number with a prime sign (e.g., C-1′, C-2′). Compared with ribose, deoxyribose has a hydrogen atom rather than a hydroxyl group at the C-2′ position. The absence of a hydroxyl group at the C-2′ position thus distinguishes DNA from RNA. In

the absence of the C-2′ hydroxyl group, the sugar is more specifically named **2-deoxyribose**.

If a molecule is composed of a purine or pyrimidine base and a ribose or deoxyribose sugar, the chemical unit is called a **nucleoside**. If a phosphate group is added to the nucleoside, the molecule is now called a **nucleotide**. Nucleosides and nucleotides are named according to the specific nitrogenous base (A, T, G, C, or U) that is part of the molecule. The structures of a nucleoside and a nucleotide and the nomenclature used in naming nucleosides and nucleotides are given in **Figure 10–8**.

The bonding between components of a nucleotide is highly specific. The C-1′ atom of the sugar is involved in the chemical linkage to the nitrogenous base. If the base is a purine, the N-9 atom is covalently bonded to the sugar; if the base is a pyrimidine, the N-1 atom bonds to the sugar. In deoxyribonucleotides, the phosphate group may be bonded to the C-2′, C-3′, or C-5′ atom of the sugar. The

Nucleoside

Nucleotide

Uridine

Deoxyadenylic acid

Ribonucleosides	Ribonucleotides
Adenosine	Adenylic acid
Cytidine	Cytidylic acid
Guanosine	Guanylic acid
Uridine	Uridylic acid
Deoxyribonucleosides	**Deoxyribonucleotides**
Deoxyadenosine	Deoxyadenylic acid
Deoxycytidine	Deoxycytidylic acid
Deoxyguanosine	Deoxyguanylic acid
Deoxythymidine	Deoxythymidylic acid

FIGURE 10–8 Structures and names of the nucleosides and nucleotides of RNA and DNA.

C-5′ phosphate configuration is shown in Figure 10–8. It is by far the prevalent form in biological systems and the one found in DNA and RNA.

Nucleoside Diphosphates and Triphosphates

Nucleotides are also described by the term **nucleoside monophosphate (NMP)**. The addition of one or two phosphate groups results in **nucleoside diphosphates (NDPs)** and **triphosphates (NTPs)**, respectively, as shown in **Figure 10–9**. The triphosphate form is significant because it serves as the precursor molecule during nucleic acid synthesis within the cell (see Chapter 11). In addition, **adenosine triphosphate (ATP)** and **guanosine triphosphate (GTP)** are important in cell bioenergetics because of the large amount of energy involved in adding or removing the terminal phosphate group. The hydrolysis of ATP or GTP to ADP or GDP and inorganic phosphate (P_i) is accompanied by the release of a large amount of energy in the cell. When these chemical conversions are coupled to other reactions, the energy produced is used to drive the reactions. As a result, both ATP and GTP are involved in many cellular activities, including numerous genetic events.

Polynucleotides

The linkage between two mononucleotides consists of a phosphate group linked to two sugars. It is called a **phosphodiester bond** because phosphoric acid has been joined to two alcohols (the hydroxyl groups on the two sugars) by an ester linkage on both sides. **Figure 10–10(a)** shows the phosphodiester bond in DNA. The same bond is found in RNA. Each structure has a **C-5′ end** and a **C-3′ end**. Two joined nucleotides form a **dinucleotide**; three nucleotides, a **trinucleotide**; and so forth. Short chains consisting of up to approximately 30 nucleotides linked together are called **oligonucleotides**; longer chains are called **polynucleotides**.

Because drawing polynucleotide structures, as shown in Figure 10–10(a), is time consuming and complex, a schematic shorthand method has been devised [**Figure 10–10(b)**]. The nearly vertical lines represent the pentose sugar; the nitrogenous base is attached at the top, in the C-1′ position. A diagonal line with the P in the middle of it is attached to the C-3′ position of one sugar and the C-5′ position of the neighboring sugar; it represents the phosphodiester bond. Several modifications of this shorthand method are in use, and they can be understood in terms of these guidelines.

Deoxynucleoside diphosphate (dNDP)

Nucleoside triphosphate (NTP)

Deoxythymidine diphosphate (dTDP)

Adenosine triphosphate (ATP)

FIGURE 10–9 Structures of nucleoside diphosphates and triphosphates. Deoxythymidine diphosphate and adenosine triphosphate are diagrammed here.

Although Levene's tetranucleotide hypothesis (described earlier in this chapter) was generally accepted before 1940, research in subsequent decades revealed it to be incorrect. It was shown that DNA does not necessarily contain equimolar quantities of the four bases. In addition, the molecular weight of DNA molecules was determined to be in the range of 10^6 to 10^9 daltons, far in excess of that of a tetranucleotide. The current view of DNA is that it consists of exceedingly long polynucleotide chains.

Long polynucleotide chains account for the large molecular weight of DNA and explain its most important property—storage of vast quantities of genetic information. If each nucleotide position in this long chain can be occupied by any one of four nucleotides, extraordinary variation is possible. For example, a polynucleotide only 1000 nucleotides in length can be arranged 4^{1000} different ways, each one different from all other possible sequences. This potential variation in molecular structure is essential if DNA is to store the vast amounts of chemical information necessary to direct cellular activities.

FIGURE 10–10 (a) Linkage of two nucleotides by the formation of a C-3′-C-5′ (3′-5′) phosphodiester bond, producing a dinucleotide. (b) Shorthand notation for a polynucleotide chain.

10.7 The Structure of DNA Holds the Key to Understanding Its Function

The previous sections in this chapter have established that DNA is the genetic material in all organisms (with certain viruses being the exception) and have provided details as to the basic chemical components making up nucleic acids. What remained to be deciphered was the precise structure of DNA. That is, how are polynucleotide chains organized into DNA, which serves as the genetic material? Is DNA composed of a single chain or more than one? If the latter is the case, how do the chains relate chemically to one another? Do the chains branch? And more important, how does the structure of this molecule relate to the various genetic functions served by DNA (i.e., storage, expression, replication, and mutation)?

From 1940 to 1953, many scientists were interested in solving the structure of DNA. Among others, Erwin Chargaff, Maurice Wilkins, Rosalind Franklin, Linus Pauling, Francis Crick, and James Watson sought information that might answer what many consider to be the most significant and intriguing question in the history of biology: *How does DNA serve as the genetic basis for life?* The answer was believed to depend strongly on the chemical structure and organization of the DNA molecule, given the complex but orderly functions ascribed to it.

In 1953, James Watson and Francis Crick proposed that the structure of DNA is in the form of a double helix. Their model was described in a short paper published in the journal *Nature*. (The article is reprinted in its entirety on page 248.) In a sense, this publication was the finish of a highly competitive scientific race. Watson's book *The Double Helix* recounts the human side of the scientific drama that eventually led to the elucidation of DNA structure.

The data available to Watson and Crick, crucial to the development of their proposal, came primarily from two sources: (1) base composition analysis of hydrolyzed samples of DNA and (2) X-ray diffraction studies of DNA. Watson and Crick's analytical success can be attributed to their focus on building a model that conformed to the existing data. If the correct solution to the structure of DNA is viewed as a puzzle, Watson and Crick, working at the Cavendish Laboratory in Cambridge, England, were the first to fit the pieces together successfully.

Before learning the details of this far-reaching discovery, you may find some of the background on James Watson and Francis Crick to be of interest. Watson began his undergraduate studies at the University of Chicago at age 15, and was originally interested in ornithology. He then pursued his Ph.D. at Indiana University, where he studied viruses. He was only 24 years old in 1953, when he and Crick proposed the double-helix theory. Crick, now considered one of the great theoretical biologists of our time, had studied undergraduate physics at University College, London, and went on to perform military research during World War II. At the time of his collaboration with Watson, he was 35 years old and was performing X-ray diffraction studies of polypeptides and proteins as a graduate student. Immediately after they made their major discovery, Crick is reputed to have walked into the Eagle Pub in Cambridge, where the two frequently lunched, and announced for all to hear, "We have discovered the secret of life." It turns out that more than 50 years later, many scientists would quite agree!

Base-Composition Studies

Between 1949 and 1953, Erwin Chargaff and his colleagues used chromatographic methods to separate the four bases in DNA samples from various organisms. Quantitative methods were then used to determine the amounts of the four bases from each source. **Table 10.3(a)** lists some of Chargaff's original data. Parts (b) and (c) of the table show

TABLE 10.3 DNA Base-Composition Data

(a) Chargaff's Data*

Organism/Source	A (1)	T (2)	G (3)	C (4)
Ox thymus	26	25	21	16
Ox spleen	25	24	20	15
Yeast	24	25	14	13
Avian tubercle bacilli	12	11	28	26
Human sperm	29	31	18	18

Molar Proportions[a]

(c) G + C Content in Several Organisms

Organism	%G + C
Phage T2	36.0
Drosophila	45.0
Maize	49.1
Euglena	53.5
Neurospora	53.7

(b) Base Compositions of DNAs from Various Sources

Organism	A (1)	T (2)	G (3)	C (4)	A/T (5)	G/C (6)	(A + G)/(C + T) (7)	(A + T)/(C + G) (8)
Human	30.9	29.4	19.9	19.8	1.05	1.00	1.04	1.52
Sea urchin	32.8	32.1	17.7	17.3	1.02	1.02	1.02	1.58
E. coli	24.7	23.6	26.0	25.7	1.04	1.01	1.03	0.93
Sarcina lutea	13.4	12.4	37.1	37.1	1.08	1.00	1.04	0.35
T7 bacteriophage	26.0	26.0	24.0	24.0	1.00	1.00	1.00	1.08

*Source: Data from Chargaff, 1950.

[a]Moles of nitrogenous constituent per mole of P. (Often, the recovery was less than 100 percent.)

more recently derived base-composition information that reinforces Chargaff's findings. As we shall see, Chargaff's data were critical to the success of Watson and Crick as they devised the double-helical model of DNA. On the basis of these data, the following conclusions may be drawn:

1. As shown in Table 10.3(b), the amount of adenine residues is proportional to the amount of thymine residues in DNA (columns 1, 2, and 5). Also, the amount of guanine residues is proportional to the amount of cytosine residues (columns 3, 4, and 6).

2. Based on this proportionality, the sum of the purines (A + G) equals the sum of the pyrimidines (C + T) as shown in column 7.

3. The percentage of (G + C) does not necessarily equal the percentage of (A + T). As you can see, this ratio varies greatly among organisms, as shown in column 8 and in part (c) of Table 10.3.

These conclusions indicate a definite pattern of base composition in DNA molecules. The data provided the initial clue to the DNA puzzle. In addition, they directly refute Levene's tetranucleotide hypothesis, which stated that all four bases are present in equal amounts.

X-Ray Diffraction Analysis

When fibers of a DNA molecule are subjected to X-ray bombardment, the X rays scatter (diffract) in a pattern that depends on the molecule's atomic structure. The pattern of diffraction can be captured as spots on photographic film and analyzed for clues to the overall shape of and regularities within the molecule. This process, **X-ray diffraction analysis**, was applied successfully to the study of protein structure by Linus Pauling and other chemists. The technique had been attempted on DNA as early as 1938 by William Astbury. By 1947, he had detected a periodicity of 3.4-angstrom unit (3.4-Å) repetitions* within the structure of the molecule, which suggested to him that the bases were stacked like coins on top of one another.

Between 1950 and 1953, Rosalind Franklin, working in the laboratory of Maurice Wilkins, obtained improved X-ray data from more purified samples of DNA (**Figure 10–11**). Her work confirmed the 3.4-Å periodicity seen by Astbury and suggested that the structure of DNA was some sort of helix. However, she did not propose a definitive model. Pauling had analyzed the work of Astbury and others and incorrectly proposed that DNA was a triple helix.

FIGURE 10–11 X-ray diffraction photograph by Rosalind Franklin using the B form of purified DNA fibers. The strong arcs on the periphery represent closely spaced aspects of the molecule, allowing scientists to estimate the periodicity of the nitrogenous bases, which are 3.4 Å apart. The inner cross pattern of spots reveals the grosser aspects of the molecule, indicating its helical nature.

The Watson–Crick Model

Watson and Crick published their analysis of DNA structure in 1953. By building models based on the above-mentioned parameters, they arrived at the double-helical form of DNA shown in **Figure 10–12(a)** on p. 246.

This model has the following major features:

1. Two long polynucleotide chains are coiled around a central axis, forming a right-handed double helix.

2. The two chains are **antiparallel**; that is, their C-5′-to-C-3′ orientations run in opposite directions.

3. The bases of both chains are flat structures lying perpendicular to the axis; they are "stacked" on one another, 3.4 Å (0.34 nm) apart, on the inside of the double helix.

4. The nitrogenous bases of opposite chains are *paired* as the result of the formation of hydrogen bonds; in DNA, only A=T and G≡C pairs occur.

5. Each complete turn of the helix is 34 Å (3.4 nm) long; thus, each turn of the helix is the length of a series of 10 base pairs.

6. A larger **major groove** alternating with a smaller **minor groove** winds along the length of the molecule.

7. The double helix has a diameter of 20 Å (2.0 nm).

The nature of the base pairing (point 4 above) is the model's most significant feature in terms of explaining

---

*Today, measurement in nanometers (nm) is favored (1 nm = 10 Å).

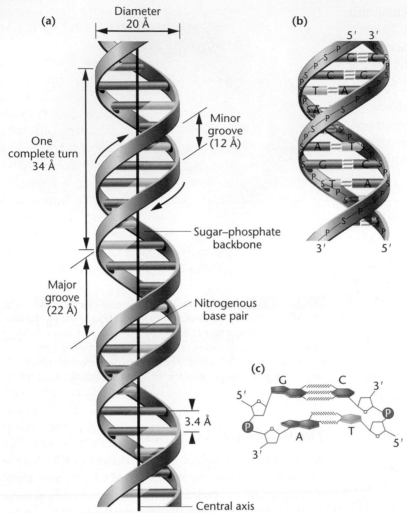

(a)

Diameter 20 Å

One complete turn 34 Å

Minor groove (12 Å)

Major groove (22 Å)

Sugar–phosphate backbone

Nitrogenous base pair

3.4 Å

Central axis

(b)

5′ 3′

3′ 5′

(c)

G ⫴ C
5′   3′
P   P
A ⫴ T
3′   5′

FIGURE 10–12 (a) The DNA double helix as proposed by Watson and Crick. The ribbon-like strands represent the sugar-phosphate backbones, and the horizontal rungs depict the nitrogenous base pairs, of which there are 10 per complete turn. The major and minor grooves are apparent. A solid vertical line shows the central axis. (b) A detailed view depicting the bases, sugars, phosphates, and hydrogen bonds of the helix. (c) A demonstration of the antiparallel arrangement of the chains and the horizontal stacking of the bases.

as shown in **Figure 10–13**. The conformation in space of the right-handed helix is most consistent with the data that were available to Watson and Crick, although an alternative form of DNA (Z-DNA) does exist as a left-handed helix, as we discuss below.

The key to the model proposed by Watson and Crick is the specificity of base pairing. Chargaff's data suggested that A was equal in amount to T and that G was equal in amount to C. Watson and Crick realized that pairing A with T and C with G would account for these proportions, and that such pairing could occur as a result of hydrogen bonds between base pairs [Figure 10–12(b)], which would also provide the chemical stability necessary to hold the two chains together. Arrangement of the components in this way produces the major and minor grooves along the molecule's length. Furthermore, a purine (A or G) opposite a pyrimidine (T or C) on each "rung of the spiral staircase" in the proposed helix accounts for the 20-Å (2-nm) diameter suggested by X-ray diffraction studies.

The specific $A{=}T$ and $G{\equiv}C$ base pairing is described as **complementarity** and results from the chemical affinity that produces the hydrogen bonds in each pair of bases. As we will see, complementarity is very important in the processes of DNA replication and gene expression.

its genetic functions. Before we discuss it, however, several other important features warrant emphasis. First, the antiparallel arrangement of the two chains is a key part of the double-helix model. While one chain runs in the 5′-to-3′ orientation (what seems right side up to us), the other chain goes in the 3′-to-5′ orientation (and thus appears upside down). This is indicated in **Figure 10–12(b)** and **(c)**. Given the bond angles in the structures of the various nucleotide components, the double helix could not be constructed easily if both chains ran parallel to one another.

Second, the right-handed nature of the helix modeled by Watson and Crick is best appreciated by comparison with its left-handed counterpart, which is a mirror image,

Right-handed double helix   **Left-handed double helix**

FIGURE 10–13 The right- and left-handed helical forms of DNA. Note that they are mirror images of one another.

Adenine-thymine base pair

C-1' of
deoxyribose

Adenine

C-1' of
deoxyribose

Thymine

Guanine-cytosine base pair

C-1' of
deoxyribose

Guanine

C-1' of
deoxyribose

Cytosine

- - - **Hydrogen bond**

FIGURE 10–14 Ball-and-stick models of A=T and G≡C base pairs. The dashes (- - -) represent the hydrogen bonds that form between bases.

Two questions are particularly worthy of discussion. First, why aren't other base pairs possible? Watson and Crick discounted the pairing of A with G or of C with T because these would represent purine–purine and pyrimidine–pyrimidine pairings, respectively. Such pairings would lead to aberrant diameters of, in one case, more than and, in the other case, less than 20 Å because of the respective sizes of the purine and pyrimidine rings. In addition, the three-dimensional configurations that would be formed by such pairings would not produce an alignment that allows sufficient hydrogen-bond formation. It is for this reason that A=C and G≡T pairings

were also discounted, even though those pairs would each consist of one purine and one pyrimidine.

The second question concerns the properties of hydrogen bonds. Just what is the nature of such a bond, and is it strong enough to stabilize the helix? A **hydrogen bond** is a very weak electrostatic attraction between a covalently bonded hydrogen atom and an atom with an unshared electron pair. The hydrogen atom assumes a partial positive charge, while the unshared electron pair—characteristic of covalently bonded oxygen and nitrogen atoms—assumes a partial negative charge. These opposite charges are responsible for the weak chemical attraction that is the basis of the hydrogen bond. As oriented in the double helix, adenine forms two hydrogen bonds with thymine, and guanine forms three hydrogen bonds with cytosine (**Figure 10–14**). Although two or three hydrogen bonds taken alone are energetically very weak, thousands of bonds in tandem (as found in long polynucleotide chains) provide great stability to the helix.

Another stabilizing factor is the arrangement of sugars and bases along the axis. In the Watson–Crick model, the hydrophobic ("water-fearing") nitrogenous bases are stacked almost horizontally on the interior of the axis and are thus shielded from the watery environment that surrounds the molecule within the cell. The hydrophilic ("water-loving") sugar-phosphate backbones are on the outside of the axis, where both components may interact with water. These molecular arrangements provide significant chemical stabilization to the helix.

A more recent and accurate analysis of the form of DNA that served as the basis for the Watson–Crick model has revealed a minor structural difference between the substance and the model. A precise measurement of the number of base pairs per turn has demonstrated a value of 10.4, rather than the 10.0 predicted by Watson and Crick. In the classic model, each base pair is rotated 36° around the helical axis relative to the adjacent base pair, but the new finding requires a rotation of 34.6°. This results in slightly more than 10 base pairs per 360° turn.

The Watson–Crick model had an instant effect on the emerging discipline of molecular biology. Even in

Molecular Structure of Nucleic Acids: A Structure for Deoxyribose Nucleic Acid

We wish to suggest a structure for the salt of deoxyribose nucleic acid (DNA). This structure has novel features which are of considerable biological interest. A structure for nucleic acid has already been proposed by Pauling and Corey.[1] They kindly made their manuscript available to us in advance of publication. Their model consists of three intertwined chains, with the phosphates near the fibre axis, and the bases on the outside. In our opinion, this structure is unsatisfactory for two reasons: (1) We believe that the material which gives the X-ray diagrams is the salt, not the free acid. Without the acidic hydrogen atoms it is not clear what forces would hold the structure together, especially as the negatively charged phosphates near the axis will repel each other. (2) Some of the van der Waals distances appear to be too small.

Another three-chain structure has also been suggested by Fraser (in the press). In his model the phosphates are on the outside and the bases on the inside, linked together by hydrogen bonds. This structure as described is rather ill-defined, and for this reason we shall not comment on it.

We wish to put forward a radically different structure for the salt of deoxyribose nucleic acid. This structure has two helical chains each coiled round the same axis. We have made the usual chemical assumptions, namely, that each chain consists of phosphate diester groups joining α-D-deoxyribofuranose residues with 3′, 5′ linkages. The two chains (but not their bases) are related by a dyad perpendicular to the fibre axis. Both chains follow right-handed helices, but owing to the dyad the sequences of the atoms in the two chains run in opposite directions. Each chain loosely resembles Furberg's[2] model No. 1; that is, the bases are on the inside of the helix and the phosphates on the outside. The configuration of the sugar and the atoms near it is close to Furberg's "standard configuration," the sugar being roughly perpendicular to the attached base. There is a residue on each chain every 3.4 Å in the z-direction. We have assumed an angle of 36° between adjacent residues in the same chain, so that the structure repeats after 10 residues on each chain, that is, after 34 Å the distance of a phosphorus atom from the fibre axis is 10 Å. As the phosphates are on the outside, cations have easy access to them.

The structure is an open one, and its water content is rather high. At lower water contents we would expect the bases to tilt so that the structure could become more compact.

The novel feature of the structure is the manner in which the two chains are held together by the purine and pyrimidine bases. The planes of the bases are perpendicular to the fibre axis. They are joined together in pairs, a single base from one chain being hydrogen-bonded to a single base from the other chain, so that the two lie side by side with identical z-coordinates. One of the pair must be a purine and the other a pyrimidine for bonding to occur. The hydrogen bonds are made as follows: purine position 1 to pyrimidine position 1; purine position 6 to pyrimidine position 6.

If it is assumed that the bases only occur in the structure in the most plausible tautomeric forms (that is, with the keto rather than the enol configurations) it is found that only specific pairs of bases can bond together. These pairs are: adenine (purine) with thymine (pyrimidine), and guanine (purine) with cytosine (pyrimidine).

In other words, if an adenine forms one member of a pair, on either chain, then on these assumptions the other member must be thymine; similarly for guanine and cytosine. The sequence of bases on a single chain does not appear to be restricted in any way. However, if only specific pairs of bases can be formed, it follows that if the sequence of bases on one chain is given, then the sequence on the other chain is automatically determined.

It has been found experimentally[3,4] that the ratio of the amounts of adenine to thymine, and the ratio of guanine to cytosine, are always very close to unity for deoxyribose nucleic acid.

It is probably impossible to build this structure with a ribose sugar in place of the deoxyribose, as the extra oxygen atom would make too close a van der Waals contact.

The previously published X-ray data[5,6] on deoxyribose nucleic acid are insufficient for a rigorous test of our structure. So far as we can tell, it is roughly compatible with the experimental data, but it must be regarded as unproved until it has been checked against more exact results. Some of these are given in the following communications. We were not aware of the details of the results presented there when we devised our structure, which rests mainly though not entirely on published experimental data and stereochemical arguments.

It has not escaped our notice that the specific pairing we have postulated immediately suggests a possible copying mechanism for the genetic material. Full details of the structure, including the conditions assumed in building it, together with a set of co-ordinates for the atoms, will be published elsewhere.

We are much indebted to Dr. Jerry Donohue for constant advice and criticism, especially on interatomic distances. We have also been stimulated by a knowledge of the general nature of the unpublished experimental results and ideas of Dr. M. H. F. Wilkins, Dr. R. E. Franklin and their co-workers at King's College, London. One of us (J. D. W.) has been aided by a fellowship from the National Foundation for Infantile Paralysis.

—J. D. **Watson**
—F.H.C. **Crick**

Medical Research Council Unit for the Study of the Molecular Structure of Biological Systems, Cavendish Laboratory, Cambridge, England.

[1]Pauling, L., and Corey, R. B., *Nature*, 171, 346 (1953); *Proc. U.S. Nat. Acad. Sci.*, 39, 84 (1953).
[2]Furberg, S., *Acta Chem. Scand.*, 6, 634 (1952).
[3]Chargaff, E. For references see Zamenhof, S., Brawerman, G., and Chargaff, E., *Biochim. et Biophys. Acta*, 9, 402 (1952).
[4]Wyatt, G. R., *J. Gen. Physiol.*, 36, 201 (1952).
[5]Astbury, W. T., *Symp. Soc. Exp. Biol. 1, Nucleic Acid*, 66 (Camb. Univ. Press, 1947).
[6]Wilkins, M.H.F., and Randall, J. T., *Biochim. et Biophys. Acta*, 10, 192 (1953).

their initial 1953 article in *Nature*, the authors observed, "It has not escaped our notice that the specific pairing we have postulated immediately suggests a possible copying mechanism for the genetic material." Two months later, Watson and Crick pursued this idea in a second article in *Nature,* suggesting a specific mechanism of replication of DNA—*the semiconservative mode of replication* (described in Chapter 11). The second article also alluded to two new concepts: (1) the storage of genetic information in the sequence of the bases and (2) the mutations or genetic changes that would result from an alteration of bases. These ideas have received vast amounts of experimental support since 1953 and are now universally accepted.

Watson and Crick's synthesis of ideas was highly significant with regard to subsequent studies of genetics and biology. The nature of the gene and its role in genetic mechanisms could now be viewed and studied in biochemical terms. Recognition of their work, along with that of Wilkins, led to all three receiving the Nobel Prize in Physiology and Medicine in 1962. Unfortunately, Rosalind Franklin had died in 1958 at the age of 37, making her contributions ineligible for consideration, since the award is not given posthumously. The Nobel Prize was to be one of many such awards bestowed for work in the field of molecular genetics.

EVOLVING CONCEPT OF THE GENE

Based on the model of DNA put forward by Watson and Crick in 1953, the gene was viewed for the first time in molecular terms as a sequence of nucleotides in a DNA helix that encodes genetic information. ∎

10.8 Alternative Forms of DNA Exist

Under different conditions of isolation, different conformations of DNA are seen. At the time when Watson and Crick performed their analysis, two forms—**A-DNA** and **B-DNA**—were known. Watson and Crick's analysis was based on Rosalind Franklin's X-ray studies of the B form, which is seen under aqueous, low-salt conditions and is believed to be the biologically significant conformation.

While DNA studies around 1950 relied on the use of X-ray diffraction, more recent investigations have been performed using **single-crystal X-ray analysis**. The earlier studies achieved resolution of about 5 Å, but single crystals diffract X rays at about 1-Å intervals, near atomic resolution. As a result, every atom is "visible," and much greater structural detail is available.

With this modern technique, A-DNA, which is prevalent under high-salt or dehydration conditions, has now been

B-DNA   **A-DNA**

FIGURE 10–15 An artist's depiction illustrating the orientation of the base pairs of B-DNA and A-DNA. Note that in B-DNA the base pairs are perpendicular to the helix, while they are tilted and pulled away from the helix in A-DNA. In comparison to B-DNA, A-DNA also displays a slightly greater diameter and contains one more base pair per turn.

scrutinized. In comparison to B-DNA, A-DNA is slightly more compact, with 9 base pairs in each complete turn of the helix, which is 23 Å (2.3 nm) in diameter (**Figure 10–15**). While it is also a right-handed helix, the orientation of the bases is somewhat different—they are tilted and displaced laterally in relation to the axis of the helix. As a result, the appearance of the major and minor grooves is modified. It seems doubtful that A-DNA occurs *in vivo* (under physiological conditions).

Still other forms of DNA right-handed helices have been discovered when investigated under various laboratory conditions. These have been designated C-, D-, E-, and most recently P-DNA. **C-DNA** is found under even greater dehydration conditions than those observed during the isolation of A- and B-DNA. Two other forms, **D-DNA** and **E-DNA**, occur in helices lacking guanine in their base composition. And most recently, it has been observed that if DNA is artificially stretched, still another conformation is assumed, called **P-DNA** (named for Linus Pauling).

Finally, still another form of DNA, called **Z-DNA**, was discovered in 1979, when a small synthetic DNA oligonucleotide containing only G≡C base pairs was studied. Z-DNA takes on the rather remarkable configuration of a *left-handed double helix*. Speculation has occasionally run high over the possibility that regions of Z-DNA exist in the chromosomes of living organisms. The unique helical arrangement has the potential to provide an important recognition site for interaction with DNA-binding molecules. However, the extent to which Z-DNA, or any of the forms mentioned above, occur *in vivo* is still not clear.

10–2 In sea urchin DNA, which is double stranded, 17.5 percent of the bases were shown to be cytosine (C). What percentages of the other three bases are expected to be present in this DNA?

■ **HINT:** *This problem asks you to extrapolate from one measurement involving a unique DNA molecule to three other values characterizing the molecule. The key to its solution is to understand the base-pairing rules in the Watson–Crick model of DNA.*

10.9 The Structure of RNA Is Chemically Similar to DNA, but Single Stranded

The structure of RNA molecules resembles DNA, with several important exceptions. Although RNA also has nucleotides linked into polynucleotide chains, the sugar ribose replaces deoxyribose, and the nitrogenous base uracil replaces thymine. Another important difference is that most RNA is single stranded, although there are two important exceptions. First, RNA molecules sometimes fold back on themselves to form double-stranded regions of complementary base pairs. Second, some animal viruses that have RNA as their genetic material contain double-stranded helices.

As established earlier (see Figure 10–1), three major classes of cellular RNA molecules function during the expression of genetic information: **ribosomal RNA (rRNA), messenger RNA (mRNA)**, and **transfer RNA (tRNA)**. These molecules all originate as complementary copies of one of the two strands of DNA segments during the process of transcription. That is, their nucleotide sequence is complementary to the deoxyribonucleotide sequence of DNA that served as the template for their synthesis. Because uracil replaces thymine in RNA, uracil is complementary to adenine during transcription and during RNA base pairing.

Table 10.4 characterizes these major forms of RNA as found in prokaryotic and eukaryotic cells. Different RNAs are distinguished according to their sedimentation behavior in a centrifugal field and by their size (the number of nucleotides each contains). Sedimentation behavior depends on a molecule's density, mass, and shape, and its measure is called the **Svedberg coefficient** (*S*). While higher *S* values almost always designate molecules of greater molecular weight, the correlation is not direct; that is, a twofold increase in molecular weight does not lead to a twofold increase in *S*. This is because,

TABLE 10.4 Principal Classes of RNA

Class	% of Total RNA*	Svedberg Coefficient	Eukaryotic (E) or Prokaryotic (P)	Number of Nucleotides
Ribosomal (rRNA)	80	5	P and E	120
		5.8	E	160
		16	P	1542
		18	E	1874
		23	P	2904
		28	E	4718
Transfer (tRNA)	15	4	P and E	75–90
Messenger (mRNA)	5	varies	P and E	100–10,000

*In *E. coli*.

in addition to a molecule's mass, the size and shape of the molecule also affect its rate of sedimentation (*S*). As you can see in Table 10.4, RNA molecules come in a wide range of sizes.

Ribosomal RNA usually constitutes about 80 percent of all RNA in an *E. coli* cell. Ribosomal RNAs are important structural components of **ribosomes**, which function as nonspecific workbenches where proteins are synthesized during translation. The various forms of rRNA found in prokaryotes and eukaryotes differ distinctly in size.

Messenger RNA molecules carry genetic information from the DNA of the gene to the ribosome. The mRNA molecules vary considerably in size, reflecting the range in the sizes of the proteins encoded by the mRNA as well as the different sizes of the genes serving as the templates for transcription of mRNA. While Table 10.4 shows that about 5 percent of RNA is mRNA in *E. coli*, this percentage varies from cell to cell and even at different times in the life of the same cell.

Transfer RNA, accounting for up to 15 percent of the RNA in a typical cell, is the smallest class (in terms of average molecule size) of these RNA molecules and carries amino acids to the ribosome during translation. Because more than one tRNA molecule interacts simultaneously with the ribosome, the molecule's smaller size facilitates these interactions.

We will discuss more detailed functions of these three classes of RNA later in the text (see Chapters 13 and 14). While these RNAs represent the major forms of the molecule involved in genetic expression, other unique RNAs exist that perform various roles, especially in eukaryotes. For example, **telomerase RNA** and **RNA primers** are involved in DNA replication at the ends of chromosomes

(Chapter 11), **small nuclear RNA (snRNA)** partici-pates in processing mRNAs (Chapter 13), and **antisense RNA, microRNA (miRNA)**, and **short interfering RNA (siRNA)** are involved in gene regulation (Chapter 17). We will also discuss still other recent findings involving RNA later in the text (see Special Topic Chapter 2—Emerging Roles of RNA).

NOW SOLVE THIS

10–3 German measles results from an infection of the rubella virus, which can cause a multitude of health prob-lems in newborns. What conclusions can you reach from a viral nucleic acid analysis that reveals an A + G/U + C ratio of 1.13?

■ **HINT:** *This problem asks you to analyze information about the chemical composition of a nucleic acid serving as the genetic mate-rial of a virus. The key to its solution is to apply your knowledge of nucleic acid chemistry, in particular your understanding of base-pairing.*

For more practice, see Problems 32 and 33.

10.10 Many Analytical Techniques Have Been Useful during the Investigation of DNA and RNA

Since 1953, the role of DNA as the genetic material and the role of RNA in transcription and translation have been clarified through detailed analysis of nucleic acids. In this section, we consider several fundamental methods that have been particularly important for accomplishing this analysis. Many of them make use of the unique nature of the hydrogen bond that is so integral to the structure of nucleic acids. Later in the text (see Chapter 20), we will consider still other techniques that have been developed for manipulating DNA in various ways, including cloning.

Absorption of Ultraviolet Light

Nucleic acids absorb ultraviolet (UV) light most strongly at wavelengths of 254 to 260 nm (Figure 10–6), due to the interaction between UV light and the ring systems of the purines and pyrimidines. In aqueous solution, peak absorption by DNA and RNA occurs at 260 nm. Thus, UV light can be used in the localization, isolation, and characterization of molecules that contain nitrogenous bases (i.e., nucleosides, nucleotides, and polynucleotides).

Ultraviolet analysis is used in conjunction with many standard procedures that separate and identify molecules. As we shall see in the next section, the use of UV absorp-tion is critical to the isolation of nucleic acids following their separation.

Denaturation and Renaturation of Nucleic Acids

Heat or other stresses can cause a complex molecule like DNA to **denature**, or lose its function due to the unfold-ing of its three-dimensional structure. In the denatur-ation of double-stranded DNA, the hydrogen bonds of the duplex (double-stranded) structure break, the helix unwinds, and the strands separate. However, no covalent bonds break. The viscosity of the DNA decreases, and both the UV absorption and the buoyant density increase. In laboratory studies, denaturation may be caused inten-tionally either by heating or chemical treatment. (Dena-turation as a result of heating is sometimes referred to as *melting*.) In such studies, the increase in UV absorp-tion of heated DNA in solution, called the **hyperchromic shift**, is the easiest change to measure. This effect is illus-trated in **Figure 10–16**.

Because $G \equiv C$ base pairs have one more hydrogen bond than do $A = T$ pairs (see Figure 10–14), they are more stable under heat treatment. Thus, DNA with a greater pro-portion of $G \equiv C$ pairs than $A = T$ pairs requires higher temperatures to denature completely. When absorption at 260 nm is monitored and plotted against temperature dur-ing heating, a **melting profile** of the DNA is obtained. The

FIGURE 10–16 A melting profile shows the increase in UV absorption versus temperature (the hyperchromic effect) for two DNA molecules with different $G \equiv C$ contents. The molecule with a melting point (T_m) of 83°C has a greater $G \equiv C$ content than the molecule with a T_m of 77°C.

midpoint of this profile, or curve, is called the **melting temperature** (T_m) and represents the point at which 50 percent of the strands are unwound, or denatured (Figure 10–16). When the curve plateaus at its maximum optical density, denaturation is complete, and only single strands exist. Analysis of melting profiles provides a characterization of DNA and an alternative method of estimating its base composition.

One might ask whether the denaturation process can be reversed; that is, can single strands of nucleic acids re-form a double helix, provided that each strand's complement is present? Not only is the answer yes, but such reassociation provides the basis for several important analytical techniques that have contributed much valuable information during genetic experimentation.

If DNA that has been denatured thermally is cooled slowly, random collisions between complementary strands will result in their reassociation. At the proper temperature, hydrogen bonds will re-form, securing pairs of strands into duplex structures. With time during cooling, more and more duplexes will form. Depending on the conditions, a complete match (that is, perfect complementarity) is not essential for duplex formation, provided there are stretches of base pairing on the two reassociating strands.

Molecular Hybridization

The denaturation and renaturation of nucleic acids are the basis for one of the most powerful and useful techniques in molecular genetics—**molecular hybridization**. This technique derives its name from the fact that single strands need not originate from the same nucleic acid source in order to combine to form duplex structures. For example, if DNA strands are isolated from two distinct organisms and a reasonable degree of base complementarity exists between them, under the proper temperature conditions, double-stranded molecular hybrids will form during renaturation. Such hybridization may also occur between single strands of DNA and RNA. A case in point is when RNA and the DNA from which it has been transcribed are mixed together (**Figure 10–17**). The RNA will find and attach to its single-stranded DNA complement. In this example, DNA molecules are heated, causing strand separation, and then the strands are slowly cooled in the presence of single-stranded RNA. If the RNA has been transcribed from the DNA used in the experiment, and is therefore complementary to it, molecular hybridization will occur, creating a DNA:RNA duplex. Several methods are available for monitoring the amount of double-stranded molecules produced following strand separation. In early studies,

radioisotopes were utilized to "tag" one of the strands and monitor its presence in the hybrid duplexes that formed.

In the 1960s, molecular hybridization techniques contributed to our increased understanding of transcriptional events occurring at the gene level. Refinements of this process have occurred continually, helping to advance the study of both molecular evolution and the organization of DNA in chromosomes. Hybridization can occur in solution or when DNA is bound either to a gel or to a specialized binding filter. Such filters are used in a variety of **DNA blotting procedures**, whereby hybridization serves as a way to "probe" for complementary nucleic acid sequences. Blotting is used routinely in modern genomic analysis. In addition, hybridization will occur even when DNA is present in tissue affixed to a slide, as in the FISH procedure (discussed in the next section), or when affixed to a glass chip, the basis of **DNA microarray analysis** (discussed in Chapter 21). Microarray analysis allows mass screening for a specific DNA sequence from among thousands of cloned genes in a single assay.

Fluorescent *in situ* Hybridization (FISH)

A refinement in the molecular hybridization technique has led to the use of DNA present in cytological preparations as the "target" for hybrid formation. When this approach is combined with the use of fluorescent probes to monitor hybridization, the technique is called **fluorescent *in situ* hybridization**, or is known simply by the acronym **FISH**. In this procedure, mitotic or interphase cells are fixed to slides and subjected to hybridization conditions. Single-stranded DNA or RNA is added, and hybridization is monitored. The added nucleic acid serves as a "probe," since it will hybridize only with the specific chromosomal areas for which it is sufficiently complementary. Before the use of fluorescent probes was refined, radioactive probes were used in these *in situ* procedures to allow detection on the slide by autoradiography.

Fluorescent probes are prepared in a unique way. When DNA is used, it is first coupled to the small organic molecule biotin (creating biotinylated DNA). Another molecule (avidin or streptavidin) that has a high binding affinity for biotin is linked with a fluorescent molecule such as fluorescein, and this complex is reacted with the cytological preparation after the *in situ* hybridization has occurred. This procedure represents an extremely sensitive method for localizing the hybridized DNA.

Figure 10–18 on p. 253 illustrates the results of using FISH to identify the DNA specific to the centromeres of human chromosomes. The resolution of FISH is great

FIGURE 10–17 Diagrammatic representation of the process of molecular hybridization between DNA fragments and RNA that has been transcribed on one strand of one of the DNA fragments (DNA-3).

enough to detect just a single gene within an entire set of chromosomes. The use of this technique to identify chromosomal locations of specific genetic information has been a valuable addition to the repertoire of experimental geneticists.

Reassociation Kinetics and Repetitive DNA

In still another extension of molecular hybridization procedures, the *rate of reassociation* of complementary single DNA strands may be analyzed. This technique, **reassociation kinetics**, was first refined and studied by Roy Britten and David Kohne.

The DNA used in such studies is first fragmented into small pieces by shearing forces introduced during its isolation. The resultant DNA fragments have an average size of several hundred base pairs. The fragments are then dissociated into single strands by heating (denatured), and when the temperature is lowered, reassociation is monitored. During reassociation, pieces of single-stranded DNA randomly collide. If they are complementary, a stable double strand is formed; if not, they separate and are free to encounter other DNA fragments. The process continues until all possible matches are made.

A great deal of information can be obtained from studies that compare the reassociation of DNA of different organisms.

FIGURE 10–18 Fluorescent *in situ* hybridization (FISH) of human metaphase chromosomes. The probe, specific to centromeric DNA, produces a yellow fluorescence signal indicating hybridization. The red fluorescence is produced by propidium iodide counterstaining of chromosomal DNA.

As genome size increases and there is more DNA, reassociation time is extended. Reassociation occurs more slowly in larger genomes because with random collisions it takes more time for all correct matches to be made. When reassociation kinetics in eukaryotic organisms with much larger genome sizes was first studied, a surprising observation was made. Rather than requiring an extended reassociation time, *some* eukaryotic DNA reassociated even more rapidly than those derived from bacteria. The remaining DNA, as expected because of its complexity, took longer to reassociate.

Based on this observation, Britten and Kohne hypothesized that the rapidly reassociating fraction might represent **repetitive DNA sequences**. This interpretation would explain why these segments reassociate so rapidly—multiple copies of the same sequence are much more likely to make matches, thus reassociating more quickly than single copies. On the other hand, the remaining DNA segments consist of **unique DNA sequences**, present only once in the genome.

It is now known that repetitive DNA is prevalent in eukaryotic genomes and is key to our understanding of how genetic information is organized in chromosomes. Careful study has shown that various levels of repetition exist. In some cases, short DNA sequences are repeated over a million times. In other cases, longer sequences are repeated only a few times, or intermediate levels of sequence redundancy are present. We will return to this topic later in the text (see Chapter 12), where we will discuss the organization of DNA in genes and chromosomes. For now, we will simply point out that the discovery of repetitive DNA was one of the first clues that much of the DNA in eukaryotes is not contained in genes that encode proteins. We will develop and elaborate on this concept as we proceed with our coverage of the molecular basis of heredity.

Electrophoresis of Nucleic Acids

We conclude the chapter by considering **electrophoresis**, a technique that has made essential contributions to the analysis of nucleic acids. Electrophoresis, also useful in protein studies, can be applied to the separation of different-sized fragments of DNA and RNA chains and is invaluable in current research investigations in molecular genetics.

In general, electrophoresis separates, or *resolves*, molecules in a mixture by causing them to migrate under the influence of an electric field. A sample to be analyzed is placed on a porous substance (a piece of filter paper or a semisolid gel) that in turn is placed in a solution that conducts electricity. If two molecules have approximately the same shape and mass, the one with the greatest net charge will migrate more rapidly toward the electrode of opposite polarity.

As electrophoretic technology developed from its initial application (which was protein separation), researchers discovered that using gels of varying pore sizes significantly improved the method's resolution. This advance is particularly useful for mixtures of molecules with a similar charge-mass ratio but different sizes. For example, two polynucleotide chains of different lengths (say, 10 vs. 20 nucleotides) are both negatively charged because of the phosphate groups of the nucleotides. Thus, both chains move to the positively charged pole (the anode), and because they have the same charge-mass ratio, the electric field moves them at similar speeds. Consequently, the separation between the two chains is minimal. However, using a porous medium such as an **agarose gel**, which can be prepared with various pore sizes, enables us to separate the two molecules. *Smaller molecules migrate at a faster rate through the gel than larger molecules* (**Figure 10–19**). The key to separation is the porous gel matrix, which restricts migration of larger molecules more than it restricts smaller molecules. The resolving power of this method is so great that polynucleotides that vary by even one nucleotide in length may be separated. Once electrophoresis is complete, bands representing the variously sized molecules are currently identified by use of a fluorescent dye that binds to nucleic acids.

Electrophoretic separation of nucleic acids is at the heart of a variety of commonly used research techniques discussed later in the text (Chapters 20 and 21). Of particular note, as you will see in those discussions, are the various "blotting" techniques (e.g., Southern blots and Northern blots), as well as DNA sequencing methods.

FIGURE 10-19 Electrophoretic separation of a mixture of DNA fragments that vary in length.

EXPLORING GENOMICS

Introduction to Bioinformatics: BLAST

MasteringGenetics™ Visit the Study Area: Exploring Genomics

In this chapter, we focused on the structural details of DNA, the genetic material for living organisms. In Chapter 20, you will learn how scientists can clone and sequence DNA—a routine technique in molecular biology and genetics laboratories. The explosion of DNA and protein sequence data that has occurred in the last 15 years has launched the field of *bioinformatics,* an interdisciplinary science that applies mathematics and computing technology to develop hardware and software for storing, sharing, comparing, and analyzing nucleic acid and protein sequence data.

A large number of sequence databases that make use of bioinformatics have been developed. An example is **GenBank** (http://www.ncbi.nlm.nih.gov/genbank/), which is the National Institutes of Health sequence database. This global resource, with access to databases in Europe and Japan, currently contains more than 152 billion base pairs of sequence data!

In the Exploring Genomics exercises for Chapter 5, you were introduced to the National Center for Biotechnology Information (NCBI) Genes and Disease site. Now we will use an NCBI application called **BLAST, Basic Local Alignment Search Tool.** BLAST is an invaluable program for searching through GenBank and other databases to find DNA- and protein-sequence similarities between cloned substances. It has many additional functions that we will explore in other exercises.

■ Exercise I – Introduction to BLAST

1. Access BLAST from the NCBI Web site at http://blast.ncbi.nlm.nih.gov/Blast.cgi.

2. Click on "nucleotide blast." This feature allows you to search DNA databases to look for a similarity between a sequence you enter and other sequences in the database. Do a nucleotide search with the following sequence:

   CCAGAGTCCAGCTGCTGCTCATA
   CTACTGATACTGCTGGG

3. Imagine that this sequence is a short part of a gene you cloned in your laboratory. You want to know if this gene or others with similar sequences have been discovered. Enter this sequence into the "Enter Query Sequence" text box at the top of the page. Near the bottom of the page, under the "Program Selection" category, choose "blastn"; then click on the "BLAST" button at the bottom of the page to run the search. It may take several minutes for results to be available because BLAST is using powerful algorithms to scroll through billions of bases of sequence data! A new page will appear with the results of your search.

4. On the search results page, below the Graphic Summary you will see a category called Descriptions and a table showing significant matches to the sequence you searched with (called the query sequence). BLAST determines significant matches based on statistical measures that consider the length of the query sequence, the number of matches with sequences in the database, and other factors. Significant *alignments,* regions of significant similarity in the query and subject sequences, typically have E values less than 1.0.

5. The top part of the table lists matches to transcripts (mRNA sequences), and the lower part lists matches to genomic DNA sequences, in order of highest to lowest number of matches.

(continued)

Exploring Genomics—continued

6. Alignments are indicated by horizontal lines. BLAST adjusts for gaps in the sequences, that is, for areas that may not align precisely because of missing bases in otherwise similar sequences. Scroll below the table to see the aligned sequences from this search, and then answer the following questions:

a. What were the top three matches to your query sequence?

b. For each alignment, BLAST also indicates the percent *identity* and the number of gaps in the match between the query and subject sequences. What was the percent identity for the top three matches? What percentage of each aligned sequence showed gaps indicating sequence differences?

c. Click on the links for the first matched sequence (far-right column). These will take you to a wealth of information, including the size of the sequence; the species it was derived from; a PubMed-linked chronology of research publications pertaining to this sequence; the complete sequence; and if the sequence encodes a polypeptide, the predicted amino acid sequence coded by the gene. Skim through the information presented for this gene. What is the gene's function?

7. A BLAST search can also be done by entering the *accession number* for a sequence, which is a unique identifying number assigned to a sequence before it can be put into a database. For example, search with the accession number NM_007305. What did you find?

8. Run a BLAST search using the sequences or accession numbers listed below. In each case, after entering the accession number or sequence in the "Enter Query Sequence" box, go to the "Choose Search Set" box and click on the "Others" button for database. Then go to the "Program Selection" box and click "megablast" before running your search. These features will allow you to align the query sequence with similar genes from a number of other species. When each search is completed, explore the information BLAST provides so that you can identify and learn about the gene encoded by the sequence.

a. NM_001006650. What is the top sequence that aligns with the query sequence of this accession number and shows 100 percent sequence identity?

b. DQ991619. What gene is encoded by this sequence?

c. NC_007596. What living animal has a sequence similar to this one?

CASE STUDY | Zigs and zags of the smallpox virus

Smallpox, a once highly lethal contagious disease, has been eradicated worldwide. However, research continues with stored samples of variola, the smallpox virus, because it is a potential weapon in bioterrorism. Human cells protect themselves from the variola virus (and other viruses) by activating genes that encode protective proteins. It has recently been discovered that in response to variola, human cells create small transitory stretches of Z-DNA at sites that regulate these genes. The smallpox virus can bypass this cellular defense mechanism by specifically targeting the segments of Z-DNA and inhibiting the synthesis of the protective proteins. This discovery raises some interesting questions:

1. What is unique about Z-DNA that might make it a specific target during viral infection?

2. How might the virus target host-cell Z-DNA formation to block the synthesis of antiviral proteins?

3. To study the interaction between viral proteins and Z-DNA, how could Z-DNA-forming DNA be synthesized in the lab?

4. How could this research lead to the development of drugs to combat infection by variola and related viruses?

Summary Points

> MasteringGenetics™ For activities, animations, and review quizzes, go to the Study Area.

1. Although both proteins and nucleic acids were initially considered as possible candidates for genetic material, proteins were initially favored.

2. By 1952, transformation studies and experiments using bacteria infected with bacteriophages strongly suggested that DNA is the genetic material in bacteria and most viruses.

3. Although initially only indirect observations supported the hypothesis that DNA controls inheritance in eukaryotes, subsequent studies involving recombinant DNA techniques and transgenic mice provided direct experimental evidence that the eukaryotic genetic material is DNA.

4. RNA serves as the genetic material in some bacteriophages as well as some plant and animal viruses.

5. As proposed by Watson and Crick, DNA exists in the form of a right-handed double helix composed of two long antiparallel polynucleotide chains held together

by hydrogen bonds formed between complementary, nitrogenous base pairs.

6. The second category of nucleic acids important in genetic function is RNA, which is similar to DNA with the exceptions that it is usually single stranded, the sugar ribose replaces the deoxyribose, and the pyrimidine uracil replaces thymine.

7. Various methods of analysis of nucleic acids, particularly molecular hybridization and electrophoresis, have led to studies essential to our understanding of genetic mechanisms.

8. Among the techniques used to study double-stranded DNA, reassociation kinetics analysis enabled geneticists to postulate the existence of repetitive DNA in eukaryotes, where certain nucleotide sequences are present many times in the genome.

INSIGHTS AND SOLUTIONS

The current chapter, in contrast to preceding chapters, does not emphasize genetic problem solving. Instead, it recounts some of the initial experimental analyses that launched the era of molecular genetics. Accordingly, our "Insights and Solutions" section shifts its emphasis to experimental rationale and analytical thinking, an approach that will continue to be used in later chapters whenever appropriate.

1. (a) Based strictly on your scrutiny of the transformation data of Avery, MacLeod, and McCarty, what objection might be made to the conclusion that DNA is the genetic material? What other conclusion might be considered?
(b) What observations, including later ones, argue against this objection?

Solution: (a) Based solely on their results, it may be concluded that DNA is essential for transformation. However, DNA might have been a substance that caused capsular formation by *directly* converting nonencapsulated cells to cells with a capsule. That is, DNA may simply have played a catalytic role in capsular synthesis, leading to cells displaying smooth type III colonies.
(b) First, transformed cells pass the trait onto their progeny cells, thus supporting the conclusion that DNA is responsible for heredity, not for the direct production of polysaccharide coats. Second, subsequent transformation studies over a period of five years showed that other traits, such as antibiotic resistance, could be transformed. Therefore, the transforming factor has a broad general effect, not one specific to polysaccharide synthesis. This observation is more in keeping with the conclusion that DNA is the genetic material.

2. If RNA were the universal genetic material, how would it have affected the Avery experiment and the Hershey–Chase experiment?

Solution: In the Avery experiment, digestion of the soluble filtrate with RNase, rather than DNase, would have eliminated transformation. Had this occurred, Avery and his colleagues would have concluded that RNA was the transforming factor. Hershey and Chase would have obtained identical results, since ^{32}P would also label RNA but not protein. Had they been using a bacteriophage with RNA as its nucleic acid, and had they known this, they would have concluded that RNA was responsible for directing the reproduction of their bacteriophage.

3. A quest to isolate an important disease-causing organism was successful, and molecular biologists were hard at work analyzing the results. The organism contained as its genetic material a remarkable nucleic acid with a base composition of A = 21 percent, C = 29 percent, G = 29 percent, U = 21 percent. When heated, it showed a major hyperchromic shift, and when the reassociation kinetics were studied, the nucleic acid of this organism reannealed more slowly than that of phage T4 and *E. coli*. T4 contains 10^5 nucleotide pairs.

Analyze this information carefully, and draw *all* possible conclusions about the genetic material of this organism, based strictly on the preceding observations. As a test of your model, make one prediction that if upheld would strengthen your hypothesis about the nature of this molecule.

Solution: First of all, because of the presence of uracil (U), the molecule appears to be RNA. In contrast to normal RNA, this one has base ratios of A/U = G/C = 1, suggesting that the molecule may be a double helix. The hyperchromic shift and reassociation kinetics support this hypothesis. In the kinetic study, since none of the nucleic acid segments reannealed more rapidly than bacterial or viral nucleic acid, there is no repetitive sequence RNA. Furthermore, the total length of unique sequence DNA is greater than that of either phage T4 (10^5 nucleotide pairs) or *E. coli*. A prediction might be made concerning the sugars. Our model suggests that ribose rather than deoxyribose should be present. If so, this observation would support the hypothesis that RNA is the genetic material in this organism.

Problems and Discussion Questions

HOW DO WE KNOW?

1. In this chapter, we first focused on the information that showed DNA to be the genetic material and then discussed the structure of DNA as proposed by Watson and Crick. We concluded the chapter by describing various techniques developed to study DNA. Along the way, we found many opportunities to consider the methods and reasoning by which much of this information was acquired. From the explanations given in the chapter, what answers would you propose to the following fundamental questions:

   (a) How were scientists able to determine that DNA, and not some other molecule, serves as the genetic material in bacteria and bacteriophages?

   (b) How do we know that DNA also serves as the genetic material in eukaryotes such as humans?

   (c) How was it determined that the structure of DNA is a double helix with the two strands held together by hydrogen bonds formed between complementary nitrogenous bases?

   (d) How do we know that G pairs with C and that A pairs with T as complementary base pairs are formed?

   (e) How do we know that repetitive DNA sequences exist in eukaryotes?

CONCEPT QUESTION

2. Review the Chapter Concepts list on p. 231. Most center around DNA and RNA and their role of serving as the genetic material. Write a short essay that contrasts these molecules, including a comparison of advantages conferred by their structure that each of them has over the other in serving in this role.

3. Discuss the reasons proteins were generally favored over DNA as the genetic material before 1940. What was the role of the tetranucleotide hypothesis in this controversy?

4. Contrast the various contributions made to an understanding of transformation by Griffith, by Avery and his colleagues, and by Taylor.

5. When Avery and his colleagues had obtained what was concluded to be the transforming factor from the IIIS virulent cells, they treated the fraction with proteases, RNase, and DNase, followed in each case by the assay for retention or loss of transforming ability. What were the purpose and results of these experiments? What conclusions were drawn?

6. Why were ^{32}P and ^{35}S chosen for use in the Hershey–Chase experiment? Discuss the rationale and conclusions of this experiment.

7. Does the design of the Hershey–Chase experiment distinguish between DNA and RNA as the molecule serving as the genetic material? Why or why not?

8. What observations are consistent with the conclusion that DNA serves as the genetic material in eukaryotes? List and discuss them.

9. What are the exceptions to the general rule that DNA is the genetic material in all organisms? What evidence supports these exceptions?

10. Draw the chemical structure of the three components of a nucleotide, and then link the three together. What atoms are removed from the structures when the linkages are formed?

11. How are the carbon and nitrogen atoms of the sugars, purines, and pyrimidines numbered?

12. Adenine may also be named 6-amino purine. How would you name the other four nitrogenous bases, using this alternative system? (O is indicated by "oxy-," and CH$_3$ by "methyl.")

13. Draw the chemical structure of a dinucleotide composed of A and G. Opposite this structure, draw the dinucleotide composed of T and C in an antiparallel (or upside-down) fashion. Form the possible hydrogen bonds.

14. Describe the various characteristics of the Watson–Crick double-helix model for DNA.

15. What evidence did Watson and Crick have at their disposal in 1953? What was their approach in arriving at the structure of DNA?

16. What might Watson and Crick have concluded had Chargaff's data from a single source indicated the following?

	A	T	G	C
%	29	19	21	31

Why would this conclusion be contradictory to Wilkins's and Franklin's data?

17. How do covalent bonds differ from hydrogen bonds? Define base complementarity.

18. List three main differences between DNA and RNA.

19. What are the three major types of RNA molecules? How is each related to the concept of information flow?

20. What component of the nucleotide is responsible for the absorption of ultraviolet light? How is this technique important in the analysis of nucleic acids?

21. What is the physical state of DNA following denaturation?

22. What is the hyperchromic effect? How is it measured? What does T_m imply?

23. Why is T_m related to base composition?

24. What is the chemical basis of molecular hybridization?

25. What did the Watson–Crick model suggest about the replication of DNA?

26. A genetics student was asked to draw the chemical structure of an adenine- and thymine-containing dinucleotide derived from DNA. His answer is shown here:

Explanations

1 Extra phosphate should not be present

The student made more than six major errors. One of them is circled, numbered 1, and explained. Find five others. Circle them, number them 2 through 6, and briefly explain each in the manner of the example given.

27. Considering the information in this chapter on B- and Z-DNA and right- and left-handed helices, carefully analyze structures (a) and (b) below and draw conclusions about their helical nature. Which is right handed and which is left handed?

(a)   (b)

28. One of the most common spontaneous lesions that occurs in DNA under physiological conditions is the hydrolysis of the amino group of cytosine, converting the cytosine to uracil. What would be the effect on DNA structure of a uracil group replacing cytosine?

29. In some organisms, cytosine is methylated at carbon 5 of the pyrimidine ring after it is incorporated into DNA. If a 5-methyl cytosine molecule is then hydrolyzed, as described in Problem 28, what base will be generated?

30. Because of its rapid turnaround time, fluorescent *in situ* hybridization (FISH) is commonly used in hospitals and laboratories as an aneuploid screen of cells retrieved from amniocentesis and chorionic villus sampling (CVS). Chromosomes 13, 18, 21, X, and Y (see Chapter 8) are typically screened for aneuploidy in this way. Explain how FISH might be accomplished using amniotic or CVS samples and why the above chromosomes have been chosen for screening.

31. Assume that you are interested in separating short (200–400 nucleotides) DNA molecules from a pool of longer molecules in the 10,000–20,000 nucleotide range. You have two recipes for making your agarose gels: one recipe uses 1.5 percent agarose and would be considered a "hard gel," while the other uses 0.5 percent agarose and would be considered a loose gel. Which recipe would you consider using and why?

Extra-Spicy Problems

MasteringGenetics™ Visit for instructor-assigned tutorials and problems.

32. A primitive eukaryote was discovered that displayed a unique nucleic acid as its genetic material. Analysis provided the following information:

(a) The general X-ray diffraction pattern is similar to that of DNA, but with somewhat different dimensions and more irregularity.

(b) A major hyperchromic shift is evident upon heating and monitoring UV absorption at 260 nm.

(c) Base-composition analysis reveals four bases in the following proportions:

Adenine	=	8%
Guanine	=	37%
Xanthine	=	37%
Hypoxanthine	=	18%

(d) About 75 percent of the sugars are deoxyribose, while 25 percent are ribose.

Postulate a model for the structure of this molecule that is consistent with the foregoing observations.

33. *Newsdate: March 1, 2030.* A unique creature has been discovered during exploration of outer space. Recently, its genetic material has been isolated and analyzed. This material is similar in some ways to DNA in its chemical makeup. It contains in abundance the 4-carbon sugar erythrose and a molar equivalent of phosphate groups. In addition, it contains six nitrogenous bases: adenine (A), guanine (G), thymine (T), cytosine (C), hypoxanthine (H), and xanthine (X). These bases exist in the following relative proportions:

$$A = T = H \text{ and } C = G = X$$

X-ray diffraction studies have established a regularity in the molecule and a constant diameter of about 30 Å. Together, these data have suggested a model for the structure of this molecule.

(a) Propose a general model of this molecule. Describe it briefly.

(b) What base-pairing properties must exist for H and for X in the model?

(c) Given the constant diameter of 30 Å, do you think that *either* (i) both H and X are purines or both pyrimidines, *or* (ii) one is a purine and one is a pyrimidine?

34. You are provided with DNA samples from two newly discovered bacterial viruses. Based on the various analytical techniques discussed in this chapter, construct a research protocol that would be useful in characterizing and contrasting the DNA of both viruses. For each technique that you include in the protocol, indicate the type of information you hope to obtain.

35. During gel electrophoresis, DNA molecules can easily be separated according to size because all DNA molecules have the same charge-to-mass ratio and the same shape (long rod). Would you expect RNA molecules to behave in the same manner as DNA during gel electrophoresis? Why or why not?

36. Electrophoresis is an extremely useful procedure when applied to analysis of nucleic acids as it can resolve molecules of different sizes with relative ease and accuracy. Large molecules migrate more slowly than small molecules in agarose gels. However, the fact that nucleic acids of the same length may exist in a variety of conformations can often complicate the interpretation of electrophoretic separations. For instance, when a single species of a bacterial plasmid is isolated from cells, the individual plasmids may exist in three forms (depending on the genotype of their host and conditions of isolation): superhelical/supercoiled (form I), nicked/open circle

(form II), and linear (form III). Form I is compact and very tightly coiled, with both DNA strands continuous. Form II exists as a loose circle because one of the two DNA strands has been broken, thus releasing the supercoil. All three have the same mass, but each will migrate at a different rate through a gel. Based on your understanding of gel composition and DNA migration, predict the relative rates of migration of the various DNA structures mentioned above.

37. Following is a table (modified from Kropinski, 1973) that presents the T_m and chemical composition (%G$\equiv$C) of DNA from certain bacteriophages. From these data develop a graph that presents %G$\equiv$C (ordinate) and T_m (abscissa). What is the relationship between T_m and %G$\equiv$C for these samples? What might be the molecular basis of this relationship?

Phage	T_m	%G $\equiv$ C
α	86.5	44.0
κ	91.5	53.8
λ	89	49.2
$\phi80$	90.5	53.0
χ	92.1	57.4
Mu-1	88	51.4
T1	89	48.0
T3	90	49.6
T7	89.5	48.0

Transmission electron micrograph of human DNA from a HeLa cell, illustrating a replication fork characteristic of active DNA replication.

11 DNA Replication and Recombination

CHAPTER CONCEPTS

- Genetic continuity between parental and progeny cells is maintained by semiconservative replication of DNA, as predicted by the Watson–Crick model.

- Semiconservative replication uses each strand of the parent double helix as a template, and each newly replicated double helix includes one "old" and one "new" strand of DNA.

- DNA synthesis is a complex but orderly process, occurring under the direction of a myriad of enzymes and other proteins.

- DNA synthesis involves the polymerization of nucleotides into polynucleotide chains.

- DNA synthesis is similar in prokaryotes and eukaryotes, but more complex in eukaryotes.

- In eukaryotes, DNA synthesis at the ends of chromosomes (telomeres) poses a special problem, overcome by a unique RNA-containing enzyme, telomerase.

- Genetic recombination, an important process leading to the exchange of segments between DNA molecules, occurs under the direction of a group of enzymes.

Following Watson and Crick's proposal for the structure of DNA, scientists focused their attention on how this molecule is replicated. Replication is an essential function of the genetic material and must be executed precisely if genetic continuity between cells is to be maintained following cell division. It is an enormous, complex task. Consider for a moment that more than 3×10^9 (3 billion) base pairs exist within the human genome. To duplicate faithfully the DNA of just one of these chromosomes requires a mechanism of extreme precision. Even an error rate of only 10^6 (one in a million) will still create 3000 errors (obviously an excessive number) during each replication cycle of the genome. Although it is not error free, and much of evolution would not have occurred if it were, an extremely accurate system of DNA replication has evolved in all organisms.

As Watson and Crick noted in the concluding paragraph of their 1953 paper (reprinted on page 248, their proposed model of the double helix provided the initial insight into how replication occurs. Called *semiconservative replication,* this mode of DNA duplication was soon to receive strong support from numerous studies of viruses, prokaryotes, and eukaryotes. Once the general *mode* of replication was clarified, research to determine the precise details of *DNA synthesis* intensified. What has since been discovered is that numerous enzymes and other proteins are needed to copy a DNA helix. Because of the complexity of the chemical events during synthesis, this subject remains an extremely active area of research.

In this chapter, we will discuss the general mode of replication, as well as the specific details of DNA synthesis. The research leading to such knowledge is another link in our understanding of life processes at the molecular level.

11.1 DNA Is Reproduced by Semiconservative Replication

Watson and Crick recognized that, because of the arrangement and nature of the nitrogenous bases, each strand of a DNA double helix could serve as a template for the synthesis of its complement (**Figure 11–1**). They proposed that, if the helix were unwound, each nucleotide along the two parent strands would have an affinity for its complementary nucleotide. As we learned earlier in the text (see Chapter 10), the complementarity is due to the potential hydrogen bonds that can be formed. If thymidylic acid (T) were present, it would "attract" adenylic acid (A); if guanidylic acid (G) were present, it would attract cytidylic acid (C); likewise, A would attract T, and C would attract G. If these nucleotides were then covalently linked into polynucleotide chains along both templates, the result would be the production of two identical double strands of DNA. Each replicated DNA molecule would consist of one "old" and one "new" strand, hence the reason for the name **semiconservative replication**.

Two other theoretical modes of replication are possible that also rely on the parental strands as a template (**Figure 11–2**). In **conservative replication**, complementary polynucleotide chains are synthesized as described earlier. Following synthesis, however, the two newly created strands then come together and the parental strands reassociate. The original helix is thus "conserved."

In the second alternative mode, called **dispersive replication**, the parental strands are dispersed into two new double helices following replication. Hence, each strand consists of both old and new DNA. This mode would involve cleavage of the parental strands during replication. It is the most complex of the three possibilities and is therefore considered to be least likely to occur. It could not, however, be ruled out as an experimental model. Figure 11–2 shows the theoretical results of a single round of replication by each of the three different modes.

New   Old   Old   New

FIGURE 11–1 Generalized model of semiconservative replication of DNA. New synthesis is shown in blue.

Conservative   Semiconservative   Dispersive

One round of replication — new synthesis is shown in blue

FIGURE 11–2 Results of one round of replication of DNA for each of the three possible modes by which replication could be accomplished.

The Meselson–Stahl Experiment

In 1958, Matthew Meselson and Franklin Stahl published the results of an experiment providing strong evidence that semiconservative replication is the mode used by bacterial cells to produce new DNA molecules. They grew *E. coli* cells for many generations in a medium that had $^{15}NH_4Cl$ (ammonium chloride) as the only nitrogen source. A "heavy" isotope of nitrogen, ^{15}N contains one more neutron than the naturally occurring ^{14}N isotope; thus, molecules containing ^{15}N are more dense than those containing ^{14}N. Unlike radioactive isotopes, ^{15}N is stable. After many generations in this medium, almost all nitrogen-containing molecules in the *E. coli* cells, including the nitrogenous bases of DNA, contained the heavier isotope.

Critical to the success of this experiment, DNA containing ^{15}N can be distinguished from DNA containing ^{14}N. The experimental procedure involves the use of a technique referred to as **sedimentation equilibrium centrifugation,** or as it is also called, *buoyant density gradient centrifugation.* Samples are forced by centrifugation through a density gradient of a heavy metal salt, such as cesium chloride. Molecules of DNA will reach equilibrium when their density equals the density of the gradient medium. In this case, ^{15}N-DNA will reach this point at a position closer to the bottom of the tube than will ^{14}N-DNA.

In this experiment (**Figure 11–3**), uniformly labeled ^{15}N cells were transferred to a medium containing only $^{14}NH_4Cl$. Thus, all "new" synthesis of DNA during replication contained only the "lighter" isotope of nitrogen. The time of transfer to the new medium was taken as time zero ($t = 0$). The *E. coli* cells were allowed to replicate over several generations, with cell samples removed after each replication cycle. DNA was isolated from each sample and subjected to sedimentation equilibrium centrifugation.

After one generation, the isolated DNA was present in only a single band of intermediate density—the expected result for semiconservative replication in which each replicated molecule was composed of one new ^{14}N-strand and one old ^{15}N-strand (**Figure 11–4**). This result was not consistent with the prediction of conservative replication, in which two distinct bands would occur; thus this mode may be rejected.

After two cell divisions, DNA samples showed two density bands—one intermediate band and one lighter band corresponding to the ^{14}N position in the gradient. Similar results occurred after a third generation, except that the proportion of the lighter band increased. This was again consistent with the interpretation that replication is semiconservative.

You may have realized that a molecule exhibiting intermediate density is also consistent with dispersive replication. However, Meselson and Stahl ruled out this mode of replication on the basis of two observations. First, after the first generation of replication in an ^{14}N-containing medium, they isolated the hybrid molecule and heat denatured it. Recall from earlier in the text (see Chapter 10), that heating will separate a duplex into single strands. When the densities of the single strands of the hybrid were determined, they exhibited *either*

FIGURE 11–3   The Meselson–Stahl experiment.

E. coli grown in ^{15}N-labeled medium

E. coli DNA becomes uniformly labeled with ^{15}N in nitrogenous bases

Generation 0

^{15}N-labeled *E. coli* added to ^{14}N medium

Generation I

Cells replicate once in ^{14}N

Generation II

Cells replicate a second time in ^{14}N

Generation III

Cells replicate a third time in ^{14}N

Gravitational force

DNA extracted and centrifuged in gradient

$^{15}N/^{15}N$ $^{15}N/^{14}N$ $^{14}N/^{14}N$ $^{15}N/^{14}N$ $^{14}N/^{14}N$ $^{15}N/^{14}N$

FIGURE 11-4 The expected results of two generations of semiconservative replication in the Meselson–Stahl experiment.

an ^{15}N profile *or* an ^{14}N profile, but *not* an intermediate density. This observation is consistent with the semiconservative mode but inconsistent with the dispersive mode.

Furthermore, if replication were dispersive, *all* generations after $t = 0$ would demonstrate DNA of an intermediate density. In each generation after the first, the ratio of ^{15}N/^{14}N would decrease and the hybrid band would become lighter and lighter, eventually approaching the ^{14}N band. This result was not observed. The Meselson–Stahl experiment provided conclusive support for semiconservative replication in bacteria and tended to rule out both the conservative and dispersive modes.

NOW SOLVE THIS

11–1 In the Meselson–Stahl experiment, which of the three modes of replication could be ruled out after one round of replication? after two rounds?

■ **HINT:** *This problem involves an understanding of the nature of the experiment as well as the difference between the three possible modes of replication. The key to its solution is to determine which mode will not create "hybrid" helices after one round of replication.*

For more practice, see Problems 3, 4, and 5.

Semiconservative Replication in Eukaryotes

In 1957, the year before the work of Meselson and Stahl was published, J. Herbert Taylor, Philip Woods, and Walter Hughes presented evidence that semiconservative replication also occurs in eukaryotic organisms. They experimented with root tips of the broad bean *Vicia faba*, which are an excellent source of dividing cells. These researchers were able to monitor the process of replication by labeling DNA with ^{3}H-thymidine, a radioactive precursor of DNA, and by performing autoradiography.

Autoradiography is a common technique that, when applied cytologically, pinpoints the location of a radioisotope in a cell. In this procedure, a photographic emulsion is placed over a histological preparation containing cellular material (root tips, in this experiment), and the preparation is stored in the dark. The slide is then developed, much as photographic film is processed. Because the radioisotope emits energy, following development the emulsion turns black at the approximate point of emission. The end result is the presence of dark spots or "grains" on the surface of the section, identifying the location of newly synthesized DNA within the cell.

Taylor and his colleagues grew root tips for approximately one generation in the presence of the radioisotope and then placed them in unlabeled medium in which cell division continued. At the conclusion of each generation, they arrested the cultures at metaphase by adding colchicine (a chemical derived from the crocus plant that poisons the spindle fibers) and then examined the chromosomes by autoradiography. They found radioactive thymidine only in association with chromatids that contained newly synthesized DNA. **Figure 11–5** illustrates the replication of a single chromosome over two division cycles, including the distribution of grains.

These results are compatible with the semiconservative mode of replication. After the first replication cycle in the presence of the isotope, both sister chromatids show radioactivity, indicating that each chromatid contains one new radioactive DNA strand and one old unlabeled strand. After the second replication cycle, *which takes place in unlabeled medium,* only one of the two sister chromatids of each chromosome should be radioactive because half of the parent strands are unlabeled. With only the minor exceptions of *sister chromatid exchanges* (discussed in Chapter 5), this result was observed.

(a)

Replication I
³H-thymidine

Unlabeled
chromosome

Both sister
chromatids labeled

Metaphase

Anaphase

Chromatids migrate into separate cells

**No sister
chromatid exchange**

Replication II
Unlabeled thymidine

**Sister chromatid
exchange**

(b)

Unlabeled
chromatid

**Only one
chromatid labeled**

(c)

**Reciprocal
regions of both
chromatids
labeled**

Metaphase II

Metaphase II

FIGURE 11–5 The Taylor–Woods–Hughes experiment, demonstrating the semiconservative mode of replication of DNA in root tips of *Vicia faba*. (a) An unlabeled chromosome proceeds through the cell cycle in the presence of ³H-thymidine. As it enters mitosis, both sister chromatids of the chromosome are labeled, as shown, by autoradiography. After a second round of replication (b), this time in the absence of ³H-thymidine, only one chromatid of each chromosome is expected to be surrounded by grains. Except where a reciprocal exchange has occurred between sister chromatids (c), the expectation was upheld. The micrographs are of the actual autoradiograms obtained in the experiment.

Together, the Meselson–Stahl experiment and the experiment by Taylor, Woods, and Hughes soon led to the general acceptance of the semiconservative mode of replication. Later studies with other organisms reached the same conclusion and also strongly supported Watson and Crick's proposal for the double-helix model of DNA.

Origins, Forks, and Units of Replication

To enhance our understanding of semiconservative replication, let's briefly consider a number of relevant issues. The first concerns the **origin of replication**. Where along the chromosome is DNA replication initiated? Is there only a single origin, or does DNA synthesis begin at more than one point? Is any given point of origin random, or is it located at a specific region along the chromosome? Second, once replication begins, does it proceed in a single direction or in both directions away from the origin? In other words, is replication *unidirectional* or *bidirectional*?

To address these issues, we need to introduce two terms. First, at each point along the chromosome where replication is occurring, the strands of the helix are unwound, creating what is called a **replication fork**. Such a fork will initially appear at the point of origin of synthesis and then move along the DNA duplex as replication proceeds. If replication is bidirectional, two such forks will be present, migrating in opposite directions away from the origin. The second term refers to the length of DNA that is replicated following one initiation event at a single origin. This is a unit referred to as the **replicon**.

The evidence is clear regarding the origin and direction of replication. John Cairns tracked replication in *E. coli*, using radioactive precursors of DNA synthesis and autoradiography. He was able to demonstrate that in *E. coli* there is only a single region, called *oriC*, where replication is initiated. The presence of only a single origin is characteristic of bacteria, which have only one circular chromosome. Since DNA synthesis in bacteria originates at a single point, the entire chromosome constitutes one replicon. In *E. coli*, the replicon consists of the entire genome of 4.6 Mb (4.6 million base pairs).

Figure 11–6 illustrates Cairns's interpretation of DNA replication in *E. coli*. This interpretation does not answer the question of unidirectional versus bidirectional synthesis. However, other results, derived from studies of bacteriophage lambda, demonstrated that replication is bidirectional, moving away from *oriC* in both

directions. Figure 11–6 therefore interprets Cairns's work with that understanding. Bidirectional replication creates two replication forks that migrate farther and farther apart as replication proceeds. These forks eventually merge, as semiconservative replication of the entire chromosome is completed, at a termination region, called *ter*.

Later in this chapter we will see that in eukaryotes, each chromosome contains multiple points of origin.

11.2 DNA Synthesis in Bacteria Involves Five Polymerases, as Well as Other Enzymes

To say that replication is semiconservative and bidirectional describes the overall *pattern* of DNA duplication and the association of finished strands with one another once synthesis is completed. However, it says little about the more complex issue of how the actual *synthesis* of long complementary polynucleotide chains occurs on a DNA template. Like most questions in molecular biology, this one was first studied using microorganisms. Research on DNA synthesis began about the same time as the Meselson–Stahl work, and the topic is still an active area of investigation. What is most apparent in this research is the tremendous complexity of the biological synthesis of DNA.

DNA Polymerase I

Studies of the enzymology of DNA replication were first reported by Arthur Kornberg and colleagues in 1957. They isolated an enzyme from *E. coli* that was able to direct DNA synthesis in a cell-free (*in vitro*) system. The enzyme is called **DNA polymerase I**, because it was the first of several similar enzymes to be isolated.

Kornberg determined that there were two major requirements for *in vitro* DNA synthesis under the direction of DNA polymerase I: (1) all four deoxyribonucleoside triphosphates (dNTPs) and (2) template DNA. If any one of the four deoxyribonucleoside triphosphates was omitted from the reaction, no measurable synthesis occurred. If derivatives of these precursor molecules other than the nucleoside triphosphate were used (nucleotides or nucleoside diphosphates), synthesis also did not occur. If no template DNA was added, synthesis of DNA occurred but was reduced greatly.

Most of the synthesis directed by Kornberg's enzyme appeared to be exactly the type required for semiconservative replication. The reaction is summarized in **Figure 11–7**, which depicts the addition of a single nucleotide. The enzyme has since been shown to consist of a single polypeptide containing 928 amino acids.

FIGURE 11–6 Bidirectional replication of the *E. coli* chromosome. The thin black arrows identify the advancing replication forks.

FIGURE 11–7 The chemical reaction catalyzed by DNA polymerase I. During each step, a single nucleotide is added to the growing complement of the DNA template, using a nucleoside triphosphate as the substrate. The release of inorganic pyrophosphate drives the reaction energetically.

The way in which each nucleotide is added to the growing chain is a function of the specificity of DNA polymerase I. As shown in **Figure 11–8**, the precursor dNTP contains the three phosphate groups attached to the 5′-carbon of deoxyribose. As the two terminal phosphates are cleaved during synthesis, the remaining phosphate attached to the 5′-carbon is covalently linked to the 3′-OH group of the deoxyribose to which it is added. Thus, **chain elongation** occurs in the **5′ to 3′ direction** by the addition of one nucleotide at a time to the growing 3′ end. Each step provides a newly exposed 3′-OH group that can participate in the next addition of a nucleotide as DNA synthesis proceeds.

Having isolated DNA polymerase I and established its catalytic activity, Kornberg next sought to demonstrate the accuracy, or fidelity, with which the enzyme replicated the DNA template. Because technology for ascertaining the nucleotide sequences of the template and newly synthesized strand was not yet available in 1957, he initially had to rely on several indirect methods.

One of Kornberg's approaches was to compare the nitrogenous base compositions of the DNA template with those of the recovered DNA product. Table 11.1 shows Kornberg's base-composition analysis of three DNA templates. Within experimental error, the base composition of each product agreed with the template DNAs used. These data, along with other types of comparisons of template and product, suggested that the templates were replicated faithfully.

DNA Polymerase II, III, IV, and V

While DNA polymerase I (DNA polymerases are abbreviated as DNA Pol I, II, etc.) clearly directs the synthesis of DNA, a serious reservation about the enzyme's true biological role was raised in 1969. Paula DeLucia and John Cairns discovered a mutant strain of *E. coli* that was deficient in polymerase I activity. The mutation was designated *polA1*. In the absence of the functional enzyme, this mutant strain of *E. coli* still duplicated its DNA and successfully

FIGURE 11–8 Demonstration of 5′ to 3′ synthesis of DNA.

TABLE 11.1 Base Composition of the DNA Template and the Product of Replication in Kornberg's Early Work

Organism	Template or Product	%A	%T	%G	%C
T2	Template	32.7	33.0	16.8	17.5
	Product	33.2	32.1	17.2	17.5
E. coli	Template	25.0	24.3	24.5	26.2
	Product	26.1	25.1	24.3	24.5
Calf	Template	28.9	26.7	22.8	21.6
	Product	28.7	27.7	21.8	21.8

Source: Kornberg (1960).

reproduced. However, the cells were deficient in their ability to repair DNA. For example, the mutant strain is highly sensitive to ultraviolet light (UV) and radiation, both of which damage DNA and are mutagenic. Nonmutant bacteria are able to repair a great deal of UV-induced damage.

These observations led to two conclusions:

1. At least one enzyme other than DNA Pol I is responsible for replicating DNA *in vivo* in *E. coli* cells.

2. DNA Pol I serves a secondary function *in vivo,* and is now believed to be critical to the maintenance of fidelity of DNA synthesis.

To date, four other unique DNA polymerases have been isolated from cells lacking polymerase I activity and from normal cells that contain DNA Pol I. Table 11.2 contrasts several characteristics of DNA Pol I with **DNA Pol II and III**. Although none of the three can *initiate* DNA synthesis on a template, all three can *elongate* an existing DNA strand, called a **primer**, and all possess 3′ to 5′ exonuclease activity, which means that they have the potential to polymerize in one direction and then pause, reverse their direction, and excise nucleotides just added. As we will later discuss, this activity provides a capacity to proofread newly synthesized DNA and to remove and replace incorrect nucleotides.

DNA Pol I also demonstrates 5′ to 3′ exonuclease activity. This activity allows the enzyme to excise nucleotides, starting at the end at which synthesis begins and proceeding in the same direction of synthesis. Two final observations probably explain why Kornberg isolated polymerase I and not polymerase III: polymerase I is present in greater amounts than is polymerase III, and it is also much more stable.

What then are the roles of the polymerases *in vivo*? DNA Pol III is the enzyme responsible for the 5′ to 3′ polymerization essential to *in vivo* replication. Its 3′ to 5′ exonuclease activity also provides a proofreading function that is activated when it inserts an incorrect nucleotide. When this occurs, synthesis stalls and the polymerase "reverses course," excising the incorrect nucleotide. Then,

it proceeds back in the 5′ to 3′ direction, synthesizing the complement of the template strand. DNA Pol I is believed to be responsible for removing the primer, as well as for the synthesis that fills gaps produced after this removal. Its exonuclease activities also allow for its participation in DNA repair. DNA Pol II, as well as **DNA Pol IV and V,** are involved in various aspects of repair of DNA that has been damaged by external forces, such as ultraviolet light. Polymerase II is encoded by a gene activated by disruption of DNA synthesis at the replication fork.

The DNA Pol III Holoenzyme

We conclude this section by emphasizing the complexity of the DNA Pol III molecule. The active form of DNA Pol III, referred to as the **holoenzyme,** is made up of unique polypeptide subunits, ten of which have been identified (Table 11.3). The largest subunit, α, along with subunits ε and θ, form a complex called the **core enzyme,** which imparts the catalytic function to the holoenzyme. In *E. coli,* each holoenzyme contains two, and possibly three, core enzyme complexes. As part of each core, the α subunit is responsible for DNA synthesis along the template strands, whereas the ε subunit possesses 3′ to 5′ exonuclease capability, essential to proofreading. The need for more than one core enzyme will soon become apparent. A second group of five subunits (γ, δ, δ', χ, and υ) are complexed to form what is called the **sliding clamp loader,** which pairs

TABLE 11.2 Properties of Bacterial DNA Polymerases I, II, and III

Properties	I	II	III
Initiation of chain synthesis	−	−	−
5′–3′ polymerization	+	+	+
3′–5′ exonuclease activity	+	+	+
5′–3′ exonuclease activity	+	−	−
Molecules of polymerase/cell	400	?	15

TABLE 11.3 Subunits of the DNA Polymerase III Holoenzyme

Subunit	Function	Groupings
α	5′–3′ polymerization	Core enzyme: Elongates polynucleotide chain and proofreads
ε	3′–5′ exonuclease	
θ	Core assembly	
γ		
δ	Loads enzyme on	
δ'	template (serves as	γ complex
χ	clamp loader)	
υ		
β	Sliding clamp structure (processivity factor)	
τ	Dimerizes core complex	

DNA Pol III holoenzyme

FIGURE 11–9 The components making up the DNA Pol III holoenzyme, as described in the text. While there may be three core enzyme complexes present in the holoenzyme, for simplicity, we illustrate only two.

with the core enzyme and facilitates the function of a critical component of the holoenzyme, called the **sliding DNA clamp.** The enzymatic function of the sliding clamp loader is dependent on energy generated by the hydrolysis of ATP. The sliding DNA clamp links to the core enzyme and is made up of multiple copies of the β subunit, taking on the shape of a donut, whereby it can open and shut, to encircle the unreplicated DNA helix. By doing so, and being linked to the core enzyme, the clamp leads the way during synthesis, maintaining the binding of the core enzyme to the template during polymerization of nucleotides. Thus, the length of DNA that is replicated by the core enzyme before it detaches from the template, a property referred to as **processivity,** is vastly increased. There is one sliding clamp per core enzyme. Finally, one τ subunit interacts with each core enzyme, linking it to the sliding clamp loader.

The DNA Pol III holoenzyme is diagrammatically illustrated in **Figure 11–9.** You should compare the diagram to the description of each component above. Note that we have shown the holoenzyme to contain two core enzyme complexes, although as stated above, a third one may be present. The components of the DNA Pol III holoenzyme will be referred to in the discussion that follows.

11.3 Many Complex Issues Must Be Resolved during DNA Replication

We have thus far established that in bacteria and viruses replication is semiconservative and bidirectional along a single replicon. We also know that synthesis is catalyzed by DNA polymerase III and occurs in the 5′ to 3′ direction. Bidirectional synthesis creates two replication forks that move in opposite directions away from the origin of synthesis. As we can see from the following list, many issues

remain to be resolved in order to provide a comprehensive understanding of DNA replication:

1. The helix must undergo localized unwinding, and the resulting "open" configuration must be stabilized so that synthesis may proceed along both strands.

2. As unwinding and subsequent DNA synthesis proceed, increased coiling creates tension further down the helix, which must be reduced.

3. A primer of some sort must be synthesized so that polymerization can commence under the direction of DNA polymerase III. Surprisingly, RNA, not DNA, serves as the primer.

4. Once the RNA primers have been synthesized, DNA polymerase III begins to synthesize the DNA complement of both strands of the parent molecule. Because the two strands are antiparallel to one another, continuous synthesis in the direction that the replication fork moves is possible along only one of the two strands. On the other strand, synthesis must be discontinuous and thus involves a somewhat different process.

5. The RNA primers must be removed prior to completion of replication. The gaps that are temporarily created must be filled with DNA complementary to the template at each location.

6. The newly synthesized DNA strand that fills each temporary gap must be joined to the adjacent strand of DNA.

7. While DNA polymerases accurately insert complementary bases during replication, they are not perfect, and, occasionally, incorrect nucleotides are added to the growing strand. A proofreading mechanism that also corrects errors is an integral process during DNA synthesis.

As we consider these points, examine Figures 11–10, 11–11, and 11–12 to see how each issue is resolved. Figure 11–13 summarizes the model of DNA synthesis.

Unwinding the DNA Helix

As discussed earlier, there is a single point of origin along the circular chromosome of most bacteria and viruses at which DNA replication is initiated. This region in *E. coli* has been particularly well studied and is called *oriC*. It consists of 245 DNA base pairs and is characterized by five repeating sequences of 9 base pairs, and three repeating sequences of 13 base pairs, called **9mers** and **13mers,** respectively. Both 9mers and 13mers are AT-rich, which renders them relatively less stable than an average double-helical sequence of DNA, which no doubt enhances helical unwinding. A specific initiator protein, called **DnaA** (because it is encoded by the *dnaA* gene), is responsible for initiating replication by binding to a region of 9mers. This newly formed complex then undergoes a slight conformational change and associates with the region of 13mers, which causes the helix to destabilize and open up, exposing single-stranded regions of DNA (ssDNA). This step facilitates the subsequent binding of another key player in the process—a protein called **DNA helicase** (made up of multiple copies of the DnaB polypeptide). DNA helicase is assembled as a hexamer of subunits around one of the exposed single-stranded DNA molecules. The helicase subsequently recruits the holoenzyme to bind to the newly formed replication fork to formally initiate replication, and it then proceeds to move along the ssDNA, opening up the helix as it progresses. Helicases require energy supplied by the hydrolysis of ATP, which aids in denaturing the hydrogen bonds that stabilize double helix.

Once the helicase has opened up the helix and ssDNA is available, base pairing must be inhibited until it can serve as a template for synthesis. This is accomplished by proteins that bind specifically to single strands of DNA, appropriately called **single-stranded binding proteins (SSBs)**.

As unwinding proceeds, a coiling tension is created ahead of the replication fork, often producing **supercoiling**. In circular molecules, supercoiling may take the form of added twists and turns of the DNA, much like the coiling you create in a rubber band by stretching it out and then twisting one end. Such supercoiling can be relaxed by **DNA gyrase**, a member of a larger group of enzymes referred to as **DNA topoisomerases**. The gyrase makes either single- or double-stranded "cuts" and also catalyzes localized movements that have the effect of "undoing" the twists and knots created during supercoiling. The strands are then resealed. These various reactions are driven by the energy released during ATP hydrolysis.

Together, the DNA, the polymerase complex, and associated enzymes make up an array of molecules that initiate DNA synthesis and are part of what we have previously called the *replisome*.

Initiation of DNA Synthesis Using an RNA Primer

Once a small portion of the helix is unwound and the holoenzyme is in place, how is synthesis initiated? As we have seen, DNA polymerase III requires a primer with a free 3′-hydroxyl group in order to elongate a polynucleotide chain. Since none is available in a circular chromosome, this absence prompted researchers to investigate how the first nucleotide could be added. It is now clear that RNA serves as the primer that initiates DNA synthesis.

A short segment of RNA (about 10 to 12 nucleotides long), complementary to DNA, is first synthesized on the DNA template. Synthesis of the RNA is directed by a form of RNA polymerase called **primase**, which is recruited to

DNA template

Initiation of RNA primer

New DNA added to RNA primer

FIGURE 11–10 The initiation of DNA synthesis. A complementary RNA primer is first synthesized, to which DNA is added. All synthesis is in the 5′ to 3′ direction. Eventually, the RNA primer is replaced with DNA under the direction of DNA polymerase I.

the replication fork by DNA helicase, and which does not require a free 3′ end to initiate synthesis. It is to this short segment of RNA that DNA Pol III begins to add deoxyribonucleotides, initiating DNA synthesis. A conceptual diagram of initiation on a DNA template is shown in **Figure 11–10**. Later, the RNA primer is clipped out and replaced with DNA. This is thought to occur under the direction of DNA Pol I. Recognized in viruses, bacteria, and several eukaryotic organisms, RNA priming is a universal phenomenon during the initiation of DNA synthesis.

Continuous and Discontinuous DNA Synthesis

We must now revisit the fact that the two strands of a double helix are **antiparallel** to each other—that is, one runs in the 5′–3′ direction, while the other has the opposite 3′–5′ polarity. Because DNA Pol III synthesizes DNA in only the 5′–3′ direction, synthesis along an advancing replication fork occurs in one direction on one strand and in the opposite direction on the other.

As a result, as the strands unwind and the replication fork progresses down the helix (**Figure 11–11**), only one strand can serve as a template for **continuous DNA synthesis**. This newly synthesized DNA is called the **leading strand**. As the fork progresses, many points of initiation are necessary on the opposite DNA template, resulting in **discontinuous DNA synthesis** of the **lagging strand**.*

Evidence supporting the occurrence of discontinuous DNA synthesis was first provided by Reiji and Tuneko Okazaki. They discovered that when bacteriophage DNA is replicated in *E. coli,* some of the newly formed DNA that is hydrogen bonded to the template strand is present as small fragments containing 1000 to 2000 nucleotides. RNA primers are part of each such fragment. These pieces, now called **Okazaki fragments**, are converted into longer and longer DNA strands of higher molecular weight as synthesis proceeds.

Discontinuous synthesis of DNA requires enzymes that both remove the RNA primers and unite the Okazaki

---

*Because DNA synthesis is continuous on one strand and discontinuous on the other, the term **semidiscontinuous synthesis** is sometimes used to describe the overall process.

FIGURE 11–11 Opposite polarity of synthesis along the two strands of DNA is necessary because they run antiparallel to one another, and because DNA polymerase III synthesizes in only one direction (5′ to 3′). On the lagging strand, synthesis must be discontinuous, resulting in the production of Okazaki fragments. On the leading strand, synthesis is continuous. RNA primers are used to initiate synthesis on both strands.

fragments into the lagging strand. As we have noted, DNA Pol I removes the primers and replaces the missing nucleotides. Joining the fragments is the work of another enzyme, **DNA ligase**, which is capable of catalyzing the formation of the phosphodiester bond that seals the nick between the discontinuously synthesized strands. The evidence that DNA ligase performs this function during DNA synthesis is strengthened by the observation of a ligase-deficient mutant strain (*lig*) of *E. coli*, in which a large number of unjoined Okazaki fragments accumulate.

Concurrent Synthesis Occurs on the Leading and Lagging Strands

Given the model just discussed, we might ask how the holoenzyme of DNA Pol III synthesizes DNA on both the leading and lagging strands. Can both strands be replicated simultaneously at the same replication fork, or are the events distinct, involving two separate copies of the enzyme? Evidence suggests that both strands are replicated simultaneously, with each strand acted upon by one of the two core enzymes that are part of the DNA Pol III holoenzyme. As **Figure 11–12** illustrates, if the lagging strand is spooled out, forming a loop, nucleotide polymerization can occur simultaneously on both template strands under the direction of the holoenzyme. After the synthesis of 1000 to 2000 nucleotides, the monomer of the enzyme on the lagging strand will encounter a completed Okazaki fragment, at which point it releases the lagging strand. A new loop of the lagging strand is spooled out, and the process is repeated. Looping inverts the orientation of the template but not the direction of actual synthesis on the lagging strand, which is always in the 5′ to 3′ direction. As mentioned above, it is believed that there is a third core enzyme associated with the DNA Pol III

FIGURE 11–12 Illustration of how concurrent DNA synthesis may be achieved on both the leading and lagging strands at a single replication fork (RF). The lagging template strand is "looped" in order to invert the physical direction of synthesis, but not the biochemical direction. The enzyme functions as a dimer, with each core enzyme achieving synthesis on one or the other strand.

holoenzyme, and that it functions in the synthesis of Okazaki fragments. For simplicity, we will include only two core enzymes in this and subsequent figures.

Another important feature of the holoenzyme that facilitates synthesis at the replication fork is the donut-shaped sliding DNA clamp that surrounds the unreplicated double helix and is linked to the advancing core enzyme. This clamp prevents the core enzyme from dissociating from the template as polymerization proceeds. By doing so, the clamp is responsible for vastly increasing the processivity of the core enzyme—that is, the number of nucleotides that may be continually added prior to dissociation from the template. This function is critical to the rapid *in vivo* rate of DNA synthesis during replication.

Proofreading and Error Correction Occurs during DNA Replication

The immediate purpose of DNA replication is the synthesis of a new strand that is precisely complementary to the template strand at each nucleotide position. Although the action of DNA polymerases is very accurate, synthesis is not perfect and a noncomplementary nucleotide is occasionally inserted erroneously. To compensate for such inaccuracies, the DNA polymerases all possess 3' to 5' exonuclease activity. This property imparts the potential for them to detect and excise a mismatched nucleotide (in the 3' to 5' direction). Once the mismatched nucleotide is removed, 5' to 3' synthesis can again proceed. This process, called **proofreading**, increases the fidelity of synthesis by a factor of about 100. In the case of the holoenzyme form of DNA polymerase III, the epsilon (ε) subunit of the core

enzyme is directly involved in the proofreading step. In strains of *E. coli* with a mutation that has rendered the ε subunit nonfunctional, the error rate (the mutation rate) during DNA synthesis is increased substantially.

11.4 A Coherent Model Summarizes DNA Replication

We can now combine the various aspects of DNA replication occurring at a single replication fork into a coherent model, as shown in **Figure 11–13**. At the advancing fork, a helicase is unwinding the double helix. Once unwound, single-stranded binding proteins associate with the strands, preventing the reformation of the helix. In advance of the replication fork, DNA gyrase functions to diminish the tension created as the helix supercoils. Each of the core enzymes of DNA Pol III holoenzyme is bound to one of the template strands by a sliding DNA clamp. Continuous synthesis occurs on the leading strand, while the lagging strand must loop around in order for simultaneous (concurrent) synthesis to occur on both strands. Not shown in the figure, but essential to replication on the lagging strand, is the action of DNA polymerase I and DNA ligase, which together replace the RNA primers with DNA and join the Okazaki fragments, respectively.

Because the investigation of DNA synthesis is still an extremely active area of research, this model will no doubt be extended in the future. In the meantime, it provides a summary of DNA synthesis against which genetic phenomena can be interpreted.

FIGURE 11–13 Summary of DNA synthesis at a single replication fork. Various enzymes and proteins essential to the process are shown.

11.5 Replication Is Controlled by a Variety of Genes

Much of what we know about DNA replication in viruses and bacteria is based on genetic analysis of the process. For example, we have already discussed studies involving the *polA1* mutation, which revealed that DNA polymerase I is not the major enzyme responsible for replication. Many other mutations interrupt or seriously impair some aspect of replication, such as the ligase-deficient and the proofreading-deficient mutations mentioned previously. Because such mutations are lethal ones, genetic analysis frequently uses **conditional mutations**, which are expressed under one condition but not under a different condition. For example, a **temperature-sensitive mutation** may not be expressed at a particular *permissive* temperature. When mutant cells are grown at a *restrictive* temperature, the mutant phenotype is expressed and can be studied. By examining the effect of the loss of function associated with

the mutation, the investigation of such temperature-sensitive mutants can provide insight into the product and the associated function of the normal, nonmutant gene.

As shown in **Table 11.4**, a variety of genes in *E. coli* specify the subunits of the DNA polymerases and encode products involved in specification of the origin of synthesis, helix unwinding and stabilization, initiation and priming, relaxation of supercoiling, repair, and ligation. The discovery of such a large group of genes attests to the complexity of the process of replication, even in the relatively simple prokaryote. Given the enormous quantity of DNA that must be unerringly replicated in a very brief time, this level of complexity is not unexpected. As we will see in the next section, the process is even more involved and therefore more difficult to investigate in eukaryotes.

TABLE 11.4 Some of the Various *E. coli* Genes and Their Products or Role in Replication

Gene	Product or Role
polA	DNA polymerase I
polB	DNA polymerase II
dnaE, N, Q, X, Z	DNA polymerase III subunits
dnaG	Primase
dnaA, I, P	Initiation
dnaB, C	Helicase at *oriC*
gyrA, B	Gyrase subunits
lig	DNA ligase
rep	DNA helicase
ssb	Single-stranded binding proteins
rpoB	RNA polymerase subunit

MODERN APPROACHES TO UNDERSTANDING GENE FUNCTION **Lethal Knockouts**

In this chapter you learned about the essential role of DNA ligase during DNA replication. Ligases also play important roles in DNA recombination and repair. Eukaryotic cells express at least three different DNA ligase genes (*Lig1*, *Lig3*, and *Lig4*). These genes have related sequences and structures, but each enzyme has different functions: DNA ligase 1 (*Lig1*) is the key ligase involved in DNA replication in mammalian cells, *Lig3* functions in the repair

Lig3 deficiency results in excessive apoptosis at day 9.5. (Left) Heterozygous (+/−) mouse embryos show wild-type embryonic development whereas Lig 3 −/− null mouse embryos (right) arrest at 9.5 dpc.

of DNA single-stranded breaks and the excision repair process (discussed at the end of Chapter 15), and *Lig4* is necessary for recombination and a process called nonhomologous end-joining. How do we know these DNA ligases exist, and how do we know their specific roles? Below we will illustrate **DNA knockout technology,** an experimental approach that reveals how organisms are affected by the designed loss of specific genes.

To understand the roles of DNA ligases, scientists have generated ligase knockout mouse strains that have each

(continued)

Modern Approaches—continued

lost a specific ligase gene. Knockout mice are made by genetically engineering parents that are heterozygous for a particular gene; one allele is wild type, and the other is a "null," or nonfunctional, allele. These animals are denoted as +/−. When the two heterozygotes are bred together, some homozygous −/− (null) offspring are created and selected for study. When −/− offspring are not produced from a mating, scientists often suspect problems with embryonic lethality. It is often a lethality in knockouts that reveals the functional significance of a gene during embryonic development.

Here we briefly highlight examples of results from ligase knockout experiments to illustrate several important interpretations that can be made when working with knockout animals.

Results:

Experiments from several different groups have shown that:

- Embryos from *Lig1* knockout mice develop normally to midterm before dying.

- *Lig3* knockout mice terminate embryonic development at 8.5 days postcoitum (dpc). Excessive cell death (apoptosis) occurs at 9.5 dpc. Thus *Lig3* null mice also show embryonic lethality. This lethality has been traced to an essential role of *Lig3* in mitochondria.

- *Lig4* knockout mice also show embryonic lethality. *Lig4−/−* cultured cell lines show increased sensitivity to damage by ionizing radiation and are deficient in nonhomologous end-joining repair of double-stranded DNA breaks.

Conclusions:

All three of these mouse knockouts resulted in embryonic lethality. How do these findings help us understand what each of the ligases do? One conclusion we can draw right away is that

each ligase is essential and plays a role independent of that of the other ligases, based on the observation that the other ligases cannot substitute for it. After reading these studies, we learn that, for example, the *Lig4−/−* experiments indicate that ligase 4 is involved in DNA repair because loss of that protein led to increased sensitivity to certain types of mutagens. We also learned that DNA ligases I and III cannot substitute for the specific functions of ligase 4. As a result, mutation or loss of any DNA ligase gene cannot be fully compensated for by another DNA ligase gene.

These experiments also demonstrate a fairly common occurrence when making knockout animals: Null mice often die at some particular stage of development. This occurrence reveals that the disrupted gene is essential to cell function, and, at least during development of the organism, that failure to express its protein product is lethal to the organism. This might not surprise you, since you might readily hypothesize that loss of a gene that is so important to an essential process such as DNA replication would cause death of an organism. Scientists have the same expectations, and time and again knockout animals have confirmed this hypothesis.

The problem of lethality when creating knockouts led geneticists to develop **conditional knockout** approaches. This method allows one to eliminate a particular gene in a specific organ instead of the whole animal. This way the animal survives and researchers can study gene function in certain cell types. Conditional knockout animals can also be used to turn gene expression back on for rescue experiments.

References:

Adachi, N., et al. 2001. DNA ligase IV-deficient cells are more resistant to ionizing radiation in the absence of Ku70: Implications for DNA double-strand break repair. *Proc. Natl. Acad. Sci. USA*, 98:12109–12113.

Bentley, D.J., et al. 2002. DNA ligase I null mouse cells show normal DNA repair activity but altered DNA replication and reduced genome stability. *J. Cell Sci.*, 115:1551–1561.

Puebla-Osorio, N., et al. 2006. Early embryonic lethality due to targeted inactivation of DNA ligase III. *Mol. Cell. Biol.*, 26:3935–3941.

Questions to Consider:

1. Sometimes making null mice for a gene thought to have important functions results in animals with *no obvious mutant phenotype*. What conclusions might you might reach about a gene that produces these results when a knockout is made?

2. How do you think it is possible for mice to develop for nine days without ligase 1—the ligase that is the "key ligase involved in DNA replication in mammalian cells"?

3. Based on the outcomes of the ligase experiments above, what might you expect if knockout mice for DNA polymerase were generated? Such mice have been produced. Follow the Exploring Genomics exercise from earlier in the text (see Chapter 2), *to* carry out a PubMed search for DNA polymerase knockouts and see what you find!

4. This *Modern Approaches to Understanding Gene Function* feature describes the role of three ligase genes, *Lig1*, *Lig3*, and *Lig4*, and their protein products. What happened to the mammalian *Lig2*? To find out, go to http://www.ncbi.nlm.nih.gov/ and type in Human Lig2 using the "Gene" database. Look at your best hit. You may need to click on a replacement record to find the answer! Read the summary to find the solution to this mystery.

11.6 Eukaryotic DNA Replication Is Similar to Replication in Prokaryotes, but Is More Complex

Eukaryotic DNA replication shares many features with replication in bacteria. In both systems, double-stranded DNA is unwound at replication origins, replication forks are formed, and bidirectional DNA synthesis creates leading and lagging strands from single-stranded DNA templates under the direction of DNA polymerase. Eukaryotic polymerases have the same fundamental requirements for DNA synthesis as do bacterial polymerases: four deoxyribonucleoside triphosphates, a template, and a primer. However, eukaryotic DNA replication is more complex, due to several features of eukaryotic DNA. Eukaryotic cells contain much more DNA, this DNA is complexed with nucleosomes, and eukaryotic chromosomes are linear rather than circular. In this section, we will describe some of the ways in which eukaryotes deal with this added complexity.

Initiation at Multiple Replication Origins

The most obvious difference between eukaryotic and prokaryotic DNA replication is that eukaryotic replication must deal with greater amounts of DNA. For example, yeast cells contain 3 times as much DNA, and *Drosophila* cells contain 40 times as much as *E. coli* cells. In addition, eukaryotic DNA polymerases synthesize DNA at a rate 25 times slower (about 2000 nucleotides per minute) than that in prokaryotes. Under these conditions, replication from a single origin on a typical eukaryotic chromosome would take days to complete. However, replication of entire eukaryotic genomes is usually accomplished in a matter of minutes to hours.

To facilitate the rapid synthesis of large quantities of DNA, eukaryotic chromosomes contain multiple replication origins. Yeast genomes contain between 250 and 400 origins, and mammalian genomes have as many as 25,000. Multiple origins are visible under the electron microscope as "replication bubbles" that form as the DNA helix opens up, each bubble providing two potential replication forks (**Figure 11–14**). Origins in yeast, called **autonomously replicating sequences (ARSs)**, consist of approximately 120 base pairs containing a **consensus sequence** (meaning a sequence that is the same, or nearly the same, in all yeast ARSs) of 11 base pairs. Origins in mammalian cells appear to be unrelated to specific sequence motifs and may be defined more by chromatin structure over a 6–55 kb region.

FIGURE 11–14 Demonstration of multiple origins of replication along a eukaryotic chromosome. DNA was isolated from a *Drosophila* nucleus and examined by electron microscopy. The DNA in this 119-kb fragment contains 23 replication bubbles, which can be located with the help of the diagram in the lower left-hand side of the electron micrograph.

Eukaryotic replication origins not only act as sites of replication initiation, but also control the timing of DNA replication. These regulatory functions are carried out by a complex of more than 20 proteins, called the **prereplication complex (pre-RC)**, which assembles at replication origins. In the early G1 phase of the cell cycle, replication origins are recognized by a six-protein complex known as an **origin recognition complex (ORC)**, which tags the origin as a site of initiation of replication. Throughout the G1 phase of the cell cycle, other proteins associate with the ORC to form the pre-RC. The presence of a pre-RC at an origin "licenses" that origin for replication. Once DNA polymerases initiate synthesis at the origin, the pre-RC is disrupted and does not reassemble again until the G1 phase of the next cell cycle. This is an important mechanism because it distinguishes segments of DNA that have completed replication from segments of unreplicated DNA, thus maintaining orderly and efficient replication. It ensures that replication occurs only once along each stretch of DNA during each cell cycle.

The initiation of DNA replication is also regulated at the pre-RC. A number of cell-cycle kinases that phosphorylate replication proteins, along with helicases that unwind DNA, associate with the pre-RC and are essential for initiation. The kinases are activated in S phase, at which time they phosphorylate other proteins that trigger the initiation of DNA replication. The end result is the unwinding of DNA at the replication forks, the stabilization of single-stranded DNA, the association of DNA polymerases with the origins, and the initiation of DNA synthesis.

TABLE 11.5 Properties of Eukaryotic DNA Polymerases

DNA Polymerase	Functions
α (alpha)	RNA/DNA primers, initiation of DNA synthesis
δ (delta)	Lagging strand synthesis, repair, recombination, proofreading
ε (epsilon)	Leading strand synthesis, repair, recombination, proofreading
γ (gamma)	Mitochondrial DNA replication and repair
β (beta)	Base-excision DNA repair
η (eta), ζ (zeta), κ (kappa), and ι (iota)	Translesion DNA synthesis
θ (theta), λ (lambda), μ (mu), ν (nu), and Rev1	DNA repair

Multiple Eukaryotic DNA Polymerases

To accommodate the increased number of replicons, eukaryotic cells contain many more DNA polymerase molecules than do bacterial cells. For example, a single *E. coli* cell contains about 15 molecules of DNA polymerase III, but a mammalian cell contains tens of thousands of DNA polymerase molecules.

Eukaryotes also utilize a larger number of different DNA polymerase types than do prokaryotes. The human genome contains genes that encode at least 14 different DNA polymerases, only three of which are involved in the majority of nuclear genome DNA replication. The nomenclature and characteristics of these DNA polymerases are summarized in **Table 11.5**.

Pol α, δ, and ε are the major forms of the enzyme involved in initiation and elongation during eukaryotic nuclear DNA synthesis, so we will concentrate our discussion on these. Two of the four subunits of the **Pol α enzyme** synthesize RNA primers on both the leading and lagging strands. After the RNA primer reaches a length of about 10 ribonucleotides, another subunit adds 10–20 complementary deoxyribonucleotides. Pol α is said to possess low **processivity**, a term that refers to the strength of the association between the enzyme and its substrate, and thus the length of DNA that is synthesized before the enzyme dissociates from the template. Once the primer is in place, an event known as **polymerase switching** occurs, whereby Pol α dissociates from the template and is replaced by Pol δ or ε. These enzymes extend the primers on opposite strands of DNA, possess much greater processivity, and exhibit 3' to 5' exonuclease activity, thus having the potential to proofread. Pol ε synthesizes DNA on the leading strand, and Pol δ synthesizes the lagging strand. Both Pol δ and ε participate in other DNA synthesizing events in the cell, including several types of DNA repair and recombination. All three DNA polymerases are essential for viability.

As in prokaryotic DNA replication, the final stages in eukaryotic DNA replication involve replacing the RNA primers with DNA and ligating the Okazaki fragments on the lagging strand. In eukaryotes, the Okazaki fragments are about ten times smaller (100 to 150 nucleotides) than in prokaryotes.

Included in the remainder of DNA-replicating enzymes is Pol γ, which is found exclusively in mitochondria, synthesizing the DNA present in that organelle. Other DNA polymerases are involved in DNA repair and replication through regions of the DNA template that contain damage or distortions (called **translesion synthesis**, or **TLS**). Although these translesion DNA polymerases are less faithful in copying DNA and thus make more errors than Pol α, δ, and ε, they are able to bypass the distortions, leaving behind gaps that may then be repaired. We will return to the topic of DNA damage and repair later in the text (see Chapter 15).

Replication through Chromatin

One of the major differences between prokaryotic and eukaryotic DNA is that eukaryotic DNA is complexed with DNA-binding proteins, existing in the cell as *chromatin*. As we will discuss later in the text (see Chapter 12), chromatin consists of regularly repeating units called nucleosomes, each of which consists of about 200 base pairs of DNA wrapped around eight histone protein molecules. Before polymerases can begin synthesis, nucleosomes and other DNA-binding proteins must be stripped away or otherwise modified to allow the passage of replication proteins. As DNA synthesis proceeds, the histones and non-histone proteins must rapidly reassociate with the newly formed duplexes, reestablishing the characteristic nucleosome pattern. Electron microscopy studies, such as the one shown in **Figure 11–15**, show that nucleosomes form immediately after new DNA is synthesized at replication forks.

FIGURE 11–15 An electron micrograph of a eukaryotic replicating fork demonstrating the presence of histone-protein-containing nucleosomes on both branches.

In order to re-create nucleosomal chromatin on replicated DNA, the synthesis of new histone proteins is tightly coupled to DNA synthesis during the S phase of the cell cycle. Research data suggest that nucleosomes are disrupted just ahead of the replication fork and that the preexisting histone proteins can assemble with newly synthesized histone proteins into new nucleosomes. The new nucleosomes are assembled behind the replication fork, onto the two daughter strands of DNA. The assembly of new nucleosomes is carried out by **chromatin assembly factors (CAFs)** that move along with the replication fork.

11.7 The Ends of Linear Chromosomes Are Problematic during Replication

A final difference between prokaryotic and eukaryotic DNA synthesis stems from the structural differences in their chromosomes. Unlike the closed, circular DNA of bacteria and most bacteriophages, eukaryotic chromosomes are linear. During replication, two special problems arise at the "ends" of these linear double-stranded DNA molecules.

The first problem is that the double-stranded "ends" of DNA molecules at the termini of linear chromosomes potentially resemble the **double-stranded breaks (DSBs)** that can occur when a chromosome becomes broken internally as a result of DNA damage. In such cases, the double-stranded loose ends can fuse, resulting in chromosome fusions and translocations. If the ends do not fuse, they are vulnerable to degradation by nucleases. The second problem occurs during DNA replication, because DNA polymerases cannot synthesize new DNA at the tips of single-stranded 5′ ends.

To deal with these two problems, linear eukaryotic chromosomes end in distinctive sequences called **telomeres** that help preserve the integrity and stability of the chromosomes. Telomeres create inert chromosome ends, protecting intact eukaryotic chromosomes from improper fusion or degradation. They also solve the 5′ end replication problem, as we will describe next.

Telomere Structure

We could speculate that there must be something unique about the DNA sequence or the proteins that bind to it that confers this protective property to telomeres. Indeed, this has been shown to be the case. First discovered by Elizabeth Blackburn and Joe Gall in their study of micronuclei—the smaller of two nuclei in the ciliated protozoan *Tetrahymena*—the DNA at the protozoan's chromosome ends consists of the short tandem repeating sequence TTGGGG. This sequence is present many times on one of the two DNA strands making up each telomere. This strand is referred to as the G-rich strand, in contrast to its complementary strand, the so-called C-rich strand, which displays the repeated sequence AACCCC. In a similar way, all vertebrates contain the sequence TTAGGG at the ends of G-rich strands, repeated several thousand times in somatic cells. Since each linear chromosome ends with two helical DNA strands running antiparallel to one another, one strand has a 3′-ending and the other has a 5′-ending. It is the 3′-strand that is the G-rich one. This has special significance during telomere replication.

But first, let's describe how this tandemly repeated DNA confers inertness to the chromosome ends. One model is based on the discovery that the 3′-ending G-rich strand extends as an overhang, lacking a complement, and thus forms a single-stranded tail at the terminus of each telomere. In *Tetrahymena*, this tail is only 12 to 16 nucleotides long. However, in vertebrates, it may be several hundred nucleotides long. The final conformation of these tails has been correlated with chromosome inertness. Though not considered complementary in the same way as A–T and G–C base pairs are, G-containing nucleotides are nevertheless capable of base pairing with one another when several are aligned opposite another G-rich sequence. Thus, the G-rich single-stranded tails are capable of looping back on themselves, forming multiple G-G hydrogen bonds to create what are referred to as **G-quartets**. The resulting loops at the chromosome ends (called **t-loops**) are much like those created when you tie your shoelaces into a bow. It is believed that these structures, in combination with specific proteins that bind to them, essentially close off the ends of chromosomes and make them resistant to nuclease digestion and DNA fusions.

Replication at the Telomere

Now let's consider the problem that semiconservative replication poses the 5′ ends of double-stranded DNA molecules. As we have learned previously in this chapter, DNA replication initiates from short RNA primers, synthesized on both leading and lagging strands (**Figure 11–16**). Primers are necessary because DNA polymerase requires a free 3′-OH on which to initiate synthesis. After replication is completed, these RNA primers are removed. The resulting gaps within the new daughter strands are filled by DNA polymerase and sealed by ligase. These internal gaps have free 3′-OH groups available at the ends of the Okazaki fragments for DNA polymerase to initiate synthesis. The problem arises at the gaps left at the 5′ ends of the newly synthesized DNA [gaps (b) and (c) in Figure 11–16]. These

(Lagging strand template)

5' ━━━━━━━━━━━━━━━━━━━━━━━ 3'
3' ━━━━━━━━━━━━━━━━━━━━━━━ 5'

(Leading strand template)

RNA primer

Discontinuous and continuous synthesis

5' ━━━━━━━━━━━━━━━━━━━━━━━ 3'
3' ◄━━━━━━━━━ ◄━━━━━━━━ 5'

5' ━━━━━━━━━━━━━━━━━━━━━━━► 3'
3' ━━━━━━━━━━━━━━━━━━━━━━━ 5'

RNA primers removed

Gaps (a), (b), and (c) created

5' ━━━━━━━━━━━━━━━━━━━━━━━ 3'
3' ◄━━━━ (a) ◄━━━━ (b)

5' (c) ━━━━━━━━━━━━━━━━━► 3'
3' ━━━━━━━━━━━━━━━━━━━━━━━ 5'

Gap (a) filled   **Gaps (b) and (c) unfilled**

5' ━━━━━━━━━━━━━━━━━━━━━━━ 3'
3' ◄━━━━━━━━━━━━━━━ (b)

5' (c) ━━━━━━━━━━━━━━━━━► 3'
3' ━━━━━━━━━━━━━━━━━━━━━━━ 5'

FIGURE 11–16 Diagram illustrating the difficulty encountered during the replication of the ends of linear chromosomes. Gaps (b) and (c) are left following synthesis both the leading and lagging strands.

gaps cannot be filled by DNA polymerase because no free 3'-OH groups are available for the initiation of synthesis.

Thus, in the situation depicted in Figure 11–16, gaps remain on newly synthesized DNA strands at each successive round of synthesis, shortening the double-stranded ends of the chromosome by the length of the RNA primer. With each round of replication, the shortening becomes more severe in each daughter cell, *eventually extending beyond the telomere and potentially deleting gene-coding regions.*

The solution to this so-called *end-replication problem* is provided by a unique eukaryotic enzyme called **telomerase**. Telomerase was first discovered by Elizabeth Blackburn and her graduate student, Carol Greider, in studies of *Tetrahymena*. As noted earlier, telomeric DNA in eukaryotes consists of many short, repeated nucleotide sequences, with the G-rich strand overhanging in the form of a single-stranded tail. In *Tetrahymena* the tail contains several repeats of the sequence 5'-TTGGGG-3'.

As we will see, telomerase is capable of adding several more repeats of this six-nucleotide sequence to the 3'end of the G-rich strand (using 5'–3' synthesis). Detailed investigation by Blackburn and Greider of how the *Tetrahymena* telomerase enzyme accomplishes this synthesis yielded an extraordinary finding. The enzyme is highly unusual in that it is a *ribonucleoprotein,* containing within its molecular structure a short piece of RNA that is essential to its catalytic activity. The telomerase RNA component (TERC) serves as both a "guide" to proper attachment of the enzyme to the telomere and a "template" for synthesis of its DNA complement. Synthesis of DNA using RNA as a template is called **reverse transcription.** The telomerase reverse transcriptase, called TERT, is the catalytic subunit of the telomerase enzyme. In addition to TERC and TERT, telomerase contains a number of accessory proteins. In *Tetrahymena,* TERC contains the sequence AACCCCAAC, within which is found the complement of the repeating telomeric DNA sequence that must be synthesized (TTGGGG).

Figure 11–17 shows one model of how researchers envision the enzyme working. Part of the RNA sequence of the enzyme (shown in green) base-pairs with the ending sequence of the single-stranded overhanging DNA, while the remainder of the RNA extends beyond the overhang. Next, reverse transcription of this extending RNA sequence—synthesizing DNA on an RNA template—extends the length of the G-rich lagging strand. It is believed that the enzyme is then translocated toward the (newly formed) end of the strand, and the same events are repeated, continuing the extension process.

Once the telomere has been lengthened by telomerase, conventional DNA synthesis ensues. Primase lays down a primer near the end of the telomere, then DNA polymerase and ligase fill most of the gap [**Figure 11–17 (d)** and **(e)**]. When the primer is removed a small gap remains. However, this gap is located well beyond the original end of the chromosome, thus preventing any chromosome shortening. Another model suggests that the DNA extension, created by telomerase, acts as a primer and facilitates DNA synthesis on the opposite C-rich strand. In this model, the single-stranded extension loops back on itself, providing the 3'-OH group necessary for initiation of synthesis to fill the gap.

Telomerase function has now been found in all eukaryotes studied. As we will discuss later in the text (see Chapter 12), telomeric DNA sequences have been highly conserved throughout evolution, reflecting the critical function of telomeres. As mentioned earlier, in humans, the telomeric DNA sequence on the lagging strand that is repeated is 5'-TTAGGG-3', differing from *Tetrahymena* by only one nucleotide.

(a) Telomerase binds to 3′ G-rich tail

Telomerase with
RNA component

(b) Telomeric DNA is synthesized on G-rich tail

(c) Telomerase is translocated and steps (a) and (b) are repeated

(d) Telomerase released; primase and DNA polymerase fill gap

Gap

Primer

(e) Primer removed; gap sealed by DNA ligase

Gap sealed

FIGURE 11–17 The predicted solution to the problem posed in Figure 11–16. The enzyme telomerase (with its RNA component shown in green) directs synthesis of repeated TTGGGG sequences, resulting in the formation of an extended 3′-overhang. This facilitates DNA synthesis on the opposite strand, filling in the gap that would otherwise have been created on the ends of linear chromosomes during each replication cycle.

In most eukaryotic somatic cells, telomerase is not active, and thus, with each cell division, the telomeres of each chromosome do shorten. After many divisions, the telomere may be seriously eroded, causing the cell to lose the capacity for further division. Most stem cells and malignant cells, on the other hand, maintain telomerase activity and this may contribute to their immortality. In the

"Genetics, Technology, and Society" feature at the end of this chapter, we will see that telomerase activity and telomere length have been linked to aging, cancer, and other diseases.

11.8 DNA Recombination, Like DNA Replication, Is Directed by Specific Enzymes

We now turn to a topic previously discussed in the text (see Chapter 5)—genetic recombination. There, we pointed out that the process of crossing over between homologs depends on the breakage and rejoining of the DNA strands, and results in the exchange of genetic information between DNA molecules. Now that we have discussed the chemistry and replication of DNA, we can consider how recombination occurs at the molecular level. In general, our discussion pertains to genetic exchange between any two homologous double-stranded DNA molecules, whether they are viral or bacterial chromosomes or eukaryotic homologs during meiosis.

Models of Homologous Recombination

Genetic exchange at equivalent positions along two chromosomes with substantial DNA sequence homology is referred to as **general**, or **homologous recombination**.

Several models attempt to explain homologous recombination, but they all have certain features in common. First, all are based on proposals first put forth independently by Robin Holliday and Harold L. K. Whitehouse in 1964. Second, they all depend on the complementarity between DNA strands to explain the precision of the exchange. Finally, each model relies on a series of enzymatic processes in order to accomplish genetic recombination.

One such model is shown in **Figure 11–18**. It begins with two paired DNA duplexes, or homologs [Step (a)], in each of which an endonuclease introduces a single-stranded nick at an identical position [Step (b)]. The internal strand endings produced by these cuts are then displaced and subsequently pair with their complements on the opposite duplex [Step (c)]. Next, a ligase seals the loose ends [Step (d)], creating hybrid duplexes called **heteroduplex DNA molecules**, held together by a cross-bridge structure. The position of this cross bridge can then move down the chromosome by a process referred to as

FIGURE 11–18 Model depicting how genetic recombination can occur as a result of the breakage and rejoining of heterologous DNA strands. Each stage is described in the text. The electron micrograph shows DNA in a χ-form structure similar to the diagram in (g); the DNA is an extended Holliday structure, derived from the *Col*E1 plasmid of *E. coli*. *David Dressler, Oxford University, England.*

branch migration [Step (e)], which occurs as a result of a zipper-like action as hydrogen bonds are broken and then reformed between complementary bases of the displaced strands of each duplex. This migration yields an increased length of heteroduplex DNA on both homologs.

If the duplexes bend [Step (f)] and the bottom portion shown in the figure rotates 180° [Step (g)], an intermediate planar structure called a χ (chi) form—or **Holliday structure**—is created. If the two strands on opposite homologs previously uninvolved in the exchange are now nicked by an endonuclease [Step (h)] and ligation occurs as in Step (i), two recombinant duplexes are created. Note that the arrangement of alleles is altered as a result of this recombination.

Whereas the model above involves *single-stranded breaks,* other recombination models have been proposed that involve *double-stranded breaks* in one of the DNA double helices. In these models, endonucleases remove nucleotides at the breakpoint, creating 3′ overhangs on each strand. One of the broken strands invades the intact double helix of the other homolog, and both strands line up with the intact homolog. DNA repair synthesis then fills all gaps, and two Holliday junctions are formed. Endonuclease cleavages and ligations finalize the exchange. The end result is the same as our original model: genetic exchange occurs between homologous DNA molecules.

Not only is homologous recombination essential for the exchange of genetic information during meiosis, but it is also important for the repair of damaged DNA. As we discuss later in the text (see Chapter 15), various types of agents can create double-stranded breaks in DNA molecules. These agents include ionizing radiation and free radicals. When cells are defective in homologous recombination mechanisms, they are prone to accumulating mutations in genes and chromosomes, which in turn may lead to the development of tumors, diseases, or even cell death.

Enzymes and Proteins Involved in Homologous Recombination

As with DNA replication, DNA recombination requires the activities of numerous enzymes and other proteins. Many of the proteins involved in recombination were identified by examining the phenotypes of gene mutations in organisms such as yeast and *E. coli.* Mutations in genes whose products regulate homologous recombination lead to sensitivity to radiation, replication failure, the development of cancer, or cell death.

Perhaps the most important proteins involved in homologous recombination are **RecA** (in *E. coli*) and **Rad51** (in eukaryotic cells). These proteins are loaded onto the single-stranded DNA ends formed after the endonuclease nicking step shown in **Figure 11–18(b)**. RecA and Rad51 then search for a homologous sequence of DNA in another DNA molecule and bring about strand invasion and displacement. Several other proteins mediate or regulate the actions of RecA and Rad51. In yeast, these mediator proteins include Rad52, Rad55, and Rad57. These proteins help to load Rad51 onto single-stranded DNA ends and to increase the stability of the DNA-protein complex. Another protein, Rad54, displaces other DNA binding proteins and stimulates branch migration, as seen in **Figure 11–18(e)**.

In higher eukaryotes, one of the most important homologous recombination mediator proteins is **BRCA2**. BRCA2 interacts directly with Rad51 and helps recruit Rad51 to single-stranded DNA. The importance of BRCA2 is revealed by its association with several types of cancer. Individuals who have mutations in the *BRCA2* gene have a predisposition to breast, ovarian, and other cancers. Mouse cells with mutations in *BRCA2* are sensitive to radiation and DNA-damaging chemicals. Those cells that survive the DNA damage accumulate chromosomal rearrangements and breaks. In this way, BRCA2 reveals the links between DNA recombination, repair, and cancer. We will return to the relationships between DNA repair and cancer later in the text (see Chapter 19).

Many other proteins are involved in homologous recombination. In *E. coli,* the **RecB**, **RecC**, and **RecD** proteins are involved with DNA cleavage and duplex unwinding. Other enzymes are responsible for the resolution of Holliday structures. DNA replication proteins, such as DNA polymerases, DNA ligases, gyrases, and single-stranded binding proteins, are also involved in homologous recombination and repair.

Gene Conversion, a Consequence of Homologous Recombination

The preceding model has helped us to understand a unique genetic phenomenon known as **gene conversion**. Gene conversion is characterized by a *nonreciprocal* genetic exchange between two DNA molecules. For example, consider a heterozygous diploid organism with the genotype *Aa* at a certain gene locus on one chromosome. When cells from this organism undergo meiosis, DNA is duplicated and four chromatids are formed; these chromatids create the haploid gametes designated as *A*, *A*, *a*, and *a*. This is the normal 2:2 ratio of gametes. In some cases, however, this 2:2 ratio becomes a 3:1 or 1:3 ratio. It appears that one of the alleles has been *converted* into the other allele.

Gene conversion is thought to be a consequence of homologous recombination. The key features of the process are summarized in **Figure 11–19**. Gene conversion begins in the same way as the first five steps of homologous recombination seen in Figure 11–18(a)–(e). However, instead of focusing on the outside markers *A* and *B*, as we did in Figure 11–18(e), we will examine the region of DNA within the heteroduplex regions, regions of two chromatids in which one single strand of DNA comes from one chromatid and the other single strand comes from another chromatid that contains a slightly different DNA sequence (TAG versus TCG in Figure 11–19). These two different sequences represent two alleles that we will represent as *G* and *g*. The resulting hybrid double-stranded

FIGURE 11–19 Mechanism of gene conversion for two alleles, *G* and *g*. Two homologous chromatids shown at the top of the diagram contain a sequence difference that defines the two alleles. Note the 5′ and 3′ ends of each single strand of DNA on each chromatid. During homologous recombination between these two nonsister chromatids, strand invasion and branch migration occur as seen in Figure 11–18. The resulting two heteroduplex regions contain mismatched nucleotide pairs. These mismatches can be excised and repaired in two different ways: either returning the heteroduplex region to the parental genotype or changing the sequence to the other genotype.

DNA molecules contain mismatches—in our example, between an A and a G nucleotide and between a T and a C nucleotide.

The next step in gene conversion involves a method of DNA repair called mismatch repair, which we will describe in more detail later in the text (see Chapter 15). Mismatch repair is a mechanism that the cell uses to correct a DNA molecule that contains a mismatch such as the A/G and T/C mismatches in Figure 11–19. During mismatch repair, specific enzymes excise one of the mismatched nucleotides and replace it with the "correct" nucleotide. Excision may occur on either one of the single strands, yielding two possible "corrections" for each heteroduplex region. In some cases, the correction results in no change to the original genotype. However,

in other cases, the correction results in gene conversion, in which the *G* allele is converted to a *g* or a *g* allele is converted to a *G*.

Gene conversion can also occur in somatic cells during DNA double-stranded break repair, as discussed later in the text (see Chapter 15). When the backbones of both strands of a DNA molecule are broken, the damaged strands are degraded at the break sites and repaired by homologous recombination using information found on a homologous DNA molecule. If the homologous DNA molecule contains a slightly different DNA sequence, this difference is copied to replace the degraded portion of the damaged DNA. The result is the conversion of a DNA sequence into another—which may create a new allele on the damaged DNA if this process occurs within a gene.

GENETICS, TECHNOLOGY, AND SOCIETY

Telomeres: The Key to Immortality?

Humans, like all multicellular organisms, grow old and die. As we age, our immune systems become less efficient, wound healing is impaired, and tissues lose resilience. Why do we go through these age-related declines, and can we reverse the march to mortality? Some recent research suggests that the answers to these questions may lie at the ends of our chromosomes.

Human cells, both those in our bodies and those growing in culture dishes, have a finite life span. When placed into tissue culture dishes, normal human fibroblasts lose their ability to grow and divide after about 50 cell divisions. Eventually, they die. Although we don't know whether cellular senescence directly causes organismal aging, the evidence is suggestive. For example, cultured cells derived from young people undergo more divisions than those from older people; cells from short-lived species stop growing after fewer divisions than those from longer-lived species; and cells from patients with premature aging syndromes undergo fewer divisions than those from normal patients.

One significant characteristic of aging cells involves their telomeres. In most mammalian somatic cells, telomeres shorten with each DNA replication because DNA polymerase cannot synthesize new DNA at the ends of each parent strand. However, cells that undergo extensive proliferation, like embryonic cells, germ cells, and adult stem cells, maintain their telomere length by using telomerase—a remarkable RNA-containing enzyme that adds telomeric DNA sequences onto the ends of linear chromosomes. However, most somatic cells in adult organisms do not contain telomerase and do not proliferate.

Could we gain perpetual youth and vitality by increasing our telomere lengths? Studies suggest that it may be possible to reverse senescence by artificially increasing the amount of telomerase in our cells. In one study, investigators introduced cloned telomerase genes into normal human cells in culture. The increase in telomerase activity caused the telomeres' lengths to increase, and the cells continued to grow past their typical senescence point. In another study, researchers created a strain of mice that was defective in the TERT subunit of telomerase. These mice showed the classic symptoms of aging, including tissue atrophy, neurodegeneration, and a shortened life span. When the researchers reactivated telomerase function in these prematurely aging adult mice, tissue atrophies and neurodegeneration were reversed and their life spans increased.

These studies suggest that some of the symptoms that accompany old age in humans might also be reversed by activating telomerase genes. However, before we use telomerase to achieve immortality, we need to consider a potential serious side effect—cancer.

Although normal cells shorten their telomeres and undergo senescence after a specific number of cell divisions, cancer cells do not. More than 80 percent of human tumor cells contain telomerase activity, maintain telomere lengths, and achieve immortality. Those that do not contain active telomerase use a less-well-understood mechanism known as ALT (for "alternative lengthening of telomeres").

These observations suggest that we should use caution before attempting to increase telomerase activity in humans. However, they also suggest that we might be able to devise new cancer therapies based on the idea that drugs that inhibit telomerase might destroy cancer cells by allowing telomeres to shorten, thereby forcing the cells into senescence. Because most normal human cells do not express telomerase, such a therapy might specifically affect tumor cells and be less toxic than most current anticancer drugs. Many such anti-telomerase drugs are currently under development, and some are in clinical trials.

Will a deeper understanding of telomeres allow us to both arrest cancers *and* reverse the descent into old age? Time will tell.

Your Turn

Take time, individually or in groups, to answer the following questions. Investigate the references and links to help you understand some of the research on telomeres, aging, and cancer.

1. Mutations in genes coding for telomerase subunits or telomere-binding proteins are associated with a number of human diseases. How do these mutations contribute to these diseases, which are characterized by a wide range of different phenotypes?

The role of telomeres and telomerase in human diseases is discussed in Calado, R.T. and Young, N.S. 2009. Telomere diseases. N. Eng. J. Med. 361: 2353–2365.

2. One anti-telomerase drug, called imetelstat (GRN163L), has being developed by Geron Corporation as a treatment for cancer. How does imetelstat work? What is the current status of imetelstat clinical trials? What are some possible side-effects of anti-telomerase drugs?

Read about this drug and its clinical trials on the Geron Web site at http://www.geron.com/imetelstat. *Search on PubMed for scientific papers dealing with GRN163L's anticancer effects.*

3. People suffering from chronic stress appear to have more health problems and to age prematurely. Is there any evidence that chronic stress, poor health, and telomere length are linked? How might stress affect telomere length or vice versa?

Some recent research suggests how these phenomena may be linked. Read about telomeres and stress in Blackburn, E.H. and Epel, E.S. 2012. Too toxic to ignore. Nature 490: 169–171.

4. The only treatment known to increase life span and to delay the development of age-related disease is calorie restriction (CR). CR is achieved by reducing food intake while maintaining adequate nutrition. Studies suggest that CR and telomere lengths may be related. How do CR and telomerase act, and interact, to prolong health and life span?

Begin your search for the relationships between telomerase activity and CR with Vera, E., et al. 2013. Telomerase reverse transcriptase synergizes with calorie restriction to increase health span and extend mouse longevity. PloS One 8: e53760.

CASE STUDY | At loose ends

A researcher was asked if his work on the genetic control of human telomere replication was related to any genetic disorders. He replied that one might think that any mutations involving replication would be lethal during early development, and thus unavailable for study. But, in fact, a rare human genetic disorder affecting telomeres is known. This disorder, dyskeratosis congenita (DKC), is associated with mutations in the protein subunits of telomerase, the enzyme responsible for replicating the ends of eukaryotic chromosomes. Initial symptoms appear in tissues derived from rapidly dividing cells, including the skin, nails, and bone marrow, and first affect children between the ages of 5 and 15 years.

This disorder raises several interesting questions.

1. How could such individuals survive?

2. Why are the tissues derived from rapidly dividing cells initially affected?

3. Is this disorder likely to impact the life span?

4. Would you predict that mutations in the RNA component of telomerase might also cause DKC?

Summary Points

1. In 1958, Meselson and Stahl resolved the question of which of three potential modes of replication is utilized by *E. coli* during the duplication of DNA in favor of semiconservative replication, showing that newly synthesized DNA consists of one old strand and one new strand.

2. Taylor, Woods, and Hughes demonstrated semiconservative replication in eukaryotes using the root tips of the broad bean as the source of dividing cells.

3. Arthur Kornberg isolated the enzyme DNA polymerase I from *E. coli* and showed that it is capable of directing *in vitro* DNA synthesis, provided that a template and precursor nucleoside triphosphates are supplied.

4. The discovery of the *polA1* mutant strain of *E. coli,* capable of DNA replication despite its lack of polymerase I activity, cast doubt on the enzyme's hypothesized *in vivo* replicative function. Polymerase III has been identified as the enzyme responsible for DNA replication *in vivo*.

5. During the initiation of DNA synthesis, the double helix unwinds, forming a replication fork at which synthesis begins. Proteins stabilize the unwound helix and assist in relaxing the coiling tension created ahead of the replication fork.

6. DNA synthesis is initiated at specific sites along each template strand by the enzyme primase, resulting in short segments of RNA that provide suitable 3′ ends upon which DNA polymerase III can begin polymerization.

7. Concurrent DNA synthesis occurs continuously on the leading strand and discontinuously on the opposite lagging strand, resulting in short Okazaki fragments that are later joined by DNA ligase.

8. DNA replication in eukaryotes is more complex than replication in prokaryotes, using multiple replication origins, multiple forms of DNA polymerases, and factors that disrupt and assemble nucleosomal chromatin.

9. Replication at the ends of linear chromosomes in eukaryotes poses a special problem that can be solved by the presence of telomeres and by a unique RNA-containing enzyme called telomerase.

10. Homologous recombination between DNA molecules relies on precise alignment of homologs and the actions of a series of enzymes that can cut, realign, and reseal DNA strands.

INSIGHTS AND SOLUTIONS

1. Predict the theoretical results of conservative and dispersive replication of DNA under the conditions of the Meselson–Stahl experiment. Follow the results through two generations of replication after cells have been shifted to a ^{14}N-containing medium, using the following sedimentation pattern.

Density ⟶

^{14}N/^{14}N ^{15}N/^{14}N ^{15}N/^{15}N

Solution:

Conservative replication

Generation I   Generation II

Dispersive replication

Generation I   Generation II

2. Mutations in the *dnaA* gene of *E. coli* are lethal and can only be studied following the isolation of conditional, temperature-sensitive mutations. Such mutant strains grow nicely and replicate their DNA at the permissive temperature of

Insights and Solutions—continued

18°C, but they do not grow or replicate their DNA at the restrictive temperature of 37°C. Two observations were useful in determining the function of the DnaA protein product. First, *in vitro* studies using DNA templates that have unwound do not require the DnaA protein. Second, if intact cells are grown at 18°C and are then shifted to 37°C, DNA synthesis continues at this temperature until one round of replication is completed and then stops. What do these observations suggest about the role of the *dnaA* gene product?

Solution: At 18°C (the permissive temperature), the mutation is not expressed and DNA synthesis begins. Following the shift to the restrictive temperature, the already initiated DNA synthesis continues, but no new synthesis can begin. Because the DnaA protein is not required for synthesis of unwound DNA, these observations suggest that, *in vivo,* the DnaA protein plays an essential role in DNA synthesis by interacting with the intact helix and somehow facilitating the localized denaturation necessary for synthesis to proceed.

Problems and Discussion Questions

MasteringGenetics™ Visit for instructor-assigned tutorials and problems.

HOW DO WE KNOW?

1. In this chapter, we focused on how DNA is replicated and synthesized. We also discussed recombination at the DNA level and the phenomenon of gene conversion. Along the way, we encountered many opportunities to consider how this information was acquired. On the basis of these discussions, what answers would you propose to the following fundamental questions?
   (a) What is the experimental basis for concluding that DNA replicates semiconservatively in both prokaryotes and eukaryotes?
   (b) How was it demonstrated that DNA synthesis occurs under the direction of DNA polymerase III and not polymerase I?
   (c) How do we know that *in vivo* DNA synthesis occurs in the 5′ to 3′ direction?
   (d) How do we know that DNA synthesis is discontinuous on one of the two template strands?
   (e) What observations reveal that a "telomere problem" exists during eukaryotic DNA replication, and how did we learn of the solution to this problem?

CONCEPT QUESTION

2. Review the Chapter Concepts list on p. 261. These are concerned with the replication and synthesis of DNA. Write a short essay that distinguishes between the terms *replication* and *synthesis*, as applied to DNA. Which of the two is most closely allied with the field of biochemistry?
3. Compare conservative, semiconservative, and dispersive modes of DNA replication.
4. Describe the role of ^{15}N in the Meselson–Stahl experiment.
5. Predict the results of the experiment by Taylor, Woods, and Hughes if replication were (a) conservative and (b) dispersive.
6. What are the requirements for *in vitro* synthesis of DNA under the direction of DNA polymerase I?
7. In Kornberg's initial experiments, it was rumored that he grew *E. coli* in Anheuser-Busch beer vats. (Kornberg was working at Washington University in St. Louis.) Why do you think this might have been helpful to the experiment?
8. How did Kornberg assess the fidelity of DNA polymerase I in copying a DNA template?
9. Which characteristics of DNA polymerase I raised doubts that its *in vivo* function is the synthesis of DNA leading to complete replication?
10. Kornberg showed that nucleotides are added to the 3′ end of each growing DNA strand. In what way does an exposed 3′-OH group participate in strand elongation?

11. What was the significance of the *polA1* mutation?
12. Summarize and compare the properties of DNA polymerase I, II, and III.
13. List and describe the function of the ten subunits constituting DNA polymerase III. Distinguish between the holoenzyme and the core enzyme.
14. Distinguish between (a) unidirectional and bidirectional synthesis, and (b) continuous and discontinuous synthesis of DNA.
15. List the proteins that unwind DNA during *in vivo* DNA synthesis. How do they function?
16. Define and indicate the significance of (a) Okazaki fragments, (b) DNA ligase, and (c) primer RNA during DNA replication.
17. Outline the current model for DNA synthesis.
18. Why is DNA synthesis expected to be more complex in eukaryotes than in bacteria? How is DNA synthesis similar in the two types of organisms?
19. Suppose that *E. coli* synthesizes DNA at a rate of 100,000 nucleotides per minute and takes 40 minutes to replicate its chromosome. (a) How many base pairs are present in the entire *E. coli* chromosome? (b) What is the physical length of the chromosome in its helical configuration—that is, what is the circumference of the chromosome if it were opened into a circle?
20. Several temperature-sensitive mutant strains of *E. coli* display the following characteristics. Predict what enzyme or function is being affected by each mutation.
   (a) Newly synthesized DNA contains many mismatched base pairs.
   (b) Okazaki fragments accumulate, and DNA synthesis is never completed.
   (c) No initiation occurs.
   (d) Synthesis is very slow.
   (e) Supercoiled strands remain after replication, which is never completed.
21. While many commonly used antibiotics interfere with protein synthesis or cell wall formation, clorobiocin, one of several antibiotics in the aminocoumarin class, inhibits the activity of bacterial DNA gyrase. Similar drugs have been tested as treatments for human cancer. How might such drugs be effective against bacteria as well as cancer?
22. Define gene conversion, and describe how this phenomenon is related to genetic recombination.
23. Many of the gene products involved in DNA synthesis were initially defined by studying mutant *E. coli* strains that could not synthesize DNA.

(a) The *dnaE* gene encodes the a subunit of DNA polymerase III. What effect is expected from a mutation in this gene? How could the mutant strain be maintained?

(b) The *dnaQ* gene encodes the ε subunit of DNA polymerase. What effect is expected from a mutation in this gene?

24. In 1994, telomerase activity was discovered in human cancer cell lines. Although telomerase is not active in human somatic tissue, this discovery indicated that humans do contain the genes for telomerase proteins and telomerase RNA. Since inappropriate activation of telomerase may contribute to cancer, why do you think the genes coding for this enzyme have been maintained in the human genome throughout evolution? Are there any types of human body cells where telomerase activation would be advantageous or even necessary? Explain.

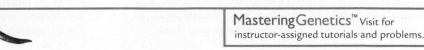

Extra-Spicy Problems

MasteringGenetics™ Visit for instructor-assigned tutorials and problems.

25. The genome of *D. melanogaster* consists of approximately 1.7×10^8 base pairs. DNA synthesis occurs at a rate of 30 base pairs per second. In the early embryo, the entire genome is replicated in five minutes. How many bidirectional origins of synthesis are required to accomplish this feat?

26. Assume a hypothetical organism in which DNA replication is conservative. Design an experiment similar to that of Taylor, Woods, and Hughes that will unequivocally establish this fact. Using the format established in Figure 11–5, draw sister chromatids and illustrate the expected results establishing this mode of replication.

27. DNA polymerases in all organisms add only 5′ nucleotides to the 3′ end of a growing DNA strand, never to the 5′ end. One possible reason for this is the fact that most DNA polymerases have a proofreading function that would not be *energetically* possible if DNA synthesis occurred in the 3′ to 5′ direction.

(a) Sketch the reaction that DNA polymerase would have to catalyze if DNA synthesis occurred in the 3′ to 5′ direction.

(b) Consider the information in your sketch and speculate as to why proofreading would be problematic.

28. An alien organism was investigated that demonstrated the "telomere problem" during DNA synthesis, but on only one end of each chromosome. Create a model of DNA that is compatible with this observation. Is this organism a prokaryote or eukaryote?

29. Assume that the sequence of bases given in this problem is present on one nucleotide chain of a DNA duplex and that the chain has opened up at a replication fork. Synthesis of an RNA primer occurs on this template starting at the base that is underlined.

(a) If the RNA primer consists of eight nucleotides, what is its base sequence?

(b) In the intact RNA primer, which nucleotide has a free 3′-OH terminus?

3′.......GGCTACC**T**GGATTCA....5′

30. Prokaryotic Okazaki fragments are in the range of 1200 nucleotides, while eukaryotic fragments are much shorter, more in the range of 100–150 nucleotides. Balakrishnan and Bambara (2013) suggest that the shorter length of Okazaki fragments is determined by nucleosome periodicity. Design an experiment to determine whether or not the length of Okazaki fragments in eukaryotes is dependent on nucleosomes being present on DNA during replication.

31. Reiji and Tuneko Okazaki conducted a now classic experiment in 1968 in which they discovered a population of short fragments synthesized during DNA replication. They introduced a short pulse of ³H-thymidine into a culture of *E. coli* and extracted DNA from the cells at various intervals. In analyzing the DNA after centrifugation in denaturing gradients, they noticed that as the interval between the time of ³H-thymidine introduction and the time of centrifugation increased, the proportion of short strands decreased and more labeled DNA was found in larger strands. What would account for this observation?

32. The following table (data adapted from Khodursky et al., 2000) presents the percentage of DNA synthesis after 15 minutes from initiation for four strains of *Escherichia coli* grown under permissive (30°C) and restrictive (42°C) temperatures and various concentrations of the gyrase inhibitor novobiocin. The strains have the following characteristics and genotypes: wild type, temperature-sensitive gyrase mutation (gyr^{ts}), novobiocin resistant (gyr^r), and the double mutant ($gyr^{ts,r}$). Based on data contained in the table, assign the appropriate genotypes to the strains labeled *A*, *B*, *C*, and *D*.

Temperature (°C)	30			42		
Novobiocin (g/ml)	0	5	40	0	5	40
Bacterial strain						
A	100	56	9	40	26	1
B	100	100	100	41	43	40
C	100	58	4	100	56	3
D	100	100	100	100	100	100

33. Consider the drawing of a dinucleotide below.

(a) Is it DNA or RNA?

(b) Is the arrow closest to the 5′ or the 3′ end?

(c) Suppose that the molecule was cleaved with the enzyme spleen diesterase, which breaks the covalent bond connecting the phosphate to C-5′. After cleavage, to which nucleoside is the phosphate now attached (A or T)?

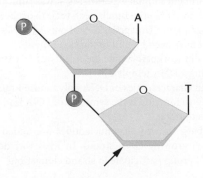

34. To gauge the fidelity of DNA synthesis, Arthur Kornberg and colleagues devised a technique called nearest-neighbor analysis, which determines the frequency with which any two bases occur adjacent to each other along the polynucleotide chain (*J. Biol. Chem.* 236: 864–875). This test relies on the enzyme spleen phosphodiesterase (see the previous problem). As we saw in Figure 11–8, DNA is synthesized by polymerization of 5'-nucleotides—that is, each nucleotide is added with the phosphate on the C-5' of deoxyribose. However, as shown in the accompanying figure, the phosphodiesterase enzyme cleaves DNA between the phosphate and the C-5' atom, thereby producing 3'-nucleotides. In this test, the phosphates on only one of the four nucleotide precursors of DNA (cytidylic acid, for example) are made radioactive with ^{32}P, and DNA is synthesized. Then the DNA is subjected to enzymatic cleavage, in which the radioactive phosphate is transferred to the base that is the "nearest neighbor" on the 5' side of all cytidylic acid nucleotides.

Following four separate experiments, in each of which a different one of the four nucleotide types is radioactive, the frequency of all 16 possible nearest neighbors can be calculated. When Kornberg applied the nearest-neighbor frequency test to the DNA template and resultant product from a variety of experiments, he found general agreement between the nearest-neighbor frequencies of the two.

Analysis of nearest-neighbor data led Kornberg to conclude that the two strands of the double helix are in opposite polarity to one another. Demonstrate this approach by determining the outcome of such an analysis if the strands of DNA shown here are (a) antiparallel versus (b) parallel:

(a)
5' ⟶ 3'
p – G – p – C – p – T – p – T – p – A – p – C – p – A
| | | | | | |
– C – p – G – p – A – p – A – p – T – p – G – p – T – p
3' ⟵ 5'

vs.

(b)
5' ⟶ 3'
p – G – p – C – p – T – p – T – p – A – p – C – p – A
| | | | | | |
p – C – p – G – p – A – p – A – p – T – p – G – p – T
5' ⟶ 3'

35. Reconsider Problem 33 in Chapter 10. In the model you proposed, could the molecule be replicated semiconservatively? Why? Would other modes of replication work?

Nucleotides prior to synthesis; cytidylic acid nucleotides are labeled with ^{32}P

DNA synthesis

Enzyme treatment

Cleavage between phosphates and 5'-carbons

^{32}P transferred to C's nearest neighbors (T and G)

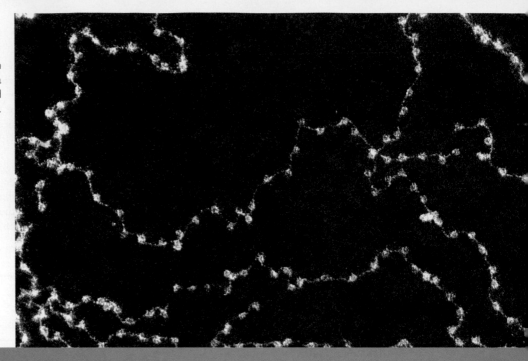

Chromatin fibers spilling out of a chicken erythrocyte, viewed using electron microscopy.

12

DNA Organization in Chromosomes

CHAPTER CONCEPTS

- Genetic information in viruses, bacteria, mitochondria, and chloroplasts, with some exceptions, is contained in a short, circular DNA molecule relatively free of associated proteins.

- Eukaryotic cells, in contrast to viruses and bacteria, contain large amounts of DNA that during most of the cell cycle is organized into nucleosomes and is present as either uncoiled chromatin fibers or more condensed structures.

- The uncoiled chromatin fibers characteristic of interphase coil up and condense into chromosomes during the stages of eukaryotic cell division.

- Whereas prokaryotic genomes consist of mostly unique DNA sequences coding for proteins, eukaryotic genomes contain a mixture of both unique and repetitive DNA sequences.

- Eukaryotic genomes consist mostly of noncoding DNA sequences.

Once geneticists understood that DNA houses genetic information, they focused their energies on discovering how DNA is organized into genes and how these basic units of genetic function are organized into chromosomes. In short, the next major questions they tackled had to do with how the genetic material is organized within the genome. These issues have a bearing on many areas of genetic inquiry. For example, the ways in which genomic organization varies has a major bearing on the regulation of genetic expression.

In this chapter, we focus on the various ways DNA is organized into chromatin, which in turn is organized into chromosomes. These structures have been studied using numerous approaches, including biochemical analysis as well as visualization by light microscopy and electron microscopy. In the first part of the chapter, after surveying what we know about chromosomes in viruses and bacteria, we examine two specialized eukaryotic structures called polytene and lampbrush chromosomes. Then, we turn to a consideration of how eukaryotic chromosomes are organized at the molecular level—for example, how DNA is complexed with proteins to form chromatin and how the chromatin fibers characteristic of interphase are condensed into chromosome structures visible during mitosis and meiosis. We conclude the chapter by examining certain aspects of DNA sequence organization in eukaryotic genomes.

Please note that some of the topics discussed in this chapter are explored in greater depth later in the text (see Special Topic Chapter 1—Epigenetics and Special Topic Chapter 2—Emerging Roles of RNA).

(a) (b)

FIGURE 12–1 Electron micrographs of (a) phage λ and (b) the DNA isolated from it. The chromosome is 17 μm long. The phages are magnified about five times more than the DNA.

12.1 Viral and Bacterial Chromosomes Are Relatively Simple DNA Molecules

The chromosomes of viruses and bacteria are much less complicated than those in eukaryotes. They usually consist of a single nucleic acid molecule quite different from the multiple chromosomes constituting the genome of higher forms. Prokaryotic chromosomes are largely devoid of associated proteins and contain relatively less genetic information. These characteristics have greatly simplified genetic analysis in prokaryotic organisms, and we now have a fairly comprehensive view of the structure of their chromosomes.

The chromosomes of viruses consist of a nucleic acid molecule—either DNA or RNA—that can be either single or double stranded. They can exist as circular structures (covalently closed circles), or they can take the form of linear molecules. The single-stranded DNA of the φX174 **bacteriophage** and the double-stranded DNA of the polyoma virus are closed circles housed within the protein coat

of the mature viruses. The **bacteriophage lambda (λ)**, on the other hand, possesses a linear double-stranded DNA molecule prior to infection, but it closes to form a ring upon infection of the host cell. Still other viruses, such as the T-even series of bacteriophages, have linear double-stranded chromosomes of DNA that do not form circles inside the bacterial host. Thus, circularity is not an absolute requirement for replication in viruses.

Viral nucleic acid molecules have been visualized with the electron microscope. **Figure 12–1** shows a mature bacteriophage λ and its double-stranded DNA molecule in the circular configuration. One constant feature shared by viruses, bacteria, and eukaryotic cells is the ability to package an exceedingly long DNA molecule into a relatively small volume. In λ, the DNA is 17 μm long and must fit into the phage head, which is less than 0.1 μm on any side. Table 12.1 compares the length of the chromosomes of several viruses with the size of their head structure. In each case, a similar packaging feat must be accomplished. Compare the dimensions given for phage T2 with the micrograph of both the DNA and the viral particle shown in

TABLE 12.1 The Genetic Material of Representative Viruses and Bacteria

Source		Nucleic Acid			Overall Size of Viral Head or Bacterial Cell (μm)
		Type	SS or DS*	Length (μm)	
Viruses	φX174	DNA	SS	2.0	0.025 × 0.025
	Tobacco mosaic virus	RNA	SS	3.3	0.30 × 0.02
	Lambda phage	DNA	DS	17.0	0.07 × 0.07
	T2 phage	DNA	DS	52.0	0.07 × 0.10
Bacteria	*Haemophilus influenzae*	DNA	DS	832.0	1.00 × 0.30
	Escherichia coli	DNA	DS	1200.0	2.00 × 0.50

*SS = single-stranded; DS = double-stranded

FIGURE 12–2 Electron micrograph of bacteriophage T2, which has had its DNA released by osmotic shock. The chromosome is 52 μm long.

FIGURE 12–3 Electron micrograph of the bacterium *Escherichia coli*, which has had its DNA released by osmotic shock. The chromosome is 1200 μm long.

Figure 12–2. Seldom does the space available in the head of a virus exceed the chromosome volume by more than a factor of two. In many cases, almost all space is filled, indicating nearly perfect packing. Once packed within the head, the virus's genetic material is functionally inert until it is released into a host cell.

Bacterial chromosomes are also relatively simple in form. They always consist of a double-stranded DNA molecule, compacted into a structure sometimes referred to as the **nucleoid**. *Escherichia coli,* the most extensively studied bacterium, has a large, circular chromosome measuring approximately 1200 μm (1.2 mm) in length. When the cell is gently lysed and the chromosome is released, the chromosome can be visualized under the electron microscope (**Figure 12–3**).

DNA in bacterial chromosomes is found to be associated with several types of DNA-binding proteins. Two, called **HU** and **H-NS (Histone-like Nucleoid Structuring) proteins,**

are small but abundant in the cell and contain a high percentage of positively charged amino acids that can bond ionically to the negative charges of the phosphate groups in DNA. These proteins function to fold and bend DNA. As such, coils are created that have the effect of compacting the DNA constituting the nucleoid. Additionally, H-NS proteins, like histones in eukaryotes, have been implicated in regulating gene activity in a nonspecific way.

12.2 Supercoiling Facilitates Compaction of the DNA of Viral and Bacterial Chromosomes

One major insight into the way DNA is organized and packaged in viral and bacterial chromosomes has come from the discovery of **supercoiled DNA**, which is particularly characteristic of closed-circular molecules. Supercoiled DNA was first proposed as a result of a study of double-stranded DNA molecules derived from the polyoma virus, which causes tumors in mice. In 1963, it was observed that when the polyoma DNA was subjected to high-speed centrifugation, it was resolved into three distinct components, each of different density and compactness. The one that was least dense and thus least compact was subsequently proposed by Jerome Vinograd to consist of linear DNA molecules. The other two fractions were more dense and both are now known to consist of circular DNA molecules. Closed-circular molecules are more compact and sediment more rapidly during centrifugation than do the same molecules in linear form. All three were of identical molecular weight.

NOW SOLVE THIS

12–1 In bacteriophages and bacteria, the DNA is almost always organized into circular (closed loops) chromosomes. Phage λ is an exception, maintaining its DNA in a linear chromosome within the viral particle. However, as soon as this DNA is injected into a host cell, it circularizes before replication begins. What advantage exists in replicating circular DNA molecules compared to linear molecules, characteristic of eukaryotic chromosomes?

■ **HINT:** *This problem involves an understanding of eukaryotic DNA replication, as discussed earlier in the text (see Chapter 11). The key to its solution is to consider why the enzyme telomerase is essential in eukaryotic DNA replication, and why bacterial and viral chromosomes can be replicated without encountering the "telomere" problem.*

Vinograd proposed further that the denser of the two fractions of circular molecules consisted of covalently closed DNA helices that are slightly *underwound* in comparison to the less dense circular molecules. Energetic forces stabilizing the double helix resist this underwinding, causing the molecule as a whole to **supercoil**, that is, to contort in a certain way, in order to retain normal base pairing. Vinograd proposed that it is the supercoiled shape that causes tighter packing and thus the increase in density.

The transitions just described are illustrated in **Figure 12–4**. Consider a double-stranded linear molecule existing in the normal Watson–Crick right-handed helix [**Figure 12–4(a)**]. This helix contains 20 complete turns, which means the **linking number** (*L*) of this molecule is 20, or *L* = 20. Suppose we were to change this linear molecule into a closed circle by bringing the opposite ends together and joining them [**Figure 12–4(b)**]. If the closed circle still has a linking number of 20 (if we haven't introduced or eliminated any turns when joining the ends), we define the molecule as being *energetically relaxed*. Now suppose that the circle were subsequently cut open, underwound by two full turns, and then resealed [**Figure 12–4(c)**]. Such a structure, in which *L* has been changed to 18, would be *energetically strained* and, as a result, would change its form to relieve the strain.

In order to assume a more energetically favorable conformation, an underwound molecule will form supercoils in the direction opposite to that of the underwinding. In our case [**Figure 12–4(d)**], two negative supercoils are introduced spontaneously, reestablishing, in total, the original number of turns in the helix. Use of the term *negative* refers to the fact that, by definition, the supercoils are left-handed (whereas the helix is right-handed). The end result is the formation of a more compact structure with enhanced physical stability.

In most closed-circular DNA molecules in bacteria and their phages, the DNA helix is slightly underwound [as in Figure 12–4(c)]. For example, the virus SV40 contains 5200 base pairs. In energetically relaxed DNA, 10.4 base pairs occupy each complete turn of the helix, and the linking number can be calculated as

$$L = \frac{5200}{10.4} = 500$$

However, analysis of circular SV40 DNA reveals that it is underwound by 25 turns, so *L* is equal to only 475. Predictably, 25 negative supercoils are observed in the molecule. In *E. coli*, an even larger number of supercoils is observed, greatly facilitating chromosome condensation in the nucleoid region.

Two otherwise identical molecules that differ only in their linking number are said to be **topoisomers** of

(a) Linear DNA

**Ends sealed
(1 to 20)**

(b) Relaxed circular DNA: *L* = (+20)

**Helix underwound
by two turns**

(c) Underwound circular DNA: *L* = (+18)

**Conformational
change**

(d) Supercoiled DNA (2 supercoils form)

FIGURE 12–4   Depictions of the transformations leading to the supercoiling of circular DNA. *L* signifies linking number.

one another. But how can a molecule convert from one topoisomer to the other if there are no free ends, as is the case in closed circles of DNA? Biologically, this may be accomplished by any one of a group of enzymes that cut one or both of the strands and wind or unwind the helix before resealing the ends.

Appropriately, these enzymes are called **topoisomerases**. First discovered by Martin Gellert and James Wang, these catalytic molecules are known as either type I or type II, depending on whether they cleave one or both strands in the helix, respectively. In *E. coli*, topoisomerase I serves to reduce the number of negative supercoils in a closed-circular DNA molecule. Topoisomerase II introduces negative supercoils into DNA. This latter enzyme is thought to bind to DNA, twist it, cleave both strands, and then pass them through the loop that it has created. Once the phosphodiester bonds are reformed, the linking number is decreased and one or more supercoils form spontaneously.

Supercoiled DNA and topoisomerases are also found in eukaryotes. While the chromosomes in these organisms are not usually circular, supercoils can occur when areas of DNA are embedded in a lattice of proteins associated with the chromatin fibers. This association creates "anchored" ends, providing the stability for the maintenance of supercoils once they are introduced by topoisomerases. In both prokaryotes and eukaryotes, DNA replication and transcription create supercoils downstream as the double helix unwinds and becomes accessible to the appropriate enzyme.

Topoisomerases may play still other genetic roles involving eukaryotic DNA conformational changes. Interestingly, these enzymes are involved in separating (decatenating) the DNA of sister chromatids following replication.

FIGURE 12–5 Polytene chromosomes derived from larval salivary gland cells of *Drosophila*.

12.3 Specialized Chromosomes Reveal Variations in the Organization of DNA

We now consider two cases of genetic organization that demonstrate specialized forms that eukaryotic chromosomes can take. Both types—*polytene chromosomes* and *lampbrush chromosomes*—are so large that their organization was discerned using light microscopy long before we understood how mitotic chromosomes form from interphase chromatin. The study of these chromosomes provided many of our initial insights into the arrangement and function of the genetic information. It is important to know that polytene and lampbrush chromosomes are unusual and not typically found in most eukaryotic cells, but the study of their structure has revealed many common themes of chromosome organization.

Polytene Chromosomes

Giant **polytene chromosomes** are found in various tissues (salivary, midgut, rectal, and malpighian excretory tubules) in the larvae of some flies, as well as in several species of protozoans and plants. They were first observed by E. G. Balbiani in 1881. The large amount of information obtained from studies of these genetic structures provided a model system for subsequent investigations of chromosomes. What is particularly intriguing about polytene chromosomes is that they can be seen in the nuclei of interphase cells.

Each polytene chromosome is 200 to 600 μm long, and when they are observed under the light microscope, they exhibit a linear series of alternating bands and interbands (**Figures 12–5** and **12–6**). The banding pattern is distinctive for each chromosome in any given species. Individual bands are sometimes called **chromomeres**, a more generalized term describing lateral condensations of material along the axis of a chromosome.

Extensive study using electron microscopy and radioactive tracers led to an explanation for the unusual appearance of these chromosomes. First, polytene chromosomes represent paired homologs. This in itself is highly unusual, since they are present in somatic cells, where, in most organisms, chromosomal material is normally dispersed as chromatin and homologs are not paired. Second, their large size and distinctive appearance result from their being composed of large numbers of identical DNA strands. The DNA of these paired homologs undergoes many rounds of replication, *but without strand separation or cytoplasmic division*. As replication proceeds, chromosomes are created, having 1000 to 5000 DNA strands that remain in precise parallel alignment with one another. Apparently, the parallel register of so many DNA strands gives rise to the distinctive band pattern along the axis of the chromosome.

The presence of bands on polytene chromosomes was initially interpreted as the visible manifestation of individual genes. The discovery that the strands present in bands undergo localized uncoiling during genetic activity further strengthened this view. Each such uncoiling event results in a bulge called a **puff**, so named because of its appearance under the microscope (Figure 12–6). That puffs are visible manifestations of a high level of gene activity (transcription that produces RNA) is evidenced by their high rate of incorporation of radioactively labeled RNA precursors, as assayed by autoradiography. Bands that are not extended into puffs incorporate fewer radioactive precursors or none at all.

The study of bands during development in insects such as *Drosophila* and the midge fly *Chironomus* reveals differential gene activity. A characteristic pattern of band formation that is equated with gene activation is observed as development proceeds. Despite attempts to resolve the issue, it is not yet clear how many genes are contained in each band. However, we do know that in *Drosophila*, which contains about 15,000 genes, there are approximately

FIGURE 12–6 Photograph of a puff within a polytene chromosome. The diagram depicts the uncoiling of strands within a band region (B) to produce a puff (P) in a polytene chromosome. Each band (B) represents a chromomere. Inter-band regions (IBs) are also labeled.

5000 bands. Interestingly, a band may contain up to 10^7 base pairs of DNA, enough DNA to encode 50 to 100 average-size genes.

NOW SOLVE THIS

12–2 After salivary gland cells from *Drosophila* are isolated and cultured in the presence of radioactive thymidylic acid, autoradiography is performed, revealing polytene chromosomes. Predict the distribution of the grains along the chromosomes.

■ **HINT:** *This problem involves an understanding of the organization of DNA in polytene chromosomes. The key to its solution is to be aware that ^{3}H-thymidine, as a molecular tracer, will only be incorporated into DNA during its replication.*

Lampbrush Chromosomes

Another specialized chromosome that has given us insight into chromosomal structure is the **lampbrush chromosome,** so named because it resembles the brushes used to clean kerosene lamp chimneys in the nineteenth century. Lampbrush chromosomes were first discovered in 1882 by Walther Flemming in salamander oocytes and then seen in 1892 by J. Ruckert in shark oocytes. They are now known to be characteristic of most vertebrate oocytes as well as the spermatocytes of some insects. Therefore, they are meiotic chromosomes. Most of the experimental work on them has been done with material taken from amphibian oocytes.

These unique chromosomes are easily isolated from oocytes in the diplotene stage of the first prophase of meiosis, where they are active in directing the metabolic activities of the developing cell. The homologs are seen as synapsed pairs held together by chiasmata. However, instead of condensing, as most meiotic chromosomes do, lampbrush chromosomes are often extended to lengths of 500 to 800 μm. Later, in meiosis, they revert to their

normal length of 15 to 20 μm. Based on these observations, lampbrush chromosomes are interpreted as being extended, uncoiled versions of the normal meiotic chromosomes.

The two views of lampbrush chromosomes in **Figure 12–7** provide significant insights into their morphology. Part (a) shows the meiotic configuration under the light microscope. The linear axis of each horizontal structure seen in the figure contains a large number of condensed areas, which, as with polytene chromosomes, are referred to as *chromomeres*. Emanating from each chromomere is a pair of lateral loops, giving the chromosome its distinctive appearance. In part (b), the scanning electron micrograph (SEM) shows many adjacent pairs of loops in detail along one of the axes. As with bands in polytene chromosomes,

(a)

(b)

Chiasma

Loops

Central axis with chromomeres

FIGURE 12–7 Lampbrush chromosomes derived from amphibian oocytes. (a) A photomicrograph. (b) A scanning electron micrograph.

much more DNA is present in each loop than is needed to encode a single gene. Such an SEM provides a clear view of the chromomeres and the chromosomal fibers emanating from them. Each chromosomal loop is thought to be composed of one DNA double helix, while the central axis is made up of two DNA helices. This hypothesis is consistent with the belief that each meiotic chromosome is composed of a pair of sister chromatids. Studies using radioactive RNA precursors reveal that the loops are active in the synthesis of RNA. The lampbrush loops, in a manner similar to puffs in polytene chromosomes, represent DNA that has been reeled out from the central chromomere axis during transcription.

TABLE 12.2	Categories and Properties of Histone Proteins	
Histone Type	Lysine-Arginine Content	Molecular Weight (Da)
H1	Lysine-rich	23,000
H2A	Slightly lysine-rich	14,000
H2B	Slightly lysine-rich	13,800
H3	Arginine-rich	15,300
H4	Arginine-rich	11,300

12.4 DNA Is Organized into Chromatin in Eukaryotes

We now turn our attention to the way DNA is organized in eukaryotic chromosomes, which are most clearly visible as highly condensed structures during mitosis. However, after chromosome separation and cell division, cells enter the interphase stage of the cell cycle, at which time the components of the chromosome uncoil and decondense into a form referred to as **chromatin**. While in interphase, the chromatin is dispersed throughout the nucleus. As the cell cycle progresses, cells may replicate their DNA and reenter mitosis, whereupon chromatin coils and condenses back into visible chromosomes once again. This condensation represents a length contraction of some 10,000 times for each chromatin fiber.

The organization of DNA during the transitions just described is much more intricate and complex than in viruses or bacteria, which never exhibit a complex process similar to mitosis. This is due to the greater amount of DNA per chromosome in eukaryotes, as well as the presence of a large number of proteins associated with eukaryotic DNA. For example, while DNA in the *E. coli* chromosome is 1200 μm long, the DNA in each human chromosome ranges from 19,000 to 73,000 μm in length. In a single human nucleus, all 46 chromosomes contain sufficient DNA to extend almost 2 meters. This genetic material, along with its associated proteins, is contained within a nucleus that usually measures about 5 to 10 μm in diameter.

Such intricacy parallels the structural and biochemical diversity of the many types of cells present in a multicellular eukaryotic organism. Different cells assume specific functions based on highly specific biochemical activity. Although all cells carry a full genetic complement, different cells activate different sets of genes. Clearly, then, a highly ordered regulatory system must exist to govern the use of

the genetic information. Such a system must in some way be imposed on or related to the molecular structure of the genetic material.

Chromatin Structure and Nucleosomes

As we have seen, the genetic material of viruses and bacteria consists of strands of DNA or RNA relatively devoid of proteins. In contrast, eukaryotic chromatin has a substantial amount of protein associated with the chromosomal DNA in all phases of the cell cycle. The associated proteins can be categorized as either positively charged **histones** or less positively charged *nonhistone proteins*. Of these two groups, the histones play the most essential structural role. Histones contain large amounts of the positively charged amino acids lysine and arginine, making it possible for them to bond electrostatically to the negatively charged phosphate groups of nucleotides. Recall that a similar interaction has been proposed for several bacterial proteins. The five main types of histones are shown in Table 12.2.

The general model for chromatin structure is based on the assumption that chromatin fibers, composed of DNA and protein, undergo extensive coiling and folding as they are condensed within the cell nucleus. Moreover, X-ray diffraction studies confirm that histones play an important role in chromatin structure. Chromatin produces regularly spaced diffraction rings, suggesting that repeating structural units occur along the chromatin axis. If the histone molecules are chemically removed from chromatin, the regularity of this diffraction pattern is disrupted.

A basic model for chromatin structure was worked out in the mid-1970s. The following observations were particularly relevant to the development of this model:

1. Digestion of chromatin by certain endonucleases, such as micrococcal nuclease, yields DNA fragments that are approximately 200 base pairs in length or multiples thereof. This enzymatic digestion is not random, for if it were, we would expect a wide range of fragment sizes. Thus, chromatin consists of some type of repeating unit, each of which protects the DNA from enzymatic cleavage except where any two units are joined. It is the area between units that is attacked and cleaved by the endonuclease.

2. Electron microscopic observations of chromatin have revealed that chromatin fibers are composed of linear arrays of spherical particles (**Figure 12–8**). Discovered by Ada and Donald Olins, the particles occur regularly along the axis of a chromatin strand and resemble beads on a string. These particles, initially referred to as *v-bodies* (*v* is the Greek letter nu), are now called **nucleosomes**. These findings conform to the above observation that suggests the existence of repeating units.

3. Studies of the chemical association between histone molecules and DNA in the nucleosomes of chromatin show that histones H2A, H2B, H3, and H4 occur as two types of tetramers, $(H2A)_2 \cdot (H2B)_2$ and $(H3)_2 \cdot (H4)_2$. Roger Kornberg predicted that each repeating nucleosome unit consists of one of each tetramer (creating an octamer) in association with about 200 base pairs of DNA. Such a structure is consistent with previous observations and provides the basis for a model that explains the interaction of histones and DNA in chromatin.

4. When nuclease digestion time is extended, some of the 200 base pairs of DNA are removed from the nucleosome, creating what is called a **nucleosome core particle** consisting of 147 base pairs. The DNA lost in the prolonged digestion is responsible for linking nucleosomes together. This **linker DNA** is associated with the fifth histone, H1.

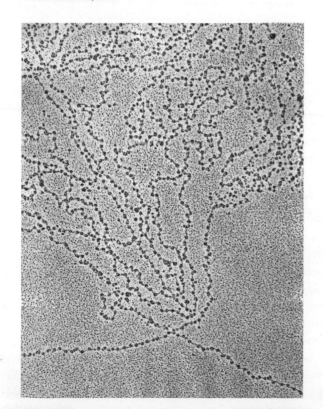

FIGURE 12–8 An electron micrograph revealing nucleosomes appearing as "beads on a string" along chromatin strands derived from *Drosophila melanogaster*.

On the basis of this information, as well as on X-ray and neutron-scattering analyses of crystallized core particles by John T. Finch, Aaron Klug, and others, a detailed model of the nucleosome was put forward in 1984, providing a basis for predicting chromatin structure and its condensation into chromosomes. In this model, illustrated in **Figure 12–9**, a 147-bp length of the 2-nm-diameter DNA molecule coils around an octamer of histones in a left-handed superhelix that completes about 1.7 turns per nucleosome. Each nucleosome, ellipsoidal in shape, measures about 11 nm at its longest point [**Figure 12–9(a)**]. Significantly, the formation of the nucleosome represents the first level of packing, whereby the DNA helix is reduced to about one-third of its original length by winding around the histones.

In the nucleus, the chromatin fiber seldom, if ever, exists in the extended form described in the previous paragraph (that is, as an extended chain of nucleosomes). Instead, the 11-nm-diameter fiber is further packed into a thicker, 30-nm-diameter structure that was initially called a *solenoid* [**Figure 12–9(b)**]. This thicker structure, which is dependent on the presence of histone H1, consists of numerous nucleosomes coiled around and stacked upon one another, creating a second level of packing. This provides a sixfold increase in compaction of the DNA. It is this structure that is characteristic of an uncoiled chromatin fiber in interphase of the cell cycle. In the transition to the mitotic chromosome, still further compaction must occur. The 30-nm structures are folded into a series of *looped domains*, which further condense the chromatin fiber into a structure that is 300 nm in diameter [**Figure 12–9(c)**]. These *coiled chromatin fibers* are then compacted into the chromosome arms that constitute a chromatid, one of the longitudinal subunits of the metaphase chromosome [**Figure 12–9(d)**]. While Figure 12–9 shows the chromatid arms to be 700 nm in diameter, this value undoubtedly varies among different organisms. At a value of 700 nm, a pair of sister chromatids comprising a chromosome measures about 1400 nm.

The importance of the organization of DNA into chromatin and of chromatin into mitotic chromosomes can be illustrated by considering that a human cell stores its genetic material in a nucleus about 5 to 10 μm in diameter. The haploid genome contains more than 3 billion base pairs of DNA distributed among 23 chromosomes. The diploid cell contains twice that amount. At 0.34 nm per base pair, this amounts to an enormous length of DNA (as stated earlier, almost 2 meters)! One estimate is that the DNA inside a typical human nucleus is complexed with roughly 25×10^6 nucleosomes.

In the overall transition from a fully extended DNA helix to the extremely condensed status of the mitotic chromosome, a packing ratio (the ratio of DNA length to the length of the structure containing it) of about 500 to 1 must be achieved. In fact, our model accounts for a ratio of only about 50 to 1. Obviously, the larger fiber can be further

(d) Metaphase chromosome

1400 nm

Chromatid
(700-nm diameter)

(c) Chromatin fiber
(300-nm diameter)

Looped domains

Nucleosome core

H1 Histone

(b) Solenoid
(30-nm diameter)

Histones

Spacer DNA
plus H1 histone

H1

Histone octamer plus
147 base pairs of DNA

DNA
(2-nm diameter)

(a) Nucleosomes
(6-nm × 11-nm flat disc)

FIGURE 12–9 General model of the association of histones and DNA to form nucleosomes, illustrating the way in which each thickness of fiber may be coiled into a more condensed structure, ultimately producing a metaphase chromosome.

bent, coiled, and packed to achieve even greater condensation during the formation of a mitotic chromosome.

NOW SOLVE THIS

12–3 If a human nucleus is 10 μm in diameter, and it must hold as much as 2 m of DNA, which is complexed into nucleosomes that during full extension are 11 nm in diameter, what percentage of the volume of the nucleus is occupied by the genetic material?

■ **HINT:** *This problem asks you to make some numerical calculations in order to see just how "filled" the eukaryotic nucleus is with a diploid amount of DNA. The key to its solution is the use of the formula* $V = (4/3)\pi r^3$, *which calculates the volume of a sphere.*

For more practice, see Problems 12, 13, and 14.

Chromatin Remodeling

As with many significant endeavors in genetics, the study of nucleosomes has answered some important questions but at the same time has opened up new ones. For example, in the preceding discussion, we established that histone proteins play an important structural role in packaging DNA into the nucleosomes that make up chromatin. While this discovery helped solve the structural problem of how the huge amount of DNA is organized within the eukaryotic nucleus, it brought another problem to the fore: *When present in several levels of compaction within the chromatin fiber, DNA is inaccessible to interaction with other important DNA-binding proteins.* For example, the various proteins that function in enzymatic and regulatory roles during the processes of replication and transcription must interact directly with DNA. To accommodate these protein–DNA interactions, chromatin must be induced to change its structure, a process now referred to as **chromatin remodeling**. To allow replication and gene expression, chromatin must relax its compact structure and expose regions of DNA to these proteins, and there must also be a mechanism for reversing the process during periods of inactivity.

Insights into how different states of chromatin structure might be achieved began to emerge in 1997, when Timothy Richmond and members of his research team were able to significantly improve the level of resolution in X-ray diffraction studies of nucleosome crystals, from 7 Å in the 1984 studies to 2.8 Å in the 1997 studies. One model based on their work is shown in **Figure 12–10**. At this resolution, most atoms are visible, thus revealing the subtle twists and turns of the superhelix of DNA encircling the histones. Recall that the double-helical ribbon in the figure represents 147 bp of DNA surrounding four pairs of histone proteins. This configuration is essentially repeated over and over in the chromatin fiber and is the principal packaging unit of DNA in the eukaryotic nucleus.

By 2003, Richmond and colleagues achieved a resolution of 1.9 Å that revealed the details of the location of each histone entity within the nucleosome. Of particular relevance to the discussion of chromatin remodeling is the observation that there are unstructured histone tails that are *not* packed into the folded histone domains within the core of the nucleosomes but instead protrude from it. For example, tails devoid of any secondary structure extending from histones H3 and H2B protrude through the minor-groove channels of the DNA helix. You should look carefully at Figure 12–10 and locate examples of such tails. Other tails of histone H4 appear to make a connection with adjacent nucleosomes. The significance of histone tails is that they provide potential targets along the chromatin fiber for a variety of chemical modifications that may be linked to genetic functions, including chromatin remodeling and the possible regulation of gene expression.

Several of these potential chemical modifications are now recognized as important to genetic function. One of the most well-studied histone modifications involves **acetylation** by the action of the enzyme *histone acetyltransferase (HAT)*. The addition of an acetyl group to the positively charged amino group present on the side chain of the amino acid lysine effectively changes the net charge of the protein by neutralizing the positive charge. Lysine is in abundance in histones, and geneticists have known for some time that acetylation is linked to gene activation. It appears that high levels of acetylation open up, or remodel, the chromatin fiber, an effect that increases in regions of active genes and decreases in inactive regions. In a well-studied example, the inactivation of the X chromosome in mammals, forming a Barr body (Chapter 7), histone H4 is known to be greatly underacetylated.

Two other important chemical modifications are the **methylation** and **phosphorylation** of amino acids that are part of histones. These chemical processes result from the action of enzymes called *methyltransferases* and *kinases*, respectively. Methyl groups can be added to both arginine and lysine residues in histones, and this change has been correlated with gene activity. Phosphate groups can be added to the hydroxyl groups of the amino acids serine and histidine, introducing a negative charge on the protein. During the cell cycle, increased phosphorylation, particularly of histone H3, is known to occur at characteristic times. Such chemical modification is believed to be related to the cycle of chromatin unfolding and condensation that occurs during and after DNA replication. It is important to note that the above chemical modifications (acetylation, methylation, and phosphorylation) are all reversible, under the direction of specific enzymes.

Interestingly, while methylation of histones *within nucleosomes* is often positively correlated with gene activity in eukaryotes, methylation of the nitrogenous base cytosine *within polynucleotide chains of DNA*, forming **5-methyl cytosine**, is usually negatively correlated with gene activity. Methylation of cytosine occurs most often when the nucleotide cytidylic acid is next to the nucleotide guanylic acid, forming what is called a **CpG island**. We must conclude, then, that methylation can have a positive or a negative impact on gene activity.

The research described above has extended our knowledge of nucleosomes and chromatin organization and serves here as a general introduction to the concept of chromatin

FIGURE 12–10 The nucleosome core particle derived from X-ray crystal analysis at 2.8 Å resolution. The double-helical DNA surrounds four pairs of histones.

remodeling. A great deal more work must be done, however, to elucidate the specific involvement of chromatin remodeling during genetic processes. In particular, the way in which the modifications are influenced by regulatory molecules within cells will provide important insights into the mechanisms of gene expression. What is clear is that the dynamic forms in which chromatin exists are vitally important to the way that all genetic processes directly involving DNA are executed. We will return to a more detailed discussion of the role of chromatin remodeling when we consider the regulation of eukaryotic gene expression later in the text (see Chapter 17). In addition, chromatin remodeling is an important topic in the discussion of **epigenetics**, the study of modifications of an organism's genetic and phenotypic expression that are *not* attributable to alteration of the DNA sequence making up a gene. This topic is discussed in depth in a future chapter (Special Topic Chapter 1—Epigenetics).

Heterochromatin

Although we know that the DNA of the eukaryotic chromosome consists of one continuous double-helical fiber along its entire length, we also know that the whole chromosome is not structurally uniform from end to end. In the early part of the twentieth century, it was observed that some parts of the chromosome remain condensed and stain deeply during interphase, while most parts are uncoiled and do not stain. In 1928, the terms **euchromatin** and **heterochromatin** were coined to describe the parts of chromosomes that are uncoiled and those that remain condensed, respectively.

Subsequent investigation revealed a number of characteristics that distinguish heterochromatin from euchromatin. Heterochromatic areas are genetically inactive because they either lack genes or contain genes that are repressed. Also, heterochromatin replicates later during the S phase of the cell cycle than does euchromatin. The discovery of heterochromatin provided the first clues that parts of eukaryotic chromosomes do not always encode proteins. For example, one particular heterochromatic region of the chromosome, the *telomere*, is thought to be involved in maintenance of the chromosome's structural integrity, and another region, the *centromere*, is involved in chromosome movement during cell division.

The presence of heterochromatin is unique to and characteristic of the genetic material of eukaryotes. In some cases, whole chromosomes are heterochromatic. A case in point is the mammalian Y chromosome, much of which is genetically inert. And, as we discussed earlier in the text (see Chapter 7), the inactivated X chromosome in mammalian females is condensed into an inert heterochromatic Barr body. In some species, such as mealy bugs, the chromosomes of one entire haploid set are heterochromatic.

When certain heterochromatic areas from one chromosome are translocated to a new site on the same or another nonhomologous chromosome, genetically active areas sometimes become genetically inert if they now lie adjacent to the translocated heterochromatin. As we saw earlier in the text (see Chapter 4), this influence on existing euchromatin is one example of what is more generally referred to as a **position effect**. That is, the position of a gene or group of genes relative to all other genetic material may affect their expression.

12.5 Chromosome Banding Differentiates Regions along the Mitotic Chromosome

Until about 1970, mitotic chromosomes viewed under the light microscope could be distinguished only by their relative sizes and the positions of their centromeres. Unfortunately, even in organisms with a low haploid number, two or more chromosomes are often visually indistinguishable from one another. Since that time, however, cytological procedures were developed that made possible differential staining along the longitudinal axis of mitotic chromosomes. Such methods are referred to as **chromosome-banding techniques,** because the staining patterns resemble the bands of polytene chromosomes.

One of the first chromosome-banding techniques was devised by Mary Lou Pardue and Joe Gall. They found that if chromosome preparations from mice were heat denatured and then treated with Giemsa stain, a unique staining pattern emerged: Only the centromeric regions of mitotic chromosomes took up the stain! The staining pattern was thus referred to as **C-banding**. Relevant to our immediate discussion, this cytological technique identifies a specific area of the chromosome composed of heterochromatin. A micrograph of the human karyotype treated in this way is shown in **Figure 12–11**. Mouse chromosomes are all telocentric, thus localizing the stain at the end of each chromosome.

Other chromosome-banding techniques were developed at about the same time. The most useful of these techniques produces a staining pattern differentially along the length of each chromosome. This method, producing **G-bands** (**Figure 12–12**), involves the digestion of the mitotic chromosomes with the proteolytic enzyme trypsin, followed by Giemsa staining. The differential staining reactions reflect the heterogeneity and complexity of the chromosome along its length.

In 1971 a uniform nomenclature for human chromosome-banding patterns was established based on G-banding. **Figure 12–13** illustrates the application of this

FIGURE 12–11 A human mitotic chromosome preparation processed to demonstrate C-banding. Only the centromeres stain (as small dark circles).

			Band
		3	p22.3
	2	2	p22.2
2		1	p22.1
p	1		p21
		4	p11.4
	1	3	p11.3
1		2	p11.2
		1	
			Centromere
		1	
	1	2	q12
		3	q13
		1	q21
q		2	q22
		3	q23
	2	4	q24
		5	q25
		6	q26
		7	q27
		8	q28

FIGURE 12–13 The regions of the human X chromosome distinguished by its banding pattern. The designations on the right identify specific bands.

nomenclature to the X chromosome. On the left of the chromosome are the various organizational levels of banding of the p and q arms that can be identified; the resulting designation for each of the specific regions is shown on the right side.

Although the molecular mechanisms involved in producing the various banding patterns are not well understood, the bands have played an important role in cytogenetic analysis, particularly in humans. The pattern of banding on each chromosome is unique, allowing a distinction to be made even between those chromosomes that are identical in size and centromere placement (e.g., human chromosomes 4 and 5 and 21 and 22). So precise is the banding pattern of each chromosome that homologs can be distinguished from one another, and when a segment of one chromosome has been translocated to another chromosome, its origin can be determined with great precision.

12.6 Eukaryotic Genomes Demonstrate Complex Sequence Organization Characterized by Repetitive DNA

Thus far, we have examined the general structure of chromosomes in bacteriophages, bacteria, and eukaryotes. We now begin an examination of what we know about the organization of DNA sequences within the chromosomes making up an organism's genome, placing our emphasis on eukaryotes. Once we establish certain general aspects of this organization, we will focus on how genes themselves are organized within chromosomes (see Chapter 21).

We learned earlier in the text (Chapter 10) that, in addition to single copies of unique DNA sequences that make up genes, a great deal of the DNA sequencing within eukaryotic chromosomes is repetitive in nature and that various levels of repetition occur within the genomes

FIGURE 12–12 G-banded karyotype of a normal human male. Chromosomes were derived from cells in metaphase.

FIGURE 12–14 An overview of the various categories of repetitive DNA.

The significance of satellite DNA remained an enigma until the mid-1960s, when Roy Britten and David Kohne developed the technique for measuring the reassociation kinetics of DNA that had previously been dissociated into single strands (Chapter 10). The researchers demonstrated that certain portions of DNA reannealed more rapidly than others, and concluded that rapid reannealing was characteristic of multiple DNA fragments composed of identical or nearly identical nucleotide sequences—the basis for the descriptive term *repetitive DNA*. Recall that, in contrast, prokaryotic DNA is nearly devoid of anything other than unique, single-copy sequences.

When satellite DNA is subjected to analysis by reassociation kinetics, it falls into the category of *highly repetitive DNA*, consisting of short sequences repeated a large number of times. Further evidence suggested that these sequences are present as tandem (meaning adjacent) repeats clustered in very specific chromosomal areas known to be heterochromatic—the regions flanking centromeres. This was discovered in 1969 when several researchers, including Mary Lou Pardue and Joe Gall, applied the technique of *in situ* hybridization to the study of satellite DNA. This technique involves molecular hybridization between an isolated fraction of labeled DNA or RNA probes and the DNA contained in the chromosomes of a cytological preparation. While fluorescent probes are standard today, radioactive probes were used by Pardue and Gall. Following the hybridization procedure, autoradiography was

of organisms. Many studies have now provided insights into **repetitive DNA**, demonstrating various classes of sequences and organization. **Figure 12–14** schematizes these categories. Some functional genes are present in more than one copy (they are referred to as **multiple-copy genes**) and so are repetitive in nature. However, the majority of repetitive sequences do not encode proteins. Nevertheless, many are transcribed, and the resultant RNAs play multiple roles in eukaryotes, including chromatin remodeling, as discussed in detail in a future chapter (see Special Topic Chapter 2—Emerging Roles of RNA). We will explore three main categories of repetitive sequences: (1) heterochromatin found to be associated with centromeres and making up telomeres; (2) tandem repeats of both short and long DNA sequences; and (3) transposable sequences that are interspersed throughout the genome of eukaryotes.

Satellite DNA

The nucleotide composition (e.g., the percentage of $G \equiv C$ versus $A = T$ pairs) of the DNA of a particular species is reflected in the DNA's density, which can be measured with a technique called sedimentation equilibrium centrifugation, which in essence determines the molecule's density. When eukaryotic DNA is analyzed in this way, the majority is present and represented as a single main band, of fairly uniform density. However, one or more additional peaks indicate the presence of DNA that differs slightly in density. This component, called **satellite DNA,** makes up a variable proportion of the total DNA, depending on the species. For example, a profile of main-band and satellite DNA from the mouse is shown in **Figure 12–15**. By contrast, prokaryotes do not contain satellite DNA.

FIGURE 12–15 Separation of main-band (MB) and satellite (S) DNA from the mouse by using ultracentrifugation in a CsCl gradient.

FIGURE 12–16 *In situ* hybridization between a radioactive probe representing mouse satellite DNA and mouse mitotic chromosomes. The grains in the autoradiograph are concentrated in chromosome regions referred to as the centromeres, revealing them to consist of and represent the location of satellite DNA sequences.

performed to locate the chromosome areas complementary to the fraction of DNA or RNA.

Pardue and Gall demonstrated that radioactive molecular probes made from mouse satellite DNA hybridize with DNA of centromeric regions of mouse mitotic chromosomes (**Figure 12–16**). Several conclusions were drawn: Satellite DNA differs from main-band DNA in its molecular composition, as established by buoyant density studies. It is composed of short repetitive sequences. Finally, satellite DNA is found in the heterochromatic centromeric regions of chromosomes.

Centromeric DNA Sequences

The separation of homologs during mitosis and meiosis depends on **centromeres**, described cytologically in the late nineteenth century as the *primary constrictions* along eukaryotic chromosomes (see Chapter 2). In this role, it is believed that the repetitive DNA sequences contained within the centromere are critical to this role. Careful analysis has confirmed this belief. The minimal region of the centromere that supports the function of chromosomal segregation is designated the **CEN region**. Within this heterochromatic region of the chromosome, the DNA binds a platform of proteins, which in multicellular organisms includes the **kinetochore** that binds to the microtubules making up the spindle fiber during division (see Figure 2–8).

The CEN regions of the yeast *Saccharomyces cerevisiae* were the first to be studied. Each centromere serves an identical function, so it is not surprising that CENs from different chromosomes were found to be remarkably similar in their DNA sequence, displaying only minor differences between chromosomes. The CEN region of yeast chromosomes consists of about 120 bp. Mutational analysis

suggests that portions near the 3′ end of this DNA region are most critical to centromere function since mutations in them, but not those nearer the 5′ end, disrupt centromere function. Thus, the DNA of this region appears to be essential to the eventual binding to the spindle fiber.

Centromere sequences of multicellular eukaryotes are much more extensive than in yeast and vary considerably in size. For example, in *Drosophila* the CEN region is found embedded within some 200 to 600 kb of DNA, much of which is highly repetitive (recall from our prior discussion that highly repetitive satellite DNA is localized in the centromere regions of mice). In humans, one of the most recognized satellite DNA sequences is the **alphoid family,** found mainly in the centromere regions. Alphoid sequences, each about 170 bp in length, are present in tandem arrays of up to 1 million base pairs. It is now believed that such repetitive DNA in eukaryotes is transcribed and that the RNA that is produced is ultimately involved in kinetochore function.

One final observation of interest is that the H3 histone, a normal part of most all eukaryotic nucleosomes, is substituted by a variant histone designated CENP-A in centromeric heterochromatin. It is believed that the unique N-terminal protein tails that make CEN-P unique are involved in the binding of kinetochore proteins that are essential to the microtubules of spindle fibers. This finding supports the supposition that the DNA sequence found only in centromeres is related to the function of this unique chromosomal structure.

Middle Repetitive Sequences: VNTRs and STRs

A brief look at still another prominent category of repetitive DNA sheds additional light on the organization of the eukaryotic genome. In addition to highly repetitive DNA, which constitutes about 5 percent of the human genome (and 10 percent of the mouse genome), a second category, **middle (or moderately) repetitive DNA,** recognized by reassociation kinetic studies, is fairly well characterized. Because we now know a great deal about the human genome, we will use our own species to illustrate this category of DNA in genome organization.

Although middle repetitive DNA does include some duplicated genes (such as those encoding ribosomal RNA), most prominent in this category are either noncoding tandemly repeated sequences or noncoding interspersed sequences. No function has been ascribed to these components of the genome. An example is DNA described as **variable number tandem repeats (VNTRs).** These repeating DNA sequences may be 15 to 100 bp long and are found within and between genes. Many such clusters are dispersed throughout the genome, and they are often referred to as **minisatellites**.

The number of tandem copies of each specific sequence at each location varies from one individual to the next, creating localized regions of 1000 to 20,000 bp (1–20 kb) in length. As we will see later in the text (see Chapter 21), the variation in size (length) of these regions between individual humans was originally the basis for the forensic technique referred to as **DNA fingerprinting**.

Another group of tandemly repeated sequences consists of di-, tri-, tetra-, and pentanucleotides, also referred to as **microsatellites** or **short tandem repeats (STRs)**. Like VNTRs, they are dispersed throughout the genome and vary among individuals in the number of repeats present at any site. For example, in humans, the most common microsatellite is the dinucleotide $(CA)_n$, where n equals the number of repeats. Most commonly, n is between 5 and 50. These clusters have served as useful molecular markers for genome analysis.

Repetitive Transposed Sequences: SINEs and LINEs

Still another category of repetitive DNA consists of sequences that are interspersed individually throughout the genome, rather than being tandemly repeated. They can be either short or long, and many have the added distinction of being **transposable sequences,** which are mobile and can potentially move to different locations within the genome. A large portion of the human genome is composed of such sequences. Transposable sequences are discussed in more detail later in the text (see Chapter 15).

For example, **short interspersed elements,** called **SINEs,** are less than 500 base pairs long and may be present 1,500,000 times or more in the human genome. The best characterized human SINE is a set of closely related sequences called the *Alu* **family** (the name is based on the presence of DNA sequences recognized by the restriction endonuclease *Alu* I). Members of this DNA family, also found in other mammals, are 200 to 300 base pairs long and are dispersed rather uniformly throughout the genome, both between and within genes. In humans, this family encompasses more than 5 percent of the entire genome.

Alu sequences are of particular interest because some members of the *Alu* family are transcribed into RNA, although the specific role of this RNA is not certain. Even so, the consequence of *Alu* sequences is their potential for transposition within the genome, which is related to chromosome rearrangements during evolution. *Alu* sequences are thought to have arisen from an RNA element whose DNA complement was dispersed throughout the genome as a result of the activity of reverse transcriptase (an enzyme that synthesizes DNA on an RNA template).

The group of **long interspersed elements (LINEs)** represents yet another category of repetitive transposable DNA sequences. LINEs are usually about 6 kb in length and in the human genome are present approximately 850,000 times. The most prominent example in humans is the **L1 family**. Members of this sequence family are about 6400 base pairs long and are present more than 500,000 times. Their 5′ end is highly variable, and their role within the genome has yet to be defined.

The general mechanism for transposition of L1 elements is now clear. The L1 DNA sequence is first transcribed into an RNA molecule. The RNA then serves as the template for synthesis of the DNA complement using the enzyme reverse transcriptase. This enzyme is encoded by a portion of the L1 sequence. The new L1 copy then integrates into the DNA of the chromosome at a new site. Because of the similarity of this transposition mechanism to that used by retroviruses, LINEs are referred to as **retrotransposons**.

SINEs and LINEs represent a significant portion of human DNA. SINEs constitute about 13 percent of the human genome, whereas LINEs constitute up to 21 percent. Within both types of elements, repeating sequences of DNA are present in combination with unique sequences.

Middle Repetitive Multiple-Copy Genes

In some cases, middle repetitive DNA includes functional genes present tandemly in multiple copies. For example, many copies exist of the genes encoding ribosomal RNA. *Drosophila* has 120 copies per haploid genome. Single genetic units encode a large precursor molecule that is processed into the 5.8*S*, 18*S*, and 28*S* rRNA components. In humans, multiple copies of this gene are clustered on the p arm of the acrocentric chromosomes 13, 14, 15, 21, and 22. Multiple copies of the genes encoding 5*S* rRNA are transcribed separately from multiple clusters found together on the terminal portion of the p arm of chromosome 1.

12.7 The Vast Majority of a Eukaryotic Genome Does Not Encode Functional Genes

Given the preceding information concerning various forms of repetitive DNA in eukaryotes, it is of interest to pose an important question: *What proportion of the eukaryotic genome actually encodes functional genes?*

We have seen that, taken together, the various forms of highly repetitive and moderately repetitive DNA comprise a substantial portion of the human genome—approximately 50 percent of all DNA sequences by most estimates. In addition to repetitive DNA, a large amount of the DNA consists of single-copy sequences that appear to be noncoding. Included are many instances of what we call **pseudogenes**. These are DNA sequences representing evolutionary vestiges of duplicated copies of genes that have undergone significant mutational alteration. As a result, although they show some homology to their parent gene, they are usually not transcribed because of insertions and deletions throughout their structure.

While the proportion of the genome consisting of repetitive DNA varies among organisms, one feature seems to be shared: *Only a very small part of the genome actually codes for proteins.* For example, the 20,000 to 30,000 genes encoding proteins in sea urchin occupy less than 10 percent of the genome. In *Drosophila*, only 5 to 10 percent of the genome is occupied by genes coding for proteins. In humans, it appears that the coding regions of the estimated 20,000 functional genes occupy only about 2 percent of the total DNA sequence making up the genome.

Study of the various forms of repetitive DNA has significantly enhanced our understanding of genome organization, which we will explore in more depth later in the text (see Chapter 21).

EXPLORING GENOMICS

Database of Genomic Variants: Structural Variations in the Human Genome

MasteringGenetics™ Visit the
Study Area: Exploring Genomics

In this chapter, we focused on structural details of chromosomes and DNA sequence organization in chromosomes. A related finding is that large segments of DNA and a number of genes can vary greatly in copy number due to duplications, creating **copy number variations (CNVs)**. Many studies are underway to identify and map CNVs and to find possible disease conditions associated with them.

Several thousand CNVs have been identified in the human genome, and estimates suggest there may be thousands more within human populations. In this Exploring Genomics exercise we will visit the **Database of Genomic Variants (DGV)**, which provides a quickly expanding summary of structural variations in the human genome including CNVs.

- **Exercise I – Database of Genomic Variants**

1. Access the DGV at http://dgv.tcag .ca/dgv/app/home. Click the "About the Project" tab to learn more about the purpose of the DGV.

2. Information in the DGV is easily viewed by clicking on a chromosome of interest using the "Find DGV Variants by Chromosome" feature. Using this feature, click on a chromosome of interest to you. A table will appear under the "Variants" tab showing several columns of data including:

- Start and Stop: Shows the locus for the CNV, including the base pairs that span the variation.
- Variation Accession: Provides a unique identifying number for each variation. Click on the variant accession number to reveal a separate page of specific details about each CNV, including the chromosomal banding location for the variation and known genes that are located in the CNV.
- Variant Type: Most variations in this database are CNVs. Variant subtypes, such as deletions or insertions, and duplications, are shown in an adjacent column.

3. Let's analyze a particular group of CNVs. Many CNVs are unlikely to affect phenotype because they involve large areas of non–protein-coding or nonregulatory sequences. But gene-containing CNVs have been identified, including variants containing genes associated with Alzheimer's disease, Parkinson's disease, and other conditions.

Defensin (*DEF*) genes are part of a large family of highly duplicated genes. To learn more about *DEF* genes and CNVs, use the Keyword Search box and search for *DEF*. A results page for the search will appear with a listing of relevant CNVs. Click on the name for any of the different

DEF genes listed, which will take you to a wealth of information (including links to Online Mendelian Inheritance in Man, OMIM) about these genes so that you can answer the following questions. Do this for several *DEF*-containing CNVs on different chromosomes to find the information you will need for your answers.

a. On what chromosome(s) did you find CNVs containing *DEF* genes?

b. What did you learn about the function of *DEF* gene products? What do DEF proteins do?

c. Variations in *DEF* genotypes and *DEF* gene expression in humans have been implicated in a number of different human disease conditions. Give examples of the kinds of disorders affected by variations in *DEF* genotypes.

d. Explore the DGV to search a chromosome of interest to you and learn more about CNVs that have been mapped to that chromosome. Try the Genome Browser feature that will show you maps of each chromosome indicating different variations. For CNVs (shown in blue), clicking on the CNV will take you to its locus on the chromosome.

CASE STUDY | Art inspires learning

A genetics student visiting a museum saw a painting by Goya showing a woman with a newborn baby in her lap who had very short arms and legs along with some facial abnormalities. Wondering whether this condition might be a genetic disorder, the student went online, learning that the baby might have Roberts syndrome (RBS), a rare autosomal recessive trait. She read that cells in RBS have mitotic errors, including the premature separation of centromeres and other heterochromatic regions of homologs in metaphase instead of anaphase. As a result, metaphase chromosomes have a rigid, or "railroad track" appearance. RBS has been shown to be caused by mutant alleles of the *ESCO2* gene, which functions during cell division.

The student wrote a list of questions to investigate in an attempt to better understand this condition. How would you answer these questions?

1. What do centromeres and other heterochromatic regions have in common that might cause this appearance?

2. What might be the role of the protein encoded by *ESCO2*, which in mutant form could cause these changes in mitotic chromosomes?

3. How could premature separation of centromeres cause the problems seen in RBS?

Summary Points

1. Bacteriophage and bacterial chromosomes, in contrast to those of eukaryotes, are largely devoid of associated proteins, are of much smaller size, and, with some exceptions, consist of circular DNA.

2. Polytene and lampbrush chromosomes are examples of specialized structures that extended our knowledge of genetic organization and function well in advance of the technology available to the modern-day molecular biologist.

3. Eukaryotic chromatin is a nucleoprotein organized into repeating units called nucleosomes, which are composed of about 200 base pairs of DNA, an octamer of four types of histones, plus one linker histone.

4. Nucleosomes provide a mechanism for compaction of chromatin within the nucleus. Several forms of chemical modification, for example, acetylation and methylation, may alter the level of compaction, a process referred to as chromatin remodeling, which is critical to replication and transcription of DNA.

5. Heterochromatin, prematurely condensed in interphase and for the most part genetically inert, is illustrated by centromeric and telomeric regions of eukaryotic chromosomes, the Y chromosome, and the Barr body.

6. Chromosome banding techniques provide a way to subdivide and identify specific regions of mitotic chromosomes.

7. Eukaryotic genomes demonstrate complex sequence organization characterized by numerous categories of repetitive DNA, consisting of either tandem repeats clustered in various regions of the genome or single sequences repeatedly interspersed at random throughout the genome.

8. The vast majority of the DNA in most eukaryotic genomes does not encode functional genes. In humans, for example, only about 2 percent of the genome is used to encode the 20,000 genes found there.

INSIGHTS AND SOLUTIONS

A previously undiscovered single-celled organism was found living at a great depth on the ocean floor. Its nucleus contains only a single, linear chromosome consisting of 7×10^6 nucleotide pairs of DNA coalesced with three types of histonelike proteins. Consider the following questions:

1. A short micrococcal nuclease digestion yielded DNA fractions consisting of 700, 1400, and 2100 base pairs. Predict what these fractions represent. What conclusions can be drawn?

   Solution: The chromatin fiber may consist of a nucleosome variant containing 700 base pairs of DNA. The 1400- and 2100-bp fractions represent two and three of these nucleosomes, respectively, linked together. Enzymatic

digestion may have been incomplete, leading to the latter two fractions.

2. The analysis of individual nucleosomes revealed that each unit contained one copy of each protein and that the short linker DNA had no protein bound to it. If the entire chromosome consists of nucleosomes (discounting any linker DNA), how many are there, and how many total proteins are needed to form them?

   Solution: Since the chromosome contains 7×10^6 base pairs of DNA, the number of nucleosomes, each containing 7×10^2 base pairs, is equal to

   $$7 \times 10^6 / 7 \times 10^2 = 10^4 \text{ nucleosomes}$$

The chromosome thus contains 10^4 copies of each of the three proteins, for a total of 3×10^4 proteins.

3. Analysis then revealed the organism's DNA to be a double helix similar to the Watson–Crick model, but containing 20 base pairs per complete turn of the right-handed helix. The physical size of the nucleosome was exactly double the volume occupied by the nucleosome found in any other known eukaryote, and the nucleosome's axis length was greater by a factor of two. Compare the degree of compaction (the number of turns per nucleosome) of this organism's nucleosome with that found in other eukaryotes.

Solution: The unique organism compacts a length of DNA consisting of 35 complete turns of the helix (700 base pairs per nucleosome/20 base pairs per turn) into each nucleosome. The normal eukaryote compacts a length of DNA consisting of 20 complete turns of the helix (200 base pairs per nucleosome/10 base pairs per turn) into a nucleosome half the volume of that in the unique organism. The degree of compaction is therefore less in the unique organism.

4. No further coiling or compaction of this unique chromosome occurs in the newly discovered organism. Compare this situation with that of a eukaryotic chromosome. Do you think an interphase human chromosome 7×10^6 base pairs in length would be a shorter or longer chromatin fiber?

Solution: The eukaryotic chromosome contains still another level of condensation in the form of solenoids, which are coils consisting of nucleosomes connected with linker DNA. Solenoids condense the eukaryotic fiber by still another factor of five. The length of the unique chromosome is compacted into 10^4 nucleosomes, each containing an axis length twice that of the eukaryotic fiber. The eukaryotic fiber consists of $7 \times 10^6/2 \times 10^2 = 3.5 \times 10^4$ nucleosomes, 3.5 times more than the unique organism. However, they are compacted by the factor of five in each solenoid. Therefore, the chromosome of the unique organism is a longer chromatin fiber.

Problems and Discussion Questions

HOW DO WE KNOW?

1. In this chapter, we focused on how DNA is organized at the chromosomal level. Along the way, we found many opportunities to consider the methods and reasoning by which much of this information was acquired. From the explanations given in the chapter, what answers would you propose to the following fundamental questions:
   (a) How do we know that viral and bacterial chromosomes most often consist of circular DNA molecules devoid of protein?
   (b) What is the experimental basis for concluding that puffs in polytene chromosomes and loops in lampbrush chromosomes are areas of intense transcription of RNA?
   (c) How did we learn that eukaryotic chromatin exists in the form of repeating nucleosomes, each consisting of about 200 base pairs and an octamer of histones?
   (d) How do we know that satellite DNA consists of repetitive sequences and has been derived from regions of the centromere?

CONCEPT QUESTION

2. Review the Chapter Concepts list on p. 288. These all relate to how DNA is organized in viral, prokaryote, and eukaryote chromosomes. Write a short essay that contrasts the major differences between the organization of DNA in viruses and bacteria versus eukaryotes.

3. Contrast the size of the single chromosome in bacteriophage λ and T2 with that of *E. coli*. How does this relate to the relative size and complexity of phages and bacteria?

4. Describe the structure of giant polytene chromosomes and how they arise.

5. What genetic process is occurring in a puff of a polytene chromosome? How do we know this experimentally?

6. During what genetic process are lampbrush chromosomes present in vertebrates?

7. Why might we predict that the organization of eukaryotic genetic material will be more complex than that of viruses or bacteria?

8. Describe the sequence of research findings that led to the development of the model of chromatin structure.

9. Describe the molecular composition and arrangement of the components in the nucleosome.

10. Describe the transitions that occur as nucleosomes are coiled and folded, ultimately forming a chromatid.

11. Provide a comprehensive definition of heterochromatin and list as many examples as you can.

12. Mammals contain a diploid genome consisting of at least 10^9 bp. If this amount of DNA is present as chromatin fibers, where each group of 200 bp of DNA is combined with 9 histones into a nucleosome and each group of 6 nucleosomes is combined into a solenoid, achieving a final packing ratio of 50, determine (a) the total number of nucleosomes in all fibers, (b) the total number of histone molecules combined with DNA in the diploid genome, and (c) the combined length of all fibers.

13. Assume that a viral DNA molecule is a 50-μm-long circular strand with a uniform 20-Å diameter. If this molecule is contained in a viral head that is a 0.08-μm-diameter sphere, will the DNA molecule fit into the viral head, assuming complete flexibility of the molecule? Justify your answer mathematically.

14. How many base pairs are in a molecule of phage T2 DNA 52 μm long?

15. Examples of histone modifications are acetylation (by histone acetyltransferase, or HAT), which is often linked to gene activation, and deacetylation (by histone deacetylases, or HDACs), which often leads to gene silencing typical of heterochromatin. Such heterochromatinization is initiated from a nucleation site and spreads bidirectionally until encountering boundaries that delimit the silenced areas. Recall from earlier in the text (see Chapter 4) the brief discussion of position effect, where

repositioning of the w^+ allele in *Drosophila* by translocation or inversion near heterochromatin produces intermittent w^+ activity. In the heterozygous state (w^+/w), a variegated eye is produced, with white and red patches. How might one explain position-effect variegation in terms of histone acetylation and/or deacetylation?

16. Contrast the structure of SINE and LINE DNA sequences. Why are LINEs referred to as retrotransposons?

17. Variable number tandem repeats (VNTRs) are repeating DNA sequences of about 15 to 100 bp in length, found both within and between genes. Why are they commonly used in forensics?

18. A number of recent studies have determined that disease pathogenesis, whether it be related to viruses, cancer, aging, or a host of other causes, is often associated with specific changes in DNA methylation. If such patterns are to be considered as biomarkers for disease diagnosis what requisite criteria would you consider essential to their use?

19. It has been shown that infectious agents such as viruses often exert a dramatic effect on their host cell's genome architecture. In many cases, viruses induce methylation of host DNA sequences in order to enhance their infectivity. What specific host gene functions would you consider as strong candidates for such methylation by infecting viruses?

20. Cancer can be defined as an abnormal proliferation of cells that defy the normal regulatory controls observed by normal cells. Recently, histone deacetylation therapies have been attempted in the treatment of certain cancers (reviewed by Delcuve et al., 2009). Specifically, the FDA has approved histone deacetylation (HDAC) inhibitors for the treatment of cutaneous T-cell lymphoma. Explain why histone acetylation might be associated with cancer and what the rationale is for the use of HDAC inhibitors in the treatment of certain forms of cancer.

Extra-Spicy Problems

MasteringGenetics™ Visit for instructor-assigned tutorials and problems.

21. In a study of *Drosophila,* two normally active genes, w^+ (wild-type allele of the *white*-eye gene) and *hsp26* (a heat-shock gene), were introduced (using a plasmid vector) into euchromatic and heterochromatic chromosomal regions, and the relative activity of each gene was assessed (Sun et al., 2002). An approximation of the resulting data is shown in the following table. Which characteristic or characteristics of heterochromatin are supported by the experimental data?

Gene	Activity (relative percentage)	
	Euchromatin	Heterochromatin
hsp26	100%	31%
w^+	100%	8%

22. While much remains to be learned about the role of nucleosomes and chromatin structure and function, recent research indicates that *in vivo* chemical modification of histones is associated with changes in gene activity. One study determined that acetylation of H3 and H4 is associated with 21.1 percent and 13.8 percent increases in yeast gene activity, respectively, and that yeast heterochromatin is hypomethylated relative to the genome average (Bernstein et al., 2000). Speculate on the significance of these findings in terms of nucleosome–DNA interactions and gene activity.

23. An article entitled "Nucleosome Positioning at the Replication Fork" states: "both the 'old' randomly segregated nucleosomes as well as the 'new' assembled histone octamers rapidly position themselves (within seconds) on the newly replicated DNA strands" (Lucchini et al., 2002). Given this statement, how would one compare the distribution of nucleosomes and DNA in newly replicated chromatin? How could one experimentally test the distribution of nucleosomes on newly replicated chromosomes?

24. The human genome contains approximately 10^6 copies of an *Alu* sequence, one of the best-studied classes of short interspersed elements (SINEs), per haploid genome. Individual

Alu units share a 282-nucleotide consensus sequence followed by a 3'-adenine-rich tail region (Schmid, 1998). Given that there are approximately 3×10^9 base pairs per human haploid genome, about how many base pairs are spaced between each *Alu* sequence?

25. Following is a diagram of the general structure of the bacteriophage λ chromosome. Speculate on the mechanism by which it forms a closed ring upon infection of the host cell.

5' GGGCGGCGACCT—double-stranded region—3'
　　　　　　　3'—double-stranded region—CCCGCCGCTGGA 5'

26. Tandemly repeated DNA sequences with a repeat sequence of one to six base pairs—for example, $(GACA)_n$—are called microsatellites and are common in eukaryotes. A particular subset of such sequences, the trinucleotide repeat, is of great interest because of the role such repeats play in human neurodegenerative disorders (Huntington disease, myotonic dystrophy, spinal-bulbar muscular atrophy, spinocerebellar ataxia, and fragile-X syndrome). Following are data (modified from Toth et al., 2000) regarding the location of microsatellites within and between genes. What general conclusions can be drawn from these data?

Percentage of Microsatellite DNA Sequences within Genes and between Genes

Taxonomic Group	Within Genes	Between Genes
Primates	7.4	92.6
Rodents	33.7	66.3
Arthropods	46.7	53.3
Yeasts	77.0	23.0
Other fungi	66.7	33.3

27. More information from the research effort in Problem 26 produced data regarding the pattern of the length of such repeats within genes. Each value in the following table represents the

number of times a microsatellite of a particular sequence length, one to six bases long, is found within genes. For instance, in primates, a dinucleotide sequence (GC, for example) is found 10 times, while a trinucleotide is found 1126 times. In fungi, a repeat motif composed of 6 nucleotides (GACACC, for example) is found 219 times, whereas a tetranucleotide repeat (GACA, for example) is found only 2 times. Analyze and interpret these data by indicating what general pattern is apparent for the distribution of various microsatellite lengths within genes. Of what significance might this general pattern be?

Distribution of Microsatellites by Unit Length within Genes

Taxonomic Group	Length of Repeated Motif (bp)					
	1	2	3	4	5	6
Primates	49	10	1126	29	57	244
Rodents	62	70	1557	63	116	620
Arthropods	12	34	1566	0	21	591
Yeasts	36	19	706	7	52	330
Other fungi	9	4	381	2	35	219

28. Microsatellites are currently exploited as markers for paternity testing. A sample paternity test is shown in the following table in which ten microsatellite markers were used to test samples from a mother, her child, and an alleged father. The name of the microsatellite locus is given in the left-hand column, and the genotype of each individual is recorded as the number of repeats he or she carries at that locus. For example, at locus D9S302, the mother carries 30 repeats on one of her chromosomes and 31 on the other. In cases where an individual carries the same number of repeats on both chromosomes, only a single number is recorded. (Some of the numbers are followed by a decimal point, for example, 20.2, to indicate a partial repeat in addition to the complete repeats.) Assuming that these markers are inherited in a simple Mendelian fashion, can

the alleged father be excluded as the source of the sperm that produced the child? Why or why not? Explain.

Microsatellite Locus-Chromosome Location	Mother	Child	Alleged Father
D9S302-9q31-q33	30	31	32
	31	32	33
D22S883-22pter-22qter	17	20.2	20.2
	22	22	
D18S535-18q12.2-q12.3	12	13	11
	14	14	13
D7SI804-7pter-7qter	27	26	26
	30	30	27
D3S2387-3p24.2.3pter	23	24	20.2
	25.2	25.2	24
D4S2386-4pter-qter	12	12	12
			16
D5S1719-5pter-5qter	11	10.3	10
	11.3	11	10.3
CSF1PO-5q33.3.q34	11	11	10
		12	12
FESFPS-15q25-15qter	11	12	10
	12	13	13
TH01-11p15.5	7	7	7
			8

29. At the end of the short arm of human chromosome 16 (16p), several genes associated with disease are present, including thalassemia and polycystic kidney disease. When that region of chromosome 16 was sequenced, gene-coding regions were found to be very close to the telomere-associated sequences. Could there be a possible link between the location of these genes and the presence of the telomere-associated sequences? What further information concerning the disease genes would be useful in your analysis?

Electron micrograph of a segment of DNA undergoing transcription.

13

The Genetic Code and Transcription

CHAPTER CONCEPTS

- Genetic information is stored in DNA by means of a triplet code that is nearly universal to all living things on Earth.

- The genetic code is initially transferred from DNA to RNA, in the process of transcription.

- Once transferred to RNA, the genetic code exists as triplet codons, which are sets of three nucleotides in which each nucleotide is one of the four kinds of ribonucleotides composing RNA.

- RNA's four ribonucleotides, analogous to an alphabet of four "letters," can be arranged into 64 different three-letter sequences. Most of the triplets in RNA encode one of the 20 amino acids present in proteins, which are the end products of most genes.

- Several codons act as signals that initiate or terminate protein synthesis.

- In eukaryotes, the process of transcription is similar to, but more complex than, that in prokaryotes and in the bacteriophages that infect them.

As we saw earlier in the text (see Chapter 10), the structure of DNA consists of a linear sequence of deoxyribonucleotides. This sequence ultimately dictates the components of proteins, the end products of most genes. A central issue is how information stored as a nucleic acid can be decoded into a protein. **Figure 13–1** provides a simple overview of how this transfer of information, resulting ultimately in gene expression, occurs. In the first step, information present on one of the two strands of DNA (the template strand) is transferred into an RNA complement through the process of transcription. Once synthesized, this RNA acts as a "messenger" molecule, transporting the coded information out of the nucleus—hence its name, *messenger RNA* (*mRNA*). The mRNAs then associate with ribosomes, where decoding into proteins occurs.

In this chapter, we will focus on the initial phases of gene expression by addressing two major questions. First, how is genetic information encoded? Second, how does the transfer from DNA to RNA occur, thus explaining the process of transcription? As you will see, ingenious analytical research has established that the genetic code is written in units of three letters—triplets of ribonucleotides in mRNA that reflect the stored information in genes. Most of the triplet code words direct the incorporation of a specific amino acid into a protein as it is synthesized. As we can predict based on the complexity of the replication of DNA (see Chapter 11), transcription is also a complex process dependent on a major polymerase enzyme and a cast of supporting proteins. We will explore what is known about transcription in bacteria and then contrast this prokaryotic model with transcription in eukaryotes.

Gene

DNA

3'   5'

TACCACAACTCG

DNA template strand

↓

Transcription

↓

mRNA   5'   3'

AUGGUGUUGAGC

Triplet code words

↓

Translation on ribosomes

↓

Met   Val   Leu   Ser

Protein

Amino acids

FIGURE 13–1 Flowchart illustrating how genetic information encoded in DNA produces protein.

We will continue our discussion of gene expression by addressing how translation occurs and then describing the structure and function of proteins (Chapter 14). Together, these chapters provide a comprehensive picture of molecular genetics, which serves as the most basic foundation for understanding living organisms.

13.1 The Genetic Code Uses Ribonucleotide Bases as "Letters"

Before we consider the various analytical approaches that led to our current understanding of the genetic code, let's summarize the general features that characterize it:

1. The genetic code is written in linear form, using as "letters" the ribonucleotide bases that compose mRNA molecules. The ribonucleotide sequence is derived from the complementary nucleotide bases in DNA.

2. Each "word" within the mRNA consists of three ribonucleotide letters, thus referred to as a **triplet code**. With several exceptions, each group of *three* ribonucleotides, called a **codon**, specifies *one* amino acid.

3. The code is **unambiguous**—each triplet specifies only a single amino acid.

4. The code is **degenerate**, meaning that a given amino acid can be specified by more than one triplet codon. This is the case for 18 of the 20 amino acids.

5. The code contains one "start" and three "stop" signals, triplets that **initiate** and **terminate** translation, respectively.

6. No internal punctuation (analogous, for example, to a comma) is used in the code. Thus, the code is said to be **commaless**. Once translation of mRNA begins, the codons are read one after the other with no breaks between them (until a stop signal is reached).

7. The code is **nonoverlapping**. After translation commences, any single ribonucleotide within the mRNA is part of only one triplet.

8. The sequence of codons in a gene is **colinear**, with the sequence of amino acids making up the encoded protein.

9. The code is nearly **universal**. With only minor exceptions, a single coding dictionary is used by almost all viruses, prokaryotes, archaea, and eukaryotes.

13.2 Early Studies Established the Basic Operational Patterns of the Code

In the late 1950s, before it became clear that mRNA serves as an intermediate in the transfer of genetic information from DNA to proteins, researchers thought that DNA might encode protein synthesis more directly. Because ribosomes had already been identified, the initial thinking was that information in DNA was transferred in the nucleus to the RNA of the ribosome, which served as the template for protein synthesis in the cytoplasm. This concept soon became untenable, as accumulating evidence indicated that there was an unstable intermediate template. The RNA of ribosomes, on the other hand, was extremely stable. In 1961, François Jacob and Jacques Monod postulated the existence of **messenger RNA (mRNA)**. After mRNA was discovered, it soon became clear that, even though genetic information is stored in DNA, the code that is translated into proteins resides in RNA. The central question then was how could only four letters—the four nucleotides—specify 20 words, the amino acids? Scientists considered the possibility that DNA codes could overlap in such a way that each nucleotide would be part of more than one code word, but accumulating evidence was inconsistent with the constraints such a code would place on the resultant amino acid sequences. We will next address some of this evidence.

The Triplet Nature of the Code

In the early 1960s, Sydney Brenner argued on theoretical grounds that the code must be a triplet, since three-letter words represent the minimal length needed for using four letters to specify 20 amino acids. A code of four nucleotides combined into two-letter words, for example, provides only 16 unique code words (4^2). A triplet code yields 64 words (4^3) and therefore is sufficient for the 20 needed but far less cumbersome than a four-letter code (4^4), which would specify 256 words.

The ingenious experimental work of Francis Crick, Leslie Barnett, Brenner, and R. J. Watts-Tobin provided the first solid evidence for a triplet code. These researchers induced insertion and deletion mutations in the *rII* locus of phage T4 (see Chapter 6). Wild-type phage cause lysis and plaque formation in strains B and K12 of *E. coli*. However, *rII* mutations prevent this infection process in strain K12, while allowing infection in strain B. Crick and his colleagues used the acridine dye *proflavin* to induce the mutations. This mutagenic agent intercalates within the double helix of DNA, causing the insertion or deletion of one or more nucleotides during replication. As shown in **Figure 13–2(a)**, an insertion of a single nucleotide causes the **reading frame** (the contiguous sequence of nucleotides encoding a polypeptide) to shift, changing all subsequent downstream codons (codons to the right of the insertion in the figure). Such mutations are referred to as frameshift mutations. Upon translation, the amino acid sequence of the encoded protein will be altered radically starting at the point where the mutation occurred. When these mutations are present at the *rII* locus, T4 will not reproduce on *E. coli* K12.

Crick and his colleagues reasoned that if phages with these induced frameshift mutations were treated again with proflavin, still other insertions or deletions would occur. A second change might result in a revertant phage, which would display wild-type behavior and successfully infect *E. coli* K12. For example, if the original mutant contained an insertion (+), a second event causing a deletion (−) close to the insertion would restore the original reading frame. In the same way, an event resulting in an insertion (+) might correct an original deletion (−).

By studying many mutations of this type, these researchers were able to compare combinations of various frameshift mutations within the same DNA sequence. They found that various combinations of one plus (+) and one minus (−) caused reversion to wild-type behavior. Still other observations shed light on the number of nucleotides constituting the genetic code. When two pluses or two minuses occurred in the same sequence, the correct reading frame *was not* reestablished. This argued against a doublet (two-letter) code. However, when three pluses [**Figure 13–2(b)**] or three minuses were present together, the original frame *was* reestablished. These observations strongly supported the triplet nature of the code.

The Nonoverlapping Nature of the Code

Work by Sydney Brenner and others soon established that the code could not be overlapping for any one transcript. For example, beginning by assuming a triplet code, Brenner deduced the restrictions that might be expected if the code were overlapping. He imagined theoretical nucleotide sequences encoding a protein consisting of three amino acids. If the nucleotide sequence were, say, GTACA, and parts of the central codon, TAC, were shared by the outer codons, GTA and ACA, then only certain amino acids (those with codons ending in TA or beginning with AC) should be found adjacent to the one encoded by the central codon. This consideration led Brenner to conclude that if the code were overlapping, the compositions of tripeptide sequences within proteins should be somewhat limited.

For example, when any particular central amino acid is considered, only 16 combinations (2^4) of three amino acids (tripeptide sequences) would theoretically be possible. Looking at the amino acid sequences of proteins that were known at that time, Brenner failed to find such restrictions in tripeptide sequences. For any central amino acid, he found many more than 16 different tripeptides. This observation led him to conclude that the code is not overlapping.

FIGURE 13–2 The effect of frameshift mutations on a DNA sequence repeating the triplet sequence GAG. (a) The insertion of a single nucleotide shifts all subsequent triplets out of the reading frame. (b) The insertion of three nucleotides changes only two triplets, after which the original reading frame is reestablished.

A second major argument against an overlapping code concerned the effect of a single-nucleotide change. With an overlapping code, two adjacent amino acids would be affected by such a point mutation. However, mutations in the genes coding for the protein coat of tobacco mosaic virus (TMV), human hemoglobin, and the bacterial enzyme tryptophan synthetase invariably revealed only single amino acid changes.

The third argument against an overlapping code was presented by Francis Crick in 1957, when he predicted that DNA would not serve as a direct template for the formation of proteins. Crick reasoned that any affinity between nucleotides and an amino acid would require hydrogen bonding. Chemically, however, such specific affinities seemed unlikely. Instead, Crick proposed that there must be an "adaptor molecule" that could covalently bind to the amino acid, yet also be capable of hydrogen bonding to a nucleotide sequence. With an overlapping code, various adaptors would somehow have to overlap one another at nucleotide sites during translation, making the translation process overly complex, in Crick's opinion, and possibly inefficient. As we will see later in this chapter, Crick's prediction was correct—*transfer RNA* (*tRNA*) serves as the adaptor in protein synthesis, and the ribosome accommodates two tRNA molecules at a time.

Crick's and Brenner's arguments, taken together, strongly suggested that, during translation, the genetic code is nonoverlapping. Without exception, this concept has been upheld.

The Commaless and Degenerate Nature of the Code

Between 1958 and 1960, information relating to the genetic code continued to accumulate. In addition to his adaptor proposal, Crick hypothesized, on the basis of genetic evidence, that the code would be *commaless*—that is, he believed no internal punctuation would occur along the reading frame. Crick also speculated that only 20 of the 64 possible codons would specify an amino acid and that the remaining 44 would carry no coding assignment.

Was Crick wrong with respect to the 44 "blank" codes? Or is the code degenerate, meaning that more than one codon specifies the same amino acid? Crick's frameshift studies (discussed earlier in this chapter) suggested that, in fact, contrary to his earlier proposal, the code is degenerate. For the cases in which wild-type function is restored—that is, (+) with (−); (++) with (−−); and (+++) with (−−−)—the original frame of reading is also restored. However, in between the insertion and deletion, there may be numerous codons that would still be out of frame. If 44 of the 64 possible codons were blank, referred to as **nonsense codons**, and did not specify an amino acid, at least one blank codon

would very likely occur in the string of nucleotides still out of frame. If such a nonsense codon was encountered during protein synthesis, the process would probably stop or be terminated at that point. If so, the product of the *rII* locus would not be made, and restoration would not occur. Because the various mutant combinations were able to reproduce on *E. coli* K12, Crick and his colleagues concluded that, in all likelihood, most, if not all, of the remaining 44 triplets were not blank. It followed that the genetic code was degenerate. As we shall see, this reasoning proved to be correct.

13.3 Studies by Nirenberg, Matthaei, and Others Led to Deciphering of the Code

In 1961, Marshall Nirenberg and J. Heinrich Matthaei became the first to characterize specific coding sequences, laying a cornerstone for the complete analysis of the genetic code. Their success, as well as that of others who made important contributions in deciphering the code, was dependent on the use of two experimental tools, an *in vitro* (cell-free in a test tube) *protein-synthesizing system* and the enzyme **polynucleotide phosphorylase**, which allowed the production of synthetic mRNAs. These mRNAs served as templates for polypeptide synthesis in the cell-free system.

Synthesizing Polypeptides in a Cell-Free System

In the cell-free protein-synthesizing system, amino acids are incorporated into polypeptide chains. The process begins with an *in vitro* mixture containing all the essential factors for protein synthesis in the cell: ribosomes, tRNAs, amino acids, and other molecules essential to translation (see Chapter 14). To allow scientists to follow (or trace) the progress of protein synthesis, one or more of the amino acids must be radioactive. Finally, an mRNA must be added, to serve as the template to be translated.

In 1961, mRNA had yet to be isolated. However, use of the enzyme polynucleotide phosphorylase allowed the artificial synthesis of RNA templates, which could be added to the cell-free system. This enzyme, isolated from bacteria, catalyzes the reaction shown in **Figure 13–3**. Discovered in 1955 by Marianne Grunberg-Manago and Severo Ochoa, the enzyme functions metabolically in bacterial cells to degrade RNA. However, *in vitro*, in the presence of high concentrations of ribonucleoside diphosphates, the reaction can be "forced" in the opposite direction, to synthesize RNA, as illustrated in the figure.

FIGURE 13–3 The reaction catalyzed by the enzyme polynucleotide phosphorylase. Note that the equilibrium of the reaction favors the degradation of RNA but that the reaction can be "forced" in the direction favoring synthesis.

In contrast to RNA polymerase (which constructs mRNA *in vivo*), polynucleotide phosphorylase does not require a DNA template. As a result, the order in which ribonucleotides are added is random, depending on the relative concentration of the four ribonucleoside diphosphates present in the reaction mixture. The probability of the insertion of a specific ribonucleotide is proportional to the availability of that molecule relative to other available ribonucleotides. *This point is absolutely critical to understanding the work of Nirenberg and others in the ensuing discussion.*

Together, the cell-free system for protein synthesis and the availability of synthetic mRNAs provided a means of deciphering the ribonucleotide composition of various codons encoding specific amino acids.

Homopolymer Codes

For their initial experiments, Nirenberg and Matthaei synthesized **RNA homopolymers**, RNA molecules containing only one type of ribonucleotide, and used them for synthesizing polypeptides *in vitro*. In other words, the mRNA they used in their cell-free protein-synthesizing system was either UUUUUU . . . , AAAAAA . . . , CCCCCC . . . , or GGGGGG. . . . They tested each of these types of mRNA to see which, if any, amino acids were consequently incorporated into newly synthesized proteins. The method they used was to conduct many experimental syntheses with each homopolymer. They always made all 20 amino acids available, but for each experiment they attached a radioactive label to a different amino acid and thus could tell when that amino acid had been incorporated into the resulting polypeptide.

For example, in experiments using ^{14}C-phenylalanine (**Table 13.1**), Nirenberg and Matthaei concluded that the RNA homopolymer UUUUU . . . (polyuridylic acid) directed the incorporation of only phenylalanine into the peptide homopolymer polyphenylalanine. Assuming the validity of a triplet code, they made the first specific codon assignment: UUU codes for phenylalanine. Using similar experiments, they quickly found that AAA codes for

TABLE 13.1 Incorporation of ^{14}C-Phenylalanine into Protein

Artificial mRNA	Radioactivity (counts/min)
None	44
Poly U	39,800
Poly A	50
Poly C	38

Source: After Nirenberg and Matthaei (1961).

lysine and CCC codes for proline. Poly G was not a functional template, probably because the molecule folds back on itself. Thus, the assignment for GGG had to await other approaches.

Note that the specific triplet codon assignments were possible only because homopolymers were used. In this method, only the general nucleotide composition of the template is known, not the specific order of the nucleotides in each triplet, but since three identical letters can have only one possible sequence (e.g., UUU), three of the actual codons for phenylalanine, lysine, and proline could be identified.

Mixed Copolymers

With the initial success of these techniques, Nirenberg and Matthaei, and Ochoa and coworkers turned to the use of **RNA heteropolymers**. In their next experiments, two or more different ribonucleoside diphosphates were used in combination to form the artificial message. The researchers reasoned that if they knew the relative proportion of each type of ribonucleoside diphosphate in their synthetic mRNA, they could predict the frequency of each of the possible triplet codons it contained. If they then added the mRNA to the cell-free system and ascertained the percentage of each amino acid present in the resulting polypeptide, they could analyze the results and predict the *composition* of the triplets that had specified those particular amino acids.

This approach is illustrated in **Figure 13–4**. Suppose that only A and C are used for synthesizing the mRNA, in

Possible compositions	Possible triplets	Probability of occurrence of any triplet	Final %
3A	AAA	$(1/6)^3 = 1/216 = 0.4\%$	0.4
1C:2A	AAC ACA CAA	$(1/6)^2(5/6) = 5/216 = 2.3\%$	$3 \times 2.3 = 6.9$
2C:1A	ACC CAC CCA	$(1/6)(5/6)^2 = 25/216 = 11.6\%$	$3 \times 11.6 = 34.8$
3C	CCC	$(5/6)^3 = 125/216 = 57.9\%$	57.9
			100.0

FIGURE 13–4 Results and interpretation of a mixed copolymer experiment in which a ratio of 1A:5C is used (1/6A:5/6C).

Chemical synthesis of message ↓

————————————————————————————————— RNA

C C C C C C C C A C C C C C C A A C C A C C C C C A C C C C C A C C C A A

Translation of message ↓

Percentage of amino acids in protein		Probable base-composition assignments
Lysine	<1	AAA
Glutamine	2	1C:2A
Asparagine	2	1C:2A
Threonine	12	2C:1A
Histidine	14	2C:1A, 1C:2A
Proline	69	CCC, 2C:1A

a ratio of 1A:5C. The insertion of a ribonucleotide at any position along the RNA molecule during its synthesis is determined by the ratio of A:C. Therefore, there is a 1/6 possibility for an A and a 5/6 chance for a C to occupy each position. On this basis, we can calculate the frequency of any given triplet appearing in the message.

For AAA, the frequency is $(1/6)^3$ or about 0.4 percent. For AAC, ACA, and CAA, the frequencies are identical—that is, $(1/6)^2(5/6)$ or about 2.3 percent for each triplet. Together, all three 2A:1C triplets account for 6.9 percent of the total three-letter sequences. In the same way, each of three 1A:2C triplets accounts for $(1/6)(5/6)^2$ or 11.6 percent (or a total of 34.8 percent); CCC is represented by $(5/6)^3$, or 57.9 percent of the triplets.

By examining the percentages of the different amino acids incorporated into the polypeptide synthesized under the direction of this message, we can propose probable base compositions for each of those amino acids (Figure 13–4). Because proline appears 69 percent of the time, we could propose that proline is encoded by CCC (57.9 percent) and also by one of the codons consisting of 2C:1A (11.6 percent). Histidine, at 14 percent, is probably coded by one 2C:1A codon (11.6 percent) and one 1C:2A codon (2.3 percent). Threonine, at 12 percent, is likely coded by only one

2C:1A codon. Asparagine and glutamine each appear to be coded by one of the 1C:2A codons, and lysine appears to be coded by AAA.

Using as many as all four ribonucleotides to construct the mRNA, the researchers conducted many similar experiments. Although the determination by this means of the *composition* of triplet code words corresponding to all 20 amino acids represented a very significant breakthrough, the *specific sequences* of triplets were still unknown—other approaches were still needed.

The Triplet-Binding Assay

It was not long before more advanced techniques for discovering codons were developed. In 1964, Nirenberg and Philip Leder developed the **triplet-binding assay**, leading to specific assignments of triplet codons. This technique took advantage of the observation that ribosomes, when presented *in vitro* with an RNA sequence as short as three ribonucleotides, will bind to it and form a complex similar to what is found *in vivo*. The triplet RNA sequence acts like a codon in mRNA, attracting a tRNA molecule containing a complementary sequence (**Figure 13–5**). Such a triplet sequence in tRNA, that is, complementary to a codon of mRNA, is known as an **anticodon**.

FIGURE 13–5 The behavior of the components during the triplet-binding assay. When the synthetic UUU triplet is positioned in the ribosome, it acts as a codon, attracting the complementary AAA anticodon of the charged tRNA^phe.

NOW SOLVE THIS

13–1 In a mixed copolymer experiment using polynucleotide phosphorylase, 3/4G:1/4C was used to form the synthetic message. The amino acid composition of the resulting protein was determined to be:

Glycine	36/64	(56 percent)
Alanine	12/64	(19 percent)
Arginine	12/64	(19 percent)
Proline	4/64	(6 percent)

From this information,

(a) indicate the percentage (or fraction) of the time each possible codon will occur in the message.
(b) determine one consistent base-composition assignment for the amino acids present.
(c) in view of the wobble hypothesis, predict as many specific codon assignments as possible.

■ **HINT:** *This problem asks you to analyze a mixed copolymer experiment and to predict codon composition assignments for the amino acids encoded by the synthetic message. The key to its solution is to first calculate the proportion of each triplet codon in the synthetic RNA and then match these to the proportions of amino acids that are synthesized.*

Although it was not yet feasible to chemically synthesize long stretches of RNA, specific triplet sequences could be synthesized in the laboratory to serve as templates. All that was needed was a method to determine which tRNA–amino acid was bound to the triplet RNA–ribosome complex. The test system Nirenberg and Leder devised was quite simple. The amino acid to be tested was made radioactive and combined with its cognate tRNA, creating a "charged" tRNA. Because codon compositions (though not exact sequences) were known, it was possible to narrow the

decision as to which amino acids should be tested for each specific triplet.

The radioactively charged tRNA, the RNA triplet, and ribosomes were incubated together on a nitrocellulose filter, which retains ribosomes (because of their larger size) but not the other, smaller components, such as charged tRNA. If radioactivity is not retained on the filter, an incorrect amino acid has been tested. If radioactivity remains on the filter, it does so because the charged tRNA has bound to the RNA triplet associated with the ribosome, which itself remains on the filter. In such a case, a specific codon assignment can be made.

Work proceeded in several laboratories, and in many cases clear-cut, unambiguous results were obtained. For example, Table 13.2 shows 26 triplet codons assigned to ten different amino acids. However, in some cases the triplet binding was inefficient, and assignments were not possible. Eventually, about 50 of the 64 triplets were assigned. These specific assignments led to two major conclusions. First, the genetic code is degenerate—that is, one amino

TABLE 13.2 Amino Acid Assignments to Specific Trinucleotides Derived from the Triplet-Binding Assay

Trinucleotides	Amino Acid
AAA AAG	Lysine
AUG	Methionine
AUU AUC AUA	Isoleucine
CCU CCC CCG CCA	Proline
CUC CUA CUG CUU	Leucine
GAA GAG	Glutamic acid
UCU UCC UCA UCG	Serine
UGU UGC	Cysteine
UUA UUG	Leucine
UUU UUC	Phenylalanine

acid may be specified by more than one triplet. Second, the code is also *unambiguous*—that is, a single codon specifies only one amino acid. As we will see later in this chapter, these conclusions have been upheld with only minor exceptions. The triplet-binding technique was a major innovation in the effort to decipher the genetic code.

Repeating Copolymers

Yet another innovative technique for deciphering the genetic code was developed in the early 1960s by Har Gobind Khorana, who was able to chemically synthesize long RNA molecules consisting of short sequences repeated many times. First, he created the individual short sequences (e.g., di-, tri-, and tetranucleotides); then he replicated them many times and finally joined them enzymatically to form the long polynucleotides. In **Figure 13–6**, a dinucleotide made in this way is converted to an mRNA with two repeating triplet codons. A trinucleotide is converted into an mRNA that can be read as containing one of three potential repeating triplets, depending on the point at which initiation occurs. Finally, a tetranucleotide creates a message with four repeating triplet sequences.

When these synthetic mRNAs were added to a cell-free system, the predicted proportions of amino acids were found to be incorporated in the resulting polypeptides. When these data were combined with data drawn from mixed copolymer and triplet binding experiments, specific assignments were possible.

One example of specific assignments made in this way will illustrate the value of Khorana's approach. Consider the following experiments in concert with one another: (1) The repeating *trinucleotide sequence* UUCUUCUUC . . . can be read as three possible repeating triplets—UUC, UCU, and CUU—depending on the initiation point. When placed in a cell-free translation system, three different polypeptide homopolymers—containing phenylalanine (phe), serine (ser), or leucine (leu)—are produced. Thus, we know that each of the three triplets encodes one of the three amino acids, but we do not know which codes which. (2) On the other hand, the *repeating dinucleotide sequence* UCUCUCUC . . . produces the triplets UCU and CUC and, when used in an experiment, leads to the incorporation of leucine and serine into a polypeptide. Thus, the triplets UCU and CUC specify leucine and serine, but we still do not know which triplet specifies which amino acid. However, when considering both sets of results in concert, we can conclude that UCU, which is common to both experiments, must encode either leucine or serine but not phenylalanine. Thus, either CUU *or* UUC encodes leucine *or* serine, while the other encodes phenylalanine. (3) To derive more specific information, we can examine the results of using the repeating tetranucleotide sequence UUAC, which produces the triplets UUA, UAC, ACU, and CUU. The CUU triplet is one of the two in which we are interested. Three amino acids are incorporated by this experiment: leucine, threonine, and tyrosine. Because CUU must specify only serine or leucine, and because, of these two, only leucine appears in the resulting polypeptide, we may conclude that CUU specifies leucine. Once this assignment is established, we can logically determine all others. Of the two triplet pairs remaining (UUC and UCU from the first experiment *and* UCU and CUC from the second experiment), whichever triplet is common to both must encode

Repeating sequence	Polynucleotides	Repeating triplets
Dinucleotide UG	5′ U G U G U G U G U G U G U 3′ — **Initiation**	UGU and GUG
Trinucleotide UUG	5′ U U G U U G U U G U U G U U G U 3′ — **Initiation**	UUG or UGU or GUU
Tetranucleotide UAUC	5′ U A U C U A U C U A U C U A U C U 3′ — **Initiation**	UAU and CUA and UCU and AUC

FIGURE 13–6 The conversion of di-, tri-, and tetranucleotides into repeating copolymers. The triplet codons produced in each case are shown.

TABLE 13.3 Amino Acids Incorporated Using Repeated Synthetic Copolymers of RNA

Repeating Copolymer	Codons Produced	Amino Acids in Resulting Polypeptides
UG	UGU	Cysteine
	GUG	Valine
AC	ACA	Threonine
	CAC	Histidine
UUC	UUC	Phenylalanine
	UCU	Serine
	CUU	Leucine
AUC	AUC	Isoleucine
	UCA	Serine
	CAU	Histidine
UAUC	UAU	Tyrosine
	CUA	Leucine
	UCU	Serine
	AUC	Isoleucine
GAUA	GAU	None
	AGA	None
	UAG	None
	AUA	None

serine. This is UCU. By elimination, UUC is determined to encode phenylalanine and CUC is determined to encode leucine. Thus, through painstaking logical analysis, four specific triplets encoding three different amino acids have been assigned from these experiments.

From these interpretations, Khorana reaffirmed the identity of triplets that had already been deciphered and filled in gaps left from other approaches. A number of examples are shown in Table 13.3. For example, the use of two

NOW SOLVE THIS

13–2 When repeating copolymers are used to form synthetic mRNAs, dinucleotides produce a single type of polypeptide that contains only two different amino acids. On the other hand, using a trinucleotide sequence produces three different polypeptides, each consisting of only a single amino acid. Why? What will be produced when a repeating tetranucleotide is used?

■ **HINT:** *This problem asks you to consider different outcomes of repeating copolymer experiments. The key to its solution is to be aware that when using a repeating copolymer of RNA, translation can be initiated at different ribonucleotides. You must simply determine the number of triplet codons produced by initiation at each of the different ribonucleotides.*

For more practice, see Problems 4, 5, and 6.

tetranucleotide sequences, GAUA and GUAA, suggested that at least two triplets were *termination codons*. Khorana reached this conclusion because neither of these repeating sequences directed the incorporation of more than a few amino acids into a polypeptide, too few to detect. There are no triplets common to both messages, and both seemed to contain at least one triplet that terminates protein synthesis. Of the possible triplets in the poly-(GAUA) sequence, shown in Table 13.3, UAG was later shown to be a termination codon.

13.4 The Coding Dictionary Reveals Several Interesting Patterns among the 64 Codons

The various techniques applied to decipher the genetic code have yielded a dictionary of 61 triplet codons assigned to amino acids. The remaining three codons are termination signals, not specifying any amino acid.

Degeneracy and the Wobble Hypothesis

A general pattern of triplet codon assignments becomes apparent when we look at the genetic coding dictionary. **Figure 13–7** displays the assignments in a particularly revealing form first suggested by Francis Crick.

Second position

	U	C	A	G	
U	UUU / UUC *phe* UUA / UUG	UCU / UCC / UCA / UCG *ser*	UAU / UAC *tyr* UAA *Stop* / UAG *Stop*	UGU / UGC *cys* UGA *Stop* / UGG *trp*	U C A G
C	CUU / CUC / CUA / CUG *leu*	CCU / CCC / CCA / CCG *pro*	CAU / CAC *his* CAA / CAG *gln*	CGU / CGC / CGA / CGG *arg*	U C A G
A	AUU / AUC *ile* AUA AUG *met*	ACU / ACC / ACA / ACG *thr*	AAU / AAC *asn* AAA / AAG *lys*	AGU / AGC *ser* AGA / AGG *arg*	U C A G
G	GUU / GUC / GUA / GUG *val*	GCU / GCC / GCA / GCG *ala*	GAU / GAC *asp* GAA / GAG *glu*	GGU / GGC / GGA / GGG *gly*	U C A G

First position (5′-end) — *Third position (3′-end)*

▢ Initiation ▢ Termination

FIGURE 13–7 The coding dictionary. AUG encodes methionine, which initiates most polypeptide chains. All other amino acids except tryptophan, which is encoded only by UGG, are represented by two to six triplets. The triplets UAA, UAG, and UGA are termination signals and do not encode any amino acids.

Most evident is that the code is degenerate, as the early researchers predicted. That is, almost all amino acids are specified by two, three, or four different codons. Three amino acids (serine, arginine, and leucine) are each encoded by six different codons. Only tryptophan and methionine are encoded by single codons.

Also evident is the *pattern* of degeneracy. Most often sets of codons specifying the same amino acid are grouped, such that the first two letters are the same, with only the third differing. For example, as you can see in Figure 13–7, the codons for phenylalanine (UUU and UUC in the top left corner of the coding table) differ only by their third letter. Either U or C in the third position specifies phenylalanine. Four codons specify valine (GUU, GUC, GUA, and GUG, in the bottom left corner), and they differ only by their third letter. In this case, all four letters in the third position specify valine.

Crick observed this pattern in the degeneracy throughout the code, and in 1966, he postulated the **wobble hypothesis**. Crick's hypothesis predicted that the initial two ribonucleotides of triplet codes are often more critical than the third member in attracting the correct tRNA. He postulated that hydrogen bonding at the third position of the codon–anticodon interaction would be *less* spatially constrained and need not adhere as strictly to the established base-pairing rules. The wobble hypothesis proposes a more flexible set of base-pairing rules at the third position of the codon (Table 13.4).

This relaxed base-pairing requirement, or "wobble," allows the anticodon of a single form of tRNA to pair with more than one triplet in mRNA. Consistent with the wobble hypothesis and the degeneracy of the code, U at the first position (the 5′ end) of the tRNA anticodon may pair with A or G at the third position (the 3′ end) of the mRNA codon, and G may likewise pair with U or C. Inosine (I), one of the modified bases found in tRNA (described in Chapter 15), may pair with C, U, or A. As a result of these wobble rules, only about 30 different tRNA species are necessary to accommodate the 61 codons specifying an amino acid. If nothing else, wobble can be considered an economy measure, assuming that the fidelity of translation is not compromised. Current estimates are that 30 to 40 tRNA species are present in bacteria and up to 50 tRNA species in animal and plant cells.

The Ordered Nature of the Code

Still another observation has been made concerning the pattern of codon sequences and their corresponding amino acids, leading to the description referred to as the **ordered genetic code**. By this is meant that *chemically similar amino acids* often share one or two "middle" bases in the different triplets encoding them. For example, either U or C is often present in the second position of triplets that specify hydrophobic amino acids, including valine and alanine, among others. Two codons (AAA and AAG) specify the positively charged amino acid lysine. If only the middle letter of these codons is changed from A to G (AGA and AGG), the positively charged amino acid arginine is specified. Hydrophilic amino acids, such as serine or threonine are specified by triplet codons with G or C in the second position.

The chemical properties of amino acids will be discussed in more detail later in the text (see Chapter 14). The end result of an "ordered" code is that it buffers the potential effect of mutation on protein function. While many mutations of the second base of triplet codons result in a change of one amino acid to another, the change is often to an amino acid with similar chemical properties. In such cases, protein function may not be noticeably altered.

Initiation, Termination, and Suppression

In contrast to the *in vitro* experiments discussed earlier, initiation of protein synthesis *in vivo* is a highly specific process. In bacteria, the initial amino acid inserted into all polypeptide chains is a modified form of methionine— *N*-formylmethionine (fmet). Only one codon, AUG, codes for methionine, and it is sometimes called the **initiator codon**. However, when AUG appears internally in mRNA, rather than at an initiating position, unformylated methionine is inserted into the polypeptide chain. Rarely, another codon, GUG, specifies methionine during initiation, though it is not clear why this happens, since GUG normally encodes valine.

In bacteria, either the formyl group is removed from the initial methionine upon completion of synthesis of a protein, or the entire formylmethionine residue is removed. In eukaryotes, unformylated methionine is the initial amino acid of polypeptide synthesis. As in bacteria, this initial methionine residue may be cleared from the polypeptide.

As mentioned in the preceding section, three other codons (UAG, UAA, and UGA) serve as **termination codons**, punctuation signals that do not code for any

TABLE 13.4 Anticodon–Codon Base-Pairing Rules	
Base at First Position (5′ End) of tRNA	**Base at Third Position (3′ End) of mRNA**
A	U
C	G
G	C or U
U	A or G
I	A, U, or C

amino acid.* They are not recognized by a tRNA molecule, and translation terminates when they are encountered. Mutations that produce any of the three codons internally in a gene also result in termination. In that case, only a partial polypeptide is synthesized, since it is prematurely released from the ribosome. When such a change occurs in the DNA, it is called a **nonsense mutation**.

13.5 The Genetic Code Has Been Confirmed in Studies of Phage MS2

The various aspects of the genetic code discussed so far yield a fairly complete picture. The code is triplet in nature, degenerate, unambiguous, and commaless, although it contains punctuation in the form of start and stop signals. These individual principles have been confirmed by the detailed analysis of the RNA-containing bacteriophage MS2 by Walter Fiers and his coworkers.

MS2 is a bacteriophage that infects *E. coli*. Its nucleic acid (RNA) contains only about 3500 ribonucleotides, making up only three genes. These genes specify a coat protein, an RNA-directed replicase, and a maturation protein (the A protein). This simple system of a small genome and few gene products allowed Fiers and his colleagues to sequence the genes and their products. The amino acid sequence of the coat protein was completed in 1970, and the nucleotide sequence of the gene encoding the protein was reported in 1972.

When the chemical constitutions of this gene and its encoded protein are compared, they are found to exhibit **colinearity** with one another. That is, the linear sequence of triplet codons formed by the nucleotides corresponds precisely with the linear sequence of amino acids in the protein. Furthermore, the codon for the first amino acid is AUG, the common initiator codon; the codon for the last amino acid is followed by two consecutive termination codons, UAA and UAG. We will return to discuss this concept later in the text (see Chapter 14).

By 1976, the other two genes of MS2 and their protein products were sequenced. The analysis clearly showed that the genetic code in this virus was identical to that established in bacterial systems. Other evidence suggests that the code is also identical in eukaryotes, thus providing confirmation of what seemed to be a universal code.

*Historically, the terms *amber* (UAG), *ochre* (UAA), and *opal* (UGA) were used to distinguish mutations producing any of the three termination codons.

13.6 The Genetic Code Is Nearly Universal

Between 1960 and 1978, it was generally assumed that the genetic code would be found to be universal, applying equally to viruses, bacteria, archaea, and eukaryotes. Certainly, the nature of mRNA and the translation machinery seemed to be very similar in these organisms. For example, cell-free systems derived from bacteria could translate eukaryotic mRNAs. Poly U stimulates synthesis of polyphenylalanine in cell-free systems when the components are derived from eukaryotes. Many recent studies involving recombinant DNA technology (Chapter 20) reveal that eukaryotic genes can be inserted into bacterial cells, which are then transcribed and translated. Within eukaryotes, mRNAs from mice and rabbits have been injected into amphibian eggs and efficiently translated. For the many eukaryotic genes that have been sequenced, notably those for hemoglobin molecules, the amino acid sequence of the encoded proteins adheres to the coding dictionary established from bacterial studies.

However, several 1979 reports on the coding properties of DNA derived from mitochondria (mtDNA) of yeast and humans undermined the hypothesis of the universality of the genetic language. Since then, mtDNA has been examined in many other organisms.

Cloned mtDNA fragments were sequenced and compared with the amino acid sequences of various mitochondrial proteins, revealing several exceptions to the coding dictionary (Table 13.5). Most surprising was that the codon UGA, normally specifying termination, specifies the insertion of tryptophan during translation in yeast and human mitochondria. In human mitochondria, AUA, which normally specifies isoleucine, directs the internal insertion of methionine. In yeast mitochondria, threonine is inserted instead of leucine when CUA is encountered in mRNA.

TABLE 13.5	Exceptions to the Universal Code		
Codon	Normal Code Word	Altered Code Word	Source
UGA	Termination	Trp	Human and yeast mitochondria; *Mycoplasma*
CUA	Leu	Thr	Yeast mitochondria
AUA	Ile	Met	Human mitochondria
AGA	Arg	Termination	Human mitochondria
AGG	Arg	Termination	Human mitochondria
UAA	Termination	Gln	*Paramecium, Tetrahymena, and Stylonychia*
UAG	Termination	Gln	*Paramecium*

In 1985, several other exceptions to the standard coding dictionary were discovered in the bacterium *Mycoplasma capricolum,* and in the nuclear genes of the protozoan ciliates *Paramecium, Tetrahymena,* and *Stylonychia.* For example, as shown in Table 13.5, one alteration converts the termination codon (UGA) to tryptophan. Several other code alterations convert a termination codon to glutamine. These changes are significant because they are seen in both a prokaryote and several eukaryotes, that is, in distinct species that have evolved separately over a long period of time.

Note the pattern apparent in several of the altered codon assignments: the change in coding capacity involves only a shift in recognition of the third, or wobble, position. For example, AUA specifies isoleucine in the cytoplasm and methionine in the mitochondrion, but in the cytoplasm, methionine is specified by AUG. In a similar example, UGA calls for termination in the cytoplasm, but for tryptophan in the mitochondrion; in the cytoplasm, tryptophan is specified by UGG. It has been suggested that such changes in codon recognition may represent an evolutionary trend toward reducing the number of tRNAs needed in mitochondria; only 22 tRNA species are encoded in human mitochondria, for example. However, until other cases are discovered, the differences must be considered to be exceptions to the previously established general coding rules.

13.7 Different Initiation Points Create Overlapping Genes

Earlier we stated that the genetic code is nonoverlapping, meaning that each ribonucleotide in the code *for a given polypeptide* is part of only one codon. However, this characteristic of the code does not rule out the possibility that a single mRNA may have multiple initiation points for translation. If so, these points could theoretically create several different reading frames within the same mRNA, thus specifying more than one polypeptide. This concept of **overlapping genes** is illustrated in **Figure 13–8(a)**. Note that gene is also referred to as an **ORF**, or **open reading frame**, which is defined as a DNA sequence that produces an RNA that has a start and stop codon, between which is a series of triplet codons specifying the amino acids making up a polypeptide. Thus, we sometimes also refer to *overlapping ORFs.*

That this might actually occur in some viruses was suspected when phage ϕX174

was carefully investigated. The circular DNA chromosome consists of 5386 nucleotides, which should encode a maximum of 1795 amino acids, sufficient for five or six proteins. However, this small virus in fact synthesizes nine proteins consisting of more than 2300 amino acids. A comparison of the nucleotide sequence of the DNA and the amino acid sequences of the polypeptides synthesized has clarified the apparent paradox. At least four instances of multiple initiation have been discovered, creating overlapping genes [**Figure 13–8(b)**].

The sequences specifying the K and B polypeptides are initiated in separate reading frames within the sequence specifying the A polypeptide. The *K* gene sequence overlaps into the adjacent sequence specifying the C polypeptide. The E sequence is out of frame with, but initiated within, that of the D polypeptide. Finally, the A′ sequence, while in frame with the A sequence, is initiated in the middle of the A sequence. They both terminate at the identical point. In all, seven different polypeptides are created from a DNA sequence that might otherwise have specified only three (A, C, and D).

A similar situation has been observed in other viruses and bacteria. The employment of overlapping reading frames optimizes the limited amount of DNA present. However, such an approach to storing information has a distinct disadvantage in that a single mutation may affect more than one protein and thus increase the chances that the change will be deleterious or lethal. In the case we just discussed [Figure 13–8(b)], a single mutation in the middle of the *B* gene could potentially affect three other proteins (the A, A′, and K proteins). It may be for this reason that, while present, overlapping genes are not the rule in other organisms.

More recently, genomic analysis has made it possible to examine extensive DNA sequence information in eukaryotes,

(a)

(b)

FIGURE 13–8 Illustration of the concept of overlapping genes. (a) Translation initiated at two different AUG positions out of frame with one another will give rise to two distinct amino acid sequences. (b) The relative positions of the sequences encoding seven polypeptides of the phage ϕX174.

revealing that the concept of overlapping genes also applies to these organisms, including mammals. For example, in one study of mouse and human DNA, over 1200 such cases were revealed. In the humans, head to tail and head to head overlap was observed as well as cases where one gene is fully embedded in the sequence of another larger gene. In the case of three human genes, *MUTYH*, *TOE1*, and *TESK2*, *TOE1* contains overlapping coding regions with *MUTYH* at the 5′ end and with *TESK2* at the 3′ end.

13.8 Transcription Synthesizes RNA on a DNA Template

Even while the genetic code was being studied, it was quite clear that proteins were the end products of many genes. Hence, while some geneticists were attempting to elucidate the code, other research efforts were directed toward the nature of genetic expression. The central question was how DNA, a nucleic acid, is able to specify a protein composed of amino acids.

The complex, multistep process begins with the transfer of genetic information stored in DNA to RNA. The process by which RNA molecules are synthesized on a DNA template is called **transcription**. It results in an mRNA molecule complementary to the gene sequence of one of the two strands of the double helix. Each triplet codon in the mRNA is, in turn, complementary to the anticodon region of its corresponding tRNA, which inserts the correct amino acid into the polypeptide chain during translation. The significance of transcription is enormous, for it is the initial step in the process of *information flow* within the cell. The idea that RNA is involved as an intermediate molecule in the process of information flow between DNA and protein is suggested by the following observations:

1. DNA is, for the most part, associated with chromosomes in the nucleus of the eukaryotic cell. However, protein synthesis occurs in association with ribosomes located outside the nucleus, in the cytoplasm. Therefore, DNA does not appear to participate directly in protein synthesis.

2. RNA is synthesized in the nucleus of eukaryotic cells, in which DNA is found, and is chemically similar to DNA.

3. Following its synthesis, most RNA migrates to the cytoplasm, in which protein synthesis (translation) occurs.

4. The amount of RNA is generally proportional to the amount of protein in a cell.

Collectively, these observations suggested that genetic information, stored in DNA, is transferred to an RNA intermediate, which directs the synthesis of the proteins. As with most new ideas in molecular genetics, the initial supporting experimental evidence for an RNA intermediate was based on studies of bacteria and bacteriophages.

13.9 Studies with Bacteria and Phages Provided Evidence for the Existence of mRNA

In two papers published in 1956 and 1958, Elliot Volkin and his colleagues reported their analysis of RNA produced immediately after bacteriophage infection of *E. coli*. Using the isotope ^{32}P to follow newly synthesized RNA, they found that its base composition closely resembled that of the phage DNA, but was different from that of bacterial RNA (Table 13.6). This newly synthesized RNA was unstable (short lived); however, its production was shown to precede the synthesis of new phage proteins. Thus, Volkin and his coworkers considered the possibility that synthesis of RNA is a preliminary step in the process of protein synthesis.

Although ribosomes were known to participate in protein synthesis, their role in this process was not clear. As we noted earlier, one possibility was that each ribosome is specific for the protein synthesized in association with it. That is, perhaps genetic information in DNA is transferred to the RNA of a ribosome (rRNA) during the latter's synthesis so that each ribosome is restricted to the production of a particular protein. The alternative hypothesis was that ribosomes are nonspecific "workbenches" for protein synthesis and that specific genetic information rests with a messenger RNA.

TABLE 13.6 Base Compositions (in mole percents) of RNA Produced Immediately Following Infection of *E. coli* by the Bacteriophages T2 and T7 in Contrast to the Composition of RNA of Uninfected *E. coli*

Source	Adenine	Thymine	Uracil	Cytosine	Guanine
Post-infection RNA in T2-infected cells	33	—	32	18	18
T2 DNA	32	32	—	17*	18
Post-infection RNA in T7-infected cells	27	—	28	24	22
T7 DNA	26	26	—	24	22
E. coli RNA	23	—	22	18	17

*5-hydroxymethyl cytosine.
Source: Volkin and Astrachan (1956); Volkin, Astrachan, and Countryman (1958).

In an elegant experiment using the *E. coli*–phage system, the results of which were reported in 1961, Sydney Brenner, François Jacob, and Matthew Meselson clarified this question. They labeled uninfected *E. coli* ribosomes with heavy isotopes and then allowed phage infection to occur in the presence of radioactive RNA precursors. By following these components during translation, the researchers demonstrated that the synthesis of phage proteins (under the direction of newly synthesized RNA) occurred on bacterial ribosomes that were present prior to infection. The ribosomes appeared to be nonspecific, strengthening the case that another type of RNA serves as an intermediary in the process of protein synthesis.

That same year, Sol Spiegelman and his colleagues reached the same conclusion when they isolated ^{32}P-labeled RNA following the infection of bacteria and used it in molecular hybridization studies. They tried hybridizing this RNA to the DNA of both phages and bacteria in separate experiments. The RNA hybridized only with the phage DNA, showing that it was complementary in base sequence to the viral genetic information.

The results of these experiments agree with the concept of a messenger RNA (mRNA) being made on a DNA template and then directing the synthesis of specific proteins in association with ribosomes. This concept was formally proposed by François Jacob and Jacques Monod in 1961 as part of a model for gene regulation in bacteria. Since then, mRNA has been isolated and thoroughly studied. There is no longer any question about its role in genetic processes.

13.10 RNA Polymerase Directs RNA Synthesis

To prove that RNA can be synthesized on a DNA template, it was necessary to demonstrate that there is an enzyme capable of directing this synthesis. By 1959, several investigators, including Samuel Weiss, had independently discovered such a molecule in rat liver. Called **RNA polymerase**, it has the same general substrate requirements as does DNA polymerase, the major exception being that the substrate nucleotides contain the ribose rather than the deoxyribose form of the sugar. Unlike DNA polymerase, no primer is required to initiate synthesis. The overall reaction summarizing the synthesis of RNA on a DNA template can be expressed as

$$n(\text{NTP}) \xrightarrow[\text{enzyme}]{\text{DNA}} (\text{NMP})_n + n(\text{PP}_i)$$

As the equation reveals, nucleoside triphosphates (NTPs) serve as substrates for the enzyme, which catalyzes the polymerization of nucleoside monophosphates (NMPs), or nucleotides, into a polynucleotide chain (NMP)*n*. Nucleotides are linked during synthesis by 5′ to 3′

phosphodiester bonds (see Figure 10–12). The energy created by cleaving the triphosphate precursor into the monophosphate form drives the reaction, and inorganic phosphates (PP$_i$) are produced.

A second equation summarizes the sequential addition of each ribonucleotide as the process of transcription progresses:

$$(\text{NMP})_n + \text{NTP} \xrightarrow[\text{enzyme}]{\text{DNA}} (\text{NMP})_{n+1} + \text{PP}_i$$

As this equation shows, each step of transcription involves the addition of one ribonucleotide (NMP) to the growing polyribonucleotide chain (NMP)$_{n+1}$, using a nucleoside triphosphate (NTP) as the precursor.

RNA polymerase from *E. coli* has been extensively characterized and shown to consist of subunits designated α, β, β', ω, and σ. The active form of the enzyme, the **holoenzyme**, contains the subunits $\alpha_2\beta\beta'\sigma$ and has a molecular weight of almost 500,000 Da. While there is some variation in the subunit composition of other bacteria, it is the β and β' polypeptides that provide the catalytic mechanism and active site for transcription. As we will see, the σ (**sigma**) **factor** [**Figure 13–9(a)**] plays a regulatory function in the initiation of RNA transcription.

While there is but a single form of the enzyme in *E. coli*, there are several different σ factors, creating variations of the polymerase holoenzyme. On the other hand, eukaryotes display three distinct forms of RNA polymerase, each consisting of a greater number of polypeptide subunits than in bacteria. In this section, we will discuss the process of transcription in prokaryotes. We will return to a discussion of eukaryotic transcription later in this chapter.

NOW SOLVE THIS

13–3 The following represent deoxyribonucleotide sequences in the template strand of DNA:

Sequence 1:	5′-CTTTTTTGCCAT-3′
Sequence 2:	5′-ACATCAATAACT-3′
Sequence 3:	5′-TACAAGGGTTCT-3′

(a) For each strand, determine the mRNA sequence that would be derived from transcription.

(b) Using Figure 13–7, determine the amino acid sequence that is encoded by these mRNAs.

(c) For Sequence 1, what is the sequence of the partner DNA strand?

■ **HINT:** *This problem asks you to consider the outcome of the transfer of complementary information from DNA to RNA and to determine the amino acids encoded by this information. The key to its solution is to remember that in RNA, uracil is complementary to adenine, and that while DNA stores genetic information in the cell, the code that is translated is contained in the RNA complementary to the template strand of DNA making up a gene.*

(a) Transcription components

(b) Template binding and initiation of transcription

(c) Chain elongation

FIGURE 13–9 The early stages of transcription in prokaryotes, showing (a) the components of the process; (b) template binding at the −10 site involving the sigma subunit of RNA polymerase and subsequent initiation of RNA synthesis; and (c) chain elongation, after the σ subunit has dissociated from the transcription complex and the enzyme moves along the DNA template.

Promoters, Template Binding, and the σ Subunit

Transcription results in the synthesis of a single-stranded RNA molecule complementary to a region along only one of the two strands of the DNA double helix. When discussing transcription, we can call the DNA strand that is transcribed the *template strand* and its complement the *partner strand*.

The initial step in prokaryotic gene transcription is referred to as **template binding** [Figure 13–9(b)]. In bacteria, the site of this initial binding is established when the RNA polymerase σ subunit recognizes specific DNA sequences called **promoters**. These sequences are located in the 5′ region, upstream from the point of initial transcription of a gene. It is believed that the enzyme "explores" a length of DNA until it encounters a promoter region and binds there to about 60 nucleotide pairs along the helix, 40 of which are upstream from the point of initial transcription. Once this occurs, the helix is denatured, or unwound, locally, making the template strand of the DNA accessible

to the action of the enzyme. The point at which transcription actually begins is called the **transcription start site**.

Because the interaction of promoters with RNA polymerase governs the efficiency of transcription—by regulating the initiation of transcription—the importance of promoter sequences cannot be overemphasized. The nature of the binding between promoter and polymerase is at the heart of future discussions concerning genetic regulation, the subject of later chapters in the text (see Chapters 16 and 17). While those chapters present more detailed information concerning promoter–enzyme interactions, we must address three points here.

The first point is the concept of **consensus sequences** of DNA, sequences that are similar (homologous) in different genes of the same organism or in one or more genes of related organisms. Their conservation during evolution attests to the critical nature of their role in biological processes. Two consensus sequences have been found in bacterial promoters. One, TATAAT, is located 10 nucleotides upstream from the site of initial transcription (the −10 region, or **Pribnow box**). The other, TTGACA, is located 35 nucleotides upstream (the −35 region). Mutations in either region diminish transcription, often severely.

Sequences such as these, in regions adjacent to the gene itself, are said to be **cis-acting elements**. The term *cis*, drawn from organic chemistry nomenclature, means "next to" or on the same side as other functional groups, in contrast to being *trans* to or "across from" them. In molecular genetics, then, *cis*-elements are those that are located on the same DNA molecule. In contrast, **trans-acting factors** are molecules that bind to these DNA elements.

The second point is that the degree of RNA polymerase binding to different promoters varies greatly, causing variable gene expression. Currently, this is attributed to sequence variation in the promoters. In bacteria, both strong promoters and weak promoters have been discovered, causing a variation in time of initiation from once every 1 to 2 seconds to as little as once every 10 to 20 minutes. Mutations in promoter sequences may severely reduce the initiation of gene expression.

A final general point to be made involves the σ subunit in bacteria. The major form is designated σ^{70} based on its molecular weight of 70 kilodaltons (kDa). The promoters of most bacterial genes recognize this form; however, several alternative forms of RNA polymerase in *E. coli* have unique σ subunits associated with them (e.g., σ^{32}, σ^{54}, σ^{S}, and σ^{E}). Each form recognizes different promoter sequences, which in turn provides specificity to the initiation of transcription.

Initiation, Elongation, and Termination of RNA Synthesis

Once RNA polymerase has recognized and bound to the promoter, DNA is converted from its double-stranded form to an open structure, exposing the template strand. The enzyme then proceeds to **initiate** RNA synthesis, whereby the first 5′-ribonucleoside triphosphate, which is complementary to the first nucleotide, is inserted at the start site. As we noted, no primer is required. Subsequent ribonucleotide complements are inserted and linked together by phosphodiester bonds as RNA polymerization proceeds. This process continues in a 5′ to 3′ direction (in terms of the nascent RNA), creating a temporary 8-bp DNA/RNA duplex whose chains run antiparallel to one another [Figure 13–9(b)].

After these ribonucleotides have been added to the growing RNA chain, the σ subunit dissociates from the holoenzyme, and **chain elongation** proceeds under the direction of the core enzyme [**Figure 13–9(c)**]. In *E. coli,* this process proceeds at the rate of about 50 nucleotides/second at 37°C. Like DNA polymerase, RNA polymerase can perform **proofreading** as it adds each nucleotide. It is capable of recognizing a mismatch where a noncomplementary base has been inserted. In such a case, the enzyme backs up and removes the mismatch. It then reverses direction and continues elongation.

The enzyme traverses the entire gene until eventually it encounters a specific nucleotide sequence that acts as a termination signal. Such termination sequences, about 40 base pairs in length, are extremely important in prokaryotes because of the close proximity of the end of one gene to the upstream sequences of the adjacent gene. An interesting aspect of termination in bacteria is that the termination sequence alluded to above is actually transcribed into RNA. The unique sequence of nucleotides in this termination region causes the newly formed transcript to fold back on itself, forming what is called a **hairpin secondary structure,** held together by hydrogen bonds. The hairpin is important to termination. In some cases, the termination of synthesis is also dependent on the **termination factor, rho (ρ).** Rho is a large hexameric protein that physically interacts with the growing RNA transcript, facilitating termination of transcription.

When the transcribed RNA molecule is released from the DNA template, termination is achieved and the core polymerase enzyme dissociates. The synthesized RNA molecule is precisely complementary to the DNA sequence of the template strand of the gene. Wherever an A, T, C, or G residue was encountered there, a corresponding U, A, G, or C residue, respectively, was incorporated into the RNA molecule. These RNA molecules ultimately provide the information leading to the synthesis of all proteins in the cell.

In bacteria, groups of genes whose protein products are involved in the same metabolic pathway are often clustered together along the chromosome. In many such cases, the genes are contiguous, and all but the last gene lack the encoded signals for termination of transcription. The result is that during transcription, a large mRNA is produced, encoding more than one protein. Since genes in bacteriophages are sometimes referred to as *complementation groups* and are called *cistrons* (see Chapter 6), the RNA is called a **polycistronic mRNA**. The products of genes transcribed in this fashion are usually all needed by the cell at the same time, so this is an efficient way to transcribe and subsequently translate the needed genetic information. In eukaryotes, **monocistronic mRNAs** are the rule, although an increasing number of exceptions are being reported.

13.11 Transcription in Eukaryotes Differs from Prokaryotic Transcription in Several Ways

Much of our knowledge of transcription has been derived from studies of prokaryotes. Most of the general aspects of the mechanics of these processes are similar in eukaryotes, but there are several notable differences:

1. Transcription in eukaryotes occurs within the nucleus under the direction of three separate forms of RNA polymerase. Unlike the prokaryotic process, in eukaryotes the RNA transcript is not free to associate with ribosomes prior to the completion of transcription. For the mRNA to be translated, it must move out of the nucleus into the cytoplasm.

2. Initiation of transcription of eukaryotic genes requires the compact chromatin fiber, characterized by nucleosome coiling, to be uncoiled and the DNA to be made accessible to RNA polymerase and other regulatory proteins. This transition, referred to as *chromatin remodeling,* reflects the dynamics involved in the conformational change that occurs as the DNA helix is opened (Chapter 12).

3. Initiation and regulation of transcription entail a more extensive interaction between *cis*-acting DNA sequences and *trans*-acting protein factors involved in stimulating and initiating transcription. Eukaryotic RNA polymerases, for example, rely on *transcription factors (TFs)* to scan and bind to DNA. In addition to promoters, other control units, called *enhancers* and *silencers*, may be located in the 5′ regulatory region upstream from the initiation point, but they have also been found within the gene or even in the 3′ downstream region, beyond the coding sequence.

4. Alteration of the primary RNA transcript to produce mature eukaryotic mRNA involves many complex stages referred to generally as "processing." An initial processing step involves the addition of a 5′ cap and a 3′ tail to most transcripts destined to become mRNAs. The initial (or primary) transcripts are most often much larger than those that are eventually translated into protein. Sometimes called **pre-mRNAs**, these primary transcripts are found only in the nucleus and referred to collectively as **heterogeneous nuclear RNA (hnRNA)**. Only about 25 percent of hnRNA molecules are converted to mRNA. From those that are converted, substantial amounts of the ribonucleotide sequence are excised, and the remaining segments are spliced back together prior to nuclear export and translation. This phenomenon has given rise to the concepts of *split genes* and *splicing* in eukaryotes (discussed in Section 13.12).

In the remainder of this chapter we will look at the basic details of transcription in eukaryotic cells. The process of transcription is highly regulated, determining which DNA sequences are copied into RNA and when and how frequently they are transcribed. We will return to topics directly related to eukaryotic gene regulation later in the text (see Chapter 17).

Initiation of Transcription in Eukaryotes

Eukaryotic RNA polymerase exists in three distinct forms. While the three forms of the enzyme share certain polypeptide subunits, each nevertheless transcribes different types of genes, as indicated in Table 13.7. Each enzyme is larger

and more complex than the single prokaryotic polymerase. For example, in yeast, the holoenzyme consists of two large subunits and 10 smaller subunits.

In regard to the initial template-binding step and promoter regions, most is known about **RNA polymerase II (RNAP II)**, which is responsible for the transcription of a wide range of genes in eukaryotes. The activity of RNAP II is dependent on both *cis*-acting elements surrounding the gene itself and a number of *trans*-acting transcription factors that bind to these DNA elements (we will return to the topic of transcription factors below). At least four *cis*-acting DNA elements regulate the initiation of transcription by RNAP II. The first of these elements, the **core promoter**, determines where RNAP II binds to the DNA and where it begins copying the DNA into RNA. The other three types of regulatory DNA sequences, called **proximal-promoter elements**, **enhancers**, and **silencers**, influence the efficiency or the rate of transcription initiation by RNAP II from the core-promoter element. Recall that in prokaryotes, the DNA sequence recognized by RNA polymerase is also called the promoter. In eukaryotes, however, transcriptional initiation is controlled by regulatory proteins that bind to a larger number of *cis*-acting DNA elements.

In many eukaryotic genes, a *cis*-acting core-promoter element is the **Goldberg–Hogness**, or **TATA**, **box**. Located about 30 nucleotide pairs upstream (−30) from the start point of transcription, TATA boxes share a consensus sequence TATA^A/$_T$AAR, where R indicates any purine nucleotide. The sequence and function of TATA boxes are analogous to those found in the −10 promoter region of prokaryotic genes. However, recall that in prokaryotes, RNA polymerase binds directly to the −10 promoter region. As we will see below, this is not the case in eukaryotes. A wide range of core-promoter and proximal-promoter elements are also found within eukaryotic gene-regulatory regions, and each can have an effect on the efficiency of transcription initiation from the start site. Many of these elements will be discussed in more detail later in the text (see Chapter 17).

Although eukaryotic promoter elements can determine the site and general efficiency of initiation, other elements, known as enhancers and silencers, have more dramatic effects on eukaryotic gene transcription. As their names suggest, enhancers increase transcription levels and silencers decrease them. The locations of these elements can vary from immediately upstream from a promoter to downstream, within, or kilobases away, from a gene. Thus they can modulate transcription from a distance. Enhancers and silencers often act to increase or decrease transcription in response to a cell's requirement for a gene product, or at a particular time during development or place within the organism. Each eukaryotic gene has its own unique arrangement of proximal promoter, enhancer, and silencer elements.

TABLE 13.7 RNA Polymerases in Eukaryotes

Form	Product	Location
I	rRNA	Nucleolus
II*	mRNA, snRNA	Nucleoplasm
III	5S rRNA, tRNA	Nucleoplasm

*RNAP II also synthesizes a variety of other RNAs, (see Special Topic Chapter 2—Emerging Roles of RNA) including miRNA and lncRNA.

Complementing the *cis*-acting regulatory sequences are various *trans*-acting factors that facilitate RNAP II binding and, therefore, the initiation of transcription. These proteins are referred to as **transcription factors**. There are two broad categories of transcription factors: the **general transcription factors** (**GTFs**) that are absolutely required for all RNAP II–mediated transcription, and the **transcriptional activators** and **repressors** that influence the efficiency or the rate of RNAP II transcription initiation. The general transcription factors are essential because RNAP II cannot bind directly to eukaryotic core-promoter sites and initiate transcription without their presence. The general transcription factors involved with human RNAP II binding are well characterized and designated **TFIIA**, **TFIIB**, and so on. One of these, **TFIID**, binds directly to the TATA-box sequence. Once initial binding of TFIID to DNA occurs, the other general transcription factors, along with RNAP II, bind sequentially to TFIID, forming an extensive **pre-initiation complex**.

The specific transcription factors (activators and repressors, above) bind to enhancer and silencer elements and regulate transcription initiation by aiding or preventing the assembly of pre-initiation complexes and the release of RNAP II from pre-initiation into full transcription elongation. They appear to supplant the role of the σ factor seen in the prokaryotic enzyme and are important in eukaryotic gene regulation. We will consider the roles of general and specific transcription factors in eukaryotic gene regulation, as well as the various DNA elements that bind these factors (Chapter 17).

Recent Discoveries Concerning RNA Polymerase Function

It is of great interest to learn how RNA polymerase II is able to achieve transcription along the chromatin fiber. The enzyme is confronted with its substrate DNA that, unlike in bacteria, is wrapped around histone proteins organized into nucleosomes. Recall that these structures have compacted the double-stranded DNA, which is a barrier to transcription (Chapter 12). Thus, the enzyme must open up the molecule and separate (denature) the two strands so that the template strand may pass through its active site during RNA synthesis. The ability to crystallize large nucleic acid–protein structures and perform X-ray diffraction analysis at a resolution below 5 Å has shed light on this issue, particularly the work of Roger Kornberg and colleagues, using RNAP II isolated from yeast. It is useful to note here that achieving a resolution below 2.8 Å allows the visualization of each amino acid of every protein in the complex!

Various discoveries have provided a highly detailed account of the most critical processes of transcription. RNAP II in yeast contains two large subunits and ten smaller ones, forming a huge three-dimensional complex with a molecular

weight of about 500 kDa. Promoter DNA initially positions itself over a cleft formed between the two large subunits of RNAP II. The subunit assemblage in fact resembles a pair of jaws that can open and partially close and at this stage is combined with TFIIB. Prior to association with DNA, the cleft is open; once associated with DNA, the cleft partially closes, securing the duplex during the initiation of transcription. The part of the enzyme that is critical for this transition is about 50 kDa in size and is called the *clamp*.

Once secured by the clamp, the strands of a small duplex region of DNA separate at a position within the enzyme referred to as the *active center,* and the template strand is scanned for the transcription start site. Complementary RNA synthesis is then initiated on the DNA template strand. However, the entire complex remains unstable, and transcription usually terminates following the incorporation of only a few ribonucleotides. It is not clear why, but this so-called *abortive transcription* is repeated a number of times before a stable DNA:RNA hybrid containing a transcript of 11 ribonucleotides is formed. Once this occurs, abortive transcription is overcome, a stable complex is achieved, and elongation of the RNA transcript proceeds in earnest. Transcription at this point is said to have achieved a level of highly processive RNA polymerization.

As transcription proceeds, the enzyme moves along the DNA, and at any given time, about 40 base pairs of DNA and 18 residues of the growing RNA chain are part of the enzyme complex. The RNA synthesized earliest runs through a groove in the enzyme and exits under a structure at the top and back designated as the *lid*. Another area, called the *pore*, has been identified at the bottom of the enzyme. It serves as the point through which RNA precursors gain entry into the complex.

Eventually, as transcription proceeds, the portion of the DNA that signals termination is encountered, and the complex once again becomes unstable, much as it was during the earlier state of abortive transcription. The clamp opens, and both DNA and RNA are released from the enzyme as transcription is terminated. This completes the cycle that constitutes transcription. In sum, an unstable complex is formed during the initiation of transcription, stability is established once elongation manages to create a duplex of sufficient size, elongation proceeds, and then instability again characterizes termination of transcription.

Clearly, Kornberg's findings extended our knowledge of transcription considerably. For this work, he was awarded the Nobel Prize in Chemistry in 2006. As you think back on this cycle, try to visualize the process mentally, from the time the DNA first associates with the enzyme until the transcript is released from the large molecular complex. If these images are clear to you, you no doubt have acquired a firm understanding of transcription in eukaryotes, which is more complex than in prokaryotes.

Processing Eukaryotic RNA: Caps and Tails

While in bacteria the base sequence of DNA is transcribed into an mRNA that is immediately and directly translated into the amino acid sequence as dictated by the genetic code, eukaryotic RNA transcripts require significant alteration before they are transported to the cytoplasm and translated. By 1970, evidence accumulated by James Darnell and others showed that eukaryotic mRNA is transcribed initially as a precursor molecule much larger than that which is translated into protein. It was proposed that this *initial transcript* of a gene must be processed in the nucleus before it appears in the cytoplasm as a *mature mRNA* molecule. The various processing steps, discussed in the sections that follow, are summarized in **Figure 13–10**.

An important **posttranscriptional modification** of eukaryotic RNA transcripts destined to become mRNAs occurs at the 5′ end of these molecules, where a **7-methylguanosine (7-mG) cap** is added. This cap, discovered by Aaron Shatkin and James Darnell, is added even before synthesis of the initial transcript is complete and appears to be important to subsequent processing within the nucleus. The cap stabilizes the mRNA by protecting the 5′ end of the molecule from nuclease attack. Subsequently, it is thought to facilitate the transport of mature mRNAs across the nuclear membrane into the cytoplasm and in the initiation of translation of the mRNA into protein. The cap is fairly complex and is distinguished by the unique 5′-5′ bonding that connects it to the initial ribonucleotide of the RNA. Some eukaryotes also acquire a methyl group (CH_3) at the 2′-carbon of the ribose sugars of the first two ribonucleotides of the RNA.

DNA template 3′ P I_1 I_2 I_3 5′
E_1 E_2 E_3

Transcription

Pre-mRNA 5′ L 3′

Cap and tail added

7-mG Poly-A

Processed pre-mRNA

Splicing

Spliced mRNA E_1 E_2 E_3

FIGURE 13–10 Posttranscriptional RNA processing in eukaryotes. Transcription produces a pre-mRNA containing a leader sequence (L), several introns (I), and several exons (E), as identified in the DNA template strand. This is processed by the addition of a 5′ 7-mG cap and a 3′ poly-A tail. The introns are then spliced out and the exons joined to create the mature mRNA. While the above figure depicts these steps sequentially, in some eukaryotic transcripts, splicing actually occurs in introns before transcription is complete and the poly-A tail has been added, leading to the concept of *cotranscriptional splicing*.

Further insights into the processing of RNA transcripts during the maturation of mRNA came from the discovery that both pre-RNAs and mRNAs contain at their 3′ end a stretch of as many as 250 adenylic acid residues. This **poly-A sequence** is added after the 3′ end of the initial transcript is cleaved enzymatically at a position some 10 to 35 ribonucleotides from a highly conserved AAUAAA sequence. Poly A has now been found at the 3′ end of almost all mRNAs studied in a variety of eukaryotic organisms. In fact, poly-A tails have also been detected in some prokaryotic mRNAs. The exceptions in eukaryotes seem to be the RNAs that encode the histone proteins.

While the AAUAAA sequence is not found on all eukaryotic transcripts, it appears to be essential to those that have it. If the sequence is changed as a result of a mutation, those transcripts that would normally have it cannot add the poly-A tail. In the absence of this tail, these RNA transcripts are rapidly degraded. Both the 5′ cap and the 3′ poly-A tail are critical if an mRNA transcript is to be transported to the cytoplasm and translated.

13.12 The Coding Regions of Eukaryotic Genes Are Interrupted by Intervening Sequences Called Introns

An explanation as to the nature of the larger initial RNA transcripts was soon forthcoming in 1977, when Susan Berget, Phillip Sharp, and Richard Roberts presented direct evidence that the genes of animal viruses contain *internal* nucleotide sequences that are not expressed in the amino acid sequence of the proteins they encode. These internal DNA sequences are represented in initial RNA transcripts, but they are removed before the mature mRNA is translated (Figure 13–10). Such nucleotide segments are called **intervening sequences**. DNA sequences that are not represented in the final mRNA product are also called **introns** ("int" for intervening), and those retained and expressed are called **exons** ("ex" for expressed). Splicing involves the removal of the corresponding ribonucleotide sequences representing introns as a result of an excision process and the rejoining of the regions representing exons.

Similar discoveries were soon made in many other eukaryotic genes. Two approaches have been most fruitful for this purpose. The first involves the molecular hybridization of purified, functionally mature mRNAs with DNA containing the genes from which the RNA was originally transcribed. Hybridization between nucleic acids that are not perfectly complementary results in **heteroduplexes**, in which introns present in the DNA but absent in the mRNA loop out and remain unpaired. Such structures

FIGURE 13–12 Intervening sequences in various eukaryotic genes. The numbers indicate the number of nucleotides present in various intron and exon regions.

FIGURE 13–11 An electron micrograph and an interpretive drawing of the hybrid molecule (heteroduplex) formed between the template DNA strand of the chicken ovalbumin gene and the mature ovalbumin mRNA. Seven DNA introns, A–G, produce unpaired loops.

can be visualized with the electron microscope, as shown in **Figure 13–11**. The chicken ovalbumin complex shown in the figure is a heteroduplex with seven loops (A through G), representing seven introns whose sequences are present in the DNA but not in the final mRNA.

The second approach provides more specific information. It involves a direct comparison of nucleotide sequences of DNA with those of mRNA and their correlation with amino acid sequences. Such an approach allows the precise identification of all intervening sequences.

Thus far, most eukaryotic genes have been shown to contain introns (**Figure 13–12**). One of the first so identified was the **β-globin gene** in mice and rabbits, studied independently by Philip Leder and Richard Flavell. The mouse gene contains an intron 550 nucleotides long, beginning immediately after the codon specifying the 104th amino acid. In the rabbit, there is an intron of 580 base pairs near the codon for the 110th amino acid. In addition, another intron of about 120 nucleotides exists earlier in both genes. Similar introns have been found in the β-globin gene in all mammals examined.

The **ovalbumin gene** of chickens has been extensively characterized by Bert O'Malley in the United States and

Pierre Chambon in France. As shown in Figure 13–12, the gene contains seven introns. In fact, the majority of the gene's DNA sequence is composed of introns and is thus "silent." The initial RNA transcript is nearly three times the length of the mature mRNA. Compare the ovalbumin gene in Figures 13–11 and 13–12. Can you match the unpaired loops in Figure 13–11 with the order of introns specified in Figure 13–12?

The list of genes containing intervening sequences is long. In fact, few eukaryotic genes seem to lack introns. An extreme example of the number of introns in a single gene is provided by the gene coding for one of the subunits of collagen, the major connective tissue protein in vertebrates. The *pro-α-2(1) collagen* gene contains 50 introns. The precision of cutting and splicing that occur must be extraordinary if errors are not to be introduced into the mature mRNA. Equally noteworthy is the difference between the size of a typical gene and the size of the final mRNA transcribed from it once introns are removed. As shown in **Table 13.8**, only about 15 percent of the collagen gene consists of exons that finally appear in mRNA. For other proteins, an even more extreme picture emerges. Only about 8 percent of the albumin gene remains to be translated, and in the largest human gene known, dystrophin (which is the protein product absent

TABLE 13.8 Contrasting Human Gene Size, mRNA Size, and Number of Introns

Gene	Gene Size (kb)	mRNA Size (kb)	Number of Introns
Insulin	1.7	0.4	2
Collagen [pro-α-2(1)]	38.0	5.0	51
Albumin	25.0	2.1	14
Phenylalanine hydroxylase	90.0	2.4	12
Dystrophin	2000.0	17.0	79

in Duchenne muscular dystrophy), less than 1 percent of the gene sequence is retained in the mRNA. Two other human genes are also contrasted in Table 13.8.

Although the vast majority of eukaryotic genes examined thus far contain introns, there are several exceptions. Notably, the genes coding for histones and for interferon appear to contain no introns. Intronless mRNAs contain specific sequences in their coding region that supplant the splicing requirement for efficient mRNA export into the cytoplasm.

Splicing Mechanisms: Self-Splicing RNAs

The discovery of introns led to intensive attempts to elucidate the mechanism by which they are excised and exons are spliced back together. A great deal of progress has already been made, relying heavily on *in vitro* studies. Interestingly, it appears that somewhat different mechanisms exist for different types of RNA, as well as for RNAs produced in mitochondria and chloroplasts.

We might envision the simplest possible mechanism for removing an intron to be as illustrated in Figure 13–10. After an endonucleolytic "cut" is made at each end of an intron, the intron is removed, and the terminal ends of the adjacent exons are ligated by an enzyme (in short, the intron is snipped out, and the exon ends are rejoined). This is apparently what happens to the introns present in transfer RNAs (tRNAs) in bacteria. A specific endonuclease recognizes the intron termini and excises the intervening sequences. Then RNA ligase seals the exon ends to complete each splicing event. However, in the studies of all other RNAs—tRNA in higher eukaryotes and rRNAs and pre-mRNAs in all eukaryotes—precise excision of introns is much more complex and a much more interesting story.

Introns in eukaryotes can be categorized into several groups based on their splicing mechanisms. Group I, an example of which is introns that are part of the primary transcript of rRNAs, require no additional components for intron excision; the intron itself is the source of the enzymatic activity necessary for removal. This amazing discovery was made in 1982 by Thomas Cech and his colleagues during a study of the ciliate protozoan *Tetrahymena*. RNAs that are capable of such catalytic activity are referred to as **ribozymes**. The self-excision process for group I introns serves to illustrate this concept and is shown in **Figure 13–13**. Chemically, two nucleophilic reactions take place—that is, reactions caused by the presence of electron-rich chemical species (in this case, they are transesterification reactions). The first is an interaction between guanosine, which acts as a cofactor in the reaction, and the primary transcript [**Figure 13–13(a)**]. The 3′-OH group of guanosine is transferred to the nucleotide adjacent to the 5′ end of the intron [**Figures 13–13(b)** and **13–13(c)**]. The

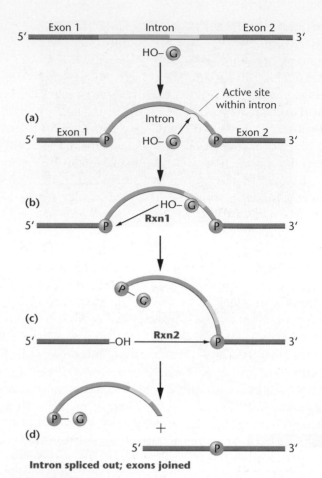

FIGURE 13–13 Splicing mechanism for removal of group I introns from the initial rRNA transcript (pre-rRNA). The process is one of self-excision involving two transesterification reactions.

second reaction involves the interaction of the newly acquired 3′-OH group on the left-hand exon and the phosphate on the 3′ end of the intron [Figure 13–13(c)]. The intron is spliced out and the two exon regions are ligated, leading to the mature RNA [**Figure 13–13(d)**].

Self-excision of group I introns, as described above, is known to occur in bacteria, lower eukaryotes, and higher plants. Self-excision also seems to govern the removal of introns from the primary mRNA and tRNA transcripts produced in mitochondria and chloroplasts. These are examples of group II introns. Splicing is somewhat different than in group I, but also involves two autocatalytic reactions leading to the excision of introns. Group II introns are found in fungi, plants, protists, and bacteria.

Splicing Mechanisms: The Spliceosome

Introns are a major component of nuclear-derived pre-mRNA transcripts of eukaryotes. Compared to the group I and group II introns discussed above, those in nuclear-derived mRNA are much larger—up to 20,000 nucleotides—and they are more plentiful. Their removal appears to require a much more complex mechanism. These splicing reactions are not autocatalytic, but instead are mediated by a huge molecular complex called a **spliceosome**, which has now been identified in extracts of yeast as well as in mammalian cells. This structure is very large, 40S in yeast and 60S in mammals, being the same size as ribosomal subunits! One set of essential components of spliceosomes is a unique set of **small nuclear RNAs (snRNAs)**. These RNAs are usually 100 to 200 nucleotides long or less and are complexed with proteins to form **small nuclear ribonucleoproteins (snRNPs, or snurps)**. Because they are rich in uridine residues, the snRNAs have been arbitrarily designated U1, U2, . . . , U6.

Figure 13–14 depicts a model illustrating the steps involved in the removal of one intron. Keep in mind that while this figure shows separate components, the process involves the huge spliceosome that envelopes the RNA being spliced. The nucleotide sequences near the ends of the intron begin at the 5′ end with a GU dinucleotide sequence, called the *donor sequence,* and terminate at the 3′ end with an AG dinucleotide, called the *acceptor sequence.* These, as well as other consensus sequences shared by introns, attract specific snRNAs of the spliceosome. For example, the snRNA U1 bears a nucleotide sequence that is complementary to the 5′-splice donor sequence end of the intron. Base pairing resulting from this homology promotes the binding that represents the initial step in the formation of the spliceosome. After the other snRNPs (U2, U4, U5, and U6) are added, splicing commences. As with group I splicing, two *transesterification reactions* occur. The first involves the interaction of the 3′-OH group from an adenine (A) residue present within the **branch point** region of the intron. The A residue attacks the 5′-splice site, cutting the RNA chain. In a subsequent step involving several other snRNPs, an intermediate structure is formed and the second reaction ensues, linking the cut 5′ end of the intron to the A. This results in the formation of a characteristic loop structure called a *lariat,* which contains the excised intron. The exons are then ligated and the snRNPs are released.

The processing involved in splicing, which occurs within the nucleus, represents a potential regulatory step in gene expression in eukaryotes. For instance, several cases are known wherein introns present in pre-mRNAs *derived from the same gene* are spliced *in more than one way,* thereby yielding different collections of exons in the mature mRNA. Such **alternative splicing** yields a group of similar but nonidentical mRNAs that, upon translation, result in a series of related proteins called **isoforms**. Many examples have been encountered in organisms ranging from viruses to *Drosophila* to humans. Alternative splicing of pre-mRNAs represents a way of producing related proteins from a single gene, increasing the number of gene products that can be derived from an organism's genome. We will return to this topic in our discussion of the regulation of gene expression in eukaryotes (see Chapter 17).

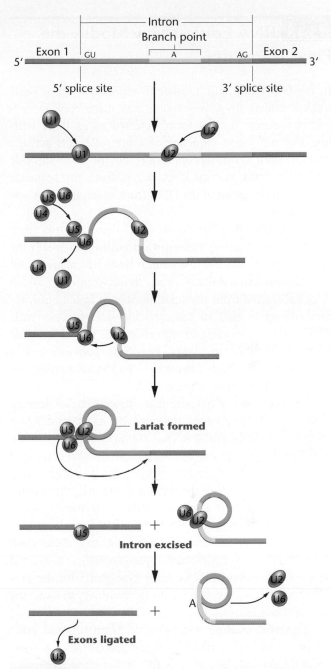

FIGURE 13–14 A model of the splicing mechanism for removal of an intron from nuclear-derived pre-mRNA. Excision is dependent on snRNAs (U1, U2, etc). The lariat structure is characteristic of this mechanism.

EVOLVING CONCEPT OF THE GENE

The elucidation of the genetic code in the 1960s supported the concept that the gene is composed of a linear series of triplet nucleotides encoding the amino acid sequence of a protein. While this is indeed the case in prokaryotes and viruses, in 1977, it became apparent that in eukaryotes, the gene is divided into coding sequences, called exons, which are interrupted by noncoding sequences, called introns (intervening sequences), which must be spliced out during production of the mature mRNA. ▪

13.13 RNA Editing May Modify the Final Transcript

In the late 1980s, still another unexpected form of post-transcriptional RNA processing was discovered in several organisms. In this form, referred to as **RNA editing**, the nucleotide sequence of a pre-mRNA is actually changed prior to translation. As a result, the ribonucleotide sequence of the mature RNA differs from the sequence encoded in the exons of the DNA from which the RNA was transcribed.

Although other variations exist, there are two main types of RNA editing: **substitution editing**, in which the identities of individual nucleotide bases are altered; and **insertion/deletion editing**, in which nucleotides are added to or subtracted from the total number of bases. Substitution editing is used in some nuclear-derived eukaryotic RNAs and is prevalent in mitochondrial and chloroplast RNAs transcribed in plants. *Physarum polycephalum,* a slime mold, uses both substitution and insertion/deletion editing for its mitochondrial mRNAs.

Trypanosoma, a parasite that causes African sleeping sickness, and its relatives use extensive insertion/deletion editing in mitochondrial RNAs. The uridines added to an individual transcript can make up more than 60 percent of the coding sequence, usually forming the initiation codon and bringing the rest of the sequence into the proper reading frame. Insertion/deletion editing in trypanosomes is directed by **gRNA (guide RNA)** templates, which are also transcribed from the mitochondrial genome. These small RNAs share a high degree of complementarity to the edited region of the final mRNAs. They base-pair with the pre-edited mRNAs to direct the editing machinery to make the correct changes.

The best-studied examples of substitutional editing occur in mammalian nuclear-encoded mRNA transcripts. One such example is the protein *apolipoprotein B (apo B)*, which exists in both a long and a short form that are encoded by the same gene. In human intestinal cells, apo B mRNA is edited by a single C-to-U change, which converts a CAA glutamine codon into a UAA stop codon and terminates the polypeptide at approximately half its genomically encoded length. The editing is performed by a complex of proteins that bind to a "mooring sequence" on the mRNA transcript just downstream of the editing site.

A second example involves the subunits constituting the *glutamate receptor channels (GluR)* in mammalian brain tissue. In this case, adenosine (A) to inosine (I) editing occurs in pre-mRNAs prior to their translation, during which I is read as guanosine (G). A family of three ADAR (*adenosine deaminase acting on RNA*) enzymes is believed to be responsible for the editing of various sites within the glutamate channel subunits. The double-stranded RNAs required for editing by the ADAR enzymes are provided by intron/exon pairing of the GluR mRNA transcripts. The editing changes alter the physiological parameters (solute permeability and desensitization response time) of the receptors containing the subunits.

A similar ADAR-editing step has more recently been reported in the voltage-dependent potassium (K^+) channel in a cephalopod. These channels are essentially gene products, and they regulate neuron function. In this interesting example, specific RNA editing occurs in the K^+ channels of squids living in near-freezing water, but not in the same species found living in more tropical environments. Thus, RNA editing has been shown to be adaptive, in this case responding to cold temperatures.

Findings such as these have established that RNA editing provides still another important mechanism of post-transcriptional modification, and that this process is not restricted to small or asexually reproducing genomes, such as those in mitochondria. These discoveries, too, have important implications for the regulation of genetic expression.

13.14 Transcription Has Been Visualized by Electron Microscopy

We conclude this chapter by presenting a striking visual demonstration of the transcription process based on the electron microscope studies of Oscar Miller, Jr., Barbara Hamkalo, and Charles Thomas. Their combined work has captured the transcription process in both prokaryotes and eukaryotes. **Figure 13–15** shows a micrograph and interpretive drawings of transcription in *E. coli.* In the micrograph, multiple strands of RNA are seen to emanate from different points along a central DNA template. Many RNA strands result because numerous transcription events are occurring simultaneously along each gene. Progressively longer RNA strands are found farther downstream from the point of initiation of transcription along a given gene, whereas the shortest strands are closest to the point of initiation.

An interesting picture emerges from study of the *E. coli* micrograph. Because prokaryotes lack nuclei, cytoplasmic ribosomes are not separated physically from the chromosome. As a result, ribosomes are free to attach to *partially* transcribed mRNA molecules and initiate

FIGURE 13–15 Electron micrograph and interpretive drawing of simultaneous transcription of genes in *E. coli*. As each transcript is forming, ribosomes attach, initiating simultaneous translation along each strand. O.L. Miller, Jr., Barbara A. Hamkalo, C.A. Thomas, Jr. *Science* 169: 392–395, 1970 by the American Association for the Advancement of Science.

translation. The longer the RNA strand, the greater the number of ribosomes attached to it. As we will see later in the text (see Chapter 14). these structures are called **polyribosomes**. Visualization of transcription confirms many of the predictions scientists had made from the biochemical analysis of this process.

CASE STUDY | A drug that sometimes works

A 30-year-old woman with β-thalassemia, a recessively inherited genetic disorder caused by absence of the hemoglobin β chain, had been treated with blood transfusions since the age of 7. However, in spite of the transfusions, her health was declining. As an alternative treatment, her physician administered 5-azacytidine to induce transcription of the fetal β hemoglobin chain to replace her missing β chain. This drug activates gene transcription by removing methyl groups from DNA. Addition of methyl groups silences genes. However, the physician expressed concern that approximately 40 percent of all human genes are normally silenced by methylation. Nevertheless, after several weeks of 5-azacytidine treatment, the patient's condition improved dramatically. Although the treatment was successful, use of this drug raises several important questions.

1. Why was her physician concerned that a high percentage of human genes are transcriptionally silenced by methylation?

2. What genes might raise the greatest concern?

3. What criteria would you use when deciding to administer a drug such as 5-azacytidine?

Summary Points

MasteringGenetics™ For activities, animations, and review quizzes, go to the Study Area.

1. Early studies of the genetic code revealed it to be triplet in nature and to be nonoverlapping, commaless, and degenerate.

2. The use of RNA homopolymers and mixed copolymers in a cell-free protein synthesizing system allowed the determination of the composition, but not the sequence, of triplet codons designating specific amino acids.

3. Use of the triplet-binding assay and of repeating copolymers allowed the determination of the specific sequences of triplet codons designating specific amino acids.

4. The complete coding dictionary reveals that of the 64 possible triplet codons, 61 encode the 20 amino acids found in proteins, while three triplets terminate translation. One of these 61 is the initiation codon and specifies methionine.

5. Confirmation for the coding dictionary, including codons for initiation and termination, was obtained by comparing the complete nucleotide sequences of phage MS2 with the amino acid sequence of the corresponding proteins. Other findings support the belief that, with only minor exceptions, the code is universal for all organisms.

6. Transcription—the initial step in gene expression—is the synthesis, under the direction of RNA polymerase, of a strand of RNA complementary to a DNA template.

7. Like DNA replication, the processes of transcription can be subdivided into the stages of initiation, elongation, and termination. Also like DNA replication, transcription relies on base-pairing affinities between complementary nucleotides.

8. Initiation of transcription is dependent on an upstream (5′) DNA region, called the promoter, that represents the initial binding site for RNA polymerase. Promoters contain specific DNA sequences, such as the TATA box, that are essential to polymerase binding.

9. The process of creating the initial transcript during transcription is more complex in eukaryotes than in prokaryotes,

including the addition of a 5′ 7-mG cap and a 3′ poly-A tail, to the pre-mRNA.

10. The primary transcript in eukaryotes reflects the presence of intervening sequences, or introns, present in DNA, which must be spliced out to create the mature mRNA.

GENETICS, TECHNOLOGY, AND SOCIETY

Fighting Disease with Antisense Therapeutics

Conventional therapeutic drugs often have toxic side effects, affecting both normal and diseased cells, with diseased or infected cells being only slightly more susceptible than the patient's normal cells. Scientists have long wished for a magic bullet that could seek out and destroy the underlying defects in diseased cells, leaving normal cells alive and healthy. Recently, a group of promising drugs has emerged, collectively described as *antisense* drugs.

Antisense therapies are based on the design and use of short synthetic single-stranded DNA molecules known as *antisense oligonucleotides (ASOs)* and have been developed through an understanding of the molecular biology of gene expression. When cells become infected with viruses, are transformed into cancer cells, or suffer from many genetic defects, their underlying disease state is determined by gene mutations or inappropriate gene expression. The mRNAs responsible for these conditions are transcribed from the template strand of DNA and therefore are known as "*sense*" RNAs. If scientists know the sequence of the sense RNA, they can synthesize a strand of DNA that is complementary to any sequence within the sense RNA. This complementary DNA is the antisense oligonucleotide. When introduced into cells, ASOs bind to the specific target sense RNA through Watson-Crick base-pairing. The binding of ASOs to sense RNAs interferes with the mRNA's translation, or causes its degradation.

The antisense approach is exciting because of its potential specificity. Because an antisense molecule has a sequence that specifically binds to a

particular sense RNA, it should be possible to inhibit synthesis of the specific protein encoded by the sense RNA. If the encoded protein causes a genetic disease or is necessary for virus reproduction or cancer cell growth—but is not necessary in normal cells—the antisense molecule should have only therapeutic effects.

In ASO-based technologies, scientists design short (about 20 nucleotides long) single-stranded antisense DNA oligonucleotides and then synthesize large amounts of these ASOs *in vitro*. Using various methods, the ASOs can be introduced into cultured cells or whole organisms.

Although the development of effective ASO drugs has been slow and often difficult, two have been approved by the FDA and are currently on the market. One of these drugs, called fomivirsen or Vitravene, targets cytomegalovirus infections in the eye. Another drug, called mipomersen or Kynamro, inhibits the synthesis of apolipoprotein B and is used to lower the levels of cholesterol lipoproteins in patients with familial hypercholesterolemia.

More than 20 ASO antisense drugs are currently in phase II and III clinical trials. These drugs are designed to treat various cancers, asthma, ulcerative colitis, renal failure, and virus infections.

Another new and promising ASO therapeutic approach involves using antisense oligonucleotides to alter mRNA splicing patterns, a therapy called "*antisense-mediated exon skipping.*" The most advanced exon-skipping therapy, now in clinical trials, is designed to treat patients with Duchenne muscular dystrophy (DMD). DMD is an X-linked recessive disorder, affecting approximately one in every 3500 newborn

males. It results in muscle degeneration, heart disease, and premature death. The disease is caused by mutations in the *dystrophin* gene, which contains 79 exons. These mutations are a variety of deletions, duplications, or other mutations that disrupt the open reading frame of the gene and result in premature translation termination and the absence of functional dystrophin protein.

Many dystrophin gene mutations occur in exon 51. Scientists have designed ASOs that target DNA sequences near the splice junctions of exon 51. These ASOs interfere with normal pre-mRNA splicing, causing exon 50 to be spliced to exon 52. This results in an internal deletion of the mutated exon 51 in the mRNA, but restores the correct reading frame to the internally deleted protein. Although missing some internal amino acid sequences, the new dystrophin protein restores partial function to the muscles. The ASO-mediated exon-skipping approach is also being applied to treatments for other conditions such as β-thalassemia, spinal muscular atrophy, and some cancers.

Your Turn

Take time, individually or in groups, to answer the following questions. Investigate the references and links to help you discuss some of the technical issues that surround the development and uses of antisense therapies.

1. What are some of the challenges in the use of ASOs as therapeutics? How are scientists addressing these challenges?

(continued)

Genetics, Technology, and Society, continued

A discussion of antisense oligonucleotide drug design is presented in: Watts, J.K. and Corey, D.R. 2012. Silencing disease genes in the laboratory and the clinic. *J. Pathol.* 226: 365-379.

2. What are some limitations in the use of ASOs for exon-skipping therapies in Duchenne muscular dystrophy? What is the status of current clinical trials for these exon-skipping therapies?

A discussion of exon skipping in DMD is presented in: Fairclough, R.J. et al. 2013. Therapy for Duchenne muscular dystrophy: Renewed optimism from genetic approaches. *Nature Rev. Genet.* 14: 373-378. *For information about clinical trials, start your search on PubMed at* http://www.ncbi.nlm.nih.gov/pubmed.

3. Mipomersen (Kynamro, Isis Pharmaceuticals) has recently been approved for use to treat familial hypercholesterolemia. How does this ASO work, and why was its use restricted to patients with a homozygous hereditary disease?

To learn about mipomersen, see Bell, D.A. et al. 2012. Mipomersen and other therapies for the treatment of severe familial hypercholesterolemia. *Vascular Health and Risk Management* 8: 651-659.

INSIGHTS AND SOLUTIONS

1. Calculate how many triplet codons would be possible had evolution seized on six bases (three complementary base pairs) rather than four bases with which to construct DNA. Would six bases accommodate a two-letter code, assuming 20 amino acids and start and stop codons?

Solution: Six bases taken three at a time would produce $(6)^3$, or 216, triplet codes. If the code was a doublet, there would be $(6)^2$, or 36, two-letter codes, more than enough to accommodate 20 amino acids and start and stop signals.

2. In a heteropolymer experiment using 1/2C : 1/4A : 1/4G, how many different triplets will occur in the synthetic RNA molecule? How often will the most frequent triplet occur?

Solution: There will be $(3)^3$, or 27, triplets produced. The most frequent will be CCC, present $(1/2)^3$ or 1/8 of the time.

3. In a regular copolymer experiment, in which UUAC is repeated over and over, how many different triplets will occur in the synthetic RNA, and how many amino acids will occur in the polypeptide when this RNA is translated? (Consult Figure 13–7.)

Solution: The synthetic RNA will repeat four triplets—UUA, CUU, ACU, and UAC—over and over. Because both UUA and CUU encode leucine, while ACU and UAC encode threonine and tyrosine, respectively, the polypeptides synthesized under the directions of such an RNA contain three amino acids in the repeating sequence leu-leu-thr-tyr.

4. Actinomycin D inhibits DNA-dependent RNA synthesis. This antibiotic is added to a bacterial culture in which a specific protein is being monitored. Compared to a control culture, into which no antibiotic is added, translation of the protein declines over a period of 20 minutes, until no further protein is made. Explain these results.

Solution: The mRNA, which is the basis for the translation of the protein, has a lifetime of about 20 minutes. When actinomycin D is added, transcription is inhibited, and no new mRNAs are made. Those already present support the translation of the protein for up to 20 minutes.

Problems and Discussion Questions

MasteringGenetics™ Visit for instructor-assigned tutorials and problems.

HOW DO WE KNOW?

1. In this chapter, we focused on the genetic code and the transcription of genetic information stored in DNA into complementary RNA molecules. Along the way, we found many opportunities to consider the methods and reasoning by which much of this information was acquired. From the explanations given in the chapter, what answers would you propose to the following fundamental questions:
   (a) Why did geneticists believe, even before direct experimental evidence was obtained, that the genetic code would turn out to be composed of triplet sequences and be nonoverlapping? Experimentally, how were these suppositions shown to be correct?
   (b) What experimental evidence provided the initial insights into the *compositions* of codons encoding specific amino acids?
   (c) How were the specific sequences of triplet codes determined experimentally?
   (d) How were the experimentally derived triplet codon assignments verified in studies using bacteriophage MS2?
   (e) What evidence do we have that the expression of the information encoded in DNA involves an RNA intermediate?
   (f) How do we know that the initial transcript of a eukaryotic gene contains noncoding sequences that must be removed before accurate translation into proteins can occur?

CONCEPT QUESTION

2. Review the Chapter Concepts list on p. 308. These all center around how genetic information is stored in DNA and transferred to RNA prior to translation into proteins. Write a short essay that summarizes the key properties of the genetic code and the process by which RNA is transcribed on a DNA template.

3. In their studies of frameshift mutations, Crick, Barnett, Brenner, and Watts-Tobin found that either three "pluses" or three "minuses" restored the correct reading frame. (a) Assuming the code is a triplet, what effect would the addition or loss of six nucleotides have on the reading frame? (b) If the code were a sextuplet (consisting of six nucleotides), would the reading frame be restored by the addition or loss of three, six, or nine nucleotides?

4. The mRNA formed from the repeating tetranucleotide UUAC incorporates only three amino acids, but the use of UAUC incorporates four amino acids. Why?

5. In studies using repeating copolymers, AC . . . incorporates threonine and histidine, and CAACAA . . . incorporates glutamine, asparagine, and threonine. What triplet code can definitely be assigned to threonine?

6. In a coding experiment using repeating copolymers (as demonstrated in Table 13.3), the following data were obtained:

Copolymer	Codons Produced	Amino Acids in Polypeptide
AG	AGA, GAG	Arg, Glu
AAG	AGA, AAG, GAA	Lys, Arg, Glu

AGG is known to code for arginine. Taking into account the wobble hypothesis, assign each of the four codons produced in the experiment to its correct amino acid.

7. In the triplet-binding technique, radioactivity remains on the filter when the amino acid corresponding to the codon is labeled. Explain the rationale for this technique.

8. When the amino acid sequences of insulin isolated from different organisms were determined, differences were noted. For example, alanine was substituted for threonine, serine for glycine, and valine for isoleucine at corresponding positions in the protein. List the single-base changes that could occur in codons of the genetic code to produce these amino acid changes.

9. In studies of the amino acid sequence of wild-type and mutant forms of tryptophan synthetase in *E. coli,* the following changes have been observed:

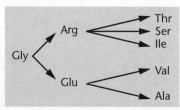

Determine a set of triplet codes in which only a single-nucleotide change produces each amino acid change.

10. Why doesn't polynucleotide phosphorylase (Ochoa's enzyme) synthesize RNA *in vivo*?

11. Refer to Table 13.1. Can you hypothesize why a mixture of poly U + poly A would not stimulate incorporation of ^{14}C-phenylalanine into protein?

12. Predict the amino acid sequence produced during translation by the following short hypothetical mRNA sequences (note that the second sequence was formed from the first by a deletion of only one nucleotide):

    Sequence 1: 5'-AUGCCGGAUUAUAGUUGA-3'
    Sequence 2: 5'-AUGCCGGAUUAAGUUGA-3'

What type of mutation gave rise to Sequence 2?

13. A short RNA molecule was isolated that demonstrated a hyperchromic shift, indicating secondary structure. Its sequence was determined to be

    5'-AGGCGCCGACUCUACU-3'

(a) Propose a two-dimensional model for this molecule.
(b) What DNA sequence would give rise to this RNA molecule through transcription?
(c) If the molecule were a tRNA fragment containing a CGA anticodon, what would the corresponding codon be?
(d) If the molecule were an internal part of a message, what amino acid sequence would result from it following translation? (Refer to the code chart in Figure 13–7.)

14. A glycine residue is in position 210 of the tryptophan synthetase enzyme of wild-type *E. coli*. If the codon specifying glycine is GGA, how many single-base substitutions will result in an amino acid substitution at position 210? What are they? How many will result if the wild-type codon is GGU?

15. Refer to Figure 13–7 to respond to the following:
(a) Shown here is a hypothetical viral mRNA sequence:

    5'-AUGCAUACCUAUGAGACCCUUGGA-3'

Assuming that it could arise from overlapping genes, how many different polypeptide sequences can be produced? What are the sequences?
(b) A base-substitution mutation that altered the sequence in (a) eliminated the synthesis of all but one polypeptide. The altered sequence is shown here:

    5'-AUGCAUACCUAUGUGACCCUUGGA-3'

Determine why.

16. Most proteins have more leucine than histidine residues, but more histidine than tryptophan residues. Correlate the number of codons for these three amino acids with this information.

17. Define the process of transcription. Where does this process fit into the central dogma of molecular genetics (DNA makes RNA makes protein)?

18. What was the initial evidence for the existence of mRNA?

19. Describe the structure of RNA polymerase in bacteria. What is the core enzyme? What is the role of the σ subunit?

20. Write a paragraph describing the abbreviated chemical reactions that summarize RNA polymerase-directed transcription.

21. Messenger RNA molecules are very difficult to isolate in prokaryotes because they are rather quickly degraded in the cell. Can you suggest a reason why this occurs? Eukaryotic mRNAs are more stable and exist longer in the cell than do prokaryotic mRNAs. Is this an advantage or a disadvantage for a pancreatic cell making large quantities of insulin?

22. Present an overview of various forms of posttranscriptional processing in eukaryotes. For each, provide an example.

23. One form of posttranscriptional modification of most eukaryotic RNA transcripts is the addition of a poly-A sequence at the 3' end. The absence of a poly-A sequence leads to rapid degradation of the transcript. Poly-A sequences of various lengths are also added to many prokaryotic RNA transcripts where, instead of promoting stability, they enhance degradation. In both cases, RNA secondary structures, stabilizing proteins, or degrading enzymes interact with poly-A sequences. Considering the activities of RNAs, what might be general functions of 3'-polyadenylation?

24. Describe the role of two forms of RNA editing that lead to changes in the size and sequence of pre-mRNAs. Briefly describe several examples of each form of editing, including their impact on respective protein products.

25. Substitution RNA editing is known to involve either C-to-U or A-to-I conversions. What common chemical event accounts for each?

Extra-Spicy Problems

MasteringGenetics™ Visit for instructor-assigned tutorials and problems.

26. It has been suggested that the present-day triplet genetic code evolved from a doublet code when there were fewer amino acids available for primitive protein synthesis.
    (a) Can you find any support for the doublet code notion in the existing coding dictionary?
    (b) The amino acids Ala, Val, Gly, Asp, and Glu are all early members of biosynthetic pathways (Taylor and Coates, 1989) and are more evolutionarily conserved than other amino acids (Brooks and Fresco, 2003). They therefore probably represent "early" amino acids. Of what significance is this information in terms of the evolution of the genetic code? Also, which base, of the first two, would likely have been the more significant in originally specifying these amino acids?
    (c) As determined by comparisons of ancient and recently evolved proteins, cysteine, tyrosine, and phenylalanine appear to be late-arriving amino acids. In addition, they are considered to have been absent in the abiotic earth (Miller, 1987). All three of these amino acids have only two codons each, while many others, earlier in origin, have more. Is this mere coincidence, or might there be some underlying explanation?

27. An early proposal by George Gamow in 1954 regarding the genetic code considered the possibility that DNA served directly as the template for polypeptide synthesis. In eukaryotes, what difficulties would such a system pose? What observations and theoretical considerations argue against such a proposal?

28. In a mixed copolymer experiment, messages were created with either 4/5C:1/5A or 4/5A:1/5C. These messages yielded proteins with the following amino acid compositions.

	4/5C:1/5A		4/5A:1/5C
Proline	63.0 percent	Proline	3.5 percent
Histidine	13.0 percent	Histidine	3.0 percent
Threonine	16.0 percent	Threonine	16.6 percent
Glutamine	3.0 percent	Glutamine	13.0 percent
Asparagine	3.0 percent	Asparagine	13.0 percent
Lysine	0.5 percent	Lysine	50.0 percent
	98.5 percent		99.1 percent

Using these data, predict the most specific coding composition for each amino acid.

29. Shown here are the amino acid sequences of the wild-type and three mutant forms of a short protein. Use this information to answer the following questions:

Wild-type:	Met-Trp-Tyr-Arg-Gly-Ser-Pro-Thr
Mutant 1:	Met-Trp
Mutant 2:	Met-Trp-His-Arg-Gly-Ser-Pro-Thr
Mutant 3:	Met-Cys-Ile-Val-Val-Val-Gln-His

(a) Using Figure 13–7, predict the type of mutation that led to each altered protein.
(b) For each mutant protein, determine the specific ribonucleotide change that led to its synthesis.
(c) The wild-type RNA consists of nine triplets. What is the role of the ninth triplet?
(d) Of the first eight wild-type triplets, which, if any, can you determine specifically from an analysis of the mutant proteins? In each case, explain why or why not.
(e) Another mutation (Mutant 4) is isolated. Its amino acid sequence is unchanged, but the mutant cells produce abnormally low amounts of the wild-type proteins. As specifically as you can, predict where this mutation exists in the gene.

30. The genetic code is degenerate. Amino acids are encoded by either 1, 2, 3, 4, or 6 triplet codons. (See Figure 13–7.) An interesting question is whether the number of triplet codes for a given amino acid is in any way correlated with the frequency with which that amino acid appears in proteins. That is, is the genetic code optimized for its intended use? Some approximations of the frequency of appearance of nine amino acids in proteins in *E. coli* are given in the following:

Amino Acid	Percentage
Met	2
Cys	2
Gln	5
Pro	5
Arg	5
Ile	6
Glu	7
Ala	8
Leu	10

(a) Determine how many triplets encode each amino acid.
(b) Devise a way to graphically compare the two sets of information (data).
(c) Analyze your data to determine what, if any, correlations can be drawn between the relative frequency of amino acids making up proteins and the number of codons for each. Write a paragraph that states your specific and general conclusions.
(d) How would you proceed with your analysis if you wanted to pursue this problem further?

31. M. Klemke et al. (2001) discovered an interesting coding phenomenon in which an exon within a neurologic hormone receptor gene in mammals appears to produce two different protein entities (XLαs, ALEX). Following is the DNA sequence of the exon's 5′ end derived from a rat. The lower-case letters represent the initial coding portion for the XLαs

protein, and the uppercase letters indicate the portion where the ALEX entity is initiated. (For simplicity, and to correspond with the RNA coding dictionary, it is customary to represent the noncoding, nontemplate strand of the DNA segment.)

5′-gtcccaaccatgcccaccgatcttccgcctgcttctgaagATGCGGGCCCAG

(a) Convert the noncoding DNA sequence to the coding RNA sequence.
(b) Locate the initiator codon within the XLαs segment.
(c) Locate the initiator codon within the ALEX segment. Are the two initiator codons in frame?
(d) Provide the amino acid sequence for each coding sequence. In the region of overlap, are the two amino acid sequences the same?
(e) Are there any evolutionary advantages to having the same DNA sequence code for two protein products? Are there any disadvantages?

32. The concept of consensus sequences of DNA was defined in this chapter as sequences that are similar (homologous) in different genes of the same organism or in genes of different organisms. Examples were the Pribnow box and the −35 region in prokaryotes and the TATA-box region in eukaryotes. One study found that among 73 isolates from the virus HIV-Type 1C (a major contributor to the AIDS epidemic), a GGGNNNNNCC consensus sequence exists (where N equals any nitrogenous base) in the promoter–enhancer region of the NF-κB transcription factor, a *cis*-acting element that is critical for initiating HIV transcription in human macrophages (Novitsky et al., 2002). The authors contend that finding this and other conserved sequences may be of value in designing an AIDS vaccine. What advantages would knowing these consensus sequences confer? Are there disadvantages as a vaccine is designed?

33. Recent observations indicate that alternative splicing is a common way for eukaryotes to expand their repertoire of gene functions. Studies indicate that approximately 50 percent of human genes exhibit alternative splicing and approximately 15 percent of disease-causing mutations involve aberrant alternative splicing. Different tissues show remarkably different frequencies of alternative splicing, with the brain accounting for approximately 18 percent of such events (Xu et al., 2002. *Nuc. Acids Res.* 30: 3754–3766).

(a) Define alternative splicing and speculate on the evolutionary strategy alternative splicing offers to organisms.
(b) Why might some tissues engage in more alternative splicing than others?

Crystal structure of a *Thermus thermophilus* 70S ribosome containing three bound transfer RNAs, bridging the two subunits. *Image provided by Dr. Albion Baucom (baucom@biology.ucsc.edu). Reprinted from the front cover of* Science, *Vol. 292, May 4, 2001.*

14

Translation and Proteins

CHAPTER CONCEPTS

- The ribonucleotide sequence of messenger RNA (mRNA) reflects genetic information stored in the DNA of genes and corresponds to the amino acid sequences in proteins encoded by those genes.

- The process of translation decodes the information in mRNA, leading to the synthesis of polypeptide chains.

- Translation involves the interactions of mRNA, tRNA, ribosomes, and a variety of translation factors essential to the initiation, elongation, and termination of the polypeptide chain.

- Proteins, the final product of most genes, achieve a three-dimensional conformation that arises from the primary amino acid sequences of the polypeptide chains making up each protein.

- The function of any protein is closely tied to its three-dimensional structure, which can be disrupted by mutation.

Earlier in the text, (see Chapter 13) we established that a genetic code stores information in the form of triplet codons in DNA and that this information is initially expressed, through the process of transcription, as a messenger RNA complementary to the template strand of the DNA helix. However, the final product of gene expression, in most instances, is a polypeptide chain consisting of a linear series of amino acids whose sequence has been prescribed by the genetic code. In this chapter, we will examine how the information present in mRNA is translated to create polypeptides, which then fold into protein molecules. We will also review the evidence confirming that proteins are the end products of genes and discuss briefly the various levels of protein structure, diversity, and function. This information extends our understanding of gene expression and provides an important foundation for interpreting how the mutations that arise in DNA can result in the diverse phenotypic effects observed in organisms.

14.1 Translation of mRNA Depends on Ribosomes and Transfer RNAs

Translation of mRNA is the biological polymerization of amino acids into polypeptide chains. This process, alluded to in our earlier discussion of the genetic code, occurs only in association with **ribosomes**, which serve as nonspecific workbenches. The central question in translation is how triplet codons of mRNA direct specific amino acids into their correct position in the polypeptide. That question was answered once **transfer RNA (tRNA)** was discovered. This class of molecules adapts genetic information present as specific triplet codons in mRNA to their corresponding amino acids. As noted in (Chapter 13), the requirement for some sort of "adaptor" was postulated by Francis Crick in 1957.

In association with a ribosome, mRNA presents a triplet codon that calls for a specific amino acid. A specific tRNA molecule contains within its nucleotide sequence three consecutive ribonucleotides complementary to the codon, called the **anticodon**, which can base-pair with the codon. Another region of this tRNA is covalently bonded to the codon's corresponding amino acid.

Hydrogen bonding of tRNAs to mRNA holds amino acids in proximity to each other so that a peptide bond can be formed between them. The process occurs over and over as mRNA runs through the ribosome, and amino acids are polymerized into a polypeptide. Before looking more closely at this process, we will first consider the structures of the ribosome and transfer RNA.

Ribosomal Structure

Because of its essential role in the expression of genetic information, the ribosome has been analyzed extensively. One bacterial cell contains about 10,000 ribosomes, and a eukaryotic cell contains many times more. Electron microscopy has revealed that the bacterial ribosome is about 40 nm at its largest diameter and consists of two subunits, one large and one small. Both subunits consist of one or more molecules of rRNA and an array of **ribosomal proteins**. When the two subunits are associated with each other in a single ribosome, the structure is sometimes called a **monosome**.

The main differences between prokaryotic and eukaryotic ribosomes are summarized in **Figure 14–1**. The subunit and rRNA components are most easily isolated and characterized on the basis of their sedimentation behavior in sucrose gradients, which is a measure of their rate of migration when centrifuged, abbreviated *S* for *Svedberg coefficient*, which reflects their density, mass, and shape. In prokaryotes, the monosome is a 70S particle, and in eukaryotes it is approximately 80S. Sedimentation coefficients, which reflect differences in the rate of migration of different-sized particles and molecules, are not additive. For example, the prokaryotic 70S monosome consists of a 50S and a 30S subunit, and the eukaryotic 80S monosome consists of a 60S and a 40S subunit.

The larger subunit in prokaryotes consists of a 23S rRNA molecule, a 5S rRNA molecule, and 31 ribosomal proteins. In the eukaryotic equivalent, a 28S rRNA molecule is accompanied by a 5.8S and a 5S rRNA molecule and 46 proteins. The smaller prokaryotic subunits consist of a 16S rRNA component and 21 proteins. In the eukaryotic equivalent, an 18S rRNA component and about 33 proteins are found. The approximate molecular weights (in daltons, or Da) and the number of nucleotides of these components are also shown in Figure 14–1.

It is now clear that the RNA components of the ribosome perform all-important catalytic functions associated with translation. The many ribosomal proteins, whose functions were long a mystery, are thought to promote

Prokaryotes Monosome 70S (2.6×10^6 Da)				**Eukaryotes** Monosome 80S (4.3×10^6 Da)			
Large subunit		**Small subunit**		**Large subunit**		**Small subunit**	
50S	1.7×10^6 Da	30S	0.9×10^6 Da	60S	2.9×10^6 Da	40S	1.4×10^6 Da
23S rRNA (2904 nucleotides) + 31 proteins + 5S rRNA (120 nucleotides)		16S rRNA (1541 nucleotides) + 21 proteins		28S rRNA (4718 nucleotides) + 46 proteins + 5S rRNA (120 nucleotides) + 5.8S rRNA (160 nucleotides)		18S rRNA (1874 nucleotides) + 33 proteins	

FIGURE 14–1 A comparison of the components in prokaryotic and eukaryotic ribosomes.

the binding of the various molecules involved in translation and, in general, to fine-tune the process. This conclusion is based on the observation that some of the catalytic functions in ribosomes still occur in experiments involving "ribosomal protein-depleted" ribosomes.

Molecular hybridization studies have established the degree of redundancy of the genes coding for the rRNA components. The *E. coli* genome contains seven copies of a single sequence that encodes all three components—23S, 16S, and 5S. The initial transcript of each set of these genes produces a 30S RNA molecule that is enzymatically cleaved into these smaller components. The coupling of the genetic information encoding these three rRNA components ensures that, following multiple transcription events, equal quantities of all three will be present as ribosomes are assembled.

In eukaryotes, many more copies of a sequence encoding the 28S, 18S, and 5.8S components are present. In *Drosophila*, approximately 120 copies per haploid genome are each transcribed into a molecule of about 45S. This is processed into the 28S, 18S, and 5.8S rRNA species. These species are homologous to the three rRNA components of *E. coli*. In *Xenopus laevis*, more than 500 copies of the 34S component are present per haploid genome. In mammalian cells, the initial transcript is 45S. The rRNA genes, called **rDNA**, are part of the moderately repetitive DNA fraction and are present in clusters at various chromosomal sites.

Each cluster in eukaryotes consists of **tandem repeats,** with each unit separated by a noncoding **spacer DNA** sequence. In humans, these gene clusters have been localized near the ends of chromosomes 13, 14, 15, 21, and 22. The unique 5S rRNA component of eukaryotes is not part of this larger transcript. Instead, genes coding for the 5S ribosomal component are distinct and located separately. In humans, a gene cluster encoding 5S rRNA has been located on chromosome 1.

Despite their detailed knowledge of the structure and genetic origin of the ribosomal components, a complete understanding of the function of these components has eluded geneticists. This is not surprising; the ribosome is the largest and perhaps the most intricate of all cellular structures. For example, the bacterial monosome has a combined molecular weight of 2.6 million Da!

tRNA Structure

Because of their small size and stability in the cell, transfer RNAs (tRNAs) have been investigated extensively and are the best characterized RNA molecules. They are composed of only 75 to 90 nucleotides, displaying a nearly identical structure in bacteria and eukaryotes. In both types of organisms, tRNAs are transcribed from DNA as larger precursors, which are cleaved into mature 4S tRNA molecules. In *E. coli,* for example, tRNA^{Tyr} (the superscript identifies the specific tRNA by the amino acid that binds to it, called its *cognate amino acid*) is composed of 77 nucleotides, yet its precursor contains 126 nucleotides.

In 1965, Robert Holley and his colleagues reported the complete sequence of tRNA^{Ala} isolated from yeast. Of great interest was their finding that a number of nucleotides are unique to tRNA, each containing a so-called *modified base.* As illustrated in **Figure 14–2**, each of these nucleotides contains a modification of one of the four nitrogenous bases expected in RNA (G, C, A, and U). Shown are inosinic acid (which contains the purine hypoxanthine), ribothymidylic acid, and pseudouridine. These modified structures are created *after* transcription of tRNA, illustrating the more general concept of **posttranscriptional modification**. In this case, an enzymatic reaction modifies the base called for by the genetic code during transcription. While it is still not clear why such modified bases are created, it is believed that their presence enhances hydrogen bonding efficiency during translation.

Holley's sequence analysis led him to propose the two-dimensional **cloverleaf model of tRNA**. It had been known that tRNA has a characteristic secondary structure created by base pairing. Holley discovered that he could arrange the linear sequence in such a way that several stretches of base pairing would result. His arrangement, with its series of paired stems and unpaired loops, resembled the shape of a cloverleaf. The loops consistently contained modified

Inosinic acid (I)   Pseudouridylic acid (Ψ)   Ribothymidylic acid (T)

FIGURE 14–2 Ribonucleotides containing unusual nitrogenous bases are found in transfer RNA.

FIGURE 14–3 Holley's two-dimensional cloverleaf model of transfer RNA. Hydrogen bonds are designated by dots (...).

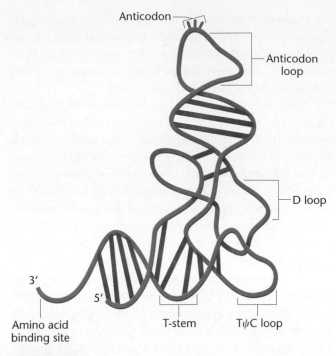

FIGURE 14–4 A three-dimensional model of transfer RNA.

bases that did not generally form base pairs. Holley's model is shown in **Figure 14–3**.

The triplets GCU, GCC, and GCA specify alanine; therefore, Holley looked for an anticodon sequence complementary to one of these codons in his tRNA^{Ala} molecule. He found it in the form of CGI (the 3' to 5' direction) in one loop of the cloverleaf. The nitrogenous base I (inosinic acid) can form hydrogen bonds with U, C, or A, the third members of the alanine triplets. Thus, the **anticodon loop** was established.

Studies of other tRNA species revealed many constant features. First, at the 3' end, all tRNAs contain the sequence (... pCpCpA-3'). At this end of the molecule, the amino acid is covalently joined to the terminal adenosine residue. All tRNAs contain the nucleotide (5'-pG...) at the other end of the molecule. In addition, the lengths of the analogous stems and loops in tRNA molecules are very similar. Each tRNA examined also contains an anticodon complementary to the known codon for the tRNA's cognate amino acid, and all anticodon loops are present in the same position of the cloverleaf.

Because the cloverleaf model was predicted strictly on the basis of nucleotide sequence, there was great interest in the three-dimensional structure that would be revealed by X-ray crystallographic examination of tRNA. By 1974, Alexander Rich and his colleagues in the United States, and J. Roberts, B. Clark, Aaron Klug, and their colleagues in England had

succeeded in crystallizing tRNA and performing X-ray crystallography at a resolution of 3 Å. At such resolution, the pattern formed by individual nucleotides is discernible.

As a result of these studies, a complete three-dimensional model of tRNA is now available (**Figure 14–4**). Both the anticodon loop and the 3'-acceptor region (to which the amino acid is covalently linked) have been located. Geneticists speculate that the shapes of the intervening loops are recognized by the enzymes responsible for attaching amino acids to tRNAs—a subject to which we now turn our attention.

Charging tRNA

Before translation can proceed, the tRNA molecules must be chemically linked to their respective amino acids. This activation process, called **charging**, or *aminoacylation*, occurs under the direction of enzymes called **aminoacyl tRNA synthetases**. Because there are 20 different amino acids, there must be at least 20 different tRNA molecules and as many different enzymes. In theory, because there are 61 triplets that encode amino acids, there could be 61 specific tRNAs and enzymes. However, because of the ability of the third member of a triplet code to "wobble," the minimum number of different tRNAs required is only 31. In actuality, there are more than this number. It is also believed that there are only 20 synthetases, one for each amino acid, regardless of the greater number of corresponding tRNAs.

The charging process is outlined in **Figure 14–5**. In the initial step, the amino acid is converted to an activated form, reacting with ATP to create an **aminoacyladenylic**

Enzyme

Aminoacyl tRNA
synthetase[x]

Amino acid   ATP

Aminoacyladenylic acid

Activated enzyme complex

tRNA[x]

3'

Aminoacyl tRNA
synthetase[x]

Charged tRNA[x]

FIGURE 14–5 Steps involved in charging tRNA. The superscript x denotes that only the corresponding specific tRNA and specific aminoacyl tRNA synthetase enzyme are involved in the charging process for each amino acid.

directly in protein synthesis. Aminoacyl tRNA synthetases are highly specific enzymes because they recognize only one amino acid and only the tRNAs corresponding to that amino acid, called **isoaccepting tRNAs**. This is a crucial point if fidelity of translation is to be maintained.

NOW SOLVE THIS

14–1 In 1962, F. Chapeville and others reported an experiment in which they isolated radioactive ^{14}C-cysteinyl-tRNA^{Cys} (charged tRNA^{Cys} + cysteine). They then removed the sulfur group from the cysteine, creating alanyl-tRNA^{Cys} (charged tRNA^{Cys} + alanine). When alanyl-tRNA^{Cys} was added to a synthetic mRNA calling for cysteine, but not alanine, a polypeptide chain was synthesized containing alanine. What can you conclude from this experiment?

■ **HINT:** *This problem is concerned with establishing whether tRNA or the amino acid added to the tRNA during charging is responsible for attracting the charged tRNA to mRNA during translation. The key to its solution is the observation that in this experiment, when the triplet codon in mRNA calls for cysteine, alanine is inserted during translation, even though it is the "incorrect" amino acid.*

For more practice, see Problems 8, 9, and 10.

acid. A covalent linkage is formed between the 5′-phosphate group of ATP and the carboxyl end of the amino acid. This reaction occurs in association with the synthetase enzyme, forming a complex that then reacts with a specific tRNA molecule. During the next step, the amino acid is transferred to the appropriate tRNA and bonded covalently to the adenine residue at the 3′ end. The charged tRNA, also referred to as *aminoacyl tRNA*, may then participate

14.2 Translation of mRNA Can Be Divided into Three Steps

Much like transcription, the process of translation can best be described by breaking it into discrete phases. We will consider three such phases, each with its own set of illustrations (Figures 14–6, 14–7, and 14–8), but keep in mind that translation is a dynamic, continuous process. As you read the following discussion, keep track of the step-by-step events depicted in the figures. Many of the protein factors and their roles in translation are presented in Table 14.1.

TABLE 14.1 Various Protein Factors Involved during Translation in *E. coli*

Process	Factor	Role
Initiation of translation	IF1	Binds to 30S subunit and prevents aminoacyl tRNA from binding to the A site
	IF2	Binds f-met-tRNA to 30S-mRNA complex and hydrolyzes GTP
	IF3	Binds to 30S subunit, preventing it from associating with the 50S subunit
Elongation of polypeptide	EF-Tu	Binds GTP; brings aminoacyl tRNA to the A site of the ribosome
	EF-Ts	Generates active EF-Tu
	EF-G	Stimulates translocation; GTP-dependent
Termination of translation and release of polypeptide	RF1	Catalyzes release of the polypeptide chain from tRNA and dissociation of the translocation complex; specific for UAA and UAG termination codons
	RF2	Behaves like RF1; specific for UGA and UAA codons
	RF3	Stimulates RF1 and RF2

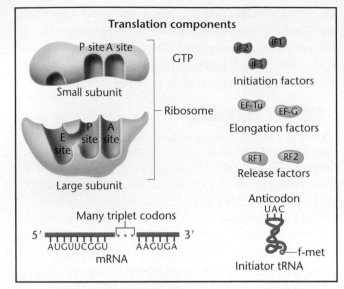

Translation components

P site A site

GTP

Small subunit

Ribosome

E site / P site / A site

Large subunit

Initiation factors

IF2 IF1 IF3

Elongation factors

EF-Tu EF-G

Release factors

RF1 RF2

Anticodon
UAC

Many triplet codons

5′ AUGUUCGGU ... AAGUGA 3′
mRNA

f-met
Initiator tRNA

FIGURE 14–6 Initiation of translation. The separate components are depicted at the left of the figure.

Initiation of Translation

1.

IF3 P A IF1

5′ AUG UUC GGU ... AAGUGA 3′

UAC

IF2 + GTP

Initiation factors bind to small subunit and attract mRNA.

2.

IF3

P A IF1

5′ AUG UUC GGU ... AAGUGA 3′
UAC

IF2 GTP

Initiation complex

tRNA^fmet binds to AUG codon of mRNA in P site, forming initiation complex; IF3 is released.

3.

IF1

P A

5′ AUG UUCGGU ... AAGUGA 3′
UAC

AAG
+ EF-Tu + GTP

IF2 + GDP

Large subunit binds to complex; IF1 and IF2 are released. Subsequent aminoacyl tRNA is poised to enter the A site.

Initiation

Initiation of prokaryotic translation is depicted in **Figure 14–6**. Recall that the ribosome serves as a nonspecific workbench for the translation process. Ribosomes, when they are not

---

involved in translation, are dissociated into their large and small subunits. Initiation of translation in *E. coli* involves the small ribosomal subunit, an mRNA molecule, a specific charged initiator tRNA, GTP, Mg^{2+}, and three proteinaceous **initiation factors (IFs)** that enhance the binding affinity of the various translational components and facilitate the process. In prokaryotes, the initiation codon of mRNA—AUG—calls for the modified amino acid *N*-**formylmethionine (f-met)**.

The three initiation factors first bind to the small ribosomal subunit, and this complex in turn binds to mRNA (Step 1). In bacteria, this binding involves a sequence of up to six ribonucleotides (AGGAGG, not shown in Figure 14–6) that *precedes* the initial AUG start codon of mRNA. This sequence—containing only purines and called the **Shine–Dalgarno sequence**—base-pairs with a region of the 16S rRNA of the small ribosomal subunit, facilitating initiation.

While IF1 primarily blocks the A site from being bound to a tRNA and IF3 serves to inhibit the small subunit from associating with the large subunit, IF2 plays a more direct role in initiation. Essentially a GTPase, IF2 interacts with the mRNA and the charged tRNA, stabilizing them in the P site (Step 2). This step "sets" the reading frame so that all subsequent groups of three ribonucleotides are translated accurately. The aggregate, upon release of IF3, then combines with the large ribosomal subunit to create the 70S initiation complex. In this process, a molecule of GTP linked to IF2 is hydrolyzed, providing the required energy, and IF1 and 2 are subsequently released (Step 3).

Elongation

The second phase of translation, elongation, is depicted in **Figure 14–7**. As per our discussion above, the initiation complex is now poised for the insertion into the A site of the second aminoacyl tRNA bearing the amino acid corresponding to the second triplet sequence on the mRNA. Charged tRNAs are transported into the complex by one of the elongation factors, EF-Tu (Step 1). Like IF2 during initiation, EF-Tu is a GTPase and is bound by a GTP, the hydrolysis of which provides energy for the process.

The next step is for the terminal amino acid in the P site (methionine in this case) to be linked to the amino acid now present on the tRNA in the A site by the formation of a peptide bond. Such lengthening of the growing polypeptide chain by one amino acid is called **elongation**. Just prior to this, the covalent bond between the tRNA occupying the P site and its cognate amino acid is hydrolyzed (broken). The newly formed dipeptide remains attached to the end of the tRNA still residing in the A site (Step 2). These reactions were initially believed to be catalyzed by an enzyme called **peptidyl transferase**, embedded in the large subunit of the ribosome. However, it is now clear that this catalytic activity is a function of the 23S rRNA of the large subunit. In such a case, as we saw with splicing of pre-mRNAs (see Chapter 13), we refer to the complex as a **ribozyme**, recognizing the catalytic role that RNA plays in the process.

Before elongation can be repeated, the tRNA attached to the P site, which is now uncharged, must be released from the large subunit. The uncharged tRNA moves briefly into a third site on the ribosome called the **E (exit) site**. The entire **mRNA–tRNA–aa₂–aa₁** complex then shifts in the direction of the P site by a distance of three nucleotides (Step 3). This event, called *translocation*, requires several protein elongation factors (EFs). While it was originally thought that the energy derived from hydrolysis of GTP was essential for translocation, the energy produced is now thought to lock the proper structures in place during each step of elongation. The result is that the third codon of mRNA has now moved into the A site and is ready to accept its specific charged tRNA (Step 4). One simple way to distinguish the two sites in your mind is to remember that, *following the shift*, the P site (*P* for peptide) contains a tRNA attached to a peptide chain, whereas the A site (*A* for amino acid) contains a charged tRNA with its amino acid attached (an aminoacyl tRNA).

The sequence of elongation and translocation is repeated over and over (Steps 4 and 5). An additional amino acid is added to the growing polypeptide chain each time the mRNA advances by three nucleotides through the ribosome. Once a polypeptide chain of reasonable size is assembled (about 30 amino acids), it begins to emerge from the base of the large subunit, as illustrated in Step 6. The large subunit contains a tunnel through which the elongating polypeptide emerges.

As we have seen, the role of the small subunit during elongation is to "decode" the codons in the mRNA, while the role of the large subunit is peptide-bond synthesis. The efficiency of the process is remarkably high: The observed error

1.   Elongation during Translation

Second charged tRNA has entered A site, facilitated by EF-Tu; first elongation step commences.

Peptide bond forms; uncharged tRNA moves to the E site and subsequently out of the ribosome; the mRNA has been translocated three bases to the left, causing the tRNA bearing the dipeptide to shift into the P site.

The first elongation step is complete, facilitated by EF-G. The third charged tRNA is ready to enter the A site.

Third charged tRNA has entered A site, facilitated by EF-Tu; second elongation step begins.

Tripeptide formed; second elongation step completed; uncharged tRNA moves to E site.

Polypeptide chain synthesized and exits the ribosome.

FIGURE 14–7   Elongation of the growing polypeptide chain during translation.

1. Termination of Translation

Termination codon enters A site; RF1 or RF2 stimulates hydrolysis of the polypeptide from peptidyl tRNA.

2.

Ribosomal subunits dissociate and mRNA is released; polypeptide folds into native 3-D conformation of protein; charged tRNA released.

FIGURE 14–8 Termination of the process of translation.

Termination

Termination, the third phase of translation, is depicted in **Figure 14–8**. The process is signaled by the presence of any one of the three possible triplet codons appearing in the A site: UAG, UAA, or UGA. These codons do not specify an amino acid, nor do they call for a tRNA in the A site. They are called **stop codons, termination codons,** or **nonsense codons.** Often, several consecutive stop codons are part of an mRNA. When one such termination stop codon is encountered, the polypeptide, now completed, is still part of the peptidyl tRNA in the P site, and the A site is empty. The termination codon signals the action of a **GTP-dependent release factor,** which stimulates hydrolysis of the polypeptide from the peptidyl tRNA, leading to its release from the translation complex (Step 1). Then, the tRNA is released from the ribosome, which then dissociates into its subunits (Step 2). In prokaryotes there are two release factors, RF1 and RF2, each specific to two of the three stop codons. If a termination codon should appear in the middle of an mRNA molecule as a result of mutation, the same process occurs, and the polypeptide chain is prematurely terminated.

Polyribosomes

As elongation proceeds and the initial portion of an mRNA molecule has passed through the ribosome, this portion of mRNA is free to associate with another small subunit to form a second initiation complex. The process can be repeated several times with a single mRNA and results in what are called **polyribosomes,** or just **polysomes.**

After cells are gently lysed in the laboratory, polyribosomes can be isolated from them and analyzed. The photos in **Figure 14–9** show these complexes as seen under the electron microscope. In **Figure 14–9(a),** you can see

rate is only about 10^{-4}. At this rate, an incorrect amino acid will occur only once in every 20 polypeptides of an average length of 500 amino acids! Elongation in *E. coli* proceeds at a rate of about 15 amino acids per second at 37°C.

(a)

(b)

FIGURE 14–9 Polyribosomes as seen under the electron microscope. (a) Examples derived from rabbit reticulocytes engaged in the translation of hemoglobin mRNA. (b) Examples taken from salivary gland cells of the midgefly, *Chironomus thummi.* Note that the nascent polypeptide chains are apparent as they emerge from each ribosome. Their length increases as translation proceeds from left to right along the mRNA.

the thin lines of mRNA between the individual ribosomes. The micrograph in **Figure 14–9(b)** is even more remarkable, for it shows the polypeptide chains emerging from the ribosomes during translation. The formation of polysome complexes represents an efficient use of the components available for protein synthesis during a unit of time. Using the analogy of a tape and a tape recorder, in polysome complexes, we would thread and play one tape (mRNA) simultaneously through several recorders (the ribosomes). At any given moment, each recorder would be playing a different part of the song (the polypeptide being synthesized in each ribosome).

14.3 High-Resolution Studies Have Revealed Many Details about the Functional Prokaryotic Ribosome

Our knowledge of the process of translation and the structure of the ribosome, as described in the previous sections, is based primarily on biochemical and genetic observations, in addition to the visualization of ribosomes under the electron microscope. To confirm and refine this information, the next step is to examine the ribosome at even higher levels of resolution. For example, X-ray diffraction analysis of ribosome crystals is one way to achieve this. However, because of its tremendous size and the complexity of molecular interactions occurring in the functional ribosome, it was extremely difficult to obtain the crystals necessary to perform X-ray diffraction studies. Nevertheless, great strides have been made over the past decade. First, the individual ribosomal subunits were crystallized and examined in several laboratories, most prominently that of V. Ramakrishnan. Then, the crystal structure of the intact 70S ribosome, complete with associated mRNA and tRNAs, was examined by Harry Noller and colleagues. In essence, the entire translational complex was seen at the atomic level. Both Ramakrishnan and Noller derived the ribosomes from the bacterium *Thermus thermophilus*.

Many noteworthy observations have been made from these investigations. For example, the sizes and shapes of the subunits, measured at atomic dimensions, are in agreement with earlier estimates based on high-resolution electron microscopy. Furthermore, the shape of the ribosome changes during different functional states, attesting to the dynamic nature of the process of translation. A great deal has also been learned about the prominence and location of the RNA components of the subunits. For example, about one-third of the 16S RNA is responsible for producing a flat projection, referred to as the *platform*,

within the smaller 30S subunit, and it modulates movement of the mRNA–tRNA complex during translocation. One of the models based on Noller's findings is shown in the opening photograph of this chapter.

Crystallographic analysis also supports the concept that RNA is the real "player" in the ribosome during translation. The interface between the two subunits, considered to be the location in the ribosome where polymerization of amino acids occurs, is composed almost exclusively of RNA. In contrast, the numerous ribosomal proteins are found mostly on the periphery of the ribosome. These observations confirm what has been predicted on genetic grounds—the catalytic steps that join amino acids during translation occur under the direction of RNA, not proteins.

Another interesting finding involves the actual location of the various sites predicted to house tRNAs during translation. All three sites (A, P, and E), have been identified in X-ray diffraction studies, and in each case, the RNA of the ribosome makes direct contact with the various loops and domains of the tRNA molecule. This observation supports the hypotheses that had been developed concerning the roles of the different regions of tRNA and helps us understand why the distinctive three-dimensional conformation that is characteristic of all tRNA molecules has been preserved throughout evolution.

Still another noteworthy observation is that the intervals between the A, P, and E sites are at least 20 Å, and perhaps as much as 50 Å, wide, thus defining the atomic distance that the tRNA molecules must shift during each translocation event. This is considered a fairly large distance relative to the size of the tRNAs themselves. Further analysis has led to the identification of molecular (RNA–protein) bridges existing between the three sites and apparently involved in the translocation events. Other such bridges are present at other key locations and have been related to ribosome function. These observations provide us with a much more complete picture of the dynamic changes that must occur within the ribosome during translation. A final observation takes us back almost 50 years, to when Francis Crick proposed the **wobble hypothesis** (as introduced in Chapter 13). The Ramakrishnan group has identified the precise location along the 16S rRNA of the 30S subunit involved in the decoding step that connects mRNA to the proper tRNA. At this location, two particular nucleotides of the 16S rRNA actually flip out and probe the codon:anticodon region, and are believed to check for accuracy of base pairing during this interaction. According to the wobble hypothesis, the stringency of this step is high for the first two base pairs but less so for the third (or wobble) base pair.

As our knowledge of the translation process in prokaryotes has continued to grow, a remarkable study was reported in 2010 by Niels Fischer and colleagues. Using a unique high-resolution approach—the technique of **time-resolved single particle cryo-electron microscopy (cryo-EM)**—the 70*S E. coli* ribosome was captured and examined while in the process of translation at a resolution of 5.5 Å. In this work, over two million images were obtained and computationally analyzed, establishing a temporal snapshot of the trajectories of tRNA during the process of translocation. This research team examined how tRNA is translocated during elongation of the polypeptide chain. They demonstrated that the trajectories are coupled with dynamic conformational changes in the components of the ribosome. Surprisingly, the work has revealed that during translation, the ribosome behaves as a complex molecular machine *powered by Brownian movement driven by thermal energy.* That is, the energetic requirement for achieving the various conformational changes essential to translocation are inherent to the ribosome itself.

Numerous questions about ribosome structure and function still remain. In particular, the precise role of the many ribosomal proteins is yet to be clarified. Nevertheless, the models that are emerging based on the work of Noller, Ramakrishnan, Fischer, and their many colleagues provide us with a much better understanding of the mechanism of translation.

14.4 Translation Is More Complex in Eukaryotes

The general features of the model we just discussed were initially derived from investigations of the translation process in bacteria. As we have seen (Figure 14–1), one main difference between prokaryotes and eukaryotes is that in the latter, translation occurs on larger ribosomes whose rRNA and protein components are more complex. Interestingly, prokaryotic and eukaryotic rRNAs do share what is called a *core sequence,* but in eukaryotes, they are lengthened by the addition of *expansion sequences* (*ES*), which presumably impart added functionality. Another significant distinction is that whereas transcription and translation are coupled in prokaryotes, in eukaryotes these two processes are separated both spatially and temporally. In eukaryotic cells transcription occurs in the nucleus and translation in the cytoplasm. This separation provides multiple opportunities for regulation of genetic expression in eukaryotic cells.

A number of aspects of the initiation of translation vary in eukaryotes. Three differences center on the mRNA that is being translated. First, the 5′ end of mRNA is capped with a 7-methylguanosine (7-mG) residue at maturation (see Chapter 13). The presence of the cap, absent in prokaryotes,

is essential for efficient initiation of translation. A second difference is that many mRNAs contain a purine (A or G) three bases upstream from the AUG initiator codon, which is followed by a G (A/GNNAUGG). Named after its discoverer, Marilyn Kozak, its presence in eukaryotes is considered to increase the efficiency of translation by interacting with the initator tRNA. This **Kozak sequence** is considered analogous to the *Shine-Dalgarno* sequence found in the upstream region of prokaryotic mRNAs.

Third, eukaryotic mRNAs require the posttranscriptional addition of a **poly-A tail** on their 3′ end; that is, they are *polyadenylated.* In the absence of poly A, these potential messages are rapidly degraded in the cytoplasm. Interestingly, histone mRNAs serve as an exception and are not polyadenylated. Still another difference related to initiation of translation is that in eukaryotes the amino acid formylmethionine is not required as it is in prokaryotes. However, the AUG triplet, which encodes methionine, is essential to the formation of the translational complex, and a unique transfer RNA ($tRNA_i^{Met}$) is used during initiation.

Still other differences are noteworthy. Eukaryotic mRNAs are much longer lived than are their prokaryotic counterparts. Most exist for hours rather than minutes prior to degradation by nucleases in the cell; thus they remain available much longer to orchestrate protein synthesis. And, during translation, protein factors similar to those in prokaryotes guide the initiation, elongation, and termination of translation in eukaryotes. Many of these eukaryotic factors are clearly homologous to their counterparts in prokaryotes. However, a greater number of factors are usually required during each step, and some are more complex than in prokaryotes. Finally, recall that in eukaryotes many, but not all, of the cell's ribosomes are found in association with the membranes that make up the endoplasmic reticulum (forming the rough ER). Such membranes are absent from the cytoplasm of prokaryotic cells. This association in eukaryotes facilitates the secretion of newly synthesized proteins from the ribosomes directly into the channels of the endoplasmic reticulum. Recent studies using electron microscopy have established how this occurs. A *tunnel* in the large subunit of the ribosome begins near the point where the two subunits interface and exits near the back of the large subunit. The location of the tunnel within the large subunit is the basis for the belief that it provides the conduit for the movement of the newly synthesized polypeptide chain out of the ribosome. In studies in yeast, newly synthesized polypeptides enter the ER through a membrane channel formed by a specific protein, Sec61. This channel is perfectly aligned with the exit point of the ribosomal tunnel. In prokaryotes, the polypeptides are released by the ribosome directly into the cytoplasm.

We conclude this section by noting that at the end of 2010, after years of work, the crystal structure of the highly complex 80S eukaryotic ribosome has now been visualized by Marat Yusupov and colleagues at the remarkable resolution of 4.15 Å. This research, focusing on the yeast ribosome, is beginning to reveal at the atomic level how many of the eukaryote-specific aspects of translation are achieved. For one, it has been established that as the mRNA shifts by three nucleotides during translation (the process of translocation), a 4°–5° CW rotation of the small subunit occurs. As expected, translation is indeed a dynamic process as the subunits shift with relationship to one another as the mRNA proceeds through the ribosome. Further analysis at such a resolution will no doubt provide greater insights into the interactions of mRNA and tRNA with the components of the ribosome, and thus a better understanding of the process in eukaryotes.

14.5 The Initial Insight That Proteins Are Important in Heredity Was Provided by the Study of Inborn Errors of Metabolism

Now, let's consider how we know that proteins are the end products of genetic expression. The first insight into the role of proteins in genetic processes was provided by observations made by Sir Archibald Garrod and William Bateson early in the twentieth century. Garrod was born into an English family of medical scientists. His father was a physician with a strong interest in the chemical basis of rheumatoid arthritis, and his eldest brother was a leading zoologist in London. As a practicing physician, Garrod himself became interested in several human disorders that seemed to be inherited. Although he also studied albinism and cystinuria, we will describe his investigation of the disorder **alkaptonuria**. Individuals afflicted with this disorder have a disruption in an important metabolic pathway (**Figure 14–10**). As a result, they cannot metabolize the alkapton 2,5-dihydroxyphenylacetic acid, also known as homogentisic acid. Homogentisic acid thus accumulates in their cells and tissues and is excreted in the urine. The molecule's oxidation products are black and easily detectable in the diapers of newborns. The unmetabolized products tend to accumulate in cartilaginous areas, causing a darkening of the ears and nose. In joints, this deposition leads to a benign arthritic condition. Alkaptonuria is a rare but not serious disease that persists throughout an individual's life.

Garrod studied alkaptonuria by looking for patterns of inheritance of this benign trait. Eventually he concluded that it was genetic in nature. Of 32 known cases, he ascertained that 19 were confined to 7 families, with one family having four affected siblings. In several instances, the parents were unaffected but known to be related as first cousins, and therefore *consanguineous*, a term describing relatives having a common recent ancestor. Parents who are so related have a higher probability than unrelated parents of producing offspring that express recessive traits, because such parents are both more likely to be heterozygous for some of the

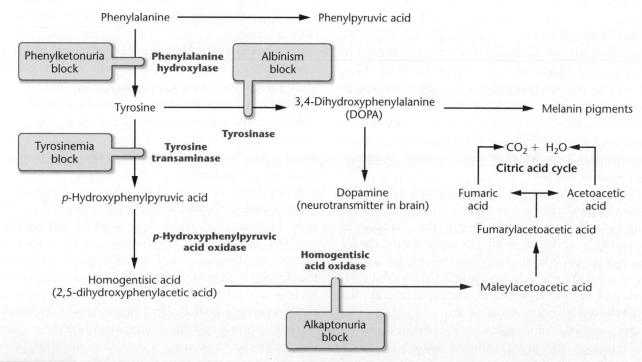

FIGURE 14–10 Metabolic pathway involving phenylalanine and tyrosine. Various metabolic blocks resulting from mutations lead to the disorders phenylketonuria, alkaptonuria, albinism, and tyrosinemia.

same recessive traits (see Chapter 25). Garrod concluded that this inherited condition was the result of an alternative mode of metabolism, thus implying that hereditary information controls chemical reactions in the body. While *genes* and *enzymes* were not familiar terms during Garrod's time, he used the corresponding concepts of *unit factors* and *ferments*. Garrod published his initial observations in 1902.

Only a few geneticists, including Bateson, were familiar with and made reference to Garrod's work. Garrod's ideas fit nicely with Bateson's belief that inherited conditions were caused by the lack of some critical substance. In 1909, Bateson published *Mendel's Principles of Heredity*, in which he linked ferments with heredity. However, for almost 30 years, most geneticists failed to see the relationship between genes and enzymes. Garrod and Bateson, like Mendel, were ahead of their time.

Phenylketonuria

It is interesting to note that the inherited human metabolic disorder **phenylketonuria (PKU)** results when another reaction in the pathway shown in Figure 14–10 is blocked. Described first in 1934, this disorder can result in mental retardation and is transmitted as an autosomal recessive disease. Afflicted individuals are unable to convert the amino acid phenylalanine to the amino acid tyrosine. These molecules differ by only a single hydroxyl group (OH), present in tyrosine but absent in phenylalanine. The reaction is catalyzed by the enzyme **phenylalanine hydroxylase**, which is inactive in affected individuals and active at a level of about 30 percent in heterozygotes. The enzyme functions in the liver. While the normal blood level of phenylalanine is about 1 mg/100 mL, people with phenylketonuria show a level as high as 50 mg/100 mL.

As phenylalanine accumulates, it may be converted to phenylpyruvic acid and, subsequently, to other derivatives. These are less efficiently resorbed by the kidney and tend to spill into the urine more quickly than phenylalanine. Both phenylalanine and its derivatives enter the cerebrospinal fluid, resulting in elevated levels in the brain. The presence of these substances during early development is thought to cause mental retardation.

Phenylketonuria occurs in approximately 1 in 11,000 births, and newborns are routinely screened for PKU throughout the United States. When the condition is detected in the analysis of an infant's blood, a strict dietary regimen is instituted in time to prevent retardation. A low-phenylalanine diet can reduce by-products such as phenylpyruvic acid, and the development of abnormalities characterizing the disease can be diminished.

Our knowledge of inherited metabolic disorders such as alkaptonuria and phenylketonuria initially caused a revolution in medical thinking and practice. Human disease, once thought to be solely attributable to the action of invading microorganisms, viruses, or parasites, clearly can have a genetic basis. We know now that hundreds of medical conditions are caused by errors in metabolism resulting from mutant genes. These human biochemical disorders include all classes of organic biomolecules.

14.6 Studies of *Neurospora* Led to the One-Gene:One-Enzyme Hypothesis

In two separate investigations beginning in 1933, George Beadle provided the first convincing experimental evidence that genes are directly responsible for the synthesis of enzymes. The first investigation, conducted in collaboration with Boris Ephrussi, involved *Drosophila* eye pigments. Together, Beadle and Ephrussi confirmed that mutant genes that altered the eye color of fruit flies could be linked to biochemical errors that, in all likelihood, involved the loss of enzyme function. Encouraged by these findings, Beadle then joined with Edward Tatum to investigate nutritional mutations in the pink bread mold *Neurospora crassa*. This investigation led to the **one-gene:one-enzyme hypothesis**.

Analysis of *Neurospora* Mutants by Beadle and Tatum

In the early 1940s, Beadle and Tatum chose to work with *Neurospora* because much was known about its biochemistry, and mutations could be induced and isolated with relative ease. By inducing mutations, they produced strains that had genetic blocks of reactions essential to the growth of the organism.

Beadle and Tatum knew that this mold could manufacture nearly every biomolecule necessary for normal development. For example, using rudimentary carbon and nitrogen sources, the organism can synthesize nine water-soluble vitamins, 20 amino acids, numerous carotenoid pigments, and all essential purines and pyrimidines. Beadle and Tatum irradiated asexual conidia (spores) with X rays to increase the frequency of mutations and then grew the spores on "complete" medium containing all the necessary growth factors (e.g., vitamins and amino acids). Under such growth conditions, a mutant strain unable to grow on minimal medium would be able to grow by ingesting the supplements present in the enriched, complete medium. All the cultures were then transferred to minimal medium. Any organisms capable of growing on the minimal medium must be able to synthesize all the necessary growth factors themselves, and the researchers could conclude that the cultures from which those organisms came did not contain a nutritional mutation. If no growth occurred, then it was concluded that the culture that had not been able to grow contained a nutritional mutation.

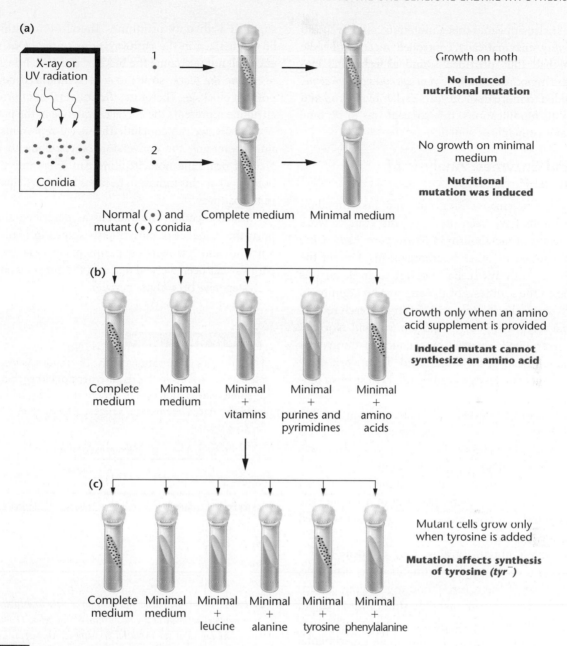

FIGURE 14–11 Induction, isolation, and characterization of a nutritional auxotrophic mutation in *Neurospora*. (a) Most conidia (blue) are not affected, but one conidium (shown in red) contains a mutation (b and c). The precise nature of the mutation is established and found to involve the biosynthesis of tyrosine.

The next task was to determine the type of nutritional mutation. The results are shown in **Figure 14–11(a)**.

Many thousands of individual spores derived by this procedure were isolated and grown on complete medium. In subsequent tests on minimal medium, many cultures failed to grow, indicating that a nutritional mutation had been induced. To identify the mutant type, the mutant strains were tested on a series of different incomplete media [**Figure 14–11(b)** and **Figure 14–11(c)**], each containing different groups of supplements, and subsequently on media containing single vitamins, amino acids, purines, or pyrimidines as supplements, until one specific supplement that permitted growth was found. Beadle and Tatum reasoned

that the supplement that restored growth was the molecule that the mutant strain could not synthesize.

The first mutant strain isolated required vitamin B_6 (pyridoxine) in the medium, and the second one required vitamin B_1 (thiamine). Using the same procedure, Beadle and Tatum eventually isolated and studied hundreds of mutants deficient in the ability to synthesize other vitamins, amino acids, nucleotides, or other substances.

The findings derived from testing more than 80,000 spores convinced Beadle and Tatum that genetics and biochemistry have much in common. It seemed likely that each nutritional mutation caused the loss of the enzymatic activity that facilitates an essential reaction in wild-type organisms. It also appeared that a mutation could be found for nearly any enzymatically controlled reaction. Beadle and Tatum had thus provided sound experimental evidence for the hypothesis that *one gene specifies one enzyme,* an idea alluded to more than 30 years earlier by Garrod and Bateson. With modifications, this concept was to become another major principle of genetics.

Genes and Enzymes: Analysis of Biochemical Pathways

The one-gene:one-enzyme concept and its attendant research methods have been used over the years to work out many details of metabolism in *Neurospora, Escherichia coli,* and a number of other microorganisms. One of the first metabolic pathways to be investigated in detail was that leading to the synthesis of the amino acid arginine in *Neurospora.* By studying seven mutant strains, each requiring arginine for growth (*arg⁻*), Adrian Srb and Norman Horowitz ascertained a partial biochemical pathway that leads to the synthesis of the amino acid. Their work demonstrates how genetic analysis can be used to establish biochemical information.

Srb and Horowitz tested each mutant strain's ability to reestablish growth if either citrulline or ornithine, two compounds with close chemical similarity to arginine, was used as a supplement to minimal medium. If either was able to substitute for arginine, they reasoned that it must be involved in the biosynthetic pathway of arginine. The researchers found that both molecules could be substituted in one or more strains.

Of the seven mutant strains, four of them (*arg 4* through *arg 7*) grew if supplied with citrulline, ornithine, or arginine. Two of them (*arg 2* and *arg 3*) grew if supplied with citrulline or arginine. One strain (*arg 1*) would grow only if arginine were supplied; neither citrulline nor ornithine could substitute for it. From these experimental observations, the following pathway and metabolic blocks for each mutation were deduced:

$$\text{Precursor} \xrightarrow[\text{Enzyme A}]{arg\,4-7} \text{Ornithine} \xrightarrow[\text{Enzyme B}]{arg\,2-3} \text{Citrulline} \xrightarrow[\text{Enzyme C}]{arg\,1} \text{Arginine}$$

The logic supporting these conclusions is as follows: If mutants *arg 4* through *arg 7* can grow regardless of which of the three molecules is supplied as a supplement to minimal medium, the mutations preventing growth must cause a metabolic block that occurs *prior* to the involvement of ornithine, citrulline, or arginine in the pathway. When any one of these three molecules is added, *its presence bypasses the block.* As a result, both citrulline and ornithine appear to be involved in the biosynthesis of arginine. However, the sequence of their participation in the pathway cannot be determined on the basis of these data.

On the other hand, both the *arg 2* and the *arg 3* mutations grow if supplied with citrulline, but not if they are supplied with only ornithine. Therefore, ornithine must be synthesized in the pathway *prior to the block.* Its presence will not overcome the block. Citrulline, however, *does overcome the block,* so it must be synthesized beyond the point of blockage. Therefore, the conversion of ornithine to citrulline represents the correct sequence in the pathway.

Finally, we can conclude that *arg 1* represents a mutation preventing the conversion of citrulline to arginine. Neither ornithine nor citrulline can overcome the metabolic block in this mutation because both participate earlier in the pathway.

Taken together, the analysis as described above supports the sequence of biosynthesis shown in **Figure 14–12.** Since Srb and Horowitz's experiments in 1944, the detailed pathway has been worked out, and the enzymes controlling each step have been characterized.

NOW SOLVE THIS

14–2 A series of mutations in the bacterium *Salmonella typhimurium* results in the requirement of either tryptophan or some related molecule in order for growth to occur. From the data shown here, suggest a biosynthetic pathway for tryptophan:

	Growth Supplement				
Mutation	Minimal Medium	Anthranilic Acid	Indole Glycerol Phosphate	Indole	Tryptophan
trp 8	−	+	+	+	+
trp 2	−	−	+	+	+
trp 3	−	−	−	+	+
trp 1	−	−	−	−	+

■ **HINT:** *This problem asks you to analyze data to establish a biochemical pathway in the bacterium Salmonella. The key to its solution is to understand the principles and to apply the same approach that was used to decipher biochemical pathways in Neurospora.*

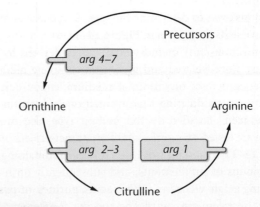

FIGURE 14–12 Abbreviated pathway describing the biosynthesis of arginine in *Neurospora.*

14.7 Studies of Human Hemoglobin Established That One Gene Encodes One Polypeptide

The one-gene:one-enzyme concept developed in the early 1940s was not immediately accepted by all geneticists. This is not surprising, since it was not yet clear how mutant enzymes could cause variation in the many different kinds of phenotypic traits. For example, *Drosophila* mutants demonstrated altered eye size, wing shape, wing vein pattern, and so on. Plants exhibited mutant varieties of seed texture, height, and fruit size. How an inactive mutant enzyme could result in such phenotypes was puzzling to many geneticists.

Two factors soon modified the one-gene:one-enzyme hypothesis. First, while *nearly all enzymes are proteins, not all proteins are enzymes*. As the study of biochemical genetics proceeded, it became clear that all proteins are specified by the information stored in genes, leading to the more accurate phraseology **one-gene:one-protein hypothesis**. Second, proteins often have a subunit structure consisting of two or more polypeptide chains. This is the basis of the quaternary structure of proteins, which we will discuss later in the chapter. Because each distinct polypeptide chain is encoded by a separate gene, a more modern statement of Beadle and Tatum's basic principle is **one-gene:one-polypeptide chain hypothesis**. The need for these modifications of the original hypothesis became apparent during the analysis of hemoglobin structure in individuals afflicted with sickle-cell anemia.

Sickle-Cell Anemia

The first direct evidence that genes specify proteins other than enzymes came from the work on mutant hemoglobin molecules derived from humans afflicted with the disorder **sickle-cell anemia**. Affected individuals have erythrocytes that, under low oxygen tension, become elongated and curved because of the polymerization of hemoglobin. The sickle shape of these erythrocytes is in contrast to the biconcave disc shape characteristic in unaffected individuals (**Figure 14–13**). Those with the disease suffer attacks when red blood cells aggregate in the venous side of capillary systems, where oxygen tension is very low. As a result, a variety of tissues are deprived of oxygen and suffer severe damage. When this occurs, an individual is said to experience a *sickle-cell crisis*. If untreated, a crisis may be fatal. The kidneys, muscles, joints, brain, gastrointestinal tract, and lungs can be affected.

In addition to suffering crises, these individuals are anemic because their erythrocytes are destroyed more rapidly than normal red blood cells. Compensatory

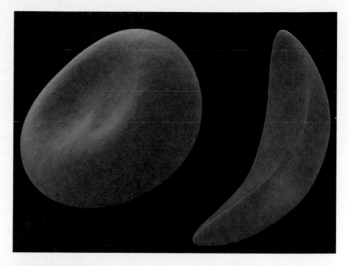

FIGURE 14–13 A comparison of a normal erythrocyte (left) with one derived from a patient with sickle-cell anemia (right).

physiological mechanisms include increased red-cell production by bone marrow and accentuated heart action. These mechanisms lead to abnormal bone size and shape as well as dilation of the heart.

In 1949, James Neel and E. A. Beet demonstrated that the disease is inherited as a Mendelian trait. Pedigree analysis revealed three genotypes and phenotypes controlled by a single pair of alleles, Hb^A and Hb^S. Unaffected and affected individuals result from the homozygous genotypes Hb^A/Hb^A and Hb^S/Hb^S, respectively. The red blood cells of heterozygotes, who exhibit the **sickle-cell trait** but not the disease, undergo much less sickling because more than half of their hemoglobin is normal. Though largely unaffected, such heterozygotes are "carriers" of the defective gene, which is transmitted on average to 50 percent of their offspring.

In the same year, Linus Pauling and his coworkers provided the first insight into the molecular basis of sickle-cell anemia. They showed that hemoglobins isolated from diseased and normal individuals differ in their rates of electrophoretic migration. In electrophoresis (described in Chapter 10), charged molecules migrate in an electric field. If the net charge of two molecules is different, their rates of migration will be different. Hence, Pauling and his colleagues concluded that a chemical difference exists between normal and sickle-cell hemoglobin. The two molecules are now designated **HbA** and **HbS**, respectively.

Figure 14–14(a) illustrates the migration pattern of hemoglobin derived from individuals of all three possible genotypes when subjected to **starch gel electrophoresis**. The gel provides the supporting medium for the molecules during migration. In this experiment, samples were placed at a point of origin between the cathode (−) and the anode

(a) Anode (+)

Starch gel → **Electrophoresis** → Migration

— Origin —

AA   AS   SS   *AA   AS   SS*

Cathode (−)

Fingerprints of peptide fragments

(b)

Altered peptide

Normal HbA   Sickle-cell HbS

(c)

NH₂ –Val–His–Leu–Thr–Pro–Glu–Glu– ---- COOH   NH₂ –Val–His–Leu–Thr–Pro–Val–Glu– ---- COOH

#6   #6

Partial amino acid sequences of β chains

FIGURE 14–14 Investigation of hemoglobin derived from Hb^AHb^A, Hb^AHb^S, and Hb^SHb^S individuals using electrophoresis, fingerprinting, and amino acid analysis. Hemoglobin from individuals with sickle-cell anemia (Hb^SHb^S): (a) migrates differently in an electrophoretic field; (b) shows an altered peptide in fingerprint analysis; and (c) shows an altered amino acid, valine, at the sixth position in the β chain. During electrophoresis, heterozygotes (Hb^AHb^S) are shown to have both forms of hemoglobin.

(+), and an electric current was applied. The migration pattern revealed that all molecules moved toward the anode, indicating a net negative charge. However, HbA migrated farther than HbS, suggesting that its net negative charge was greater. The electrophoretic pattern of hemoglobin derived from individuals who were carriers revealed the presence of both HbA and HbS, and confirmed their heterozygous genotype.

Pauling's findings suggested two possibilities. It was known that hemoglobin consists of four nonproteinaceous, iron-containing *heme groups* and a *globin portion* that contains four polypeptide chains. The alteration in net charge in HbS had to be due, theoretically, to a chemical change in one of these components.

Work carried out between 1954 and 1957 by Vernon Ingram resolved this question. He demonstrated that the chemical change occurs in the primary structure of the globin portion of the hemoglobin molecule. Using the **fingerprinting technique** shown in **Figure 14–14(b)**, Ingram showed that HbS differs in amino acid composition

compared to HbA. Human adult hemoglobin contains two identical α chains of 141 amino acids and two identical β chains of 146 amino acids in its quaternary structure.

The fingerprinting technique involves the enzymatic digestion of the protein into peptide fragments. The mixture is then placed on absorbent paper and exposed to an electric field, where migration occurs according to net charge. The paper is next turned at a right angle to its first exposure and placed in a solvent, in which chromatographic action causes the migration of the peptides in the second direction. The end result is a two-dimensional separation of the peptide fragments into a distinctive pattern of spots, or a "fingerprint." Ingram's work revealed that HbS and HbA differed by only a single peptide fragment [Figure 14–14(b)]. Further analysis then revealed a single amino acid change: Valine was substituted for glutamic acid at the sixth position of the β chain, accounting for the peptide difference [**Figure 14–14(c)**].

The significance of this discovery has been multifaceted. It clearly establishes that a single gene provides the genetic information for a single polypeptide chain. Studies of HbS also demonstrate that a mutation can affect the phenotype by directing a single amino acid substitution. Also, by providing the explanation for sickle-cell anemia, the concept of inherited **molecular disease** was firmly established. Finally, this work led to a thorough study of human hemoglobins, which has provided valuable genetic insights.

In the United States, sickle-cell anemia is found almost exclusively in the African-American population. It affects about 1 in every 625 African-American infants. Currently, about 50,000 to 75,000 individuals are afflicted. In about 1 of every 145 African-American married couples, both partners are heterozygous carriers. In these cases, each of their children has a 25 percent chance of having the disease.

Human Hemoglobins

Having introduced human hemoglobins in a historical context, we now end the discussion by providing an update of what is currently known about these molecules in our species. Molecular analysis reveals that an individual human produces different types of hemoglobin molecules at different stages of the life cycle. All are tetramers consisting of different combinations of seven distinct polypeptide chains, each encoded by a separate gene. The expression of these various genes is developmentally regulated.

Almost all adult hemoglobin consists of **HbA**, which contains two α and two β **chains**. Recall that the mutation in sickle-cell anemia involves the β chain. HbA represents about 98 percent of all hemoglobin found in an adult's erythrocytes after the age of six months. The remaining 2 percent consists of **HbA$_2$**, a minor adult component. This molecule contains two α chains and two **delta (δ) chains**. The δ chain is very similar to the β chain, consisting of 146 amino acids.

During embryonic and fetal development, quite a different set of hemoglobins is found. The earliest set to develop is called **Gower 1**, containing two **zeta (ζ) chains**, which are most similar to α chains, and two **epsilon (ε) chains**, which are similar to β chains. By eight weeks' gestation, the embryonic form is gradually replaced by still another hemoglobin molecule with still different chains. This molecule is called **HbF**, or **fetal hemoglobin**, and consists of two α chains and two **gamma (γ) chains**. There are two types of γ chains, designated $^G\gamma$ and $^A\gamma$. Both are similar to β chains and differ from each other by only a single amino acid. These persist until birth, after which HbF is, again gradually, replaced with HbA and HbA$_2$. The nomenclature and sequence of appearance of the five tetramers we have described are summarized in Table 14.2.

TABLE 14.2 Chain Compositions of Human Hemoglobins from Conception to Adulthood

Hemoglobin Type	Chain Composition
Embryonic-Gower 1	$\zeta_2 \varepsilon_2$
Fetal-HbF	$\alpha_2\, ^G\gamma_2$
	$\alpha_2\, ^A\gamma_2$
Adult-HbA	$\alpha_2\, \beta_2$
Minor adult-HbA$_2$	$\alpha_2\, \delta_2$

EVOLVING CONCEPT OF THE GENE

In the 1940s, a time when the molecular nature of the gene had yet to be defined, groundbreaking work of Beadle and Tatum provided the first experimental evidence concerning the product of genes, their "one-gene:one-enzyme" hypothesis. This idea received further support and was later modified to indicate that one gene specifies one polypeptide chain. ∎

14.8 The Nucleotide Sequence of a Gene and the Amino Acid Sequence of the Corresponding Protein Exhibit Colinearity

Once it was established that genes specify the synthesis of polypeptide chains, the next logical question was how the genetic information contained in the nucleotide sequence of a gene can serve as the basis for creating the amino acid sequence of a polypeptide chain. It seemed most likely that a colinear relationship would exist between the two molecules. That is, the order of nucleotides in the DNA of a gene would correlate directly with the order of amino acids in the corresponding polypeptide—the concept of **colinearity**.

The initial experimental evidence in support of this concept was derived from Charles Yanofsky's studies of the *trpA* gene that encodes the A subunit of the enzyme *tryptophan synthetase* in *E. coli*. Yanofsky isolated many independent mutants that had lost the activity of the enzyme. He then mapped the various mutations, establishing their location with respect to one another within the gene. He also determined where the amino acid substitution had occurred in each mutant protein. When the two sets of data were compared, the colinear relationship was apparent. The location of each mutation in the *trpA* gene correlated with the position of the altered amino acid in the A polypeptide of tryptophan synthetase. This comparison is illustrated in **Figure 14–15**.

trpA mutation	A446 A487	A223	A23 A187	A78 A169
trpA gene map	⊢.04⊣——.30———	———.44———	⊢.061⊣———.50———	⊢.016⊣
Normal amino acid	tyr leu	tyr	gly gly	gly ser
Substitution	cys arg	ile	arg val	cys leu
Amino acid position	175 177	183	211 213	234 235

FIGURE 14–15 Demonstration of colinearity between the genetic map of various *trpA* mutations in *E. coli* and the affected amino acids in the protein product. The numbers shown between mutations represent linkage distances.

14.9 Variation in Protein Structure Provides the Basis of Biological Diversity

In contrast to nucleic acids, which store and express genetic information, proteins, as end products of genetic expression, are more closely aligned with biological function. It is the variation in biological function that provides the basis of diversity between cell types and between organisms. What is it about proteins that enable them to perform or control enormous numbers of complex and important cellular activities in an organism? As we will see, the secret of the complexity of protein function lies in the incredible structural diversity of proteins.

At the outset of our discussion, we should differentiate between **polypeptides** and **proteins**. Polypeptides, most simply, are precursors of proteins. Thus, as the amino acid polymer is assembled on and then released from the ribosome during translation, it is called a *polypeptide*. Once a polypeptide subsequently folds up and assumes a functional three-dimensional conformation, it is called a *protein*. In most cases, several polypeptides combine during this process to produce an even higher order of protein structure. It is its three-dimensional conformation in space that is essential to a protein's specific function and that distinguishes it from other proteins.

Like nucleic acids, the polypeptide chains comprising proteins are linear, nonbranched polymers. In the vast majority of organisms, there are 20 amino acids that serve as the subunits (the building blocks) of proteins.* Each amino acid has a **carboxyl group**, an **amino group**, and a **radical (R) group** (a side chain that determines the type of amino acid) bound covalently to a **central carbon (C) atom**. **Figure 14–16** shows the 20 R groups that define the 20 amino acids in proteins. The R groups are varied in structure

and can be divided into four main classes: (1) **nonpolar (hydrophobic)**, (2) **polar (hydrophilic)**, (3) **positively charged**, and (4) **negatively charged**. Because polypeptides are often long polymers, and because each unit in the polymer may be any 1 of 20 amino acids, each with unique chemical properties, enormous variation in the molecule's final conformation and chemical activity is possible. For example, if an average polypeptide is composed of 200 amino acids (a molecular weight of about 20,000 Da), 20^{200} different molecules, each with a unique sequence, can be created from the 20 different building blocks.

Around 1900, German chemist Emil Fischer determined the manner in which the amino acids are bonded together. He showed that the amino group of one amino acid can react with the carboxyl group of another amino acid in a dehydration (condensation) reaction, releasing a molecule of H_2O. The resulting covalent bond is called a **peptide bond** (**Figure 14–17**). Two amino acids linked together constitute a *dipeptide*, three a *tripeptide*, and so on. Once ten or more amino acids are linked by peptide bonds, the chain is referred to as a *polypeptide*. Generally, no matter how long a polypeptide is, it will have an amino group at one end (the N-terminus) and a carboxyl group at the other end (the C-terminus).

---

*Two other amino acids are exceptions to this rule of 20: **selenocysteine (Sec)** and **pyrrolysine (Pyl)**, modified versions of cysteine and lysine, respectively. Sec is found in the active sites of a small number of proteins in the three domains of life (archaea, bacteria, and eukaryotes). The insertion of Sec into polypeptides requires a molecular process that recodes UGA codons, which normally function as stop signals, to serve as Sec codons. Similarly, Pyl is inserted into polypeptide chains in response to the stop codon, UAG, when it is present internally in an mRNA. Pyl is found in several methane-loving bacteria and, as discovered more recently, in a bacterium that lives symbiotically under the skin of an annelid worm.

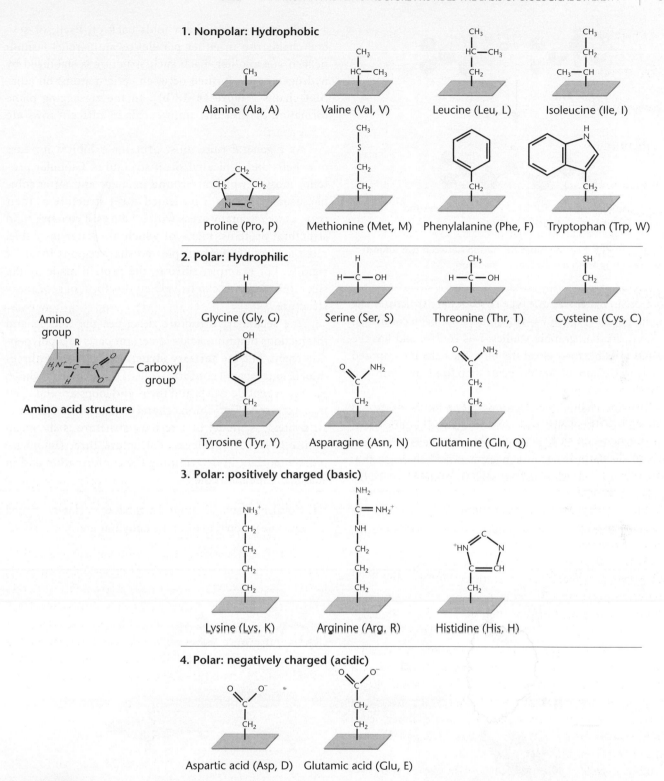

FIGURE 14–16 Chemical structures and designations of the 20 amino acids encoded by living organisms, divided into four major categories. Each amino acid has two abbreviations in universal use; for example, alanine is designated either Ala or A.

Four levels of protein structure are recognized: primary, secondary, tertiary, and quaternary. The sequence of amino acids in the linear backbone of the polypeptide constitutes its **primary structure**. This sequence is specified by the sequence of deoxyribonucleotides in DNA through an mRNA intermediate. The primary structure of a polypeptide helps determine the specific characteristics of the higher orders of organization as a protein is formed.

Secondary structures are certain regular or repeating configurations in space assumed by amino acids lying close to one another in the polypeptide chain. In 1951, Linus Pauling and Robert Corey predicted, on theoretical

Amino end   Carboxyl end

Peptide bond

FIGURE 14–17 Peptide bond formation between two amino acids, resulting from a dehydration reaction.

grounds, an **α helix** as one type of secondary structure. The α-helix model [**Figure 14–18(a)**] has since been confirmed by X-ray crystallographic studies. It is rodlike and has the greatest possible theoretical stability. The helix is composed of a spiral chain of amino acids stabilized by hydrogen bonds.

The side chains (the R groups) of amino acids extend outward from the helix, and each amino acid residue occupies a distance of 1.5 Å in the length of the helix. There are 3.6 residues per turn. Although left-handed helices are theoretically possible, all α helices seen in proteins are right-handed.

Also in 1951, Pauling and Corey proposed another secondary structure, the **β-pleated sheet**. In this model,

a single polypeptide chain folds back on itself, or several chains run in either parallel or antiparallel fashion next to one another. Each such structure is stabilized by hydrogen bonds formed between certain atoms on adjacent chains [**Figure 14–18(b)**]. In the zigzagging plane formation that results, amino acids in adjacent rows are 3.5 Å apart.

As a general rule, most proteins exhibit a mixture of α-helix and β-pleated sheet structures. Globular proteins, most of which are round in shape and water soluble, usually contain a β-pleated sheet structure at their core, as well as many areas with α helices. The more rigid structural proteins, many of which are water insoluble, rely on more extensive β-pleated sheet regions for their rigidity. For example, **fibroin**, the protein made by the silk moth, depends extensively on this form of secondary structure.

The secondary structure describes the folding and interactions of amino acids in certain parts of a polypeptide chain, but the **tertiary structure** defines the three-dimensional spatial conformation of the chain as a whole. Each polypeptide twists and turns and loops around itself in a very specific fashion, characteristic of the particular protein. A model of a tertiary structure is shown in **Figure 14–19.** At this level of structure, three factors are most important in determining the conformation and in stabilizing the molecule:

1. Covalent disulfide bonds form between closely aligned cysteine residues to form the unique amino acid cystine.

(a) α helix   **(b) β-pleated sheet**

Key

Hydrogen bond ——————⫶ O atom

Covalent bond —————— C atom of carboxyl group

Central C atom —————— N atom

R group —————— H atom

⫶—— Hydrogen bond

FIGURE 14–18 (a) The right-handed α helix, which represents one form of secondary structure of a polypeptide chain. (b) The β-pleated sheet, an alternative form of secondary structure of polypeptide chains. To maintain clarity, not all atoms are shown.

FIGURE 14–19 The tertiary level of protein structure for the respiratory pigment myoglobin. The bound oxygen atom is shown in red.

β chain

β chain

α chain

α chain

Heme group

FIGURE 14–20 The quaternary level of protein structure as seen in hemoglobin. Four chains (two α and two β) interact with four heme groups to form the functional molecule.

2. Usually, the polar hydrophilic R groups are located on the surface of the configuration, where they can interact with water.

3. The nonpolar hydrophobic R groups are usually located on the inside of the molecule, where they interact with one another, avoiding interaction with water.

It is important to emphasize that the three-dimensional conformation achieved by any protein is a product of the *primary structure* of the polypeptide. Thus, the genetic code need only specify the sequence of amino acids in order ultimately to produce the final configuration of proteins. The effects of the three stabilizing factors depend on the location of each amino acid relative to all others in the chain. As folding occurs, the most thermodynamically stable conformation results. This level of organization is extremely important because the specific function of any protein is directly related to its tertiary structure.

The concept of **quaternary structure** of proteins applies only to those composed of more than one polypeptide chain and refers to the position of the various chains in relation to one another. This type of protein is *oligomeric*, and each chain in it is a *protomer*, or, less formally, a *subunit*. Protomers have conformations that facilitate their fitting together in a specific complementary fashion. Hemoglobin, an oligomeric protein consisting of four protomers (two α and two β chains), has been studied in great detail. Its quaternary structure is shown in **Figure 14–20**. Most enzymes, including DNA and RNA polymerase, demonstrate quaternary structure.

NOW SOLVE THIS

14–3 HbS results from the substitution of valine for glutamic acid at the number 6 position in the β chain of human hemoglobin. HbC is the result of a change at the same position in the β chain, but in this case lysine replaces glutamic acid. Return to the genetic code table (Figure 13–7) and determine whether single-nucleotide changes can account for these mutations. Then view Figure 14–16 and examine the R groups in the amino acids glutamic acid, valine, and lysine. Describe the chemical differences between the three amino acids. Predict how the changes might alter the structure of the molecule and lead to altered hemoglobin function.

■ **HINT:** *This problem asks you to consider the potential impact of several amino acid substitutions that result from mutations in one of the genes encoding one of the chains making up human hemoglobin. The key to its solution is to consider and compare the structure of the three amino acids (glutamic acid, lysine, and valine) and their net charge.*

14.10 Posttranslational Modification Alters the Final Protein Product

Before we turn to a discussion of protein function, it is important to point out that polypeptide chains, like RNA transcripts, are often modified once they have been synthesized. This additional processing is broadly described as **posttranslational modification**. Although many of these alterations are detailed biochemical transformations and beyond the scope of our discussion, you should be aware that they occur and that they are critical to the functional capability of the final protein product. Several examples of posttranslational modification are as follows:

1. *The N-terminal amino acid is usually removed or modified.* For example, either the formyl group or the entire formylmethionine residue in bacterial polypeptides is usually removed enzymatically. In eukaryotic polypeptide chains, the amino group of the initial methionine residue is often removed, and the amino group of the N-terminal residue may be modified (acetylated).

2. *Individual amino acid residues are sometimes modified.* For example, phosphates may be added to the hydroxyl groups of certain amino acids, such as tyrosine. Modifications such as these create negatively charged residues that may form an ionic bond with other molecules. The process of phosphorylation is extremely important in regulating many cellular activities and is a result of the action of enzymes called *kinases*. At other amino acid residues, methyl groups or acetyl groups may be added enzymatically, which can affect the function of the modified polypeptide chain.

3. *Carbohydrate side chains are sometimes attached.* These are added covalently, producing *glycoproteins*, an important category of cell-surface molecules, such as those specifying the antigens in the ABO blood-type system in humans.

4. *Polypeptide chains may be trimmed.* For example, the insulin gene is first translated into a longer molecule that is enzymatically trimmed to insulin's final 51-amino-acid form.

5. *Signal sequences are removed.* At the N-terminal end of some proteins is a sequence of up to 30 amino acids that plays an important role in directing the protein to the location in the cell in which it functions. This is called a **signal sequence**, and it determines the final destination of a protein in the cell. The process is called **protein targeting**. For example, proteins whose fate involves secretion or proteins that are to become part of the plasma membrane are dependent on specific sequences for their initial transport into the lumen of the endoplasmic reticulum. While the signal sequence of various proteins with a common destination might differ in their primary amino acid sequence, they share many chemical properties. For example, those destined for secretion all contain a string of up to 15 hydrophobic amino acids preceded by a positively charged amino acid at the N-terminus of the signal sequence. Once the polypeptides are transported, but before they achieve their functional status as proteins, the signal sequence is enzymatically removed from them.

6. *Polypeptide chains are often complexed with metals.* The tertiary and quaternary levels of protein structure often include and are dependent on metal atoms. The functional protein is thus a molecular complex that includes both polypeptide chains and metal atoms. Hemoglobin, which contains four iron atoms along with its four polypeptide chains, is a good example.

Protein Folding and Misfolding

It was long thought that **protein folding** was a spontaneous process whereby a linear molecule exiting the ribosome achieved a three-dimensional, thermodynamically stable conformation based solely on the combined chemical properties inherent in the amino acid sequence. This indeed is the case for many proteins. However, numerous studies have shown that for other proteins, correct folding is dependent on members of a family of molecules called **chaperones**. Chaperones are themselves proteins (sometimes called *molecular chaperones* or *chaperonins*) that function by mediating the folding process by excluding the formation of alternative, incorrect patterns. While they may bind to the protein in question, like enzymes, they do not become part of the final product. Initially discovered in *Drosophila*, in which they are called **heat-shock proteins**, chaperones are ubiquitous, having now been discovered in all organisms. They are even present in mitochondria and chloroplasts.

In eukaryotic cells, chaperones are particularly important when translation occurs on membrane-bound ribosomes, where the newly translated polypeptide is extruded into the lumen of the endoplasmic reticulum. Even in their presence, misfolding may still occur, and one more system of "quality control" exists. As misfolded proteins are transported out of the endoplasmic reticulum to the cytoplasm, they are "tagged" by another class of small proteins called **ubiquitins**. A *polyubiquitin–protein complex* is formed that moves to a cellular structure called the **proteasome,** within which the ubiquitins are released and the misfolded proteins are degraded by proteases.

Protein folding is a critically important process, not only because misfolded proteins may be nonfunctional, but also because improperly folded proteins can accumulate and be detrimental to cells and the organisms that contain them. For example, a group of transmissible brain disorders in mammals—scrapie in sheep, **bovine spongiform encephalopathy** (**mad cow disease**) in cattle, and **Creutzfeldt–Jakob disease** in humans—are caused by the presence in the brain of **prions**, which are aggregates of a misfolded protein. The misfolded protein (called PrP^{Sc}) is an altered version of a normal cellular protein (called PrP^{C}) synthesized in neurons and found in the brains of all adult animals. The difference between PrP^{C} and PrP^{Sc} lies in their secondary protein structures. Normal, noninfectious PrP^{C} folds into an α helix, whereas infectious PrP^Sc folds into a β-pleated sheet. When an abnormal PrP^Sc molecule contacts a PrP^C molecule, the normal protein refolds into the abnormal conformation. The process continues as a chain reaction, with potentially devastating results—the formation of prion particles that eventually destroy the brain. Hence, this group of disorders can be considered diseases of secondary protein structure. Currently, many laboratories are studying protein folding and misfolding, particularly as related to genetics. Numerous inherited human disorders are caused by misfolded proteins that form abnormal aggregates. **Sickle-cell anemia,** discussed earlier in this chapter, is a case in point, where the β chains of hemoglobin are altered as the result of a single amino acid change, causing the molecules to aggregate within erythrocytes, with devastating results. An autosomal dominant inherited form of **Creutzfeldt–Jakob disease** is known in which the mutation alters the PrP amino acid sequence, leading to prion formation. And various progressive neurodegenerative diseases such as **Huntington disease, Alzheimer disease**, and **Parkinson disease** are linked to the formation of abnormal protein aggregate in the brain. Huntington disease is inherited as an autosomal dominant trait, whereas less clearly defined genetic components are associated with Alzheimer and Parkinson diseases.

14.11 Proteins Function in Many Diverse Roles

The essence of life on Earth resides at the level of diversity of cellular function. While DNA and RNA serve as vehicles for storing and expressing genetic information, proteins are the *means* of cellular function. And it is the capability of cells to assume diverse structures and functions that distinguishes most eukaryotes from less evolutionarily advanced organisms such as bacteria. Therefore, an introductory understanding of protein function is critical to a complete view of genetic processes.

Proteins are the most abundant macromolecules found in cells. As the end products of genes, they play many diverse roles. For example, the respiratory pigments **hemoglobin** and **myoglobin** transport oxygen, which is essential for cellular metabolism. **Collagen** and **keratin** are structural proteins associated with the skin, connective tissue, and hair of organisms. **Actin** and **myosin** are

contractile proteins, found in abundance in muscle tissue, while **tubulin** is the basis of the function of microtubules in mitotic and meiotic spindles. Still other examples are the **immunoglobulins**, which function in the immune system of vertebrates; **transport proteins**, involved in the movement of molecules across membranes; some of the **hormones** and their **receptors**, which regulate various types of chemical activity; **histones**, which bind to DNA in eukaryotic organisms; and **transcription factors** that regulate gene expression.

Nevertheless, the most diverse and extensive group of proteins (in terms of function) are the **enzymes**, to which we have referred throughout this chapter. Enzymes specialize in catalyzing chemical reactions within living cells. Like all catalysts, they increase the rate at which a chemical reaction reaches equilibrium, but they do not alter the endpoint of the chemical equilibrium. Their remarkable, highly specific catalytic properties largely determine the metabolic capacity of any cell type and provide the underlying basis of what we refer to as **biochemistry**. The specific functions of many enzymes involved in the genetic and cellular processes of cells are described throughout the text.

Biological catalysis is a process whereby enzymes lower the **energy of activation** for a given reaction (**Figure 14–21**). The energy of activation is the increased kinetic energy state that molecules must usually reach before they react with one another. This state can be attained as a result of elevated temperatures, but enzymes allow biological reactions to occur at lower, physiological temperatures. Thus, enzymes make life as we know it possible.

The catalytic properties of an enzyme are determined by the chemical configuration of the molecule's **active site**. This site is associated with a crevice, a cleft, or a pit on the

E = Enzyme
S = Substrate
P = Product

FIGURE 14–21 Energy requirements of an uncatalyzed versus an enzymatically catalyzed chemical reaction. The energy of activation (E_a) necessary to initiate the reaction is substantially lower as a result of catalysis.

surface of the enzyme that binds the reactants, or substrates, and facilitates their interaction. Enzymatically catalyzed reactions control metabolic activities in the cell. Each reaction is either *catabolic* or *anabolic*. **Catabolism** is the degradation of large molecules into smaller, simpler ones with the release of chemical energy. **Anabolism** is the synthetic phase of metabolism, building the various components that make up nucleic acids, proteins, lipids, and carbohydrates.

14.12 Proteins Are Made Up of One or More Functional Domains

We conclude this chapter by briefly discussing the important discovery that distinct regions made up of specific amino acid sequences are associated with unique functions in protein molecules. Such sequences, usually between 50 and 300 amino acids, constitute **protein domains** and represent modular portions of the protein that fold into stable, unique conformations independently of the rest of the molecule. Different domains impart different functional capabilities. Some proteins contain only a single domain, while others contain two or more.

The significance of domains resides in the tertiary structures of proteins. Each domain can contain a mixture of secondary structures, including α helices and β-pleated sheets. The unique conformation of a given domain imparts a specific function to the protein. For example, a domain may serve as the catalytic site of an enzyme, or it may impart an ability to bind to a specific ligand. Thus, discussions of proteins may mention *catalytic domains, DNA-binding domains,* and so on. In short, a protein must be seen as being composed of a series of structural and functional modules. Obviously, the presence of multiple domains in a single protein increases the versatility of each molecule and adds to its functional complexity.

Exon Shuffling

An interesting hypothesis concerning the genetic origin of protein domains was put forward by Walter Gilbert in 1977. Gilbert suggested that the functional regions of genes in higher organisms consist of collections of exons originally present in ancestral genes and brought together through recombination during the course of evolution. Referring to the process as **exon shuffling**, Gilbert proposed that exons, like protein domains, are also modular, and that during evolution exons may have been reshuffled between genes in eukaryotes, with the result that different genes have similar domains.

Several observations lend support to this proposal. Most exons are fairly small, averaging about 150 base pairs and encoding about 50 amino acids, consistent with the sizes of many functional domains in proteins. Second, recombinational events that during evolution may lead to exon shuffling would be expected to occur within areas of genes represented by introns. Because introns are free to accumulate mutations without harm to the organism, recombinational events would tend to further randomize their nucleotide sequences. Over extended evolutionary periods, sequence diversity would increase. This is, in fact, what is observed: Introns range from 50 to 20,000 bases in length and exhibit fairly random base sequences.

Since 1977, a serious research effort has been aimed at analyzing gene structure. In 1985, more direct evidence in favor of Gilbert's proposal of exon modules was presented. For example, the human gene encoding the membrane receptor for low-density lipoproteins (LDLs) was isolated and sequenced. The *LDL receptor protein* is essential to the transport of plasma cholesterol into the cell. It mediates endocytosis and is expected to have numerous functional domains. These include domains capable of binding specifically to the LDL substrates and interacting with other proteins located at different depths within the membrane as the LDL is being transported across it. In addition, the receptor molecule is modified posttranslationally by the addition of a carbohydrate; a domain must exist that links to this carbohydrate. Given these functional constraints, one would predict that the LDL receptor polypeptide would contain several distinct domains.

Detailed analysis of the gene encoding the LDL receptor supports the concept of exon modules and their shuffling during evolution. The gene is quite large—45,000 base pairs—and contains 18 exons, which in turn contain only slightly less than 2600 nucleotides. These exons code the various functional domains of the protein *and* appear to have been recruited from other genes during evolution.

Figure 14–22 shows these relationships. The first exon encodes a signal sequence that is removed from the protein before the LDL receptor becomes part of the membrane. The next five exons, collectively, represent the domain specifying the binding site for cholesterol. This domain is made up of a 40-amino-acid sequence repeated seven

FIGURE 14–22 The 18 exons making up the gene encoding the LDL receptor protein are organized into five functional domains and one signal sequence.

times. The next domain, encoded by eight exons, consists of a sequence of 400 amino acids bearing a striking homology to the peptide-hormone *epidermal growth factor* (*EGF*) in mice (a similar sequence is also found in three blood-clotting proteins). This region contains three repetitive sequences of 40 amino acids. The 15th exon specifies the domain for the posttranslational addition of the carbohydrate, while the next two specify regions of the protein that are integrated into the membrane, anchoring the receptor to specific sites called *coated pits* on the cell surface.

These observations concerning the LDL exons are fairly compelling in support of the theory of exon shuffling during evolution. Certainly, there is no disagreement concerning the concept of protein domains being responsible for specific molecular interactions.

The Origin of Protein Domains

What remains controversial and evocative in the exon-shuffling theory is the question of when introns first appeared on the evolutionary scene. In 1978, W. Ford Doolittle proposed that these intervening sequences were part of the genome of the most primitive ancestors of modern-day eukaryotes. In support of this "intron-early" idea, Gilbert has argued that if similarities in intron DNA sequences are found in identical positions within genes shared by distantly related eukaryotes (such as humans, chickens, and corn), they must have also been present in primitive ancestral genomes.

If Doolittle's proposal is correct, why are introns absent in most prokaryotes and infrequent in yeast? Gilbert argues that they were present at one point during evolution, but as the genome of these primitive organisms evolved, they were lost. The loss resulted from strong selection pressure to streamline chromosomes so as to minimize the energy expenditure on replication and gene expression. Furthermore, streamlining led to fewer errors in mRNA production. However, supporters of the opposing "intron-late" school, including Jeffrey Palmer, argue that introns first appeared much later in evolution, when they were acquired by a single group of eukaryotes that are ancestral to modern-day eukaryotes but not to prokaryotes.

The advent of large-scale genome sequencing has served to increase the controversy. We now have the ability to decipher the complete nucleotide sequence of all DNA in specific organisms. By comparing the amino acid coding and the noncoding DNA sequences from evolutionarily spaced species, geneticists hope to gain insight into how these sequences evolved. Currently, no indisputable evidence in support of either the "intron-early" or the "intron-late" theory has been found, and the question has remained difficult to resolve.

EXPLORING GENOMICS

Translation Tools and Swiss-Prot for Studying Protein Sequences

MasteringGenetics™ Visit the Study Area: Exploring Genomics

Many of the databases and bioinformatics programs we have used for Exploring Genomics exercises have focused on manipulating and analyzing DNA and RNA sequences. Scientists working on various aspects of translation and protein structure and function also have a wide range of bioinformatics tools and databases at their disposal via the Internet. Many of these sites were developed through *proteomics,* the study of all the proteins expressed in a cell or tissue. We will discuss proteomics in more detail later in the text (see Chapter 21).

In this Exploring Genomics exercise, we will use a program from **ExPASy (Expert Protein Analysis System)** to translate a segment of a gene into a possible polypeptide. We will then explore databases for learning more about this polypeptide.

■ **Exercise I – Translating a Nucleotide Sequence and Analyzing a Polypeptide**

ExPASy (Expert Protein Analysis System), hosted by the Swiss Institute of Bioinfor-matics, provides a wealth of resources for studies in proteomics. We will use a program from ExPASy called **Translate Tool** to translate a nucleotide sequence to a polypeptide sequence. Although many other programs are available on the Web for this purpose, ExPASy is one of the more student-friendly tools. Translate Tool allows you to make a predicted polypeptide sequence from a cloned gene and then look for open reading frames and variations in possible polypeptides.

(continued)

Exploring Genomics—continued

1. At the Web site we provide a partial sequence for a human gene based on a complementary DNA (cDNA) sequence. Later in the text (see Chapter 20), you will learn that cDNA sequences are DNA copies complementary to mRNA molecules expressed in a cell. Before you translate this sequence in ExPASy, run a nucleotide–nucleotide BLAST search from the NCBI Web site (http://blast.ncbi.nlm.nih.gov/Blast.cgi) to identify the gene corresponding to this sequence. Refer to the Exploring Genomics exercise in Chapter 10 if you need help with BLAST searches.

ACATTTGCTTCTGACACAATTGTGT
TCACTAGCAACCTCAAACAGACAC
CATGGTGCATCTGACTCCTGAGGAG
AAGTCTGCCGTTACTGCCCTGTGGG
GCAAGGTGAACGTGGATGAAGTTG
GTGGTGAGGCCCTGGGCAG

2. Access the ExPASy Translate Tool program at http://web.expasy.org/translate/. Copy and paste the cDNA sequence into Translate Tool and click "Translate Sequence" to generate possible polypeptide sequences encoded by this cDNA.

3. Review the translation results and then answer the following questions:

   a. Did Translate Tool provide one or multiple possible polypeptide sequences?

   b. If the translation results showed multiple polypeptide sequences, what does this mean? Explain.

   c. Refer to Figure 14–14 in the chapter. Based on this figure, which reading frame generated by Translate Tool appears to be correct?

4. ExPASy also provides access to a wealth of information about this polypeptide by connecting to a large number of different databases such as **UniProt KB/Swiss-Prot**, a protein sequence database maintained by the Swiss Institute for Bioinformatics (SIB) and the European Bioinformatics Institute (EBI), and a database called the Protein Data Bank. UniProt KB/Swiss-Prot is widely used by scientists around the world.

5. To learn more about the features of this polypeptide, it is best to work with a complete sequence. To obtain a complete sequence, click on the link for the reading frame you believe is correct.

6. To retrieve the amino acid sequence for the entire polypeptide, click "M" for methionine as the first amino acid in the polypeptide and then use the "BLAST" submission on ExPASy/SIB link near the bottom of the next page to run a BLAST search. From the BLAST results page, locate UniProtKB/Swiss-Prot entry P68871; this is an accession number for the protein sequence, similar to the accession numbers assigned to DNA and RNA sequences, and it is the correct match for this sequence.

Click on this link to reveal a comprehensive report about the protein. Be sure the identity of this protein agrees with what you discovered in Step 1.

7. Scroll down the Swiss-Prot report; then explore the following features:

   a. Use the "Protein Attributes" and "General Annotation (comments)" section to learn more about this polypeptide.

   b. Under the "Sequence Annotations" feature, find the links for Natural Variants to learn more about naturally occurring mutations related to this polypeptide.

   c. Under the "Cross-References" category, find 3D Structure Databases—presents 3D modeling representations showing polypeptide folding arrangements.

   d. Under "Cross-References" locate 2D Gel Databases; use the Swiss-2D PAGE link to view 2D gels of this polypeptide from different tissue samples. Refer to Figure 21–21 for a representation of 2D gels. When viewing a 2D gel image with this feature, click on links under "Map Locations" to identify specific spots on a gel that correspond to this polypeptide.

   e. Under "Cross-References" the Family and Domain databases links will take you to a wealth of information about this polypeptide and related polypeptides and proteins.

   f. Under "Cross-References" explore the "Other" category and visit the DrugBank link that provides information on drugs that bind to and affect this polypeptide.

CASE STUDY | Crippled ribosomes

Diamond Blackfan anemia (DBA) is a rare, dominantly inherited syndrome characterized by bone marrow failure, birth defects, and a significant predisposition to cancer. Those affected with DBA usually develop anemia in the first year of life, have abnormal numbers of cell types in their bone marrow, and have an increased risk of developing leukemia and bone cancer. At the molecular level, DBA is caused by a mutation in any of 11 genes that encode ribosomal proteins. The common feature of all these mutations is the disruption of ribosome formation, ultimately affecting the stability or function of ribosomes.

Many questions about this disorder remain to be answered.

1. Given the central importance of ribosomes in maintaining life, how is it possible that individuals carrying mutations in ribosomal protein genes survive?

2. Why might some cells in the body, such as those in bone marrow, be more susceptible to ribosomal protein mutations than other cell types?

3. DBA exhibits variable penetrance with significant differences in the clinical symptoms. How does this provide a way of studying the molecular events that cause this disorder?

Summary Points

1. Translation is the synthesis of polypeptide chains under the direction of mRNA in association with ribosomes.
2. Translation depends on tRNA molecules that serve as adaptors between triplet codons in mRNA and the corresponding amino acids.
3. Translation occurs in association with ribosomes and, like transcription, is subdivided into the stages of initiation, elongation, and termination and relies on base-pairing affinities between complementary nucleotides.
4. Inherited metabolic disorders are most often due to the loss of enzyme activity resulting from mutations in genes encoding those proteins.
5. Beadle and Tatum's work with nutritional mutations in *Neurospora* led them to propose that one gene encodes one enzyme.
6. Pauling and Ingram's investigations of hemoglobin from patients with sickle-cell anemia led to the modification of the one-gene:one-enzyme hypothesis to indicate that one gene encodes one polypeptide chain.
7. Proteins, the end products of genes, demonstrate four levels of structural organization that together describe their three-dimensional conformation, which is the basis of each molecule's function.
8. Of the myriad functions performed by proteins, the most influential role belongs to enzymes, which serve as highly specific biological catalysts that play a central role in the production of all classes of molecules in living systems.
9. In eukaryotes, proteins contain one or more functional domains, each prescribed by exon regions interspersed within genes. Specific domains impart specific functional capacities to proteins and appear to have been "shuffled" between genes during evolution.

INSIGHTS AND SOLUTIONS

The growth responses in the following chart were obtained by growing four mutant strains of *Neurospora* on different media, each containing one of four related compounds, A, B, C, and D. None of the mutations grows on minimal medium. Draw all possible conclusions from this data.

Mutation	Growth Supplement			
	A	B	C	D
1	−	−	−	−
2	+	+	−	+
3	+	+	−	−
4	−	+	−	−

Solution: Nothing can be concluded about mutation *1* except that it is lacking some essential factor, perhaps even unrelated to any biochemical pathway in which A, B, C, and D participate. Nor can anything be concluded about compound C. If it is involved in a pathway with the other compounds, it is a product synthesized prior to the synthesis of A, B, and D. We must now analyze these three compounds and the control of their synthesis by the enzymes encoded by genes *2*, *3*, and *4*. Because product B allows growth in all three cases, it may be considered the "end product"—it bypasses the block in all three instances. Similar reasoning suggests that product A precedes B in the pathway, since A bypasses the block in two of the three steps. Product D precedes B, yielding a partial solution:

$$C(?) \longrightarrow D \longrightarrow A \longrightarrow B$$

Now let's determine which mutations control which steps. Since mutation *2* can be alleviated by products D, B, and A, it must control a step prior to all three products, perhaps the direct conversion to D, although we cannot be certain. Mutation *3* is alleviated by B and A, so its effect must precede theirs in the pathway. Thus, we will assign it a role controlling the conversion of D to A. Likewise, we can provisionally assign mutation *4* to the conversion of A to B, leading to the following more complete solution.

$$C(?) \xrightarrow{2(?)} D \xrightarrow{3} A \xrightarrow{4} B$$

Problems and Discussion Questions

HOW DO WE KNOW?

1. In this chapter, we focused on the translation of mRNA into proteins as well as on protein structure and function. Along the way, we found many opportunities to consider the methods and reasoning by which much of this information was acquired. From the explanations given in the chapter, what answers would you propose to the following fundamental questions:

(a) What experimentally derived information led to Holley's proposal of the two-dimensional cloverleaf model of tRNA?
(b) What experimental information verifies that certain codons in mRNA specify chain termination during translation?
(c) How do we know, based on studies of *Neurospora* nutritional mutations, that one gene specifies one enzyme?

(d) On what basis have we concluded that proteins are the end products of genetic expression?

(e) What experimental information directly confirms that the genetic code, as shown in Figure 13–7, is correct?

(f) How do we know that the structure of a protein is intimately related to the function of that protein?

CONCEPT QUESTION

2. Review the Chapter Concepts list on p. 337. These all relate to the translation of genetic information stored in mRNA into proteins and how chemical information in proteins impart function to those molecules. Write a brief essay that discusses the role of ribosomes in the process of translation as it relates to these concepts.

3. Contrast the roles of tRNA and mRNA during translation and list all enzymes that participate in the transcription and translation process.

4. Francis Crick proposed the "adaptor hypothesis" for the function of tRNA. Why did he choose that description?

5. During translation, what molecule bears the codon? the anticodon?

6. The α chain of eukaryotic hemoglobin is composed of 141 amino acids. What is the minimum number of nucleotides in an mRNA coding for this polypeptide chain?

7. Assuming that each nucleotide is 0.34 nm long in the mRNA, how many triplet codes can occupy at one time the space in a ribosome that is 20 nm in diameter?

8. Summarize the steps involved in charging tRNAs with their appropriate amino acids.

9. To carry out its role, each transfer RNA requires at least four specific recognition sites that must be inherent in its tertiary structure. What are they?

10. What are isoaccepting tRNAs? Assuming that there are only 20 different aminoacyl tRNA synthetases but 31 different tRNAs, speculate on parameters that might be used to ensure that each charged tRNA has received the correct amino acid.

11. Discuss the potential difficulties of designing a diet to alleviate the symptoms of phenylketonuria.

12. Phenylketonurics cannot convert phenylalanine to tyrosine. Why don't these individuals exhibit a deficiency of tyrosine?

13. Phenylketonurics are often more lightly pigmented than are normal individuals. Can you suggest a reason why this is so?

14. Early detection and adherence to a strict dietary regime have prevented much of the mental retardation that used to occur in those afflicted with phenylketonuria (PKU). Affected individuals now often lead normal lives and have families. For various reasons, such individuals adhere less rigorously to their diet as they get older. Predict the effect that mothers with PKU who neglect their diets might have on newborns.

15. The synthesis of flower pigments is known to be dependent on enzymatically controlled biosynthetic pathways. For the crosses shown here, postulate the role of mutant genes and their products in producing the observed phenotypes:
(a) P₁: white strain A × white strain B
F₁: all purple
F₂: 9/16 purple: 7/16 white
(b) P₁: white × pink
F₁: all purple
F₂: 9/16 purple: 3/16 pink: 4/16 white

16. The study of biochemical mutants in organisms such as *Neurospora* has demonstrated that some pathways are branched. The data shown here illustrate the branched nature of the pathway resulting in the synthesis of thiamine:

Mutation	Minimal Medium	Pyrimidine	Thiazole	Thiamine
thi-1	−	−	+	+
thi-2	−	+	−	+
thi-3	−	−	−	+

Why don't the data support a linear pathway? Can you postulate a pathway for the synthesis of thiamine in *Neurospora*?

17. Explain why the one-gene:one-enzyme concept is not considered totally accurate today.

18. Why is an alteration of electrophoretic mobility interpreted as a change in the primary structure of the protein under study?

19. Contrast the polypeptide-chain components of each of the hemoglobin molecules found in humans.

20. Using sickle-cell anemia as an example, describe what is meant by a molecular or genetic disease. What are the similarities and dissimilarities between this type of a disorder and a disease caused by an invading microorganism?

21. Contrast the contributions of Pauling and Ingram to our understanding of the genetic basis for sickle-cell anemia.

22. Hemoglobins from two individuals are compared by electrophoresis and by fingerprinting. Electrophoresis reveals no difference in migration, but fingerprinting shows an amino acid difference. How is this possible?

23. HbS results in anemia and resistance to malaria, whereas in those with HbA, the parasite *Plasmodium falciparum* invades red blood cells and causes the disease. Predict whether those with HbC are likely to be anemic and whether they would be resistant to malaria.

24. Shown below are several amino acid substitutions in the α and β chains of human hemoglobin:

Hb Type	Normal Amino Acid	Substituted Amino Acid
Hb Toronto	Ala	Asp (α-5)
HbJ Oxford	Gly	Asp (α-15)
Hb Mexico	Gln	Glu (α-54)
Hb Bethesda	Tyr	His (β-145)
Hb Sydney	Val	Ala (β-67)
HbM Saskatoon	His	Tyr (β-63)

Using the code table (Figure 13–7), determine how many of them can occur as a result of a single-nucleotide change.

25. Certain mutations called *amber* in bacteria and viruses result in premature termination of polypeptide chains during translation. Many *amber* mutations have been detected at different points along the gene coding for a head protein in phage T4. How might this system be further investigated to demonstrate and support the concept of colinearity?

26. Describe what colinearity means. Of what significance is the concept of colinearity in the study of genetics?

27. Does Yanofsky's work with the *trpA* locus in *E. coli* (discussed in this chapter) constitute more or less direct evidence in support of colinearity than Fiers's work with phage MS2 (discussed in Chapter 13)? Explain.

28. Define and compare the four levels of protein organization.
29. List as many different categories of protein functions as you can. Wherever possible, give an example of each category.
30. How does an enzyme function? Why are enzymes essential for living organisms on Earth?

31. Exon shuffling is a proposal that relates exons in DNA to the repositioning of functional domains in proteins. What evidence exists in support of exon shuffling? Two schools of thought have emerged concerning the origin of exons, "intron-early" and "intron-late." Briefly describe both theories and present support for each.

Extra-Spicy Problems

MasteringGenetics™ Visit for instructor-assigned tutorials and problems.

32. Three independently assorting genes are known to control the following biochemical pathway that provides the basis for flower color in a hypothetical plant:

$$\text{Colorless} \xrightarrow{A-} \text{yellow} \xrightarrow{B-} \text{green} \xrightarrow{C-} \text{speckled}$$

Three homozygous recessive mutations are also known, each of which interrupts a different one of these steps. Determine the phenotypic results in the F_1 and F_2 generations resulting from the P_1 crosses of true-breeding plants listed here:

(a) speckled ($AABBCC$) × yellow ($AAbbCC$)
(b) yellow ($AAbbCC$) × green ($AABBcc$)
(c) colorless ($aaBBCC$) × green ($AABBcc$)

33. How would the results vary in cross (a) of Problem 32 if genes A and B were linked with no crossing over between them? How would the results of cross (a) vary if genes A and B were linked and 20 map units (mu) apart?

34. Deep in a previously unexplored South American rain forest, a species of plants was discovered with true-breeding varieties whose flowers were pink, rose, orange, or purple. A very astute plant geneticist made a single cross, carried to the F_2 generation, as shown:

P_1:	purple × pink
F_1:	all purple
F_2:	27/64 purple
	16/64 pink
	12/64 rose
	9/64 orange

Based solely on these data, he was able to propose both a mode of inheritance for flower pigmentation and a biochemical pathway for the synthesis of these pigments.

Carefully study the data. Create a hypothesis of your own to explain the mode of inheritance. Then propose a biochemical pathway consistent with your hypothesis. How could you test the hypothesis by making other crosses?

35. The emergence of antibiotic-resistant strains of *Enterococci* and transfer of resistant genes to other bacterial pathogens have highlighted the need for new generations of antibiotics to combat serious infections. To grasp the range of potential sites for the action of existing antibiotics, sketch the components of the translation machinery (e.g., see Step 3 of Figure 14–6), and using a series of numbered pointers, indicate the specific location for the action of the antibiotics shown in the following table.

Antibiotic	Action
1. Streptomycin	Binds to 30S ribosomal subunit
2. Chloramphenicol	Inhibits peptidyl transferase of 70S ribosome
3. Tetracycline	Inhibits binding of charged tRNA to ribosome
4. Erythromycin	Binds to free 50S particle and prevents formation of 70S ribosome
5. Kasugamycin	Inhibits binding of tRNA^{fmet}
6. Thiostrepton	Prevents translocation by inhibiting EF-G

36. The development of antibiotic resistance by pathogenic bacteria represents a major health concern. One potential new antibiotic is evernimicin, which was isolated from *Micromonospora carbonacea*? Evernimicin is an oligosaccharide with antibiotic activity against a broad range of gram-positive pathogenic bacteria. To determine the mode of action of this drug, researchers have analyzed 23S ribosomal DNA mutants that showed reduced sensitivity to evernimicin (e.g., Adrian et al., 2000. *Antimicrob. Ag. and Chemo.* 44: 3101–3106). They discovered two classes of mutants that conferred resistance: In one class, the mutation occurs in 23S rRNA nucleotides 2475–2483; in the other class, it occurs in ribosomal protein L16. This suggests that these two ribosomal components are structurally and functionally linked. It turns out that the tRNA anticodon stem-loop appears to bind to the A site of the ribosome at rRNA bases 2465–2485. This finding conforms to the proposed function of L16, which appears to be involved in attracting the aminoacyl stem of the tRNA to the ribosome at its A site. Using your sketch of the translation machinery from Problem 35 along with this information, designate where the proposed antibacterial action of evernimicin is likely to occur.

37. The flow of genetic information from DNA to protein is mediated by messenger RNA. If you introduce short DNA strands (called antisense oligonucleotides) that are complementary to mRNAs, hydrogen bonding may occur and "label" the DNA/RNA hybrid for ribonuclease-H degradation of the RNA. One study compared the effect of different-length antisense oligonucleotides upon ribonuclease-H–mediated degradation of tumor necrosis factor (*TNFα*) mRNA. *TNFα* exhibits antitumor and proinflammatory activities (Lloyd et al., 2001. *Nuc.*

Acids Res. 29: 3664–3673). The following graph indicates the efficacy of various-sized antisense oligonucleotides in causing ribonuclease-H cleavage.

(a) Describe how antisense oligonucleotides interrupt the flow of genetic information in a cell.

(b) What general conclusion can be drawn from the graph?

(c) What factors other than oligonucleotide length are likely to influence antisense efficacy *in vivo*?

38. The fidelity of translation is dependent on the reliable action of aminoacyl tRNA synthetases that ensure the association of only one type of amino acid with a specific tRNA. Two relatively rare human conditions, Charcot-Marie-Tooth disease 2D (CMT2D) and distal spinal muscular atrophy type V (dSMA-V), are neuropathologies of the peripheral axons that map to a well-defined region of the short arm of chromosome 7, as does the gene for glycyl tRNA synthetase. Families with CMT2D or dSMA-V have been identified with missense mutations in the gene for glycyl tRNA synthetase; and the mutations present in CMT2D and dSMA-V have been found to result in a loss of activity of glycyl tRNA synthetase (Antonellis et al., 2003). A sample pedigree (from Antonellis et al., 2003) is presented here (to maintain anonymity, sexes are not provided).

(a) Considering the following pedigree and the function of aminoacyl tRNA synthetases in general, would you conclude that the genes causing these diseases are dominant or recessive in their action?

(b) Considering the vital role that synthetases play in protein synthesis, speculate as to how individuals might survive with such a defect in translational efficiency.

(c) Why might some tissues (neural) be more affected than others?

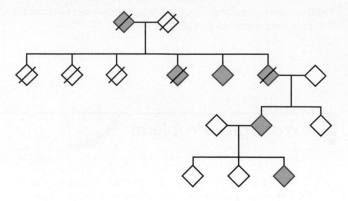

39. Knowing the quaternary structure of proteins, specifically their surface properties, provides novel opportunities for enhancing the development of targeted drug therapies.

(a) Referring to Figure 14–16 and the accompanying discussion, predict the class(es) of amino acids likely to reside on the surface of a protein within a cell.

(b) Assuming that Glu, Arg, and Asp exist in a functional site of a receptor molecule on the surface of a cell, provide an amino acid sequence that is likely to be effective in blocking that site.

(c) The androgen receptor associated with prostate cancer has recently been targeted using synthetic molecules known generally as peptidomimetics, many of which incorporate D-amino acid stereoisomers rather than the more naturally occurring L-amino acid stereoisomers. Why might D-amino acid stereoisomers be especially useful for inhibiting a functional site of the androgen receptor, or any deleterious functional site for that matter?

(d) Rational drug design is a relatively recent approach to the design of targeted therapeutic agents. Predict how knowledge of protein structure, especially surface properties, might be used in rational drug design as compared with the more classical "trial-and-error" approach.

Pigment mutations within an ear of corn, caused by transposition of the *Ds* element.

15 Gene Mutation, DNA Repair, and Transposition

CHAPTER CONCEPTS

- Mutations comprise any change in the base-pair sequence of DNA.

- Mutations are a source of genetic variation and provide the raw material for natural selection. They are also the source of genetic damage that contributes to cell death, genetic diseases, and cancer.

- Mutations have a wide range of effects on organisms depending on the type of base-pair alteration, the location of the mutation within the chromosome, and the function of the affected gene product.

- Mutations can occur spontaneously as a result of natural biological and chemical processes, or they can be induced by external factors, such as chemicals or radiation.

- Single-gene mutations cause a wide variety of human diseases.

- Organisms rely on a number of DNA repair mechanisms to counteract mutations. These mechanisms range from proofreading and correction of replication errors to base excision and homologous recombination repair.

- Mutations in genes whose products control DNA repair lead to genome hypermutability, human DNA repair diseases, and cancers.

- Transposable elements may move into and out of chromosomes, causing chromosome breaks and inducing mutations both within coding regions and in gene-regulatory regions.

The ability of DNA molecules to store, replicate, transmit, and decode information is the basis of genetic function. But equally important are the changes that occur to DNA sequences. Without the variation that arises from changes in DNA sequences, there would be no phenotypic variability, no adaptation to environmental changes, and no evolution. Gene mutations are the source of new alleles and are the origin of genetic variation within populations. On the downside, they are also the source of genetic changes that can lead to cell death, genetic diseases, and cancer.

Mutations also provide the basis for genetic analysis. The phenotypic variations resulting from mutations allow geneticists to identify and study the genes responsible for the modified trait. In genetic investigations, mutations act as identifying "markers" for genes so that they can be followed during their transmission from parents to offspring. Without phenotypic variability, classical genetic analysis would be impossible. For example, if all pea plants displayed a uniform phenotype, Mendel would have had no foundation for his research.

As discussed earlier in the text (see Chapter 8), we examined mutations in large regions of chromosomes—chromosomal mutations. In contrast, the mutations we will now explore are those occurring primarily in the base-pair sequence of DNA within individual genes—**gene mutations**. We will also describe how the cell defends itself from such mutations using various mechanisms of DNA repair.

15.1 Gene Mutations Are Classified in Various Ways

A mutation can be defined as an alteration in DNA sequence. Any base-pair change in any part of a DNA molecule can be considered a mutation. A mutation may comprise a single base-pair substitution, a deletion or insertion of one or more base pairs, or a major alteration in the structure of a chromosome.

Mutations may occur within regions of a gene that code for protein or within noncoding regions of a gene such as introns and regulatory sequences. Mutations may or may not bring about a detectable change in phenotype. The extent to which a mutation changes the characteristics of an organism depends on which type of cell suffers the mutation and the degree to which the mutation alters the function of a gene product or a gene-regulatory region.

Mutations can occur in somatic cells or within germ cells. Those that occur in germ cells are heritable and are the basis for the transmission of genetic diversity and evolution, as well as genetic diseases. Those that occur in somatic cells are not transmitted to the next generation but may lead to altered cellular function or tumors.

Because of the wide range of types and effects of mutations, geneticists classify mutations according to several different schemes. These organizational schemes are not mutually exclusive. In this section, we outline some of the ways in which gene mutations are classified.

Classification Based on Type of Molecular Change

Geneticists often classify gene mutations in terms of the nucleotide changes that constitute the mutation. A change of one base pair to another in a DNA molecule is known as a **point mutation**, or **base substitution** (**Figure 15–1**). A change of one nucleotide of a triplet within a protein-coding portion of a gene may result in the creation of a new triplet that codes for a different amino acid in the protein product. If this occurs, the mutation is known as a **missense mutation**. A second possible outcome is that the triplet will be changed into a stop codon, resulting in the termination of translation of the protein. This is known as a **nonsense mutation**. If the point mutation alters a codon but does not result in a change in the amino acid at that position in the protein (due to degeneracy of the genetic code), it can be considered a **silent mutation**.

You will often see two other terms used to describe base substitutions. If a pyrimidine replaces a pyrimidine or a purine replaces a purine, a **transition** has occurred. If a purine replaces a pyrimidine, or vice versa, a **transversion** has occurred.

Another type of change is the insertion or deletion of one or more nucleotides at any point within the gene. As illustrated in Figure 15–1, the loss or addition of a single nucleotide causes all of the subsequent three-letter codons to be changed. These are called **frameshift mutations** because the frame of triplet reading during translation is altered. A frameshift mutation will occur when any number of bases are added or deleted, except multiples of three, which would reestablish the initial frame of reading. It is possible that one of the many altered triplets will be UAA, UAG, or UGA, the translation termination codons. When one of these triplets is encountered during translation, polypeptide synthesis is terminated at that point. Obviously, the results of frameshift mutations can be very severe, especially if they occur early in the coding sequence.

FIGURE 15–1 Analogy showing the effects of substitution, deletion, and insertion of one letter in a sentence composed of three-letter words to demonstrate point and frameshift mutations.

Classification Based on Phenotypic Effects

Depending on their type and location, mutations can have a wide range of phenotypic effects, from none to severe.

As discussed earlier in the text (see Chapter 4), a **loss-of-function mutation** is one that reduces or eliminates the function of the gene product. Any type of mutation, from a point mutation to deletion of the entire gene, may lead to a loss of function. Mutations that result in complete loss of function are known as **null mutations**.

Most loss-of-function mutations are recessive. A **recessive mutation** results in a wild-type phenotype when present in a diploid organism and the other allele is wild type. In this case, the presence of less than 100 percent of the gene product is sufficient to bring about the wild-type phenotype.

Some loss-of-function mutations can be dominant. A **dominant mutation** results in a mutant phenotype in a diploid organism, even when the wild-type allele is also present. Dominant mutations can have two different types of effects. **Haploinsufficiency** occurs when the single wild-type copy of the gene does not produce enough gene product to bring about a wild-type phenotype. In humans, Marfan syndrome is an example of a disorder caused by haploinsufficiency—in this case as a result of a loss-of-function mutation in one copy of the *FBN1* gene. In contrast, a **dominant gain-of-function mutation** results in a gene product with enhanced, negative, or new functions. This may be due to a change in the amino acid sequence of the protein that confers a new activity, or it may result from a mutation in a regulatory region of the gene, leading to expression of the gene at higher levels or at abnormal times or places. A **dominant negative mutation** may directly interfere with the function of the product of the wild-type allele. Often this occurs when the mutant nonfunctional gene product binds to the wild-type gene product, inactivating it.

The most easily observed mutations are those affecting a morphological trait. These mutations are known as **visible mutations** and are recognized by their ability to alter a normal or wild-type visible phenotype. For example, all of Mendel's pea characteristics and many genetic variations encountered in *Drosophila* fit this designation, since they cause obvious changes to the morphology of the organism.

Some mutations give rise to nutritional or biochemical effects. In bacteria and fungi, a typical **nutritional mutation** results in a loss of ability to synthesize an amino acid or vitamin. In humans, sickle-cell anemia and hemophilia are examples of diseases resulting from **biochemical mutations**. Although such mutations do not always affect morphological characters, they affect the function of proteins that can affect the well-being and survival of the affected individual.

Still another category consists of mutations that affect the behavior patterns of an organism. The primary effect of **behavioral mutations** is often difficult to analyze. For example, the mating behavior of a fruit fly may be impaired if it cannot beat its wings. However, the defect may be in the flight muscles, the nerves leading to them, or the brain, where the nerve impulses that initiate wing movements originate.

Another group of mutations—**regulatory mutations**—affect the regulation of gene expression. A mutation in a regulatory gene or a gene control region can disrupt normal regulatory processes and inappropriately activate or inactivate expression of a gene. For example, as we will see with the *lac* operon discussed later in the text (see Chapter 16), a regulatory gene produces a product that controls the transcription of the entire *lac* operon. Mutations within this regulatory gene can lead to the production of a regulatory protein with abnormal effects on the *lac* operon. Our knowledge of genetic regulation has been dependent on the study of such regulatory mutations. Regulatory mutations may also occur in regions such as splice junctions, promoters, or other regulatory regions of a gene that affect many aspects of gene regulation including transcription initiation, mRNA splicing, and mRNA stability.

It is also possible that a mutation may adversely affect a gene product that is essential to the survival of the organism. In this case, it is referred to as a **lethal mutation**. Various inherited human biochemical disorders are examples of lethal mutations. For example, Tay–Sachs disease and Huntington disease are caused by mutations that result in lethality, but at different points in the life cycle of humans.

Another interesting class of mutations exerts effects on the organism in ways that depend on the environment in which the organism finds itself. Such mutations are called **conditional mutations** because these mutations are present in the genome of an organism but can be detected only under certain conditions. Among the best examples of conditional mutations are **temperature-sensitive mutations**. At a "permissive" temperature, the mutant gene product functions normally, but it loses its function at a different, "restrictive" temperature. Therefore, when the organism is shifted from the permissive to the restrictive temperature, the effect of the mutation becomes apparent. The temperature-sensitive coat color variations in Siamese cats and Himalayan rabbits, discussed earlier in the text (see Chapter 4), are striking examples of the effects of conditional mutations.

A **neutral mutation** is a mutation that can occur either in a protein-coding region or in any part of the genome, and its effect on the genetic fitness of the organism is negligible. For example, a neutral mutation within a gene may change a lysine codon (AAA) to an arginine codon (AGA). The two amino acids are chemically similar; therefore, this change may be insignificant to the function of the protein. Because eukaryotic genomes consist mainly of noncoding regions, the vast majority of mutations are likely to occur in the large portions of the genome that do not contain genes. These may be considered neutral mutations, if they do not affect gene products or gene expression.

Classification Based on Location of Mutation

Mutations may be classified according to the cell type or chromosomal locations in which they occur. **Somatic mutations** are those occurring in any cell in the body except germ cells. **Autosomal mutations** are mutations within genes located on the autosomes, whereas **X-linked** and **Y-linked mutations** are those within genes located on the X or Y chromosome, respectively.

Mutations arising in somatic cells are not transmitted to future generations. When a recessive autosomal mutation occurs in a somatic cell of a diploid organism, it is unlikely to result in a detectable phenotype. The expression of most such mutations is likely to be masked by expression of the wild-type allele within that cell. Somatic mutations will have a greater impact if they are dominant or, in males, if they are X-linked, since such mutations are most likely to be immediately expressed. Similarly, the impact of dominant or X-linked somatic mutations will be more noticeable if they occur early in development, when a small number of undifferentiated cells replicate to give rise to several differentiated tissues or organs. Dominant mutations that occur in cells of adult tissues are often masked by the activity of thousands upon thousands of nonmutant cells in the same tissue that perform the nonmutant function.

Mutations in germ cells are of greater significance because they may be transmitted to offspring as gametes. They have the potential of being expressed in all cells of an offspring. Inherited dominant autosomal mutations will be expressed phenotypically in the first generation. X-linked recessive mutations arising in the gametes of a **homogametic** female may be expressed in hemizygous male offspring. This will occur provided that the male offspring receives the affected X chromosome. Because of heterozygosity, the occurrence of an autosomal recessive mutation in the gametes of either males or females (even one resulting in a lethal allele) may go unnoticed for many generations, until the resultant allele has become widespread in the population. Usually, the new allele will become evident only when a chance mating brings two copies of it together into the homozygous condition.

NOW SOLVE THIS

15–1 If one spontaneous mutation occurs within a human egg cell genome, and this mutation changes an A to a T, what is the most likely effect of this mutation on the phenotype of an offspring that develops from this mutated egg?

■ **HINT:** *This problem asks you to predict the effects of a single base-pair mutation on phenotype. The key to its solution involves an understanding of the organization of the human genome as well as the effects of mutations on coding and noncoding regions of genes, and the effects of mutations on development.*

For more practice, see Problems 3, 4, 5, 6, and 7.

15.2 Mutations Occur Spontaneously and Randomly

When we think about gene mutations, we sometimes assume that genetic errors are predominantly the result of environmental assaults from factors such as toxic chemicals or radiation. Although environmental influences do affect mutation rates, much of the genetic alterations within a genome arise from unknown and endogenous factors. In addition, mutations are not stimulated by evolutionary pressures, but are nondirected. To explore these characteristics of gene mutation, the following subsections describe categories of spontaneous, induced, and random mutations as well as the rates of spontaneous mutations in humans and other organisms.

Spontaneous and Induced Mutations

Mutations can be classified as either spontaneous or induced, although these two categories overlap to some degree. **Spontaneous mutations** are changes in the nucleotide sequence of genes that appear to occur naturally. No specific agents are associated with their occurrence, and they are generally assumed to be accidental. Many of these mutations arise as a result of normal biological or chemical processes in the organism that alter the structure of nitrogenous bases. Often, spontaneous mutations occur during the enzymatic process of DNA replication, as we discuss later in this chapter.

In contrast to spontaneous mutations, mutations that result from the influence of extraneous factors are considered to be **induced mutations**. Induced mutations may be the result of either natural or artificial agents. For example, radiation from cosmic and mineral sources and ultraviolet radiation from the sun are energy sources to which most organisms are exposed and, as such, may be factors that cause induced mutations.

The earliest demonstration of the artificial induction of mutations occurred in 1927, when Hermann J. Muller reported that X rays could cause mutations in *Drosophila*. In 1928, Lewis J. Stadler reported that X rays had the same effect on barley. In addition to various forms of radiation, numerous natural and synthetic chemical agents are also mutagenic.

Several generalizations can be made regarding spontaneous mutation rates in organisms. The **mutation rate** is defined as the likelihood that a gene will undergo a mutation in a single generation or in forming a single gamete. First, the rate of spontaneous mutation is exceedingly low for all organisms. Second, the rate varies between different organisms. Third, even within the same species, the spontaneous mutation rate varies from gene to gene.

TABLE 15.1 Spontaneous Mutation Rates at Various Loci in Different Organisms

Organism	Character	Locus	Rate*
Bacteriophage T2	Lysis inhibition	$r \rightarrow r^+$	1×10^{-8}
	Host range	$h^+ \rightarrow h$	4×10^{-9}
Escherichia coli	Lactose fermentation	$lac^- \rightarrow lac^+$	2×10^{-7}
	Streptomycin sensitivity	$str\text{-}d \rightarrow str\text{-}s$	1×10^{-8}
Zea mays	Shrunken seeds	$sh^+ \rightarrow sh^-$	1×10^{-6}
	Purple	$pr^+ \rightarrow pr^-$	1×10^{-5}
Drosophila melanogaster	Yellow body	$y^+ \rightarrow y$	1.2×10^{-6}
	White eye	$w^+ \rightarrow w$	4×10^{-5}
Mus musculus	Piebald coat	$s^+ \rightarrow s$	3×10^{-5}
	Brown coat	$b^+ \rightarrow b$	8.5×10^{-4}

*Rates are expressed per gene replication (T2), per cell division (*Escherichia coli*), or per gamete per generation (*Zea mays, Drosophila melanogaster, and Mus musculus*).

Viral and bacterial genes undergo spontaneous mutation at an average of about 1 in 100 million (10^{-8}) replications or cell divisions (Table 15.1). Maize and *Drosophila* demonstrate rates several orders of magnitude higher. The genes studied in these groups average between 1 in 1,000,000 (10^{-6}) and 1 in 100,000 (10^{-5}) mutations per gamete formed. Some mouse genes are another order of magnitude higher in their spontaneous mutation rate, 1 in 100,000 to 1 in 10,000 (10^{-5} to 10^{-4}). It is not clear why such large variations occur in mutation rates. The variation between genes in a given organism may be due to inherent differences in mutability in different regions of the genome. Some DNA sequences appear to be highly susceptible to mutation and are known as **mutation hot spots**. The variation between organisms may, in part, reflect the relative efficiencies of their DNA proofreading and repair systems. We will discuss these systems later in the chapter.

Spontaneous Mutation Rates in Humans

The rates at which spontaneous mutations occur in the human genome and the potential effects of these new mutations are an ongoing focus of genetic research. Until recently, scientists have studied human germ-line mutation rates by examining individual genes or small regions of the genome. Now that whole-genome sequencing is becoming both rapid and economical, it is possible to examine entire genomes, both coding and noncoding regions, and to compare genomes from parents and offspring. These methods provide a more accurate estimate of mutation rates across the entire genome.

In 2012, a research group in Iceland sequenced the genomes of 78 parent/offspring sets, comprising 219 individuals, and compared the single-nucleotide polymorphisms (SNPs) throughout their genomes.[1] Their data revealed that a newborn baby's genome contains an average of 60 new mutations, compared with those of his or her parents. Their research also revealed that the number of new mutations depends significantly on the age of the father at the time of conception. For example, when the father is 20 years old, he contributes approximately 25 new mutations to the child. When he is 40 years old, he contributes approximately 65 new mutations. In contrast, the mother contributes about 15 new mutations, at any age. The researchers estimated that the father contributes approximately 2 mutations per year of his age, with the mutation rate doubling every 16.5 years. The large proportion of mutations contributed by fathers is likely due to the fact that male germ cells go through more cell divisions during a lifetime than do female germ cells.

Of the 4933 new SNP mutations that were identified in this study, only 73 occurred within gene exons. Other studies have suggested that about 10 percent of single-nucleotide mutations lead to negative phenotypic changes. If so, then an average spontaneous mutation rate of 60 new mutations might yield about six deleterious phenotypic effects per generation. This study points out the difficulties in determining spontaneous mutation rates in humans; as factors such as demographic features and parental ages must be taken into account in arriving at accurate estimates.

The Fluctuation Test: Are Mutations Random or Adaptive?

One of the basic concepts in genetics is that mutations occur randomly and are not directed by the environment

[1] Kong, A., et al. 2012. Rate of de novo mutations and the importance of father's age to disease risk. *Nature* 488: 471–475.

in which the organism finds itself—that is, mutations arise spontaneously in the absence of selective pressure rather than being the consequence of selective pressure. This concept has been verified by many experiments, including the classic Luria–Delbrück Fluctuation Test.

In 1943, Salvador Luria and Max Delbrück presented the first direct evidence that mutations do not occur as part of an adaptive mechanism, but instead take place spontaneously and randomly. Their experiment, known as the **Luria–Delbrück fluctuation test**, is an example of exquisite analytical and theoretical work.

Luria and Delbrück carried out their experiments using the *Escherichia coli*-T1 system. The T1 bacteriophage is a bacterial virus that infects *E. coli* cells and lyses the infected bacteria. Mutations can occur in *E. coli* cells that make the cells resistant to T1. To begin their experiment, Luria and Delbruck inoculated a large flask and a number of individual culture tubes with a few *E. coli* cells and grew all the cultures for several generations in the absence of any T1 bacteriophage. After growth, each small flask contained about 20 million cells, and the large flask was allowed to grow to a higher density. At this point, the bacteria in the smaller individual tubes were spread onto the surface of growth media containing T1 bacteriophage, in a petri dish. Similarly, several portions of the large flask (each portion also containing about 20 million cells) were spread onto T1-containing media in petri plates. After incubation, any individual cells of *E. coli* that were resistant to the T1 bacteriophage grew and formed colonies. All other *E. coli* cells that were not resistant would die. The colonies present on the plates were then counted.

The experimental rationale for distinguishing between the two hypotheses (adaptive versus random mutation) was as follows:

Hypothesis 1: Adaptive Mutations. If mutations occur adaptively, in response to the presence of T1 bacteriophage in the growth medium, every *E. coli* cell that is grown on the T1-containing growth medium would have a constant probability of acquiring a mutation that would give it resistance to T1. Therefore, the number of resistant cells (colonies) would depend only on the number of *E. coli* cells and bacteriophages present on the petri plates. In this case, because a constant number of cells and T1 were present on each plate, there would be a fairly constant number of resistant colonies from plate to plate and from experiment to experiment.

Hypothesis 2: Random Mutations. If mutations occur randomly and are not affected by the presence or absence of bacteriophage, mutations leading to resistance would occur at a low rate at any time during incubation even in the absence of T1 bacteriophage. If a mutation occurred early in the incubation process in the culture tubes, the subsequent growth of the mutant bacteria would produce

TABLE 15.2 The Luria–Delbrück Experiment Demonstrating That Mutations Are Spontaneous

Sample No.	Number of T1-Resistant Bacteria	
	Same Culture (Control)	Different Cultures
1	14	6
2	15	5
3	13	10
4	21	8
5	15	24
6	14	13
7	26	165
8	16	15
9	20	6
10	13	10
Mean	16.7	26.2
Variance	15.0	2178.0

Source: After Luria and Delbrück (1943).

a large number of resistant cells in the culture. If a mutation occurred later in the incubation process, there would be fewer resistant colonies. The random mutation hypothesis predicts that the number of resistant cells would fluctuate from experiment to experiment, and from tube to tube, reflecting the varying times at which the resistance mutations occurred in liquid culture. In contrast, each portion of the large culture flask (containing a stirred and homogeneous mixture of resistant and susceptible cells) would produce a constant number of resistant colonies from plate to plate.

Table 15.2 shows a representative set of data from the Luria–Delbrück experiments. The middle column shows the number of mutant colonies recovered from a series of aliquots derived from the large liquid culture. These data serve as a control, and, as predicted, little fluctuation is observed in these samples. In contrast, the right-hand column shows the number of resistant colonies recovered from each of 10 independently incubated liquid cultures. These data reveal a great deal of fluctuation between independently incubated cultures, supporting the hypothesis that mutations arise randomly, even in the absence of selective pressure, and are inherited in a stable fashion.

Although the concept of spontaneous mutation has been accepted for some time, the possibility that organisms might also be capable of inducing specific mutations as a result of environmental pressures has long intrigued geneticists. Some recent and controversial research has suggested that under some stressful nutritional conditions such as starvation, bacteria may be capable of activating mechanisms that create a hypermutable state in genes that would, when mutated, enhance survival. The conclusions from these studies are still a source of debate, but they keep alive the interest in the possibility of adaptive mutation.

15.3 Spontaneous Mutations Arise from Replication Errors and Base Modifications

In this section, we will outline some of the processes that lead to spontaneous mutations. It is useful to keep in mind, however, that many of the DNA changes that occur during spontaneous mutagenesis also occur, at a higher rate, during induced mutagenesis.

DNA Replication Errors and Slippage

As we learned earlier in the text (see Chapter 11), the process of DNA replication is imperfect. Occasionally, DNA polymerases insert incorrect nucleotides during replication of a strand of DNA. Although DNA polymerases can correct most of these replication errors using their inherent 3′ to 5′ exonuclease proofreading capacity, misincorporated nucleotides may persist after replication. If these errors are not detected and corrected by DNA repair mechanisms, they may lead to mutations. Replication errors due to mispairing predominantly lead to point mutations. The fact that bases can take several forms, known as **tautomers**, increases the chance of mispairing during DNA replication, as we explain next.

In addition to mispairing and point mutations, DNA replication can lead to the introduction of small insertions or deletions. These mutations can occur when one strand of the DNA template loops out and becomes displaced during replication, or when DNA polymerase slips or stutters

during replication. If a loop occurs in the template strand during replication, DNA polymerase may miss the looped-out nucleotides, and a small deletion in the new strand will be introduced. If DNA polymerase repeatedly introduces nucleotides that are not present in the template strand, an insertion of one or more nucleotides will occur, creating an unpaired loop on the newly synthesized strand. Insertions and deletions may lead to frameshift mutations, or amino acid insertions or deletions in the gene product.

Replication slippage can occur anywhere in the DNA but seems distinctly more common in regions containing tandemly repeated sequences. Repeat sequences are hot spots for DNA mutation and in some cases contribute to hereditary diseases, such as fragile-X syndrome and Huntington disease. The hypermutability of repeat sequences in noncoding regions of the genome is the basis for current methods of forensic DNA analysis.

Tautomeric Shifts

Purines and pyrimidines can exist in tautomeric forms—that is, in alternate chemical forms that differ by only a single proton shift in the molecule. The biologically important tautomers are the keto–enol forms of thymine and guanine and the amino–imino forms of cytosine and adenine. These shifts change the bonding structure of the molecule, allowing hydrogen bonding with noncomplementary bases. Hence, **tautomeric shifts** may lead to permanent base-pair changes and mutations. **Figure 15–2** compares normal base-pairing relationships with rare unorthodox pairings. Anomalous T≡G and C=A pairs, among others, may be formed.

(a) Standard base-pairing arrangements

Thymine (keto)   Adenine (amino)   Cytosine (amino)   Guanine (keto)

(b) Anomalous base-pairing arrangements

Thymine (enol)   Guanine (keto)   Cytosine (imino)   Adenine (amino)

FIGURE 15–2 Standard base-pairing relationships (a) compared with examples of the anomalous base-pairing that occurs as a result of tautomeric shifts (b). The long triangle indicates the point at which the base bonds to the pentose sugar.

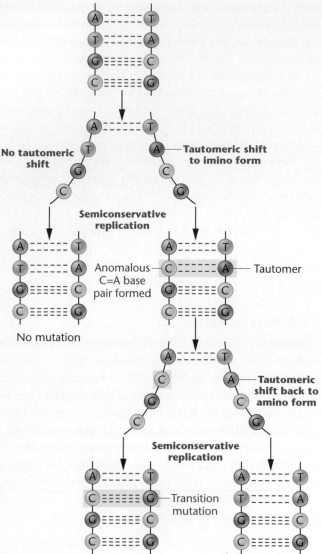

FIGURE 15–3 Formation of an A═T to G≡C transition mutation as a result of a tautomeric shift in adenine.

A mutation occurs during DNA replication when a transiently formed tautomer in the template strand pairs with a noncomplementary base. In the next round of replication, the "mismatched" members of the base pair are separated, and each becomes the template for its normal complementary base. The end result is a point mutation (**Figure 15–3**).

Depurination and Deamination

Some of the most common causes of spontaneous mutations are two forms of DNA base damage: depurination and deamination. **Depurination** is the loss of one of the nitrogenous bases in an intact double-helical DNA molecule. Most frequently, the base is a purine—either guanine or adenine. These bases may be lost if the glycosidic bond linking the 1′-C of the deoxyribose and the number 9 position of the purine

ring is broken, leaving an **apurinic site** on one strand of the DNA. Geneticists estimate that thousands of such spontaneous lesions are formed daily in the DNA of mammalian cells in culture. If apurinic sites are not repaired, there will be no base at that position to act as a template during DNA replication. As a result, DNA polymerase may introduce a nucleotide at random at that site.

In **deamination**, an amino group in cytosine or adenine is converted to a keto group (**Figure 15–4**). In these cases, cytosine is converted to uracil, and adenine is changed to hypoxanthine. The major effect of these changes is an alteration in the base-pairing specificities of these two bases during DNA replication. For example, cytosine normally pairs with guanine. Following its conversion to uracil, which pairs with adenine, the original G≡C pair is converted to an A═U pair and then, in the next replication, is converted to an A═T pair. When adenine is deaminated, the original A═T pair is converted to a G≡C pair because hypoxanthine pairs naturally with cytosine. Deamination may occur spontaneously or as a result of treatment with chemical mutagens such as nitrous acid (HNO_2).

Oxidative Damage

DNA may also suffer damage from the by-products of normal cellular processes. These by-products include reactive oxygen species (electrophilic oxidants) that are generated during normal aerobic respiration. For example, superoxides (O_2^-), hydroxyl radicals (·OH), and hydrogen peroxide (H_2O_2) are created during cellular metabolism and are constant threats to the integrity of

Cytosine   Uracil   Adenine

Adenine   Hypoxanthine   Cytosine

FIGURE 15–4 Deamination of cytosine and adenine, leading to new base pairing and mutation. Cytosine is converted to uracil, which base-pairs with adenine. Adenine is converted to hypoxanthine, which base-pairs with cytosine.

DNA. Such **reactive oxidants**, also generated by exposure to high-energy radiation, can produce more than 100 different types of chemical modifications in DNA, including modifications to bases, loss of bases, and single-stranded breaks.

Transposable Elements

Transposable genetic elements, or **transposons**, are DNA elements that can move within, or between, genomes. These elements are present in the genomes of all organisms, from bacteria to humans, and often comprise large portions of these genomes. Transposons can act as naturally occurring mutagens. If in moving to a new location they insert themselves into the coding region of a gene, they can alter the reading frame or introduce stop codons. If they insert into the regulatory region of a gene, they can disrupt proper expression of the gene. Transposons can also create chromosomal damage, including double-stranded breaks, inversions, and translocations. Transposable genetic elements are described in detail later in this chapter (Section 15.8).

NOW SOLVE THIS

15–2 One of the most famous cases of an X-linked recessive mutation in humans is that of hemophilia found in the descendants of Britain's Queen Victoria. The pedigree of the royal family indicates that Victoria was heterozygous for the trait; however, her father was not affected, and there is no evidence that her mother was a carrier. What are some possible explanations of how the mutation arose? What types of mutations could lead to the disease?

■ **HINT:** *This problem asks you to determine the sources of new mutations. The key to its solution is to consider the ways in which mutations occur, the types of cells in which they can occur, and how they are inherited.*

15.4 Induced Mutations Arise from DNA Damage Caused by Chemicals and Radiation

Induced mutations are those that increase the rate of mutation above the spontaneous background. All cells on Earth are exposed to a plethora of agents called **mutagens**, which have the potential to damage DNA and cause induced mutations. Some of these agents, such as some fungal toxins, cosmic rays, and ultraviolet light, are natural components of our environment. Others, including some industrial pollutants, medical X rays, and chemicals within tobacco smoke, can be considered as unnatural or human-made additions to our modern world. On the positive side, geneticists harness some

mutagens for use in analyzing genes and gene functions. The mechanisms by which some of these natural and unnatural agents lead to mutations are outlined in this section.

Base Analogs

One category of mutagenic chemicals is **base analogs**, compounds that can substitute for purines or pyrimidines during nucleic acid biosynthesis. For example, **5-bromouracil (5-BU)**, a derivative of uracil, behaves as a thymine analog but is halogenated at the number 5 position of the pyrimidine ring. If 5-BU is chemically linked to deoxyribose, the nucleoside analog **bromodeoxyuridine (BrdU)** is formed. **Figure 15–5** compares the structure of this analog with that of thymine. The presence of the bromine atom in place of the methyl group increases the probability that a tautomeric shift will occur. If 5-BU is incorporated into DNA in place of thymine and a tautomeric shift to the enol form occurs, 5-BU base-pairs with guanine. After one round of replication, an $A = T$ to $G \equiv C$ transition results. Furthermore, the presence of 5-BU within DNA increases the sensitivity of the molecule to ultraviolet (UV) light, which itself is mutagenic.

There are other base analogs that are mutagenic. For example, **2-amino purine (2-AP)** can act as an analog of adenine. In addition to its base-pairing affinity with thymine, 2-AP can also base-pair with cytosine, leading to possible transitions from $A = T$ to $G \equiv C$ following replication.

Alkylating, Intercalating, and Adduct-Forming Agents

A number of naturally occurring and human-made chemicals alter the structure of DNA and cause mutations. The sulfur-containing mustard gases, discovered during World War I, were some of the first chemical mutagens identified in chemical warfare studies. Mustard gases are **alkylating agents**—that is, they donate an alkyl group, such as CH_3 or CH_3CH_2, to amino or keto groups in nucleotides. Ethylmethane sulfonate (EMS), for example, alkylates the keto groups in the number 6 position of guanine and in the number 4 position of thymine. As with base analogs, base-pairing affinities are altered, and transition mutations result. For example, 6-ethylguanine acts as an analog of adenine and pairs with thymine (**Figure 15–6**).

Intercalating agents are chemicals that have dimensions and shapes that allow them to wedge between the base pairs of DNA. When bound between base pairs, intercalating agents cause base pairs to distort and DNA strands to unwind. These changes in DNA structure affect many functions including transcription, replication, and repair. Deletions and insertions occur during DNA replication and repair, leading to frame-shift mutations.

Some intercalating agents are used as DNA stains. An example is ethidium bromide, a fluorescent compound that

FIGURE 15–5 Similarity of the chemical structure of 5-bromouracil (5-BU) and thymine. In the common keto form, 5-BU base-pairs normally with adenine, behaving as a thymine analog. In the rare enol form, it pairs anomalously with guanine.

frequently than noncancer cells, they are more sensitive than normal cells to the mutagenic and damaging effects of these chemotherapeutic agents.

Another group of chemicals that cause mutations are known as adduct-forming agents. A DNA adduct is a substance that covalently binds to DNA, altering its conformation and interfering with replication and repair. Two examples of adduct-forming substances are acetaldehyde (a component of cigarette smoke) and heterocyclic amines (HCAs). HCAs are cancer-causing chemicals that are created during the cooking of meats such as beef, chicken, and fish. HCAs are formed at high temperatures from amino acids and creatine. Many HCAs covalently bind to guanine bases. At least 17 different HCAs have been linked to the development of cancers, such as those of the stomach, colon, and breast.

Ultraviolet Light

All electromagnetic radiation consists of energetic waves that we define by their different wavelengths (**Figure 15–7**). The full range of wavelengths is referred to as the **electromagnetic spectrum**, and the energy of any radiation in the spectrum varies inversely with its wavelength. Waves in the range of visible light and longer are benign when they interact with most organic molecules. However, waves of shorter length than visible light, being inherently more energetic, have the potential to disrupt organic molecules. As we know, purines and pyrimidines absorb **ultraviolet (UV) radiation** most intensely at a wavelength of about 260 nm. Although Earth's ozone layer absorbs the most dangerous types of UV radiation, sufficient UV radiation can induce thousands of DNA lesions per hour in any cell exposed to this radiation. One major effect of UV radiation on DNA is the creation of **pyrimidine**

is commonly used in molecular biology laboratories to visualize DNA during purifications and gel electrophoresis. The mutagenic characteristics of both ethidium bromide and the ultraviolet light used to visualize its fluorescence mean that this chemical must be used with caution. Other intercalating agents are used for cancer chemotherapy. Examples are doxorubicin, which is used to treat Hodgkin lymphoma, and dactinomycin, which is used to treat a variety of sarcomas. Because cancer cells undergo DNA replication more

FIGURE 15–6 Conversion of guanine to 6-ethylguanine by the alkylating agent ethylmethane sulfonate (EMS). The 6-ethylguanine base-pairs with thymine.

Visible spectrum (wavelength)

750 nm 700 nm 650 nm 600 nm 550 nm 500 nm 450 nm   380 nm

FIGURE 15–7 The regions of the electromagnetic spectrum and their associated wavelengths.

| Radio waves | Microwaves | Infrared | | UV | X rays | Gamma rays | Cosmic rays |

10^3 m 10^9 nm 10^6 nm 10^3 nm   1 nm 10^{-3} nm 10^{-5} nm
(1 m)

Decreasing wavelength →

Increasing energy →

dimers—chemical species consisting of two identical pyrimidines—particularly ones consisting of two thymine residues (**Figure 15–8**). The dimers distort the DNA conformation and inhibit normal replication. As a result, errors can be introduced in the base sequence of DNA during replication. When UV-induced dimerization is extensive, it is responsible (at least in part) for the killing effects of UV radiation on cells.

Ionizing Radiation

As noted above, the energy of radiation varies inversely with wavelength. Therefore, **X rays, gamma rays,** and **cosmic rays** are more energetic than UV radiation (Figure 15–7). As a result, they penetrate deeply into tissues, causing ionization of the molecules encountered along the way. Hence, this type of radiation is called **ionizing radiation**.

As ionizing radiation penetrates cells, stable molecules and atoms are transformed into **free radicals**—chemical species containing one or more unpaired electrons. Free radicals

can directly or indirectly affect the genetic material, altering purines and pyrimidines in DNA, breaking phosphodiester bonds, disrupting the integrity of chromosomes, and producing a variety of chromosomal aberrations, such as deletions, translocations, and chromosomal fragmentation.

Given the capacity of ionizing radiation to cause serious genetic damage, it is important to consider what levels of radiation are mutagenic in humans and what sources of ionizing radiation cause the most damage in everyday life. **Figure 15–9** shows a graph of the percentage of induced X-linked recessive lethal mutations versus the dose of X rays administered. There is a linear relationship between X-ray dose and the induction of mutation; for each doubling of the dose, twice as many mutations are induced. Because the

Dimer formed between adjacent thymidine residues along a DNA strand

FIGURE 15–8 Induction of a thymine dimer by UV radiation, leading to distortion of the DNA. The covalent crosslinks occur between the atoms of the pyrimidine ring.

FIGURE 15–9 Plot of the percentage of X-linked recessive mutations induced in *Drosophila* by increasing doses of X rays. If extrapolated, the graph intersects the zero axis as shown by the dashed line.

Nuclear power waste 0.2%
Nuclear weapons fallout 0.4%
Occupational exposure 0.4%
Consumer products 3%
Radioactive pharmaceuticals 3.8%
Diagnostic X rays 10.5%
Cosmic rays 7.4%
Soil radioactivity 7.5%
Natural isotopes in body 10.3%
Radon gas 56.5%

FIGURE 15–10 Chart showing average yearly dose of radiation from natural and human-made sources.

line intersects near the zero axis, this graph suggests that even very small doses of radiation are mutagenic.

Although it is often assumed that radiation from artificial sources such as nuclear power plant waste and medical X rays are the most significant sources of radiation exposure for humans, scientific data indicate otherwise. Scientists estimate that less than 20 percent of human radiation exposure arises from human-made sources. **Figure 15–10** summarizes the annual radiation exposure for humans residing in the United States. As these data indicate, the greatest radiation exposure comes from radon gas, cosmic rays, and natural soil radioactivity. More than half of human-made radiation exposure comes from medical X rays and radioactive pharmaceuticals.

NOW SOLVE THIS

15–3 The cancer drug melphalan is an alkylating agent of the mustard gas family. It acts in two ways: by causing alkylation of guanine bases and by cross linking DNA strands together. Describe two ways in which melphalan might kill cancer cells. What are two ways in which cancer cells could repair the DNA-damaging effects of melphalan?

■ **HINT:** *This problem asks you to consider the effect of the alkylation of guanine on base pairing during DNA replication. The key to its solution is to consider the effects of mutations on cellular processes that allow cells to grow and divide. In Section 15.6, you will learn about the ways in which cells repair the types of mutations introduced by alkylating agents.*

15.5 Single-Gene Mutations Cause a Wide Range of Human Diseases

Now that the human genome has been sequenced and genome-wide techniques are available to pinpoint disease-associated genes and the mutations within them, scientists are rapidly accumulating information about how specific types of mutations contribute to human disorders.

Although most human genetic diseases are **polygenic**—that is, caused by variations in several genes—even a single base-pair change in one of the approximately 20,000 human genes can lead to a serious inherited disorder. These **monogenic** diseases can be caused by many different types of single-gene mutations. **Table 15.3** lists some examples of the types of single-gene mutations that can lead to serious genetic diseases. A comprehensive database of human genes, mutations, and disorders is available in the Online Mendelian Inheritance in Man (OMIM) database, which is described in the "Exploring Genomics" feature earlier in the text (see Chapter 3). As of 2014, the OMIM database has catalogued over 4000 human phenotypes for which the molecular basis is known.

Geneticists estimate that approximately 30 percent of mutations that cause human diseases are single base-pair changes that create nonsense mutations. These mutations not only code for a prematurely terminated protein product, but also trigger rapid decay of the mRNA. Many more mutations are missense mutations that alter the amino acid sequence of a protein and frameshift mutations that alter the protein sequence and create internal nonsense codons. Other common disease-associated mutations affect the sequences of gene promoters, mRNA splicing signals, and other noncoding sequences that affect transcription, processing, and stability of mRNA or protein. One recent study showed that about 15 percent of all point mutations that cause human genetic diseases result in abnormal mRNA splicing. Approximately 85 percent of these splicing mutations alter the sequence of 5′ and 3′ splice signals. The remainder create new splice sites within the gene. Splicing defects often result in degradation of the abnormal mRNA or creation of abnormal protein products.

TABLE 15.3 Examples of Human Disorders Caused by Single-Gene Mutations

Type of DNA Mutation	Disorder	Molecular Change
Missense	Achondroplasia	Glycine to arginine at position 380 of *FGFR2* gene
Nonsense	Marfan syndrome	Tyrosine to STOP codon at position 2113 of *fibrillin-1* gene
Insertion	Familial hypercholesterolemia	Various short insertions throughout the *LDLR* gene
Deletion	Cystic fibrosis	Three-base-pair deletion of phenylalanine codon at position 508 of *CFTR* gene
Trinucleotide repeat expansions	Huntington disease	>40 repeats of (CAG) sequence in coding region of *Huntingtin* gene

Single Base-Pair Mutations and β-Thalassemia

Although some genetic diseases, such as sickle-cell anemia, are caused by one specific base-pair change within a single gene, most are caused by any of a large number of different mutations. The mutation profile associated with β-thalassemia provides an example of how one inherited disease can arise from a large number of possible mutations.

β-thalassemia is an inherited autosomal recessive blood disorder resulting from a reduction or absence of hemoglobin. It is the most common single-gene disease in the world, affecting people worldwide, but especially populations in Mediterranean, North African, Middle Eastern, Central Asian, and Southeast Asian countries.

People with β-thalassemia have varying degrees of anemia—from severe to mild—with symptoms including weakness, delayed development, jaundice, enlarged organs, and often a need for frequent blood transfusions.

Mutations in the β-*globin* gene (*HBB* gene) cause β-thalassemia. The *HBB* gene encodes the 146-amino-acid β-globin polypeptide. Two β-globin polypeptides associate with two α-globin polypeptides to form the adult hemoglobin tetramer. The *HBB* gene spans 1.6 kilobases of DNA on the short arm of chromosome 11. It is made up of three exons and two introns.

Scientists have discovered over 250 different mutations in the *HBB* gene that cause β-thalassemia, although most cases worldwide are associated with about 20 of these mutations. Most mutations change a single nucleotide within or surrounding the *HBB* gene, or create small insertions and deletions. In addition, each population affected by β-thalassemia has a unique mix of mutations. For example, the most prevalent mutation in a Sardinian population—a mutation that accounts for more than 95 percent of cases—is a single base-pair change at codon 39, creating a nonsense mutation and premature termination of the β-globin polypeptide. In contrast, a study of β-thalassemia mutations in a population from the former Yugoslavia revealed 14 different mutations, with only three (all in intron 1 splice signals) accounting for 75 percent of cases.

The types of mutations that cause β-thalassemia not only affect the β-globin amino acid sequence (missense, nonsense, and frameshift mutations), but also alter *HBB* transcription efficiency, mRNA splicing and stability, translation, and protein stability.

Table 15.4 provides a summary of the types of single-gene mutations that cause β-thalassemia. More than half of these mutations are single base-pair changes, and the remainder are short insertions, deletions, and duplications.

Mutations Caused by Expandable DNA Repeats

Beginning in about 1990, molecular analyses of the genes responsible for a number of inherited human disorders revealed a remarkable set of observations. Researchers discovered that some mutant genes contain expansion

TABLE 15.4	Types of Mutations in the *HBB* Gene That Cause β-Thalassemia	
Number of Mutations Known	**Gene Region Affected**	**Description**
22	5′ upstream region	Single base-pair mutations occur between −101 and −25 upstream from transcription start site. For example, a T→A transition in the TATA sequence at −30 results in decreased gene transcription and severe disease.
1	mRNA CAP site	Single base-pair mutation (A→C transversion) at +1 position leads to decreased levels of mRNA.
3	5′ untranslated region	Single base-pair mutations at +20, +22, and +33 cause decreases in transcription and translation and mild disease.
7	ATG translation initiation codon	Single base-pair mutations alter the mRNA AUG sequence, resulting in no translation and severe disease.
36	Exons 1, 2, and 3 coding regions	Single base-pair missense and nonsense mutations, and mutations that create abnormal mRNA splice sites. Disease severity varies from mild to extreme.
38	Introns 1 and 2	Single base-pair transitions and transversions that reduce or abolish mRNA splicing and create abnormal splice sites that affect mRNA stability. Most cause severe disease.
6	Polyadenylation site	Single base-pair changes in the AATAAA sequence reduce the efficiency of mRNA cleavage and polyadenylation, yielding long mRNAs or unstable mRNAs. Disease is mild.
> 100	Throughout and surrounding the *HBB* gene	Short insertions, deletions, and duplications that alter coding sequences, create frameshift stop codons, and alter mRNA splicing.

of **trinucleotide repeat sequences**—specific short DNA sequences repeated many times. Normal individuals have a low number of repetitions of these sequences; however, individuals with over 20 different human disorders appear to have abnormally large numbers of repeat sequences—in some cases, over 200—within and surrounding specific genes.

Examples of diseases associated with these trinucleotide repeat expansions are fragile-X syndrome (discussed in detail in Chapter 8), myotonic dystrophy, and Huntington disease (discussed in Chapter 4). When trinucleotide repeats such as $(CAG)_n$ occur within a coding region, they can be translated into long tracks of glutamine. These glutamine tracks may cause the proteins to aggregate abnormally. When the repeats occur outside coding regions, but within the mRNA, it is thought that the mRNAs may act as "toxic" RNAs that bind to important regulatory proteins, sequestering them away from their normal functions in the cell. Another possible consequence of long trinucleotide repeats is that the regions of DNA containing the repeats may become abnormally methylated, leading to silencing of gene transcription.

The mechanisms by which the repeated sequences expand from generation to generation are of great interest. It is thought that expansion may result from either errors during DNA replication or errors during DNA damage repair. Whatever the cause may be, the presence of these short and unstable repeat sequences seems to be prevalent in humans and in many other organisms.

15.6 Organisms Use DNA Repair Systems to Counteract Mutations

Living systems have evolved a variety of elaborate repair systems that counteract both spontaneous and induced DNA damage. These **DNA repair** systems are absolutely essential to the maintenance of the genetic integrity of organisms and, as such, to the survival of organisms on Earth. The balance between mutation and repair results in the observed mutation rates of individual genes and organisms. Of foremost interest in humans is the ability of these systems to counteract genetic damage that would otherwise result in genetic diseases and cancer. The link between defective DNA repair and cancer susceptibility is described in detail later in the text (see Chapter 19).

We now embark on a review of some systems of DNA repair, with the emphasis on the major approaches that organisms use to counteract genetic damage.

Proofreading and Mismatch Repair

Some of the most common types of mutations arise during DNA replication when an incorrect nucleotide is inserted by DNA polymerase. The major DNA synthesizing enzyme in bacteria (**DNA polymerase III**) makes an error approximately once every 100,000 insertions, leading to an error rate of 10^{-5}. Fortunately, DNA polymerase proofreads each step, catching 99 percent of those errors. If an incorrect nucleotide is inserted during polymerization, the enzyme can recognize the error and "reverse" its direction. It then behaves as a 3' to 5' exonuclease, cutting out the incorrect nucleotide and replacing it with the correct one. This improves the efficiency of replication 100-fold, creating only 1 mismatch in every 10^7 insertions, for a final error rate of 10^{-7}.

To cope with errors such as base–base mismatches, small insertions, and deletions that remain after proofreading, another mechanism, called **mismatch repair**, may be activated. During mismatch repair, the mismatches are detected, the incorrect nucleotide is removed, and the correct nucleotide is inserted in its place. But how does the repair system recognize which nucleotide is correct (on the template strand) and which nucleotide is incorrect (on the newly synthesized strand)? If the mismatch is recognized but no such discrimination occurs, the excision will be random, and the strand bearing the correct base will be clipped out 50 percent of the time. Hence, strand discrimination is a critical step.

The process of strand discrimination has been elucidated in some bacteria, including *E. coli,* and is based on **DNA methylation**. These bacteria contain an enzyme, **adenine methylase**, which recognizes the DNA sequence

$$5' \text{—— GATC —— } 3'$$
$$3' \text{—— CTAG —— } 5'$$

as a substrate, adding a methyl group to each of the adenine residues during DNA replication.

Following replication, the newly synthesized DNA strand remains temporarily unmethylated, as the adenine methylase lags behind the DNA polymerase. Prior to methylation, the repair enzyme recognizes the mismatch and binds to the unmethylated (newly synthesized) DNA strand. An **endonuclease** enzyme creates a nick in the backbone of the unmethylated DNA strand, either 5' or 3' to the mismatch. An **exonuclease** unwinds and degrades the nicked DNA strand, until the region of the mismatch is reached. Finally, DNA polymerase fills in the gap created by the exonuclease, using the correct DNA strand as a template. DNA ligase then seals the gap.

A series of *E. coli* gene products, MutH, MutL, and MutS, as well as exonucleases, DNA polymerase III and ligase, are involved in mismatch repair. Mutations in the *MutH, MutL,* and *MutS* genes result in bacterial strains deficient in mismatch repair. While the preceding mechanism occurs in *E. coli,* similar mechanisms involving homologous proteins exist in yeast and in mammals.

In humans, mutations in genes that code for DNA mismatch repair proteins (such as the *hMSH2* and *hMLH1,* which are the human equivalents of the *MutS* and *MutL* genes of

E. coli) are associated with the hereditary nonpolyposis colon cancer. Mismatch repair defects are commonly found in other cancers, such as leukemias, lymphomas, and tumors of the ovary, prostate, and endometrium. Cells from these cancers show genome-wide increases in the rate of spontaneous mutation. The link between defective mismatch repair and cancer is supported by experiments with mice. Mice that are engineered to have deficiencies in mismatch repair genes accumulate large numbers of mutations and are cancer-prone.

Postreplication Repair and the SOS Repair System

Another DNA repair system, called **postreplication repair**, responds *after* damaged DNA has escaped repair and has failed to be completely replicated. As illustrated in **Figure 15–11**,

Postreplication repair

DNA unwound prior to replication

Replication skips over lesion and continues

Undamaged complementary region of parental strand is recombined

New gap formed

Recombined complement

New gap is filled by DNA polymerase and DNA ligase

FIGURE 15–11 Postreplication repair occurs if DNA replication has skipped over a lesion such as a thymine dimer. Through the process of recombination, the correct complementary sequence is recruited from the parental strand and inserted into the gap opposite the lesion. The new gap is filled by DNA polymerase and DNA ligase.

when DNA bearing a lesion of some sort (such as a pyrimidine dimer) is being replicated, DNA polymerase may stall at the lesion and then skip over it, leaving an unreplicated gap on the newly synthesized strand. To correct the gap, the RecA protein directs a recombinational exchange with the corresponding region on the undamaged parental strand of the same polarity (the "donor" strand). When the undamaged segment of the donor strand DNA replaces the gapped segment, a gap is created on the donor strand. The gap can be filled by repair synthesis as replication proceeds. Because a recombinational event is involved in this type of DNA repair, it is considered to be a form of **homologous recombination repair**.

Still another repair pathway, the *E. coli* **SOS repair system**, also responds to damaged DNA, but in a different way. In the presence of a large number of unrepaired DNA mismatches and gaps, bacteria can induce the expression of about 20 genes (including *lexA*, *recA*, and *uvr*) whose products allow DNA replication to occur even in the presence of these lesions. This type of repair is a last resort to minimize DNA damage, hence its name. During SOS repair, DNA synthesis becomes error-prone, inserting random and possibly incorrect nucleotides in places that would normally stall DNA replication. As a result, SOS repair itself becomes mutagenic—although it may allow the cell to survive DNA damage that would otherwise kill it.

Photoreactivation Repair: Reversal of UV Damage

As illustrated in Figure 15–8, UV light is mutagenic as a result of the creation of pyrimidine dimers. UV-induced damage to *E. coli* DNA can be partially reversed if, following irradiation, the cells are exposed briefly to light in the blue range of the visible spectrum. The process is dependent on the activity of a protein called **photoreactivation enzyme (PRE)**. The enzyme's mode of action is to cleave the bonds between thymine dimers, thus directly reversing the effect of UV radiation on DNA (**Figure 15–12**). Although the enzyme will associate with a thymine dimer in the dark, it must absorb a photon of light to cleave the dimer. In spite of its ability to reduce the number of UV-induced mutations, **photoreactivation repair** is not absolutely essential in *E. coli*; we know this because a mutation creating a null allele in the gene coding for PRE is not lethal. Nonetheless, the enzyme is detectable in many organisms, including bacteria, fungi, plants, and some vertebrates—though not in humans. Humans and other organisms that lack photoreactivation repair must rely on other repair mechanisms to reverse the effects of UV radiation.

Base and Nucleotide Excision Repair

A number of light-independent DNA repair systems exist in all prokaryotes and eukaryotes. The basic mechanisms involved in these types of repair—collectively referred to as

Photoreactivation repair

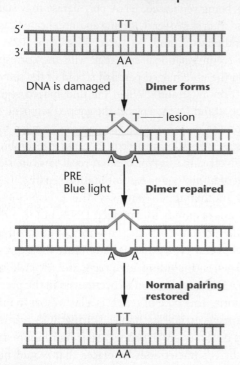

FIGURE 15-12 Damaged DNA repaired by photoreactivation repair. The bond creating the thymine dimer is cleaved by the photoreactivation enzyme (PRE), which must be activated by blue light in the visible spectrum.

Base excision repair

FIGURE 15-13 Base excision repair (BER) accomplished by uracil DNA glycosylase, AP endonuclease, DNA polymerase, and DNA ligase. Uracil is recognized as a noncomplementary base, excised, and replaced with the complementary base (C).

excision repair or cut-and-paste mechanisms—consist of the following three steps.

1. The distortion or error present on one of the two strands of the DNA helix is recognized and enzymatically clipped out by an endonuclease. Excisions in the phosphodiester backbone usually include a number of nucleotides adjacent to the error as well, leaving a gap on one strand of the helix.

2. A DNA polymerase fills in the gap by inserting nucleotides complementary to those on the intact strand, which it uses as a replicative template. The enzyme adds these nucleotides to the free 3'-OH end of the clipped DNA. In *E. coli*, this step is usually performed by DNA polymerase I.

3. DNA ligase seals the final "nick" that remains at the 3'-OH end of the last nucleotide inserted, closing the gap.

There are two types of excision repair: base excision repair and nucleotide excision repair. **Base excision repair (BER)** corrects DNA that contains a damaged DNA base. The first step in the BER pathway in *E. coli* involves the recognition of the altered base by an enzyme called **DNA glycosylase**. There are a number of DNA glycosylases, each of which recognizes a specific base (**Figure 15–13**). For example, the enzyme uracil DNA

glycosylase recognizes the presence of uracil in DNA. DNA glycosylases first cut the glycosidic bond between the base and the sugar, creating an **apyrimidinic** or **apurinic site**. The sugar with the missing base is then recognized by an enzyme called **AP endonuclease**. The AP endonuclease makes a cut in the phosphodiester backbone at the apyrimidinic or apurinic site. Endonucleases then remove the deoxyribose sugar, and the gap is filled by DNA polymerase and DNA ligase.

Although much has been learned about the mechanisms of BER in *E. coli*, BER systems have also been detected in eukaryotes from yeast to humans. Experimental evidence shows that both mouse and human cells that are defective in BER activity are hypersensitive to the killing effects of gamma rays and oxidizing agents.

Nucleotide excision repair (NER) pathways repair "bulky" lesions in DNA that alter or distort the double helix. These lesions include the UV-induced pyrimidine dimers and DNA adducts discussed previously.

The NER pathway (**Figure 15–14**) was first discovered in *E. coli* by Paul Howard-Flanders and coworkers, who isolated several independent mutants that are sensitive to UV radiation. One group of genes was designated *uvr* (ultraviolet repair) and included the *uvrA*, *uvrB*, and *uvrC* mutations. In the NER pathway, the *uvr* gene products are involved in recognizing and clipping out lesions in the

Nucleotide excision repair

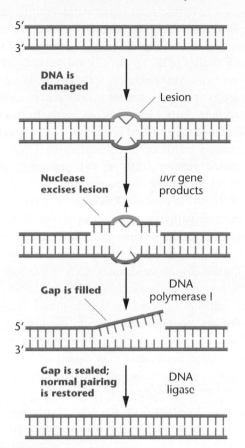

DNA is damaged

Lesion

Nuclease excises lesion

uvr gene products

Gap is filled

DNA polymerase I

Gap is sealed; normal pairing is restored

DNA ligase

FIGURE 15–14 Nucleotide excision repair (NER) of a UV-induced thymine dimer. During repair, 13 nucleotides are excised in prokaryotes, and 28 nucleotides are excised in eukaryotes.

FIGURE 15–15 Two individuals with xeroderma pigmentosum. These XP patients show characteristic XP skin lesions induced by sunlight, as well as mottled redness (erythema) and irregular pigment changes to the skin, in response to cellular injury.

DNA. Usually, a specific number of nucleotides is clipped out around both sides of the lesion. In *E. coli,* usually a total of 13 nucleotides is removed, including the lesion. The repair is then completed by DNA polymerase I and DNA ligase, in a manner similar to that occurring in BER. The undamaged strand opposite the lesion is used as a template for the replication, resulting in repair.

Nucleotide Excision Repair and Xeroderma Pigmentosum in Humans

The mechanism of NER in eukaryotes is much more complicated than that in prokaryotes and involves many more proteins, encoded by about 30 genes. Much of what is known about the system in humans has come from detailed studies of individuals with **xeroderma pigmentosum (XP),** a rare recessive genetic disorder that predisposes individuals to severe skin abnormalities, skin cancers, and a wide range of other symptoms including developmental and neurological defects. Patients with XP are extremely sensitive to UV radiation in sunlight. In addition, they have a 2000-fold higher rate of cancer, particularly skin cancer,

than the general population. The condition is severe and may be lethal, although early detection and protection from sunlight can arrest it (**Figure 15–15**).

The repair of UV-induced lesions in XP has been investigated *in vitro,* using human fibroblast cell cultures derived from normal individuals and those with XP. (Fibroblasts are undifferentiated connective tissue cells.) The results of these studies suggest that the XP phenotype is caused by defects in NER pathways and by mutations in more than one gene.

In 1968, James Cleaver showed that cells from XP patients were deficient in DNA synthesis other than that occurring during chromosome replication—a phenomenon known as **unscheduled DNA synthesis**. Unscheduled DNA synthesis is elicited in normal cells by UV radiation. Because this type of synthesis is thought to represent the activity of DNA polymerization during NER, the lack of unscheduled DNA synthesis in XP patients suggested that XP may be a deficiency in NER.

The involvement of multiple genes in NER and XP was further investigated by studies using **somatic cell hybridization**. Fibroblast cells from any two unrelated XP patients, when grown together in tissue culture, can fuse together, forming heterokaryons. A **heterokaryon** is a single cell with two nuclei from different organisms but a common cytoplasm. NER in the heterokaryon can be measured by the level of unscheduled DNA synthesis. If the mutation in each of the two XP cells occurs in the same gene, the heterokaryon, like the cells that fused to form it, will still be unable to undergo NER. This is because there is no normal copy of the relevant gene present in the heterokaryon. However, if NER does occur in the heterokaryon, the mutations in the two XP cells must have been present in two different genes. Hence, the two mutants are said to demonstrate **complementation**, a concept also discussed earlier in the text (see Chapter 4). Complementation occurs because the heterokaryon has at least one normal copy of each gene in the fused cell. By fusing XP cells from a large number of XP patients, researchers were able to determine how many genes contribute to the XP phenotype.

Based on these and other studies, XP patients were divided into seven complementation groups, indicating that at least seven different genes are involved in nucleotide excision repair in humans. A gene representing each of these complementation groups, *XPA* to *XPG* (*Xeroderma Pigmentosum gene A to G*), has now been identified, and a homologous gene for each has been identified in yeast. Approximately 20 percent of XP patients do not fall into any of the seven complementation groups. Cells from most of these patients have mutations in the gene coding for DNA polymerase H and are defective in repair DNA synthesis. Approximately 6 percent of XP patients do not have mutations in either the seven complementation group genes or the *polymerase H* gene, suggesting that other genes or mutations outside of coding regions may be involved in XP.

As a result of the study of defective genes in XP, a great deal is now known about how NER counteracts DNA damage in normal cells. The first step in humans is recognition of the damaged DNA by proteins encoded by the *XPC, XPE,* and *XPA* genes. These proteins then recruit the remainder of the repair proteins to the site of DNA damage. The *XPB* and *XPD* genes encode helicases, and the *XPF* and *XPG* genes encode nucleases. The excision repair complex containing these and other factors is responsible for the excision of an approximately 28-nucleotide-long fragment from the DNA strand that contains the lesion.

Two other rare autosomal recessive diseases are associated with defects in NER pathways—Cockayne syndrome (CS) and trichothiodystrophy (TTD). The symptoms of CS include developmental and neurological defects and sensitivity to sunlight, but not an increase in cancers. Patients with CS age prematurely and usually die before the age of 20. Patients with TTD suffer from dwarfism, retardation, brittle hair and skin, and facial deformities. Like CS, these patients are sensitive to sunlight but do not have higher than normal rates of cancer. TTD patients have a median life span of six years.

Both CS and TTD arise from mutations in some of the same genes involved in XP (such as *XPB* and *XPD*), as well as other genes that encode proteins involved in NER within transcribed regions of the genome. It is not known why such a wide variety of different symptoms result from mutations in the same genes or DNA repair pathways; however, it may reflect the fact that products of many NER genes are also involved in other essential processes.

Double-Strand Break Repair in Eukaryotes

Thus far, we have discussed repair pathways that deal with damage or errors within one strand of DNA. We conclude our discussion of DNA repair by considering what happens when both strands of the DNA helix are cleaved—as a result of exposure to ionizing radiation, for example. These types of damage are extremely dangerous to cells, leading to chromosome rearrangements, cancer, or cell death. In this section, we will discuss double-strand breaks in eukaryotic cells.

Specialized forms of DNA repair, the DNA **double-strand break repair (DSB repair)** pathways, are activated and are responsible for reattaching two broken DNA strands. Recently, interest in DSB repair has grown because defects in these pathways are associated with X-ray hypersensitivity and immune deficiency. Such defects may also underlie familial disposition to breast and ovarian cancer. Several human disease syndromes, such as Fanconi anemia and ataxia telangiectasia, result from defects in DSB repair.

One pathway involved in double-strand break repair is **homologous recombination repair**. The first step in this process involves the activity of an enzyme that recognizes the double-strand break, and then digests back the 5′ ends of the broken DNA helix, leaving overhanging 3′ ends (**Figure 15–16**). One overhanging end searches for a region of sequence complementarity on the sister chromatid and then invades the homologous DNA duplex, aligning the complementary sequences. Once aligned, DNA synthesis proceeds from the 3′ overhanging ends, using the undamaged DNA strands as templates. The interaction of two sister chromatids is necessary because, when both strands of one helix are broken, there is no undamaged parental DNA strand available to use as a source of the complementary template DNA sequence during repair. After DNA repair synthesis, the resulting heteroduplex molecule is resolved and the two chromatids separate, as previously discussed earlier in the text (see Chapter 11).

DSB repair usually occurs during the late S or early G2 phase of the cell cycle, after DNA replication, a time when sister chromatids are available to be used as repair templates. Because an undamaged template is used during repair synthesis, homologous recombination repair is an accurate process.

A second pathway, called **nonhomologous end joining**, also repairs double-strand breaks. However, as the name implies, the mechanism does not recruit a homologous region of DNA during repair. This system is activated in G1, prior to DNA replication. End joining involves a complex of many proteins, and may include the DNA-dependent protein kinase and the breast cancer susceptibility gene product, BRCA1. These and other proteins bind to the free ends of the broken DNA, trim the ends, and ligate them back together. Because some nucleotide sequences are lost in the process of end joining, it is an error-prone repair system. In addition, if more than one chromosome suffers

FIGURE 15–16 Steps in homologous recombination repair of double-stranded breaks.

a double-strand break, the wrong ends could be joined together, leading to abnormal chromosome structures, such as those discussed earlier in the text (see Chapter 8).

NOW SOLVE THIS

15–4 Geneticists often use ethylmethane sulfonate (EMS) to induce mutations in *Drosophila*. Why is EMS a mutagen of choice for genetic research? What would be the effects of EMS in a strain of *Drosophila* lacking functional mismatch repair systems?

■ **HINT:** *This problem asks you to evaluate EMS as a useful mutagen and to determine its effects in the absence of DNA repair. The key to its solution is to consider the chemical effects of EMS on DNA. Also, consider the types of DNA repair that may operate on EMS-mutated DNA and the efficiency of these processes.*

15.7 The Ames Test Is Used to Assess the Mutagenicity of Compounds

There is great concern about the possible mutagenic properties of any chemical that enters the human body, whether through the skin, the digestive system, or the respiratory tract. Examples of synthetic chemicals that concern us are those found in air and water pollution, food preservatives, artificial sweeteners, herbicides, pesticides, and pharmaceutical products. Mutagenicity can be tested in various organisms, including fungi, plants, and cultured mammalian cells; however, one of the most common tests, which we describe here, uses bacteria.

The **Ames test** uses a number of different strains of the bacterium *Salmonella typhimurium* that have been selected for their ability to reveal the presence of specific types of mutations. For example, some strains are used to detect base-pair substitutions, and other strains detect various frameshift mutations. Each strain contains a mutation in one of the genes of the histidine operon. The mutant strains are unable to synthesize histidine (his^- strains) and therefore require histidine for growth (**Figure 15–17**). The assay measures the frequency of reverse mutations that occur within the mutant gene, yielding wild-type bacteria (his^+ revertants). These *Salmonella* strains also have an increased sensitivity to mutagens due to the presence of mutations in genes involved in both DNA damage repair and the synthesis of the lipopolysaccharide barrier that coats bacteria and protects them from external substances.

Many substances entering the human body are relatively innocuous until activated metabolically, usually in the liver, to more chemically reactive products. Thus, the Ames test includes a step in which the test compound is incubated *in vitro* in the presence of a mammalian liver extract. Alternatively, test compounds may be injected into a mouse where they are modified by liver enzymes and then recovered for use in the Ames test.

In the initial use of Ames testing in the 1970s, a large number of known **carcinogens**, or cancer-causing agents, were examined, and more than 80 percent of these were shown to be strong mutagens. This is not surprising, as the transformation of cells to the malignant state occurs as a result of mutations. For example, more than 60 compounds found in cigarette smoke test positive in the Ames test and cause cancer in animal tests. Although a positive response in the Ames test does not prove that a compound is carcinogenic, the Ames test is useful as a preliminary screening device. The Ames test is used extensively during the development of industrial and pharmaceutical chemical compounds.

FIGURE 15–17 The Ames test, which screens compounds for potential mutagenicity.

his⁻ auxotrophs plus liver enzymes

Potential mutagen plus liver enzymes

Add mixture to filter paper disk

Spread bacteria on agar medium without histidine

Place disk on surface of medium

Incubate at 37°C

Spontaneous *his⁺* revertants (control)

his⁺ revertants induced by mutagen

15.8 Transposable Elements Move within the Genome and May Create Mutations

Transposable elements, also known as **transposons** or "jumping genes," can move or transpose within and between chromosomes, inserting themselves into various locations within the genome.

Transposable elements are present in the genomes of all organisms from bacteria to humans. Not only are they ubiquitous, but they also comprise large portions of some eukaryotic genomes. For example, almost 50 percent of the human genome is derived from transposable elements. Some organisms with unusually large genomes, such as salamanders and barley, contain hundreds of thousands of copies of various types of transposable elements. Although the function of these elements is unknown, data from human genome sequencing suggest that some genes may have evolved from transposable elements and that the presence of these elements may help to modify and reshape the genome. Transposable elements are also valuable tools in genetic

research. Geneticists harness transposons as mutagens, as cloning tags, and as vehicles for introducing foreign DNA into model organisms. One use of transposons in genetic research is described in the Modern Approaches to Gene Function feature on page 389.

In this section, we discuss transposable elements as naturally occurring mutagens. The movement of transposable elements from one place in the genome to another has the capacity to disrupt genes and cause mutations, as well as to create chromosomal damage such as double-strand breaks.

Insertion Sequences and Bacterial Transposons

There are two types of transposable elements in bacteria: insertion sequences and bacterial transposons. **Insertion sequences (IS elements)** can move from one location to another and, if they insert into a gene or gene-regulatory region, may cause mutations.

IS elements were first identified during analyses of mutations in the *gal* operon of *E. coli*. Researchers discovered that certain mutations in this operon were due to the presence of several hundred base pairs of extra DNA inserted into the beginning of the operon. Surprisingly, the segment of mutagenic DNA could spontaneously excise from this location, restoring wild-type function to the *gal* operon. Subsequent research revealed that several other DNA elements could behave in a similar fashion, inserting into bacterial chromosomes and affecting gene function.

IS elements are relatively short, not exceeding 2000 bp (2 kb). The first insertion sequence to be characterized in *E. coli*, IS1, is about 800 bp long. Other IS elements such as IS2, 3, 4, and 5 are about 1250 to 1400 bp in length. IS elements are present in multiple copies in bacterial genomes. For example, the *E. coli* chromosome contains five to eight copies of IS1, five copies each of IS2 and IS3, as well as copies of IS elements on plasmids such as F factors.

All IS elements contain two features that are essential for their movement. First, they contain a gene that encodes an enzyme called **transposase**. This enzyme is responsible for making staggered cuts in chromosomal DNA, into which the IS element can insert. Second, the ends of IS elements contain **inverted terminal repeats (ITRs)**. ITRs are short segments of DNA that have the same nucleotide sequence as each other but are oriented in the opposite direction (**Figure 15–18**). Although Figure 15–18 shows the ITRs to consist of only a few nucleotides, IS ITRs usually contain about 20 to 40 nucleotide pairs. ITRs are essential for transposition and act as recognition sites for the binding of the transposase enzyme.

Bacterial transposons (**Tn elements**) are larger than IS elements and contain protein-coding genes that are unrelated to their transposition. Some Tn elements, such as Tn10, are composed of a drug-resistance gene flanked by two IS

FIGURE 15–18 An insertion sequence (IS), shown in purple. The terminal sequences are perfect inverted repeats of one another.

elements present in opposite orientations. The IS elements encode the transposase enzyme that is necessary for transposition of the Tn element. Other types of Tn elements, such as Tn3, have shorter inverted repeat sequences at their ends and encode their transposase enzyme from a transposase gene located in the middle of the Tn element. Like IS elements, Tn elements are mobile in both bacterial chromosomes and in plasmids and can cause mutations if they insert into genes or gene-regulatory regions.

Tn elements are currently of interest because they can introduce multiple drug resistance onto bacterial plasmids. These plasmids, called **R factors**, may contain many Tn elements conferring simultaneous resistance to heavy metals, antibiotics, and other drugs. These elements can move from plasmids onto bacterial chromosomes and can spread multiple drug resistance between different strains of bacteria.

The *Ac–Ds* System in Maize

About 20 years before the discovery of transposons in bacteria, Barbara McClintock discovered mobile genetic elements in corn plants (maize). She did this by analyzing the genetic behavior of two mutations, **Dissociation (Ds)** and **Activator (Ac)**, expressed in either the endosperm or aleurone layers. She then correlated her genetic observations with cytological examinations of the maize chromosomes. Initially, McClintock determined that *Ds* was located on chromosome 9. If *Ac* was also present in the genome, *Ds* induced breakage at a point on the chromosome adjacent to its own location. If chromosome breakage occurred in somatic cells during their development, progeny cells often lost part of the broken chromosome, causing a variety of phenotypic effects. The chapter-opening photo illustrates the types of phenotypic effects caused by *Ds* mutations in kernels of corn.

Subsequent analysis suggested to McClintock that both *Ds* and *Ac* elements sometimes moved to new chromosomal locations. While *Ds* moved only if *Ac* was also present, *Ac* was capable of autonomous movement. Where *Ds* came to reside determined its genetic effects—that is, it might cause chromosome breakage, or it might inhibit expression of a certain gene. In cells in which *Ds* caused a gene mutation, *Ds* might move again, restoring the gene mutation to wild type.

Figure 15–19 illustrates the types of movements and effects brought about by *Ds* and *Ac* elements. In McClintock's original observation, pigment synthesis was restored in cells in which the *Ds* element jumped out of chromosome 9. McClintock concluded that the *Ds* and *Ac* genes were **mobile controlling elements**. We now commonly refer to them as transposable elements, a term coined by another great maize geneticist, Alexander Brink.

Several *Ac* and *Ds* elements have now been analyzed, and the relationship between the two elements has been clarified. The first *Ds* element studied (*Ds9*)

(a) In absence of *Ac*, *Ds* is not transposable.

(b) When *Ac* is present, *Ds* may be transposed.

(c) *Ds* can move into and out of another gene.

FIGURE 15–19 Effects of *Ac* and *Ds* elements on gene expression. (a) If *Ds* is present in the absence of *Ac*, there is normal expression of a distantly located hypothetical gene *W*. (b) In the presence of *Ac*, *Ds* may transpose to a region adjacent to *W*. *Ds* can induce chromosome breakage, which may lead to loss of a chromosome fragment bearing the *W* gene. (c) In the presence of *Ac*, *Ds* may transpose into the *W* gene, disrupting *W*-gene expression. If *Ds* subsequently transposes out of the *W* gene, *W*-gene expression may return to normal.

is nearly identical to *Ac* except for a 194-bp deletion within the transposase gene. The deletion of part of the transposase gene in the *Ds9* element explains its dependence on the *Ac* element for transposition. Several other *Ds* elements have also been sequenced, and each contains an even larger deletion within the transposase gene. In each case, however, the ITRs are retained.

Although the significance of Barbara McClintock's mobile controlling elements was not fully appreciated following her initial observations, molecular analysis has since verified her conclusions. She was awarded the Nobel Prize in Physiology or Medicine in 1983.

Copia and P Elements in *Drosophila*

There are more than 30 families of transposable elements in *Drosophila,* each of which is present in 20 to 50 copies in the genome. Together, these families constitute about 5 percent of the *Drosophila* genome and over half of the middle repetitive DNA of this organism. One study suggests that 50 percent of all visible mutations in *Drosophila* are the result of the insertion of transposons into otherwise wild-type genes.

In 1975, David Hogness and his colleagues David Finnegan, Gerald Rubin, and Michael Young identified a class of DNA elements in *Drosophila melanogaster* that they designated as *copia*. These elements are transcribed into "copious" amounts of RNA (hence their name). *Copia* elements are present in 10 to 100 copies in the genomes of *Drosophila* cells. Mapping studies show that they are transposable to different chromosomal locations and are dispersed throughout the genome.

Each *copia* element consists of approximately 5000 to 8000 bp of DNA, including a long **direct terminal repeat (DTR)** sequence of 267 bp at each end. Within each DTR is an inverted terminal repeat (ITR) of 17 bp (**Figure 15–20**). The short ITR sequences are characteristic of *copia* elements. The DTR sequences are found in other transposons in other organisms, but they are not universal.

Insertion of *copia* is dependent on the presence of the ITR sequences and seems to occur preferentially at specific target sites in the genome. The *copia*-like elements demonstrate regulatory effects at the point of their insertion in the chromosome. Certain mutations, including those affecting

eye color and segment formation, are due to *copia* insertions within genes. For example, the eye-color mutation *white-apricot* is caused by an allele of the *white* gene, which contains a *copia* element within the gene. Transposition of the *copia* element out of the *white-apricot* allele can restore the allele to wild type.

Perhaps the most significant *Drosophila* transposable elements are the **P elements**. These were discovered while studying the phenomenon of **hybrid dysgenesis**, a condition characterized by sterility, elevated mutation rates, and chromosome rearrangements in the offspring of crosses between certain strains of fruit flies. Hybrid dysgenesis is caused by high rates of *P* element transposition in the germ line, in which transposons insert themselves into or near genes, thereby causing mutations. *P* elements range from 0.5 to 2.9 kb long, with 31-bp ITRs. Full-length *P* elements encode at least two proteins, one of which is the transposase enzyme that is required for transposition, and another is a repressor protein that inhibits transposition. The transposase gene is expressed only in the germ line, accounting for the tissue specificity of *P* element transposition. Strains of flies that contain full-length *P* elements inserted into their genomes are resistant to further transpositions due to the presence of the repressor protein encoded by the *P* elements.

Mutations can arise from several kinds of insertional events. If a *P* element inserts into the coding region of a gene, it can terminate transcription of the gene and destroy normal gene expression. If it inserts into the promoter region of a gene, it can affect the level of expression of the gene. Insertions into introns can affect splicing or cause the premature termination of transcription.

Geneticists have harnessed *P* elements as tools for genetic analysis. One of the most useful applications of *P* elements is as vectors to introduce transgenes into *Drosophila*—a technique known as **germ-line transformation**. *P* elements are also used to generate mutations and to clone mutant genes. In addition, researchers are perfecting methods to target *P* element insertions to precise single-chromosomal sites, which should increase the precision of germ-line transformation in the analysis of gene activity.

Transposable Elements in Humans

The human genome, like that of other eukaryotes, is riddled with DNA derived from transposons. Recent genomic sequencing data reveal that approximately half of the human genome is composed of transposable element DNA. As discussed earlier in the text (see Chapter 8), the major families of human transposable elements are the long interspersed elements and short interspersed elements (**LINEs** and **SINEs**, respectively). Together, they comprise over 30 percent of the human genome. Other families of

FIGURE 15–20 Structural organization of a *copia* transposable element in *Drosophila melanogaster,* showing the terminal repeats.

MODERN APPROACHES TO UNDERSTANDING GENE FUNCTION

Transposon-Mediated Mutations Reveal Genes Involved in Colorectal Cancer

In this chapter you learned about transposons and how they can move within a genome. Scientists have taken advantage of transposons, using them as a tool for mutagenesis of specific and random DNA sequences in the genome. This represents a **forward genetics** approach to create transgenic and knockout animals to learn about gene function.

Human colorectal cancers (CRCs) arise from complex underlying genetic and epigenetic alterations. Some genes are thought to be *drivers of tumorigenesis*; that is, they cause tumor formation. Other mutations are thought to be *passenger mutations*: They appear at some point during the progression of CRCs, but they have little to no direct effect on the origin of a tumor. To develop novel, targeted therapies for treating CRCs, it is essential that scientists distinguish driver mutations from passenger mutations. Here we profile a landmark study in which transposons were used to reveal CRC driver genes in a mouse model.

Researchers used a **conditional knockout** strategy involving a mating between different transgenic animals. One transgenic mouse strain contained a transposase gene coupled to a promoter sequence for the *Villin* gene, a gene that is expressed in the small intestine. As a result, these animals mainly express high levels of transposase in the epithelial cells of the GI tract. Another transgenic strain, called *T2/Onc*, contains a transposon. This transposon will not move in this parent strain, as it lacks the correct transposase. Crossing these mice resulted in offspring with active transposase confined to cells of the GI tract. The transposase allows the transposition of the *T2/Onc* transposon into other positions within the mouse genome. In theory, transposition mutagenesis of driver genes involved in CRCs would produce mice with mutant phenotypes resembling CRCs.

Results:

It was found that 72 percent of transgenic mice offspring expressing transposase in the GI tract had intestinal tumors (see photo). These animals died at a faster rate than control animals and at a younger age. Analysis of intestinal lesions confirmed characteristics of CRC tumor types. DNA from tumors was sequenced to identify the locations of transposon insertions, and an analysis of over 16,000 transposons revealed 77 candidate genes for CRC. The genes revealed in this study were compared to a recent large-scale exon sequencing project that analyzed mutations in genes from human CRC tumor samples. Sixty of the mouse genes identified in this study were shown to be mutated or improperly expressed in human CRC. This transposon screen also revealed 17 candidate genes that had not been previously implicated in CRC.

Conclusions:

This transposon screen produced mice with identified mutations resulting in tumors of the GI tract and revealed candidate genes that may be drivers of CRC tumor formation in humans. It suggests that tumorigenesis of CRC is driven by a small subset of mutated genes. Discovering significant overlap between mouse candidate genes and human genes known to be involved in CRC suggests that this mouse model will be useful for developing drug-based and other strategies for treating CRC in humans.

Reference:

Starr, T. K. 2009. A transposon-based genetic screen in mice identifies genes altered in colorectal cancer. *Science*, 323:1747-1750.

Questions to Consider:

1. The *T2/Onc* transposon system in this paper is sometimes called "Sleeping Beauty." Why do you think that is a good name? Do a Google search to learn more about this system to help you answer this question.
2. What do you think are limitations to this type of screening approach?
3. *Apc, Tcf12,* and *Fbxw7* were among the top-ranked driver genes identified in this study based on the number of transposon insertions in transgenic mice and their mutant or aberrant expression in human CRCs. Search Online Mendelian Inheritance in Man (OMIM, http://www.omim.org) to reveal what is known about the function of these genes.

(a)

(b)

Photomicrographs of hematoxylin and eosin-stained tissue from the small intestine of transgenic animals showing an adenocarcinoma [(a), arrow; 500 μm] and a cluster of tumors that has invaded the GI epithelium [(b), arrow; 100 μm].

TABLE 15.5	Transposable Elements in the Human Genome		
Element Type	Length	Copies in Genome	% of Genome
LINEs	1–6 kb	850,000	21
SINEs	100–500 bp	1,500,000	13
LTR Elements	<5 kb	443,000	8
DNA Elements	80–300 bp	294,000	3
Unclassified	–	3,000	0.1

transposable elements account for a further 11 percent (Table 15.5). As coding sequences comprise only about 1 percent of the human genome, there is about 40 to 50 times more transposable element DNA in the human genome than DNA in functional genes.

Although most human transposable elements appear to be inactive, the potential mobility and mutagenic effects of these elements have far-reaching implications for human genetics, as can be seen in a recent example of a transposable element "caught in the act." The case involves a male child with hemophilia. One cause of hemophilia is a defect in blood-clotting factor VIII, the product of an X-linked gene. Haig Kazazian and his colleagues found LINEs inserted at two points within the gene. Researchers were interested in determining if one of the mother's X chromosomes also contained this specific LINE. If so, the unaffected mother would be heterozygous and pass the LINE-containing chromosome to her son. The surprising finding was that the LINE sequence was *not* present on either of her X chromosomes but *was* detected on chromosome 22 of both parents. This suggests that this mobile element may have transposed from one chromosome to another in the gamete-forming cells of the mother, prior to being transmitted to the son.

LINE insertions into the human *dystrophin* gene have resulted in at least two separate cases of Duchenne muscular dystrophy. In one case, a LINE inserted into exon 48, and in another case, it inserted into exon 44, both leading to frameshift mutations and premature termination of translation of the dystrophin protein. There are also reports that LINEs have inserted into the *APC* and *c-myc* genes, leading to mutations that may have contributed to the development of some colon and breast cancers. In the latter cases, the transposition had occurred within one or a few somatic cells. As of 2009, researchers have determined that cases of at least 11 human diseases are due to insertions of LINE elements.

SINE insertions are also responsible for more than 30 cases of human disease. In one case, an ***Alu* element** integrated into the *BRCA2* gene, inactivating this tumor suppressor gene and leading to a familial case of breast cancer. Other genes that have been mutated by *Alu* integrations are the *factor IX* gene (leading to hemophilia B), the *ChE* gene (leading to acholinesterasemia), and the *NF1* gene (leading to neurofibromatosis).

Transposons, Mutations, and Evolution

Transposons can have a wide range of effects on genes. The insertion of a transposon into the coding region of a gene may disrupt the gene's normal translation reading frame or may induce premature termination of translation of the mRNA transcribed from the gene. Many transposable elements contain their own promoters and enhancers, as well as splice sites and polyadenylation signals. The presence of these regulatory sequences can have effects on nearby genes. The insertion of a transposable element containing polyadenylation or transcription termination signals into a gene's intron may bring about termination of the gene's transcription within the element. In addition, it can cause aberrant splicing of an RNA transcribed from the gene. Insertions of a transposon into a gene's transcription regulatory region may disrupt the gene's normal regulation or may cause the gene to be expressed differently as a result of the presence of the transposon's own promoter or enhancer sequences. The presence of two or more identical transposons in a genome creates the potential for recombination between the transposons, leading to duplications, deletions, inversions, or chromosome translocations. Any of these rearrangements may bring about phenotypic changes or disease.

It is thought that about 0.2 percent of detectable human mutations may be due to transposable element insertions. Other organisms appear to suffer more damage due to transposition. About 10 percent of new mouse mutations and 50 percent of *Drosophila* mutations are caused by insertions of transposable elements in or near genes.

Because of their ability to alter genes and chromosomes, transposons may contribute to the variability that underlies evolution. For example, the Tn elements of bacteria carry antibiotic resistance genes between organisms, conferring a survival advantage to the bacteria under certain conditions. Another example of a transposon's contribution to evolution is provided by *Drosophila* telomeres. LINE-like elements are present at the ends of *Drosophila* chromosomes, and these elements act as telomeres, maintaining the length of *Drosophila* chromosomes over successive cell divisions. Other examples of evolved transposons are the *RAG1* and *RAG2* genes in humans. These genes encode **recombinase** enzymes that are essential to the development of the immune system. These two genes appear to have evolved from transposons.

Transposons may also affect the evolution of genomes by altering gene-expression patterns in ways that are subsequently retained by the host. For example, the human *amylase* gene contains an enhancer that causes the gene to be expressed in the parotid gland. This enhancer evolved from transposon sequences that were inserted into the gene-regulatory region early in primate evolution. Other examples of gene-expression patterns that were affected by the presence of transposon sequences are T-cell-specific expression of the *CD8* gene and placenta-specific expression of the *leptin* and *CYP19* genes.

Sequence Alignment to Identify a Mutation

MasteringGenetics™ Visit the
Study Area: Exploring Genomics

In this chapter, we examined the causes of different types of mutations and how mutations affect phenotype by altering the structure and function of proteins. The emergence of genomics, bioinformatics, and proteomics as key disciplines in modern genetics has provided geneticists with an unprecedented set of tools for identifying and analyzing mutations in gene and protein sequences.

In this exercise we will use the **ExPASy (Expert Protein Analysis System)** site, which is hosted by the Swiss Institute for Bioinformatics and provides a wealth of resources for studying proteins. Here we will use an ExPASy program called SIM (for "similarity" in sequence) to compare two polypeptide sequences so as to pinpoint a mutation. Once the mutation has been identified, you will learn more about the gene encoding these polypeptides and about a human disease condition associated with this gene.

■ **Exercise I — Identifying a Missense Mutation Affecting a Protein in Humans**

1. Begin this exercise by accessing the ExPASy site at http://web.expasy.org/sim/. The SIM feature is an algorithm-based software program that allows us to compare multiple polypeptide sequences by looking for amino acid similarity in the sequences.

2. Go to the Companion Web site for *Concepts of Genetics* and open the Exploring Genomics exercise for this chapter. At the Web site we provide amino acid sequences for polypeptides expressed in two different people (Person A and Person B). Note that the amino acid sequence is provided using the single-letter code for each amino acid (see the accompanying table for amino acid names and single-letter codes).

3. Copy and paste each sequence into separate "SEQUENCE" text boxes in SIM. Use the Person A sequence for sequence 1 and the Person B sequence for sequence 2. Click the "User-entered sequence" button for each. Name the sequences Person A and Person B as appropriate. Submit the sequences for comparison and then answer the following questions:

    a. How many amino acids (called "residues" in the SIM results report) are in each polypeptide sequence that was analyzed?

    b. Look carefully at the alignment results. Can you find any differences in amino acid sequence when comparing these two polypeptides? What did you find?

■ **Exercise II – Identifying the Genetic Basis for a Human Genetic Disease Condition**

1. From the ExPASy site use the BLAST link (http://web.expasy.org/blast/) and run a protein BLAST (blastp) search to identify which polypeptide you have been studying. Explore the BLAST reports for the top three protein sequences that aligned with your query sequence by clicking on the link for each sequence. Pay particular attention to the "Comment" section of each report to help you answer the questions in the following part.

2. Now that you know what gene you are working with, go to PubMed (http://www.ncbi.nlm.nih.gov/pubmed) and search for a review article from the authors Vajo, Z., Francomano, C. A., and Wilkin, D. J.

3. Answer the following questions:

    a. What gene codes for the polypeptides have you been studying?

    b. What is the function of this protein?

    c. Based on what you learned from the alignment results you analyzed in Exercise I, the BLAST reports, and your PubMed search, what human disease is caused by the mutation you identified in Exercise I? Explain your answer and briefly describe phenotypes associated with the disease.

CASE STUDY | Genetic dwarfism

Seven months pregnant, an expectant mother was undergoing a routine ultrasound. While prior tests had been normal, this one showed that the limbs of the fetus were unusually short. The doctor suspected that the baby might have a genetic form of dwarfism called achondroplasia. He told her that the disorder was due to an autosomal dominant mutation and occurred with a frequency of about 1 in 25,000 births. The expectant mother had studied genetics in college and immediately raised several questions. How would you answer them?

1. How could her baby have a dominantly inherited disorder if there was no history of this condition on either side of the family?

2. Is the mutation more likely to have come from the mother or the father?

3. If this child has achondroplasia, is there an increased chance that their next child would also have this disorder?

4. Could this disorder have been caused by X rays or ultrasounds she had earlier in pregnancy?

Summary Points

1. Mutations can be spontaneous or induced, somatic or germ-line, autosomal or sex-linked. Mutations can have many different effects on gene function depending on the type of nucleotide changes that comprise the mutation and the location of those mutations.

2. Spontaneous mutations occur in many ways, ranging from errors during DNA replication to damage caused to DNA bases as a result of normal cellular metabolism.

3. Mutations can be induced by many types of chemicals and radiation. These agents can damage both bases and the sugar-phosphate backbone of DNA molecules.

4. Single-gene mutations in humans cause a wide range of diseases. These mutations may be base-pair changes, insertions, deletions, and expanded DNA repeats.

5. Organisms counteract mutations using DNA repair systems including proofreading, mismatch repair, postreplication repair, photoreactivation repair, SOS repair, base excision repair, nucleotide excision repair, and double-strand break repair.

6. The Ames test allows scientists to estimate the mutagenicity and cancer-causing potential of chemical agents.

7. Transposable elements can move within a genome, creating mutations and altering gene expression. In addition, transposons may contribute to evolution.

INSIGHTS AND SOLUTIONS

1. The base analog 2-amino purine (2-AP) substitutes for adenine during DNA replication, but it may base-pair with cytosine. The base analog 5-bromouracil (5-BU) substitutes for thymidine, but it may base-pair with guanine. Follow the double-stranded trinucleotide sequence shown here through three rounds of replication, assuming that, in the first round, both analogs are present and become incorporated wherever possible. Before the second and third round of replication, any unincorporated base analogs are removed. What final sequences occur?

Solution:

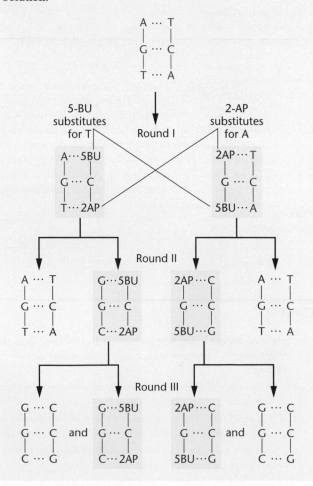

2. A rare dominant mutation expressed at birth was studied in humans. Records showed that six cases were discovered in 40,000 live births. Family histories revealed that in two cases, the mutation was already present in one of the parents. Calculate the spontaneous mutation rate for this mutation. What are some underlying assumptions that may affect our conclusions?

Solution: Only four cases represent a new mutation. Because each live birth represents two gametes, the sample size is from 80,000 meiotic events. The rate is equal to

$$4/80,000 = 1/20,000 = 5 \times 10^{-5}$$

We have assumed that the mutant gene is fully penetrant and is expressed in each individual bearing it. If it is not fully penetrant, our calculation may be an underestimate because one or more mutations may have gone undetected. We have also assumed that the screening was 100 percent accurate. One or more mutant individuals may have been "missed," again leading to an underestimate. Finally, we assumed that the viability of the mutant and nonmutant individuals is equivalent and that they survive equally *in utero*. Therefore, our assumption is that the number of mutant individuals at birth is equal to the number at conception. If this were not true, our calculation would again be an underestimate.

3. Consider the following estimates:
   a. There are 7×10^9 humans living on this planet.
   b. Each individual has about 20,000 (0.2×10^5) genes.
   c. The average mutation rate at each locus is 10^{-5}.

How many spontaneous mutations are currently present in the human population? Assuming that these mutations are equally distributed among all genes, how many new mutations have arisen in each gene in the human population?

Solution: First, since each individual is diploid, there are two copies of each gene per person, each arising from a separate gamete. Therefore, the total number of spontaneous mutations is
($2 \times 0.2 \times 10^5$ genes/individual)
   $\times$ (7×10^9) − individuals (10^{-5} mutations/gene)
= (0.4×10^5) $\times$ (7×10^9) $\times$ (10^{-5}) mutations
= 2.8×10^9 mutations in the population
2.8×10^9 mutations/0.2×10^5 genes
   = 14×10^4 mutations per gene in the population

Problems and Discussion Questions

HOW DO WE KNOW?

1. In this chapter, we focused on how gene mutations arise and how cells repair DNA damage. At the same time, we found opportunities to consider the methods and reasoning by which much of this information was acquired. From the explanations given in the chapter,
   (a) How do we know that mutations occur spontaneously?
   (b) How do we know that certain chemicals and wavelengths of radiation induce mutations in DNA?
   (c) How do we know that DNA repair mechanisms detect and correct the majority of spontaneous and induced mutations?

CONCEPT QUESTION

2. Review the Chapter Concepts list on page 367. These concepts relate to how gene mutations occur, their phenotypic effects, and how mutations can be repaired. The first four concepts focus on the effects of gene mutations in diploid organisms. Write a short essay describing how these concepts would apply, or not apply, to a haploid organism such as *E. coli*.

3. What is a spontaneous mutation, and why are spontaneous mutations rare?

4. Why would a mutation in a somatic cell of a multicellular organism escape detection?

5. Most mutations are thought to be deleterious. Why, then, is it reasonable to state that mutations are essential to the evolutionary process?

6. Why is a random mutation more likely to be deleterious than beneficial?

7. Most mutations in a diploid organism are recessive. Why?

8. What is meant by a conditional mutation?

9. Describe a tautomeric shift and how it may lead to a mutation.

10. Contrast and compare the mutagenic effects of deaminating agents, alkylating agents, and base analogs.

11. Acridine dyes induce frameshift mutations. Why are frameshift mutations likely to be more detrimental than point mutations, in which a single pyrimidine or purine has been substituted?

12. Why are X rays more potent mutagens than UV radiation?

13. DNA damage brought on by a variety of natural and artificial agents elicits a wide variety of cellular responses involving numerous signaling pathways. In addition to the activation of DNA repair mechanisms, there can be activation of pathways leading to apoptosis (programmed cell death) and cell-cycle arrest. Why would apoptosis and cell-cycle arrest often be part of a cellular response to DNA damage?

14. Contrast the various types of DNA repair mechanisms known to counteract the effects of UV radiation. What is the role of visible light in repairing UV-induced mutations?

15. Mammography is an accurate screening technique for the early detection of breast cancer in humans. Because this technique uses X rays diagnostically, it has been highly controversial. Can you explain why? What reasons justify the use of X rays for such a medical screening technique?

16. A significant number of mutations in the *HBB* gene that cause human β-thalassemia occur within introns or in upstream noncoding sequences. Explain why mutations in these regions often lead to severe disease, although they may not directly alter the coding regions of the gene.

17. Describe how the Ames test screens for potential environmental mutagens. Why is it thought that a compound that tests positively in the Ames test may also be carcinogenic?

18. What genetic defects result in the disorder xeroderma pigmentosum (XP) in humans? How do these defects create the phenotypes associated with the disorder?

19. Compare several transposable elements in bacteria, maize, *Drosophila*, and humans. What properties do they share?

20. Speculate on how improved living conditions and medical care in the developed nations might affect human mutation rates, both neutral and deleterious.

21. In maize, a *Ds* or *Ac* transposon can cause mutations in genes at or near the site of transposon insertion. It is possible for these elements to transpose away from their original site, causing a reversion of the mutant phenotype. In some cases, however, even more severe phenotypes appear, due to events at or near the mutant allele. What might be happening to the transposon or the nearby gene to create more severe mutations?

22. It is estimated that about 0.2 percent of human mutations are due to transposon insertions, and a much higher degree of mutational damage is known to occur in some other organisms. In what way might transposons contribute positively to evolution?

23. In a bacterial culture in which all cells are unable to synthesize leucine (*leu⁻*), a potent mutagen is added, and the cells are allowed to undergo one round of replication. At that point, samples are taken, a series of dilutions is made, and the cells are plated on either minimal medium or minimal medium containing leucine. The first culture condition (minimal medium) allows the growth of only *leu⁺* cells, while the second culture condition (minimal medium with leucine added) allows growth of all cells. The results of the experiment are as follows:

Culture Condition	Dilution	Colonies
Minimal medium	10^{-1}	18
Minimal medium + leucine	10^{-7}	6

What is the rate of mutation at the locus associated with leucine biosynthesis?

Extra-Spicy Problems

24. Presented here are hypothetical findings from studies of het-erokaryons formed from seven human xeroderma pigmento-sum cell strains:

	XP1	XP2	XP3	XP4	XP5	XP6	XP7
XP1	−						
XP2	−	−					
XP3	−	−	−				
XP4	+	+	+	−			
XP5	+	+	+	+	−		
XP6	+	+	+	+	−	−	
XP7	+	+	+	+	−	−	−

Note: + = complementation; − = no complementation

These data are measurements of the occurrence or nonoccur-rence of unscheduled DNA synthesis in the fused heterokaryon. None of the strains alone shows any unscheduled DNA synthesis. Which strains fall into the same complementation groups? How many different groups are revealed based on these data? What can we conclude about the genetic basis of XP from these data?

25. Imagine yourself as one of the team of geneticists who launches a study of the genetic effects of high-energy radiation on the surviving Japanese population immediately following the atom bomb attacks at Hiroshima and Nagasaki in 1945. Demonstrate your insights into both chromosomal and gene mutation by outlining a short-term and long-term study that addresses these radiation effects. Be sure to include strategies for considering the effects on both somatic and germ-line tissues.

26. With the knowledge that radiation causes mutations, many assume that human-made forms of radiation are the major contributors to the mutational load in humans. What evidence suggests otherwise?

27. Human equivalents of bacterial DNA mismatch repair pro-teins are subject to mutational damage just as are other pro-teins. What evidence indicates that mutations in human DNA mismatch repair genes are related to certain forms of cancer?

28. Among Betazoids in the world of *Star Trek*®, the ability to read minds is under the control of a gene called *mindreader* (abbre-viated *mr*). Most Betazoids can read minds, but rare recessive mutations in the *mr* gene result in two alternative phenotypes: *delayed-receivers* and *insensitives*. Delayed-receivers have some mind-reading ability but perform the task much more slowly than normal Betazoids. Insensitives cannot read minds at all. Betazoid genes do not have introns, so the gene only contains coding DNA. It is 3332 nucleotides in length, and Betazoids use a four-letter genetic code.

The following table shows some data from five unrelated *mr* mutations.

Mutation	Description of Mutation	Phenotype
mr-1	Nonsense mutation in codon 829	Delayed-receiver
mr-2	Missense mutation in codon 52	Delayed-receiver
mr-3	Deletion of nucleotides 83–150	Delayed-receiver
mr-4	Missense mutation in codon 192	Insensitive
mr-5	Deletion of nucleotides 83–93	Insensitive

For each mutation, provide a plausible explanation for why it gives rise to its associated phenotype and not to the other phenotype. For example, hypothesize why the *mr-1* nonsense mutation in codon 829 gives rise to the milder delayed-receiv-er phenotype rather than the more severe insensitive pheno-type. Then repeat this type of analysis for the other mutations. (More than one explanation is possible, so be creative within *plausible* bounds!)

29. Skin cancer carries a lifetime risk nearly equal to that of all other cancers combined. Following is a graph (modified from Kraemer, 1997. *Proc. Natl. Acad. Sci. (USA)* 94: 11–14) depict-ing the age of onset of skin cancers in patients with or without XP, where the cumulative percentage of skin cancer is plot-ted against age. The non-XP curve is based on 29,757 cancers surveyed by the National Cancer Institute, and the curve rep-resenting those with XP is based on 63 skin cancers from the Xeroderma Pigmentosum Registry.
(a) Provide an overview of the information contained in the graph.
(b) Explain why individuals with XP show such an early age of onset.

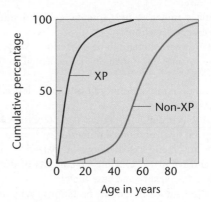

30. The initial discovery of IS elements in bacteria revealed the presence of an element upstream (5′) of three genes control-ling galactose metabolism. All three genes were affected simul-taneously, although there was only one IS insertion. Offer an explanation as to why this might occur.

31. It has been noted that most transposons in humans and other organisms are located in noncoding regions of the genome—regions such as introns, pseudogenes, and stretches of particu-lar types of repetitive DNA. There are several ways to interpret this observation. Describe two possible interpretations. Which interpretation do you favor? Why?

32. Mutations in the *IL2RG* gene cause approximately 30 per-cent of severe combined immunodeficiency disorder (SCID) cases. These mutations result in alterations to a protein com-ponent of cytokine receptors that are essential for proper development of the immune system. The *IL2RG* gene is com-posed of eight exons and contains upstream and downstream sequences that are necessary for proper transcription and translation. Below are some of the mutations observed. For

each, explain its likely influence on the *IL2RG* gene product (assume its length to be 375 amino acids).

(a) Nonsense mutation in coding regions

(b) Insertion in Exon 1, causing frameshift

(c) Insertion in Exon 7, causing frameshift

(d) Missense mutation

(e) Deletion in Exon 2, causing frameshift

(f) Deletion in Exon 2, in frame

(g) Large deletion covering Exons 2 and 3

33. A variety of neural and muscular disorders are associated with expansions of trinucleotide repeat sequences. The table below lists several disorders, the repeat motifs, their locations, the normal number of repeats, and the number of repeats in the full mutations.

(a) Most disorders attributable to trinucleotide repeats result from expansion of the repeats. Two mechanisms are often proposed to explain repeat expansion: (1) unequal synapsis and crossing over and (2) errors in DNA replication where single-stranded, base-paired loops are formed that conflict with linear replication. Present a simple sketch of each mechanism.

(b) Notice that some of the repeats occur in areas of the gene that are not translated. How can a mutation occur if the alteration is not reflected in an altered amino acid sequence?

(c) In the two cases where the repeat expansions occur in exons, the extent of expansion is considerably less than when the expansion occurs outside exons. Present an explanation for this observation.

Disorder	Repeat	Location	Normal Number	Full Mutation
Fragile X	CCG	5′ untranslated region	6–230	>230
Huntington	CAG	Exon	6–35	36–120
Myotonic dystrophy	CTG	3′ untranslated region	5–37	37–1500
Oculopharyngeal muscular dystrophy	GCG	Exon	6	8–13
Friedreich ataxia	AAG	Intron	20	200–900

Model showing how the *lac* repressor (red) and catabolite-activating protein (dark blue in center of DNA loop) bind to the *lac* operon promoter, creating a 93-base-pair repression loop in the *lac* regulatory DNA.

16 Regulation of Gene Expression in Prokaryotes

CHAPTER CONCEPT

- In bacteria, regulation of gene expression is often linked to the metabolic needs of the cell.

- Efficient expression of genetic information in bacteria is dependent on intricate regulatory mechanisms that exert control over transcription.

- Mechanisms that regulate transcription are categorized as exerting either positive or negative control of gene expression.

- Prokaryotic genes that encode proteins with related functions tend to be organized in clusters and are often under coordinated control. Such clusters, including their adjacent regulatory sequences, are called operons.

- Transcription of genes within operons is either inducible or repressible.

- Often, the metabolic end product of a biosynthetic pathway induces or represses gene expression in that pathway.

Previous chapters have discussed how DNA is organized into genes, how genes store genetic information, and how this information is expressed through the processes of transcription and translation. We now consider one of the most fundamental questions in molecular genetics: *How is genetic expression regulated?* It is clear that not all genes are expressed at all times in all situations. For example, detailed analysis of proteins in *Escherichia coli* shows that concentrations of the 4000 or so polypeptide chains encoded by the genome vary widely. Some proteins may be present in as few as 5 to 10 molecules per cell, whereas others, such as ribosomal proteins and the many proteins involved in the glycolytic pathway, are present in as many as 100,000 copies per cell. Although most prokaryotic gene products are present continuously at a basal level (a few copies), the concentration of these products can increase dramatically when required. Clearly, fundamental regulatory mechanisms must exist to control the expression of the genetic information.

In this chapter, we will explore regulation of gene expression in prokaryotes. As we have seen in a number of previous chapters, bacteria have been especially useful research organisms in genetics for a number of reasons. For one thing, they have extremely short reproductive cycles, and literally hundreds of generations, giving rise to billions of genetically identical bacteria, can be produced in overnight cultures. In addition, they can be studied in "pure culture," allowing mutant strains of genetically unique bacteria to be isolated and investigated separately.

Relevant to our current topic, bacteria also serve as an excellent model system for studies involving the induction of genetic transcription in response to changes in environmental conditions. While our primary focus will involve regulation of transcription, we will also consider instances where mRNAs contain sequences that serve as sensors that modulate their translation.

Please note that some of the topics discussed in this chapter are explored in greater depth later in the text (see Special Topic Chapter 2—Emerging Roles of RNA.)

16.1 Prokaryotes Regulate Gene Expression in Response to Environmental Conditions

Regulation of gene expression has been extensively studied in prokaryotes, particularly in *E. coli*. Geneticists have learned that highly efficient genetic mechanisms have evolved in these organisms to turn transcription of specific genes on and off, depending on the cell's metabolic need for the respective gene products. Not only do bacteria respond to changes in their environment, but they also regulate gene activity associated with a variety of cellular activities, including the replication, recombination, and repair of their DNA, and with cell division.

The idea that microorganisms regulate the synthesis of their gene products is not a new one. As early as 1900, it was shown that when lactose (a galactose and glucose-containing disaccharide) is present in the growth medium of yeast, the organisms synthesize enzymes required for lactose metabolism. When lactose is absent, synthesis diminishes to a basal level. Soon thereafter, investigators were able to generalize that bacteria also adapt to their environment, producing certain enzymes only when specific chemical substrates are present. These are now referred to as **inducible enzymes**. In contrast, enzymes that are produced continuously, regardless of the chemical makeup of the environment, are called **constitutive enzymes**.

More recent investigation has revealed a contrasting system, whereby the presence of a specific molecule *inhibits* gene expression. Such molecules are usually end products of anabolic biosynthetic pathways. For example, the amino acid tryptophan can be synthesized by bacterial cells. If a sufficient supply of tryptophan is present in the environment or culture medium, then there is no reason for the organism to expend energy in synthesizing the enzymes necessary for tryptophan production. A mechanism has therefore evolved whereby tryptophan plays a role in repressing the transcription of mRNA needed for producing tryptophan-synthesizing enzymes. In contrast to the inducible system controlling lactose metabolism, the system governing tryptophan expression is said to be **repressible**.

Regulation, whether of the inducible or repressible type, may be under either **negative** or **positive control**.

Under negative control, genetic expression occurs *unless it is shut off by some form of a regulator molecule*. In contrast, under positive control, transcription occurs *only if a regulator molecule directly stimulates RNA production*. In theory, either type of control or a combination of the two can govern inducible or repressible systems. Our discussion in the ensuing sections of this chapter will help clarify these contrasting systems of regulation. The enzymes involved in lactose digestion and tryptophan synthesis are under negative control.

16.2 Lactose Metabolism in *E. coli* Is Regulated by an Inducible System

Beginning in 1946 with the studies of Jacques Monod and continuing through the next decade with significant contributions by Joshua Lederberg, François Jacob, and André Lwoff, genetic and biochemical evidence concerning lactose metabolism was amassed. Research provided insights into the way in which the gene activity is repressed when lactose is absent but induced when it is available. In the presence of lactose, the concentration of the enzymes responsible for its metabolism increases rapidly from a few molecules to thousands per cell. The enzymes responsible for lactose metabolism are thus inducible, and lactose serves as the inducer.

In prokaryotes, genes that code for enzymes with related functions (for example, the set of genes involved with lactose metabolism) tend to be organized in clusters on the bacterial chromosome, and transcription of these genes is often under the coordinated control of a single regulatory region. The location of this regulatory region is almost always upstream (5′) of the gene cluster it controls. Because the regulatory region is on the same strand as those genes, we refer to it as a ***cis*-acting site**. *Cis*-acting regulatory regions bind molecules that control transcription of the gene cluster. Such molecules are called ***trans*-acting elements**. Events at the regulatory site determine whether the genes are transcribed into mRNA and thus whether the corresponding enzymes or other protein products may be synthesized from the genetic information in the mRNA. Binding of a *trans*-acting element at a *cis*-acting site can regulate the gene cluster either negatively (by turning off transcription) or positively (by turning on transcription of genes in the cluster). In this section, we discuss how transcription of such bacterial gene clusters is coordinately regulated.

The discovery of a regulatory gene and a regulatory site that are part of the gene cluster was paramount to the understanding of how gene expression is controlled in

FIGURE 16–1 A simplified overview of the genes and regulatory units involved in the control of lactose metabolism. (The regions within this stretch of DNA are not drawn to scale.) A more detailed model will be developed later in this chapter. (See Figure 16–10.)

the system. Neither of these regulatory elements encodes enzymes necessary for lactose metabolism—the function of the three genes in the cluster. As illustrated in **Figure 16–1**, the three structural genes and the adjacent regulatory site constitute the **lactose**, or **lac**, **operon**. Together, the entire gene cluster functions in an integrated fashion to provide a rapid response to the presence or absence of lactose.

Structural Genes

Genes coding for the primary structure of an enzyme are called **structural genes**. There are three structural genes in the *lac* operon. The *lacZ* gene encodes **β-galactosidase**, an enzyme whose primary role is to convert the disaccharide lactose to the monosaccharides glucose and galactose (**Figure 16–2**). This conversion is essential if lactose is to serve as the primary energy source in glycolysis. The second gene, *lacY*, specifies the primary structure of **permease**, an enzyme that facilitates the entry of lactose into the bacterial cell. The third gene, *lacA*, codes for the enzyme

transacetylase. While its physiological role is still not completely clear, it may be involved in the removal of toxic by-products of lactose digestion from the cell.

To study the genes coding for these three enzymes, researchers isolated numerous mutations that lacked the function of one or the other enzyme. Such *lac⁻* mutants were first isolated and studied by Joshua Lederberg. Mutant cells that fail to produce active β-galactosidase (*lacZ⁻*) or permease (*lacY⁻*) are unable to use lactose as an energy source. Mutations were also found in the transacetylase gene. Mapping studies by Lederberg established that all three genes are closely linked or contiguous to one another on the bacterial chromosome, in the order *Z–Y–A* (see Figure 16–1).

Knowledge of their close linkage led to another discovery relevant to what later became known about the regulation of structural genes: All three genes are transcribed as a single unit, resulting in a so-called *polycistronic mRNA* (**Figure 16–3**; recall that *cistron* refers to the part of a

FIGURE 16–2 The catabolic conversion of the disaccharide lactose into its monosaccharide units, galactose and glucose.

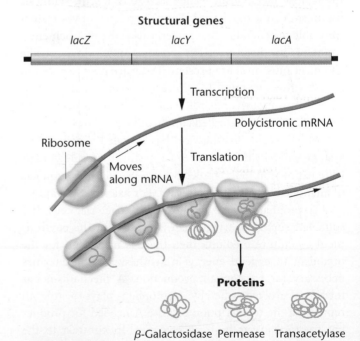

FIGURE 16–3 The structural genes of the *lac* operon are transcribed into a single polycistronic mRNA, which is translated simultaneously by several ribosomes into the three enzymes encoded by the operon.

nucleotide sequence coding for a single gene). This results in the coordinate regulation of all three genes, since a single-message RNA is simultaneously translated into all three gene products.

The Discovery of Regulatory Mutations

How does lactose stimulate transcription of the *lac* operon and induce the synthesis of the enzymes for which it codes? A partial answer came from studies using **gratuitous inducers**, chemical analogs of lactose such as the sulfur-containing analog **isopropylthiogalactoside (IPTG)**, shown in **Figure 16–4**. Gratuitous inducers behave like natural inducers, but they do not serve as substrates for the enzymes that are subsequently synthesized. Their discovery provides strong evidence that the primary induction event does *not* depend on the interaction between the inducer and the enzyme.

What, then, is the role of lactose in induction? The answer to this question requires the study of another class of mutations described as **constitutive mutations**. In cells bearing these types of mutations, enzymes are produced regardless of the presence or absence of lactose. Studies of the constitutive mutation *lacI⁻* mapped the mutation to a site on the bacterial chromosome close to, but not part of, the structural genes *lacZ*, *lacY*, and *lacA*. This mutation led researchers to discover the *lacI* gene, which is appropriately called a **repressor gene**. A second set of constitutive mutations producing effects identical to those of *lacI⁻* is present in a region immediately adjacent to the structural genes. This class of mutations, designated *lac O^C*, is located in the **operator region** of the operon. In both types of constitutive mutants, the enzymes are produced continually, inducibility is eliminated, and gene regulation has been lost.

The Operon Model: Negative Control

Around 1960, Jacob and Monod proposed a hypothetical mechanism involving negative control that they called the **operon model**, in which a group of genes is regulated and expressed together as a unit. As we saw in Figure 16–1, the *lac* operon they proposed consists of the *Z*, *Y*, and *A* structural genes, as well as the adjacent sequences of DNA referred to as the *operator region*. They argued that the *lacI* gene regulates the transcription of the structural genes by

producing a **repressor molecule**, and that the repressor is **allosteric**, meaning that the molecule reversibly interacts with another molecule, undergoing both a conformational change in three-dimensional shape and a change in chemical activity. **Figure 16–5** illustrates the components of the *lac* operon as well as the action of the *lac* repressor in the presence and absence of lactose.

Jacob and Monod suggested that the repressor normally binds to the DNA sequence of the operator region. When it does so, it inhibits the action of RNA polymerase, effectively repressing the transcription of the structural genes [**Figure 16–5(b)**]. However, when lactose is present, this sugar binds to the repressor and causes an allosteric (conformational) change. The change alters the binding site of the repressor, rendering it incapable of interacting with operator DNA [**Figure 16–5(c)**]. In the absence of the repressor–operator interaction, RNA polymerase transcribes the structural genes, and the enzymes necessary for lactose metabolism are produced. Because transcription occurs only when the repressor *fails* to bind to the operator region, regulation is said to be under *negative control*.

To summarize, the operon model invokes a series of molecular interactions between proteins, inducers, and DNA to explain the efficient regulation of structural gene expression. In the absence of lactose, the enzymes encoded by the genes are not needed, and expression of genes encoding these enzymes is repressed. When lactose is present, it indirectly induces the activation of the genes by binding with the repressor.* If all lactose is metabolized, none is available to bind to the repressor, which is again free to bind to operator DNA and to repress transcription.

Both the *I⁻* and *O^C* constitutive mutations interfere with these molecular interactions, allowing continuous transcription of the structural genes. In the case of the *I⁻* mutant, seen in **Figure 16–6(a)**, the repressor protein is altered or absent and cannot bind to the operator region, so the structural genes are always turned on. In the case of the *O^C* mutant [**Figure 16–6(b)**], the nucleotide sequence of the operator DNA is altered and will not bind with a normal repressor molecule. The result is the same: The structural genes are always transcribed.

Genetic Proof of the Operon Model

The operon model is a good one because it leads to three major predictions that can be tested to determine its validity. The major predictions to be tested are that (1) the *I* gene produces a diffusible product (that is, a *trans*-acting product); (2) the *O* region is involved in regulation but

FIGURE 16–4 The gratuitous inducer isopropylthiogalactoside (IPTG).

---

*Technically, the inducer is allolactose, an isomer of lactose. When lactose enters the bacterial cell, some of it is converted to allolactose by the β-galactosidase enzyme.

(a) Components

Repressor gene *(I)*   Promoter *(P)*   Operator gene *(O)*   Leader *(L)*   Structural genes   Z   Y   A

Operator-binding site

Repressor protein

RNA polymerase

Lactose-binding site

Lactose

(b) $I^+ O^+ Z^+ Y^+ A^+$ (wild type) — no lactose present — **Repressed**

I   P   O   L   Z   Y   A

Repressor binds to operator, blocking transcription

No transcription

No enzymes

(c) $I^+ O^+ Z^+ Y^+ A^+$ (wild type) — lactose present — **Induced**

I   P   O   L   Z   Y   A

No binding occurs; transcription proceeds

Transcription

Operator-binding region is altered when bound to lactose

mRNA

Translation

Enzymes

FIGURE 16–5 The components of the wild-type *lac* operon and the response in the absence and presence of lactose.

does not produce a product (it is *cis*-acting); and (3) the *O* region must be adjacent to the structural genes in order to regulate transcription.

The creation of partially diploid bacteria allows us to assess these assumptions, particularly those that predict the presence of *trans*-acting regulatory elements. For example, the F plasmid may contain chromosomal genes (Chapter 6), in which case it is designated F′. When an F⁻ cell acquires such a plasmid, it contains its own chromosome plus one or more additional genes present in the plasmid. This host cell is thus a **merozygote**, a cell that is diploid for certain added genes (but not for the rest of the chromosome). The use of such a plasmid makes it possible, for example, to introduce an I^+ gene into a host cell whose genotype is I^-,

or to introduce an O^+ region into a host cell of genotype O^C. The Jacob–Monod operon model predicts how regulation should be affected in such cells. Adding an I^+ gene to an I^- cell should restore inducibility, because the normal wild-type repressor, which is a *trans*-acting factor, would be produced by the inserted I^+ gene. In contrast, adding an O^+ region to an O^C cell should have no effect on constitutive enzyme production, since regulation depends on an O^+ region being located immediately adjacent to the structural genes—that is, O^+ is a *cis*-acting regulator.

Results of these experiments are shown in **Table 16.1**, where *Z* represents the structural genes (and the inserted genes are listed after the designation F′). In both cases described above, the Jacob–Monod model is upheld (part B

(a) $I^- O^+ Z^+ Y^+ A^+$ (mutant repressor gene) — no lactose present — **Constitutive**

(b) $I^+ O^C Z^+ Y^+ A^+$ (mutant operator gene) — no lactose present — **Constitutive**

FIGURE 16–6 The response of the *lac* operon in the absence of lactose when a cell bears either the I^- or the O^C mutation.

of Table 16.1). Part C of the table shows the reverse experiments, where either an I^- gene or an O^C region is added to cells of normal inducible genotypes. As the model predicts, inducibility is maintained in these partial diploids.

Another prediction of the operon model is that certain mutations in the I gene should have the opposite effect of I^-. That is, instead of being constitutive because the repressor can't bind the operator, mutant repressor molecules should be produced that cannot interact with the inducer, lactose. As a result, these repressors would always bind to the operator sequence, and the structural genes would be permanently repressed. In cases like this, the presence of an additional I^+ gene would have little or no effect on repression.

In fact, such a mutation, I^S, was discovered wherein the operon, as predicted, is "superrepressed," as shown in part D of Table 16.1 (and depicted in **Figure 16–7**). An additional I^+ gene does not effectively relieve repression of gene activity. These observations are consistent with the idea that the repressor contains separate DNA-binding domains and inducer-binding domains.

TABLE 16.1 A Comparison of Gene Activity (+ or −) in the Presence or Absence of Lactose for Various *E. coli* Genotypes

Genotype	Presence of β-Galactosidase Activity	
	Lactose Present	Lactose Absent
A. $I^+O^+Z^+$	+	−
$I^+O^+Z^-$	−	−
$I^-O^+Z^+$	+	+
$I^+O^CZ^+$	+	+
B. $I^-O^+Z^+/F'I^+$	+	−
$I^+O^CZ^+/F'O^+$	+	+
C. $I^+O^+Z^+/F'I^-$	+	−
$I^+O^+Z^+/F'O^C$	+	−
D. $I^SO^+Z^+$	−	−
$I^SO^+Z^+/F'I^+$	−	−

Note: In parts B to D, most genotypes are partially diploid, containing an F factor plus attached genes (F′).

Isolation of the Repressor

Although Jacob and Monod's operon theory succeeded in explaining many aspects of genetic regulation in prokaryotes,

$I^S\ O^+\ Z^+\ Y^+\ A^+$ (mutant repressor gene) — lactose present — **Repressed**

Repressor always bound to operator, blocking transcription

Lactose-binding region is altered; no binding to lactose

FIGURE 16–7 The response of the *lac* operon in the presence of lactose in a cell bearing the I^S mutation.

the nature of the repressor molecule was not known when their landmark paper was published in 1961. While they had assumed that the allosteric repressor was a protein, RNA was also a viable candidate because the activity of the molecule required the ability to bind to DNA. Despite many attempts to isolate and characterize the hypothetical repressor molecule, no direct chemical evidence was forthcoming. A single *E. coli* cell contains no more than ten or so copies of the *lac* repressor, and direct chemical identification of ten molecules in a population of millions of proteins and RNAs in a single cell presented a tremendous challenge.

In 1966, Walter Gilbert and Benno Müller-Hill reported the isolation of the *lac* repressor in partially purified form. To achieve the isolation, they used a *regulator quantity* (I^q) mutant strain that contains about ten times as much repressor as do wild-type *E. coli* cells. Also instrumental in their success was the use of the gratuitous inducer IPTG, which binds to the repressor, and the technique of **equilibrium dialysis**. In this technique, extracts of I^q cells were placed in a dialysis bag and allowed to attain equilibrium with an external solution of radioactive IPTG, a molecule small enough to diffuse freely in and out of the

bag. At equilibrium, the concentration of radioactive IPTG was higher inside the bag than in the external solution, indicating that an IPTG-binding material was present in the cell extract and was too large to diffuse across the wall of the bag.

Ultimately, the IPTG-binding material was purified and shown to have various characteristics of a protein. In contrast, extracts of I^- constitutive cells having no *lac* repressor activity did not exhibit IPTG binding, strongly suggesting that the isolated protein was the repressor molecule.

To confirm this thinking, Gilbert and Müller-Hill grew *E. coli* cells in a medium containing radioactive sulfur and then isolated the IPTG-binding protein, which was labeled in its sulfur-containing amino acids. Next, this protein was mixed with DNA from a strain of phage lambda (λ) carrying the *lacO*$^+$ gene. When the two substances are not mixed together, the DNA sediments at 40S, while the IPTG-binding protein sediments at 7S. However, when the DNA and protein were mixed and sedimented in a gradient, using ultracentrifugation, the radioactive protein sedimented at the same rate as did DNA, indicating that the protein binds to the DNA. Further experiments showed that the IPTG-binding, or repressor, protein binds only to DNA containing the *lac* region and does not bind to *lac* DNA containing an operator-constitutive O^C mutation.

NOW SOLVE THIS

16–1 Even though the *lac Z, Y,* and *A* structural genes are transcribed as a single polycistronic mRNA, each gene contains the initiation and termination signals essential for translation. Predict what will happen when a cell growing in the presence of lactose contains a deletion of one nucleotide (a) early in the *Z* gene and (b) early in the *A* gene.

■ **HINT:** *This problem requires you to combine your understanding of the genetic expression of the lac operon with that of the genetic code, frameshift mutations, and termination of transcription. The key to its solution is to consider the effect of the loss of one nucleotide within a polycistronic mRNA.*

For more practice, see Problems 5, 6, and 7.

16.3 The Catabolite-Activating Protein (CAP) Exerts Positive Control over the *lac* Operon

As described in the preceding discussion of the *lac* operon, the role of β-galactosidase is to cleave lactose into its components, glucose and galactose. Then, in order to be used by the cell, the galactose, too, must be converted to glucose. What if the cell found itself in an environment that contained ample amounts of both lactose *and* glucose? Given that glucose is the preferred carbon source for *E. coli*, it would not be energetically efficient for a cell to induce transcription of the *lac* operon, since what it really needs—glucose—is already present. As we will see next, still another molecular component, called the **catabolite-activating protein (CAP)**, is involved in diminishing the expression of the *lac* operon when glucose is present. This inhibition is called **catabolite repression**.

To understand CAP and its role in regulation, let's backtrack for a moment to review the system depicted in Figure 16–5. When the *lac* repressor is bound to the inducer (lactose), the *lac* operon is activated, and RNA polymerase transcribes the structural genes. As stated earlier in the text (see Chapter 14), transcription is initiated as a result of the binding that occurs between RNA polymerase and the nucleotide sequence of the **promoter region**, found upstream (5′) from the initial coding sequences. Within the *lac* operon, the promoter is found between the *I* gene and the operator region (*O*) (see Figure 16–1). Careful examination has revealed that polymerase binding is never very efficient unless CAP is also present to facilitate the process.

The mechanism is summarized in **Figure 16–8**. In the absence of glucose and under inducible conditions, CAP exerts positive control by binding to the CAP site, facilitating RNA-polymerase binding at the promoter, and thus

transcription. Therefore, for maximal transcription of the structural genes, the repressor must be bound by lactose (so as not to repress operon expression), *and* CAP must be bound to the CAP-binding site.

This leads to the central question about CAP: How does the presence of glucose inhibit CAP binding? The answer involves still another molecule, **cyclic adenosine monophosphate (cAMP)**, upon which CAP binding is dependent. *In order to bind to the promoter, CAP must be bound to cAMP.* The level of cAMP is itself dependent on an enzyme, **adenyl cyclase**, which catalyzes the conversion of ATP to cAMP (see **Figure 16–9**).* The role of glucose in catabolite repression is now clear. It inhibits the activity of adenyl cyclase, causing a decline in the level of cAMP in the cell. Under this condition, CAP cannot form the cAMP–CAP complex essential to the positive control of transcription of the *lac* operon.

Like the *lac* repressor, CAP and cAMP–CAP have been examined by X-ray crystallography. CAP is a dimer

---

*Because of its involvement with cAMP, CAP is also called *cyclic AMP receptor protein (CRP)*, and the gene encoding the protein is named *crp*. Since the protein was first named CAP, we will adhere to the initial nomenclature.

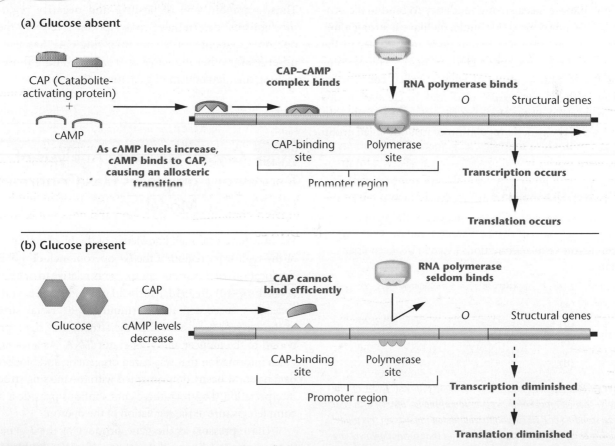

(a) Glucose absent

CAP (Catabolite-activating protein)
+
cAMP

As cAMP levels increase, cAMP binds to CAP, causing an allosteric transition

CAP–cAMP complex binds

CAP-binding site

Promoter region

RNA polymerase binds

Polymerase site

O   Structural genes

Transcription occurs

Translation occurs

(b) Glucose present

Glucose

CAP

cAMP levels decrease

CAP cannot bind efficiently

CAP-binding site

Promoter region

RNA polymerase seldom binds

Polymerase site

O   Structural genes

Transcription diminished

Translation diminished

FIGURE 16–8 Catabolite repression. (a) In the absence of glucose, cAMP levels increase, resulting in the formation of a cAMP–CAP complex, which binds to the CAP site of the promoter, stimulating transcription. (b) In the presence of glucose, cAMP levels decrease, cAMP–CAP complexes are not formed, and transcription is not stimulated.

FIGURE 16–9 The formation of cAMP from ATP, catalyzed by adenyl cyclase.

that inserts into adjacent regions of a specific nucleotide sequence of the DNA making up the *lac* promoter. The cAMP–CAP complex, when bound to DNA, bends it, causing it to assume a new conformation.

Binding studies in solution further clarify the mechanism of gene activation. Alone, neither cAMP–CAP nor RNA polymerase has a strong tendency to bind to *lac* promoter DNA, nor does either molecule have a strong affinity for the other. However, when both are together in the presence of the *lac* promoter DNA, a tightly bound complex is formed, an example of what is called **cooperative binding**. In the case of cAMP–CAP and the *lac* operon, this phenomenon illustrates the high degree of specificity that is involved in the genetic regulation of just one small group of genes.

Regulation of the *lac* operon by catabolite repression results in efficient energy use, because the presence of glucose will override the need for the metabolism of lactose, should the lactose also be available to the cell. In contrast to the negative regulation conferred by the *lac* repressor, the action of cAMP–CAP constitutes positive regulation. Thus, a combination of positive and negative regulatory mechanisms determines transcription levels of the *lac* operon. Catabolite repression involving CAP has also been observed for other inducible operons, including those controlling the metabolism of galactose and arabinose.

16.4 Crystal Structure Analysis of Repressor Complexes Has Confirmed the Operon Model

We now have thorough knowledge of the biochemical nature of the regulatory region of the *lac* operon, including the precise locations of its various components relative to one another (**Figure 16–10**). In 1996, Mitchell Lewis, Ponzy Lu, and their colleagues succeeded in determining the crystal structure of the *lac* repressor, as well as the structure of the repressor bound to the inducer and to operator DNA. As a result, previous information that was based on genetic and biochemical data has now been complemented with the missing structural interpretation. Together, these contributions provide a nearly complete picture of the regulation of the operon.

The repressor, as the gene product of the *I* gene, is a monomer consisting of 360 amino acids. Within this monomer, the region of inducer binding has been identified [**Figure 16–11(a)**]. While dimers [**Figure 16–11(b)**] can

NOW SOLVE THIS

16–2 Predict the level of genetic activity of the *lac* operon as well as the status of the *lac* repressor and the CAP protein under the cellular conditions listed in the accompanying table.

	Lactose	Glucose
(a)	–	–
(b)	+	–
(c)	–	+
(d)	+	+

■ **HINT:** *This problem asks you to combine your knowledge of the Jacob–Monod model of the regulation of the lac operon with your understanding of how catabolite repression impacts on this model. The key to its solution is to keep in mind that regulation involving lactose is a negative control system, while regulation involving glucose and catabolite repression is a positive control system.*

Repressor loop region

FIGURE 16–10 The various regulatory regions involved in the control of genetic expression of the *lac* operon, as described in the text. The numbers on the bottom scale represent nucleotide sites upstream and downstream from the initiation of transcription.

also bind the inducer, the functional repressor is a homotetramer (that is, it contains four copies of the monomer). The tetramer can be cleaved with a protease under controlled conditions to yield five fragments. Four are derived from the N-terminal ends of the tetramer subunits, and they bind to operator DNA. The fifth fragment is the remaining core of the tetramer, derived from the COOH-terminal ends; it binds to lactose and gratuitous inducers such as IPTG.

Analysis has revealed that each tetramer can bind to two symmetrical operator DNA helices at a time.

The operator DNA that was previously defined by mutational studies ($lacO^C$) and confirmed by DNA-sequencing analysis is located just upstream from the beginning of the actual coding sequence of the *lacZ* gene. Crystallographic studies show that the actual region of repressor binding of this primary operator, O_1, consists of 21 base pairs. Two other auxiliary operator regions have been identified, as shown in Figure 16–10. One, O_2, is 401 base pairs downstream from the primary operator, within the *lacZ* gene. The other, O_3, is 93 base pairs upstream from O_1, just beyond the CAP site. *In vivo*, all three operators must be bound for maximum repression.

Binding by the repressor simultaneously at two operator sites distorts the conformation of DNA, causing it to bend away

FIGURE 16–11 Models of the *lac* repressor and its binding to operator sites in DNA, as generated from crystal structure analysis. (a) The repressor monomer, showing the inducer-binding site. The DNA-binding region is shown in red. (b) The repressor dimer bound to two 21-base-pair segments of operator DNA (shown in dark blue). (c) The repressor (shown in pink) and CAP (shown in dark blue) bound to the *lac* DNA. Binding to operator regions O_1 and O_3 creates a 93-base-pair repression loop of promoter DNA.

from the repressor. When a model is created to demonstrate dual binding of operators O_1 and O_3 [**Figure 16–11(c)**], the 93 base pairs of DNA that intervene must jut out, forming what is called a **repression loop**. This model positions the promoter region that binds RNA polymerase on the inside of the loop, which prevents access by the polymerase during repression. In addition, the repression loop positions the CAP-binding site in a way that facilitates CAP interaction with RNA polymerase upon subsequent induction. The DNA looping caused by repression in this model is similar to configuration changes that are predicted to occur in eukaryotic systems (see Chapter 17).

Studies have also defined the three-dimensional conformational changes that accompany the interactions with the inducer molecules. Taken together, the crystallographic studies have brought a new level of understanding of the regulatory process occurring within the *lac* operon, confirming the findings and predictions of Jacob and Monod in their model set forth over 40 years ago, which was based strictly on genetic observations.

16.5 The Tryptophan (*trp*) Operon in *E. coli* Is a Repressible Gene System

Although the process of induction had been known for some time, it was not until 1953 that Monod and colleagues discovered a repressible operon. Wild-type *E. coli* are capable of producing the enzymes necessary for the biosynthesis of amino acids as well as other essential macromolecules. Focusing his studies on the amino acid tryptophan and the enzyme **tryptophan synthetase**, Monod discovered that if tryptophan is present in sufficient quantity in the growth medium, the enzymes necessary for its synthesis are not produced. It is energetically advantageous for bacteria to repress expression of genes involved in tryptophan synthesis when ample tryptophan is present in the growth medium.

Further investigation showed that a series of enzymes encoded by five contiguous genes on the *E. coli* chromosome are involved in tryptophan synthesis. These genes are part of an operon, and in the presence of tryptophan, all are coordinately repressed, and none of the enzymes is produced. Because of the great similarity between this repression and the induction of enzymes for lactose metabolism, Jacob and Monod proposed a model of gene regulation analogous to the *lac* system (the updated version is shown in **Figure 16–12**).

To account for repression, Jacob and Monod suggested the presence of a *normally inactive repressor* that alone cannot interact with the operator region of the operon. However, the repressor is an allosteric molecule that can bind to tryptophan. When tryptophan is present, the resultant complex of repressor and tryptophan attains a new conformation

that binds to the operator, repressing transcription. Thus, when tryptophan, the end product of this anabolic pathway, is present, the system is repressed and enzymes are not made. Since the regulatory complex inhibits transcription of the operon, this repressible system is under negative control. And as tryptophan participates in repression, it is referred to as a **corepressor** in this regulatory scheme.

Evidence for the *trp* Operon

Support for the concept of a repressible operon was soon forthcoming, based primarily on the isolation of two distinct categories of constitutive mutations. The first class, *trpR⁻*, maps at a considerable distance from the structural genes. This locus represents the gene coding for the repressor. Presumably, the mutation inhibits either the repressor's interaction with tryptophan or repressor formation entirely. Whichever the case, no repression ever occurs in cells with the *trpR⁻* mutation. As expected, if the *trpR⁺* gene encodes a functional repressor molecule, the presence of a copy of this gene will restore repressibility.

The second constitutive mutation is analogous to that of the operator of the lactose operon, because it maps immediately adjacent to the structural genes. Furthermore, the insertion of a plasmid bearing a wild-type operator gene into mutant cells does not restore repression. This is what would be predicted if the mutant operator no longer interacts with the repressor–tryptophan complex.

The entire *trp* operon has now been well defined, as shown in Figure 16–12. The five contiguous structural genes (*trpE, D, C, B,* and *A*) are transcribed as a polycistronic message directing translation of the enzymes that catalyze the biosynthesis of tryptophan. As in the *lac* operon, a promoter region (*trpP*) represents the binding site for RNA polymerase, and an operator region (*trpO*) binds the repressor. In the absence of binding, transcription is initiated within the *trpP–trpO* region and proceeds along a **leader sequence** 162 nucleotides prior to the first structural gene (*trpE*). Within that leader sequence, still another regulatory site has been demonstrated, called an *attenuator*—the subject of the next section. As we will see, this regulatory unit is an integral part of this operon's control mechanism.

EVOLVING CONCEPT OF THE GENE

The groundbreaking work of Jacob, Monod, and Lwoff in the early 1960s, which established the operon model for the regulation of gene expression in bacteria, expanded the concept of the gene to include noncoding regulatory sequences that are present upstream (5′) from the coding region. In bacterial operons, the transcription of several contiguous structural genes whose products are involved in the same biochemical pathway are regulated by a single set of regulatory sequences. ∎

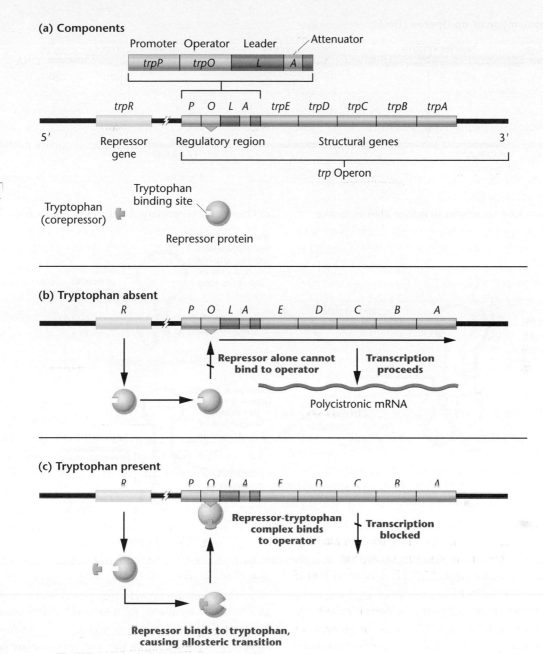

FIGURE 16–12 A repressible operon. (a) The components involved in regulation of the tryptophan operon. (b) In the absence of tryptophan, an inactive repressor is made that cannot bind to the operator (*O*), thus allowing transcription to proceed. (c) When tryptophan is present, it binds to the repressor, causing an allosteric transition to occur. This complex binds to the operator region, leading to repression of the operon.

16.6 Alterations to RNA Secondary Structure Contribute to Prokaryotic Gene Regulation

In the preceding sections of this chapter we focused on gene regulation brought about by DNA-binding regulatory proteins that interact with promoter and operator regions of the genes to be regulated. These regulatory proteins, such as the *lac* repressor and the CAP protein, act to decrease or increase

transcription initiation from their target promoters by affecting the binding of RNA polymerase to the promoter.

Gene regulation in prokaryotes can also occur through the interactions of regulatory molecules with specific regions of a nascent mRNA, after transcription has been initiated. The binding of these regulatory molecules alters the secondary structure of the mRNA, leading to premature transcription termination or repression of translation. We will discuss two types of regulation by RNA secondary structure—*attenuation* and *riboswitches*.

(a) Transcription of *trp* Operon (DNA)

(b) Stem-loop structures in leader RNA sequence

(c) Alternative secondary structures of leader RNA

FIGURE 16–13 The attenuation model regulating the tryptophan operon.

Both types of regulation help to fine-tune prokaryotic gene regulation.

Attenuation

Charles Yanofsky, Kevin Bertrand, and their colleagues observed that, when tryptophan is present and the *trp* operon is repressed, initiation of transcription still occurs at a low level, but is subsequently terminated at a point about 140 nucleotides along the transcript. They called this process **attenuation,** as it "weakens or impairs" expression of the operon. In contrast, when tryptophan is absent or present in very low concentrations, transcription is initiated but is *not* subsequently terminated, instead continuing beyond the leader sequence into the structural genes.

Based on the above observations, Yanofsky and colleagues presented a model to explain how attenuation occurs and is regulated (**Figure 16–13**). They proposed that the initial DNA sequence that is transcribed gives rise to an mRNA sequence that has the potential to fold into two mutually exclusive stem-loop structures referred to as "hairpins." If tryptophan is scarce, an mRNA secondary structure referred to as the **antiterminator hairpin** is formed. Transcription proceeds past the antiterminator hairpin region, and the entire mRNA is subsequently produced. Alternatively, in the presence of excess tryptophan, the mRNA structure that is formed is referred to as a **terminator hairpin**, and transcription is almost always terminated prematurely, just beyond the attenuator.

A key point in Yanofsky's model is that the transcript of the leader sequence in the 5′-untranslated region (5′-UTR) of the mRNA must be translated in order for the antiterminator hairpin to form. This leader transcript contains two triplets (UGG) that encode tryptophan, and these are present just downstream of the initial AUG sequence that signals the initiation of translation by ribosomes. When adequate tryptophan is present, charged tRNA^{Trp} is present in the cell. As a result, ribosomes translate these UGG triplets, proceed through the attenuator, and allow the *terminator hairpin* to form. The terminator hairpin signals RNA polymerase to prematurely terminate transcription, and the operon is not transcribed. If cells are starved of tryptophan, charged tRNA^{Trp} is unavailable. As a result, ribosomes "stall" during translation of the UGG triplets. The presence of ribosomes in this region of the mRNA interferes with the formation of the terminator hairpin, but allows the formation of the anti-terminator hairpin within the leader transcript. As a result, transcription proceeds, leading to expression of the entire set of structural genes.

Many other bacterial operons use attenuation to control gene expression. These include operons that encode enzymes involved in the biosynthesis of amino acids such as threonine, histidine, leucine, and phenylalanine. As with the *trp* operon, attenuation occurs in a leader sequence that contains an attenuator region.

Riboswitches

Since the elucidation of attenuation in the *trp* operon, numerous cases of gene regulation that also depend on alternative forms of mRNA secondary structure have been documented. These are examples of what are more generally referred to as **riboswitches**. As with attenuation of the *trp* operon discussed above, the mechanism of riboswitch regulation involves short ribonucleotide sequences (or elements) present in the 5′-UTR of mRNAs. These RNA elements are capable of binding with small molecule ligands, such as metabolites, whose synthesis or activity is controlled by the genes encoded by the mRNA. Such binding causes a conformational change in one domain of the riboswitch element, which induces another change at a second RNA domain, most often creating a transcription *terminator structure*. This terminator structure interfaces directly with the transcriptional machinery and shuts it down.

Riboswitches can recognize a broad range of ligands, including amino acids, purines, vitamin cofactors, amino sugars, and metal ions, among others. They are widespread in bacteria. In *Bacillus subtilis,* for example, approximately 5 percent of this bacterium's genes are regulated by riboswitches. They are also found in archaea, fungi, and plants, and may prove to be present in animals as well.

The two important domains within a riboswitch are the ligand-binding site, called the **aptamer**, and the **expression platform**, which is capable of forming the terminator structure. **Figure 16–14** illustrates the principles involved in riboswitch control. The 5′-UTR of an mRNA is shown on the left side of the figure in the absence of the ligand (metabolite). RNA polymerase has transcribed the unbound ligand-binding site, and in the *default conformation*, the expression domain adopts an *antiterminator conformation*. Thus, transcription continues through the expression platform and into the coding region. On the right side of the figure, the presence of the ligand on the ligand-binding site induces an alternative conformation in the expression platform, creating the *terminator conformation*. RNA polymerase is effectively blocked and transcription ceases.

While the above description fits the majority of riboswitches that have been studied, there are two variations from this model that complete our coverage of the topic. First, it is possible for the default position of a riboswitch to be in the terminator conformation. For example, consider

Antiterminator conformation — Ligand-binding site — RNA polymerase — + Ligand — Ligand binds, inducing conformational changes — **Terminator conformation** — Transcription is terminated

FIGURE 16–14 Illustration of the mechanism of riboswitch regulation of gene expression, where the default position (left) is in the antiterminator conformation. Upon binding by the ligand, the mRNA adopts the terminator conformation (right).

the 5'-UTRs representing genes encoding aminoacyl tRNA synthetases, the enzymes that charge tRNAs with their cognate amino acid (see Chapter 14). In these cases, uncharged tRNAs serve as the ligand and bind to the aptamer of the 5'-UTR, inducing the *antiterminator conformation*. This allows the transcription of the genes, leading to the subsequent translation of the enzymes that are required to charge tRNAs. When charged tRNAs are in abundance and uncharged tRNAs are not present to bind to the aptamer, the riboswitch, in the default condition, adapts the *terminator conformation*, effectively shutting down transcription. As predicted, charged tRNAs are unable to bind to the aptamer.

Finally, there are examples of bacterial riboswitches where, like attenuation of the *trp* operon discussed earlier, the alternative 5'-UTR conformations allow transcription to be completed, but ligand binding to the aptamer induces a conformation that inhibits translation by ribosomes. In such cases, regulation of gene expression has been invoked at the level of translation.

We will discuss other recent findings involving RNA later in the text (Special Topic Chapter 2—Emerging Roles of RNA).

16.7 The *ara* Operon Is Controlled by a Regulator Protein That Exerts Both Positive and Negative Control

We conclude this chapter with a brief discussion of the **arabinose (*ara*) operon** as analyzed in *E. coli*. This inducible operon is unique because the same regulatory protein is capable of exerting both positive and negative control, and as a result, at some times induces and at others represses gene expression. **Figure 16–15(a)** shows the operon components, and **Figures 16–15(b)** and **(c)** show, respectively, the conditions under which the operon is active or inactive.

1. The metabolism of the sugar arabinose is governed by the enzymatic products of three structural genes, *araB, A,* and *D* [Figure 16–15(a)]. Their transcription is controlled by the regulatory protein AraC, encoded by the *araC* gene, which interacts with two regulatory regions, *araI* and *araO₂*.* These sites can be bound individually or coordinately by the AraC protein.

---

*An additional operator O_1 region is also present, but is not involved in the regulation of the *ara* structural gene.

(a) Components of *ara* operon

(b) Arabinose present; operon is induced — positive regulation

(c) Arabinose absent; operon is repressed — negative regulation

FIGURE 16–15 Genetic regulation of the *ara* operon. The regulatory protein of the *araC* gene acts as either an inducer (in the presence of arabinose) or a repressor (in the absence of arabinose).

2. The *I* region bears that designation because when it is the only region bound by AraC, the system is induced [Figure 16–15(b)]. For this binding to occur, both arabinose and cAMP must be present. Thus, like induction of the *lac* operon, a CAP-binding site is present in the promoter region that modulates catabolite repression in the presence of glucose.

3. In the absence of both arabinose and cAMP, the AraC protein binds coordinately to both the *I* site *and* the O_2 site (so named because it was the second operator region to be discovered in this operon). When both *I* and O_2 are bound by AraC, a conformational change occurs in the DNA to form a tight loop [Figure 16–15(c)], and the structural genes are repressed.

4. The O_2 region is located about 200 nucleotides upstream from the *I* region. Binding at either regulatory region involves a dimer of AraC. When both regions are bound, the dimers interact, producing the loop that causes repression. Presumably, this loop inhibits the access of RNA polymerase to the promoter region. The region of DNA that loops out (the stretch between *I* and O_2) is critical to the formation of the repression complex. Genetic alteration here by insertion or deletion of even a few nucleotides is sufficient to interfere with loop formation and, therefore, repression.

Our observations involving the *ara* operon illustrate the degree of complexity that may be seen in the regulation of a group of related genes. As we mentioned at the beginning of this chapter, the development of regulatory mechanisms has provided evolutionary advantages that allow bacterial systems to adjust to a range of natural environments. Without question, these systems are well equipped genetically not only to survive under varying physiological conditions but to do so with great biochemical efficiency.

CASE STUDY | Food poisoning and bacterial gene expression

At a Midwestern university, several undergraduates reported to the health service with fever, muscle aches, and vomiting. Blood tests showed they had bacterial food poisoning, caused by *Listeria monocytogenes*. One student, a biology major, asked how the bacteria were able to get from the intestine into the bloodstream. The physician explained that *Listeria* cells that express a cell-surface protein, InlA, are able to use receptors on the surface of intestinal cells to gain entry and spread from there to the blood. Once in the blood, the bacteria reach the liver, where they use another cell-surface protein, InlB, to enter liver cells, which are the main sites of infection. She further explained that transcriptional levels of the *inlA* and *inlB* genes determine the infective ability of different *Listeria* strains.

Later, the student discussed this information with her genetics instructor, and together they pondered several questions about how bacteria are able to hijack the normal functions of receptors on human cells as part of their life cycle.

1. How can we tell if the *inlA* and *inlB* genes are expressed constitutively or are induced in the presence of the human receptors?

2. Might these genes be normally expressed at low levels, but undergo increased transcription once in contact with intestinal epithelial cells? How could this be determined?

3. Are the *inlA* and *inlB* genes part of an operon, or do they use a common promoter? What experiments might show this?

4. How might an understanding of the regulation of these bacterial genes be used to treat infections?

Summary Points

MasteringGenetics™ For activities, animations, and review quizzes, go to the Study Area.

1. Research on the *lac* operon in *E. coli* pioneered our understanding of gene regulation in bacteria.

2. Genes involved in the metabolism of lactose are coordinately regulated by a negative control system that responds to the presence or absence of lactose.

3. The catabolite-activating protein (CAP) exerts positive control over *lac* gene expression by interacting with RNA polymerase at the *lac* promoter and by responding to the levels of cyclic AMP in the bacterial cell.

4. The *lac* repressor of *E. coli* has been isolated and studied. Crystal structure analysis has shown how it interacts with the DNA of the operon as well as with inducers, revealing conformational changes in DNA leading to the formation of a repression loop that inhibits binding between RNA polymerase and the promoter region of the operon.

5. Unlike the inducible *lac* operon, the *trp* operon is repressible. In the presence of tryptophan, the repressor binds to the regulatory region of the *trp* operon and represses transcription initiation.

6. The process of attenuation, which regulates operons based on the presence of an end product, involves alterations to mRNA secondary structure, leading to premature termination of transcription.

7. Riboswitches regulate gene expression by virtue of conformational changes in the secondary structure of the 5'-UTR leader region of mRNAs.

8. The *ara* operon in *E. coli* is unique in that the regulator protein exerts both positive and negative control over expression of the genes specifying the enzymes that metabolize the sugar arabinose.

GENETICS, TECHNOLOGY, AND SOCIETY

Quorum Sensing: Social Networking in the Bacterial World

For decades, scientists regarded bacteria as independent single-celled organisms, incapable of cell-to-cell communication. However, recent research is revealing that many bacteria can regulate gene expression and coordinate group behavior through a form of communication termed *quorum sensing*. Through this process, bacteria send and receive chemical signals called autoinducers that relay information about population size. When the population size reaches a "quorum," defined in the business world as the minimum number of members of an organization that must be present to conduct business, the autoinducers regulate gene expression in a way that benefits the group as a whole. Quorum sensing has been described in more than 70 species of bacteria, and its uses range from controlling bioluminescence in marine bacteria to regulating the expression of virulence factors in pathogenic bacteria. Our understanding of quorum sensing has altered our perceptions of prokaryotic gene regulation and is leading to the development of practical applications, including new antibiotic drugs.

Quorum sensing was discovered in the 1960s, during research on the bioluminescent bacterium *Vibrio fischeri* which lives in a symbiotic relationship with the Hawaiian bobtail squid *Euprymna scolopes*. While hunting for food at night, the squid uses light emitted by the *V. fischeri* present in its light organ to illuminate the ocean floor and to counter the shadows created by moonlight that normally act as a beacon for the squid's predators. In return, the bacteria gain a protected, nutrient-rich environment in the squid's light organ. During the day, the bacteria do not glow as a result of the squid's ability to reduce the concentration of bacteria in its light organ, which in turn prevents expression of the bacterial luciferase (*lux*) operon.

What turns the bacteria's *lux* genes on in response to high cell density and off in response to low cell density? In *V. fischeri*, the responsible autoinducer is a secreted homoserine lactone molecule. At a critical population size, these molecules accumulate, are taken up by bacteria within the population, and regulate the *lux* operon by binding directly to transcription factors that stimulate *lux* gene expression.

Since the discovery of quorum sensing in *Vibrio fischeri*, scientists have identified similar microbial communication systems in other bacteria, including significant human pathogens such as pseudomonal, staphylococcal, and streptococcal species. The expression of as many as 15 percent of bacterial genes may be regulated by quorum sensing.

Quorum sensing molecules may also mediate communication among members of different species. In 1994, Bonnie Bassler and her colleagues at Princeton University discovered an autoinducer molecule in the marine bacterium *Vibrio harveyi* that was also present in many diverse types of bacteria. This molecule, autoinducer-2 (AI-2), has the potential to mediate "quorum-sensing cross talk" between species and thus serve as a universal language for bacterial communication. Because the accumulation of AI-2 is proportional to cell number, and because the structure of AI-2 may vary slightly between different species, the current hypothesis is that AI-2 can transmit information about both the cell density and species composition of a bacterial community.

Pathogenic bacteria use quorum sensing to regulate the expression of genes whose products help these bacteria invade a host and avoid immune system detection. For example, *Vibrio cholerae*, the causative agent of cholera, uses AI-2 and an additional species-specific autoinducer to activate the genes controlling the production of cholera toxin. *Pseudomonas aeruginosa*, the Gram-negative bacterium that often affects cystic fibrosis patients, uses quorum sensing to regulate the production of elastase, a protease that disrupts the respiratory epithelium and interferes with ciliary function. *P. aeruginosa* also uses autoinducers to control the production of biofilms, tough protective shells that resist host defenses and make treatment with antibiotics nearly impossible. Other bacteria determine cell density through quorum sensing to delay the production of toxic substances until the colony is large enough to overpower the host's immune system and establish an infection. Because many bacteria rely on quorum sensing to regulate disease-causing genes, therapeutics that block quorum sensing may help combat infections. Research into these

potential therapies is now in progress, and several are now approaching the clinical trial phase. Thus, what began as a fascinating observation in the glowing squid has launched an exciting era of research in bacterial genetics that may one day prove of great clinical significance.

Your Turn

Take time, individually or in groups, to answer the following questions. Investigate the references and links to help you understand the mechanisms and potential uses of quorum sensing in bacteria.

1. Inhibitors of quorum sensing molecules have potential as antibacterial agents. What are some ways in which quorum sensing inhibitors could work to combat bacterial infections? Have any of these therapeutics reached clinical trials?

A recent review of quorum sensing therapeutics can be found in Njoroge, J. and Sperandio, V. 2009. Jamming bacterial communication: New approaches for the treatment of infectious diseases. *EMBO Mol. Med.* 1(4): 201–210.

2. Regulation of bacterial gene expression by autoinducer molecules involves several different mechanisms. Describe these mechanisms and how each could be used as a target for the control of bacterial infections.

The mechanisms by which autoinducers regulate gene expression are summarized in Asad, S. and Opal, S.M. 2008. Bench-to-bedside review: Quorum sensing and the role of cell-to-cell communication during invasive bacterial infection. *Critical Care* 12: 236–247.

3. Quorum sensing systems are also capable of detecting and responding to chemical signals given off by host cells. Explain how this works and how this might benefit pathogenic bacteria.

A review article dealing with interkingdom communication and quorum sensing can be found at Wagner, V.E. et al. 2006. Quorum sensing: dynamic response of *Pseudomonas aeruginosa* to external signals. *Trends Microbiol.* 14(2): 55–58.

INSIGHTS AND SOLUTIONS

A hypothetical operon (*theo*) in *E. coli* contains several structural genes encoding enzymes that are involved sequentially in the biosynthesis of an amino acid. Unlike the *lac* operon, in which the repressor gene is separate from the operon, the gene encoding the regulator molecule is contained within the *theo* operon. When the end product (the amino acid) is present, it combines with the regulator molecule, and this complex binds to the operator, repressing the operon. In the absence of the amino acid, the regulatory molecule fails to bind to the operator, and transcription proceeds.

Categorize and characterize this operon, then consider the following mutations, as well as the situation in which the wild-type gene is present along with the mutant gene in partially diploid cells (F′):

(a) Mutation in the operator region.

(b) Mutation in the promoter region.

(c) Mutation in the regulator gene.

In each case, will the operon be active or inactive in transcription, assuming that the mutation affects the regulation of the *theo* operon? Compare each response with the equivalent situation for the *lac* operon.

Solution: The *theo* operon is repressible and under negative control. When there is no amino acid present in the medium (or the environment), the product of the regulatory gene cannot bind to the operator region, and transcription proceeds under the direction of RNA polymerase. The enzymes necessary for the synthesis of the amino acid are produced,

as is the regulator molecule. If the amino acid *is* present, either initially or after sufficient synthesis has occurred, the amino acid binds to the regulator, forming a complex that interacts with the operator region, causing repression of transcription of the genes within the operon.

The *theo* operon is similar to the tryptophan system, except that the regulator gene is within the operon rather than separate from it. Therefore, in the *theo* operon, the regulator gene is itself regulated by the presence or absence of the amino acid.

(a) As in the *lac* operon, a mutation in the *theo* operator gene inhibits binding with the repressor complex, and transcription occurs constitutively. The presence of an F′ plasmid bearing the wild-type allele would have no effect, since it is not adjacent to the structural genes.

(b) A mutation in the *theo* promoter region would no doubt inhibit binding to RNA polymerase and therefore inhibit transcription. This would also happen in the *lac* operon. A wild-type allele present in an F′ plasmid would have no effect.

(c) A mutation in the *theo* regulator gene, as in the *lac* system, may inhibit either its binding to the repressor or its binding to the operator gene. In both cases, transcription will be constitutive, because the *theo* system is repressible. Both cases result in the failure of the regulator to bind to the operator, allowing transcription to proceed. In the *lac* system, failure to bind the corepressor lactose would permanently repress the system. The addition of a wild-type allele would restore repressibility, provided that this gene was transcribed constitutively.

Problems and Discussion Questions

MasteringGenetics™ Visit for instructor-assigned tutorials and problems.

HOW DO WE KNOW?

1. In this chapter, we focused on the regulation of gene expression in prokaryotes. Along the way, we found many opportunities to consider the methods and reasoning by which much of this information was acquired. From the explanations given in the chapter, what answers would you propose to the following fundamental questions?
   (a) How do we know that bacteria regulate the expression of certain genes in response to the environment?
   (b) What evidence established that lactose serves as the inducer of a gene whose product is related to lactose metabolism?
   (c) What led researchers to conclude that a repressor molecule regulates the lac operon?
   (d) How do we know that the *lac* repressor is a protein?
   (e) How do we know that the *trp* operon is a repressible control system, in contrast to the *lac* operon, which is an inducible control system?

CONCEPT QUESTION

2. Review the Chapter Concepts list on p. 396. These all relate to the regulation of gene expression in prokaryotes. Write a brief essay that discusses why you think regulatory systems evolved

in bacteria (i.e., what advantages do regulatory systems provide to these organisms?), and, in the context of regulation, discuss why genes related to common functions are found together in operons.

3. Contrast positive versus negative control of gene expression.
4. Contrast the role of the repressor in an inducible system and in a repressible system.
5. For the *lac* genotypes shown in the accompanying table, predict whether the structural genes (Z) are constitutive, permanently repressed, or inducible in the presence of lactose.

Genotype	Constitutive	Repressed	Inducible
$I^+O^+Z^+$			×
$I^-O^+Z^+$			
$I^-O^cZ^+$			
$I^-O^cZ^+/F'O^+$			
$I^+O^cZ^+/F'O^+$			
$I^sO^+Z^+$			
$I^sO^+Z^+/F'I^+$			

6. For the genotypes and conditions (lactose present or absent) shown in the following table, predict whether functional enzymes, nonfunctional enzymes, or no enzymes are made.

Genotype	Condition	Functional Enzyme Made	Nonfunctional Enzyme Made	No Enzyme Made
$I^+O^+Z^+$	No lactose			×
$I^+O^CZ^+$	Lactose			
$I^-O^+Z^-$	No lactose			
$I^-O^+Z^-$	Lactose			
$I^-O^+Z^+/F'I^+$	No lactose			
$I^+O^CZ^+/F'O^+$	Lactose			
$I^+O^+Z^-/F'I^+O^+Z^+$	Lactose			
$I^-O^+Z^-/F'I^+O^+Z^+$	No lactose			
$I^SO^+Z^+/F'O^+$	No lactose			
$I^+O^CZ^+/F'O^+Z^+$	Lactose			

7. The locations of numerous $lacI^-$ and $lacI^S$ mutations have been determined within the DNA sequence of the $lacI$ gene. Among these, $lacI^-$ mutations were found to occur in the 5′-upstream region of the gene, while $lacI^S$ mutations were found to occur farther downstream in the gene. Are the locations of the two types of mutations within the gene consistent with what is known about the function of the repressor that is the product of the $lacI$ gene?

8. Describe the experimental rationale that allowed the *lac* repressor to be isolated.

9. What properties demonstrate the *lac* repressor to be a protein? Describe the evidence that it indeed serves as a repressor within the operon system.

10. Predict the effect on the inducibility of the *lac* operon of a mutation that disrupts the function of (a) the *crp* gene, which encodes the CAP protein, and (b) the CAP-binding site within the promoter.

11. Erythritol, a natural sugar abundant in fruits and fermenting foods, is about 65 percent as sweet as table sugar and has about 95 percent fewer calories. It is "tooth friendly" and generally devoid of negative side effects as a human consumable product. Pathogenic *Brucella* strains that catabolize erythritol contain four closely spaced genes, all involved in erythritol metabolism. One of the four genes (*eryD*) encodes a product that represses the expression of the other three genes. Erythritol catabolism is stimulated by erythritol. Present a simple regulatory model to account for the regulation of erythritol

catabolism in *Brucella*. Does this system appear to be under inducible or repressible control?

12. Describe the role of attenuation in the regulation of tryptophan biosynthesis.

13. Attenuation of the *trp* operon was viewed as a relatively inefficient way to achieve genetic regulation when it was first discovered in the 1970s. Since then, however, attenuation has been found to be a relatively common regulatory strategy. Assuming that attenuation is a relatively inefficient way to achieve genetic regulation, what might explain its widespread occurrence?

14. Neelaredoxin is a 15-kDa protein that is a gene product common in anaerobic prokaryotes. It has superoxide-scavenging activity, and it is *constitutively expressed*. In addition, its expression is not further *induced* during its exposure to O_2 or H_2O_2 (Silva, G., et al. 2001. *J. Bacteriol.* 183: 4413–4420). What do the terms *constitutively expressed* and *induced* mean in terms of neelaredoxin synthesis?

15. Milk products such as cheeses and yogurts are dependent on the conversion by various anaerobic bacteria, including several *Lactobacillus* species, of lactose to glucose and galactose, ultimately producing lactic acid. These conversions are dependent on both permease and β-galactosidase as part of the *lac* operon. After selection for rapid fermentation for the production of yogurt, one *Lactobacillus* subspecies lost its ability to regulate *lac* operon expression (Lapierre, L., et al. 2002. *J. Bacteriol.* 184: 928–935). Would you consider it likely that in this subspecies the *lac* operon is "on" or "off"? What genetic events would likely contribute to the loss of regulation as described above?

16. Assume that the structural genes of the *lac* operon have been fused, through recombinant DNA techniques, to the regulatory apparatus of the *ara* operon. If arabinose is provided in a minimal medium to *E. coli* carrying this gene fusion, would you expect β-galactosidase to be produced at induced levels? Explain.

17. Both attenuation of the *trp* operon in *E. coli* and riboswitches in *B. subtilis* rely on changes in the secondary structure of the leader regions of mRNA to regulate gene expression. Compare and contrast the specific mechanisms in these two types of regulation.

18. Keeping in mind the life cycle of bacteriophages discussed earlier in the text (see Chapter 6), consider the following problem: During the reproductive cycle of a temperate bacteriophage, the viral DNA inserts into the bacterial chromosome where the resultant prophage behaves much like a Trojan horse. It can remain quiescent, or it can become lytic and initiate a burst of progeny viruses. Several operons maintain the prophage state by interacting with a repressor that keeps the lytic cycle in check. Insults (ultraviolet light, for example) to the bacterial cell lead to a partial breakdown of the repressor, which in turn causes the production of enzymes involved in the lytic cycle. As stated in this simple form, would you consider this system of regulation to be operating under positive or negative control?

Extra-Spicy Problems

MasteringGenetics™ Visit for instructor-assigned tutorials and problems.

19. Bacterial strategies to evade natural or human-imposed antibiotics are varied and include membrane-bound efflux pumps that export antibiotics from the cell. A review of efflux pumps (Grkovic, S., et al., 2002) states that, because energy is required

to drive the pumps, activating them in the absence of the antibiotic has a selective disadvantage. The review also states that a given antibiotic may play a role in the regulation of efflux by interacting with either an activator protein or a repressor protein, depending on the system involved. How might such systems be categorized in terms of *negative control* (*inducible* or *repressible*) or *positive control* (*inducible* or *repressible*)?

20. In a theoretical operon, genes *A*, *B*, *C*, and *D* represent the repressor gene, the promoter sequence, the operator gene, and the structural gene, *but not necessarily in the order named*. This operon is concerned with the metabolism of a theoretical molecule (tm). From the data provided in the accompanying table, first decide whether the operon is inducible or repressible. Then assign *A*, *B*, *C*, and *D* to the four parts of the operon. Explain your rationale. (AE = active enzyme; IE = inactive enzyme; NE = no enzyme)

Genotype	tm Present	tm Absent
$A^+B^+C^+D^+$	AE	NE
$A^-B^+C^+D^+$	AE	AE
$A^+B^-C^+D^+$	NE	NE
$A^+B^+C^-D^+$	IE	NE
$A^+B^+C^+D^-$	AE	AE
$A^-B^+C^+D^+/F'A^+B^+C^+D^+$	AE	AE
$A^+B^-C^+D^+/F'A^+B^+C^+D^+$	AE	NE
$A^+B^+C^-D^+/F'A^+B^+C^+D^+$	AE + IE	NE
$A^+B^+C^+D^-/F'A^+B^+C^+D^+$	AE	NE

21. A bacterial operon is responsible for the production of the biosynthetic enzymes needed to make the hypothetical amino acid tisophane (tis). The operon is regulated by a separate gene, *R*, deletion of which causes the loss of enzyme synthesis. In the wild-type condition, when tis is present, no enzymes are made; in the absence of tis, the enzymes are made. Mutations in the operator gene (O^-) result in repression regardless of the presence of tis. Is the operon under positive or negative control? Propose a model for (a) repression of the genes in the presence of tis in wild-type cells and (b) the mutations.

22. A marine bacterium is isolated and shown to contain an inducible operon whose genetic products metabolize oil when it is encountered in the environment. Investigation demonstrates that the operon is under positive control and that there is a *reg* gene whose product interacts with an operator region (*o*) to regulate the structural genes, designated *sg*.

In an attempt to understand how the operon functions, a constitutive mutant strain and several partial diploid strains were isolated and tested with the results shown here:

Host Chromosome	F′ Factor	Phenotype
wild type	none	inducible
wild type	*reg* gene from mutant strain	inducible
wild type	operon from mutant strain	constitutive
mutant strain	*reg* gene from wild type	constitutive

Draw all possible conclusions about the mutation as well as the nature of regulation of the operon. Is the constitutive mutation in the *trans*-acting *reg* element or in the *cis*-acting *o* operator element?

23. The SOS repair genes in *E. coli* (discussed in Chapter 15) are negatively regulated by the *lexA* gene product, called the LexA repressor. When a cell sustains extensive damage to its DNA, the LexA repressor is inactivated by the *recA* gene product (RecA), and transcription of the SOS genes is increased dramatically.

One of the SOS genes is the *uvrA* gene. You are a student studying the function of the *uvrA* gene product in DNA repair. You isolate a mutant strain that shows constitutive expression of the UvrA protein. Naming this mutant strain $uvrA^C$, you construct the following diagram showing the *lexA* and *uvrA* operons:

(a) Describe two different mutations that would result in a *uvrA* constitutive phenotype. Indicate the actual genotypes involved.

(b) Outline a series of genetic experiments that would use partial diploid strains to determine which of the two possible mutations you have isolated.

24. A fellow student considers the issues in Problem 23 and argues that there is a more straightforward, nongenetic experiment that could differentiate between the two types of mutations. The experiment requires no fancy genetics and would allow you to easily assay the products of the other SOS genes. Propose such an experiment.

25. Figure 16–13 depicts numerous critical regions of the leader sequence of mRNA that play important roles during the process of attenuation in the *trp* operon. A closer view of the leader sequence, which begins at about position 30 downstream from the 5′ end, is given at the bottom of the page, running across both columns.

Within this molecule are the sequences that cause the formation of the alternative hairpins. It also contains the successive triplets that encode tryptophan, where stalling during translation occurs. Take a large piece of paper (such as manila wrapping paper) and, along with several other students from your genetics class, work through the base sequence to identify the *trp* codons and the parts of the molecule representing the base-pairing regions that form the terminator and antiterminator hairpins shown in Figure 16–13.

26. One of the most prevalent sexually transmitted diseases is caused by the bacterium *Chlamydia trachomatis* and leads to blindness if left untreated. Upon infection, metabolically inert cells differentiate, through gene expression, to become metabolically active cells that divide by binary fission. It has been proposed that release from the inert state is dependent on heat-shock proteins that both activate the reproductive cycle and facilitate the binding of chlamydiae to host cells. Researchers made the following observations regarding the heat-shock regulatory system in *Chlamydia trachomatis*: (1) a regulator protein (call it R) binds to a *cis*-acting DNA element (call it D); (2) R and D function as a repressor–operator pair; (3) R functions as a negative regulator of transcription; (4) D is composed of an inverted-repeat sequence; (5) repression by R is dependent on D being supercoiled (Wilson & Tan, 2002).

(a) Based on this information, devise a model to explain the heat-dependent regulation of metabolism in *Chlamydia trachomatis*.

AUGAAAGCAAUUUUCGUACUGAAAGGUUGGUGGCGCACUUCCUGAAACGGGCAGUGUAUUCACCAUGCGUAAAGCAAUCAGAUACCCAGCCCGCCUAAUGAGCGGGCUUUUUUUU

(Leader sequence for Problem 25. above)

(b) Some bacteria, like *E. coli*, use a heat-shock sigma factor to regulate heat-shock transcription. Are the above findings in *Chlamydia* compatible with use of a heat-sensitive sigma factor?

27. A reporter gene—that is, a gene whose activity is relatively easy to detect—is commonly used to study promoter activity under a variety of investigative circumstances. Recombinant DNA technology is used to attach such a reporter gene to the promoter of interest, after which the recombinant molecule is inserted by transformation or transfection into the cell or host organism of choice. Green fluorescent protein (GFP) from the jellyfish *Aequorea victoria* fluoresces green when exposed to blue light. Assume that you wished to study the regulatory apparatus of the *lac* operon and you developed a plasmid (*p*) that contained all the elements of the *lac* operon except that you replaced the *lac* structural genes with the *GFP* gene (your reporter gene). You used this plasmid to transform *E. coli*. Considering the following genotypes, under which of the following conditions would you expect

β-galactosidase production and/or green colonies when examined under blue light?

| | Medium Condition | | Response | |
Genotype	Lactose	Glucose	β-galactosidase	Green Colonies
$I^+O^+Z^+/p-I^+O^+GFP$	−	+	−	−
	+	+		
	+	−		
$I^+O^+Z^-/p-I^+O^cGFP$	−	+		
	+	−		
$I^+O^+Z^+/p-I^sO^cGFP$	−	+		
	+	−		
$I^+O^cZ^+/p-I^sO^+GFP$	−	+		
	+	−		

Chromosome territories in a chicken cell nucleus. Each chromosome is stained with a different-colored probe.

17 Regulation of Gene Expression in Eukaryotes

CHAPTER CONCEPTS

- Expression of genetic information is regulated by mechanisms that exert control over transcription, mRNA processing, export from the nucleus, mRNA stability, translation, and posttranslational modifications.

- Chromatin remodeling, as well as modifications to DNA and histones, play important roles in regulating gene expression in eukaryotes.

- Eukaryotic transcription initiation requires the assembly of transcription regulatory proteins at *cis*-acting DNA sites known as promoters, enhancers, and silencers.

- Transcription activators and repressors stimulate the association of the general transcription factors into pre-initiation complexes at gene promoters.

- Eukaryotic gene expression is also regulated by multiple posttranscriptional mechanisms, including alternative splicing of pre-mRNA, export from the nucleus, control of mRNA stability, translation regulation, and posttranslational processing.

- RNA-induced gene silencing controls gene expression in several ways and is being harnessed for scientific research and medical treatments.

- Programmed DNA rearrangements contribute to gene regulation in a small number of genes.

Virtually all cells in a eukaryotic organism contain a complete genome; however, only a subset of genes is expressed in any particular cell type. For example, some white blood cells express genes encoding certain immunoglobulins, allowing these cells to synthesize antibodies that defend the organism from infection and foreign agents. However, skin, kidney, and liver cells do not express immunoglobulin genes. Pancreatic islet cells synthesize and secrete insulin in response to the presence of blood sugars; however, they do not manufacture immunoglobulins. In addition, they do not synthesize insulin when it is not required. Eukaryotic cells, as part of multicellular organisms, do not grow solely in response to the availability of nutrients. Instead, they regulate their growth and division to occur at appropriate places in the body and at appropriate times during development. The loss of gene regulation that controls normal cell growth and division may lead to developmental defects or cancer.

Eukaryotic gene regulation is one of the most rapidly advancing fields in genetic research. Our ever-increasing understanding about the mechanisms that regulate gene expression in eukaryotes is contributing knowledge that is fascinating and often surprising. It is also leading to practical applications, such as potential therapies for many human diseases.

In this chapter, we will explore the regulation of gene expression in eukaryotes. We will outline some of the general features of gene regulation, from DNA rearrangements and chromatin modifications to transcriptional and posttranscriptional mechanisms.

Please note that some of the topics discussed in this chapter are explored in greater depth later in the text (see Special Topic Chapter 1—Epigenetics and Special Topic Chapter 2—Emerging Roles of RNA.)

17.1 Eukaryotic Gene Regulation Can Occur at Any of the Steps Leading from DNA to Protein Product

In eukaryotes, gene expression is tightly controlled in order to express the required levels of gene products at specific times, in specific cell types, and in response to complex changes in the environment. To achieve this degree of fine-tuning, eukaryotes employ a wide range of mechanisms for altering the expression of genes. In contrast to prokaryotic gene regulation, which occurs primarily at the level of transcription initiation, regulation of gene expression in eukaryotes can occur at many different levels. These include alterations in the DNA template, initiation of transcription, mRNA modifications and stability, and synthesis, modification, and stability of the protein product (**Figure 17–1**). Several features of eukaryotic cells make it possible for them to use more types of gene regulation than are possible in prokaryotic cells:

- Eukaryotic cells contain a much greater amount of DNA than do prokaryotic cells, and this DNA is associated with histones and other proteins to form highly compact chromatin structures within an enclosed nucleus. Eukaryotic cells modify this structural organization in order to influence gene expression.
- The mRNAs of most eukaryotic genes must be spliced, capped, and polyadenylated prior to transport from the nucleus. Each of these processes can be regulated in order to influence the numbers and types of mRNAs available for translation.
- Eukaryotic genes are located on many chromosomes (rather than just one), and these chromosomes are enclosed within a double-membrane-bound nucleus. After transcription, transport of RNAs into the cytoplasm can be regulated in order to modulate the availability of mRNAs for translation.
- Eukaryotic mRNAs can have a wide range of half-lives ($t_{1/2}$). In contrast, the majority of prokaryotic mRNAs decay very rapidly. Rapid turnover of mRNAs allows prokaryotic cells to rapidly respond to environmental changes. In eukaryotes, the types and quantities of mRNAs in each cell type can be more subtly manipulated by altering mRNA decay rates over a larger range.

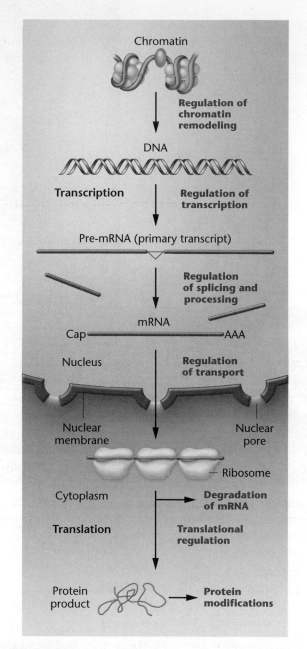

FIGURE 17–1 Regulation can occur at any stage in the expression of genetic material in eukaryotes. All these forms of regulation affect the degree to which a gene is expressed.

- In eukaryotes, translation rates can be modulated, as can the way proteins are processed, modified, and degraded.

In the following sections, we examine some of the major ways in which eukaryotic gene expression is regulated. We will limit our discussion to regulation of genes transcribed by RNA polymerase II (RNAP II). As discussed earlier in the text (see chapter 13), eukaryotes use three different RNA polymerases for transcription. RNAP II transcribes genes that encode all mRNAs and some small nuclear RNAs, whereas RNA polymerases I and III transcribe genes that code for ribosomal RNAs, some small nuclear RNAs, and transfer RNAs. The genes transcribed by RNA polymerase I and III are regulated differently than those transcribed by RNAP II. The promoters recognized by each type of RNA polymerase have different nucleotide sequences and bind different transcription factors. In addition, genes transcribed by each polymerase have different transcription termination signals and mRNA processing mechanisms.

17.2 Eukaryotic Gene Expression Is Influenced by Chromatin Modifications

Two structural features of eukaryotic genes distinguish them from the genes of prokaryotes. First, eukaryotic genes are situated on chromosomes that occupy a distinct location within the cell—the nucleus. This sequestering of genetic information in a discrete compartment allows the proteins that directly regulate transcription to be kept apart from those involved with translation and other aspects of cellular metabolism. Second, as described earlier in the text (see Chapter 12), eukaryotic DNA is combined with histones and nonhistone proteins to form chromatin. Chromatin's basic structure is characterized by repeating units called nucleosomes that are wound into 30-nm fibers, which in turn form other, even more compact structures. The presence of these compact chromatin structures is inhibitory to many processes, including transcription, replication, and DNA repair.

In this section, we outline some of the ways in which eukaryotic cells modify chromatin in order to regulate gene expression.

Chromosome Territories and Transcription Factories

The development of chromosome-painting techniques has revealed that the interphase nucleus is not a bag of tangled chromosome arms, but has a highly organized structure. In the interphase nucleus, each chromosome occupies a discrete domain called a **chromosome territory** and stays separate from other chromosomes. Channels between chromosomes contain little or no DNA and are called **interchromosomal domains**.

Research suggests that transcriptionally active genes are located at the edges of chromosome territories next to interchromosomal domain channels. Scientists hypothesize that this organization may bring actively expressed genes into closer association with transcription factors, or with other actively expressed genes, thereby facilitating their coordinated expression.

Another feature within the nucleus—the **transcription factory**—may also contribute to regulating gene expression. Transcription factories are nuclear sites that contain most of the active RNA polymerase and transcription regulatory molecules. Scientists have used live cell imaging to show that transcription factories are dynamic structures that can form rapidly, then disassemble, as transcription is stimulated and repressed. It is not yet clear whether the formation of transcription factories is a prerequisite or a consequence of transcription initiation; however, by concentrating transcription proteins and actively transcribed genes in specific locations in the nucleus, the cell may enhance the expression of these genes.

Open and Closed Chromatin

The tight association of DNA with nucleosomes and other chromatin-binding proteins inhibits access of the DNA to the proteins involved in many functions including transcription. This inhibitory structure is often referred to as "closed" chromatin. Before transcription can be initiated within nucleosomal chromatin, the structure of chromatin must become "open" to transcription regulatory factors and enzymes such as RNA polymerases.

One of the first demonstrations of a link between open chromatin configurations and active transcription was reported in a study by Mark Groudine and Harold Weintraub in 1976. In this study, Groudine and Weintraub isolated nuclei from chicken red blood cells, fibroblasts, and brain cells. They then treated the nuclei with low levels of the enzyme DNase I. This enzyme digests DNA to varying degrees, depending on the DNA's conformation within chromatin. DNA that is tightly bound within nucleosomes is resistant to DNase I, and DNA that is associated loosely with nucleosomes is rapidly digested. After treating the nuclei with DNase I, they isolated DNA from the nuclei and probed it for the presence of sequences from three genes: β-globin (which is transcribed only in red blood cells), avian tumor virus (which is transcribed in all three cell types), and ovalbumin (which is not transcribed in any of these cell types). They found that β-globin DNA was digested in red blood cell nuclei, but not in nuclei of fibroblasts or brain. In contrast, the avian tumor virus DNA was digested in nuclei from all three cell types, and ovalbumin DNA was not digested in any of the cell nuclei. In addition, by using staphylococcal DNase digestion assays, they determined that all three genes in all three cell-type nuclei remained in association with nucleosomes.

From these studies, Weintraub and Groudine concluded that both transcriptionally active and transcriptionally inactive genes are associated with nucleosomes, but that the nucleosomes associated with transcriptionally active genes are in an altered conformation.

Since Weintraub and Groudine's study, scientists have defined more clearly the nature of the altered chromatin conformations that are associated with transcriptionally active and inactive states. These include histone modifications, chromatin remodeling, and DNA modifications such as methylation.

Histone Modifications and Nucleosomal Chromatin Remodeling

One way in which nucleosomes can be modified is by changing their composition. For example, most nucleosomes contain the normal histone H2A. Some gene promoter regions may be flanked by nucleosomes containing variant histones, such as H2A.Z. The presence of the H2A.Z variant within these nucleosomes affects nucleosome mobility and positioning on DNA. As a result, a gene promoter associated with these variant nucleosomes may be either transcriptionally activated or repressed depending on the nucleosome position.

A second mechanism of chromatin alteration involves histone modification. Histone modification involves the covalent bonding of functional groups onto the N-terminal tails of histone proteins. The most common histone modifications are the addition of acetyl, methyl, or phosphate groups onto the basic amino acids of histone tails.

Acetylation decreases the positive charge on histones, resulting in a reduced affinity of the histone for DNA. In turn, this may assist the formation of open chromatin conformations which would allow the binding of transcription regulatory proteins to DNA.

Histone acetylation is catalyzed by **histone acetyl-transferase enzymes (HATs).** In some cases, HATs are recruited to genes by the presence of certain transcription activator proteins that bind to transcription regulatory regions. In other cases, transcription activator proteins themselves have HAT activity. Of course, what can be opened can also be closed. In that case, **histone deacetylases (HDACs)** remove acetate groups from histone tails. HDACs can be recruited to genes by the presence of certain repressor proteins on regulatory regions.

The third mechanism is chromatin remodeling, which involves the repositioning or removal of nucleosomes on DNA, brought about by chromatin remodeling complexes. Chromatin remodeling complexes are large multi-subunit complexes that use the energy of ATP hydrolysis to move and rearrange nucleosomes along the DNA. Repositioned nucleosomes make regions of the chromosome accessible to transcription regulatory proteins, such as transcription activators and RNAP II. One of the best-studied remodeling complexes is the **SWI/SNF** complex. Remodelers such as SWI/SNF can act in several different ways (**Figure 17–2**). They may loosen the attachment between histones and DNA, resulting in the nucleosome sliding along the DNA and exposing regulatory regions. Alternatively, they may loosen the DNA strand from the nucleosome core, or they may cause reorganization of the internal nucleosome components. In all cases, the DNA is left transiently exposed to association with transcription factors and RNA polymerase. Like HATs, chromatin remodeling complexes can

(a) Alteration of DNA-histone contacts

(b) Alteration of the DNA path

(c) Remodeling of nucleosome core particle

FIGURE 17–2 Three ways by which chromatin remodelers, such as the SWI/SNF complex, alter the association of nucleosomes with DNA. (a) The DNA-histone contacts may be loosened, allowing the nucleosomes to slide along the DNA, exposing DNA regulatory regions. (b) The path of the DNA around a nucleosome core particle may be altered. (c) Components of the core nucleosome particle may be rearranged, resulting in a modified nucleosome structure.

be recruited to DNA by transcription activator proteins that are bound to specific regions of DNA. The interactions of remodeling complexes are also affected by the presence or absence of histone modifications.

DNA Methylation

Another type of change in chromatin that plays a role in gene regulation is the enzyme-mediated addition or removal of methyl groups to or from bases and sugars in DNA. **DNA methylation** most often occurs at position 5 of cytosine (**5-methylcytosine**), causing the methyl group to protrude into the major groove of the DNA helix. Methylation occurs most often on the cytosine of CG doublets in DNA, usually on both strands:

$$5'-{}^{m}CpG-3'$$

$$3'-GpC^{m}-5'$$

Methylatable CpG sequences are not randomly distributed throughout the genome, but tend to be concentrated in CpG-rich regions, called **CpG islands**, located at the 5′ ends of genes, usually in promoter regions. In the genome of eukaryotic species, approximately 5 percent of the cytosine residues are methylated.

Evidence of a role for methylation in eukaryotic gene expression is based on a number of observations. First, an inverse relationship exists between the degree of methylation and the degree of expression. Large transcriptionally inert regions of the genome, such as the inactivated X chromosome in mammalian female cells, are often heavily methylated.

Second, methylation patterns are tissue specific and, once established, are heritable for all cells of that tissue. It appears that proper patterns of DNA methylation are essential for normal mammalian development. Despite this heritability, DNA methylation in specific gene regions can be altered by methylase and demethylase enzymes in order to activate or silence regions of DNA.

Perhaps the most direct evidence of a role for methylation in gene expression comes from studies using base analogs. The nucleoside **5-azacytidine** can be incorporated into DNA in place of cytidine during DNA replication. This analog cannot be methylated, causing the undermethylation of the sites where it is incorporated. The incorporation of 5-azacytidine into DNA changes the pattern of gene expression and stimulates expression of alleles on inactivated X chromosomes. In addition, the presence of 5-azacytidine in DNA can induce the expression of genes that would normally be silent in certain differentiated cells.

How might methylation affect gene regulation? Data from *in vitro* studies suggest that methylation can repress transcription by inhibiting the binding of transcription factors to DNA. Methylated DNA may also recruit repressive chromatin remodeling complexes and HDACs to gene-regulatory regions.

NOW SOLVE THIS

17–1 Cancer cells often have abnormal patterns of chromatin modifications. In some cancers, the DNA repair genes *MLH1* and *BRCA1* are hypermethylated on their promoter regions. Explain how this abnormal methylation pattern could contribute to cancer.

■ **HINT:** *This problem involves an understanding of the types of genes that are mutated in cancer cells. The key to its solution is to consider how DNA methylation affects gene expression of cancer-related genes.*

17.3 Eukaryotic Transcription Initiation Requires Specific *Cis*-Acting Sites

Eukaryotic transcription regulation requires the binding of many regulatory factors to specific DNA sequences located in and around genes, as well as to sequences located at great distances. Although these sequences do not, by themselves, regulate transcription, they are essential because they position regulatory proteins in regions where those proteins can act to stimulate or repress transcription of the associated gene. In this section, we will discuss some of the DNA sequences known as *cis*-acting sequences—that are required for the accurate and regulated transcription of genes transcribed by RNAP II. As defined earlier in the text (see Chapter 13), a ***cis*-acting sequence** is one that is located on the same chromosome as the gene that it regulates. This is in contrast to ***trans*-acting factors** (such as DNA-binding proteins or small RNA molecules) that can influence the expression of a gene on any chromosome.

Promoter Elements

A **promoter** is a region of DNA that recognizes the transcription machinery and binds one or more proteins that regulate transcription initiation. Promoters are necessary in order for transcription to be initiated accurately and at a basal level. Promoters are located immediately adjacent to the genes they regulate. They specify the site or sites at which transcription begins and the direction of transcription along the DNA. Within promoters are a number of **promoter elements**—short nucleotide sequences that bind specific regulatory factors.

There are two subcategories within eukaryotic promoters. First, the **core promoter** determines the accurate initiation of transcription by RNAP II. Second, **proximal-promoter elements** are those that modulate the efficiency of basal levels of transcription.

Recent bioinformatic and genomic research has introduced new complexities to our understanding of promoters and how they work. This research reveals that there is a great deal of diversity in eukaryotic promoters, in terms of both their structures and functions. Promoters are now thought to be either *focused* or *dispersed*. **Focused promoters** specify transcription initiation at a single specific nucleotide (the **transcription start site**). In contrast, **dispersed promoters** direct initiation from a number of weak transcription start sites located over a 50- to 100-nucleotide region (**Figure 17–3**). Focused transcription initiation is the major type of initiation for most genes of lower eukaryotes, but for only about 30 percent of vertebrate genes. Focused promoters are usually associated with genes whose transcription levels are highly regulated, whereas dispersed promoters are associated with genes that are transcribed constitutively.

Little is known about the DNA elements that make up dispersed promoters. These promoters are usually found within CpG islands, suggesting that chromatin modifications may influence initiation from these promoters. In addition, some data suggest that dispersed promoters contain the same types of elements as focused promoters and

(a) Focused promoter

One major transcript

(b) Dispersed promoter

Multiple transcripts

FIGURE 17–3 Focused and dispersed promoters. Focused promoters (a) specify one specific transcription initiation site. Dispersed promoters (b) specify weak transcription initiation at multiple start site positions over an approximately 100-bp region. Dispersed promoters are common in vertebrates and are associated with housekeeping genes. Transcription start sites and the directions of transcription are indicated with arrows.

that they bind the same transcription initiation proteins. However, these elements contain multiple mismatches to the element consensus sequences, perhaps accounting for the low levels of transcription initiation from these types of promoters.

Much more is known about the structure of focused promoters. These promoters are made up of one or more DNA sequence elements, including the Initiator (Inr), TATA box, TFIIB recognition element (BRE), downstream promoter element (DPE), and motif ten element (MTE). The locations and consensus sequences of these elements are summarized in **Figure 17–4**. Versions of the BRE, TATA, and Inr elements appear to be universal components of all focused promoters; however, the MTEs and DPEs are found in only some of these promoters. The role of these core-promoter elements is to bind to specific

transcription initiation proteins, and these will be discussed in the next section.

The **Inr element** encompasses the transcription start site, from approximately nucleotides −2 to +4, relative to the start site. In humans, the Inr consensus sequence is YYAN^A/$_T$YY (where Y indicates any pyrimidine nucleotide and N indicates any nucleotide). The transcription start site is the first A residue at +1. The **TATA-box** element is located at approximately −30 relative to the transcription start site and has the consensus sequence TATA^A/$_T$AAR (where R indicates any purine nucleotide). The **BRE** is found in core promoters at positions either immediately upstream or downstream from the TATA box. The **MTE** and **DPE** sequence motifs are located downstream of the transcription start site, at approximately +18 to +27 and +28 to +33, respectively.

In addition to core-promoter elements, many promoters also contain proximal-promoter elements located upstream of the TATA box and BRE. Proximal-promoter elements act along with the core-promoter elements to increase the levels of basal transcription. For example, the CAAT box is a common proximal-promoter element. The **CAAT box** has the consensus sequence CAAT or CCAAT and is usually located about 70 to 80 base pairs upstream from the start site. Mutational analysis suggests that CAAT boxes (when present) are critical to the promoter's ability to initiate transcription. Mutations on either side of this element have no effect on transcription, whereas mutations within the CAAT sequence dramatically lower the rate of transcription. **Figure 17–5** summarizes the transcriptional effects of mutations in the CAAT box and other promoter elements. The **GC box** is another element often found in promoter regions and has the consensus sequence GGGCGG. It is located, in one or more copies, at about position −110.

Enhancers and Silencers

Transcription of eukaryotic genes is regulated not only at promoter sequences but also at DNA sequences called **enhancers**. Enhancers can be located on either side of a

FIGURE 17–4 Core-promoter elements found in focused promoters. Core-promoter elements are usually located between −40 and +40 nucleotides, relative to the transcription start site, indicated as +1. BRE is the TFIIB recognition element, which can be found on either side of the TATA box. TATA is the TATA box, Inr is the Initiator element, MTE is the motif ten element, and DPE is the downstream promoter element.

FIGURE 17–5 Summary of the effects on transcription levels of different point mutations in the promoter region of the β-globin gene. Each line represents the level of transcription produced in a separate experiment by a single-nucleotide mutation (relative to wild type) at a particular location. Dots represent nucleotides for which no mutation was tested. Note that mutations within specific elements of the promoter have the greatest effects on the level of transcription.

gene, at some distance from the gene, or even within the gene. Some studies show that enhancers can be located as far away as a million base pairs from the genes they regulate. Like promoters, they are *cis* regulators because they function when located on the same chromosome as the structural genes they regulate. While promoter sequences are essential for basal-level transcription, enhancers are necessary for achieving the maximum level of transcription. In addition, enhancers are responsible for time- and tissue-specific gene expression. Thus, some degree of analogy exists between enhancers and operator regions in prokaryotes; however, enhancers are more complex in both structure and function.

Scientists have studied promoters and enhancers by analyzing the effects that specific mutations have on the transcription of cloned genes introduced into cultured cells. They have also studied enhancers by introducing cloned enhancer elements in various orientations relative to a cloned reporter gene, then testing the expression of these constructs in tissue culture cells. These *in vitro* studies have revealed several features that distinguish promoters from enhancers:

1. The position of an enhancer need not be fixed relative to the gene it regulates; it will function whether it is upstream, downstream, or within a gene.

2. The orientation of an enhancer element can be inverted without significant effect on its action.

3. If an enhancer is cloned next to a cloned gene that it does not normally regulate *in vivo*, the transcription of the gene is enhanced.

An example of an enhancer located *within* the gene it regulates is the immunoglobulin heavy-chain gene

enhancer, which is located in an intron between two exons. This enhancer is active only in cells expressing the immunoglobulin genes, indicating that tissue-specific gene expression can be modulated through the enhancer. An example of a downstream enhancer is the β-globin gene enhancer. In chickens, an enhancer located between the β-globin gene and the ε-globin gene works in one direction to control transcription of the ε-globin gene during embryonic development and in the opposite direction to regulate expression of the β-globin gene during adult life.

Enhancers are modular and often contain several different short DNA sequences. For example, the enhancer of the SV40 virus (which is transcribed inside a eukaryotic cell) has a complex structure consisting of two adjacent sequences of approximately 100 bp each, located some 200 bp upstream from a transcriptional start point. Each of the two 100-bp regions contains multiple sequence motifs that contribute to achieving the maximum rate of transcription. If one or the other of these regions is deleted, there is no effect on transcription; but if both are deleted, *in vivo* transcription is greatly reduced.

Another type of *cis*-acting transcription regulatory element, the **silencer,** acts upon eukaryotic genes to repress the level of transcription initiation. Silencers, like enhancers, are *cis*-acting short DNA sequence elements that affect the rate of transcription initiated from an associated promoter. They often act in tissue- or temporal-specific ways to control gene expression.

Our understanding of promoters, enhancers, and other DNA elements has been expanded by data recently reported by the ENCODE project. We will describe the significance of the ENCODE data in Section 17.10.

17.4 Eukaryotic Transcription Initiation Is Regulated by Transcription Factors That Bind to *Cis*-Acting Sites

It is generally accepted that *cis*-acting regulatory sites—including promoters, enhancers, and silencers—influence transcription initiation by acting as binding sites for transcription regulatory proteins. These transcription regulatory proteins, known as **transcription factors**, can have diverse and complicated effects on transcription. Some transcription factors increase the levels of transcription initiation and are known as **activators**, whereas others reduce transcription levels and are known as **repressors**.

The effects of activators and repressors can be finely tuned to the appropriate cell type, as a response to environmental cues, or during the correct time in development. To do this, some transcription factors may be present in only certain types of cells, thereby regulating their target genes for tissue-specific levels of expression. Some transcription factors are expressed in cells only at certain times during development or in response to certain external or internal signals. In some cases, a transcription factor that binds to a *cis*-acting site and regulates a certain gene may be present in a cell and may even bind to its appropriate *cis*-acting site but will only become active when modified structurally (for example, by phosphorylation) or by binding to another molecule such as a hormone. These modifications to transcription factors may also be regulated in tissue- or temporal-specific ways. In addition, different transcription factors may compete for binding to the same DNA sequence or to one of two overlapping sequences. Transcription factor concentrations in the cell and the strength with which each factor binds to the DNA will dictate which factor binds and hence will determine the level of transcription initiation dictated by the factor that binds. Finally, multiple transcription factors that bind to several different enhancers and promoter elements within a gene-regulatory region can interact with each other to fine-tune the levels and timing of transcription initiation.

The Human Metallothionein IIA Gene: Multiple *Cis*-Acting Elements and Transcription Factors

The human **metallothionein IIA gene** (*hMTIIA*) provides an example of how the transcription of one gene can be regulated by the interplay of multiple promoter and enhancer elements and the transcription factors that bind to them. The product of the *hMTIIA* gene is a protein that binds to heavy metals such as zinc and cadmium, thereby protecting cells from the toxic effects of high levels of these metals. It is also implicated in protecting cells from the effects of oxidative stress. The gene is expressed at low levels in all cells but is transcribed at high levels when cells are exposed to heavy metals or to steroid hormones such as glucocorticoids.

The *cis*-acting regulatory elements controlling transcription of the *hMTIIA* gene include promoter, enhancer, and silencer elements (**Figure 17–6**). Each *cis*-acting element is a short DNA sequence that has specificity for binding to one or more transcription factors.

The *hMTIIA* gene contains the core-promoter elements TATA box and Inr, which specify the start of transcription. The factors that bind to core promoters will be described in the next section of this chapter. The proximal-promoter element, GC, binds the SP1 factor, which is present at all times in most eukaryotic cells and stimulates transcription at low levels in most cells. Expression levels are also regulated by the BLE (basal element) and ARE (AP factor response element) regions, which can be considered enhancer elements. These *cis*-elements bind the activator proteins 1, 2, and 4 (AP1, AP2, and AP4), which are present at various levels in different cell types and can be activated in response to extracellular growth signals. The BLE contains overlapping binding sites for the AP1 and AP4 factors, providing some degree of selectivity in how these factors stimulate transcription of *hMTIIA* when bound to the BLE in different cell types. High levels of transcription are stimulated by the presence of the enhancers MRE (metal response element) and GRE (glucocorticoid response element). The metal-inducible transcription factor (MTF1) binds to the MRE in

FIGURE 17–6 The human metallothionein IIA gene promoter and enhancer regions, containing multiple *cis*-acting regulatory sites. The transcription factors controlling both basal and induced levels of *hMTIIA* transcription are indicated below the gene, with arrows showing their binding sites.

response to the presence of heavy metals. The presence of excess heavy metals within cells is thought to displace zinc from metallothionein proteins, which are present at low levels in all cells. The free zinc ions bind to zinc-finger motifs within the DNA-binding domains of the MTF1 transcription factors, altering their conformation. After binding to zinc ions, MTF1 moves from the cytoplasm to the nucleus and binds to MREs upstream of the *hMTIIA* gene, activating metallothionein gene transcription. The glucocorticoid receptor protein binds to the GRE, but only when the receptor protein is in a complex with the glucocorticoid steroid hormone. The glucocorticoid receptor is normally located in the cytoplasm of the cell; however, when glucocorticoid hormone enters the cytoplasm, it binds to the receptor and causes a conformational change that allows the receptor to enter the nucleus, bind to the GRE, and stimulate *hMTIIA* gene transcription. In addition to activation, transcription of the *hMTIIA* gene can be repressed by the actions of the repressor protein PZ120, which binds over the transcription start region.

The presence of multiple regulatory elements and transcription factors that bind to them allows the *hMTIIA* gene to be transcriptionally activated or repressed in response to subtle changes in both extracellular and intracellular conditions.

Functional Domains of Eukaryotic Transcription Factors

We have described transcription factors as proteins that bind to DNA and activate or repress transcription initiation. These actions are achieved through the presence of two functional domains (clusters of amino acids that carry out a specific function) within each of these proteins. One domain, the **DNA-binding domain**, binds to specific DNA sequences present in the *cis*-acting regulatory site. The other domain, the ***trans*-activating** or ***trans*-repression domain**, activates or represses transcription. The *trans*-activating and *trans*-repression domains bring about their effects by interacting with other transcription factors or RNA polymerase, as we will discuss in the next section.

The DNA-binding domains of eukaryotic transcription factors have various characteristic three-dimensional structural motifs. Examples include the helix–turn–helix (HTH), zinc-finger, and basic leucine zipper (bZIP) motifs.

The **helix–turn–helix (HTH)** motif, present in both prokaryotic and eukaryotic transcription factors, is characterized by a certain geometric conformation rather than a distinctive amino acid sequence. The presence of two adjacent α-helices separated by a "turn" of several amino acids (hence the name of the motif) enables the protein to bind to DNA.

Zinc-finger motifs (such as those present in the MTF1 transcription factor) are found in a wide range of transcription factors that regulate gene expression. A typical zinc-finger protein contains clusters of two cysteines and two histidines at repeating intervals. These clusters bind zinc atoms, fold into loops, and interact with specific DNA sequences.

The **basic leucine zipper (bZIP)** motif contains a region called a leucine zipper that allows protein–protein dimerization. When two bZIP-containing molecules dimerize, the leucine residues "zip" together. The resulting dimer contains two basic α-helical regions adjacent to the zipper that bind to the phosphate residues and specific bases in their DNA-binding site.

Transcription factors also contain *trans*-activating or *trans*-repressing domains that are distinct from their DNA-binding domains. These domains can occupy from 30 to 100 amino acids. The amino acid sequences within *trans*-activating or *trans*-repressing domains vary considerably between transcription factors. The ways in which they activate transcription initiation are also varied and are discussed in the next section.

17.5 Activators and Repressors Interact with General Transcription Factors and Affect Chromatin Structure

We have now discussed two of the steps involved in eukaryotic transcription regulation: first, chromatin must be remodeled and modified to allow transcription regulatory proteins to bind to their specific *cis*-acting sites; second, transcription factors bind to *cis*-acting sites and bring about positive and negative effects on the transcription initiation rate—often in response to extracellular signals or in tissue- or time-specific ways. The next question for us to consider is how do these *cis*-acting regulatory elements and their DNA-binding factors act to influence transcription initiation? To answer this question, we must first discuss how eukaryotic RNAP II and its general transcription factors assemble at promoters.

Formation of the RNA Polymerase II Transcription Initiation Complex

A number of proteins called **general transcription factors** are needed at a promoter in order to initiate either basal-level or enhanced levels of transcription. These proteins assemble in a specific order, forming a transcription **preinitiation complex (PIC)** that provides a platform for RNAP II to recognize transcription start sites and to initiate transcription.

The general transcription factors that assist RNAP II at a core promoter are called **TFIID** (*Transcription Factor* for RNAP *IID*). **TFIIB, TFIIA, TFIIE, TFIIF, TFIIH,** and

FIGURE 17-7 The assembly of general transcription factors required for the initiation of transcription by RNAP II.

Mediator. The general transcription factors and their interactions with the core promoter and RNAP II are outlined in **Figure 17–7**.

The first step in the formation of a PIC is the binding of TFIID to the TATA box of the core promoter. TFIID is a multi-subunit complex that contains **TBP** (*TATA Binding Protein*) and approximately 13 proteins called **TAFs** (*TBP Associated Factors*). In addition, a subset of TAFs binds to Inr elements, as well as DPEs and MTEs. TFIIA interacts with TFIID and assists the binding of TFIID to the core promoter. Once TFIID has made contact with the core promoter, TFIIB binds to BREs on one or both sides of the TATA box. Once TFIID and TFIIB have bound the core promoter, the other general transcription factors interact with RNAP II and help recruit it to the promoter. The fully formed PIC mediates the unwinding

of promoter DNA at the start site and the transition of RNAP II from transcription initiation to elongation. On many promoters of higher eukaryotes, RNAP II remains paused at about 50 bp downstream of the transcription start site, awaiting signals that release it into transcription elongation. In other gene promoters of higher eukaryotes and in all promoters in yeast, RNAP II immediately leaves the promoter region and proceeds down the DNA template in an **elongation complex**. Several of the general transcription factors, specifically TFIID, TFIIE, TFIIH, and Mediator, remain on the core promoter to help set up the next PIC.

Mechanisms of Transcription Activation and Repression

Researchers have proposed several models to explain how transcription activators and repressors bring about changes to RNAP II transcription. In most cases, these models involve the formation of DNA loops that bring distant enhancer or silencer elements into close physical contact with the promoter regions of genes that they regulate.

Evidence supporting the formation of DNA loops comes from two types of assays: formaldehyde cross linking and direct visualization. When cells are treated with formaldehyde, proteins become crosslinked to DNA or other proteins with which they are closely associated. Formaldehyde cross linking shows that enhancer regions and promoter regions, even when separated by millions of base pairs, are in close proximity when promoters are active—presumably through the interactions of proteins bound to each region. Direct visualization assays use fluorescence *in situ* hybridization (FISH) techniques to reveal that enhancers and promoters are located in close physical proximity within the nucleus.

In one model of transcription activation and repression, DNA looping may deliver activators, repressors, and general transcription factors to the vicinity of promoters that must be activated or repressed. In this *recruitment model*, enhancer and silencer elements act as donors that increase the concentrations of important regulatory proteins at gene promoters. By enhancing the rate of PIC assembly or stability, or by accelerating the release of RNAP II from a promoter, transcription activators bound at enhancers may stimulate the rate of transcription initiation. In order to make contact with promoter-bound factors, activators are thought to interact with other proteins called **coactivators** that form a complex known as an **enhanceosome** (**Figure 17–8**). Enhanceosomes may directly contact the PIC through subunits of the mediator and TFIID. In a similar way, repressors bound at silencer elements may decrease the rate of PIC assembly and the release of RNAP II.

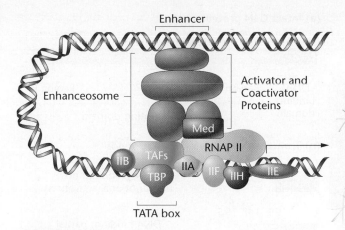

Enhancer

Enhanceosome

Activator and Coactivator Proteins

Med

RNAP II

IIB   TAFs   IIA   IIF   IIH   IIE

TBP

TATA box

FIGURE 17–8 Formation of a DNA loop allows factors that bind to an enhancer or silencer at a distance from a promoter to interact with general transcription factors in the pre-initiation complex and to regulate the level of transcription.

In a second model, DNA looping may result in *chromatin alterations* that either stimulate or repress transcription of target genes. Chromatin remodeling complexes or chromatin modifiers, once delivered to the vicinity of a promoter, may open or close the promoter to interactions with general transcription factors and RNAP II, or may inhibit the release of paused RNAP II from pre-initiation complexes.

A third model of transcription activation and repression states that enhancer or repressor looping may relocate a target gene to a nuclear region that is favorable or inhibitory to transcription. This *nuclear relocation* model would be consistent with the presence of the transcription factories—regions of the nucleus that contain concentrations of RNAP II and transcription regulatory factors.

17.6 Gene Regulation in a Model Organism: Transcription of the *GAL* Genes of Yeast

One of the first model systems used to study eukaryotic gene regulation was the **GAL gene system** in yeast. The *GAL* system comprises four structural genes (*GAL1, GAL10, GAL2,* and *GAL7*) and three regulatory genes (*GAL4, GAL80,* and *GAL3*). The products of the structural genes transport galactose into the cell and metabolize the sugar. The products of the regulatory genes positively and negatively control the transcription of the structural genes.

Transcription of the *GAL* structural genes is **inducible**—that is, transcription is regulated by the presence or absence of the substrate, galactose. In the absence of galactose, the *GAL* structural genes are not transcribed. If galactose is added to the growth medium, transcription begins immediately, and the mRNA concentration increases a thousand-fold. Null mutations in the regulatory gene *GAL4* prevent activation, indicating that transcription is under **positive control**—that is, the activator protein must be present to turn on gene transcription. In this section, we will examine how transcription of two *GAL* genes, *GAL1* and *GAL10*, is positively regulated [**Figure 17–9(a)**]

Transcription of these two genes is controlled by a control region called **UAS$_G$** (*upstream activating sequence* of *GAL* genes), of approximately 170 bp. In yeast, UAS elements are functionally similar to the enhancers found in higher eukaryotes. The chromatin structure of the UAS$_G$ is constitutively open, or **DNase hypersensitive**, meaning that it is loosely associated with nucleosomes. Within the UAS$_G$ are four binding sites for the Gal4 protein (**Gal4p**), which is encoded by the *GAL4* gene. These sites are permanently occupied by Gal4p, whether or not the *GAL1* and *GAL10* genes are transcribed. Gal4p is, in turn, negatively regulated by the Gal80 protein (**Gal80p**), which is the product of the *GAL80* gene.

In the absence of galactose, Gal80p is always bound to Gal4p, covering Gal4p's transcription activation domain, which is shown in **Figure 17–9(b)** as a dark patch. Transcription activation occurs when galactose interacts with the Gal3 protein (**Gal3p**), encoded by the *GAL3* gene. When bound to galactose, the Gal3p molecule undergoes a conformational change that allows it to interact with the UAS$_G$-bound Gal4p/Gal80p complex. This interaction disrupts the association of Gal4p with Gal80p, exposing the Gal4p activation domain.

Gal4p is a protein consisting of 881 amino acids. It includes a DNA-binding domain that recognizes and binds

(a) *GAL* gene cluster

(b)

FIGURE 17–9 Model of *GAL1* and *GAL10* transcriptional activation. (a) The structure of the yeast genome region containing three of the *GAL* genes—*GAL7, GAL10,* and *GAL1.* Arrows indicate transcription start sites and the directions of transcription. Promoter regions are indicated as "P"s. (b) The *GAL10* and *GAL1* gene UAS_G region. The UAS_G region has four binding sites for Gal4p, shown as purple boxes. Gal4p molecules are shown as blue circles, and Gal80p molecules are shown as red triangles or squares. Induction is indicated by a change in the conformation of Gal80p, and its association with Gal4p, which exposes the transcription activation domain of Gal4p.

to DNA sequences in the UAS_G and a *trans*-activating domain that activates transcription [**Figure 17–10(a)**]. Researchers have identified these functional domains by making deletions in the *GAL4* gene and assaying the gene products for their ability to bind DNA and to activate transcription [**Figure 17–10(b)**].

Data from many studies suggest that transcription activation results from contacts between the activating domain of Gal4p and other proteins. Research shows that the first factor to interact with the Gal promoter is a coactivator known as SAGA, which associates directly with Gal4p. Following the recruitment of SAGA, the general transcription factor Mediator interacts with Gal4p and enters the complex. Finally, the remaining general transcription factors, as well as RNAP II, are recruited into a PIC on *GAL* promoters. Another step that is stimulated by Gal4p is nucleosome remodeling. Gal4p recruits the nucleosome-remodeling complex SWI/SNF to *GAL* promoters, followed by the removal of promoter-bound nucleosomes.

(a) Intact Gal4 protein

(b) Truncated and deleted Gal4 proteins

FIGURE 17–10 Structure and function of the Gal4p activator. (a) Gal4p contains a DNA-binding domain, shown in dark blue, and two transcriptional activation regions, shown in light blue. The Gal80p binding region resides in the amino acid region 851–881. (b) Effects of various deletions on the activity of Gal4p.

17.7 Posttranscriptional Gene Regulation Occurs at Many Steps from RNA Processing to Protein Modification

We have noted that regulation of gene expression occurs at many points along the pathway from DNA to protein. Although transcriptional control exerts the primary effect on gene regulation in eukaryotes, **posttranscriptional regulation** plays an equal, if not more significant, role. Prior to translation, eukaryotic mRNA transcripts can be processed by the removal of noncoding introns, the precise splicing together of the remaining exons, the addition of a cap at the mRNA 5′ end, and the synthesis of a poly-A tail at its 3′ end. In addition, RNA molecules can be edited and bases can be modified. The mature messenger RNA is then exported to the cytoplasm, where it is translated and degraded. Each of these steps can be regulated to control the quantity of a protein product. In addition, the stability, modifications, and activities of the protein product can be regulated.

In this section, we examine several mechanisms of posttranscriptional gene regulation that are especially important in eukaryotes—control of alternative splicing, mRNA stability, and translation. In a subsequent section, we will discuss another method of posttranscriptional gene regulation—RNA silencing.

Alternative Splicing of mRNA

Alternative splicing can generate different forms of mRNA from identical pre-mRNA molecules, so that expression of one gene can give rise to a number of proteins, with similar or different functions.

Changes in splicing patterns can have many different effects on the translated protein. Even small changes can alter the protein's enzymatic activity, receptor-binding capacity, or protein localization in the cell.

Figure 17–11 presents the example of alternative splicing of the pre-mRNA transcribed from the **calcitonin/calcitonin gene-related peptide gene (CT/CGRP gene)**. In thyroid cells, the *CT/CGRP* primary transcript is spliced in such a way that the mature mRNA contains the first four exons only. In these cells, the exon 4 polyadenylation signal is used to process the mRNA and add the poly-A tail. This mRNA is translated into the calcitonin peptide, a 32-amino-acid peptide hormone that

FIGURE 17–11 Alternative splicing of the *CT/CGRP* gene transcript. The primary transcript, which is shown in the middle of the diagram, contains six exons. The primary transcript can be spliced into two different mRNAs, both containing the first three exons but differing in their final exons. The *CT* mRNA contains exon 4, with polyadenylation occurring at the end of the fourth exon. The *CGRP* mRNA contains exons 5 and 6, with polyadenylation occurring at the end of exon 6. The *CT* mRNA is produced in thyroid cells. After translation, the resulting protein is processed into the calcitonin peptide. In contrast, the *CGRP* mRNA is produced in neuronal cells, and after translation, its protein product is processed into the CGRP peptide.

is involved in regulating calcium. In the brain and peripheral nervous system, the *CT/CGRP* primary transcript is spliced to include exons 5 and 6, but not exon 4. In these cells, the exon 6 polyadenylation site is recognized. The *CGRP* mRNA encodes a 37-amino-acid peptide with hormonal activities in a wide range of tissues. Through alternative splicing, two peptide hormones with different structures, locations, and functions are synthesized from the same gene.

Alternative splicing increases the number of proteins that can be made from each gene. As a result, the number of proteins that an organism can make—its **proteome**—is not the same as the number of genes in the genome, and protein diversity can exceed gene number by an order of magnitude. Alternative splicing is found in all metazoans but is especially common in vertebrates, including humans. Scientists estimate that at least two-thirds of protein-coding genes in the human genome can undergo alternative splicing. Thus, humans can produce several hundred thousand different proteins (or perhaps more) from the approximately 20,000 genes in the haploid genome.

Given the existence of alternative splicing, how many different polypeptides can be derived from the same pre-mRNA? One answer to that question comes from research on the *Dscam* gene in *Drosophila melanogaster*. During development, cells of the nervous system must accurately connect with each other. Even in *Drosophila*, with only about 250,000 neurons, this is a formidable task. Neurons have cellular processes called axons that form connections with other nerve cells. The *Drosophila* **Dscam gene** encodes a protein that guides axon growth, ensuring that neurons are correctly wired together. In *Dscam* pre-mRNA, exons 4, 6, 9, and 17 each consist of an array of possible alternatives (**Figure 17–12**). These are spliced into the mature mRNA in an exclusive fashion, so that each exon is represented by no more than one of its possible alternatives. There are 12 alternatives for exon 4; 48 alternatives for exon 6; 33 alternatives for exon 9; and 2 alternatives for exon 17. The number of possible combinations that could be formed in this way suggests that, theoretically, the *Dscam* gene can produce 38,016 different proteins. Although this is an impressive number of possible different mRNAs and protein isoforms, does the *Drosophila* nervous system require all these alternatives? Recent research suggests that it does.

Scientists have shown that each neuron expresses a different subset of Dscam protein isoforms. In addition, *in vitro* studies show that each Dscam protein isoform can bind to the same Dscam protein isoform but not to others. Even a small change in amino acid sequence reduces or eliminates the binding between two Dscam molecules. *In vivo* studies show that cells expressing the same isoforms of Dscam interact with each other. Therefore, it appears that the diversity of Dscam protein isoforms in neurons

FIGURE 17–12 Alternative splicing of the *Dscam* gene mRNA. (Top) Organization of the *Dscam* gene in *Drosophila melanogaster* and the transcribed pre-mRNA. The *Dscam* gene encodes a protein that guides axon growth during development. Each mRNA will contain one of the 12 possible exons for exon 4 (red), one of the 48 possible exons for exon 6 (blue), one of the 33 possible exons for exon 9 (green), and one of the 2 possible exons for exon 17 (yellow). Counting all possible combinations of these exons, the *Dscam* gene could encode 38,016 different versions of the Dscam protein.

provides a kind of molecular identity tag for each neuron, helping to guide it to the correct target and preventing the tangling of extensions from different neurons.

A more extreme example is provided by *para*, another gene expressed in the nervous system of *Drosophila*. *Para* not only has at least 6 sites of alternative splicing, leading to 48 possible different mRNA variants, but also undergoes another posttranscriptional modification called RNA editing, at 11 positions. **RNA editing** involves base substitutions made after transcription and splicing. With both alternative splicing and editing, the *para* gene can theoretically produce more than 1 million different transcripts.

The *Drosophila* genome contains about 13,000 genes, but the *Dscam* gene alone can produce 2.5 times that many proteins. Because alternative splicing is far more common in vertebrates, the combinations of proteins that can be produced from the human genome may be astronomical.

Alternative Splicing and Human Diseases

Mutations that affect regulation of splicing contribute to several genetic disorders. One of these disorders, **myotonic dystrophy**, provides an example of how defects in alternative RNA splicing can lead to a wide range of symptoms. Myotonic dystrophy (DM) is the most common form of adult muscular dystrophy, affecting 1 in 8000 individuals. It is an autosomal dominant disorder that occurs in two forms—DM1 and DM2. Both of these diseases show a wide range of symptoms, including muscle wasting, **myotonia** (difficulty relaxing muscles), insulin resistance, cataracts, testicular atrophy, behavior and cognitive defects, cardiac muscle problems, and hair follicle tumors.

DM1 is caused by the expansion of the trinucleotide repeat CTG in the 3′-untranslated region of the **DMPK gene**. In unaffected individuals, the *DMPK* gene contains between 5 and 35 copies of the CTG repeat sequence, whereas in DM1 patients, the gene contains between 150 and 2000 copies. The severity of the symptoms is directly related to the number of copies of the repeat sequence. DM2 is caused by an expansion of the repeat sequence CCTG within the first intron of the **ZNF9 gene**. Affected individuals may have up to 11,000 copies of the repeat sequence in the *ZNF9* intron. In DM2, the severity of symptoms is not related to the number of repeats.

Recently, scientists have discovered that DM1 and DM2 are caused not by changes in the protein products of the *DMPK* or *ZNF9* genes, but by the toxic effects of their repeat-containing RNAs. These RNAs accumulate and form inclusions within the nucleus. In the case of *ZNF9*, only the CCUG sequence repeat itself accumulates in the nucleus, as the remainder of the intron is degraded after splicing of the gene. It appears that the accumulated RNAs bind to, and sequester, proteins that would normally be involved in regulating the alternative splicing patterns of a large number of other RNAs. These RNAs include those whose products are required for the proper functioning of muscle and neural tissue. So far, scientists have discovered over 20 genes that are inappropriately spliced in DM1 muscle, heart, and brain. Often, the fetal splicing patterns occur in DM1 and DM2 patients, and the normal transitions to adult splicing patterns are lacking. Such defects in the regulation of RNA splicing are known as **spliceopathies**.

Sex Determination in *Drosophila*: A Model for Regulation of Alternative Splicing

As outlined earlier in the text (see chapter 7), sex in *Drosophila* is determined by the ratio of X chromosomes to sets of autosomes (X:A). When the ratio is 0.5 (1X:2A), males are produced, even when no Y chromosome is present; when the ratio is 1.0 (2X:2A), females are produced. Intermediate ratios (2X:3A) produce intersexes. Chromosomal ratios are interpreted by a small number of genes that initiate a cascade of splicing events, resulting in the production of male or female somatic cells and the corresponding male or female phenotypes. Three major genes in this pathway are *Sex lethal*

(*Sxl*), *transformer* (*tra*), and *doublesex* (*dsx*). We will review some of the key steps in this process.

The regulatory gene at the beginning of this cascade (**Figure 17–13**) is the gene **Sex lethal (Sxl)**, which encodes an RNA-binding protein. In females, transcription factors encoded by genes on the X chromosome are thought to activate transcription of the *Sxl* gene. In males, the lower concentration of these transcription factors is not sufficient to activate transcription of *Sxl*. As a result of this differential regulation of transcription, the SXL protein is expressed only in female embryos. The presence (in females) or absence (in males) of SXL protein begins cascades of pre-mRNA splicing events that are specific for females or males. In the presence of SXL, female splicing patterns are expressed, which override the default male splicing patterns.

One of the targets of SXL protein is the pre-mRNA encoded by the **transformer (tra)** gene. This pre-mRNA is transcribed in both male and female cells. When SXL protein is present, *tra* pre-mRNAs are spliced to produce mature mRNAs that are translated into functional TRA protein. If SXL is absent, *tra* pre-mRNAs are spliced in such a way that a translation stop codon remains in the mature mRNA. Translation of this mRNA results in a truncated, nonfunctional protein. SXL alters the splicing pattern of *tra* pre-mRNA by binding to the pre-mRNA and altering recognition of splicing signals by the splicing machinery.

The next gene in the cascade, **doublesex (dsx)**, is a critical control point in the development of sexual phenotype. It produces a functional mRNA and protein in both females and males. However, the pre-mRNA is processed in a sex-specific manner to produce different transcripts and hence different DSX proteins. In females, the functional TRA protein acts as a splicing factor that binds to the *dsx* pre-mRNA and directs splicing in a female-specific pattern. In males, no TRA protein is present, and splicing of the *dsx* pre-mRNA results in a male-specific mRNA and protein. The female DSX protein (DSX-F) and the male protein (DSX-M) are both transcription factors, but act in different ways. DSX-F represses the transcription of genes whose products control male sexual development, whereas DSX-M activates the transcription of genes whose products control male sexual development. In addition, DSX-M represses the transcription of genes that control female sexual development.

In sum, the product of the *Sxl* gene acts as a switch that selects the pathway of sexual development by controlling splicing of the *dsx* transcript. The SXL protein is produced only in embryos with an X:A ratio of 1. Failure to control the splicing of the *dsx* transcript in a female mode results in the default splicing of the transcript in a male mode, leading to the production of a male phenotype.

FIGURE 17–13 Regulation of pre-mRNA splicing that determines male and female sexual development in *Drosophila*. The ratio of X chromosomes to autosomes (AA) affects transcription of the *Sxl* gene. The presence of SXL protein begins a cascade of pre-mRNA splicing events that culminate in female-specific gene expression and production of the DSX-F transcription factor. In the absence of SXL protein, a male-specific pattern of pre-mRNA splicing results in male-specific patterns of gene expression induced by the DSX-M protein.

NOW SOLVE THIS

17–3 Some mutations in the *tra* gene of *Drosophila* cause XX females to appear as males. In contrast, other mutations in *tra* cause XY male flies to appear as normal females. Which of these phenotypes would you expect if a mutation in *tra* resulted in a null allele? Which would you expect if the mutation produced a constitutively active *tra* gene product?

■ **HINT:** *This problem involves an understanding of the SXL pathway in* Drosophila. *The key to its solution is to review the functions of the normal TRA protein in* Drosophila *males and females.*

Control of mRNA Stability

The **steady-state level** of an mRNA is its amount in the cell as determined by a combination of the rate at which the gene is transcribed and the rate at which the mRNA is degraded. The steady-state level determines the amount of mRNA that is available for translation. All mRNA molecules are degraded at some point after their synthesis, but the lifetime of an mRNA, defined in terms of its **half-life** or $t_{1/2}$, can vary widely between different mRNAs and can be regulated in response to the needs of the cell.

An mRNA may be degraded along three general pathways. First, an mRNA may be targeted for degradation by enzymes that shorten the length of the poly-A tail. In newly synthesized mRNAs, the poly-A tail is about 200 nucleotides long and binds a protein known as the **poly-A binding protein**. The binding of this protein to the poly-A tail helps to stabilize the mRNA. If the poly-A tail is shortened to less than about 30 nucleotides, the mRNA becomes unstable and acts as a substrate for exonucleases that degrade the RNA in either a 5′ to 3′ or 3′ to 5′ direction. Second, **decapping enzymes** can remove the 7-methylguanosine cap, which also renders the mRNA unstable. Third, an mRNA may be cleaved internally by an endonuclease, providing unprotected ends at which exonuclease degradation may proceed. Examples of endonucleolytic cleavages are those that occur during **nonsense-mediated decay** and those triggered by RNA interference (which will be discussed in Section 17.8). Nonsense-mediated mRNA decay occurs when translation terminates at premature stop codons. Endonucleases attack the mRNA near the stop codon, leaving unprotected ends that are then degraded by exonucleases. Nonsense-mediated decay is an important mechanism for removing mutated mRNA molecules that could, if efficiently translated, result in accumulations of aberrant protein products.

What are the mechanisms by which mRNA stability can be regulated? One way that an mRNA's half-life can be altered is through specific RNA-sequence elements that recruit degrading or stabilizing complexes. One well-studied mRNA stability element is the **adenosine-uracil rich element (ARE)**—a stretch of ribonucleotides that consist of A and U ribonucleotides. These AU-rich elements are usually located in the 3′ untranslated regions of mRNAs that have short, regulated half-lives. These ARE-containing mRNAs encode proteins that are involved in cell growth or transcription control and need to be rapidly modulated in abundance. In cells that are not growing or require low levels of gene expression, specific complexes bind to the AREs of these mRNA molecules, bringing about shortening of the poly-A tail and rapid mRNA degradation. It is estimated that approximately 10 percent of mammalian mRNAs contain these instability elements.

Translational and Posttranslational Regulation

The ultimate end-point of gene expression is the presence of an active gene product. There are many ways by which the quantity and activity of a gene product can be regulated. In some cases, the translation of an mRNA can be regulated to produce the correct quantity of protein product. In other cases, the stability of a protein can be modulated or the protein can be modified after translation to change its structure and affect its activity.

An important example of posttranslational regulation is that of the **p53 protein.** The p53 protein is essential to protect normal cells from the effects of DNA damage and other stresses. It is a transcription factor that increases the transcription of a number of genes whose products are involved in cell-cycle arrest, DNA repair, and programmed cell death. Under normal conditions, the levels of p53 are extremely low in cells, and the p53 that is present is inactive. When cells suffer DNA damage or metabolic stress, the level of p53 protein increases dramatically. In addition, p53 becomes an active transcription factor.

The changes in the levels and activity of p53 are due to a combination of increased protein stability and modifications to the protein. In unstressed cells, p53 is bound by another protein called **Mdm2**. The Mdm2 protein binds to the transcriptional activation domain of the p53 molecule, blocking its ability to induce transcription. In addition, Mdm2 acts as a ubiquitin ligase, adding ubiquitin residues onto the p53 protein. **Ubiquitin** (a "ubiquitous" molecule) is a small protein that tags other proteins for degradation by proteolytic enzymes. The presence of ubiquitin on p53 results in p53 degradation. When cells are stressed, Mdm2 and p53 are modified by phosphorylation and acetylation, resulting in the release of Mdm2 from p53. As a consequence, p53 proteins are stabilized, the levels of p53 increase, and the protein is able to act as a transcription factor. An added level of control is that p53 is a transcription factor that induces the transcription of the *Mdm2* gene. Hence, the presence of active p53 triggers a negative feedback loop that creates more Mdm2 protein, which rapidly returns p53 to its rare and inactive state.

17.8 RNA Silencing Controls Gene Expression in Several Ways

In the last decade, the discovery that small RNA molecules control gene expression has given rise to a new field of research. First discovered in plants, short RNA molecules, ~21 nucleotides long, are now known to regulate gene expression in the cytoplasm of plants, animals, and fungi by repressing translation and triggering the degradation of mRNAs. This form of sequence-specific posttranscriptional regulation is known as **RNA interference (RNAi)**. More recently, researchers have discovered that short RNAs act in the nucleus to alter chromatin structure and bring about repression of transcription. Together, these phenomena are known as **RNA-induced gene silencing**. We will outline some basic features of RNA-induced gene silencing, while keeping in mind that this field is rapidly expanding and advancing. Later in the text (see Special Topic Chapter 2—Emerging Roles of RNA), we present a more comprehensive description of gene regulation by various types of RNA molecules, including those discussed here.

RNAi was first discovered during laboratory research, in studies of plant and animal gene expression. In one research project, Andrew Fire and Craig Mello injected roundworm (*Caenorhabditis elegans*) cells with either single-stranded or double-stranded RNA molecules—both containing sequences complementary to the mRNA of the *unc-22* gene. Although they expected that the single-stranded antisense RNA molecules would suppress *unc-22* gene expression by binding to the endogenous sense mRNA, they were surprised to discover that the injection of double-stranded *unc-22* RNA was 10- to 100-fold more powerful in repressing expression of the *unc-22* mRNA. They studied the phenomenon further and published their results in the journal *Nature* in 1998. They reported that the presence of double-stranded RNA acts to degrade the mRNA if the mRNA is complementary in sequence to one strand of the double-stranded RNA. Only a few molecules of double-stranded RNA are needed to bring about the degradation of large amounts of mRNA. Fire and Mello's research opened up an entirely new and surprising branch of molecular biology, with far-reaching implications for practical applications. For their insights into RNAi, they were awarded the Nobel Prize for Physiology or Medicine in 2006.

The Molecular Mechanisms of RNA-Induced Gene Silencing

Two major types of short RNA molecules are involved in RNA-induced gene silencing: The **small interfering RNAs (siRNAs)** and the **microRNAs (miRNAs)**. Although they arise from different sources, their mechanisms of action are similar. Both types of RNA are short, double-stranded molecules, between 20 and 25 ribonucleotides long. The siRNAs are derived from longer RNA molecules that are linear, double-stranded, and located in the cell cytoplasm. In nature, these siRNA precursors arise within cells as a result of virus infection or the expression of transposons—both of which synthesize double-stranded RNA molecules as part of their life cycles. RNAi may be a method by which cells recognize these double-stranded RNAs and inactivate them, protecting the organism from external or internal assaults. Another source of siRNA molecules is in the research lab. Scientists are now able to introduce double-stranded RNAs into cells for research or therapeutic purposes. In the cytoplasm, double-stranded RNA molecules are recognized by an enzyme complex known as **Dicer** and are cleaved by Dicer into siRNAs.

The miRNAs are derived from single-stranded RNAs that are transcribed within the nucleus from the cell's own genome and that contain a double-stranded stem-loop structure. Nuclease enzymes within the nucleus recognize these stem-loop structures and cleave them from the longer single-stranded RNA. The stem-loop RNA fragments are exported from the nucleus into the cytoplasm where they are further processed by the Dicer complex into short, linear, double-stranded miRNAs. Over the last few years, scientists have discovered that significant amounts of eukaryotic genomes are transcribed by RNAP II into RNA products that contain no open reading frames and are not translated into protein products. These RNAs are transcribed from sequences within the introns of other protein-coding genes or from their own promoters located within noncoding regions of the genome. So far, more than 1500 miRNAs have been discovered in the human genome. This is probably an underestimate, and scientists speculate that eukaryotic genomes may contain thousands of genes that are transcribed into short noncoding RNAs, which may regulate the expression of more than half of all protein-coding genes.

How do these noncoding RNAs work to negatively regulate gene expression? Two pathways involved in RNA-induced gene silencing are outlined in **Figure 17–14**.

The RNAi pathway involves several steps. First, siRNA or miRNA molecules associate with an enzyme complex called the **RNA-induced silencing complex (RISC)**. Second, within the RISC, the short double-stranded RNA is denatured and the sense strand is degraded. Third, the RNA/RISC complex becomes a functional and highly specific agent of RNAi, seeking out mRNA molecules that are complementary to the antisense RNA contained in the RISC. At this point, RNAi can take one of two different pathways. If the antisense RNA in the RISC is perfectly complementary to the mRNA, the RISC will cleave the mRNA. The cleaved mRNA is then degraded by ribonucleases. If the antisense RNA within the RISC is not exactly complementary to the mRNA, the RISC complex stays bound to the mRNA, interfering with the ability of ribosomes to translate the mRNA. Hence, RNAi can silence gene expression by affecting either mRNA stability or translation.

In addition to repressing mRNA translation and triggering mRNA degradation, siRNAs and miRNAs can also repress the transcription of specific genes and larger regions of the genome. They do this by associating with a different complex—the **RNA-induced transcription silencing complex (RITS)**. The antisense RNA strand within the RITS

CYTOPLASM   NUCLEUS

FIGURE 17-14 Mechanisms of gene regulation by RNA-induced gene silencing. The siRNA or miRNA precursors are processed into short double-stranded RNA molecules by the Dicer complex in the cytoplasm. They are then recognized by either the RISC complex or the RITS complex, and one strand is degraded. In the RNAi pathway, the RISC complex, guided by the antisense single-stranded RNA, recognizes target mRNA substrates, marking them for degradation or translation inhibition. In the transcription silencing pathway, the RITS complex acts in the nucleus, by recognizing genomic DNA that is complementary to the single strands of the miRNAs or siRNAs. The RITS complex recruits enzymes that modify chromatin and repress transcription.

cell, transcription of genes whose expression depends on these factors is also repressed.

Recent studies are demonstrating that RNA-induced gene-silencing mechanisms operate during normal development and control the expression of batteries of genes involved in tissue-specific cellular differentiation. In addition, scientists have discovered that abnormal activities of miRNAs contribute to the occurrence of cancers, diabetes, and heart disease.

RNA-Induced Gene Silencing in Biotechnology and Medicine

Recently, geneticists have applied RNAi as a powerful research tool. RNAi technology allows investigators to specifically create single-gene defects without having to induce inherited gene mutations. RNAi-mediated gene silencing is relatively specific and inexpensive, and it allows scientists to rapidly analyze gene function. Several dozen scientific supply companies now manufacture synthetic siRNA molecules of specific ribonucleotide sequence for use in research. These molecules can be introduced into cultured cells to knock out specific gene products.

In addition to its use in laboratory research, RNAi is being developed as a potential pharmaceutical agent. In theory, any disease caused by overexpression of a specific gene, or even normal expression of an abnormal gene product, could be attacked by therapeutic RNAi. Viral infections are an obvious target, and scientists have had promising results using RNAi in tissue cultures to reduce the severity of infection by several types of viruses such as HIV, influenza, and polio. In animal models, siRNA molecules have successfully treated virus infections, eye diseases, cancers, and inflammatory bowel disease. In these studies, the synthetic siRNA molecules were applied to the surfaces of mucous membranes, or into eyes, brain tissues, or the lower intestine. Research into RNAi pharmaceuticals has made rapid progress, and the Phase I (toxicity) stages of the first human clinical trials have been completed. Phase II and III (efficacy) clinical trials have begun to test the use of siRNAs directed against the product of the vascular endothelial growth factor gene, as a drug to treat age-related macular degeneration. Clinical trials have also been started to test RNAi in the treatment of hepatitis B and respiratory syncytial virus infections. Other clinical trials are planned for

targets the RITS complex to specific gene promoters or larger regions of chromatin. RITS then recruits chromatin modifying enzymes to these regions. These enzymes methylate histones and DNA, resulting in heterochromatin formation and subsequent transcriptional silencing. As a result of their effects on chromatin-mediated gene silencing, miRNA molecules are thought to be involved in epigenetic phenomena such as gene imprinting and X chromosome inactivation.

RNAi pathways are also able to repress transcription in indirect ways. Transcription factor mRNAs are frequent targets for RNAi-mediated silencing. When the levels of specific transcription factors are reduced in a siRNA treatment of influenza and hepatitis C virus infections, as well as some solid tumors.

Scientists are particularly enthusiastic about the potential uses of RNAi in the diagnosis and treatment of cancers. Recent studies show that the expression profiles of miRNA genes are characteristic of each tumor type. This observation may lead to more precise methods of diagnosing tumors, predicting their course, and planning treatments. In addition, certain cancers appear to have defects in miRNA gene expression. Treatment of these tumors with synthetic siRNAs may be able to correct these defects and reverse the cancer phenotype. Finally, some cancers are characterized by overexpression or abnormal expression of one or several key proto-oncogenes. If RNAi methods can target these specific gene products, they might help treat cancers that have become resistant to other methods such as radiation or chemotherapy.

New as it is, the science of RNAi holds powerful promise for molecular medicine. Analysts expect the first RNAi drugs to be available within the next decade.

MODERN APPROACHES TO UNDERSTANDING GENE FUNCTION

MicroRNAs Regulate Ovulation in Female Mice

In this chapter you learned about microRNAs (miRNAs) and their roles in silencing gene expression. When miRNAs were first identified it was unclear what role, if any, they played in the post-transcriptional regulation of gene expression. Using the same methods for knocking out protein-coding genes, scientists have created knockouts to study the functions of miRNAs. We will discuss in detail how knockout animals are generated later in the text (see Chapter 20). Through these studies we now know that miRNAs have important roles during development and adult life.

Here we consider a recent study of two miRNAs, miR-200b and miR-429. MiR-429 is in the miR-200 family of related sequences, and it differs from miR-200b by a single nucleotide. MiRNA-200b was detected in the mouse testis; its expression peaked at about 2 weeks of age and continued through adulthood. Because of this finding, scientists hypothesized that miRNA-200b might play a role in male fertility. To test this hypothesis, miRNA-200b and 429 double knockouts (DKOs) were generated.

Results:

Researchers were surprised that no abnormalities were found in the testis and there were no fertility defects in DKO male mice. But miR-DKO female mice showed greatly reduced fertility when mated to males heterozygous for both miRNA-200b and 429. The pregnancy rate of miR-DKO females was at best 9 percent compared to 85 percent in wild-type females (see panel a below). This fertility difference persisted even after 3 months of attempted mating with male mice. A substantial decrease in serum levels of luteinizing hormone (LH), a hormone essential for ovulation, was observed in miR-DKO females. When the ovaries of these mice were examined, they showed a reduced number of ovulated oocytes (see panel b below). But when miR-DKO mice were treated with hormones (gonadotropins) to stimulate ovulation, they produced a similar number of oocytes as heterozygous females. Finally, a series of experiments were carried out to demonstrate that loss of miR-200b and 429 led to increased expression of the *Zeb1* gene in the pituitary gland, which directly resulted in decreased expression of the *Lhb* gene, which encodes the LH protein. *Zeb1* encodes a transcription factor thought to regulate expression of the *Lhb* gene.

(a)

(b)

(a) Pregnancy rate of wild-type, miR-200b and 429 heterozygous females and miR-DKO female mice crossed with miR-200b and 429 heterozygous male mice. (b) Number of ovulated eggs derived from heterozygous and miR-DKO mice naturally or following induced ovulation.

Conclusions:

The ovulation experiment demonstrated that miR-DKO females could undergo normal oogenesis and ovulate when supplemented with hormones. This suggests that knocking out miR-200b and 429 impairs some aspect of the hormonal regulation of ovulation, most likely involving LH. Because the miRNA-200b cluster is present in humans and is adjacent to the human *ZEB* and *LHB* genes, it is possible that miR-200b and 429 play a role in regulating ovulation in humans.

Reference:

Hasuwa, H., Ueda, J., Ikawa, M., and Okabe, M. 2013. MiR-200b and miR-429 function in mouse ovulation and are essential for female fertility. *Science,* 341:71–73.

Questions to Consider:

1. Based on the results described above, draw a diagram to explain possible relationships between miR-220b and 429, the *Zeb1* and *Lhb* genes, and ovulation in miR-DKO female mice.

2. In this study, miR-DKO female mice were mated with male mice overexpressing transgenes for miR-200b and miR-429. Would you expect that the pregnancy rate of miR-DKO females would increase, decrease, or stay the same as miR-DKO female mice crossed with heterozygous males? Refer to the reference to examine the results produced by this mating.

3. Using OMIM, identify the human homolog for *Zeb1*, and find out if there are any human disorders associated with problems with this gene. Do these results surprise you?

17.9 Programmed DNA Rearrangements Regulate Expression of a Small Number of Genes

Except for the occurrence of sequence alterations due to mutations, genomic DNA in most organisms remains remarkably stable. However, despite this genomic stability, some significant examples of gene regulation by DNA rearrangement exist. Earlier in the text (see Chapter 8) we were introduced to DNA amplification and learned how amplification of specific genes, such as the *rRNA* genes in *Xenopus* oocytes, allows expression of these genes at times during development when high levels of these gene products are required.

Besides gene amplifications, several other types of programmed DNA rearrangements occur during developmental regulation of some eukaryotic genes. One type of rearrangement results in the creation of new genes from gene fragments located at various positions in the genome. Another type of rearrangement results in a switch in expression of genes as a result of a recombination or DNA copying event. In these cases, these DNA rearrangements are programmed and essential for normal expression of the genes involved. In addition, rearrangements that lead to loss of some DNA sequences occur only in particular types of somatic cells in higher eukaryotes; hence, these changes are not passed on to progeny.

In this section, we present an example of gene regulation by **programmed DNA rearrangements**: the immunoglobulin system in humans.

The Immune System and Antibody Diversity

The immune system protects organisms against infections and the presence of foreign substances that may enter blood or body tissues. It does this by recognizing molecules on the surface of these foreign substances, and by physically binding to them in a kind of lock-and-key configuration—a phenomenon known as **antigen recognition**. **Antigens** are defined as molecules, usually proteins, which bring about an immune response. Although the immune system has many components, we will focus on **humoral immunity**, which involves the production of proteins called **immunoglobulins**, or **antibodies**, that bind directly to antigens.

Immunoglobulins are synthesized by a type of blood cell known as the **B lymphocyte**, or **B cell**, which undergoes development and maturation in the bone marrow. Immunoglobulin molecules consist of four polypeptide chains, held together by disulfide bonds. Two of these polypeptides are identical **light (L) chains**, and two are identical **heavy (H) chains** (**Figure 17–15**). Together, they form a Y-shaped immunoglobulin structure. Each of the light and heavy chains contains a **constant region** at the C-terminus of the polypeptide and a **variable region** at the N-terminus. The four variable regions, when combined together into the immunoglobulin molecule, form a unique structure that recognizes one specific antigen. Each B cell synthesizes only one type of immunoglobulin.

Mammals are capable of producing hundreds of millions of different types of antibodies in response to the presence of a wide variety of antigens—in fact, more types of antibodies than there are genes in the genome. How can such immense diversity arise from a limited number of genes? The answer lies in the fact that the DNA encoding

(a)

(b)

FIGURE 17–15 Structure of immunoglobulin molecules. (a) Immunoglobulin molecules are Y-shaped and consist of four polypeptide chains. Each chain contains a constant region (purple), a variable region (red), and a hypervariable region (blue). The variable and hypervariable regions form an antigen-recognition site that interacts with a specific antigen in a lock-and-key arrangement. The chains are joined by disulfide bonds. (b) This colored scanning electron micrograph reveals the Y-shaped structure of immunoglobulin molecules, which have been negatively stained prior to electron microscopy.

the immunoglobulin genes is not fixed but undergoes multiple programmed changes, including deletions, translocations, and random mutations.

Gene Rearrangements in the κ Light-Chain Gene

To illustrate how DNA rearrangements contribute to antibody diversity, we will describe the formation of one type of the immunoglobulin light-chain gene (the κ **light-chain gene**) in humans.

The human κ light-chain gene is assembled during B-cell development, from multiple DNA regions located along chromosome 2. In most somatic cells, as well as in germ cells, these DNA regions are organized as shown in **Figure 17–16**. There are 70 to 100 different **L (leader)** and **V (variable) regions**, about half of which are functional and can encode the variable (V) portion of the κ light-chain molecule. Each LV region is preceded by transcription initiation sequences. The LV regions are located about 6 kilobases away from the **J (joining) region**, a region that contains five possible J-encoding exons. Adjacent to the J region is an enhancer sequence that stimulates transcription from any promoter located nearby, and a single **C exon** that encodes the constant region of the κ light-chain molecule.

During development of a mature B cell, one of the LV regions (L_2V_2 in Figure 17–16), along with its promoter, is randomly joined by a recombination event to one of the five J regions (J_3 in our example). This recombination event deletes the entire intervening DNA on chromosome 2. After this somatic

FIGURE 17–16 Assembly of a κ light-chain gene in a B cell, followed by its transcription, mRNA processing, translation, and posttranslational modification. The B-cell gene contains one LV region (L_2V_2) recombined with one J region (J_3). The remaining J regions and the enhancer-containing intron are removed from the transcript by intron splicing. Following translation, the leader sequence (L_2) is cleaved off as the mature polypeptide chain crosses the cell membrane.

recombination event, the LV promoter is activated by the nearby presence of the immunoglobulin enhancer, resulting in transcription of the gene. The resulting RNA is spliced to remove the introns between the L and V regions, and between the J and C regions. After translation of the mature mRNA, the polypeptide is processed by removal of the leader (L) amino acids. The rearranged κ gene is then maintained and passed on to all progeny of that B cell.

Antibody diversity results in part from the random recombination of one of 35 to 50 different functional LV regions with any one of five different J regions. Two other mechanisms further increase the level of diversity. The recombination event that joins an LV region to a J region is not precise and can occur anywhere within a region containing several base pairs. Because of this imprecision, the recombination between any particular pair of LV and J regions still shows considerable variation. In addition, V regions are susceptible to high rates of random somatic mutation—**hypermutation**—during B-cell development. Hypermutation introduces even more variation into the LVJ region's sequence. The mechanisms of DNA rearrangements described here for the human κ light-chain genes also occur during the formation of the gene that encodes another type of light-chain gene (called the λ light-chain gene) as well as the gene that encodes the immunoglobulin heavy chains.

17.10 ENCODE Data Are Transforming Our Concepts of Eukaryotic Gene Regulation

We conclude this chapter by reviewing a project that has revolutionized our thinking about the human genome and eukaryotic gene regulation. In 2003, the U.S. National Human Genome Research Institute launched the **Encyclopedia of DNA Elements (ENCODE) Project**. The goal of ENCODE is to identify all of the functional DNA sequences that lie within the 3.1 billion nucleotides of the human genome and to determine how these elements act to regulate gene expression. This massive endeavor, which is occupying more than 400 scientists from around the world, is approximately half completed. Even half done, the data that have emerged are seriously challenging our views about gene regulation.

One of the most surprising discoveries of ENCODE research is that more than 80 percent of the human genome contains some type of regulatory element or participates in active transcription. This is in contrast to the approximately 20,000 protein-coding genes that occupy less than 2 percent of the genome. Within the 80 percent of the genome once considered "junk DNA," ENCODE has catalogued

thousands of enhancers, promoters, sequences encoding RNA transcripts, and sites of specific chromatin modifications. The abundance of elements as well as the discovery of the extent of their interactions promises to alter our definition of a gene and our understanding of how the information in DNA is transformed into phenotype.

In this section, we present a brief glimpse of ENCODE data as they relate to eukaryotic gene regulation. We also speculate on how these new data modify our concepts of genetic regulation. Implications of data from the ENCODE project are also presented later in the text (see Chapter 21).

Enhancer and Promoter Elements

By examining chromatin features such as DNase hypersensitivity and histone modifications that are characteristic of DNA involved in regulatory-factor binding, ENCODE researchers discovered more than 1 million binding sites for gene-regulation proteins, including transcription factors that bind to enhancers and promoters. These binding sites include approximately 400,000 enhancer elements and 100,000 promoters. Within the 125 cell types examined, approximately 30 percent of these DNA sites are bound by transcription factors in any one cell type. Only 3700 DNA sites are bound by transcription factors in all cell types.

Another interesting discovery was the location of promoter elements. Approximately 30,000 of the promoter regions found by examining chromatin features were located *within* protein-coding genes, and 17,000 of these were oriented in an antisense direction. These data suggest the potential for large amounts of antisense and overlapping transcription initiation through protein-coding and noncoding genes, the consequences of which are not known.

As we learned in Section 17.5, transcription factors bound to enhancer and silencer elements are thought to work by interacting with other transcription proteins located at promoters. These interactions result in the formation of DNA loops of up to 1 million base pairs in length. ENCODE has examined the interactions between enhancers and promoters, with more surprising results. Although researchers examined only 1 percent of the genome, they identified more than 1000 direct physical interactions between promoters and distal regulatory elements such as enhancers in each cell type examined. Approximately 60 percent of these interactions were specific to only one cell type.

ENCODE data show that enhancers can influence the transcription of several different promoters, and not necessarily the closest one. Only about 7 percent of looping interactions occur between an enhancer and the nearest promoter. Approximately 50 percent of promoters physically interact with more than one distal regulatory element, and some have as many as 20 different interactions. Similarly, approximately 10 percent of enhancers interact with more than one promoter and sometimes with as many as ten different promoters.

The researchers speculate that all of these multiple interactions between enhancers and promoters likely do not occur simultaneously within the same cell, but reflect the sum of interactions that are occurring within a population of cells that are assayed together in individual experiments. These data suggest that genes and their regulatory elements likely interact in complex and fluid networks. Because enhancer interactions often skip the nearest gene promoter, unknown mechanisms must exist to allow regulatory elements to target the appropriate gene at the right times and places to allow appropriate gene expression.

These data also indicate that major differences exist between cell types as to how their genomes are regulated, with each cell type using different combinations of regulatory elements and binding proteins in order to determine the cell's gene-expression phenotype.

Transcripts and RNA Processing

Perhaps the most surprising finding of the ENCODE project is that up to 75 percent of the human genome can be transcribed. A total of 128,000 transcript species were identified, and more than 70,000 of these transcripts arise either from DNA in intergenic regions or from antisense transcription within protein-coding genes. More than 7000 small RNAs were identified, including small nuclear (sn) RNAs, small nucleolar (sno)RNAs, micro (mi)RNAs, and transfer (t)RNAs. Many of these small RNAs originate within mRNAs and other long noncoding RNAs. Another interesting type of RNA is the **enhancer RNA**. Enhancer elements often contain bona fide promoter elements that initiate transcription from the enhancer element and

extend outward for several kilobases. The most active enhancers in a cell type produce the most enhancer RNA. Overall, the vast majority of transcripts in a cell do not code for proteins and remain within the nucleus.

ENCODE experiments demonstrate that RNA splicing occurs during transcription. Introns were seen to be spliced in primary transcripts that were still in the process of being transcribed. Another observation is that genes express many splicing variants simultaneously. Approximately two-thirds of protein-coding genes express at least two different splicing variants, with an average of four alternative transcripts per locus. Splicing variants expressed by each gene are expressed at different levels, with one variant being the predominant one.

The functional relevance of this enormous amount of transcription throughout the genome is intriguing but controversial. Some scientists argue that it may be simply "noise" without significance to cellular phenotype. If this is the case, substantial regulation of gene expression must occur at posttranscriptional levels in eukaryotic cells. As regulatory roles are being discovered for many of the small noncoding RNAs as well as some long noncoding RNAs, it is still possible that functions will be discovered for more of these RNAs.

Another consequence of the ENCODE data is that it will be necessary to alter our concept of a gene as the discrete unit of inheritance. ENCODE scientists propose that the transcript be considered the basic *unit of inheritance*, rather than the DNA from which it is transcribed. In this case, the term *gene* would encompass a higher-order concept that includes all of the sequences encoding RNAs that contribute to a specific phenotype.

As more data emerge from the ENCODE project, it is certain to continue challenging our views of eukaryotic gene regulation.

EXPLORING GENOMICS

Tissue-Specific Gene Expression

MasteringGenetics™ Visit the Study Area: Exploring Genomics

I n this chapter, we discussed how gene expression can be regulated in many complex ways. One aspect of gene-expression regulation we considered is the way promoter, enhancer, and silencer sequences can govern transcriptional initiation of genes to allow for tissue-specific gene expression. All cells and tissues of an organism possess the same genome, and many genes are expressed in all cell and tissue types. However, muscle cells, blood cells, and all other tissue types express genes that are largely tissue-specific (i.e., they have limited or no expression in other tissue types). In this exercise, we return to

(continued)

Exploring Genomics—continued

the National Center for Biotechnology Information (NCBI) site and use the search tool BLAST (Basic Local Alignment Search Tool), which you were introduced to in the "Exploring Genomics" exercise for Chapter 10. We will use BLAST to learn more about tissue-specific gene-expression patterns.

■ **Exercise – Tissue-Specific Gene Expression**

1. Access BLAST from the NCBI Web site at http://blast.ncbi.nlm.nih.gov /Blast.cgi

2. The following are GenBank accession numbers for four different genes that show tissue-specific expression patterns. You will perform your searches on these genes.

    NM_021588.1
    NM_00739.1
    AY260853.1
    NM_004917

3. For each gene, carry out a nucleotide BLAST search using the accession numbers for your sequence query. Refer to the "Exploring Genomics" feature in Chapter 10 to refresh your memory

on BLAST searches. Because the accession numbers are for nucleotide sequences, be sure to use the "nucleotide blast" (blastn) program when running your searches. Once you enter "blastn," under the "Choose Search Set" category, you should set the database to "Others (nr etc.)," so that you are not searching an organismspecific database.

4. Once your BLAST search results appear, look at the top alignments for each gene. Clicking on the link for the top alignment will take you to the page showing the sequence alignment for this gene. To the far right of the page you will see a section called "Related Information." The "Gene" link provides a report on details related to this gene.

    Some alignments will display a link for "Map Viewer," which will take you to genome mapping information about the gene. The "UniGene" link will show you a UniGene report. For some genes, upon entering UniGene you may need to click a link above the gene name or the gene name itself before retrieving a UniGene report. Be

sure to explore the "EST Profile" link under the "Gene Expression" category in each UniGene report. EST profiles will show a table of gene-expression patterns in different tissues.

    Also explore the "GEO Profiles" link under the "Gene Expression" category of the UniGene reports, when available. These links will take you to a number of gene-expression studies related to each gene of interest. Explore these resources for each gene, and then answer the following questions:

a. What is the identity of each sequence, based on sequence alignment? How do you know this?

b. What species was each gene cloned from?

c. Which tissue(s) are known to express each gene?

d. Does this gene show regulated expression during different times of development?

e. Which gene shows the most restricted pattern of expression by being expressed in the fewest tissues?

CASE STUDY │ A mysterious muscular dystrophy

A man in his early 30s suddenly developed weakness in his hands and neck, followed a few weeks later by burning muscle pain—all symptoms of late-onset muscular dystrophy. His internist ordered genetic tests to determine whether he had one of the inherited muscular dystrophies, focusing on Becker muscular dystrophy, myotonic dystrophy Type I, and myotonic dystrophy Type II. These tests were designed to detect mutations in the related *dystrophin, DMPK,* and *ZNF9* genes. The testing ruled out Becker muscular dystrophy. While awaiting the results of the *DMPK* and *ZNF9* gene tests, the internist explained that the possible mutations were due to expanded tri- and tetranucleotide repeats, but not in the protein-coding portions of the genes. She went on to say that the resulting disorders were the result not of changes in the encoded proteins, which appear to be normal, but instead of altered RNA splic-

ing patterns, whereby the RNA splicing remnants containing the nucleotide repeats disrupt normal splicing of the transcripts of other genes. This discussion raises several interesting questions about the diagnosis and genetic basis of the disorders.

1. What is alternative splicing, where does it occur, and how could disrupting it affect the expression of the affected gene(s)?

2. What role might the expanded tri- and tetranucleotide repeats play in the altered splicing?

3. How does this contrast with other types of muscular dystrophy, such as Becker muscular dystrophy and Duchenne muscular dystrophy?

Summary Points

MasteringGenetics™ For activities, animations, and review quizzes, go to the Study Area.

1. In eukaryotes, gene regulation can occur at any of the steps involved in gene expression, from DNA rearrangements and chromatin modification to transcription initiation and post-transcriptional processing.

2. Eukaryotic gene regulation at the chromatin level may involve gene-specific chromatin remodeling, histone modifications, or DNA modifications.

3. Eukaryotic transcription is regulated at gene-specific promoter, enhancer, and silencer elements.
4. Transcription factors influence transcription rates by binding to *cis*-acting regulatory sites located within promoters, enhancers, and silencers.
5. Transcription factors are thought to act by enhancing or repressing the association of general transcription factors with the core promoter. They may also remodel and modify chromatin.
6. Posttranscriptional gene regulation includes alternative splicing of nascent RNA, RNA transport, or changes in mRNA stability.
7. Alternative splicing increases the number of gene products encoded by a single gene.
8. Posttranscriptional gene regulation at the levels of translation and protein stability also affect the levels of active gene product.
9. RNA-induced gene silencing is a posttranscriptional mechanism of gene regulation that affects the translatability or stability of mRNA as well as transcription.
10. Programmed DNA rearrangements occur in some genes in specific cell types. These rearrangements are necessary for normal regulated expression of these genes.

INSIGHTS AND SOLUTIONS

1. As a research scientist, you have decided to study transcription regulation of a gene whose DNA has been cloned and sequenced. To begin your study, you obtain the DNA clone of the gene, which includes the gene and at least 1 kb of upstream DNA. You then create a number of subclones of this DNA, containing various deletions in the gene's upstream region. These deletion templates are shown in the figure below. To test these DNA templates for their ability to direct transcription of the gene, you prepare two different types of *in vitro* transcription systems. The first is a defined system containing purified RNAP II and the purified general transcription factors TFIID, TFIIB, TFIIE, TFIIF, and TFIIH. The second system consists of a crude nuclear extract, which is made by extracting most of the proteins from the nuclei of cultured cells. When you test your two transcription systems using each of your templates, you obtain the following results:

Undeleted template

Deleted templates

DNA added	Nuclear extract	Purified system
undeleted	++++	+
−127 deletion	++++	+
−81 deletion	++++	+
−50 deletion	+	+
−11 deletion	o	o

```
  +    Low-efficiency transcription
++++   High-efficiency transcription
  o    No transcription
```

(a) Why is there no transcription from the −11 deletion template in both the crude extract and the purified system?

(b) How do the results for the nuclear extract and the purified system differ, for the *undeleted* template? How would you interpret this result?

(c) For each of the various deletion templates, compare the results obtained from both the nuclear extract and the purified systems.

(d) What do these data tell you about the transcription regulation of this gene?

Solution:

(a) The lack of transcription from the −11 template suggests that some essential DNA sequences are missing from this deletion template. As the −50 template does show some transcription in both the crude extract and purified system, it is likely that the essential missing sequences, at least for basal levels of transcription, lie between −50 and −11. As the TATA box is located in this region, its absence in the −11 template may be the reason for the lack of transcription.

(b) The undeleted template containing large amounts of upstream DNA is sufficient to promote high levels of transcription in a nuclear extract, but only low levels in a purified system. These data suggest that something is missing in the purified system, compared with the nuclear extract, and this component is important for high levels of transcription from this promoter. As crude nuclear extracts are not defined in content, it would not be clear from these data what factors in the extract are the essential ones.

(c) Both the −127 and −81 templates act the same way as the undeleted template in both the nuclear extract and the purified system—high levels of transcription in nuclear extracts but low levels in a purified system. In contrast, the −50 template shows only low levels of transcription in both systems. These results indicate that all of the sequences necessary for high levels of transcription in a crude system are located between −81 and −50.

(d) First, these data tell you that general transcription factors alone are not sufficient to specify high efficiencies of

(continued)

Insights and Solutions—continued

transcription from this promoter. The DNA sequence elements through which the general transcription factors work are located within 50 bp of the transcription start site. Second, the data tell you that the promoter for this gene is likely a member of the "focused" class of promoters, with one defined transcription start site and an essential TATA box. Third, high levels of transcription require sequences between −81 and −50 relative to the transcription start site. These sequences interact with some component(s) of crude nuclear extracts.

2. Scientists estimate that more than 15 percent of disease-causing mutations involve errors in alternative splicing. However, there is an interesting case in which an exon deletion appears to enhance dystrophin production in muscle cells of Duchenne muscular dystrophy (DMD) patients. A deletion of exon 45 of the *dystrophin* gene is the most frequent DMD-causing mutation. But some individuals with Becker muscular dystrophy (BMD), a milder form of muscular dystrophy, have deletions of both exons 45 and 46 (van Deutekom and van Ommen, 2003. *Nat. Rev. Genetics* 4: 774–783). Provide a possible explanation for why BMD patients, with a deletion of both exon 45 and 46, produce more dystrophin than DMD patients do.

Solution: Having a deletion of one exon has several possible effects on a gene product. One possibility is that the mRNA transcribed from the exon-deleted *dystrophin* gene is unstable, leading to a lack of dystrophin protein production. Even if the mRNA is stable, the resulting mutated dystrophin protein could be targeted for rapid degradation, leading to the absence of stable active protein. Another possibility is that the deletion of one exon creates a frameshift mutation, which creates a premature translation stop codon. As the dystrophin gene has 79 exons spanning over 2.6 million base pairs of DNA, a frameshift mutation in exon 45 could create a stop codon near the middle of the gene. The mRNA transcribed from this gene could be targeted for nonsense-mediated mRNA degradation, due to the presence of the premature stop codon. Any mRNA escaping degradation would encode a shorter than normal dystrophin protein, which likely would be rapidly degraded.

It is possible that a deletion encompassing both exon 45 and 46 could restore the reading frame of the dystrophin protein in exon 47. The protein product of this gene would be missing amino acid sequences encoded by the two missing exons; however, the protein itself could still have some activity, partially restoring the wild-type phenotype.

As described in the van Deutekom and van Ommen paper, about 60 percent of all DMD mutations involve deletions of an exon. One strategy being considered for DMD gene therapy is to restore the normal reading frame by causing other exons to be skipped during pre-mRNA splicing. If successful, this type of therapy could convert a severe DMD phenotype into a milder form of the disease, similar to BMD.

Problems and Discussion Questions

MasteringGenetics™ Visit for instructor-assigned tutorials and problems.

HOW DO WE KNOW?

1. In this chapter, we focused on how eukaryotic genes are regulated at different steps in their expression, from chromatin modifications to control of protein stability. At the same time, we found many opportunities to consider the methods and reasoning by which much of this information was acquired. From the explanations given in the chapter,
   (a) How do we know that promoter and enhancer sequences control the initiation of transcription in eukaryotes?
   (b) How do we know that eukaryotic transcription factors bind to DNA sequences at or near promoter regions?
   (c) How do we know that double-stranded RNA molecules can control gene expression?

CONCEPT QUESTION

2. Review the Chapter Concepts list on page 417. These concepts relate to the many different regulatory steps that contribute to gene expression in eukaryotic organisms. The fifth concept summarizes several of the steps in posttranscriptional regulation. Write a short essay describing how the recent data emerging from the ENCODE project influence our views of the relative importance of transcriptional and posttranscriptional gene regulation in humans.

3. Why is gene regulation more complex in a multicellular eukaryote than in a prokaryote? Why is the study of this phenomenon in eukaryotes more difficult?

4. Provide a definition of chromatin remodeling, and give two examples of this phenomenon.

5. Describe the organization of the interphase nucleus. Include in your presentation a description of chromosome territories, interchromosomal domains, and transcription factories.

6. A number of experiments have demonstrated that areas of the genome that are relatively inert transcriptionally are resistant to DNase I digestion; however, those areas that are transcriptionally active are DNase I sensitive. Describe how DNase I resistance or sensitivity might indicate transcriptional activity.

7. Provide a brief description of two different types of histone modification.

8. Present an overview of the manner in which chromatin can be remodeled. Describe the manner in which these remodeling processes influence transcription.

9. Distinguish between the *cis*-acting regulatory elements referred to as promoters and enhancers.

10. Describe the manner in which activators and repressors influence the rate of transcription initiation. How might chromatin structure be involved in such regulation?

11. Compare the control of gene regulation in eukaryotes and prokaryotes at the level of initiation of transcription. How do the regulatory mechanisms work? What are the similarities and differences in these two types of organisms in terms of the specific components of the regulatory mechanisms?

12. Many promoter regions contain CAAT boxes containing consensus sequences CAAT or CCAAT approximately 70 to 80 bases upstream from the transcription start site. How might one determine the influence of CAAT boxes on the transcription rate of a given gene?

13. Recent research indicates that promoters may fall into one of two classes: *focused* or *dispersed*. How do these differ, and which genes tend to be associated with each?

14. Present an overview of RNA-induced gene silencing achieved through RNA interference (RNAi). How do the silencing processes begin, and what major components participate?

15. How does the inherent imprecision of recombination events during immunoglobulin gene rearrangement contribute to the diversity of the immune response?

16. Explain the structural features of the Initiator (Inr) elements, BREs, DPEs, and MTEs of focused promoters.

17. DNA supercoiling, which occurs when coiling tension is generated ahead of the replication fork, is relieved by DNA gyrase. Supercoiling may also be involved in transcription regulation. Researchers discovered that transcriptional enhancers operating over a long distance (2500 base pairs) are dependent on DNA supercoiling, while enhancers operating over shorter distances (110 base pairs) are not so dependent (Liu et al., 2001. *Proc. Natl. Acad. Sci. [USA]* 98: 14,883–14,888). Using a diagram, suggest a way in which supercoiling may positively influence enhancer activity over long distances.

18. In some organisms, including mammals, there is an inverse relationship between the presence of 5-methylcytosine (m^5C) in CpG sequences and gene activity. In addition, m^5C may be involved in the recruitment of proteins that convert chromatin regions from transcriptionally active to inactive states. Overall, genomic DNA is relatively poor in CpG sequences due to the conversion of m^5C to thymine; however, unmethylated CpG islands are often associated with active genes. Researchers have determined that patterns of DNA methylation in spermatozoa vary with age in rats and suggest that such age-related alterations in DNA methylation may be one mechanism underlying age-related abnormalities in mammals (Oakes et al., 2003. *Proc. Natl. Acad. Sci.* 100: 1775–1780). In light of the above information, provide an explanation that relates paternal age-related alterations in DNA methylation to birth abnormalities.

19. In the hypothetical extraterrestrial organism, the Quagarre, the immunoglobulin genes undergo rearrangements similar to those in humans, with two main differences. One difference is that the κ light-chain V regions are located on chromosome 4 and the other κ light-chain regions are located on chromosome 10. Another difference is that the Quagarre immunoglobulin genes do not rearrange until the creature is 13 years old. By examining a mitotic spread of chromosomes from a Quagarre B cell, how could you estimate the creature's age?

Extra-Spicy Problems

20. Because the degree of DNA methylation appears to be a relatively reliable genetic marker for some forms of cancer, researchers have explored the possibility of altering DNA methylation as a form of cancer therapy. Initial studies indicate that while hypomethylation suppresses the formation of some tumors, other tumors thrive. Why would one expect different cancers to respond differently to either hypomethylation or hypermethylation therapies?

21. Explain how the following mutations would affect the transcription of the yeast *GAL1* gene.
    (a) A deletion within the *GAL4* gene that removes the region encoding amino acids 1 to 100.
    (b) A deletion of the entire *GAL3* gene.
    (c) A mutation within the *GAL80* gene that blocks the ability of Gal80 protein to interact with Gal3p.
    (d) A deletion of one of the four UAS_G elements upstream from the *GAL1* gene.
    (e) A point mutation in the *GAL1* core promoter that alters the sequence of the TATA box.

22. The interphase nucleus appears to be a highly structured organelle with chromosome territories, interchromosomal domains, and transcription factories. In cultured human cells, researchers have identified approximately 8000 transcription factories per cell, each containing an average of eight tightly associated RNAP II molecules actively transcribing RNA. If each RNAP II molecule is transcribing a different gene, how might such a transcription factory appear? Provide a simple diagram that shows eight different genes being transcribed in a transcription factory and include the promoters, structural genes, and nascent transcripts in your presentation.

23. A particular type of anemia in humans, called β-thalassemia, results from a severe reduction or absence of a normal β chain of hemoglobin. A variety of studies have explored the use of 5-azacytidine for the treatment of such patients. How might administration of 5-azacytidine be an effective treatment for β-thalassemia? Would you consider adverse side-effects likely? Why?

24. The addition of a "5′-cap" and a "3′ poly-A" tail to many nuclear RNA species occurs prior to export of mature mRNAs to the cytoplasm. Such modifications appear to influence mRNA stability. Many assays for gene regulation involve the use of reporter genes such as luciferase from the North American firefly (*Photinus pyralis*). When the luciferase gene is transcribed and translated, the protein product can be easily assayed in a test tube. In the presence of luciferin, ATP, and oxygen, the luciferase enzyme produces light that can be easily quantified. Assuming that luciferase mRNA can be obtained and differentially modified (5′-capped, poly-A tailed) in a test tube, suggest an assay system that would allow you to determine the influence of 5′-capping and poly-A tail addition on mRNA stability.

25. DNA methylation is commonly associated with a reduction of transcription. The following data come from a study of the impact of the location and extent of DNA methylation on gene activity in human cells. A bacterial gene, luciferase, was cloned next to eukaryotic promoter fragments that were methylated to various degrees, *in vitro*. The chimeric plasmids

were then introduced into tissue culture cells, and the luciferase activity was assayed. These data compare the degree of expression of luciferase with differences in the location of DNA methylation (Irvine et al., 2002. *Mol. and Cell. Biol.* 22: 6689–6696). What general conclusions can be drawn from these data?

DNA Segment	Patch Size of Methylation (kb)	Number of Methylated CpGs	Relative Luciferase Expression
Outside transcription unit (0–7.6 kb away)	0.0	0	490X
	2.0	100	290X
	3.1	102	250X
	12.1	593	2X
Inside transcription unit	0.0	0	490X
	1.9	108	80X
	2.4	134	5X
	12.1	593	2X

26. Incorrectly spliced RNAs often lead to human pathologies. Scientists have examined human cancer cells for splice-specific changes and found that many of the changes disrupt tumor-suppressor gene function (Xu and Lee, 2003. *Nucl. Acids Res.* 31: 5635–5643). In general, what would be the effects of splicing changes on these RNAs and the function of tumor-suppressor gene function? How might loss of splicing specificity be associated with cancer?

27. In a classical genetic analysis, scientists create mutations within or surrounding cloned gene sequences. They then introduce these mutated gene sequences into cell cultures or model organisms and examine the phenotypes. Geneticists are now adding RNA-induced gene silencing to their gene-analysis toolbox. Describe how you would use RNA-induced gene silencing to study the role of the *Drosophila tra* gene in sex determination. Next, describe how you would study *tra* function, using a classical genetic analysis. What are the advantages and limitations of each research approach?

28. Approximately 75 percent of all breast cancers are "ER positive" in that they grow when exposed to estrogen. In addition, over half of these ER-positive cancers are also "PR positive" in that they grow in response to progesterone. Suggest steps by which hormones such as estrogen or progesterone might enhance cell proliferation. Tamoxifen is commonly used to treat ER-positive cancer patients. Speculate on the role of Tamoxifen at the molecular level.

29. During an examination of the genomic sequences surrounding the human β-globin gene, you discover a region of DNA that bears sequence resemblance to the GRE of the human metallothionein IIA (*hMTIIA*) gene. Describe experiments that you would design to test (1) whether this sequence was necessary for accurate β-globin gene expression and (2) whether this sequence acted in the same way as the *hMTIIA* gene's GRE.

30. Transcription factors play key roles in the regulation of gene expression, but to do so, they must act within the nucleus. Like most proteins, however, transcription factors are translated in the cytoplasm. To enter the nucleus, transcription factors contain nuclear location signals, which in some cases can only work when bound to some other molecule such as a steroid hormone. After entering the nucleus, transcription factors must bind to appropriate DNA sites and must interact with other transcription proteins at promoters, enhancers, and silencers. Transcription factors then activate or repress transcription through their activation or repression domains. Many drug therapies target transcription factors. Based on the information provided above, suggest three specific mechanisms through which a successful drug therapy, targeted to a transcription factor, might work.

This unusual four-winged *Drosophila* has developed an extra set of wings as a result of a mutation in a homeotic selector gene.

18

Developmental Genetics

CHAPTER CONCEPTS

- Gene expression during development is based on the differential transcription of selected genes.

- Animals use a small number of shared signaling systems and regulatory networks to construct a wide range of adult body forms from the zygote. These shared properties make it possible to use animal models to study human development.

- Differentiation is controlled by cascades of gene expression that are a consequence of events that specify and determine the developmental fate of cells.

- Plants independently evolved developmental regulatory mechanisms that parallel those of animals.

- In many organisms, binary switch genes program the developmental fate of embryonic cells.

O ver the last two decades, genetic analysis, molecular biology, and genomics have shown that, in spite of wide diversity in the size and shape of adult animals and plants, multicellular organisms share many genes, genetic pathways, and molecular signaling mechanisms that control developmental events leading from the zygote to the adult. At the cellular level, development is marked by three important events: **specification**, when the first cues confer spatially distinct identity, **determination**, the

time when a specific developmental fate for a cell becomes fixed, and **differentiation**, the process by which a cell achieves its final adult form and function. Thanks to newly developed methods of analysis including microarrays, high-throughput sequencing, epigenetics, proteomics, and systems biology, we are beginning to understand how the expression and interaction of genes with environmental factors control developmental processes in eukaryotes.

In this chapter, the primary emphasis will be on how genetic analysis has been used to study development. This field, called developmental genetics, laid the foundation for our understanding of developmental events at the molecular and cellular levels, which contribute to the continually changing phenotype of the newly formed organism.

18.1 Differentiated States Develop from Coordinated Programs of Gene Expression

Animal genomes contain tens of thousands of genes, but only a small subset of these control the events that shape the adult body (**Figure 18–1**).

Developmental geneticists study mutant alleles of these genes to ask important questions about development:

(a)

(b)

FIGURE 18–1 (a) A *Drosophila* embryo and (b) the adult fly that develops from it.

- What genes are expressed?
- When are they expressed?
- In what parts of the developing embryo are they expressed?
- How is the expression of these genes regulated?
- What happens when these genes are defective?

These questions provide a foundation for exploring the molecular basis of developmental processes such as determination, induction, cell–cell communication, and cellular differentiation. Genetic analysis of mutant alleles is used to establish a causal relationship between the presence or absence of inducers, receptors, transcriptional events, cell and tissue interactions, and the observable structural changes that accompany development.

A useful way to define **development** is to say that it is the *attainment of a differentiated state* by all the cells of an organism (except for stem cells). For example, a cell in a blastula-stage embryo (when the embryo is just a ball of uniform-looking cells) is undifferentiated, while a red blood cell synthesizing hemoglobin in the adult body is

differentiated. How do cells get from the undifferentiated to the differentiated state? The process involves progressive activation of different groups of gene sets in different cells of the embryo. From a genetics perspective, one way of defining the different cell types that form during development in multicellular organisms is to identify and catalog the genes that are active in each cell type. In other words, development depends on patterns of differential gene expression.

The idea that differentiation is accomplished by activating and inactivating genes at different times and in different cell types is called the **variable gene activity hypothesis**. Its underlying assumptions are, first, that each cell contains an entire genome and, second, that differential transcription of selected genes controls the development and differentiation of each cell. In multicellular organisms, the genes involved with development have been conserved throughout evolution, along with the patterns of differential transcription, and the ensuing developmental mechanisms. As a result, scientists are able to learn about development in complex multicellular organisms including humans by dissecting these mechanisms in a small number of genetically well-characterized model organisms.

18.2 Evolutionary Conservation of Developmental Mechanisms Can Be Studied Using Model Organisms

Genetic analysis of development across a wide range of organisms has shown that the size and shape of all animal bodies are controlled by a common set of genes and developmental mechanisms. For example, most of the differences in shape between zebras and zebrafish and thousands of other organisms are the result of different patterns of expression in a single gene set, called the homeotic (abbreviated as *Hox*) genes, and not by species-specific genes. Genome-sequencing projects have confirmed that homeotic genes from a wide range of organisms have a common ancestry; this homology means that many aspects of normal human embryonic development and associated genetic disorders can be studied in model organisms such as *Drosophila melanogaster*, where genetic methods including mutagenesis, genetic crosses, and large-scale experiments involving hundreds of offspring can be conducted (see Chapter 1 for a discussion of model organisms in genetics).

Results from a field called evo-devo, which combines evolutionary and developmental biology, have revealed that although many developmental mechanisms are common to all animals, evolution has generated several new and unique ways of transforming a zygote into an adult. These evolutionary changes result from several genetic mechanisms including mutation, gene duplication and evolutionary divergence, the assignment of new functions to old genes, and the recruitment of genes to new developmental pathways. However, the emphasis in this chapter will be on the similarities in genes and developmental mechanisms among species.

Analysis of Developmental Mechanisms

In the space of this chapter, we cannot survey all aspects of development, nor can we explore in detail how developmental mechanisms triggered by the fusion of sperm and egg were identified. Instead, we will focus on a number of general processes in development:

- how the adult body plan of animals is laid down in the embryo
- the program of gene expression that turns undifferentiated cells into differentiated cells
- the role of cell–cell communication in development

We will use three model systems—the fruit fly *Drosophila melanogaster,* the flowering plant *Arabidopsis thaliana,* and the nematode *Caenorhabditis elegans*—to illustrate these developmental processes and related topics. We will examine how patterns of differential gene expression lead to the progressive restriction of developmental options resulting in the formation of the adult body plan in *Drosophila* and *Arabidopsis.* We will then expand the discussion to consider how our knowledge of events in these organisms has contributed to our understanding of developmental defects in humans. Finally, we will consider the role of cell–cell communication in the development of adult structures in *C. elegans.*

18.3 Genetic Analysis of Embryonic Development in *Drosophila* Reveals How the Body Axis of Animals Is Specified

How does a given cell at a precise position in the embryo switch on or switch off specific genes at timed stages of development? This is a central question in developmental biology. To answer this question, we will examine the sequence of gene expression in the embryo of the model organism *Drosophila.* Although development in a fruit fly appears to have little in common with humans, recall that the same genes regulate development in both species.

Overview of *Drosophila* Development

The life cycle of *Drosophila* is about 10 days long with a number of distinct phases: the embryo, three larval stages, the pupal stage, and the adult stage (**Figure 18–2**). Internally, the cytoplasm of the unfertilized egg is organized into

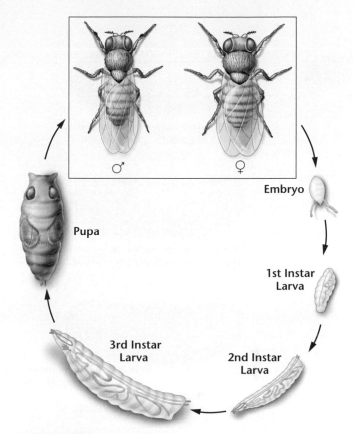

FIGURE 18–2 *Drosophila* life cycle.

a series of maternally constructed molecular gradients that play a key role in determining the developmental fates of nuclei located in specific regions of the embryo.

Immediately after fertilization, the zygote nucleus undergoes a series of nuclear divisions without cytokinesis [**Figure 18–3 (a)** and **(b)**]. The resulting cell, with multiple nuclei, is called a syncytium. At about the tenth division, nuclei move to the periphery of the egg, where the cytoplasm contains localized gradients of maternally derived mRNA transcripts and proteins [**Figure 18–3(c)**]. After several more divisions, the nuclei become enclosed in plasma membranes [**Figure 18–3(d)**], forming a cellular layer around the outside edge of the embryo. Interactions between the nuclei and the cytoplasmic components of these cells initiate and direct the pattern of embryonic gene expression.

Germ cells, which in the adult, are destined to undergo meiosis and produce gametes, form at the posterior pole of the embryo [Figure 18–3(c) and (d)]. Nuclei in other regions of the embryo normally form somatic cells. In experiments where nuclei from these regions are transplanted into the posterior cytoplasm, they will form germ cells and not somatic cells, confirming that the cytoplasm at the posterior pole of the embryo contains maternal components that direct nuclei to form germ cells.

Transcriptional programs activated by cytoplasmic components in somatic (non–germ-cell) nuclei form the

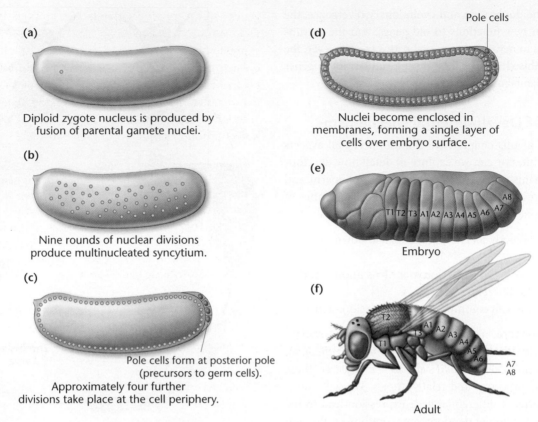

FIGURE 18–3 Early stages of embryonic development in *Drosophila*. (a) Fertilized egg with zygotic nucleus (2*n*), shortly after fertilization. (b) Nuclear divisions occur about every 10 minutes. Nine rounds of division produce a multinucleate cell, the syncytial blastoderm. (c) At the tenth division, the nuclei migrate to the periphery or cortex of the egg, and four additional rounds of nuclear division occur. A small cluster of cells, the pole cells, form at the posterior pole about 2.5 hours after fertilization. These cells will form the germ cells of the adult. (d) About 3 hours after fertilization, the nuclei become enclosed in membranes, forming a single layer of cells over the embryo surface, creating the cellular blastoderm. (e) The embryo at about 10 hours after fertilization. At this stage, the segmentation pattern of the body is clearly established. Behind the segments that will form the head, T1–T3 are thoracic segments, and A1–A8 are abdominal segments. (f) The adult fly showing the structures formed from each segment of the embryo.

embryo's anterior–posterior (front to back) and dorsal–ventral (upper to lower) axes of symmetry, leading to the formation of a segmented embryo [**Figure 18–3(e)**]. Under control of the *Hox* genes (discussed in a later section), these segments will give rise to the differentiated structures of the adult fly [**Figure 18–3(f)**].

Genetic Analysis of Embryogenesis

Two different gene sets control embryonic development in *Drosophila*: maternal-effect genes and zygotic genes (**Figure 18–4**). Products of maternal-effect genes (mRNA and/or proteins) are placed in the developing egg by the "mother" fly. Many of these products are distributed in a gradient or concentrated in specific regions of the egg cytoplasm. Female flies homozygous for deleterious recessive mutations of maternal-effect genes are sterile. None of their embryos receive wild-type maternal gene products, so all of the embryos develop abnormally and die. Maternal-effect genes encode transcription factors, receptors, and proteins that regulate gene expression. During development,

these gene products activate or repress time- and location-specific programs of gene expression in the embryo.

Zygotic genes are those transcribed in the embryonic nuclei formed after fertilization. These products of the embryonic genome are differentially transcribed in specific regions of the embryo in response to the distribution of maternal-effect proteins. Deleterious recessive mutations in these genes can lead to embryonic lethality in homozygotes.

Much of our knowledge about the genes that regulate *Drosophila* development is based on the work of Ed Lewis, Christiane Nüsslein-Volhard, and Eric Wieschaus, who were awarded the 1995 Nobel Prize for Physiology or Medicine. Ed Lewis initially identified and studied one of these regulatory genes in the 1970s. In the late 1970s, Nüsslein-Volhard and Wieschaus devised a strategy to identify all the genes that control development in *Drosophila*. Their scheme required examining thousands of offspring of mutagenized flies, looking for recessive embryonic lethal mutations with defects in external structures. The parents were

FIGURE 18–4 The hierarchy of genes involved in establishing the segmented body plan in *Drosophila*. Gene products from the maternal genes regulate the expression of the first three groups of zygotic genes (gap, pair-rule, and segment polarity, collectively called the segmentation genes), which in turn control expression of the homeotic genes.

thus identified as heterozygous carriers of these mutations, which the researchers grouped into three classes based on their phenotypes: **gap, pair-rule,** and **segment polarity** genes. In 1980, on the basis of their observations, Nüsslein-Volhard and Wieschaus proposed a model in which embryonic development is initiated by gradients of maternal-effect gene products. The positional information laid down by these molecular gradients is interpreted by two sets of zygotic (embryonic) genes: (1) **segmentation genes** (gap, pair-rule, and segment polarity genes) and (2) **homeotic selector** (*Hox*) **genes.** Segmentation genes divide the embryo into a series of stripes or segments and define the number, size, and polarity of each segment. The homeotic genes specify the developmental fate of cells within each segment as well as the adult structures that will be formed from each segment (Figure 18–4).

Their model is shown in **Figure 18–5.** Most maternal-effect gene products placed in the egg during oogenesis are activated immediately after fertilization and help establish the anterior–posterior axis of the embryo by activating position-specific patterns of gene expression in the embryo's nuclei [**Figure 18–5(a)**]. Many maternal gene products are involved in specification and determination. These maternal genes encode transcription factors that activate gap genes, whose expression divides the embryo into a series of regions corresponding to the head, thorax, and abdomen of the adult [**Figure 18–5(b)**]. Gap genes encode other transcription factors that activate pair-rule

genes, whose products divide the embryo into smaller regions about two segments wide [**Figure 18–5(c)**]. In turn, expression of the pair-rule genes activates the segment polarity genes, which divide each segment into anterior and posterior regions [**Figure 18–5(d)**]. The collective action of the maternal genes and the segmentation genes define the anterior–posterior axis, which is the field of action for the homeotic (*Hox*) genes [**Figure 18–5(e)**].

NOW SOLVE THIS

18–1 Suppose you initiate a screen for maternal-effect mutations in *Drosophila* affecting external structures of the embryo and you identify more than 100 mutations that affect these structures. From their screenings, other researchers concluded that there are only about 40 maternal-effect genes. How do you reconcile these different results?

■ **HINT:** *This problem involves an understanding of how mutants are identified when adult* Drosophila *have been exposed to mutagens. The key to its solution is an understanding of the differences between genes and alleles.*

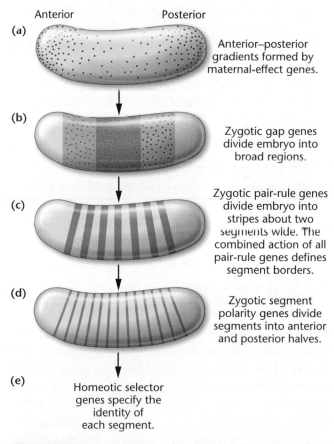

FIGURE 18–5 (a) Progressive restriction of cell fate during development in *Drosophila*. Gradients of maternal proteins are established along the anterior–posterior axis of the embryo. (b–d) Three groups of segmentation genes progressively define the body segments. (e) Individual segments are given identity by the homeotic genes.

18.4 Zygotic Genes Program Segment Formation in *Drosophila*

Over 20 segmentation genes (Table 18.1), have been identified, and they are classified on the basis of their mutant phenotypes: (1) mutations in gap genes delete a group of adjacent segments, causing gaps in the normal body plan of the embryo, (2) mutations in pair-rule genes affect every other segment and eliminate a specific part of each affected segment, and (3) mutations in segment polarity genes cause defects in portions of each segment.

In addition to these three sets of genes that determine the anterior–posterior axis of the developing embryo, another set of genes determines the dorsal–ventral axis of the embryo. Our discussion will be limited to the gene sets involved in the anterior–posterior axis. Let us now examine members of each group in greater detail.

Gap Genes

Transcription of **gap genes** in the embryo is controlled by maternal gene products laid down in gradients in the egg. Gap genes also cross-regulate each other to define the early stage of the body plan. Transcription of wild-type gap genes (which encode transcription factors) divides the embryo into a series of broad regions that become the head, thorax, and abdomen. Within these regions, different combinations of gene activity eventually specify both the type of segment that forms and the proper order of segments in the body of the larva, pupa, and adult. Mutant alleles of these genes produce large gaps in the embryo's segmentation pattern. *Hunchback* mutants lose head and thorax structures, *Krüppel* mutants lose thoracic and abdominal structures, and *knirps* mutants lose most abdominal structures. Expression domains of the gap genes in different parts of the embryo correlate roughly

Yellow stripe contains both hunchback and Krüppel proteins

Hunchback protein

Krüppel protein

Anterior

Posterior

FIGURE 18–6 Visualization of gap gene expression in a *Drosophila* embryo. The hunchback protein is shown in orange, and Krüppel is indicated in green. The yellow stripe is created when cells contain both hunchback and Krüppel proteins. Each dot in the embryo is a nucleus.

with the location of their mutant phenotypes: *hunchback* at the anterior, *Krüppel* in the middle (**Figure 18–6**), and *knirps* at the posterior. As mentioned earlier, gap genes encode transcription factors that control the expression of pair-rule genes.

Pair-Rule Genes

Pair-rule genes are expressed in a series of seven narrow bands or stripes of nuclei extending around the circumference of the embryo. The expression of this gene set does two things: first it establishes the boundaries of segments, and then it programs the developmental fate of the cells within each segment by controlling expression of the segment polarity genes. Mutations in pair-rule genes eliminate segment-size sections of the embryo at every other segment. At least eight pair-rule genes act to divide the embryo into a series of stripes. The transcription of the pair-rule genes is mediated by the action of maternal gene products and gap gene products. Initially, the boundaries of these stripes overlap, so that in each area of overlap, cells express a different combination of pair-rule genes (**Figure 18–7**). The resolution of boundaries in this segmentation pattern results from the combined activity of different transcription factors in adjacent segments (**Figure 18–8**).

Segment Polarity Genes

Expression of **segment polarity genes** is controlled by transcription factors encoded by pair-rule genes. Within each of the segments created by pair-rule genes, segment polarity genes become active in a single band of cells that extends around the embryo's circumference (**Figure 18–9**).

TABLE 18.1 Segmentation Genes in *Drosophila*

Gap Genes	Pair-Rule Genes	Segment Polarity Genes
Krüppel	*hairy*	*engrailed*
knirps	*even-skipped*	*wingless*
hunchback	*runt*	*cubitis*
giant	*fushi-tarazu*	*hedgehog*
tailless	*paired*	*fused*
buckebein	*odd-paired*	*armadillo*
caudal	*odd-skipped*	*patched*
	sloppy-paired	*gooseberry*
		paired
		naked
		disheveled

(a)

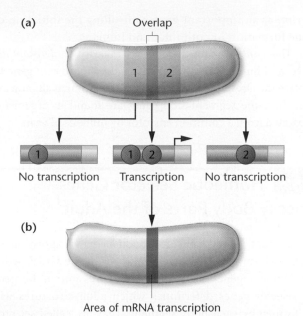

(b)

Area of mRNA transcription

FIGURE 18–7 New patterns of gene expression can be generated by overlapping regions containing two different gene products. (a) Transcription factors 1 and 2 are present in an overlapping region of expression. If both transcription factors must bind to the promoter of a target gene to trigger expression, the gene will be active only in cells containing both factors (most likely in the zone of overlap). (b) The expression of the target gene in the restricted region of the embryo.

This divides the embryo into 14 segments. The products of the segment polarity genes control the cellular identity within each of them and establish the anterior–posterior pattern (the polarity) within each segment.

Segmentation Genes in Mice and Humans

We have seen that segment formation in *Drosophila* depends on the action of three sets of segmentation genes. Are these genes found in humans and other mammals, and do they control aspects of embryonic development in these organisms? To answer this question, let's examine *runt*, one of the pair-rule genes in *Drosophila*. Later in development, it controls aspects of sex determination and formation of the nervous system. The gene encodes a protein that regulates transcription of its target genes. Runt contains a 128-amino-acid DNA-binding region (called the runt domain) that is highly conserved in *Drosophila*, mouse, and human proteins. In fact, *in vitro* experiments show that the *Drosophila* and mouse runt proteins are functionally interchangeable. In mice, *runt* is expressed early in development and controls formation of blood cells, bone, and the genital system. Although the target gene sets controlled by *runt* are different in *Drosophila* and the mouse, in both organisms, expression of *runt* specifies the fate of uncommitted cells in the embryo by regulating transcription of target genes.

(a)

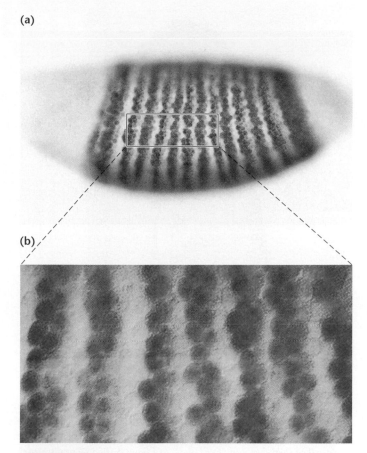

(b)

FIGURE 18–8 Stripe pattern of pair-rule gene expression in a *Drosophila* embryo. This embryo is stained to show patterns of expression of the genes *even skipped* and *fushi-tarazu*; (a) low-power view and (b) inset: high-power view of the same embryo.

In humans, mutations in *RUNX2*, a human homolog of *runt*, causes cleidocranial dysplasia (CCD), an autosomal dominantly inherited trait. Those affected with CCD have a hole in the top of their skull because bone does not form in the membranous gap known as the fontanel. Their collar bones (clavicles) do not develop, enabling affected individuals to fold their shoulders across their chest (**Figure 18–10**). Mice with one mutant copy of the *runt* homolog have a phenotype similar to that seen in

FIGURE 18–9 The 14 stripes of expression of the segment polarity gene *engrailed* in a *Drosophila* embryo.

FIGURE 18-10 A boy affected with cleidocranial dysplasia (CCD). This disorder, inherited as an autosomal dominant trait, is caused by mutation in a human *runt* gene, *RUNX2*. Affected heterozygotes have a number of skeletal defects, including a hole in the top of the skull where the infant fontanel fails to close, and collar bones that do not develop or form only small stumps. Because the collar bones do not form, CCD individuals can fold their shoulders across their chests. *Reprinted by permission from Macmillan Publishers Ltd.: Fig 1 on p. 244 from: British Dental Journal 195: 243–248 2003. Greenwood, M. and Meechan, J. G. "General medicine and surgery for dental practitioners." Copyright © Macmillan Magazines Limited.*

humans; mice with two mutant copies of the gene have no bones at all. Their skeletons contain only cartilage (**Figure 18–11**), much like sharks, emphasizing the role

FIGURE 18-11 Bone formation in normal mice and mutants for the *runt* gene *Cbfa1*. (a) Normal mouse embryos at day 17.5 show cartilage (blue) and bone (brown). (b) The skeleton of a 17.5-day homozygous mutant embryo. Only cartilage has formed in the skeleton. There is complete absence of bone formation in the mutant mouse. Expression of a normal copy of the *Cbfa1* gene is essential for specifying the developmental fate of bone-forming osteoblasts.

of *runt* as an important gene controlling the initiation of bone formation in both mice and humans.

The *runt* domain sequence similarity in *Drosophila*, mice, and humans and the ability of the mouse *runt* gene to replace the *Drosophila* version in fly development all indicate that the same segmentation genes are found in organisms separated from a common ancestor by millions of years.

18.5 Homeotic Selector Genes Specify Body Parts of the Adult

As segment boundaries are established by expression of segmentation genes, the homeotic (from the Greek word for "same") genes are activated. Expression of homeotic selector genes determines which adult structures will be formed by each body segment. They are called selector genes because action of these genes selects one developmental pathway appropriate for a given segment from several alternatives. In *Drosophila*, these pathways lead to the formation of the antennae, mouth parts, legs, wings, thorax, and abdomen. Mutants of these genes are called **homeotic mutants** because one segment is transformed so that it forms the same structure as another segment. For example, the wild-type allele of *Antennapedia (Antp)* specifies the developmental pathway leading to formation of a leg on the second segment of the thorax. Dominant gain-of-function *Antp* mutations cause this gene to be expressed in the head *and* the thorax. The result is that mutant flies have a leg on their head instead of an antenna (**Figure 18–12**).

Hox Genes in Drosophila

The *Drosophila* genome contains two clusters of homeotic selector genes (called *Hox* genes) on chromosome 3 that encode transcription factors (**Table 18.2**). The *Antennapedia (ANT-C)* cluster contains five genes that specify structures in the head and first two segments of the thorax [**Figure 18–13(a)**]. The second cluster, the *bithorax (BX-C)* complex, contains three genes that specify structures in the posterior portion of the second thoracic segment, the entire third thoracic segment, and the abdominal segments [**Figure 18–13(b)**].

TABLE 18.2 *Hox* Genes of *Drosophila*

Antennapedia **Complex**	*Bithorax* **Complex**
labial	*Ultrabithorax*
Antennapedia	*abdominal A*
Sex combs reduced	*Abdominal B*
Deformed	
proboscipedia	

(a)

(b)

FIGURE 18–12 *Antennapedia (Antp)* mutation in *Drosophila*. (a) Head from wild-type *Drosophila*, showing the antenna and other head parts. (b) Head from an *Antp* mutant, showing the replacement of normal antenna structures with legs. This is caused by activation of the *Antp* gene in the head region.

Hox genes (listed in Table 18.2) from a wide range of species have two properties in common. First, each contains a highly conserved 180-bp nucleotide sequence known as a **homeobox.** (*Hox* is a contraction of homeobox.) The homeobox encodes a DNA-binding region of 60 amino acids known as a **homeodomain.** Second, in most species, expression of *Hox* genes is colinear with the anterior to posterior organization of the body. In other words, genes at one end of the cluster (the 3′ end) are expressed at the anterior end of the embryo, those in the middle are expressed in the middle of the embryo, and genes at the other end of a cluster (the 5′ end) are expressed at the embryo's posterior region (**Figure 18–14**). Although first identified in *Drosophila*, *Hox* genes are found in the genomes of most eukaryotes with segmented body plans, including nematodes, sea urchins, zebrafish, frogs, mice, and humans (**Figure 18–15**).

To summarize, genes that control development in *Drosophila* act in a temporally and spatially ordered cascade, beginning with the genes that establish the anterior–posterior (and dorsal–ventral) axis of the early embryo. Gradients of maternal mRNAs and proteins along the anterior–posterior axis activate gap genes, which subdivide the embryo into broad bands. Gap genes in turn activate pair-rule genes, which divide the embryo into segments. The final group of segmentation genes, the segment polarity genes, divides each segment into anterior and posterior regions arranged linearly along the anterior–posterior axis. The segments are then given identity by action of the *Hox* genes. Therefore, this progressive

(a)

(b)

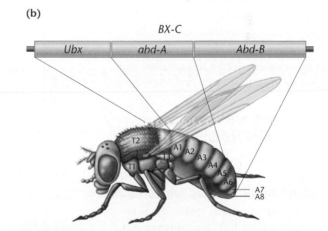

FIGURE 18–13 Genes of the *Antennapedia* complex and the adult structures they specify. (a) In the *ANT-C* complex, the *labial* (*lab*) and *Deformed* (*Dfd*) genes control the formation of head segments. The *Sex comb reduced* (*Scr*) and *Antennapedia* (*Antp*) genes specify the identity of the first two thoracic segments, T1 and T2. The remaining gene in the complex, *proboscipedia* (*pb*), may not act during embryogenesis but may be required to maintain the differentiated state in adults. In mutants, the labial palps are transformed into legs. (b) In the *BX-C* complex, *Ultrabithorax* (*Ubx*) controls formation of structures in the posterior compartment of T2 and structures in T3. The two other genes, *abdominal A* (*abdA*) and *Abdominal B* (*AbdB*), specify the segmental identities of the eight abdominal segments (A1–A8).

(a) Expression domains of homeotic genes

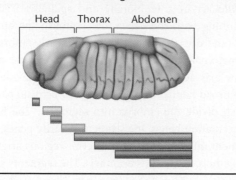

Head | Thorax | Abdomen

(b) Chromosomal locations of homeotic genes

3′ lab pb Dfd Scr Antp Ubx abd-A Abd-B 5′

FIGURE 18–14 The colinear relationship between the spatial pattern of expression and chromosomal locations of homeotic genes in *Drosophila*. (a) *Drosophila* embryo and the domains of homeotic gene expression in the embryonic epidermis and central nervous system. (b) Chromosomal location of homeotic selector genes. Note that the order of genes on the chromosome correlates with the sequential anterior borders of their expression domains.

restriction of developmental potential of the *Drosophila* embryo's cells (all of which occurs during the first third of embryogenesis) involves a cascade of gene action, with regulatory proteins acting on transcription, translation, and signal transduction.

Hox Genes and Human Genetic Disorders

Although first described in *Drosophila*, *Hox* genes are found in the genomes of all animals, where they play a fundamental role in shaping the body and its appendages. In vertebrates, the conservation of sequence, the order of genes in the *Hox* clusters, and their pattern of expression in vertebrates suggest that, as in *Drosophila*, these genes control development along the anterior–posterior and the formation of appendages. However, in vertebrates, there are four clusters of *Hox* genes—*HOXA, HOXB, HOXC,* and *HOXD* due to cluster duplication during vertebrate evolution—instead of a single cluster as in *Drosophila*. This means that in vertebrates, not just one, but a combination of two to four

Hox genes is involved in forming specific structures. As a result, in vertebrates, mutations in individual *Hox* genes do not produce complete transformation as in *Drosophila*, where mutation of a single *Hox* gene can transform a haltere into a wing (see the photo at the beginning of this chapter). The role of *HOXD* genes in human development was confirmed by the discovery that several inherited limb malformations are caused by mutations in *HOXD* genes. For example, mutations in *HOXD13* cause synpolydactyly (SPD), a malformation characterized by extra fingers and toes, and abnormalities in bones of the hands and feet (**Figure 18–16**).

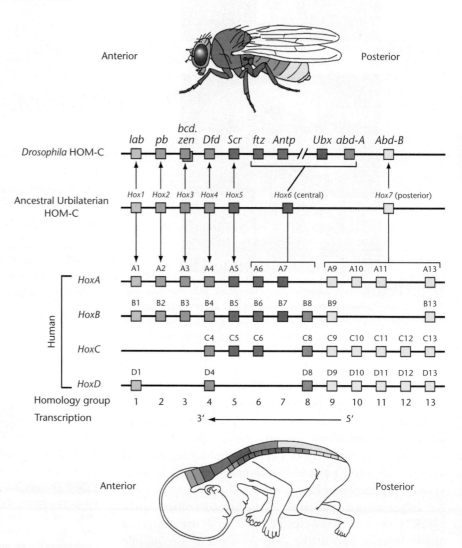

FIGURE 18–15 Conservation of organization and patterns of expression in *Hox* genes. (Top) The structures formed in adult *Drosophila* are shown, with the colors corresponding to members of the *Hox* cluster that control their formation. (Bottom) The arrangement of the *Hox* genes in an early human embryo. As in *Drosophila*, genes at the (3′ end) of the cluster form anterior structures, and genes at the (5′ end) of the cluster form posterior structures.

FIGURE 18-16 Mutations in posterior *Hox* genes (*HOXD13* in this case) in humans result in malformations of the limbs, shown here as extra toes. This condition is known as synpolydactyly. Mutations in *HOXD13* are also associated with abnormalities of the bones in the hands and feet.

NOW SOLVE THIS

18-2 In *Drosophila*, both *fushi tarazu* (*ftz*) and *engrailed* (*eng*) genes encode homeobox transcription factors and are capable of eliciting the expression of other genes. Both genes work at about the same time during development and in the same region to specify cell fate in body segments. To discover if *ftz* regulates the expression of *engrailed*; if *engrailed* regulates *ftz*; or if both are regulated by another gene, you perform a mutant analysis. In *ftz* embryos (*ftz/ftz*) engrailed protein is absent; in *engrailed* embryos (*eng/eng*) *ftz* expression is normal. What does this tell you about the regulation of these two genes—does the *engrailed* gene regulate *ftz*, or does the *ftz* gene regulate *engrailed*?

■ **HINT:** *This problem involves an understanding of how genes are regulated at different stages of preadult development in* Drosophila. *The key to its solution lies in using the results of the mutant analysis to determine the timing of expression of the two genes being examined.*

For more practice, see Problems 15, 16, and 18.

18.6 Plants Have Evolved Developmental Regulatory Systems That Parallel Those of Animals

Plants and animals diverged from a common ancestor about 1.6 billion years ago, after the origin of eukaryotes and probably before the rise of multicellular organisms. Genetic analysis of mutants and genome sequencing in plants and animals indicate that basic mechanisms of

FIGURE 18-17 The flowering plant *Arabidopsis thaliana,* used as a model organism in plant genetics.

developmental pattern formation evolved independently in animals and plants. We have already examined the genetic systems that control development and pattern formation in animals, using *Drosophila* as a model organism, and will now briefly examine these systems in plants.

In plants, pattern formation has been extensively studied using flower development in *Arabidopsis thaliana* (**Figure 18-17**), a small plant in the mustard family, as a model organism. A cluster of undifferentiated cells, called the *floral meristem*, gives rise to flowers (**Figure 18-18**). Each flower consists of four organs—sepals, petals, stamens, and carpels—that develop from concentric rings of cells within the meristem [**Figure 18-19(a)**]. Each organ develops from a different concentric ring, or whorl of cells.

Homeotic Genes in *Arabidopsis*

Three classes of floral homeotic genes control the development of these organs (Table 18.3). Acting alone, class A genes specify sepals; class A and class B genes expressed together specify petals. Acting together, class B and class C genes control stamen formation. Class C genes acting

TABLE 18.3 Homeotic Selector Genes in *Arabidopsis**

Class A	APETALA1 (AP1)
	APETALA2 (AP2)
Class B	APETALA3 (AP3)
	PISTILLATA (P1)
Class C	AGAMOUS (AG)

*By convention, wild-type genes in *Arabidopsis* use capital letters.

FIGURE 18–18 (a) Parts of the *Arabidopsis* flower. The floral organs are arranged concentrically. The sepals form the outermost ring, followed by petals and stamens, with carpels on the inside. (b) View of the flower from above.

alone specify carpels. During flower development [**Figure 18–19(b)**], class A genes are active in whorls 1 and 2 (sepals and petals), class B genes are expressed in whorls 2 and 3 (petals and stamens), and class C genes are expressed in whorls 3 and 4 (stamens and carpels). The organ formed depends on the expression pattern of the three gene classes. In whorl 1, expression of class A genes alone causes sepals to form. Expression of class A *and* class B genes in whorl 2 leads to petal formation. Expression of class B and class C genes in whorl 3 leads to stamen formation. In whorl 4, expression of class C genes alone causes carpel formation.

As in *Drosophila*, mutations in homeotic genes cause organs to form in abnormal locations. For example, in *APETALA2* mutants (*AP2*), the order of organs is carpel, stamen, stamen, and carpel instead of the normal order, sepal, petal, stamen, and carpel [**Figure 18–20(a) and (b)**]. In class B loss-of-function mutants (*AP3*, *P1*), petals become sepals, and stamens are transformed into carpels [**Figure 18–20(c)**], and the order of organs becomes sepal, sepal, carpel, carpel. Plants carrying a mutation for the class C gene *AGAMOUS* will have petals in whorl 3 (instead of stamens) and sepals in whorl 4 (instead of carpels), and the order of organs will be sepal, petal, petal, and sepal [**Figure 18–20(d)**].

Evolutionary Divergence in Homeotic Genes

Drosophila and *Arabidopsis* use different sets of nonhomologous master regulatory genes to establish the body axis and specify the identity of structures along the axis. In *Drosophila*, this task is accomplished in part by the *Hox* genes, which encode a set of transcription factors sharing a homeobox domain. In *Arabidopsis*, the floral homeotic genes belong to a different family of transcription factors, called the **MADS-box proteins**, characterized by a common sequence of 58 amino acids with no similarity in amino acid sequence or protein structure with the *Hox* genes. Both gene sets encode transcription factors, both sets are master regulators of development expressed in a pattern of overlapping domains, and both specify identity of structures.

Reflecting their evolutionary origin from a common ancestor, the genomes of both *Drosophila* and *Arabidopsis* contain members of the homeobox and MADS-box genes, but these genes have been adapted for different uses in the plant and animal kingdoms. This indicates that developmental mechanisms evolved independently in each group.

In both plants and animals, the action of transcription factors depends on changes in chromatin structure that make genes available for expression. Mechanisms of transcription initiation are conserved in plants and animals, as is reflected in the homology of genes in *Drosophila* and *Arabidopsis* that maintain patterns of expression initiated by

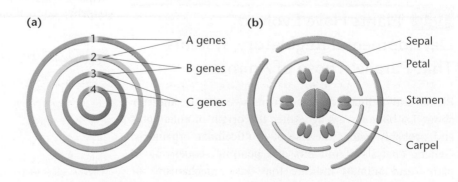

FIGURE 18–19 Cell arrangement in the floral meristem. (a) The four concentric rings, or whorls, labeled 1–4, give rise to (b) arrangement of the sepals, petals, stamens, and carpels, respectively, in the mature flower.

FIGURE 18–20   (a) Wild-type flowers of *Arabidopsis* have (from outside to inside) sepals, petals, stamens, and carpels. (b) A homeotic *APETALA2* mutant flower has carpels, stamens, stamens, and carpels. (c) *PISTILLATA* mutants have sepals, sepals, carpels, and carpels. (d) *AGAMOUS* mutants have petals and sepals at places where stamens and carpels should form.

regulatory gene sets. Action of the floral homeotic genes is controlled by a gene called *CURLY LEAF*. This gene shares significant homology with members of a *Drosophila* gene family called *Polycomb*. This family of regulatory genes controls expression of homeobox genes during development. Both *CURLY LEAF* and *Polycomb* encode proteins that alter chromatin conformation and shut off gene expression. Thus, although different genes are used to control development, both plants and animals use an evolutionarily conserved mechanism to regulate expression of these gene sets.

and incorporates multi-branched pathways involved in basic basic aspects of animal development. Many parts of this system are being explored by researchers in the hope that understanding how Wnt/β-catenin signaling controls development will result in treatments for disorders associated with pathway malfunctions.

Here, we will focus on an introduction to the components and interactions of another signaling system the **Notch signaling pathway**—and examine its role in the development of the vulva in the nematode *Caenorhabditis elegans*.

18.7   *C. elegans* Serves as a Model for Cell–Cell Interactions in Development

During development in multicellular organisms, cell–cell interactions influence the transcriptional programs and developmental fate of the interacting cells and surrounding cells. Cell–cell interaction is an important process in the embryonic development of most eukaryotic organisms, including *Drosophila*, mice, and humans.

Signaling Pathways in Development

In early development, animals use a number of signaling pathways to regulate development; after organ formation begins, additional pathways are added to those already in use. These newly activated pathways act both independently and in coordinated networks to generate specific transcriptional patterns. Signal networks establish anterior–posterior polarity and body axes, coordinate pattern formation, and direct the differentiation of tissues and organs. The signaling pathways used in early development and some of the developmental processes they control are listed in Table 18.4. The Wnt/β-catenin signaling system arose early in animal evolution. It is complex, highly conserved,

TABLE 18.4   Signaling Pathways Used in Early Embryonic Development

Wnt Pathway
Dorsalization of body
Female reproductive development
Dorsal–ventral differences
TGF-β Pathway
Mesoderm induction
Left–right asymmetry
Bone development
Hedgehog Pathway
Notochord induction
Somitogenesis
Gut/visceral mesoderm
Receptor Tyrosine Kinase Pathway
Mesoderm maintenance
Notch Signaling Pathway
Blood cell development
Neurogenesis
Retina development

Source: *Taken from* Gerhart, J. 1999. 1998 Warkany lecture: Signaling pathways in development. *Teratology* 60: 226–239. © 1998 John Wiley & Sons, Inc.

MODERN APPROACHES TO UNDERSTANDING GENE FUNCTION

Single-Gene Signaling Mechanism Reveals Secrets to Head Regeneration in Planaria

The regenerative properties of some organisms are truly remarkable. Animals such as hydra, planaria, and salamanders can regenerate organs and entire body parts after they have been damaged or even fully amputated. Developmental biologists and other scientists have been very interested in understanding why these organisms possess regenerative properties. What are the evolutionary mechanisms that have ultimately determined why some organisms can regenerate and others cannot? This information is also relevant when applied to humans for the benefits of tissue and organ repair and replacement.

In 2013, *Nature* published papers from three teams identifying a molecular signaling pathway that is responsible for head regeneration from stem cells called neoblasts. In many species of *Planaria*, animals can regenerate a head from a tail piece. However, this work focused on planarian species that are regeneration-deficient and unable to regenerate a head from a tail fragment. The logic for using these species is that if scientists can determine why such planarians cannot regenerate heads, it will likely provide important clues about the genetic pathways necessary for regeneration in flatworms and other animals.

In this chapter you were introduced to the Wnt/β-catenin pathway and its roles in early embryonic development in multicellular organisms, including humans. Wnt protein causes an accumulation of β-catenin, which regulates expression of genes important for development and tissue repair and maintenance. Mutations of the Wnt/β-catenin pathway are associated with developmental defects and other phenotypes such as tumor formation. Previous studies on

(a) A timed photo series showing the effect of control (top) or β-catenin1 RNAi treated tail pieces (bottom). Control pieces fail to regenerate heads. 16 of 24 tail pieces treated with RNAi formed heads. (b) β-catenin1 RNAi treated tail pieces (yellow) but not control pieces (gray) developed heads that could ingest phenol-red labeled food particles, demonstrating functionality of the regenerated heads.

regeneration-capable planarians have shown that enhanced activation of the Wnt/β-catenin pathway results in tail growth from anterior wounds, producing animals with two tails. Conversely, in posterior wounds reduced activity of the pathway results in head growth, instead of a tail, creating animals with two heads.

One hypothesis to explain the inability of planaria to regenerate a head from tail fragments is that specific levels of Wnt/β-catenin pathway activation are required for head regeneration. To test this hypothesis we highlight a particular experiment that applied **RNA interference (RNAi)**. Recall from earlier in the text (see Chapter 17), that RNAi is a sequence-specific method for silencing RNA molecules. Using the regeneration-deficient planaria species *Dugesia lacteum* (*D. lacteum*), researchers tried a head "rescue" experiment (see figure panel a). They removed tail pieces of *D. lacteum* and injected these segments with double-stranded RNA (dsRNA) designed to silence *β-catenin1* mRNA by RNAi.

Results:

β-catenin1 RNAi treatment rescued head regeneration in 16 out of 24 tail pieces (figure panel a). Researchers analyzed marker genes associated with head and central nervous system structures to assess

head structure. They tested functionality of rescued heads by demonstrating that *β-catenin1* RNAi regenerated planaria could ingest dye-labeled food particles.

In separate experiments, the authors noted that a failure to upregulate expression of a Wnt inhibitor gene called *notum* in *D. lacteum* tail pieces may possibly explain failed head regeneration.

Conclusions:

Researchers concluded that in regeneration-deficient species such as *D. lacteum* there is insufficient downregulation (inhibition) of the Wnt/β-catenin to allow heads to regenerate. Thus downregulating this pathway by RNAi leads to head regeneration. These results suggest that regeneration-capable species can downregulate the Wnt/β-catenin when necessary. Most impressive is the finding that a single signaling pathway is sufficient to induce regeneration of functioning heads. Understanding which genes regulate the Wnt/β-catenin pathway in both regeneration-capable and regeneration-deficient species is an important next step in this research. There is every reason to expect that learning about molecular mechanisms involved in regeneration in planaria will help scientists improve regenerative capabilities in humans.

References:

Umesono, Y., et al. (2013). The molecular logic for planarian regeneration along the anterior posterior axis. *Nature* 500: 73–76.

Sikes, J.M. and Newmark P.A. (2013). Restoration of anterior regeneration in a planarian with limited regenerative ability. *Nature* 500: 77–80.

Liu, S-Y., et al. (2013). Reactivating head regrowth in a regeneration-deficient planarian species. *Nature* 500: 81–84.

Questions to Consider:

1. It is thought that high levels of the protein ERK are required for head formation in *D. lacteum* and that the Wnt/ß-catenin pathway may suppress ERK. Propose an experiment to test this hypothesis. Based on the experimental approach shown above, what experiments could you do to determine if ERK is involved in head regeneration?

2. One reason why scientists are excited about this result is that it suggests that regenerating complex body parts may not always require a detailed understanding of many different individual signaling pathways. Defend or refute this statement keeping in mind potential species-specific applications (not just human tissue repair) of repairing regeneration defects.

The Notch Signaling Pathway

The genes in the Notch pathway are named after the *Drosophila* mutants that were used to identify components of this signal transduction system (*Notch* mutants have an indentation or notch in their wings). The Notch signal system works through direct cell–cell contact to control the developmental fate of interacting cells. The *Notch* gene (and the equivalent gene in other organisms) encodes a signal receptor protein embedded in the plasma membrane (**Figure 18–21**). The signal is another membrane protein encoded by the *Delta* gene (and its equivalents). Because both the signal and receptor are membrane proteins, the Notch signal system works only between adjacent cells. When the Delta protein from one cell binds to the Notch receptor protein on a neighboring cell, the cytoplasmic tail of the Notch protein is cleaved off and binds to a cytoplasmic protein encoded by the *Su(H)* (suppressor of *Hairless*) gene. This protein complex moves into the nucleus and binds to transcriptional cofactors, activating transcription of a gene set that controls a specific developmental pathway (Figure 18–21).

One of the main roles of the Notch signal system is to specify different developmental fates for equivalent cells in a population. In its simplest form, this interaction involves two neighboring cells that are developmentally equivalent. We will explore the role of the Notch signaling system in development of the vulva in *C. elegans,* after a brief introduction to nematode embryogenesis.

Overview of *C. elegans* Development

The nematode *C. elegans* is widely used to study the genetic control of development. There are several advantages in using this organism: (1) its genetics are well known, (2) its genome has been sequenced, and (3) adults contain a small number of cells that follow a highly deterministic developmental program. Adult nematodes are about 1 mm long and develop from a fertilized egg in about two days

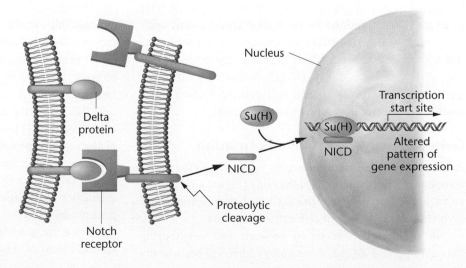

FIGURE 18–21 Components of the Notch signaling pathway in *Drosophila*. The cell carrying the Delta transmembrane protein is the sending cell; the cell carrying the transmembrane Notch protein receives the signal. Binding of Delta to Notch triggers a proteolytic-mediated activation of transcription. The fragment cleaved from the cytoplasmic side of the Notch protein, called the Notch intracellular domain (NICD), combines with the Su(H) protein and moves to the nucleus where it activates a program of gene transcription.

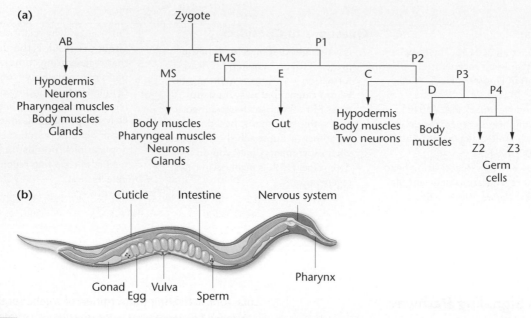

FIGURE 18–22 (a) A truncated cell lineage chart for *C. elegans,* showing early divisions and the tissues and organs formed from these lineages. Each vertical line represents a cell division, and horizontal lines connect the two cells produced. For example, the first division of the zygote creates two new cells, AB and P1. During embryogenesis, cell divisions will produce the 959 somatic cells of the adult hermaphrodite worm. (b) An adult *C. elegans* hermaphrodite. This nematode, about 1 mm in length, consists of 959 cells and is widely used as a model organism to study the genetic control of development.

(Figure 18–22). The life cycle includes an embryonic stage (about 16 hours), four larval stages (L1 through L4), and the adult stage. Adults are of two sexes: XX self-fertilizing hermaphrodites that can make both eggs and sperm, and XO males. Self-fertilization of mutagen-treated hermaphrodites is used to develop homozygous stocks of mutant strains, and hundreds of such mutants have been generated, cataloged, and mapped.

Adult hermaphrodites have 959 somatic cells (and about 2000 germ cells). The lineage of each cell, from fertilized egg to adult, has been mapped (Figure 18–22) and is invariant from individual to individual. Knowing the lineage of each cell, we can easily follow altered cell fates generated by mutations or by killing specific cells with laser microbeams or ultraviolet irradiation. In hermaphrodites, the developmental fate of cells in the reproductive system is determined by cell–cell interaction, illustrating how gene expression and cell–cell interaction work together to specify developmental outcomes.

Genetic Analysis of Vulva Formation

Adult *C. elegans* hermaphrodites lay eggs through the vulva, an opening near the middle of the body (Figure 18–22). The vulva is formed in stages during larval development and involves several rounds of cell–cell interactions.

In *C. elegans,* interaction between two neighboring cells, Z1.ppp and Z4.aaa, determines which will become the

gonadal anchor cell (from which the vulva forms) and which will become a precursor to the uterus **(Figure 18–23)**. The determination of which cell becomes which occurs during the second larval stage (L2) and is controlled by the Notch receptor gene, *lin-12*. In recessive *lin-12(0)* mutants (a loss-of-function mutant), no functional receptor protein is present, and both cells become anchor cells. The dominant mutation *lin-12(d)* (a gain-of-function mutation) causes both to become uterine precursors. Thus, expression of *lin-12* directs selection of the uterine pathway, because in the absence of the LIN-12 (Notch) receptor, both cells become anchor cells.

However, the situation is more complex than it first appears. Initially, the two neighboring cells are developmentally equivalent. Each synthesizes low levels of the Notch signal protein (encoded by the *lag-2* gene) *and* the Notch receptor protein. By chance, one cell ends up secreting more of the signal (LAG-2 or Delta protein) than the other cell. This causes the neighboring cell to increase production of the receptor (LIN-12 protein). The cell producing more of the receptor protein becomes the uterine precursor, and the other cell, producing more signal protein, becomes the anchor cell. The critical factor in this first round of cell–cell interaction is the balance between the LAG-2 (Delta) signal gene product and the LIN-12 (Notch) receptor gene product.

Once the gonadal anchor cell has been determined, a second round of cell–cell interaction leads to formation of

(a)

During L2, both cells begin secreting
signal for uterine differentiation

(b)

By chance, Z1.ppp
secretes more signal

Becomes anchor cell

In response to signal, Z4.aaa
increases production of LIN-12
receptor protein, triggering
determination as uterine
precursor cell

Becomes ventral uterine
precursor cell

FIGURE 18–23 Cell–cell interaction in anchor cell determination. (a) During L2, two neighboring cells begin the secretion of chemical signals for the induction of uterine differentiation. (b) By chance, cell Z1.ppp produces more of these signals, causing cell Z4.aaa to increase production of the receptor for signals. The action of increased signals causes Z4.aaa to become the ventral uterine precursor cell and allows Z1.ppp to become the anchor cell.

the vulva. This interaction involves the anchor cell (located in the gonad) and six neighboring cells (called precursor cells) located in the skin (**Figure 18–24**). The precursor cells, named P3.p to P8.p, are called Pn.p cells. The developmental fate of each Pn.p cell is specified by its position relative to the anchor cell.

During vulval development, the LIN-3 signal protein is synthesized by the anchor cell; this signal is received and processed by three adjacent Pn.p precursor cells (Pn.p 5–7). The cell closest to the anchor cell (usually Pn.p 6) becomes the primary vulval precursor cell, and the adjacent cells (Pn.p 5 and 7) become secondary precursor cells. A signal protein from the primary vulval precursor cell activates the *lin-12* receptor gene in the secondary cells, preventing them from becoming primary precursor cells. The other precursor cells (Pn.p 3, 4, and 8) receive no signal from the anchor cell and become skin cells.

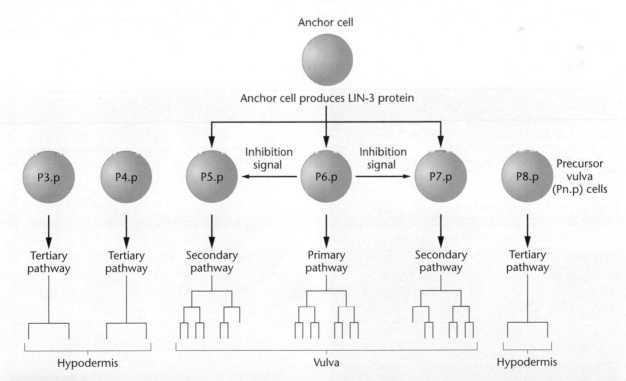

FIGURE 18–24 Cell lineage determination in *C. elegans* vulva formation. A signal from the anchor cell in the form of LIN-3 protein is received by three precursor cells (Pn.p cells). The cell closest to the anchor cell becomes the primary vulval precursor cell and adjacent cells become secondary precursor cells. The primary cell produces a signal that activates the *lin-12* gene in secondary cells, preventing them from becoming primary cells. Flanking precursor cells, which receive no signal from the anchor cell, become skin (hypodermis) cells, instead of vulval cells.

18.8 Binary Switch Genes and Signaling Pathways Program Genomic Expression

During development, certain genes act as switches, decreasing the number of alternative developmental pathways that a cell can follow. Each decision point is usually binary—that is, there are two alternative developmental fates for a cell at a given time—and the action of a switch gene programs the cell to follow only one of these pathways. These genes are called **binary switch genes**. They are defined by their ability to initiate complete development of an organ or a tissue type, and in combination with signaling pathways, form **gene-regulatory networks (GRNs)**. We will briefly describe how a binary switch gene controls the formation of the eye and how this regulatory pathway is used in all organisms with eyes.

The Control of Eye Formation

Drosophila adults have compound eyes [**Figure 18–25(a)**] that develop in preadult stages. Action of the wild-type allele of the binary switch gene *eyeless* programs cells to follow the developmental pathway for eye formation instead of the pathway for antenna formation. In flies homozygous for the recessive mutant allele *eyeless*, the eyes are reduced in size and have irregular facets.

[**Figure 18–25(b)**]. In developmental pathways that normally specify the formation of other organs such as legs, wings, and antennae, abnormal expression of *eyeless* results in eye formation in other parts of the body [**Figure 18–26(a)**]. This indicates that switching on the *eyeless* gene during development of these structures overrides the normal program of determination and differentiation, causing cells to follow the developmental program for eye formation instead of the normal pathway followed by neighboring cells.

The *eyeless* gene is part of a network of seven genes [**Figure 18–26(b)**], which is the master regulator of eye formation. These seven genes encode transcription factors, which in turn regulate the expression of many other genes that control cell determination and specification during development of the eye. The key regulators in this network are *twin of eyeless* (*toy*) and *eyeless* (*ey*). These control activity of the downstream transcription factors *sine oculis* (*so*) and *eyes absent* (*eya*), which, in turn, activate the gene *dachshund* (*dac*). The network also receives input from the genes *eyegone* (*eyg*) and *optix* (*opt*). During the stages of eye formation, this network interacts with several signaling pathways, including *Notch* (*N*), hedgehog (hh), and decapentaplegic (dpp), to form the retinal determination gene network (RDGN).

The *eyeless* allele and the other genes in this network have been highly conserved during evolution and are used by all animals, including humans, to make eyes. The human

(a)

(b)

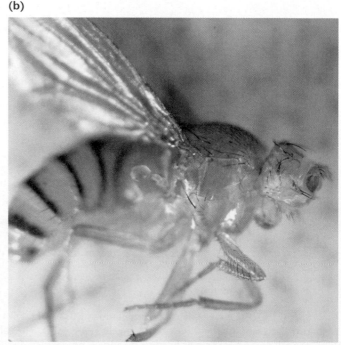

FIGURE 18–25 (a) The normal compound eye of adult *Drosophila*. (b) In flies homozygous for the *eyeless* (*ey*) mutation, eye development is abnormal, and adults have no eyes. The *ey* gene is a binary switch gene regulating eye development in all animals.

TABLE 18.5 Eye Genes in *Drosophila* and Vertebrates

Vertebrate Gene	*Drosophila* Homolog	Expression in Vertebrate Eye	Loss of Function
Pax6	eyeless, twin of eyeless	Lens placode, optic vesicle	Aniridia (human), *small eye* (mouse)
Bmp4	dpp	Optic vesicle, head ectoderm	No lens (mouse)
Bmp7	60A	Optic vesicle, head ectoderm	No lens (mouse)
EYA4	clift (eyes absent)	Perioptic mesenchyme, weak lens expression	No eye phenotype (human) or (mouse), some human mutations lead to cataracts and anterior defects
Six3	sine oculis	Lens placode, optic vesicle	Very small eyes (human)
Optx2	optix	Optic vesicle	No eyes (human)
Dach1	dachshund	Optic vesicle	*n.d.

*n.d., not determined
Source: Wawersik, S. and Maas, R.L. 2000. Vertebrate eye development as modelled in *Drosophila*. *Hum. Mol. Genet.* 9:917–925, Table 1, p. 921.

and fly genes in this network are compared in Table 18.5. The discovery that *eyeless* directs the formation of eyes in vertebrates forced reevaluation of the long-held belief that the compound eye of insects and the single-lens eye of vertebrates evolved independently. This assumption was based on the observation that the compound insect eye and the vertebrate camera eye have different embryonic origins, develop by different pathways, and are structurally very different. However, at the molecular level, the *eyeless* gene and its vertebrate equivalent, *Pax6*, have a high degree of sequence homology in encoded regions critical for DNA binding, and both are expressed in the development of the eye.

Walter Gehring and his colleagues examined the relationship between *eyeless* and *Pax6* by generating transgenic *Drosophila* that carried copies of the mouse *Pax6* gene. The striking results led to two conclusions: (1) the vertebrate version of this binary switch gene was capable of triggering the formation of extra eyes on the antennae of flies [**Figure 18–27(a)**], and (2) because the mouse gene works in flies, the invertebrate and vertebrate eyes *are* in fact homologous at the molecular level. Therefore, the eyes of *Drosophila* and the mouse are related evolutionarily. The downstream targets of these transcription factors are also conserved, indicating that steps in the genetic control of eye development are shared between species that diverged over half a billion years ago from a common ancestor. This evolutionary conservation makes it possible to use genetic analysis in *Drosophila* to study the development of eyes and to explore the molecular basis for inherited eye defects in humans.

(a)

(b)

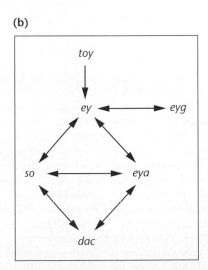

FIGURE 18–26 (a) Eye formation on the leg of a fly. This abnormal location (ectopic eye) is the result of eyeless expression in cells normally destined to form a leg. (b) The network of genes that regulate eye formation in *Drosophila*. *toy, twin of eyeless; ey, eyeless; so, sine oculis; eya, eyes absent; dac, dachshund; opt, optix; eyg, eyegone.*

(a)   (b)

FIGURE 18–27 (a) Eye formation on the antenna (arrow) of *Drosophila* induced by action of the mouse version of the *eyeless* gene (*Small eye*). (b) High magnification of the induced eye showing that the eye structure on the antenna is normal.

GENETICS, TECHNOLOGY, AND SOCIETY

Stem Cell Wars

Stem cell research may be the most controversial research area since the beginning of recombinant DNA technology in the 1970s. Although stem cell research is the focus of presidential proclamations, media campaigns, and ethical debates, few people understand it sufficiently to evaluate its pros and cons.

Stem cells are primitive cells that replicate indefinitely and have the capacity to differentiate into cells with specialized functions, such as the cells of heart, brain, liver, and muscle tissue. All the cells that make up the approximately 200 distinct types of tissues in our bodies are descended from stem cells. Some types of stem cells are defined as *totipotent,* meaning that they have the ability to differentiate into any mature cell type in the body, as well as tissues associated with the developing embryo, such as placenta. Other types of stem cells are *pluripotent,* meaning that they are able to differentiate into any of a smaller number of mature cell types. In contrast, mature, fully differentiated cells do not replicate or undergo transformations into different cell types.

In the last few years, several research teams have isolated and cultured human pluripotent stem cells. These cells remain undifferentiated and grow indefinitely in culture dishes—a process known as self-renewal. When treated with growth factors or hormones, these pluripotent stem cells differentiate into cells that have the characteristics of neural, bone, kidney, liver, heart, or pancreatic cells.

The fact that pluripotent stem cells grow prolifically in culture and differentiate into more specialized cells has created great excitement. Some foresee a day when stem cells may be a cornucopia from which to harvest unlimited numbers of specialized cells to replace cells in damaged and diseased tissues. Hence, stem cells could be used to treat Parkinson disease, type 1 diabetes, chronic heart disease, Alzheimer disease, and spinal cord injuries. Some predict that stem cells will be genetically modified to eliminate transplant rejection or to deliver specific gene products, thereby correcting genetic defects or treating cancers. The excitement about stem cell therapies has been fueled by reports of dramatically successful experiments in animals. For example, mice with spinal cord injuries regained their mobility and bowel and bladder control after they were injected with human stem cells. Both proponents and critics of stem cell research agree that stem cell therapies could be revolutionary. Why, then, should stem cell research be so contentious?

The answer to that question lies in the source of the pluripotent stem cells. Until recently, all pluripotent stem cell lines were derived from five-day-old embryonic blastocysts. Blastocysts at this stage consist of 50–150 cells, most of which will develop into placental and supporting tissues for the early embryo. The inner cell mass of the blastocyst consists of about 30 to 40 pluripotent stem cells that can develop into all the embryo's tissues. *In vitro* fertilization clinics grow fertilized eggs to the five-day blastocyst stage prior to uterine transfer. Embryonic stem cell (ESC) lines are created by taking the inner cell mass out of five-day blastocysts and growing the cells in culture dishes.

The fact that early embryos are destroyed in the process of establishing human ESC lines disturbs people who believe that preimplantation embryos are persons with rights; however, it does not disturb people who believe that these embryos are too primitive to have the status of a human being. Both sides in the debate invoke fundamental questions of what constitutes a human being.

Recently, scientists have developed several types of pluripotent stem cells without using embryos. One of the most promising types—known as *induced pluripotent stem (iPS) cells*—uses adult somatic cells as the source of pluripotent stem cell lines. To prepare iPS cells, scientists isolate somatic cells (such as cells from skin) and infect them with engineered retroviruses that integrate into the cells' DNA. These retroviruses contain several cloned human genes that encode products responsible for converting the somatic cells into immortal, pluripotent stem cells.

The development of iPS cell lines has generated renewed enthusiasm for stem cell research, as these cells bypass the ethical problems associated with the use of human embryos. In addition, they may become sources of patient-specific pluripotent stem cell lines that can be used for transplantation, without immune system rejection.

At the present time, it is unknown whether stem cells of any type will be as miraculous as predicted; however, if stem cell research progresses at its current rapid pace, we won't have long to wait.

Your Turn

Take time, individually or in groups, to answer the following questions. Investigate the references and links to help you understand the technologies and controversies surrounding stem cell research.

1. In 2013, a research group reported that they had created a human blastocyst after transferring a somatic cell nucleus into an enucleated human egg and activating the egg. They used the blastocyst to isolate ESCs that were a genetic match to the nucleus donor. How did these researchers do this, and why did they use this method rather than derive iPS cells from the donor?

   Read about this study in Tachibana, M., et al. 2013. Human embryonic stem cells derived by somatic cell nuclear transfer. *Cell* 153: 1–11. *A discussion of the ethical issues can be found in* "Cloning is used to create embryonic stem cells" *on the New York Times Web site:* http://www.nytimes.com/2013/05/16/science/scientists-use-cloning-to-create-embryonic-stem-cells.html?ref=science&_r=0.

2. The technologies that give rise to iPS cells and ESCs using nuclear transfer are based on the work of Drs. John Gurdon and Shinya Yamanaka. In 2012, these scientists were awarded the Nobel Prize in Physiology or Medicine for their work in reprogramming adult cells to stem cells. Describe their key discoveries on which stem cell therapies are based.

   A summary of their work can be found on the Nobel Prize Web site: http://www.nobelprize.org/nobel_prizes/medicine/laureates/2012/advanced.html.

3. At the present time, stem cell therapies have been tested in only three human Phase I clinical trials. Despite these promising but modest beginnings, human stem cell therapies are advertised and offered by many unregulated clinics throughout the world. Which clinical trials are presently being offered and what is the status of unregulated stem cell therapy?

   Begin your search with information from the International Society for Stem Cell Research: http://www.closerlookatstemcells.org.

CASE STUDY | One foot or another

In humans the *HOXD* homeotic gene cluster plays a critical role in limb development. In one large family, 16 of 36 members expressed one of two dominantly inherited malformations of the feet known as rocker bottom foot (CVT) or claw foot (CMT). One individual had one foot with CVT and the other with CMT. Genomic analysis identified a missense mutation in the *HOXD10* gene, resulting in a single amino acid substitution in the homeodomain of the encoded transcription factor. This region is crucial for making contact and binding to the target genes controlled by this protein. All family members with the foot malformations were heterozygotes; all unaffected members were homozygous for the normal allele.

1. Given that affected heterozygotes carry one normal allele of the *HOXD10* gene, how might a dominant mutation in a gene encoding a transcription factor lead to a developmental malformation?

2. How can two clinically different disorders result from the same mutation?

3. What might we learn about the control of developmental processes from an understanding of how this mutation works?

Summary Points

1. Developmental genetics, which explores the mechanisms by which genetic information controls development and differentiation, is one of the major areas of study in biology. Geneticists are investigating this topic by isolating developmental mutations and identifying the genes involved in developmental processes.

2. During embryogenesis, the activity of specific genes is controlled by the internal environment of the cell, including localized cytoplasmic components. In flies, the regulation of early events is mediated by the maternal cytoplasm, which then influences zygotic gene expression. As development

proceeds, both the cell's internal environment and its external environment become further altered by the presence of early gene products and communication with other cells.

3. In *Drosophila*, both genetic and molecular studies have confirmed that the egg contains information specifying the body plan of the larva and adult.

4. Extensive genetic analysis of embryonic development in *Drosophila* has led to the identification of maternal-effect genes whose products establish the anterior—posterior axis of the embryo. In addition, these maternal-effect genes activate sets of zygotic segmentation genes, initiating a cascade of gene

regulation that ends with the determination of segment identity by the homeotic selector genes. These same gene sets control aspects of embryonic development in all bilateral animals, including humans.

5. Flower formation in *Arabidopsis* is controlled by homeotic genes, but these gene sets are from a different gene family than the homeotic selector genes of *Drosophila* and other animals.

6. During development, major transitions are often controlled by binary switch genes whose action results in the selection of a pathway that results in the formation of an organ or tissue type.

INSIGHTS AND SOLUTIONS

1. In the slime mold *Dictyostelium,* experimental evidence suggests that cyclic AMP (cAMP) plays a central role in the developmental program leading to spore formation. The genes encoding the cAMP cell-surface receptor have been cloned, and the amino acid sequence of the protein components is known. To form reproductive structures, free-living individual cells aggregate together and then differentiate into one of two cell types, prespore cells or prestalk cells. Aggregating cells secrete waves or oscillations of cAMP to foster the aggregation of cells and then continuously secrete cAMP to activate genes in the aggregated cells at later stages of development. It has been proposed that cAMP controls cell–cell interaction and gene expression. It is important to test this hypothesis by using several experimental techniques. What different approaches can you devise to test this hypothesis, and what specific experimental systems would you employ to test them?

Solution: Two of the most powerful forms of analysis in biology involve the use of biochemical analogs (or inhibitors) to block gene transcription or the action of gene products in a predictable way, and the use of mutations to alter genes and their products. These two approaches can be used to study the role of cAMP in the developmental program of *Dictyostelium.* First, compounds chemically related to cAMP, such as GTP and GDP, can be used to test whether they have any effect on the processes controlled by cAMP. In fact, both GTP and GDP lower the affinity of cell-surface receptors for cAMP, effectively blocking the action of cAMP.

Mutational analysis can be used to dissect components of the cAMP receptor system. One approach is to use transformation with wild-type genes to restore mutant function. Similarly, because the genes for the receptor proteins have been cloned, it is possible to construct mutants with known

alterations in the component proteins and transform them into cells to assess their effects.

2. In the sea urchin, early development may occur even in the presence of actinomycin D, which inhibits RNA synthesis. However, if actinomycin D is present early in development but is removed a few hours later, all development stops. In fact, if actinomycin D is present only between the sixth and eleventh hours of development, events that normally occur at the fifteenth hour are arrested. What conclusions can be drawn concerning the role of gene transcription between hours 6 and 15?

Solution: Maternal mRNAs are present in the fertilized sea urchin egg. Thus, a considerable amount of development can take place without transcription of the embryo's genome. Because development past 15 hours is inhibited by prior treatment with actinomycin D, it appears that transcripts from the embryo's genome are required to initiate or maintain these events. This transcription must take place between the sixth and fifteenth hours of development.

3. If it were possible to introduce one of the homeotic genes from *Drosophila* into an *Arabidopsis* embryo homozygous for a homeotic flowering gene, would you expect any of the *Drosophila* genes to negate (rescue) the *Arabidopsis* mutant phenotype? Why or why not?

Solution: The *Drosophila* homeotic genes belong to the *Hox* gene family, whereas *Arabidopsis* homeotic genes belong to the MADS-box protein family. Both gene families are present in *Drosophila* and *Arabidopsis,* but they have evolved different functions in the animal and the plant kingdoms. As a result, it is unlikely that a transferred *Drosophila Hox* gene would rescue the phenotype of a MADS-box mutant, but only an actual experiment would confirm this.

Problems and Discussion Questions

MasteringGenetics™ Visit for instructor-assigned tutorials and problems.

HOW DO WE KNOW?

1. In this chapter, we have focused on large-scale as well as the inter- and intracellular events that take place during embryogenesis and the formation of adult structures. In particular, we discussed how the adult body plan is laid down by a cascade of gene expression, and the role of cell–cell communication

in development. Based on your knowledge of these topics, answer several fundamental questions:
(a) How do we know how many genes control development in an organism like *Drosophila*?
(b) What experimental evidence demonstrates that molecular gradients in the egg control development?

(c) How did we discover that selector genes specify which adult structures will be formed by body segments?

(d) How did we learn about the levels of gene regulation involved in vulval development in *C. elegans*?

(e) How do we know that eye formation in all animals is controlled by a binary switch gene?

CONCEPT QUESTION

2. Review the Chapter Concepts list on page 445. These all center around concepts related to stages of development. Write a short essay based on these concepts that outlines the role of differential transcription, gene control of cell fate, and the role of signaling systems in development.

3. Carefully distinguish between the terms *differentiation* and *determination*. Which phenomenon occurs initially during development?

4. Nuclei from almost any source may be injected into *Xenopus* oocytes. Studies have shown that these nuclei remain active in transcription and translation. How can such an experimental system be useful in developmental genetic studies?

5. Distinguish between the syncytial blastoderm stage and the cellular blastoderm stage in *Drosophila* embryogenesis.

6. (a) What are maternal-effect genes?
(b) When are gene products from these genes made, and where are they located?
(c) What aspects of development do maternal-effect genes control?
(d) What is the phenotype of maternal-effect mutations?

7. (a) What are zygotic genes, and when are their gene products made?
(b) What is the phenotype associated with zygotic gene mutations?
(c) Does the maternal genotype contain zygotic genes?

8. List the main classes of zygotic genes. What is the function of each class of these genes?

9. Experiments have shown that any nuclei placed in the polar cytoplasm at the posterior pole of the *Drosophila* egg will differentiate into germ cells. If polar cytoplasm is transplanted into the anterior end of the egg just after fertilization, what will happen to nuclei that migrate into this cytoplasm at the anterior pole?

10. How can you determine whether a particular gene is being transcribed in different cell types?

11. You observe that a particular gene is being transcribed during development. How can you tell whether the expression of this gene is under transcriptional or translational control?

12. The homeotic mutation *Antennapedia* causes mutant *Drosophila* to have legs in place of antennae and is a dominant gain-of-function mutation. What are the properties of such mutations? How does the *Antennapedia* gene change antennae into legs?

13. The *Drosophila* homeotic mutation *spineless aristapedia* (*ssᵃ*) results in the formation of a miniature tarsal structure (normally part of the leg) on the end of the antenna. What insight is provided by (*ssᵃ*) concerning the role of genes during determination?

14. Embryogenesis and oncogenesis (generation of cancer) share a number of features including cell proliferation, apoptosis, cell migration and invasion, formation of new blood vessels, and differential gene activity. Embryonic cells are relatively undifferentiated, and cancer cells appear to be undifferentiated or dedifferentiated. Homeotic gene expression directs early development, and mutant expression leads to loss of the differentiated state or an alternative cell identity. M. T. Lewis (2000. *Breast Can. Res.* 2: 158–169) suggested that breast cancer may be caused by the altered expression of homeotic genes. When he examined 11 such genes in cancers, 8 were underexpressed while 3 were overexpressed compared with controls. Given what you know about homeotic genes, could they be involved in oncogenesis?

15. Early development depends on the temporal and spatial interplay between maternally supplied material and mRNA and the onset of zygotic gene expression. Maternally encoded mRNAs must be produced, positioned, and degraded (Surdej and Jacobs-Lorena, 1998. *Mol. Cell Biol.* 18: 2892–2900). For example, transcription of the *bicoid* gene that determines anterior–posterior polarity in *Drosophila* is maternal. The mRNA is synthesized in the ovary by nurse cells and then transported to the oocyte, where it localizes to the anterior ends of oocytes. After egg deposition, *bicoid* mRNA is translated and unstable bicoid protein forms a decreasing concentration gradient from the anterior end of the embryo. At the start of gastrulation, *bicoid* mRNA has been degraded. Consider two models to explain the degradation of *bicoid* mRNA: (1) degradation may result from signals within the mRNA (intrinsic model), or (2) degradation may result from the mRNA's position within the egg (extrinsic model). Experimentally, how could one distinguish between these two models?

16. Formation of germ cells in *Drosophila* and many other embryos is dependent on their position in the embryo and their exposure to localized cytoplasmic determinants. Nuclei exposed to cytoplasm in the posterior end of *Drosophila* eggs (the pole plasm) form cells that develop into germ cells under the direction of maternally derived components. R. Amikura et al. (2001. *Proc. Nat. Acad. Sci. (USA)* 98: 9133–9138) consistently found mitochondria-type ribosomes outside mitochondria in the germ plasm of *Drosophila* embryos and postulated that they are intimately related to germ-cell specification. If you were studying this phenomenon, what would you want to know about the activity of these ribosomes?

17. One of the most interesting aspects of early development is the remodeling of the cell cycle from rapid cell divisions, apparently lacking G1 and G2 phases, to slower cell cycles with measurable G1 and G2 phases and checkpoints. During this remodeling, maternal mRNAs that specify cyclins are deadenylated, and zygotic genes are activated to produce cyclins. Audic et al. (2001. *Mol. and Cell. Biol.* 21: 1662–1671) suggest that deadenylation requires transcription of zygotic genes. Present a diagram that captures the significant features of these findings.

Extra-Spicy Problems

MasteringGenetics™ Visit for instructor-assigned tutorials and problems.

18. A number of genes that control expression of *Hox* genes in *Drosophila* have been identified. One of these homozygous mutants is *extra sex combs,* where some of the head and all of the thorax and abdominal segments develop as the last abdominal segment. In other words, all affected segments develop as posterior segments. What does this phenotype tell you about which set of *Hox* genes is controlled by the *extra sex combs* gene?

19. The *apterous* gene in *Drosophila* encodes a protein required for wing patterning and growth. It is also known to function in nerve development, fertility, and viability. When human and

mouse genes whose protein products closely resemble *apterous* were used to generate transgenic *Drosophila* (Rincon-Limas et al. 1999. *Proc. Nat. Acad. Sci. [USA]* 96: 2165–2170), the *apterous* mutant phenotype was *rescued*. In addition, the whole-body expression patterns in the transgenic *Drosophila* were similar to normal *apterous*.

(a) What is meant by the term *rescued* in this context?

(b) What do these results indicate about the molecular nature of development?

20. In *Arabidopsis,* flower development is controlled by sets of homeotic genes. How many classes of these genes are there, and what structures are formed by their individual and combined expression?

21. The floral homeotic genes of *Arabidopsis* belong to the MADS-box gene family, while in *Drosophila,* homeotic genes belong to the homeobox gene family. In both *Arabidopsis* and *Drosophila,* members of the *Polycomb* gene family control expression of these divergent homeotic genes. How do *Polycomb* genes control expression of two very different sets of homeotic genes?

22. The identification and characterization of genes that control sex determination has been a focus of investigators working with *C. elegans*. As with *Drosophila*, sex in this organism is determined by the ratio of X chromosomes to sets of autosomes. A diploid wild-type male has one X chromosome and a diploid wild-type hermaphrodite has two X chromosomes. Many different mutations have been identified that affect sex determination. Loss-of-function mutations in a gene called *her-1* cause an XO nematode to develop into a hermaphrodite and have no effect on XX development. (That is, XX nematodes are normal hermaphrodites.) In contrast, loss-of-function mutations in a gene called *tra-1* cause an XX nematode to develop into a male. Deduce the roles of these genes in wild-type sex determination from this information.

23. Vulval development in *C. elegans* is dependent on the response of some of the central epidermal progenitor cells in the region of the developing vulva to a chemical signal from the gonad. Signaling from the gonad is blocked by action of the vulvaless mutant *let-23* so that none of the central progenitor cells form vulval structures. In the vulvaless mutant, *n300*, the central progenitor cells do not form.

(a) Which gene is likely to act earlier in the vulval developmental pathway?

(b) What phenotype (vulva formed or vulvaless) would you expect from the double mutant? Why?

24. Based on the information in Problem 22 and the analysis of the phenotypes of single- and double-mutant strains, a model for sex determination in *C. elegans* has been generated. This model proposes that the *her-1* gene controls sex determination by establishing the level of activity of the *tra-1* gene, which, in turn, controls the expression of genes involved in generating the various sexually dimorphic tissues. Given this information,

(a) does the *her-1* gene product have a negative or a positive effect on the activity of the *tra-1* gene?

(b) What would be the phenotype of a *tra-1, her-1* double mutant?

25. Much of what we know about gene interactions in development has been learned using nematodes, yeast, flies, and bacteria.

This is due, in part, to the relative ease of genetic manipulation of these well-characterized genomes. However, of great interest are gene interactions involving complex diseases in humans. Wang and White (2011. *Nature Methods* 8(4) 341–346) describe work using RNAi to examine the interactive proteome in mammalian cells. They mention that knockdown inefficiencies and off-target effects of introduced RNAi species are areas that need particular improvement if the methodology is to be fruitful.

(a) How might one use RNAi to study developmental pathways?

(b) Comment on how "knockdown inefficiencies" and "off-target effects" would influence the interpretation of results.

26. Below is a microarray analysis of gene expression among developmentally significant categories (tissues and organs) in the model organism *Arabidopsis thaliana* (Schmid et al., 2005). Relative gene activities are presented on the ordinate, while several tissue types are presented on the abscissa.

(a) Are gene-expression patterns reasonably compatible with expectations?

(b) The general developmental program of plants contrasts with that of animals in that plants develop continuously, with new organs being added throughout their life span. How much does such a developmental program help explain the expression of photosynthetic genes in flowers and seeds?

(c) Typically, single or small numbers of genes are studied to determine their impact on development. Here, genome-wide analysis reveals output from general classes containing many genes. How might such a global approach further our understanding of the role of genes in development?

27. Dominguez et al. (2004) suggest that by studying genes that determine growth and tissue specification in the eye of *Drosophila*, much can be learned about human eye development.

(a) What evidence suggests that genetic eye determinants in *Drosophila* are also found in humans? Include a discussion of orthologous genes in your answer.

(b) What evidence indicates that the *eyeless* gene is part of a developmental network?

(c) Are genetic networks likely to specify developmental processes in general? Explain fully and provide an example.

Colored scanning electron micrograph of two prostate cancer cells in the final stages of cell division (cytokinesis). The cells are still joined by strands of cytoplasm.

9

Cancer and Regulation of the Cell Cycle

CHAPTER CONCEPTS

- Cancer is characterized by genetic defects in fundamental aspects of cellular function, including DNA repair, chromatin modification, cell-cycle regulation, apoptosis, and signal transduction.

- Most cancer-causing mutations occur in somatic cells; only about 5 percent of cancers have a hereditary component.

- Mutations in cancer-related genes lead to abnormal proliferation and loss of control over how cells spread and invade surrounding tissues.

- The development of cancer is a multistep process requiring mutations in genes controlling many aspects of cell proliferation and metastasis.

- Cancer cells show high levels of genomic instability, leading to the accumulation of multiple mutations, some in cancer-related genes.

- Epigenetic effects such as DNA methylation and histone modifications play significant roles in the development of cancers.

- Mutations in proto-oncogenes and tumor-suppressor genes contribute to the development of cancers.

- Cancer-causing viruses introduce oncogenes into infected cells and stimulate cell proliferation.

- Environmental agents contribute to cancer by damaging DNA.

Cancer is the leading cause of death in Western countries. It strikes people of all ages, and one out of three people will experience a cancer diagnosis sometime in his or her lifetime. Each year, more than 1 million cases of cancer are diagnosed in the United States, and more than 500,000 people die from the disease.

Over the last 30 years, scientists have discovered that cancer is a genetic disease at the somatic cell level, characterized by the presence of gene products derived from mutated or abnormally expressed genes. The combined effects of numerous abnormal gene products lead to the uncontrolled growth and spread of cancer cells. Although some mutated cancer genes may be inherited, most are created within somatic cells that then divide and form tumors. Completion of the Human Genome Project and numerous large-scale rapid DNA sequencing studies have opened the door to a wealth of new information about the mutations that trigger a cell to become cancerous. This new understanding of cancer genetics is also leading to new gene-specific treatments, some of which are now entering clinical trials. Some scientists predict that gene-targeted therapies will replace chemotherapies within the next 25 years.

The goal of this chapter is to highlight our current understanding of the nature and causes of cancer. As we will see, cancer is a genetic disease that arises from the accumulation of mutations in genes controlling many basic aspects of cellular function. We will examine the relationship between genes and cancer, and consider how mutations, chromosomal changes, epigenetics, and environmental agents play roles in the development of cancer. Please note that some of the topics discussed in this chapter are explored in greater depth later in the text (see Special Topic Chapter 1—Epigenetics and Special Topic Chapter 4—Genomics and Personalized Medicine).

19.1 Cancer Is a Genetic Disease at the Level of Somatic Cells

Perhaps the most significant development in understanding the causes of cancer is the realization that cancer is a genetic disease. Genomic alterations that are associated with cancer range from single-nucleotide substitutions to large-scale chromosome rearrangements, amplifications, and deletions (**Figure 19–1**). However, unlike other genetic diseases, cancer is caused by mutations that arise predominantly in somatic cells. Only about 5 percent of cancers are associated with germ-line mutations that increase a person's susceptibility to certain types of cancer. Another important difference between cancers and other genetic diseases is that cancers rarely arise from a single mutation in a single gene, but from the accumulation of many mutations. The mutations that lead to cancer affect multiple cellular functions, including repair of DNA damage, cell division, apoptosis, cellular differentiation, migratory behavior, and cell–cell contact.

What Is Cancer?

Clinically, cancer is defined as a large number of complex diseases, up to a hundred, that behave differently depending on the cell types from which they originate and the types of genetic alterations that occur within each cancer type. Cancers vary in their ages of onset, growth rates, invasiveness, prognoses, and responsiveness to treatments. However, at the molecular level, all cancers exhibit common characteristics that unite them as a family.

All cancer cells share two fundamental properties: (1) abnormal cell growth and division (**proliferation**), and (2) defects in the normal restraints that keep cells from spreading and colonizing other parts of the body (**metastasis**). In normal cells, these functions are tightly controlled by genes that are expressed appropriately in time and place. In cancer cells, these genes are either mutated or are expressed inappropriately.

It is this combination of uncontrolled cell proliferation and metastatic spread that makes cancer cells dangerous. When a cell simply loses genetic control over cell growth, it may grow into a multicellular mass, a **benign tumor**. Such a tumor can often be removed by surgery and may cause no serious harm. However, if cells in the tumor also have the ability to break loose, enter the bloodstream, invade other tissues, and form secondary tumors (**metastases**), they become malignant. **Malignant tumors** are often difficult to treat and may become life threatening. As we will see later in the chapter, there are multiple steps and genetic mutations that convert a benign tumor into a dangerous malignant tumor.

The Clonal Origin of Cancer Cells

Although malignant tumors may contain billions of cells, and may invade and grow in numerous parts of the body, all cancer cells in the primary and secondary tumors are clonal, meaning that they originated from a common ancestral cell that accumulated specific cancer-causing mutations. This is an important concept in understanding the molecular causes of cancer and has implications for its diagnosis.

Numerous data support the concept of cancer clonality. For example, reciprocal chromosomal translocations are characteristic of many cancers, including leukemias and lymphomas (two cancers involving white blood cells). Cancer cells from patients with **Burkitt lymphoma** show reciprocal translocations between chromosome 8 (with translocation breakpoints at or near the *c-myc* gene) and chromosomes 2, 14, or 22 (with translocation breakpoints at or near one of the immunoglobulin genes). Each Burkitt lymphoma patient exhibits unique breakpoints in his or her *c-myc* and

(a)

(b)

FIGURE 19–1 (a) Spectral karyotype of a normal cell. (b) Karyotype of a cancer cell showing translocations, deletions, and aneuploidy—characteristic features of cancer cells.

immunoglobulin gene DNA sequences; however, all lymphoma cells within that patient contain identical translocation breakpoints. This demonstrates that all cancer cells in each case of Burkitt lymphoma arise from a single cell, and this cell passes on its genetic aberrations to its progeny.

Another demonstration that cancer cells are clonal is their pattern of X-chromosome inactivation. As explained earlier in the text (see Chapter 7), female humans are mosaic, with some cells containing an inactivated paternal X chromosome and other cells containing an inactivated maternal X chromosome. X-chromosome inactivation occurs early in development and takes place at random. All cancer cells within a tumor, both primary and metastatic, within one female individual, contain the same inactivated X chromosome. This supports the concept that all the cancer cells in that patient arose from a common ancestral cell.

The Cancer Stem Cell Hypothesis

A concept that is related to the clonal origin of cancer cells is that of the cancer stem cell. Many scientists now believe that most of the cells within tumors do not proliferate. Those that do proliferate and give rise to all the cells within the tumor are known as **cancer stem cells**. Stem cells are undifferentiated cells that have the capacity for self-renewal—a process in which the stem cell divides unevenly, creating one daughter cell that goes on to differentiate into a mature cell type and one that remains a stem cell. Stem cells are also discussed earlier in the text (see Chapter 18). The cancer stem cell hypothesis contrasts the random or stochastic model. This model predicts that every cell within a tumor has the potential to form a new tumor.

Although scientists still actively debate the existence of cancer stem cells, evidence is accumulating that cancer stem cells do exist, at least in some tumors. Cancer stem cells have been identified in leukemias as well as in solid tumors of the brain, breast, colon, ovary, pancreas, and prostate. It is still not clear what fraction of any tumor is composed of cancer stem cells. For example, human acute myeloid leukemias contain less than 1 cancer stem cell in 10,000. In contrast, some solid tumors may contain as many as 40 percent cancer stem cells.

Scientists are also not sure about the origins of cancer stem cells. It is possible that they may arise from normal adult stem cells within a tissue, or they may be created from more differentiated somatic cells that acquire properties similar to stem cells after accumulating numerous mutations and changes to chromatin structure.

Cancer as a Multistep Process, Requiring Multiple Mutations

Although we know that cancer is a genetic disease initiated by mutations that lead to uncontrolled cell proliferation and metastasis, a single mutation is not sufficient to transform a normal cell into a tumor-forming (tumorigenic),

malignant cell. If it were sufficient, then cancer would be far more prevalent than it is. In humans, mutations occur spontaneously at a rate of about 10^{-6} mutations per gene, per cell division, mainly due to the intrinsic error rates of DNA replication. Because there are approximately 10^{16} cell divisions in a human body during a lifetime, a person might suffer up to 10^{10} mutations per gene somewhere in the body, during his or her lifetime. However, only about one person in three will suffer from cancer.

The phenomenon of age-related cancer is another indication that cancer develops from the accumulation of several mutagenic events in a single cell. The incidence of most cancers rises exponentially with age. If a single mutation were sufficient to convert a normal cell to a malignant one, then cancer incidence would appear to be independent of age. The age-related incidence of cancer suggests that many independent mutations, occurring randomly and with a low probability, are necessary before a cell is transformed into a malignant cancer cell. Another indication that cancer is a multistep process is the delay that occurs between exposure to **carcinogens** (cancer-causing agents) and the appearance of the cancer. For example, an incubation period of five to eight years separated exposure of people to the radiation of the atomic explosions at Hiroshima and Nagasaki and the onset of leukemias.

The multistep nature of cancer development is supported by the observation that cancers often develop in progressive steps, beginning with mildly aberrant cells and progressing to cells that are increasingly tumorigenic and malignant.

Each step in **tumorigenesis** (the development of a malignant tumor) appears to be the result of two or more genetic alterations that release the cells progressively from the controls that normally operate on proliferation and malignancy. This observation suggests that the progressive genetic alterations that create a cancer cell confer selective advantages to the cell and are propagated through cell divisions during the creation of tumors.

The progressive nature of cancer is illustrated by the development of colorectal cancer. Colorectal cancers are known to proceed through several clinical stages that are characterized by the stepwise accumulation of genetic defects in several genes (**Figure 19–2**). The first step is the conversion of a normal epithelial cell into a small cluster of cells known as an **adenoma** or **polyp**. This step requires inactivating mutations in the **adenomatous polyposis coli (APC)** gene, a gene that encodes a protein involved in the normal differentiation of intestinal cells. The *APC* gene is a tumor-suppressor gene, which will be discussed later in the chapter. The resulting adenoma grows slowly and is considered benign.

The second step in the development of colorectal cancer is the acquisition of a second genetic alteration in one of the cells within the small adenoma. This is usually a mutation in the *Kras* gene, a gene whose product is normally

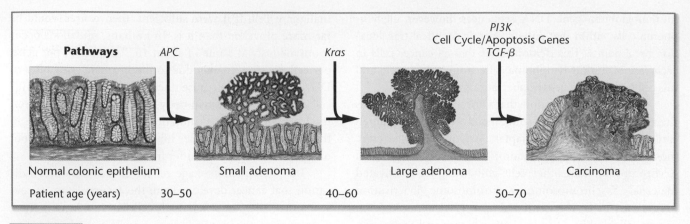

FIGURE 19-2 Steps in the development of colorectal cancers. Some of the genes that acquire driver mutations and cause the progressive development of colorectal cancer are shown at the top of the figure. These driver mutations accumulate over time and can take 40 years or more to result in the formation of a malignant tumor.

involved with regulating cell growth. The mutations in *Kras* that contribute to colorectal cancer cause the Kras protein to become constitutively active, resulting in unregulated cell division. The cell containing the *APC* and *Kras* mutations grows and expands to form a larger intermediate adenoma of approximately 1 cm in diameter—in a process known as **clonal expansion**. The cells of the original small adenoma (containing the *APC* mutation) are now vastly outnumbered by cells containing the two mutations.

The third step, which transforms a large adenoma into a malignant tumor (**carcinoma**), requires several more waves of clonal expansions triggered by the acquisition of defects in several genes, including *p53*, *PI3K*, and *TGF-β*. The products of these genes control several important aspects of normal cell growth and division, such as apoptosis, growth signaling, and cell-cycle regulation—all of which we will discuss in more detail later in the chapter. The resulting carcinoma is able to further grow and invade the underlying tissues of the colon. A few cells within the carcinoma acquire one or more new mutations that allow them to break free of the tumor, migrate to other parts of the body, and form metastases.

Driver Mutations and Passenger Mutations

Scientists are now applying some of the recent advances in DNA sequencing in order to identify all of the somatic mutations that occur during the development of a cancer cell. These studies compare the DNA sequences of genomes from cancer cells and normal cells derived from the same patient. Data from these studies are revealing that tens of thousands of somatic mutations can be present in cancer cells. Solid tumors such as those of the colon or breast may contain as many as 70 mutated genes. Some other cancers, such as lung cancer and melanomas, may contain several hundred mutations. Researchers believe that only a handful

of mutations in each tumor—called **driver mutations**—give a growth advantage to a tumor cell. The remainder of the mutations may be acquired over time, perhaps as a result of the increased levels of DNA damage that accumulate in cancer cells, but these mutations have no direct contribution to the cancer phenotype. These are known as **passenger mutations**. The total number of driver mutations that occur in any particular cancer is small—between 2 and 8.

As we will discover in subsequent sections of this chapter, the genes that acquire driver mutations that lead to cancer (called oncogenes and tumor-suppressor genes) are those that control a large number of essential cellular functions including DNA damage repair, chromatin modification, cell-cycle regulation, and programmed cell death. We will now investigate these fundamental processes, the genes that control them, and how mutations in these genes may lead to cancer.

19.2 Cancer Cells Contain Genetic Defects Affecting Genomic Stability, DNA Repair, and Chromatin Modifications

Cancer cells contain higher than normal numbers of mutations and chromosomal abnormalities. Many researchers believe that the fundamental defect in cancer cells is a derangement of the cells' normal ability to repair DNA damage. This loss of genomic integrity leads to a general increase in the mutation rate for every gene in the genome, including those whose products control aspects of cell proliferation, programmed cell death, and metastasis. The high level of genomic instability seen in cancer cells is known as the **mutator phenotype**. In addition, recent research has

(a) Double minutes

(b) Heterogeneous staining region

FIGURE 19-3 DNA amplifications in neuroblastoma cells. (a) Two cancer genes (*MYCN* in red and *MDM2* in green) are amplified as small DNA fragments that remain separate from chromosomal DNA within the nucleus. These units of amplified DNA are known as double minute chromosomes. Normal chromosomes are stained blue. (b) Multiple copies of the *MYCN* gene are amplified within one large region called a heterogeneous staining region (green). Single copies of the *MYCN* gene are visible as green dots at the ends of the normal parental chromosomes (white arrows). Normal chromosomes are stained red.

revealed that cancer cells contain aberrations in the types and locations of chromatin modifications, particularly DNA and histone methylation patterns.

Genomic Instability and Defective DNA Repair

Genomic instability in cancer cells is characterized by the presence of gross defects such as translocations, aneuploidy, chromosome loss, DNA amplification, and chromosome deletions (Figures 19–1 and **19–3**). Cancer cells that are grown in cultures in the lab also show a great deal of genomic instability—duplicating, losing, and translocating chromosomes or parts of chromosomes. Often cancer cells show specific chromosomal defects that are used to diagnose the type and stage of the cancer. For example, leukemic white blood cells from patients with **chronic myelogenous leukemia (CML)** bear a specific translocation, in which the *C-ABL* gene on chromosome 9 is translocated into the *BCR* gene on chromosome 22. This translocation creates a structure known as the **Philadelphia chromosome (Figure 19–4)**. The *BCR-ABL* fusion gene codes for a chimeric BCR-ABL protein. The normal ABL protein is a **protein kinase** that acts within signal transduction pathways, transferring growth factor signals from the external environment to the nucleus. The BCR-ABL protein is an abnormal signal transduction molecule in CML cells, which stimulates these cells to proliferate even in the absence of external growth signals.

In keeping with the concept of the cancer mutator phenotype, a number of inherited cancers are caused by defects in genes that control DNA repair. For example, xeroderma pigmentosum (XP) is a rare hereditary disorder that is characterized by extreme sensitivity to ultraviolet light and other carcinogens. Patients with XP often develop skin cancer. Cells from patients with XP are defective in nucleotide excision repair, with mutations appearing in any one of seven genes whose products are necessary to carry out DNA repair. XP cells are impaired in their ability to repair DNA lesions such as thymine dimers induced by UV light. The relationship between XP and genes controlling nucleotide excision repair is also described earlier in the text (see Chapter 17).

Another example is hereditary nonpolyposis colorectal cancer (HNPCC), which is caused by mutations in genes controlling DNA repair. HNPCC is an autosomal dominant syndrome, affecting about one in every 200 to 1000 people. Patients affected by HNPCC have an increased risk of developing colon, ovary, uterine, and kidney cancers. Cells from patients with HNPCC show higher than normal mutation rates and genomic instability. At least eight genes are associated with HNPCC, and four of these genes control aspects of DNA mismatch repair. Inactivation of any of these four genes—*MSH2, MSH6, MLH1*, and *MLH3*—causes a rapid accumulation of genome-wide mutations and the subsequent development of cancers.

The observation that hereditary defects in genes controlling nucleotide excision repair and DNA mismatch repair lead to high rates of cancer lends support to the idea that the mutator phenotype is a significant contributor to the development of cancer.

Normal chromosome 9

Normal chromosome 22

Translocation t(9;22)

q11.2 (*BCR*)

q34.1 (*C-ABL*)

(*BCR*)
(*ABL*)

Philadelphia chromosome

FIGURE 19-4 A reciprocal translocation involving the long arms of chromosomes 9 and 22 results in the formation of a characteristic chromosome, the Philadelphia chromosome, which is associated with chronic myelogenous leukemia (CML). The t(9;22) translocation results in the fusion of the *C-ABL* proto-oncogene on chromosome 9 with the *BCR* gene on chromosome 22. The fusion protein is a powerful hybrid molecule that allows cells to escape control of the cell cycle, contributing to the development of CML.

Chromatin Modifications and Cancer Epigenetics

The field of cancer epigenetics is providing new perspectives on the genetics of cancer. **Epigenetics** is the study of factors that affect gene expression but that do not alter the nucleotide sequence of DNA. Epigenetic effects can be inherited from one cell to its progeny cells and may be present in either somatic or germ-line cells. DNA methylation and histone modifications such as acetylation and phosphorylation are examples of epigenetic modifications. The genomic patterns and locations of these modifications can affect gene expression. For example, DNA methylation is thought to be responsible for the gene silencing associated with parental imprinting, heterochromatin gene repression, and X-chromosome inactivation. The effects of chromatin modifications and epigenetic factors on gene expression and hereditary disease are discussed in more detail later in the text (see Chapter 17 and Special Topic Chapter 1—Epigenetics).

Cancer cells contain altered DNA methylation patterns. Overall, there is much less DNA methylation in cancer cells than in normal cells. At the same time, the promoters of some genes are hypermethylated in cancer cells. These changes are thought to result in the release of transcription repression over the bulk of genes that would be silent in normal cells—including cancer-causing genes—while at the same time repressing transcription of genes that would regulate normal cellular functions such as DNA repair and cell-cycle control.

Histone modifications are also disrupted in cancer cells. Genes that encode histone acetylases, deacetylases, methyltransferases, and demethylases are often mutated or aberrantly expressed in cancer cells. The large numbers of epigenetic abnormalities in tumors have prompted some scientists to speculate that there may be more epigenetic defects in cancer cells than there are gene mutations. In addition, because epigenetic modifications are reversible, it may be possible to treat cancers using epigenetic-based therapies.

NOW SOLVE THIS

19–1 In chronic myelogenous leukemia (CML), leukemic blood cells can be distinguished from other cells of the body by the presence of a functional BCR-ABL hybrid protein. Explain how this characteristic provides an opportunity to develop a therapeutic approach to a treatment for CML.

■ **HINT:** *This problem asks you to imagine a therapy that is based on the unique genetic characteristics of CML leukemic cells. The key to its solution is to remember that the BCR-ABL fusion protein is found only in CML white blood cells and that this unusual protein has a specific function thought to directly contribute to the development of CML. To help you answer this problem, you may wish to learn more about the cancer drug Gleevec (see http://www.cancer.gov/cancertopics/druginfo/imatinibmesylate).*

19.3 Cancer Cells Contain Genetic Defects Affecting Cell-Cycle Regulation

One of the fundamental aberrations in all cancer cells is a loss of control over cell proliferation. Cell proliferation is the process of cell growth and division that is essential for all development and tissue repair in multicellular organisms. Although some cells, such as epidermal cells of the skin or blood-forming cells in the bone marrow, continue to grow and divide throughout an organism's lifetime, most cells in adult multicellular organisms remain in a nondividing, quiescent, and differentiated state. **Differentiated cells** are those that are specialized for specific functions, such as photoreceptor cells of the retina or muscle cells of the heart. The most extreme examples of nonproliferating cells are nerve cells, which divide little, if at all, even to replace damaged tissue. In contrast, many differentiated cells, such as those in the liver and kidney, are able to grow and divide when stimulated by extracellular signals and growth factors. In this way, multicellular organisms are able to replace dead and damaged tissue. However, the growth and differentiation of cells must be strictly regulated; otherwise, the integrity of organs and tissues would be compromised by the presence of inappropriate types and quantities of cells. Normal regulation over cell proliferation involves a large number of gene products that control steps in the cell cycle, programmed cell death, and the response of cells to external growth signals. In cancer cells, many of the genes that control these functions are mutated or aberrantly expressed, leading to uncontrolled cell proliferation.

In this section, we will review steps in the cell cycle, some of the genes that control the cell cycle, and how these genes, when mutated, lead to cancer.

The Cell Cycle and Signal Transduction

The cellular events that occur in sequence from one cell division to the next comprise the **cell cycle** (**Figure 19–5**). The **interphase** stage of the cell cycle is the interval between mitotic divisions. During this time, the cell grows and replicates its DNA. During **G1**, the cell prepares for DNA synthesis by accumulating the enzymes and molecules required for DNA replication. G1 is followed by **S phase**, during which the cell's chromosomal DNA is replicated. During **G2**, the cell continues to grow and prepare for division. During **M phase**, the duplicated chromosomes condense, sister chromosomes separate to opposite poles, and the cell divides in two. These phases of the cell cycle are also discussed in more detail earlier in the text (see Chapter 2).

In early to mid-G1, the cell makes a decision either to enter the next cell cycle or to withdraw from the cell cycle into quiescence. Continuously dividing cells do not exit the

FIGURE 19–5 Checkpoints and proliferation decision points monitor the progress of the cell through the cell cycle.

cell cycle but proceed through G1, S, G2, and M phases; however, if the cell receives signals to stop growing, it enters the **G0** phase of the cell cycle. During G0, the cell remains metabolically active but does not grow or divide. Most differentiated cells in multicellular organisms can remain in this G0 phase indefinitely. Some, such as neurons, never reenter the cell cycle. In contrast, cancer cells are unable to enter G0, and instead, they continuously cycle. Their *rate* of proliferation is not necessarily any greater than that of normal proliferating cells; however, they are not able to become quiescent at the appropriate time or place.

Cells in G0 can often be stimulated to reenter the cell cycle by external growth signals. These signals are delivered to the cell by molecules such as growth factors and hormones that bind to cell-surface receptors, which then relay the signal from the plasma membrane to the cytoplasm. The process of transmitting growth signals from the external environment to the cell nucleus is known as **signal transduction**. Ultimately, signal transduction initiates a program of gene expression that propels the cell out of G0 back into the cell cycle. Cancer cells often have defects in signal transduction pathways. Sometimes, abnormal signal transduction molecules send continuous growth signals to the nucleus even in the absence of external growth signals. An example of abnormal signal transduction due to mutations in the *ras* gene is described in Section 19.4. In addition, malignant cells may not respond to external signals from surrounding cells—signals that would normally inhibit cell proliferation within a mature tissue.

Cell-Cycle Control and Checkpoints

In normal cells, progress through the cell cycle is tightly regulated, and each step must be completed before the next step can begin. There are at least three distinct points in the cell cycle at which the cell monitors external signals and internal equilibrium before proceeding to the next stage. These are the **G1/S**, the **G2/M**, and **M checkpoints** (Figure 19–5). At the G1/S checkpoint, the cell monitors its size and determines whether its DNA has been damaged. If the cell has not achieved an adequate size, or if the DNA has been damaged, further progress through the cell cycle is halted until these conditions are corrected. If cell size and DNA integrity are normal, the G1/S checkpoint is traversed, and the cell proceeds to S phase. The second important checkpoint is the G2/M checkpoint, where physiological conditions in the cell are monitored prior to mitosis. If DNA replication or repair of any DNA damage has not been completed, the cell cycle arrests until these processes are complete. The third major checkpoint occurs during mitosis and is called the M checkpoint. At this checkpoint, both the successful formation of the spindle-fiber system and the attachment of spindle fibers to the kinetochores associated with the centromeres are monitored. If spindle fibers are not properly formed or attachment is inadequate, mitosis is arrested.

In addition to regulating the cell cycle at checkpoints, the cell controls progress through the cell cycle by means of two classes of proteins: **cyclins** and **cyclin-dependent kinases (CDKs)**. The cell accumulates and destroys cyclin proteins in a precise pattern during the cell cycle (**Figure 19–6**). When a cyclin is present, it binds to a specific CDK, triggering activity

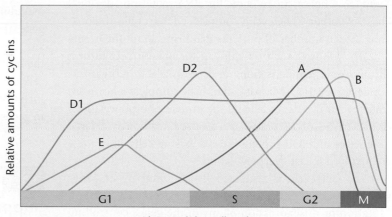

FIGURE 19–6 Relative expression times and amounts of cyclins during the cell cycle. Cyclin D1 accumulates early in G1 and is expressed at a constant level through most of the cycle. Cyclin E accumulates in G1, reaches a peak, and declines by mid-S phase. Cyclin D2 begins accumulating in the last half of G1, reaches a peak just after the beginning of S, and then declines by early G2. Cyclin A appears in late G1, accumulates through S phase, peaks at the G2/M transition, and is rapidly degraded. Cyclin B peaks at the G2/M transition and declines rapidly in M phase.

FIGURE 19–7 CDK1 and cyclin B control the transition from G2 to M phase. In late G2 phase, cyclin B accumulates and forms complexes with inactive CDK1 molecules. CDK1 is activated within the complexes and adds phosphate groups to cellular components. These phosphorylated molecules bring about the structural and biochemical changes that are necessary for M phase. In late M phase, cyclin B is degraded, CDK1 becomes inactive, and M phase phosphorylations are reversed.

of the CDK/cyclin complex. The CDK/cyclin complex then selectively phosphorylates and activates other proteins that in turn bring about the changes necessary to advance the cell through the cell cycle. For example, in G1 phase, CDK4/cyclin D complexes activate proteins that stimulate transcription of genes whose products (such as DNA polymerase δ and DNA ligase) are required for DNA replication during S phase. Another CDK/cyclin complex, CDK1/cyclin B, phosphorylates a number of proteins that bring about the events of early mitosis, such as nuclear membrane breakdown, chromosome condensation, and cytoskeletal reorganization (**Figure 19–7**). Mitosis can only be completed, however, when cyclin B is degraded and the protein phosphorylations characteristic of M phase are reversed. Although a large number of different protein kinases exist in cells, only a few are involved in cell-cycle regulation.

The cell cycle is regulated by an interplay of genes whose products either promote or suppress cell division. Mutation or misexpression of any of the genes controlling the cell cycle can contribute to the development of cancer. For example, if genes that control the G1/S or G2/M checkpoints are mutated, the cell may continue to grow and divide without repairing DNA damage. As these cells continue to divide, they accumulate mutations in genes whose products control cell proliferation or metastasis. Similarly, if genes that control progress through the cell cycle, such as those that encode the cyclins, are expressed at the wrong

time or at incorrect levels, the cell may grow and divide continuously and may be unable to exit the cell cycle into G0. The result in both cases is that the cell loses control over proliferation and is on its way to becoming cancerous.

Control of Apoptosis

As already described, if DNA replication, repair, or chromosome assembly is defective, normal cells halt their progress through the cell cycle until the condition is corrected. This reduces the number of mutations and chromosomal abnormalities that accumulate in normal proliferating cells. However, if DNA or chromosomal damage is so severe that repair is impossible, the cell may initiate a second line of defense—a process called **apoptosis**, or **programmed cell death**. Apoptosis is a genetically controlled process whereby the cell commits suicide. Besides its role in preventing cancer, apoptosis is also initiated during normal multicellular development in order to eliminate certain cells that do not contribute to the final adult organism. The steps in apoptosis are the same for damaged cells and for cells being eliminated during development: nuclear DNA becomes fragmented, internal cellular structures are disrupted, and the cell dissolves into small spherical structures known as apoptotic bodies **Figure 19–8(a)**. In the final step, the apoptotic bodies are engulfed by the immune system's phagocytic cells. A series of proteases called **caspases** are responsible for initiating apoptosis and for digesting intracellular components.

Apoptosis is genetically controlled in that regulation of the levels of specific gene products such as Bcl2 and BAX [**Figure 19–8(b)**] can trigger or prevent apoptosis. By removing damaged cells, programmed cell death reduces the number of mutations that are passed to the next generation, including those in cancer-causing genes. Some of the same genes that control cell-cycle checkpoints can trigger apoptosis. These genes are mutated in many cancers. As a result of the mutation or inactivation of these checkpoint genes, the cell is unable to repair its DNA or undergo apoptosis. This inability leads to the accumulation of even more mutations in genes that control growth, division, and metastasis.

19.4 Proto-oncogenes and Tumor-Suppressor Genes Are Altered in Cancer Cells

Two general categories of genes are mutated or misexpressed in cancer cells—the proto-oncogenes and the tumor-suppressor genes (**Table 19.1**). **Proto-oncogenes** encode transcription factors that stimulate expression of other genes, signal transduction molecules that stimulate cell division, and cell-cycle regulators that move the cell through

(a)

(b)

FIGURE 19–8 (a) Normal white blood cell (bottom) and a white blood cell undergoing apoptosis (top). Apoptotic bodies appear as grape-like clusters on the cell surface. (b) The relative concentrations of the Bcl2 and BAX proteins regulate apoptosis. A normal cell contains a balance of Bcl2 and BAX, which form inactive heterodimers. A relative excess of Bcl2 results in the formation of Bcl2 homodimers, which prevent apoptosis. Cancer cells with Bcl2 overexpression are resistant to chemotherapies and radiation therapies. A relative excess of BAX results in the formation of BAX homodimers, which induce apoptosis. In normal cells, activated p53 protein induces transcription of the *BAX* gene and inhibits transcription of the *Bcl2* gene, leading to cell death. In many cancer cells, p53 is defective, preventing the apoptotic pathway from removing the cancer cells.

the cell cycle. Their products are important for normal cell functions, especially cell growth and division. When normal cells become quiescent and cease division, they repress the expression of most proto-oncogenes or modify the activities of their products. In cancer cells, one or more proto-oncogenes are altered in such a way that the activities of their products cannot be regulated in a normal fashion. This is sometimes due to mutations that result in an abnormal protein product. In other cases, proto-oncogenes may be overexpressed or expressed at an incorrect time due to mutations within gene-regulatory regions such as enhancer

elements or due to alterations in chromatin structure that affect gene expression. If a proto-oncogene is continually in an "on" state, its product may constantly stimulate the cell to divide. When a proto-oncogene is mutated or abnormally expressed and contributes to the development of cancer, it is known as an **oncogene**—a cancer-causing gene. Oncogenes are proto-oncogenes that have experienced a gain-of-function alteration. As a result, only one allele of a proto-oncogene needs to be mutated or misexpressed in order to contribute to cancer. Hence, oncogenes confer a dominant cancer phenotype.

TABLE 19.1 Some Proto-oncogenes and Tumor-Suppressor Genes

Proto-oncogene	Normal Function	Alteration in Cancer	Associated Cancers
c-myc	Transcription factor, regulates cell cycle, differentiation, apoptosis	Translocation, amplification, point mutations	Lymphomas, leukemias, lung cancer, many types
c-kit	Tyrosine kinase, signal transduction	Mutation	Sarcomas
RARα	Hormone-dependent transcription factor, differentiation	Chromosomal translocations with *PML* gene, fusion product	Acute promyelocytic leukemia
E6	Human papillomavirus encoded oncogene, inactivates p53	HPV infection	Cervical cancer
Cyclins	Bind to CDKs, regulate cell cycle	Gene amplification, overexpression	Lung, esophagus, many types

Tumor-Suppressor	Normal Function	Alteration in Cancer	Associated Cancers
RB1	Cell-cycle checkpoints, binds E2F	Mutation, deletion, inactivation by viral oncogene products	Retinoblastoma, osteosarcoma, many types
APC	Cell–cell interaction	Mutation	Colorectal cancers, brain, thyroid
p53	Transcription regulation	Mutation, deletion, viruses	Many types
BRCA1, BRCA2	DNA repair	Point mutations	Breast, ovarian, prostate cancers

Tumor-suppressor genes are genes whose products normally regulate cell-cycle checkpoints or initiate the process of apoptosis. In normal cells, proteins encoded by tumor-suppressor genes halt progress through the cell cycle in response to DNA damage or growth-suppression signals from the extracellular environment. When tumor-suppressor genes are mutated or inactivated, cells are unable to respond normally to cell-cycle checkpoints, or are unable to undergo programmed cell death if DNA damage is extensive. This leads to the accumulation of more mutations and the development of cancer. When both alleles of a tumor-suppressor gene are inactivated through mutation or epigenetic modifications, and other changes in the cell keep it growing and dividing, cells may become tumorigenic.

The following are examples of proto-oncogenes and tumor-suppressor genes that contribute to cancer when mutated or abnormally expressed. Approximately 400 oncogenes and tumor-suppressor genes are now known, and more will likely be discovered as cancer research continues.

The *ras* Proto-oncogenes

Some of the most frequently mutated genes in human tumors are those in the **ras gene family**. These genes are mutated in more than 30 percent of human tumors. The *ras* gene family encodes signal transduction molecules that are associated with the cell membrane and regulate cell growth and division. Ras proteins normally transmit signals from the cell membrane to the nucleus, stimulating the cell to divide in response to external growth factors (**Figure 19–9**). Ras proteins alternate between an inactive (switched off) and an active (switched on) state by binding either guanosine diphosphate (GDP) or guanosine triphosphate (GTP). When a cell encounters a growth factor (such as platelet-derived growth factor or epidermal growth factor), growth factor receptors on the cell membrane bind to the growth factor, resulting in autophosphorylation of the cytoplasmic portion of the growth factor receptor. This causes recruitment of proteins known as nucleotide exchange factors to the plasma membrane. These nucleotide exchange factors cause Ras to release GDP and bind GTP, thereby activating Ras. The active, GTP-bound form of Ras then sends its signals through cascades of protein phosphorylations in the cytoplasm. The end-point of these cascades is activation of nuclear transcription factors that stimulate expression of genes whose products drive the cell from quiescence into the cell cycle. Once Ras has sent its signals to the nucleus, it hydrolyzes GTP to GDP and becomes inactive. Mutations that convert the *ras* proto-oncogene to an oncogene prevent the Ras protein from hydrolyzing GTP to GDP and hence freeze the Ras protein into its "on" conformation, constantly stimulating the cell to divide.

FIGURE 19–9 A signal transduction pathway mediated by Ras.

The *p53* Tumor-Suppressor Gene

The most frequently mutated gene in human cancers— mutated in more than 50 percent of all cancers —is the **p53 gene**. This gene encodes a transcription factor that represses or stimulates transcription of more than 50 different genes.

Normally, the p53 protein is continuously synthesized but is rapidly degraded and therefore is present in cells at low levels. In addition, the p53 protein is normally bound to another protein called **MDM2**, which has several effects on p53. The presence of MDM2 on the p53 protein tags p53 for degradation and sequesters the transcriptional activation domain of p53. It also prevents the phosphorylations and acetylations that convert the p53 protein from an inactive to an active form.

Several types of cellular stress events bring about rapid increases in the nuclear levels of activated p53 protein. These include chemical damage to DNA, double-stranded breaks in DNA induced by ionizing radiation, and the presence of DNA-repair intermediates generated by exposure of cells to ultraviolet light. In response to these signals, MDM2 dissociates from p53, making p53 more stable and unmasking its transcription activation domain. Increases in the levels of activated p53 protein also result from increases in protein phosphorylation, acetylation, and other posttranslational modifications (**Figure 19–10**). Activated p53 protein acts as a transcription factor that

(a) p53 in unstressed cells

(b) After DNA damage and cell stress

FIGURE 19–10 Steps in the regulation of p53 levels and activity. (a) In normal unstressed cells, p53 is kept inactive and at low abundance by MDM2, which binds to the transactivation domain (TAD) and stimulates the addition of ubiquitin onto lysine residues in the carboxy-terminal domain (CTD). The presence of ubiquitin promotes p53 degradation. (b) After various types of cellular stress including DNA damage, cellular kinases add phosphates (P's) to serines and threonines in the TAD, leading to dissociation of MDM2 and subsequent loss of ubiquitin. As the levels of p53 increase in the nucleus, acetyl transferases add acetyl groups (A's) to lysines in the CTD, which increases p53 stability and affinity for specific DNA sequences within the promoter regions of target genes. Examples of genes that are transcriptionally stimulated by p53 are *p21* (leading to G1/S cell cycle arrest), *BAX* (stimulating apoptosis), *GADD45* (contributing to DNA repair), and *MDM2* (returning p53 to an inactive and low abundance state).

stimulates expression of the *MDM2* gene. As the levels of MDM2 increase, p53 protein is again bound by MDM2, returned to an inactive state, and targeted for degradation, in a negative feedback loop.

The activated p53 protein initiates several different responses to DNA damage including cell-cycle arrest followed by DNA repair and apoptosis if DNA cannot be repaired. These responses are accomplished by p53 acting as a transcription factor that stimulates or represses the expression of genes involved in each response.

In normal cells, activated p53 can arrest the cell cycle at the G1/S and G2/M checkpoints, as well as retarding the progression of the cell through S phase. To arrest the cell cycle at the G1/S checkpoint, activated p53 protein stimulates transcription of a gene encoding the p21 protein. The p21 protein inhibits the CDK4/cyclin D1 complex, hence preventing the cell from moving from G1 phase into S phase. Activated p53 protein also regulates expression of genes that retard the progress of DNA replication, thus allowing time for DNA damage to be repaired during S phase. By regulating expression of other genes, activated p53 can block cells at the G2/M checkpoint, if DNA damage occurs during S phase.

Activated p53 can also instruct a damaged cell to commit suicide by apoptosis. It does so by activating the transcription of the *Bax* gene and repressing transcription of the *Bcl2* gene. In normal cells, the BAX protein is present in a heterodimer with the Bcl2 protein, and the cell remains viable (Figure 19–8). But when the levels of BAX protein increase in response to p53 stimulation of *Bax* gene transcription, BAX homodimers are formed, and these homodimers activate the cellular changes that lead to apoptosis. In cancer cells that lack functional p53, BAX protein levels do not increase in response to cell damage, and apoptosis may not occur.

Cells lacking functional p53 are unable to arrest at cell-cycle checkpoints or to enter apoptosis in response to DNA damage. As a result, they move unchecked through the cell cycle, regardless of the condition of the cell's DNA. Cells lacking p53 have high mutation rates and accumulate the types of mutations that lead to cancer. Because of the importance of the *p53* gene to genomic integrity, it is often referred to as the "guardian of the genome."

The *RB1* Tumor-Suppressor Gene

The loss or mutation of the *RB1* (**retinoblastoma 1**) tumor-suppressor gene contributes to the development of many cancers, including those of the breast, bone, lung, and bladder. The *RB1* gene was originally identified as a result of studies on **retinoblastoma**, an inherited disorder in which tumors develop in the eyes of young children. Retinoblastoma occurs with a frequency of about 1 in 15,000 individuals. In the familial form of the disease, individuals

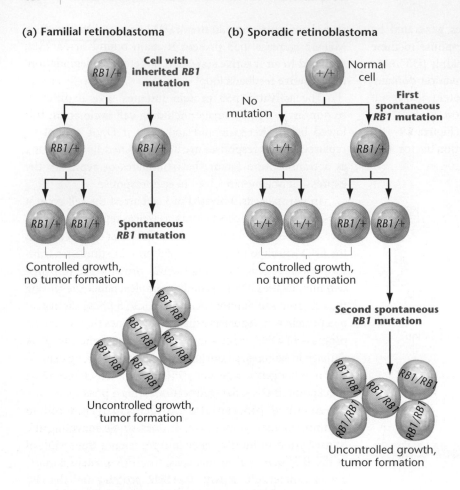

(a) Familial retinoblastoma

Cell with inherited *RB1* mutation

RB1/+

RB1/+   *RB1/+*

No mutation

RB1/+   *RB1/+*

Controlled growth, no tumor formation

Spontaneous *RB1* mutation

RB1/RB1

Uncontrolled growth, tumor formation

(b) Sporadic retinoblastoma

Normal cell

+/+

No mutation

First spontaneous *RB1* mutation

+/+   *RB1/+*

+/+   *+/+*   *RB1/+*   *RB1/+*

Controlled growth, no tumor formation

Second spontaneous *RB1* mutation

RB1/RB1

Uncontrolled growth, tumor formation

FIGURE 19–11 (a) In familial retinoblastoma, one mutation (designated as *RB1*) is inherited and present in all cells. A second mutation at the retinoblastoma locus in any retinal cell contributes to uncontrolled cell growth and tumor formation. (b) In sporadic retinoblastoma, independent mutations in both alleles of the retinoblastoma gene within a single cell are acquired sequentially, also leading to tumor formation.

inherit one mutated allele of the *RB1* gene and have an 85 percent chance of developing retinoblastomas as well as an increased chance of developing other cancers. All somatic cells of patients with hereditary retinoblastoma contain one mutated allele of the *RB1* gene. However, it is only when the second normal allele of the *RB1* gene is lost or mutated in certain retinal cells that retinoblastoma develops. In individuals who do not have this hereditary condition, retinoblastoma is extremely rare, as it requires at least two separate somatic mutations in a retinal cell in order to inactivate both copies of the *RB1* gene (**Figure 19–11**).

The **retinoblastoma protein (pRB)** is a tumor-suppressor protein that controls the G1/S cell-cycle checkpoint. The pRB protein is found in the nuclei of all cell types at all stages of the cell cycle. However, its activity varies throughout the cell cycle, depending on its phosphorylation state. When cells are in the G0 phase of the cell cycle, the pRB protein is nonphosphorylated and binds to transcription factors such as E2F, inactivating them (**Figure 19–12**). When the cell is stimulated by growth factors, it enters G1 and approaches S phase. Throughout the G1 phase, the pRB protein becomes phosphorylated by the CDK4/cyclin D1 complex. Phosphorylated pRB releases its bound regulatory proteins. When E2F and other regulators

FIGURE 19–12 During G0 and early G1, pRB interacts with and inactivates transcription factor E2F. As the cell moves from G1 to S phase, a CDK4/cyclin D1 complex forms and adds phosphate groups to pRB. As pRB becomes phosphorylated, E2F is released and becomes transcriptionally active, allowing the cell to pass through S phase. Phosphorylation of pRB is transitory; as CDK/cyclin complexes are degraded and the cell moves through the cell cycle to early G1, pRB phosphorylation declines, allowing pRB to reassociate with E2F.

are released by pRB, they are free to induce the expression of over 30 genes whose products are required for the transition from G1 into S phase. After cells traverse S, G2, and M phases, pRB reverts to a nonphosphorylated state, binds to regulatory proteins such as E2F, and keeps them sequestered until required for the next cell cycle. In normal quiescent cells, the presence of the pRB protein prevents passage into S phase. In many cancer cells, including retinoblastoma cells, both copies of the *RB1* gene are defective, inactive, or absent, and progression through the cell cycle is not regulated.

NOW SOLVE THIS

19–2 People with a genetic condition known as Li–Fraumeni syndrome inherit one mutant copy of the *p53* gene. These people have a high risk of developing a number of different cancers, such as breast cancer, leukemia, bone cancer, adrenocortical tumors, and brain tumors. Explain how mutations in one cancer-related gene can give rise to such a diverse range of tumors.

■ **HINT:** *This problem involves an understanding of how tumor-suppressor genes regulate cell growth and behavior. The key to its solution is to consider which cellular functions are regulated by the p53 protein and how the absence of p53 could affect each of these functions. Also, read about loss of heterozygosity in Section 19.6.*

For more practice, see Problems 25, 26, and 27.

19.5 Cancer Cells Metastasize and Invade Other Tissues

As discussed at the beginning of this chapter, uncontrolled growth alone is insufficient to create a malignant and life-threatening cancer. Cancer cells must also become malignant, acquiring the ability to disengage from the original tumor site, to enter the blood or lymphatic system, to invade surrounding tissues, and to develop into secondary tumors. In order to leave the site of the primary tumor and invade other tissues, tumor cells must dissociate from the primary tumor and secrete proteases that digest components of the **extracellular matrix** and **basal lamina**, which normally surround and separate the body's tissues. The extracellular matrix and basal lamina are composed of proteins and carbohydrates. They surround and separate body tissues, form the scaffold for tissue growth, and inhibit the migration of cells. The ability to invade the extracellular matrix is also a property of some normal cell types. For example, implantation of the embryo in the uterine wall

during pregnancy requires cell migration across the extracellular matrix. In addition, white blood cells reach sites of infection by penetrating capillary walls. The mechanisms of invasion are probably similar in these normal cells and in cancer cells. The difference is that, in normal cells, the invasive ability is tightly regulated, whereas in tumor cells, this regulation has been lost.

Once cancer cells have disengaged from the primary tumor and traversed tissue barriers, they enter the blood or lymphatic system and may become lodged in microvessels of other tissues. At this point the cells may undergo a second round of invasion to enter the new tissue and grow into new (metastatic) tumors. Only a small percentage of circulating cancer cells—about 0.01 percent—survive to establish metastatic tumors. Other important features of metastatic cells are increased cell motility, the capacity to stimulate new blood vessel formation, and the ability to escape detection by the host's immune system.

Metastasis is controlled by a large number of gene products, including cell-adhesion molecules, cytoskeleton regulators, and proteolytic enzymes. For example, epithelial tumors have a lower than normal level of the **E-cadherin glycoprotein**, which is responsible for cell–cell adhesion in normal tissues. Also, proteolytic enzymes such as **metalloproteinases** are present at higher than normal levels in many highly malignant tumors. For example, breast cancer cells that metastasize to bone abnormally express the metalloproteinase gene *MMP1*. Those that spread to the lungs overexpress the *MMP1* and *MMP2* genes. It has been shown that the level of aggressiveness of a tumor correlates positively with the levels of proteolytic enzymes expressed by the tumor. In addition, malignant cells are not susceptible to the normal controls conferred by regulatory molecules such as **tissue inhibitors of metalloproteinases (TIMPs)**.

Like the tumor-suppressor genes that are mutated in primary cancers, **metastasis-suppressor genes** are mutated or disrupted in metastatic tumors. Less than a dozen of these metastasis-suppressor genes have been identified so far, but all appear to affect the growth and development of metastatic tumors and not the primary tumor. One example is the CD82 protein, encoded by the *CD82* gene. This protein normally inhibits functions related to metastasis such as invasiveness and cell motility. It does this by directly interacting with proteins involved in these functions. In metastatic tumors, the expression of *CD82* is reduced or lost. The expression of *CD82* and other metastasis-suppressor genes is reduced by epigenetic mechanisms rather than by mutation. This observation provides hope that researchers can develop antimetastasis therapies that target the epigenetic silencing of metastasis-suppressor genes.

19.6 Predisposition to Some Cancers Can Be Inherited

Although the vast majority of human cancers are sporadic, a small fraction (approximately 5 percent) have a hereditary or familial component. At present, about 50 forms of hereditary cancer are known (Table 19.2).

Most inherited cancer-susceptibility alleles occur in tumor-suppressor genes, and though transmitted in a Mendelian dominant fashion, are not sufficient in themselves to trigger development of a cancer. At least one other somatic mutation in the other copy of the gene must occur in order to drive a cell toward tumorigenesis. In addition, mutations in still other genes are usually necessary to fully express the cancer phenotype. As mentioned earlier, inherited mutations in the *RB1* gene predispose individuals to developing various cancers. Although the normal somatic cells of these patients are heterozygous for the *RB1* mutation, cells within their tumors contain mutations in both copies of the gene. The phenomenon whereby the second, wild-type, allele is mutated in a tumor is known as **loss of heterozygosity**. Although loss of heterozygosity is an essential first step in expression of these inherited cancers, further mutations in other proto-oncogenes, tumor-suppressor genes, or chromatin-modifying genes are necessary for the tumor cells to become fully malignant.

The development of hereditary colon cancer illustrates how inherited mutations in one allele of a gene contribute only one step in the multistep pathway leading to malignancy. In Section 19.1, we described how colorectal cancers develop through the accumulation of mutations in several genes, leading to a stepwise clonal expansion of cells and the development of carcinomas. Although the vast majority of colorectal cancers are sporadic, about 1 percent of cases result from a genetic predisposition to cancer known as **familial adenomatous polyposis (FAP)**. In FAP, individuals inherit one mutant copy of the *APC* (adenomatous polyposis) gene located on the long arm of chromosome 5. Mutations include deletions, frameshift, and point mutations. The normal function of the *APC* gene product is to act as a tumor suppressor controlling growth and differentiation. The presence of a heterozygous *APC* mutation causes the epithelial cells of the colon to partially escape cell-cycle control, and the cells divide to form small clusters of cells called **polyps** or adenomas. People who are heterozygous for this condition develop hundreds to thousands of colon and rectal polyps early in life. Although it is not necessary for the second allele of the *APC* gene to be mutated in polyps at this stage, in the majority of cases, the second *APC* allele becomes mutant in a later stage of cancer development. The remaining steps in development of colorectal carcinoma follow the same order as that shown in Figure 19–2.

NOW SOLVE THIS

19–3 Although tobacco smoking is responsible for a large number of human cancers, not all smokers develop cancer. Similarly, some people who inherit mutations in the tumor-suppressor genes *p53* or *RB1* never develop cancer. Explain these observations.

■ **HINT:** *This problem asks you to consider the reasons why only some people develop cancer as a result of environmental factors or mutations in tumor-suppressor genes. The key to its solution is to consider the steps involved in the development of cancer and the number of abnormal functions in cancer cells. Also, consider how genetics may affect DNA repair functions.*

19.7 Viruses Contribute to Cancer in Both Humans and Animals

Viruses that cause cancer in animals have played a significant role in the search for knowledge about the genetics of human cancer. Most cancer-causing animal viruses are RNA viruses known as **retroviruses**. In humans, most of the known cancer viruses are DNA viruses.

To understand how retroviruses cause cancer in animals, it is necessary to know how these viruses replicate in cells. When a retrovirus infects a cell, its RNA genome is copied into DNA by the **reverse transcriptase** enzyme, which is brought into the cell with the infecting virus. The DNA copy then enters the nucleus of the infected cell, where it integrates at random into the host cell's genome. The integrated DNA copy

TABLE 19.2 Some Inherited Predispositions to Cancer

Tumor Predisposition Syndrome	Chromosome	Gene Affected
Early-onset familial breast cancer	17q	BRCA1
Familial adenomatous polyposis	5q	APC
Familial melanoma	9p	CDKN2
Gorlin syndrome	9q	PTCH1
Hereditary nonpolyposis colon cancer	2p	MSH2, 6
Li-Fraumeni syndrome	17p	p53
Multiple endocrine neoplasia, type 1	11q	MEN1
Multiple endocrine neoplasia, type 2	10q	RET
Neurofibromatosis, type 1	17q	NF1
Neurofibromatosis, type 2	22q	NF2
Retinoblastoma	13q	pRb
Von Hippel–Lindau syndrome	3p	VHL
Wilms tumor	11p	WT1

FIGURE 19–13 The genome of a typical retrovirus is shown at the top of the diagram. The genome contains repeats at the termini (R), the U5 and U3 regions that contain promoter and enhancer elements, and the three major genes that encode viral structural proteins (*gag* and *env*) and the viral reverse transcriptase (*pol*). RNA transcripts of the entire viral genome comprise the new viral genomes. If the retrovirus acquires all or part of a host-cell proto-oncogene (*c-onc*), this gene (now known as a *v-onc*) is expressed along with the viral genes, leading to overexpression or inappropriate expression of the *v-onc* gene. The *v-onc* gene may also acquire mutations that enhance its transforming ability.

of the retroviral RNA is called a **provirus**. The proviral DNA contains powerful enhancer and promoter elements in its U5 and U3 sequences at the ends of the provirus (**Figure 19–13**). The proviral promoter uses the host cell's transcription proteins, directing transcription of the viral genes (*gag, pol,* and *env*). The products of these genes are the proteins and RNA genomes that make up the new retroviral particles. Because the provirus is integrated into the host genome, it is replicated along with the host's DNA during the cell's normal cell cycle. A retrovirus may not kill a cell, but it may continue to use the cell as a factory to replicate more viruses that will then infect surrounding cells.

A retrovirus may cause cancer in three different ways. First, the proviral DNA may integrate by chance near one of the cell's normal proto-oncogenes. The strong promoters and enhancers in the provirus then stimulate high levels or inappropriate timing of transcription of the proto-oncogene, leading to stimulation of host-cell proliferation. Second, a retrovirus may pick up a copy of a host proto-oncogene and integrate it into its genome (Figure 19–13). The cellular proto-oncogene may be mutated during the process of transfer into the virus, or it may be expressed at abnormal levels because it is now under the control of viral promoters. Retroviruses that carry these cell-derived oncogenes can infect and transform normal cells into tumor cells, and are known as **acute transforming retroviruses**. Through the study of many acute transforming viruses of animals, scientists have identified dozens of proto-oncogenes. Third, a retrovirus may contain a normal viral gene whose product can either stimulate the cell cycle or act as a gene-expression regulator for both cellular and viral genes. As a result, expression of such a viral gene may lead to inappropriate cell growth or to abnormal expression of cancer-related cellular genes.

So far, no acute transforming retroviruses have been identified in humans; however, several human retroviruses, such as **human immunodeficiency virus (HIV)** and the **human**

T-cell leukemia virus (HTLV-1), are associated with human cancers. These retroviruses are thought to stimulate cancer development through the third mechanism, described in the previous paragraph.

DNA viruses also contribute to the development of human cancers in a variety of ways. Because viruses are composed solely of a nucleic acid genome surrounded by a protein coat, they must utilize the host cell's biosynthetic machinery in order to reproduce themselves. To access the host's DNA-synthesizing enzymes, viruses require the host cell to be in an actively growing state. Thus, many DNA viruses contain genes encoding products that stimulate the cell cycle. These products often interact with tumor-suppressor proteins, inactivating them. If the host cell survives the infection, it may lose control of the cell cycle and begin its journey to carcinogenesis.

It is thought that, worldwide, about 15 percent of human cancers are associated with viruses, making virus infection the second greatest risk factor for cancer, next to tobacco smoking. The most significant contributors to virus-induced cancers are listed in Table 19.3. Like other risk factors for cancer, including hereditary predisposition

TABLE 19.3 Human Viruses Associated with Cancers

Virus		Associated Cancers
DNA Viruses		
Epstein-Barr virus	EBV	Burkitt lymphoma, nasopharyngeal carcinoma, Hodgkin lymphoma
Hepatitis B virus	HBV	Hepatocellular carcinoma
Hepatitis C virus	HCV	Hepatocellular carcinoma, non-Hodgkin lymphoma
Human papilloma viruses 16, 18	HPV16, 18	Cervical cancer, ano-genital cancers, oral cancers
Kaposi sarcoma-associated herpesvirus	KSHV	Kaposi sarcoma, primary effusion lymphoma
Retroviruses		
Human T-cell lymphotropic virus type 1	HTLV-1	Adult T-cell leukemia and lymphoma
Human immunodeficiency virus type-1	HIV-1	Immune suppression, leading to cancers caused by other viruses (KSHV, EBV, HPV)

to certain cancers, virus infection alone is not sufficient to trigger human cancers. Other factors, including DNA damage or the accumulation of mutations in one or more of a cell's oncogenes and tumor-suppressor genes, are required to move a cell down the multistep pathway to cancer.

19.8 Environmental Agents Contribute to Human Cancers

Any substance or event that damages DNA has the potential to be carcinogenic. Unrepaired or inaccurately repaired DNA introduces mutations, which, if they occur in proto-oncogenes or tumor-suppressor genes, can lead to abnormal regulation of the cell cycle or disruption of controls over apoptosis or metastasis.

Our environment, both natural and human-made, contains abundant carcinogens. These include chemicals, radiation, some viruses, and chronic infections. Perhaps the most significant carcinogen in our environment is tobacco smoke, which contains at least 60 chemicals that interact with DNA and cause mutations. Epidemiologists estimate that about 30 percent of human cancer deaths are associated with cigarette smoking. Smokers have a 20-fold increased risk of developing lung cancer, which kills more than one million people, worldwide, each year.

Diet is often implicated in the development of cancer. Consumption of red meat and animal fat is associated with some cancers, such as colon, prostate, and breast cancer. The mechanisms by which these substances may contribute to carcinogenesis may involve stimulation of cell division through hormones or creation of carcinogenic chemicals during cooking. Alcohol may cause inflammation of the liver and contribute to liver cancer.

Although most people perceive the human-made, industrial environment to be a highly significant contributor to cancer, it may account for only a small percentage of total cancers, and only in special situations. Some of the most mutagenic agents, and hence potentially the most carcinogenic, are natural substances and natural processes. For example, **aflatoxin**, a component of a mold that grows on peanuts and corn, is one of the most carcinogenic chemicals known. Most chemical carcinogens, such as **nitrosamines**, are components of synthetic substances and are found in some preserved meats; however, many are naturally occurring. For example, natural pesticides and antibiotics found in plants may be carcinogenic, and the human body itself creates alkylating agents in the acidic environment of the gut. Nevertheless, these observations do not diminish the serious cancer risks to specific populations who are exposed to human-made carcinogens such as synthetic pesticides or asbestos.

DNA lesions brought about by natural radiation (X rays, ultraviolet light), dietary substances, and substances in the external environment contribute the majority of environmentally caused mutations that lead to cancer. In addition, normal metabolism creates oxidative end products that can damage DNA, proteins, and lipids. It is estimated that the human body suffers about 10,000 damaging DNA lesions per day due to the actions of oxygen free radicals. DNA repair enzymes deal successfully with most of this damage; however, some damage may lead to permanent mutations. The process of DNA replication itself is mutagenic. Hence, substances such as growth factors or hormones that stimulate cell division are ultimately mutagenic and perhaps carcinogenic. Chronic inflammation due to infection also stimulates tissue repair and cell division, resulting in DNA lesions accumulating during replication. These mutations may persist, particularly if cell-cycle checkpoints are compromised due to mutations or inactivation of tumor-suppressor genes such as *p53* or *RB1*.

Both ultraviolet (UV) light and ionizing radiation (such as X rays and gamma rays) induce DNA damage. UV in sunlight is well accepted as an inducer of skin cancers. Ionizing radiation has clearly shown itself to be a carcinogen in studies of populations exposed to neutron and gamma radiation from atomic blasts such as those in Hiroshima and Nagasaki. Another significant environmental component, radon gas, may be responsible for about 50 percent of the ionizing radiation exposure of the U.S. population and could contribute to lung cancers in some populations.

NOW SOLVE THIS

19–4 Cancer can arise spontaneously, but can also be induced as a result of environmental factors such as sun exposure, infections, and tobacco smoking. If you were asked to help allocate resources to cancer research, what emphasis would you place on research to find cancer cures, compared to that placed on education about cancer prevention?

■ **HINT:** *This problem asks you to consider the outcomes of two different approaches to cancer research. The key to its solution is to think about the relative rates of environmentally induced and spontaneous cancers. (An interesting source of information on this topic is Ames, B. N. et al. 1995. The causes and prevention of cancer. Proc. Natl. Acad. Sci. USA 92: 5258–5265.)*

The Cancer Genome Anatomy Project (CGAP)

MasteringGenetics™ Visit the
Study Area: Exploring Genomics

A research group headed by Dr. Victor Velculescu of Johns Hopkins University reported that breast and colon cancers contain about 11 gene mutations that may contribute to the cancer phenotype. The research group analyzed 13,023 of the 21,000 known genes in the human genome, comparing the DNA sequences from normal cells and cancer cells. Most of the mutations that were specific to cancer cells were not previously known to be associated with cancer.

Dr. Velculescu's study was one of the first in *The Cancer Genome Atlas (TCGA)* project, a $1.5 billion federal project designed to systematically scan the human genome to find genes that are mutated in many different cancers. In this exercise, we will explore aspects of Dr. Velculescu's research by mining information available in the online database **Cancer Genome Anatomy Project (CGAP)**. The purpose of the CGAP is to understand the expression profiles of genes from normal, precancer, and cancer cells.

■ **Exercise – Colon Cancer and the *TBX22* Gene**

One gene that Dr. Velculescu's research group discovered to be mutated in colon cancers—*TBX22*—was not previously suspected to contribute to this cancer. What is *TBX22*, and how do you think a mutated *TBX22* gene would contribute to the development of colon cancer?

1. To begin your search for the answers, go to CGAP at http://cgap.nci.nih .gov/cgap.html.

2. Click the "Genes" button near the top of the page.

3. From the list of "Gene Tools" in the left-hand margin, select "Gene Finder."

4. Select "Homo sapiens" in the "Select organism" box, and type TBX22 in the "Enter a unique identifier" box. Submit the query.

5. Select "Gene Info" in the right-hand column of the table.

6. Explore the many sources of information about *TBX22* from various database links listed on this page.

Prepare a brief written or verbal report on what you learned during your explorations and which sources you used to reach your conclusions about *TBX22*.

CASE STUDY | I thought it was safe

A middle-aged woman taking the breast cancer drug Tamoxifen for ten years became concerned when she saw a news report with disturbing information. In some women, the drug made their cancer more aggressive and more likely to spread. Other women with breast cancer, the report stated, do not respond to Tamoxifen at all, and 30 to 40 percent of women who take the drug eventually become resistant to chemotherapy. The woman contacted her oncologist to ask some questions:

1. How can some people react one way to a cancer treatment and others react a different way?

2. Why do most cancers eventually become resistant to a specific chemotherapeutic drug?

3. Why does it seem that some drugs are thought to be safe one day and declared unsafe the next day?

Summary Points

MasteringGenetics™ For activities, animations, and review quizzes, go to the Study Area.

1. Cancer cells show two fundamental properties: abnormal cell proliferation and a propensity to spread and invade other parts of the body.

2. Cancers are clonal, meaning that all cells within a tumor originate from a single cell that contained a number of mutations.

3. The development of cancer is a multistep process, requiring mutations in several cancer-related genes.

4. Cancer cells contain gene mutations, chromosomal abnormalities, genomic instability, and abnormal patterns of chromatin modifications.

5. Cancer cells have defects in DNA damage repair, chromatin modifications, cell-cycle regulation, and programmed cell death.

6. Proto-oncogenes are normal genes that promote cell growth and division. When proto-oncogenes are mutated or misexpressed in cancer cells, they are known as oncogenes.

7. Tumor-suppressor genes normally regulate cell-cycle checkpoints and apoptosis. When tumor-suppressor genes are mutated or inactivated, cells cannot correct DNA damage. This leads to accumulations of mutations that may cause cancer.

8. The ability of cancer cells to metastasize requires defects in gene products that control a number of functions such as cell adhesion, proteolysis, and tissue invasion.

9. Inherited mutations in cancer-susceptibility genes are not sufficient to trigger cancer. Other somatic mutations in proto-oncogenes or tumor-suppressor genes are necessary for the development of hereditary cancers.

10. Tumor viruses contribute to cancers by introducing viral oncogenes, interfering with tumor-suppressor proteins, or altering expression of a cell's proto-oncogenes.

11. Environmental agents such as chemicals, radiation, viruses, and chronic infections contribute to the development of cancer. The most significant environmental factors that affect human cancers are tobacco smoke, chronic infections, diet, and natural radiation.

INSIGHTS AND SOLUTIONS

1. In disorders such as retinoblastoma, a mutation in one allele of the *RB1* gene can be inherited from the germ line, causing an autosomal dominant predisposition to the development of eye tumors. To develop tumors, a somatic mutation in the second copy of the *RB1* gene is necessary, indicating that the mutation itself acts as a recessive trait. Given that the first mutation can be inherited, in what ways can a second mutational event occur?

Solution: In considering how this second mutation arises, we must look at several types of mutational events, including changes in nucleotide sequence and events that involve whole chromosomes or chromosome parts. Retinoblastoma results when both copies of the *RB1* locus are lost or inactivated. With this in mind, you must first list the phenomena that can result in a mutational loss or the inactivation of a gene.

One way the second *RB1* mutation can occur is by a nucleotide alteration that converts the remaining normal *RB1* allele to a mutant form. This alteration can occur through a nucleotide substitution or through a frameshift mutation caused by the insertion or deletion of nucleotides during replication. A second mechanism involves the loss of the chromosome carrying the normal allele. This event would take place during mitosis, resulting in chromosome 13 monosomy and leaving the mutant copy of the gene as the only *RB1* allele. This mechanism does not necessarily involve loss of the entire chromosome; deletion of the long arm (*RB1* is on 13q) or an interstitial deletion involving the *RB1* locus and some surrounding material would have the same result. Alternatively, a chromosome aberration involving loss of the normal copy of the *RB1* gene might be followed by duplication of the chromosome carrying the mutant allele. Two copies of chromosome 13 would be restored to the cell, but the normal *RB1* allele would not be present. Finally, a recombination event followed by chromosome segregation could produce a homozygous combination of mutant *RB1* alleles.

2. Proto-oncogenes can be converted to oncogenes in a number of different ways. In some cases, the proto-oncogene itself becomes amplified up to hundreds of times in a cancer cell. An example is the *cyclin D1* gene, which is amplified in some

cancers. In other cases, the proto-oncogene may be mutated in a limited number of specific ways, leading to alterations in the gene product's structure. The *ras* gene is an example of a proto-oncogene that becomes oncogenic after suffering point mutations in specific regions of the gene. Explain why these two proto-oncogenes (*cyclin D1* and *ras*) undergo such different alterations in order to convert them into oncogenes.

Solution: The first step in solving this question is to understand the normal functions of these proto-oncogenes and to think about how either amplification or mutation would affect each of these functions.

The cyclin D1 protein regulates progression of the cell cycle from G1 into S phase, by binding to CDK4 and activating this kinase. The cyclin D1/CDK4 complex phosphorylates a number of proteins including pRB, which in turn activate other proteins in a cascade that results in transcription of genes whose products are necessary for DNA replication in S phase. The simplest way to increase the activity of cyclin D1 would be to increase the number of cyclin D1 molecules available for binding to the cell's endogenous CDK4 molecules. This can be accomplished by several mechanisms, including amplification of the *cyclin D1* gene. In contrast, a point mutation in the *cyclin D1* gene would most likely interfere with the ability of the cyclin D1 protein to bind to CDK4; hence, mutations within the gene would probably repress cell-cycle progression rather than stimulate it.

The *ras* gene product is a signal transduction protein that operates as an on/off switch in response to external stimulation by growth factors. It does so by binding either GTP (the "on" state) or GDP (the "off" state). Oncogenic mutations in the *ras* gene occur in specific regions that alter the ability of the Ras protein to exchange GDP for GTP. Oncogenic Ras proteins are locked in the "on" conformation, bound to GTP. In this way, they constantly stimulate the cell to divide. An amplification of the *ras* gene would simply provide more molecules of normal Ras protein, which would still be capable of on/off regulation. Hence, simple amplification of *ras* would less likely be oncogenic.

Problems and Discussion Questions

MasteringGenetics™ Visit for instructor-assigned tutorials and problems.

HOW DO WE KNOW?

1. In this chapter, we focused on cancer as a genetic disease, with an emphasis on the relationship between cancer, the cell cycle, and DNA damage, as well as on the multiple steps that lead to cancer.

At the same time, we found many opportunities to consider the methods and reasoning by which much of this information was acquired. From the explanations given in the chapter,

(a) How do we know that malignant tumors arise from a single cell that contains mutations?

(b) How do we know that cancer development requires more than one mutation?

(c) How do we know that cancer cells contain defects in DNA repair?

CONCEPT QUESTION

2. Review the Chapter Concepts list on page 469. These concepts relate to the multiple ways in which genetic alterations lead to the development of cancers. The sixth concept states that epigenetic effects including DNA methylation and histone modifications contribute to the genetic alterations leading to cancer. Write a short essay describing how epigenetic changes in cancer cells contribute to the development of cancers.

3. Where are the major regulatory points in the cell cycle?

4. List the functions of kinases and cyclins, and describe how they interact to cause cells to move through the cell cycle.

5. (a) How does pRB function to keep cells at the G1 checkpoint? (b) How do cells get past the G1 checkpoint to move into S phase?

6. What is the difference between saying that cancer is inherited and saying that the predisposition to cancer is inherited?

7. As a genetic counselor, you are asked to assess the risk for a couple with a family history of retinoblastoma who are thinking about having children. Both the husband and wife are phenotypically normal, but the husband has a sister with familial retinoblastoma in both eyes. What is the probability that this couple will have a child with retinoblastoma? Are there any tests that you could recommend to help in this assessment?

8. What is apoptosis, and under what circumstances do cells undergo this process?

9. Define tumor-suppressor genes. Why is a mutated single copy of a tumor-suppressor gene expected to behave as a recessive gene?

10. A genetic variant of the retinoblastoma protein, called PSM-RB (phosphorylation site mutated RB), is not able to be phosphorylated by the action of CDK4/cyclin D1 complex. Explain why PSM-RB is said to have a constitutive growth-suppressing action on the cell cycle.

11. Part of the Ras protein is associated with the plasma membrane, and part extends into the cytoplasm. How does the Ras protein transmit a signal from outside the cell into the cytoplasm? What happens in cases where the *ras* gene is mutated?

12. If a cell suffers damage to its DNA while in S phase, how can this damage be repaired before the cell enters mitosis?

13. Distinguish between oncogenes and proto-oncogenes. In what ways can proto-oncogenes be converted to oncogenes?

14. Of the two classes of genes associated with cancer, tumor-suppressor genes and oncogenes, mutations in which group can be considered gain-of-function mutations? In which group are the loss-of-function mutations? Explain.

15. How do translocations such as the Philadelphia chromosome contribute to cancer?

16. Explain why many oncogenic viruses contain genes whose products interact with tumor-suppressor proteins.

17. DNA sequencing has provided data to indicate that cancer cells may contain tens of thousands of somatic mutations, only some of which confer a growth advantage to a cancer cell. How do scientists describe and categorize these recently discovered populations of mutations in cancer cells?

18. How do normal cells protect themselves from accumulating mutations in genes that could lead to cancer? How do cancer cells differ from normal cells in these processes?

19. Describe the difference between an acute transforming virus and a virus that does not cause tumors.

20. Epigenetics is a relatively new area of genetics with a focus on phenomena that affect gene expression but do not affect DNA sequence. Epigenetic effects are quasi-stable and may be passed to progeny somatic or germ-line cells. What are known causes of epigenetic effects, and how do they relate to cancer?

21. Radiotherapy (treatment with ionizing radiation) is one of the most effective current cancer treatments. It works by damaging DNA and other cellular components. In which ways could radiotherapy control or cure cancer, and why does radiotherapy often have significant side effects?

22. Genetic tests that detect mutations in the *BRCA1* and *BRCA2* oncogenes are widely available. These tests reveal a number of mutations in these genes—mutations that have been linked to familial breast cancer. Assume that a young woman in a suspected breast cancer family takes the *BRCA1* and *BRCA2* genetic tests and receives negative results. That is, she does not test positive for the mutant alleles of *BRCA1* or *BRCA2*. Can she consider herself free of risk for breast cancer?

23. Explain the apparent paradox that both hypermethylation and hypomethylation of DNA are often found in the same cancer cell.

24. As part of a cancer research project, you have discovered a gene that is mutated in many metastatic tumors. After determining the DNA sequence of this gene, you compare the sequence with those of other genes in the human genome sequence database. Your gene appears to code for an amino acid sequence that resembles sequences found in some serine proteases. Conjecture how your new gene might contribute to the development of highly invasive cancers.

25. Describe the steps by which the *p53* gene responds to DNA damage and/or cellular stress to promote cell-cycle arrest and apoptosis. Given that *p53* is a recessive gene and is not located on the X chromosome, why would people who inherit just one mutant copy of a recessive tumor-suppressor gene be at higher risk of developing cancer than those without the recessive gene?

Extra-Spicy Problems

MasteringGenetics™ Visit for instructor-assigned tutorials and problems.

26. Mutations in tumor-suppressor genes are associated with many types of cancers. In addition, epigenetic changes (such as DNA methylation) of tumor-suppressor genes are also associated with tumorigenesis (Otani et al., 2013. *Expert Rev Mol Diagn* 13: 445–455).

(a) How might hypermethylation of the *p53* gene promoter influence tumorigenesis?

(b) Knowing that tumors release free DNA into certain surrounding body fluids through necrosis and apoptosis (Kloten et al., 2013. *Breast Cancer Res.* 15(1): R4), outline an experimental protocol for using human blood as a biomarker for cancer and as a method for monitoring the progression of cancer in an individual.

27. Vanderbilt University Medical Center maintains a Web site (http://bioinfo.mc.vanderbilt.edu/TSGene/) that contains descriptions of tumor-suppressor genes, including 637 protein-coding genes and 79 noncoding segments of DNA. How can noncoding segments of DNA function or produce products that function as tumor suppressors?

28. A study by Bose and colleagues (1998. *Blood* 92: 3362–3367) and a previous study by Biernaux and others (1996. *Bone Marrow Transplant* 17: (Suppl. 3) S45–S47) showed that *BCR-ABL* fusion gene transcripts can be detected in 25 to 30 percent of healthy adults who do not develop chronic myelogenous leukemia (CML). Explain how these individuals can carry a fusion gene that is transcriptionally active and yet do not develop CML.

29. Those who inherit a mutant allele of the *RB1* gene are at risk for developing a bone cancer called osteosarcoma. You suspect that in these cases, osteosarcoma requires a mutation in the second *RB1* allele, and you have cultured some osteosarcoma cells and obtained a cDNA clone of a normal human *RB1* gene. A colleague sends you a research paper revealing that a strain of cancer-prone mice develop malignant tumors when injected with osteosarcoma cells, and you obtain these mice. Using these three resources, what experiments would you perform to determine (a) whether osteosarcoma cells carry two *RB1* mutations, (b) whether osteosarcoma cells produce any pRB protein, and (c) if the addition of a normal *RB1* gene will change the cancer-causing potential of osteosarcoma cells?

30. The table in this problem summarizes some of the data that have been collected on *BRCA1* mutations in families with a high incidence of both early-onset breast cancer and ovarian cancer.

Predisposing Mutations in *BRCA1*

Kindred	Codon	Nucleotide Change	Coding Effect	Frequency in Control Chromosomes
1901	24	−11 bp	Frameshift or splice	0/180
2082	1313	C → T	Gln → Stop	0/170
1910	1756	Extra C	Frameshift	0/162
2099	1775	T → G	Met → Arg	0/120
2035	NA*	?	Loss of transcript	NA*

Source: 1994. *Science* 266: 66–71. © AAAS.
*NA indicates not applicable, as the regulatory mutation is inferred, and the position has not been identified.

(a) Note the coding effect of the mutation found in kindred group 2082. This results from a single base-pair substitution. Draw the normal double-stranded DNA sequence for this codon (with the 5′ and 3′ ends labeled), and show the sequence of events that generated this mutation, assuming that it resulted from an uncorrected mismatch event during DNA replication.
(b) Examine the types of mutations that are listed in the table and determine if the *BRCA1* gene is likely to be a tumor-suppressor gene or an oncogene.

(c) Although the mutations listed in the table are clearly deleterious and cause breast cancer in women at very young ages, each of the kindred groups had at least one woman who carried the mutation but lived until age 80 without developing cancer. Name at least two different mechanisms (or variables) that could underlie variation in the expression of a mutant phenotype and propose an explanation for the incomplete penetrance of this mutation. How do these mechanisms or variables relate to this explanation?

31. The following table shows neutral polymorphisms found in control families (those with no increased frequency of breast and ovarian cancer).

Neutral Polymorphisms in *BRCA1*

Name	Codon Location	Base in Codon†	Frequency in Control Chromosomes* A	C	G	T
PM1	317	2	152	0	10	0
PM6	878	2	0	55	0	100
PM7	1190	2	109	0	53	0
PM2	1443	3	0	115	0	58
PM3	1619	1	116	0	52	0

*The number of chromosomes with a particular base at the indicated polymorphic site (A, C, G, or T) is shown.
†Position 1, 2, or 3 of the codon.

Examine the data in the table and answer the following questions:
(a) What is meant by a neutral polymorphism?
(b) What is the significance of this table in the context of examining a family or population for *BRCA1* mutations that predispose an individual to cancer?
(c) Is the PM2 polymorphism likely to result in a neutral missense mutation or a silent mutation?
(d) Answer part (c) for the PM3 polymorphism.

32. Prostate cancer is a major cause of cancer-related deaths among men. Epigenetic changes that regulate gene expression are involved in both the initiation and progression of such cancers. Following is a table that lists the number of genes known to be hypermethylated in prostate cancer cells (modified from Long-Cheng, L. et al., 2005. *J. Natl. Cancer Inst.* 97: 103–115). For each category of genes, speculate on the mechanism(s) by which cancer initiation or progression might be influenced by hypermethylation.

DNA Hypermethylation of	Number of Known Genes
Hormonal response genes	5
Cell-cycle control genes	2
Tumor cell invasion genes	8
DNA damage repair genes	2
Signal transduction genes	4

A researcher examines an agarose gel containing separated DNA fragments stained with the DNA-binding dye ethidium bromide and visualized under ultraviolet light.

20

Recombinant DNA Technology

CHAPTER CONCEPTS

- Recombinant DNA technology creates combinations of DNA sequences from different sources.

- A common application of recombinant DNA technology is to clone a DNA segment of interest.

- For some cloning applications, specific DNA segments are inserted into vectors to create recombinant DNA molecules that are transferred into eukaryotic or prokaryotic host cells, where the recombinant DNA replicates as the host cells divide.

- DNA libraries are collections of cloned DNA and were historically used to isolate specific genes.

- DNA segments can be quickly amplified and cloned millions of times using the polymerase chain reaction (PCR).

- DNA, RNA, and proteins can be analyzed using a range of molecular techniques.

- DNA sequencing reveals the nucleotide composition of cloned DNA, and major improvements in sequencing technologies have rapidly advanced many areas of modern genetics research, particularly genomics.

- Gene knockout methods and transgenic animals have become invaluable for studying gene function *in vivo*.

- Recombinant DNA technology has revolutionized our ability to investigate the genomes of diverse species and has led to the modern revolution in genomics.

I n 1971, a paper published by Kathleen Danna and Daniel Nathans marked the beginning of the recombinant DNA era. The paper described the isolation of an enzyme from a bacterial strain and the use of the enzyme to cleave viral DNA at specific nucleotide sequences. It contained the first published photograph of DNA cut with such an enzyme, now called a restriction enzyme.

Using restriction enzymes and a number of other resources, researchers of the mid- to late 1970s developed various techniques to create, replicate, and analyze **recombinant DNA** molecules—DNA created by joining together pieces of DNA from different sources. The methods used to copy or **clone** DNA, called **recombinant DNA technology** and often known as "gene splicing" in the early days, marked a major advance in research in molecular biology and genetics, allowing scientists to isolate and study specific DNA sequences. For their contributions to the development of this technology, Nathans, Hamilton Smith, and Werner Arber were awarded the 1978 Nobel Prize in Physiology or Medicine.

The power of recombinant DNA technology is astonishing, enabling geneticists to identify and isolate a single gene or DNA segment of interest from a genome. Through cloning, large quantities of identical copies of this specific DNA molecule can be produced. These identical copies, or clones, can then be manipulated for numerous purposes, including conducting research on the structure and organization of the DNA, studying gene expression, studying protein products to understand their structure and function, and producing important commercial products from the protein encoded by a gene. The fundamental techniques involved in recombinant DNA technology subsequently led to the field of genomics, enabling scientists to sequence and analyze entire genomes. Note that some of the topics discussed in this chapter are explored in greater depth later in the text (see Special Topic Chapters 3—DNA Forensics, 5—Genetically Modified Foods, and 6—Gene Therapy). In this chapter, we review basic methods of recombinant DNA technology used to isolate, replicate, and analyze DNA.

20.1 Recombinant DNA Technology Began with Two Key Tools: Restriction Enzymes and DNA Cloning Vectors

Although natural genetic processes such as crossing over produce recombined DNA molecules, the term *recombinant DNA* is generally reserved for molecules produced by artificially joining DNA obtained from different sources. We begin our discussion of recombinant DNA technology by considering two important tools used to construct and amplify recombinant DNA molecules: DNA-cutting enzymes called **restriction enzymes** and **DNA cloning vectors**. The use of restriction enzymes and cloning vectors was largely responsible for advancing the field of molecular biology because a wide range of laboratory techniques are based on recombinant DNA technology.

Restriction Enzymes Cut DNA at Specific Recognition Sequences

Restriction enzymes are produced by bacteria as a defense mechanism against infection by bacteriophage. They restrict or prevent viral infection by degrading the DNA of invading viruses. More than 3500 restriction enzymes have been identified, and over 250 are commercially produced and available for use by researchers. A restriction enzyme recognizes and binds to DNA at a specific nucleotide sequence called a **recognition sequence** or **restriction site** (Figure 20–1). The enzyme then cuts both strands of the DNA within that sequence by cleaving the phosphodiester backbone of DNA. Scientists commonly refer to this as "digestion" of DNA. The usefulness of restriction enzymes in cloning derives from their ability to accurately and reproducibly cut genomic DNA into fragments. Restriction enzymes represent sophisticated molecular scissors for cutting DNA into fragments of desired sizes.

Restriction sites are present randomly in the genome. The number of DNA restriction fragments produced by digesting DNA with a particular enzyme can be estimated from the number of times a given restriction enzyme cuts the DNA. Enzymes with a four-base recognition sequence—such as the enzyme *Alu*I, which recognizes the sequence AGCT—will cut, on average, every 256 base pairs ($4^n = 4^4 = 256$) if all four nucleotides are present in equal proportions,

Enzyme	Recognition Sequence	DNA Fragments Produced	Source Microbe
*Hind*III	A-A-G-C-T-T / T-T-C-G-A-A	A / T-T-C-G-A A-G-C-T-T / A — Cohesive Ends	*Haemophilus influenzae* Rd
*Bam*HI	G-G-A-T-C-C / C-C-T-A-G-G	G / C-C-T-A-G G-A-T-C-C / G — Cohesive Ends	*Bacillus amyloliquefaciens* H
*Alu*I	A-G-C-T / T-C-G-A	A-G / T-C C-T / G-A — Blunt Ends	*Arthrobacter luteus*
*Sau*3AI	G-A-T-C / C-T-A-G	G-A-T-C / C-T-A-G — Cohesive Ends	*Staphylococcus aureus* 3A

FIGURE 20–1 Common restriction enzymes, with their recognition sequence, DNA cutting patterns, and sources. Arrows indicate the location in the DNA cut by each enzyme.

producing many small fragments. The actual fragment sizes produced by DNA digestion with a given restriction enzyme vary because the number and location of recognition sequences are not always distributed randomly in DNA.

Recognition sequences exhibit a form of symmetry described as a **palindrome**: the nucleotide sequence reads the same on both strands of the DNA when read in the 5′ to 3′ direction. Each restriction enzyme recognizes its particular recognition sequence and cuts the DNA in a characteristic cleavage pattern. The most common recognition sequences are four or six nucleotides long, but some contain eight or more nucleotides. Enzymes such as *Eco*RI and *Hind*III make offset cuts in the DNA strands, thus producing fragments with single-stranded overhanging ends called **cohesive ends** (or "sticky" ends), while others such as *Alu*I and *Bal*I cut both strands at the same nucleotide pair, producing DNA fragments with double-stranded ends called **blunt-end** fragments. Four common restriction enzymes, their restriction sites, and source microbes are shown in Figure 20–1.

One of the first restriction enzymes to be identified was isolated from *Escherichia coli* strain R and was designated *Eco*RI. DNA fragments produced by *Eco*RI digestion (**Figure 20–2**) have cohesive ends because they can base-pair with complementary single-stranded ends on other DNA fragments cut using *Eco*RI. When mixed together, single-stranded ends of DNA fragments from different sources cut with the same restriction enzyme can **anneal**, or stick together, by hydrogen bonding of complementary base pairs in single-stranded ends. Addition of the enzyme **DNA ligase**—recall the role of DNA ligase in DNA replication as discussed earlier in the text (see Chapter 11)—to DNA fragments will seal the phosphodiester backbone of DNA to covalently join the fragments together to form recombinant DNA molecules (Figure 20–2).

Scientists often use restriction enzymes that create cohesive ends since the overhanging ends make cloning less technically challenging. Blunt-end ligation is more technically challenging because it is not facilitated by hydrogen bonding, but a scientist can ligate fragments digested at different sequences by different blunt-end generating enzymes.

DNA Vectors Accept and Replicate DNA Molecules to Be Cloned

Scientists recognized that DNA fragments produced by restriction-enzyme digestion could be copied or cloned if they had a technique for replicating the fragments. The second key tool that allowed DNA cloning was the development of **cloning vectors**, DNA molecules that accept DNA fragments and replicate these fragments when vectors are introduced into host cells.

Many different vectors are available for cloning. Vectors differ in terms of the host cells they are able to enter and in the size of DNA fragment inserts they can carry, but most DNA vectors have several key properties.

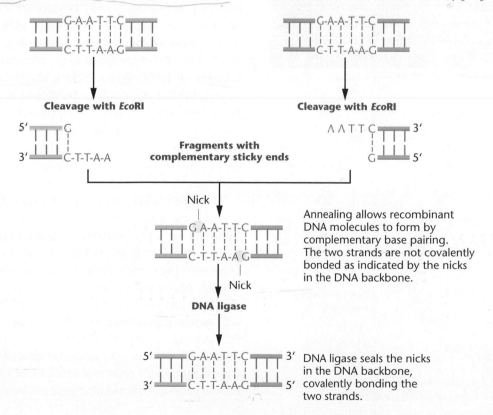

FIGURE 20–2 DNA from different sources is cleaved with *Eco*RI and mixed to allow annealing. The enzyme DNA ligase forms phosphodiester bonds between these fragments to create an intact recombinant DNA molecule.

- A vector contains several restriction sites that allow insertion of the DNA fragments to be cloned.
- Vectors must be capable of replicating in host cells to allow for independent replication of the vector DNA and any DNA fragment it carries.
- To distinguish host cells that have taken up vectors from host cells that have not, the vector should carry a **selectable marker gene** (usually an antibiotic resistance gene or a gene that encodes a protein which produces a visible product, such as color or fluorescent light).
- Many vectors incorporate specific sequences that allow for sequencing inserted DNA.

Bacterial Plasmid Vectors

Genetically modified bacterial **plasmids** were the first vectors developed, and they are still widely used for cloning. Plasmid cloning vectors were derived from naturally occurring

(a)

(b)

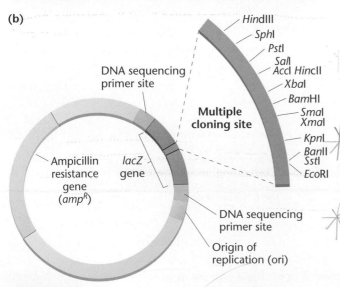

FIGURE 20–3 (a) A color-enhanced electron micrograph of circular plasmid molecules isolated from *E. coli*. Genetically engineered plasmids are used as vectors for cloning DNA. (b) A diagram of a typical DNA cloning plasmid.

plasmids. Recall from earlier discussions (see Chapter 6) that plasmids are extrachromosomal, double-stranded DNA molecules that replicate independently from the chromosomes within bacterial cells [**Figure 20–3(a)**]. Plasmids have been extensively modified by genetic engineering to serve as cloning vectors. Many commercially prepared plasmids are readily available with a range of useful features [**Figure 20–3(b)**]. Plasmids are introduced into bacteria by the process of **transformation** (see Chapter 6). Two main techniques are widely used for bacterial transformation. One approach involves treating cells with calcium ions and using a brief heat shock to pulse DNA into cells. The other technique, called **electroporation**, uses a brief, but high-intensity, pulse of electricity to move DNA into bacterial cells.

Only one or a few plasmids generally enter a bacterial host cell by transformation. Because plasmids have an *origin of replication* (*ori*) that allows for plasmid replication, many plasmids can increase their copy number to produce several hundred copies in a single host cell. These plasmids greatly enhance the number of DNA clones that can be produced. Plasmid vectors have also been genetically engineered to contain a number of restriction sites for commonly used restriction enzymes in a region called the **multiple cloning site**. Multiple cloning sites allow scientists to clone a range of different fragments generated by many commonly used restriction enzymes.

Cloning DNA with a plasmid generally begins by cutting both the plasmid DNA and the DNA to be cloned with the same restriction enzyme (**Figure 20–4**). Typically the plasmid is cut once within the multiple cloning site to produce a linear vector. DNA restriction fragments from the DNA to be cloned are added to the linearized vector in the presence of DNA ligase. Sticky ends of DNA fragments anneal, joining the DNA to be cloned and the plasmid. DNA ligase is then used to create phosphodiester bonds to seal nicks in the DNA backbone, thus producing recombinant DNA, which is then introduced into bacterial host cells by transformation. Once inside the cell, plasmids replicate quickly to produce multiple copies.

However, when cloning DNA using plasmids, not all plasmids will incorporate DNA to be cloned. For example, a plasmid cut with a particular restriction enzyme can close back on itself (self-ligation) if cut ends of the plasmid rejoin. Obviously then, such nonrecombinant plasmids are not desired. Also, during transformation, not all host cells will take up plasmids. Therefore it is important that bacterial cells containing recombinant DNA can be readily identified in a cloning experiment. One way this is accomplished is through the use of selectable marker genes described earlier. Genes that provide resistance to antibiotics such as ampicillin and genes such as the *lacZ* gene are very effective selectable marker genes. **Figure 20–5** provides an example of how these genes can be used to identify bacteria containing

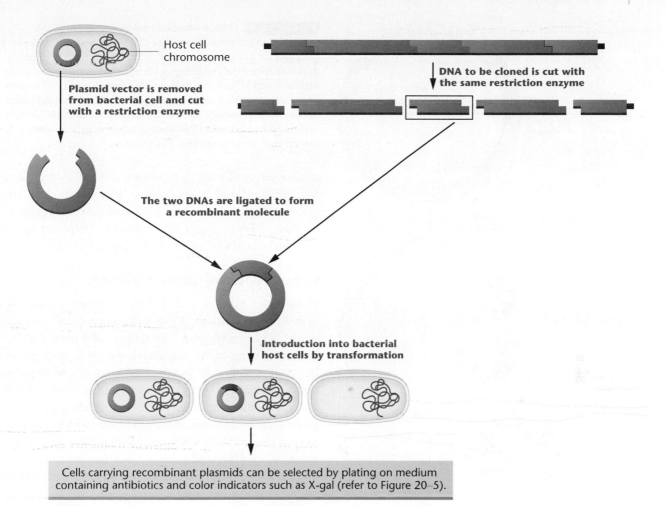

Host cell chromosome

Plasmid vector is removed from bacterial cell and cut with a restriction enzyme

DNA to be cloned is cut with the same restriction enzyme

The two DNAs are ligated to form a recombinant molecule

Introduction into bacterial host cells by transformation

Cells carrying recombinant plasmids can be selected by plating on medium containing antibiotics and color indicators such as X-gal (refer to Figure 20–5).

FIGURE 20–4 Cloning with a plasmid vector involves cutting both plasmid and the DNA to be cloned with the same restriction enzyme. The DNA to be cloned is ligated into the vector and transferred to a bacterial host for replication. Bacterial cells carrying plasmids with DNA inserts can be identified by selection and then isolated. The cloned DNA is then recovered from the bacterial host for further analysis.

recombinant plasmids. This process is often referred to as **"blue-white" selection** for a reason that will soon become obvious. In blue-white selection a plasmid is used that contains the *lacZ* gene incorporated into the multiple cloning site. The *lacZ* gene encodes the enzyme β-galactosidase, which, as you learned earlier in the text (see Chapter 16), is used to cleave the disaccharide lactose into its component monosaccharides glucose and galactose. Blue-white selection takes advantage of the enzymatic activity of β-galactosidase.

Using this approach, one can easily identify transformed bacterial cells containing recombinant or nonrecombinant plasmids. If a DNA fragment is inserted anywhere in the multiple cloning site, the *lacZ* gene is disrupted and will not produce functional copies of β-galactosidase. Transformed bacteria in this experiment are plated on agar plates that contain an antibiotic—ampicillin in this case. Nontransformed bacteria cannot grow well on these plates because they do not have the *amp*^R gene and so the ampicillin kills these cells. These agar plates

also contain a substance called X-gal (technically 5-bromo-4-chloro-3-indolyl-β-D-galactopyranoside). X-gal is similar to lactose in structure. It is a substrate for β-galactosidase, and when it is cleaved by β-galactosidase it turns blue. As a result, bacterial cells carrying nonrecombinant plasmids (those that have self-ligated and thus do not contain inserted DNA) have a functional *lacZ* gene and produce β-galactosidase, which cleaves X-gal in the medium, and these cells turn blue. However, recombinant bacteria with plasmids containing an inserted DNA fragment will form white colonies when they grow on X-gal medium because the plasmids in these cells are not producing functional β-galactosidase (Figure 20–5). Bacteria in these white colonies are clones of each other—genetically identical cells with copies of recombinant plasmids. White colonies can be transferred to flasks of bacterial culture broth and grown in large quantities, after which it is relatively easy to isolate and purify recombinant plasmids from these cells.

Plasmids are still the workhorses for many applications of recombinant DNA technology, but they have a major

1. Multiple cloning site of plasmid is cut with restriction enzyme.

2. DNA to be cloned cut with same restriction enzyme.

3. DNA ligase joins together plasmid DNA and DNA to be cloned to create recombinant plasmid.

DNA insertion disrupts *lacZ* gene

4. Transform bacteria with plasmids. Grow cells on media with ampicillin and X-gal.

Bacteria with nonrecombinant plasmids are blue

Bacteria with recombinant plasmids are white

FIGURE 20–5 In blue-white selection procedures, DNA inserted into multiple cloning site of a plasmid disrupts the *lacZ* gene so that bacteria containing recombinant DNA are unable to metabolize X-gal, resulting in white colonies that allow direct identification of bacterial colonies carrying cloned DNA inserts. Photo of a petri dish showing the growth of bacterial cells after uptake of recombinant plasmids. Cells in blue colonies contain vectors without cloned DNA inserts, whereas cells in white colonies contain vectors carrying DNA inserts.

smaller pieces. Therefore as recombinant DNA technology has developed and it has become desirable to clone large pieces of DNA, other vectors have been developed primarily for their ability to accept larger pieces of DNA and because they can be used with other types of host cells beside bacteria.

Other Types of Cloning Vectors

Phage vector systems were among the earliest vectors used in addition to plasmids. These included genetically modified strains of bacteriophage λ. The genome of λ phage has been completely mapped and sequenced, and the λ phage genome has been modified to incorporate many of the important features of cloning vectors described earlier in this chapter, including a multiple cloning site. Phage vectors were popular for quite some time and are still in use today because they can carry inserts up to 45 kb, more than twice as long as DNA inserts in most plasmid vectors. DNA fragments are ligated into the phage vector to produce recombinant λ vectors that are subsequently packaged into phage protein heads *in vitro* and introduced into bacterial host cells growing on petri plates. Inside the bacteria, the vectors replicate and form many copies of infective phage, each of which carries a DNA insert. As they reproduce, they lyse their bacterial host cells, forming the clear spots known as plaques (described in Chapter 6), from which phage can be isolated and the cloned DNA can be recovered.

Bacterial artificial chromosomes (BACs) and yeast artificial chromosomes (YACs) are two other examples of vectors that can be used to clone large fragments of DNA. For example, the mapping and analysis of large eukaryotic genomes such as the human genome required cloning vectors that could carry very large DNA fragments such as segments of an entire chromosome. BACs are essentially very large but low copy number (typically one or two copies/bacterial cell) plasmids that can accept DNA inserts in the 100- to 300-kb range. Like natural chromosomes, a YAC has telomeres at each end, origins of replication, and a centromere. These components are joined to selectable marker genes and to a cluster of restriction-enzyme recognition sequences for insertion of foreign DNA. Yeast chromosomes range in size from 230 kb to over 1900 kb, making it possible to clone DNA inserts from 100 to 1000 kb in YACs. The ability to clone large pieces of DNA in these vectors made them an important tool in the Human Genome Project (see Chapter 21).

limitation: because they are small, they can only accept inserted pieces of DNA up to about 25 kilobases (kb) in size, and most plasmids can often only accept substantially

Unlike the vectors described so far, **expression vectors** are designed to ensure mRNA expression of a cloned gene with the purpose of producing many copies of the gene's encoded protein in a host cell. This is an important distinction since most plasmid, phage vectors and YACs only carry DNA and do not signal for the cell to transcribe it into mRNA. Expression vectors are available for both prokaryotic and eukaryotic host cells and contain the appropriate sequences to initiate both transcription and translation of the cloned gene. For many research applications that involve studies of protein structure and function, producing a recombinant protein in bacteria (or other host cells) and purifying the protein is a routine approach, although it is not always easy to properly express a protein that maintains its biological function. The biotechnology industry also relies heavily on expression vectors to produce commercially valuable protein products from cloned genes, a topic we will discuss later in the text (see Chapter 22).

Ti Vectors for Plant Cells

Introducing genes into plants is a common application that can be done in many ways, and we will discuss aspects of genetic engineering of food plants later in the text (see Special Topic Chapter 5—Genetically Modified Foods). One widely used approach to insert genes into plant cells involves the soil bacterium *Rhizobium radiobacter,* which infects plant cells and produces tumors (called crown galls) in many species of plants. Formerly *Agrobacterium tumefaciens*, this bacterium was renamed based on genomic analysis. *Rhizobium* contains a plasmid called the **Ti plasmid** (tumor-inducing). In the wild, when Ti plasmid-carrying bacteria infect plant cells, a segment of the Ti plasmid, known as *T-DNA*, is transferred into the genome of the host plant cell. Genes in the T-DNA segment control tumor formation and the synthesis of compounds required for growth of the infecting bacteria. Restriction sites in Ti plasmids can be used to insert foreign DNA, and recombinant vectors are introduced into *Rhizobium* by transformation. Tumor-inducing genes from Ti plasmids are removed from the vector so that the recombinant vector does not result in tumor production. *Rhizobium* containing recombinant DNA is mixed with plant cells (not all types of plant cells can be infected by *Rhizobium*). Once inside the cell, the plasmid is inserted into the plant genome when the T-DNA integrates into a host-cell chromosome. Plant cells carrying a recombinant Ti plasmid can be grown in tissue culture. The presence of certain compounds in the culture medium plant cells stimulates the formation of roots and shoots, and eventually a mature plant carrying a foreign gene.

Host Cells for Cloning Vectors

Besides deciding which DNA cloning vector to use, another cloning consideration worthy of discussion is which host cells are used to accept recombinant DNA for cloning. There are many different reasons why particular host cells are chosen for a recombinant DNA experiment, depending on the purpose of the work. Whereas *E. coli* is widely used as a prokaryotic host cell of choice when working with plasmids to manipulate short fragments of DNA, the yeast *Saccharomyces cerevisiae* is extensively used as a host cell for the cloning and expression of eukaryotic genes. There are several reasons for choosing yeast: (1) Although yeast is a eukaryotic organism, it can be grown and manipulated in much the same way as bacterial cells. (2) The genetics of yeast has been intensively studied, providing a large catalog of mutants and a highly developed genetic map (prior to completion of the yeast genome). (3) The entire yeast genome has been sequenced, and genes in the organism have been identified. (4) To study the function of some eukaryotic proteins, it is necessary to use a host cell that can modify the protein, by adding carbohydrates, for example, after it has been synthesized, to convert it to a functional form (bacteria cannot

NOW SOLVE THIS

20–1 An ampicillin-resistant, tetracycline-resistant plasmid, pBR322, is cleaved with *Pst*I, which cleaves within the ampicillin resistance gene. The cut plasmid is ligated with *Pst*I-digested *Drosophila* DNA to prepare a genomic library, and the mixture is used to transform *E. coli* K12.

(a) Which antibiotic should be added to the medium to select cells that have incorporated a plasmid?

(b) If recombinant cells were plated on medium containing ampicillin or tetracycline and medium with both antibiotics, on which plates would you expect to see growth of bacteria containing plasmids with *Drosophila* DNA inserts?

(c) How can you explain the presence of colonies that are resistant to both antibiotics?

■ **HINT:** *This problem involves an understanding of antibiotic selectable marker genes in plasmids and antibiotic DNA selection for identifying bacteria transformed with recombinant plasmid DNA. The key to its solution is to recognize that inserting foreign DNA into the plasmid vector disrupts one of the antibiotic resistance genes in the plasmid.*

carry out most of these modifications). (5) Yeast has been used for centuries in the baking and brewing industries and is considered to be a safe organism for producing proteins for vaccines and therapeutic agents.

The choice of host cells also extends to a number of other cell types, including insect cells. A variety of different human cell types can be grown in culture and used to express genes and proteins. Such cell lines can also then be subjected to various approaches for gene or protein functional analysis, including drug testing for effectiveness at blocking or influencing a particular recombinant protein being expressed, particularly if the cell lines are of a human disease condition such as cancer.

20.2 DNA Libraries Are Collections of Cloned Sequences

Only relatively small DNA segments—representing just a single gene or even a portion of a gene—are produced by cloning DNA into vectors, particularly plasmids. Even when several hundred genes are introduced into larger vectors such as BACs or YACs, one still needs a method for identifying the DNA pieces that were cloned. Consider this: in the cloning discussions we have had so far, we have described *how* DNA can be inserted into vectors and cloned—a relatively straightforward process—but we have not discussed how one knows what particular DNA sequence they have cloned. Simply cutting DNA and inserting into vectors does not tell you what gene or sequences have been cloned.

During the first several decades of DNA cloning, scientists created **DNA libraries**, which represent a collection of cloned DNA. Depending on how a library is constructed, it may contain genes and noncoding regions of DNA. Generally, there are two main types of libraries, genomic DNA libraries and complementary DNA (cDNA) libraries.

Genomic Libraries

Ideally, a **genomic library** consists of many overlapping fragments of the genome, with at least one copy of every DNA sequence in an organism's genome, which in summary span the entire genome. In making a genomic library, DNA is extracted from cells or tissues and cut randomly with restriction enzymes, and the resulting fragments are inserted into vectors using techniques that we discussed in the previous section. Since some vectors (such as plasmids) can carry only a few thousand base pairs of inserted DNA, selecting the vector so that the library contains the whole genome in the smallest number of clones is an important consideration. Because genomic DNA is the foreign DNA introduced into vectors, genomic libraries contain coding and noncoding

segments of DNA such as introns, and vectors in the library may contain more than one gene or only a portion of a gene.

When working with large genomes such as the human genome, the choice of a vector is a primary consideration when making such libraries. As a result, YACs were commonly used to accommodate large sizes of DNA necessary to span the approximately 3 billion bp of DNA in the human genome. If, for example, a human genome library was constructed using plasmid vectors with an average insert size of 5 kb, then more than 2.4 million clones would be required for a 99 percent probability of recovering any given sequence from the genome. Because of its size, this library would be difficult to use efficiently. However, if the library was constructed in a YAC vector with an average insert size of 1 Mb, then the library would only need to contain about 14,000 YACs, making it relatively easy to use. Vectors with large cloning capacities such as YACs were essential tools for the Human Genome Project.

As you will learn later in the text (see Chapter 21), **whole-genome shotgun cloning** approaches (see Figure 21–1) and new sequencing methodologies are readily replacing traditional genomic DNA libraries because they effectively allow one to sequence an entire genomic DNA sample without the need for inserting DNA fragments into vectors and cloning them in host cells. Later in the text (see Chapter 21), we will also consider how DNA sequence analysis using bioinformatics allows one to identify protein-coding and noncoding sequences in cloned DNA.

Complementary DNA (cDNA) Libraries

Complementary DNA (cDNA) libraries offer certain advantages over genomic libraries and continue to be a useful methodology for gene cloning. This is primarily because a cDNA library contains DNA copies—called cDNA—which are made from mRNA molecules isolated from cultured cells or a tissue sample and therefore represent the genes being expressed in cells at the time the library was made. cDNA is complementary to the nucleotide sequence of the mRNA, and so unlike a genomic library, which contains all of the DNA in a genome— gene coding and noncoding sequences—a cDNA library contains only expressed genes. As a result, cDNA libraries have been particularly useful for identifying and studying genes expressed in certain cells or tissues under certain conditions: for example, during development, cell death, cancer, and other biological processes. One can also use these libraries to compare expressed genes from normal tissues and diseased tissues. For instance, this approach has been used to identify genes involved in cancer formation, such as those genes that contribute to progression from a normal cell to a cancer cell and genes involved in cancer cell metastasis (spreading).

A cDNA library is prepared by isolating mRNA from a population of cells of interest. Typically, one picks cells that

FIGURE 20–6 Producing cDNA from mRNA. Because most eukaryotic mRNAs have a poly-A tail at the 3′ end, a short oligo(dT) molecule annealed to this tail serves as a primer for the enzyme reverse transcriptase. Reverse transcriptase uses the mRNA as a template to synthesize a complementary DNA strand (cDNA) and forms an mRNA/cDNA double-stranded duplex. The mRNA is digested with the enzyme RNAse H, producing gaps in the RNA strand. The 3′ ends of the remaining RNA serve as primers for DNA polymerase I, which synthesizes a second DNA strand. The result is a double-stranded cDNA molecule that can be cloned into a suitable vector or used directly as a probe for library screening.

express an abundance of mRNA for the genes to be cloned. Nearly all mRNA isolated from eukaryotic cells has a string of adenines on the 3′ end called the poly-A tail (recall this from Chapter 13), and we can take advantage of this structural feature of mRNA. The next step in making a cDNA library is to mix mRNAs with oligo(dT) primers—short, single-stranded sequences of T nucleotides that anneal to the poly-A tail (**Figure 20–6**). The enzyme **reverse transcriptase** extends the oligo(dT) primer and synthesizes a complementary DNA copy of the mRNA sequence. The product of this reaction is an mRNA–DNA double-stranded hybrid molecule. The RNA

in the hybrid molecule can be enzymatically digested or chemically degraded and a second, opposing strand of DNA synthesized by DNA polymerase. Over time all of the RNA in hybrid molecules is replaced with DNA, creating double-stranded cDNA molecules that are complementary to the mRNA. As an alternative, cDNA can also be synthesized using primers that bind randomly to mRNA and the first strand of cDNA to eventually create double-stranded cDNA from the original mRNA strand.

The cDNA molecules are now ready to be inserted into vectors, usually plasmids. Because one typically wouldn't know what restriction enzymes could be used to cut this DNA, to insert cDNA into a plasmid one usually needs to attach linker sequences to the ends of the cDNA. Linkers are short double-stranded oligonucleotides containing a restriction-enzyme recognition sequence (e.g., *Eco*RI). After attachment to the cDNAs, the linkers are cut with *Eco*RI and ligated to vectors treated with the same enzyme. Transfer of vectors carrying cDNA molecules to host cells and cloning is used to make a cDNA library.

These libraries provide a snapshot of the genes that were transcriptionally active in a tissue at a particular time because the relative amount of cDNA in a particular library is equivalent to the amount of starting mRNA isolated from the tissue and used to make the library. Many different cDNA libraries are available from cells and tissues in specific stages of development, different organs such as brain, muscle, and kidney, and tissues from different disease states such as cancer. These libraries provide an instant catalog of all the genes active in a cell at a specific time and have been very valuable tools for scientists isolating and studying genes in particular tissues.

Specific Genes Can Be Recovered from a Library by Screening

Genomic and cDNA libraries often consist of several hundred thousand different DNA clones, much like a large book library may have many books but only a few of interest to your studies in genetics. So how can libraries be used to locate a specific gene of interest in a library? To find a specific gene, we need to identify and isolate only the clone or clones containing that gene. We must also determine whether a given clone contains all or only part of the gene we are studying. Several methods allow us to sort through a library and isolate specific genes of interest, and this approach is called **library screening**. The choice of method often depends on available information about the gene being sought.

Often, probes are used to screen a library to recover clones of a specific gene. A **probe** is any DNA or RNA sequence that is complementary to some part of a cloned sequence present in the library—the target gene or sequence to be identified. A probe must be labeled or tagged in different ways so that it can be identified. When used in a hybridization reaction, the probe binds to any complementary DNA sequences present in one or more clones. Probes can be labeled with radioactive isotopes, or increasingly these days probes are labeled with nonradioactive compounds that undergo chemical or color reactions to indicate the location of a specific clone in a library.

Probes are derived from a variety of sources—often related genes isolated from another species can be used if enough of the DNA sequence is conserved. For example, genes from rats, mice, or even *Drosophila* that have conserved sequence similarity to human genes can be used as probes to identify human genes during library screening.

To screen a library with a probe, bacterial clones from the library are grown on agar plates, where they form hundreds or thousands of colonies (**Figure 20–7**). A replica of the colonies on each plate is made by gently pressing a nylon or nitrocellulose membrane onto the plate's surface; this transfers the pattern of bacterial colonies from the plate to the membrane. The membrane is processed to lyse the bacterial cells, denature the double-stranded DNA released from the cells into single strands, and bind these strands to the membrane.

The DNA on the membrane is screened by incubation with a labeled nucleic acid probe. First, the probe is heated and quickly cooled to form single-stranded molecules, and then it is added to a solution containing the membrane. If the nucleotide sequence of any of the DNA on the membrane is complementary to the probe, a double-stranded DNA–DNA hybrid molecule will form (one strand from the probe and the other from the cloned DNA on the membrane). This step is called **hybridization**.

After incubation of the probe and the membrane, unbound probe molecules are washed away, and the membrane is assayed to detect the hybrid molecules that remain. If a radioactive probe has been used, the membrane is overlaid with a piece of X-ray film. Radioactivity from the probe molecules bound to DNA on the membrane will expose the film, producing dark spots on the film—a process known as *autoradiography*. These spots represent colonies on the plate containing the cloned gene of interest (Figure 20–7). The positions of spots on the film are used as a guide to identify and recover the corresponding colonies on the plate. The cloned DNA contained in these cells can be used in further experiments. With some nonradioactive probes, a chemical reaction emits photons of light (*chemiluminescence*) to expose photographic film, or the light can be captured with a digital camera and an image produced to reveal the location of colonies carrying the gene of interest.

As we have discussed here, libraries enable scientists to clone DNA and then identify individual genes in the library. Cloning DNA from libraries is still a technique with valuable

applications. However, as you will learn later in the text (see Chapter 21), the basic methods of recombinant DNA technology were the foundation for the development of powerful techniques for whole-genome cloning and sequencing, which led to the **genomics** era of modern genetics and molecular biology. Genomic techniques, in which entire genomes are being sequenced without creating libraries, are replacing many traditional recombinant DNA approaches that cloned or identified individual or a few genes at a time.

NOW SOLVE THIS

20–2 A colleague provided you with a cDNA library of human genes cloned into bacterial plasmid vectors. Armed with the cloned yeast gene that encodes EF-1a, a protein that is highly conserved among eukaryotes, you use the yeast gene as a probe to isolate a cDNA clone containing the human EF-1a gene. You sequence the human gene and find that it is 1384 nucleotide pairs long. Using this cDNA clone as a probe, you isolate the DNA encoding EF-1a from a human genomic library. The genomic clone is sequenced and found to be 5282 nucleotides long. What accounts for the difference in length observed between the cDNA clone and the genomic clone?

■ **HINT:** *This problem asks you to use a cDNA library to isolate the human EF-1a gene when you have access to the yeast EF-1a gene. The key to its solution is to remember that cDNA clones do not have all the sequences of a genomic library, but do contain coding sequences (exons) and they can be identified with the proper probe.*

20.3 The Polymerase Chain Reaction Is a Powerful Technique for Copying DNA

As we will discuss later in the text (see Chapter 22), the recombinant DNA techniques developed in the early 1970s gave birth to the biotechnology industry because these methods enabled scientists to clone human genes, such as the insulin gene, whose protein product could be used for therapeutic purposes. However, cloning DNA using vectors and host cells is labor intensive and time consuming. In 1986, another technique, called the **polymerase chain reaction (PCR)**, was developed. This advance revolutionized recombinant DNA methodology and further accelerated the pace of biological research. The significance of this method was underscored by the awarding of the 1993 Nobel Prize in Chemistry to Kary Mullis, who developed the technique.

PCR is a rapid method of DNA cloning that extends the power of recombinant DNA research and in many cases eliminates the need to use host cells for cloning. PCR

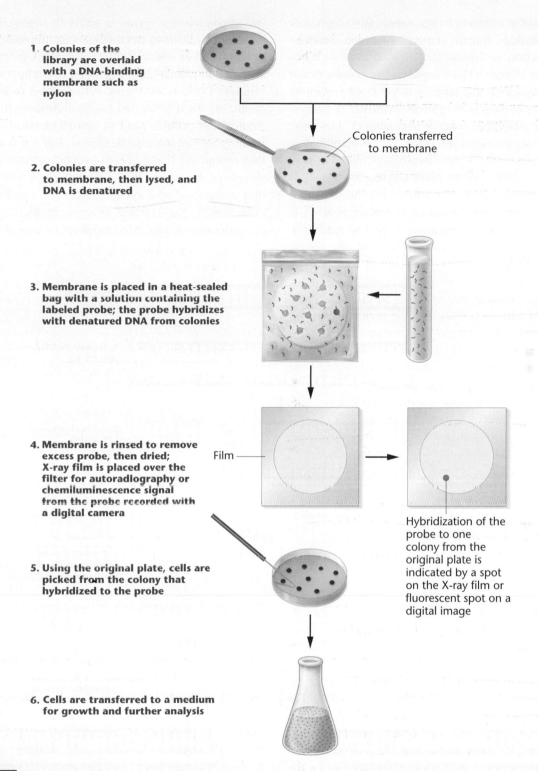

1. Colonies of the library are overlaid with a DNA-binding membrane such as nylon

Colonies transferred to membrane

2. Colonies are transferred to membrane, then lysed, and DNA is denatured

3. Membrane is placed in a heat-sealed bag with a solution containing the labeled probe; the probe hybridizes with denatured DNA from colonies

4. Membrane is rinsed to remove excess probe, then dried; X-ray film is placed over the filter for autoradiography or chemiluminescence signal from the probe recorded with a digital camera

Film

Hybridization of the probe to one colony from the original plate is indicated by a spot on the X-ray film or fluorescent spot on a digital image

5. Using the original plate, cells are picked from the colony that hybridized to the probe

6. Cells are transferred to a medium for growth and further analysis

FIGURE 20–7 Screening a library to recover a specific gene. The library, present in bacteria on petri plates, is overlaid with a DNA-binding membrane, and colonies are transferred to the membrane. Colonies on the membrane are lysed, and the DNA is denatured to single strands. The membrane is placed in a hybridization bag along with buffer and a labeled single-stranded DNA probe. During incubation, the probe forms a double-stranded hybrid with any complementary sequences on the membrane. The membrane is removed from the bag and washed to remove excess probe. Hybrids are detected by placing a piece of X-ray film over the membrane and exposing it for a short time or by chemiluminescence detection and image capture using a digital camera. Colonies containing the cloned DNA that hybridized to the probe are identified from the orientation of the spots. Cells are picked from this colony for growth and further analysis.

is also a method of choice for many applications, whether in molecular biology, human genetics, evolution, development, conservation, or forensics.

By copying a specific DNA sequence through a series of *in vitro* reactions, PCR can amplify target DNA sequences that are initially present in very small quantities in a population of other DNA molecules. When using PCR to clone DNA, double-stranded target DNA to be amplified is placed in a tube with DNA polymerase, Mg^{2+} (as an important cofactor for DNA polymerase), and the four deoxyribonucleoside triphosphates. In addition, some information about the nucleotide sequence of the target DNA is required. This sequence information is used to synthesize two oligonucleotide **primers**: short (typically about 20 nt long) single-stranded DNA sequences, one complementary to the 5′ end of one strand of target DNA to be amplified and another primer complementary to the opposing strand of target DNA at its 3′ end. When added to a sample of double-stranded DNA that has been denatured into single strands, the primers bind to complementary nucleotides flanking the sequence to be cloned. DNA polymerase can then extend the 3′ end of each primer to synthesize second strands of the target DNA. Therefore, one complete reaction process, called a **cycle**, doubles the number of DNA molecules in the reaction (**Figure 20–8**). Repetition of the process produces large numbers of copied DNA very

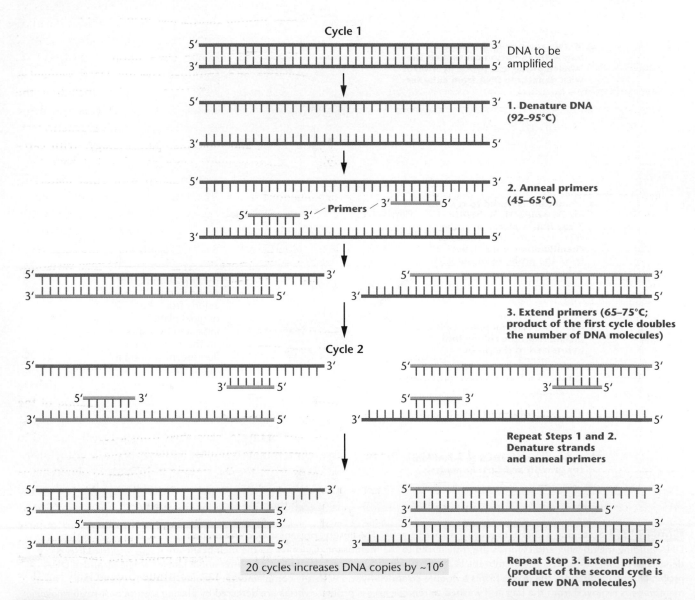

FIGURE 20–8 In the polymerase chain reaction (PCR), the target DNA is denatured into single strands; each strand is then annealed to short, complementary primers. DNA polymerase extends the primers in the 5′ to 3′ direction, using the single-stranded DNA as a template. The result after one round of replication is a doubling of DNA molecules to create two newly synthesized double-stranded DNA molecules. Repeated cycles of PCR can quickly amplify the original DNA sequence more than a millionfold.

Note: shown here is a relatively short sequence of DNA being amplified. Typically much longer segments of DNA are used for PCR, and the primers bind somewhere within the DNA molecule and not so close to the end of the actual molecule.

quickly. If desired, the PCR products can be cloned into plasmid vectors for further use.

The amount of amplified DNA produced is theoretically limited only by the number of times these cycles are repeated, although several factors prevent PCR reactions from amplifying very long stretches of DNA or amplifying DNA indefinitely. Most routine PCR applications involve a series of three reaction steps in a cycle. These three steps are as follows:

1. **Denaturation:** The double-stranded DNA to be cloned is *denatured* into single strands. The DNA can come from many sources, including genomic DNA, mummified remains, fossils, or forensic samples such as dried blood or semen, single hairs, or dried samples from medical records. Heating to 92–95°C for about 1 minute denatures the double-stranded DNA into single strands.

2. **Hybridization/Annealing:** The temperature of the reaction is lowered to a temperature between 45°C and 65°C, which causes the primer binding, also called hybridization or annealing, to the denatured, single-stranded DNA. As described earlier, the primers are short oligonucleotides complementary to sequences flanking the target DNA. The primers serve as starting points for DNA polymerase to synthesize new DNA strands complementary to the target DNA. Factors such as primer length, base composition of primers (GC-rich primers are more thermally stable than AT-rich primers), and whether or not all bases in a primer are complementary to bases in the target sequence are among primary considerations when selecting a hybridization temperature for an experiment.

3. **Extension:** The reaction temperature is adjusted to between 65°C and 75°C, and DNA polymerase uses the primers as a starting point to synthesize new DNA strands by adding nucleotides to the ends of the primers in a 5′ to 3′ direction.

PCR is a chain reaction because the number of new DNA strands is doubled in each cycle, and the new strands, along with the old strands, serve as templates in the next cycle. Each cycle takes 2 to 5 minutes and can be repeated immediately, so that in less than 3 hours, 25 to 30 cycles result in over a million-fold increase in the amount of DNA (Figure 20–8). This process is automated by instruments called *thermocyclers,* or simply PCR machines, that can be programmed to carry out a predetermined number of cycles. As a result, large amounts of a specific DNA sequence are produced that can be used for many purposes, including cloning into plasmid vectors, DNA sequencing, clinical diagnosis, and genetic screening.

A key requirement for PCR is the type of DNA polymerase used in PCR reactions. Multiple PCR cycles involve repetitive heating and cooling of samples, which eventually lead to heat denaturation and loss of activity of most proteins. PCR reactions rely on thermostable forms of DNA polymerase capable of withstanding multiple heating and cooling cycles without significant loss of activity. PCR became a major tool when DNA polymerase was isolated from *Thermus aquaticus,* a bacterium living in the hot springs of Yellowstone National Park. Called *Taq Polymerase,* this enzyme is capable of tolerating extreme temperature changes and was the first thermostable polymerase used for PCR.

PCR-based DNA cloning has several advantages over library cloning approaches. PCR is rapid and can be carried out in a few hours, rather than the days required for making and screening DNA libraries. PCR is also very sensitive and amplifies specific DNA sequences from vanishingly small DNA samples, including the DNA in a single cell. This feature of PCR is invaluable in several kinds of applications, including genetic testing, forensics, and molecular paleontology. With carefully designed primers, DNA samples that have been partially degraded, contaminated with other materials, or embedded in a matrix (such as amber) can be recovered and amplified, when conventional cloning would be difficult or impossible. A wide variety of PCR-based techniques involve different variations of the basic technique described here. Several commonly used variations are discussed below.

Limitations of PCR

Although PCR is a valuable technique, it does have limitations: some information about the nucleotide sequence of the target DNA must be known in order to synthesize primers. In addition, even minor contamination of the sample with DNA from other sources can cause problems. For example, cells shed from a researcher's skin can contaminate samples gathered from a crime scene or taken from fossils, making it difficult to obtain accurate results. PCR reactions must always be performed in parallel with carefully designed and appropriate controls. Also, PCR typically cannot amplify particularly long segments of DNA. Normally, DNA polymerase in a PCR reaction only extends primers for relatively short distances and does not continue processively until it reaches the other end of long template strands of DNA. Because of this characteristic, scientists often use PCR to amplify pieces of DNA that are several thousand nucleotides in length, which is fine for most routine applications.

Applications of PCR

Cloning DNA by PCR has been one of the most widely used techniques in genetics and molecular biology for over 20 years. PCR and its variations have many other applications as well. In short, PCR is one of the most versatile techniques in modern genetics. As you will learn later in the text (see Chapter 22), gene-specific primers provide a way of using PCR for screening mutations involved in genetic disorders, allowing the location and nature of a mutation to be determined quickly. Primers can be designed to distinguish between target sequences that differ by only a single nucleotide. This makes it possible to synthesize allele-specific probes for genetic testing; thus PCR is important for diagnosing genetic disorders. PCR is also a key diagnostic methodology for detecting bacteria and viruses (such as hepatitis or HIV) in humans, and pathogenic bacteria such as *E. coli* and *Staphylococcus aureus* in contaminated food.

PCR techniques are particularly advantageous when studying samples from single cells, fossils, or a crime scene, where a single hair or even a saliva-moistened postage stamp is the source of the DNA. Later in the text (see Special Topic Chapter 3—DNA Forensics), we will discuss how PCR is used in human identification, including remains identification, and in forensic applications. Using PCR, researchers can also explore uncharacterized DNA regions adjacent to known regions and even sequence DNA.

Reverse transcription PCR (RT-PCR) is a powerful methodology for studying gene expression, that is, mRNA production by cells or tissues. In RT-PCR, RNA is isolated from cells or tissues to be studied, and reverse transcriptase is used to generate double-stranded cDNA molecules, as described earlier when we discussed preparation of cDNA libraries. This reaction is followed by PCR to amplify cDNA with a set of primers specific for the gene of interest. Amplified cDNA fragments are then separated and visualized on an agarose gel. Because the amount of amplified cDNA in RT-PCR is based on the relative number of mRNA molecules in the starting reaction, RT-PCR can be used to evaluate relative levels of gene expression in different samples. The amplified cDNA can be inserted into plasmid vectors, which are replicated to produce a cDNA library. RT-PCR is more sensitive than conventional cDNA preparation and is a powerful tool for identifying mRNAs that may be present in only one or two copies per cell.

Finally, in discussing PCR approaches, one of the most valuable modern PCR techniques involves a method called **quantitative real-time PCR (qPCR)** or simply real-time PCR. This approach makes it possible to determine the amount of PCR product made during an experiment, which enables researchers to quantify amplification reactions as they occur in "real time" (**Figure 20–9**). There are several ways to run qPCR experiments, but the basic procedure involves the use of specialized thermal cyclers that use a laser to scan a beam of light through the top or bottom of each PCR tube. Each reaction tube contains either a dye-containing probe or a DNA-binding dye that emits fluorescent light when illuminated by the laser. The light emitted by these dyes correlates to the amount of PCR product amplified. Light from each tube is captured by a detector

1. Hybridization. Forward and reverse PCR primers bind to denatured target DNA. TaqMan probe with reporter (R) and quencher (Q) dye binds to target DNA between the primers. When probe is intact, emission by the reporter dye is quenched.

2. Extension. As DNA polymerase extends the forward primer, it reaches the TaqMan probe and cleaves the reporter dye from the probe. Released from the quencher, the reporter can now emit light excited by a laser.

3. Detection. Emitted light from the reporter is detected and interpreted to produce a plot that quantitates the amount of PCR product produced with each cycle.

FIGURE 20–9 The TaqMan approach to quantitative real-time PCR (qPCR) involves a pair of PCR primers along with a probe sequence complementary to the target gene. The probe contains a reporter dye (R) at one end and a quencher dye (Q) at the other end. When the quencher dye is close to the reporter dye, it interferes with fluorescence released by the reporter dye. When *Taq* DNA polymerase extends a primer to synthesize a strand of DNA, it cleaves the reporter dye off of the probe allowing the reporter to give off energy. (b) Each subsequent PCR cycle removes more reporter dyes so that increased light emitted from the dye can be captured by a computer to produce a readout of fluorescence intensity with each cycle.

that relays information to a computer to provide a readout on the amount of fluorescence produced after each cycle and the precise number of molecules in the original sample.

Two commonly used approaches for qPCR involve the use of a dye called SYBR Green and TaqMan probes. SYBR Green is a dye that binds double-stranded DNA. As more double-stranded DNA is copied with each round of real-time PCR, there are more DNA copies to bind SYBR Green, which increases the amount of fluorescent light emitted. TaqMan probes are complementary to specific regions of the target DNA between where the forward and reverse primers for PCR bind (Figure 20–9). TaqMan probes contain two dyes. One dye, the reporter, is located at the 5′ end of the probe and can release fluorescent light when excited by laser light from the thermal cycler. The other dye, called a quencher, is attached to the 3′ end of the probe. When these two dyes are close to each other, the quencher dye interferes with the fluorescent light released from the reporter dye.

As *Taq* DNA polymerase extends each primer, it removes the reporter dye from the end of the probe (and eventually removes the entire probe). TaqMan is a useful option with primers that could amplify more than one sequence, since the probe confers additional sequence specificity. Now that the reporter dye is separated from the quencher, the fluorescent light released by the reporter can be detected by the thermal cycler. A computer analyzes the detected light to produce a plot displaying the amount of fluorescence emitted with each cycle. Because qPCR does not involve running gels, it is a powerful and rapid technique for measuring and quantitating changes in gene expression, particularly when multiple samples and different genes are being analyzed.

NOW SOLVE THIS

20–3 You have just created the world's first genomic library from the African okapi, a relative of the giraffe. No genes from this genome have been previously isolated or described. You wish to isolate the gene encoding the oxygen-transporting protein β-globin from the okapi library. This gene has been isolated from humans, and its nucleotide sequence and amino acid sequence are available in databases. Using the information available about the human β-globin gene, what two strategies can you use to isolate this gene from the okapi library?

■ **HINT:** *This problem asks you to design PCR primers to amplify the β-globin gene from a species whose genome you just sequenced. The key to its solution is to remember that you have at your disposal sequence data for the human β-globin gene and consider that PCR experiments require the use of primers that bind to complementary bases in the DNA to be amplified.*

For more practice, see Problems 16 and 18.

20.4 Molecular Techniques for Analyzing DNA

The identification of genes and other DNA sequences by cloning or by PCR plays a very powerful role in analyzing genomic structure and function. In addition to cloning and PCR methods, a wide range of molecular techniques are available to geneticists, molecular biologists, and almost anyone who does research involving DNA and RNA, particularly those who study the structure, expression, and regulation of genes. In the following sections, we consider some of the most commonly used molecular methods that provide information about the organization and function of cloned sequences. Throughout later sections of the text you will see these and other techniques discussed in the context of certain applications in modern genetics.

Restriction Mapping

Historically, one of the first steps in characterizing a DNA clone was the construction of a **restriction map**. A restriction map establishes the number of, order of, and distances between restriction-enzyme cleavage sites along a cloned segment of DNA, thus providing information about the length of the cloned insert and the location of restriction-enzyme cleavage sites within the clone. The data the maps provide can be used to reclone fragments of a gene or compare its internal organization with that of other cloned sequences.

Before DNA sequencing and bioinformatics became popular, restriction maps were created experimentally by cutting DNA with different restriction enzymes and separating DNA fragments by gel electrophoresis, a method that separates fragments by size, with the smallest pieces moving farthest through the gel (see Chapter 10; refer to Figure 10–20). The fragments form a series of bands that can be visualized by staining the DNA with DNA binding stains such as *ethidium bromide* and illuminating it with ultraviolet light (**Figure 20–10**). The digestion pattern of fragments generated can then be interpreted to determine the location of restriction sites for different enzymes.

Because of advances in DNA sequencing and the use of bioinformatics, most restriction maps are now created by simply using software to identify restriction-enzyme cutting sites in sequenced DNA. The Exploring Genomics exercise in this chapter involves a Web site, Webcutter, which is commonly used for generating restriction maps. Restriction maps were an important way of characterizing cloned DNA and could be constructed in the absence of any other information about the DNA, including whether or not it encodes a gene or has other functions. In the Human Genome Project, restriction maps of the human genome were important for digesting the genome into pieces that could be sequenced.

FIGURE 20–10 An agarose gel containing separated DNA fragments stained with the DNA-binding dye (ethidium bromide) and visualized under ultraviolet light. Smaller fragments migrate faster and farther than do larger fragments, resulting in the distribution shown. Molecular techniques involving agarose gel electrophoresis are routinely used in a wide range of applications.

In addition, if a restriction site maps close to a mutant allele, this site can be used as a marker in genetic testing to identify carriers of recessively inherited disorders or to prenatally diagnose a fetal genotype. This topic will be discussed later in the text (see Chapter 22).

Nucleic Acid Blotting

Several of the techniques described in this chapter rely on hybridization between complementary nucleic acid (DNA or RNA) molecules. One of the most widely used methods for detecting such hybrids is called Southern blotting (after Edwin Southern, who devised it). The **Southern blot** method can be used to identify which clones in a library contain a given DNA sequence (such as the β-globin gene) and to characterize the size of the fragments. Southern blots can also be used to identify fragments carrying specific genes in genomic DNA digested with a restriction enzyme. Fragments of genomic clones identified by Southern blots can in turn be isolated and recloned, providing a way to study parts of a gene. Southern blotting has also been a valuable tool for identifying the number of copies of a particular sequence or gene that are present in a genome.

Southern blotting has two components: separation of DNA fragments by gel electrophoresis and hybridization of the fragments using labeled probes. Gel electrophoresis can be used, as shown above, to characterize the number of fragments produced by restriction digestion and to estimate their molecular weights. However, restriction-enzyme digestion of large genomes—such as the human genome, with more than 3 billion nucleotides—will produce so many different fragments that they will run together on a gel to produce a continuous smear. The identification of specific fragments in these cases is

accomplished in the next step: hybridization characterizes the DNA sequences present in the fragments.

To make a Southern blot, DNA is cut into fragments with one or more restriction enzymes, and the fragments are separated by gel electrophoresis (**Figure 20–11**). Sometimes if smaller pieces of DNA are being analyzed (for example, plasmid DNA), undigested DNA may be used for Southern blot. In preparation for hybridization, the DNA in the gel is denatured with alkaline treatment to form single-stranded fragments. The gel is then overlaid with a DNA-binding membrane, usually nylon. Transfer of the DNA fragments to the membrane is accomplished by placing the membrane and gel on a wick sitting in a buffer solution. Layers of paper towels or blotting paper are placed on top of the membrane and held in place with a weight. Capillary action draws buffer up through the gel, and in the process transferring the DNA fragments from the gel to the membrane.

The membrane is incubated with a labeled, single-stranded DNA probe for hybridization. For many years Southern blots were primarily carried out with radioactively labeled probes, but as was mentioned when describing library screening, probes that use fluorescent and chemiluminescent labels are now commonly used. DNA fragments on the membrane that are complementary to the probe's nucleotide sequence bind to the probe to form double-stranded hybrids. Excess probe is then washed away, and the hybridized fragments are visualized on a piece of film (Figures 20–11 and **20–12**).

To produce Figure 20–12, researchers cut samples of genomic DNA with several restriction enzymes. The pattern of fragments obtained for each restriction enzyme is shown in **Figure 20–12(a)**. A Southern blot of this gel is illustrated in **Figure 20–12(b)**. The probe hybridized to complementary sequences, identifying fragments of interest.

Southern blotting led to the development of other blotting approaches. RNA blotting was subsequently called **Northern blot analysis** or simply **Northern blotting**, and following a naming scheme that correlates with the directionality of a compass, a related blotting technique involving proteins is known as **Western blotting**. Western blotting is a widely used technique for analyzing proteins. Thus part of the historical significance of Southern blotting is that it led to the development of other blotting methods that are key tools for studying nucleic acids and proteins.

Prior to the development of RT-PCR and real-time PCR, a common approach used to study gene expression was Northern blotting. To determine whether a gene is actively being expressed in a given cell or tissue type, Northern blotting probes for the presence of mRNA complementary to a cloned gene (**Figure 20–13**). To do this, mRNA is extracted from a specific cell or tissue type and

1. **DNA samples cut with restriction enzymes are loaded on agarose gel for electrophoresis**

Lane 1: DNA size markers
Lane 2: DNA cut with restriction enzyme A
Lane 3: DNA cut with restriction enzyme B

2. **DNA is separated by electrophoresis**

DNA is denatured

Gel is placed on sponge wick

Weight
Paper towels
DNA-binding filter
Gel
Wick (sponge)
Buffer

3. **DNA-binding filter, paper towels, and weight are placed on gel; buffer passes upward through sponge by capillary action, transferring DNA fragments to filter**

Radioactive or nonradioactively labeled probe

4. **The filter is placed in heat-sealed bag or a tube with solution containing labeled probe; probe hybridizes with complementary sequences**

5. **Bound probe detected by film or probe signal captured with a digital camera**

All size markers appear because they are labeled; in lanes 2 and 3, only those bands that hybridize with probe are visible

FIGURE 20–11 In the Southern blotting technique, samples of the DNA to be probed are cut with restriction enzymes and the fragments are separated by gel electrophoresis. The pattern of fragments is visualized and photographed under ultraviolet illumination. Then the gel is placed on a sponge wick that is in contact with a buffer solution and covered with a DNA-binding membrane. Layers of paper towels or blotting paper are placed on top of the membrane and held in place with a weight. Capillary action draws the buffer through the gel, transferring the pattern of DNA fragments from the gel to the membrane. The DNA fragments on the membrane are then denatured into single strands and hybridized with a labeled DNA probe. The membrane is washed to remove excess probe and overlaid with a piece of X-ray film for autoradiography or chemiluminescence from the probe detected with a digital camera. The hybridized fragments show up as bands on the X-ray film.

separated by gel electrophoresis. The resulting pattern of RNA bands is transferred to a membrane, as in Southern blotting. The membrane is then exposed to a labeled single-stranded DNA or RNA probe derived from a cloned copy of the gene. If mRNA complementary to the DNA probe is present, the complementary sequences will hybridize and be detected as a band on the film. Northern blots provide information about the expression of specific genes and are

(a)   (b)

FIGURE 20–12 (a) Agarose gel stained with ethidium bromide to show DNA fragments. (b) Exposed X-ray film of a Southern blot prepared from the gel in part (a). Only those bands containing DNA sequences complementary to the probe show hybridization.

used to study patterns of gene expression in embryonic tissues, cancer, and genetic disorders. Northern blots also detect alternatively spliced mRNAs (multiple types of transcripts derived from a single gene) and are used to derive other information about transcribed mRNAs such as the size of a gene's mRNA transcripts. Measuring band density gives an estimate of the relative transcriptional activity of the gene. Thus, Northern blots characterize and quantify the transcriptional activity of genes in different cells, tissues, and organisms. Northern blots are occasionally still used to study RNA expression, but because PCR-based techniques are faster and more sensitive than blotting methods, techniques such as RT-PCR are often the preferred approach, particularly for measuring changes in gene expression.

Finally, as noted earlier in the text (see Chapter 10), **fluorescent *in situ* hybridization**, or **FISH**, is a powerful tool that involves hybridizing a probe directly to a chromosome or RNA without blotting (see Figure 10–18 and Figures 18–8 and 18–9). FISH can be carried out with isolated chromosomes on a slide or directly *in situ* in tissue sections or entire organisms, particularly when embryos are used for various studies in developmental genetics (**Figure 20–14**). For example, in developmental studies one can identify which cell types in an embryo express different genes during specific stages of development.

For *in situ* hybridization, a probe for a particular sequence is labeled with nucleotides tagged with a particular dye that will fluoresce under fluorescent light. When hybridized to a chromosome, for example, the probe can reveal the specific location of a gene on a particular chromosome. Variations of the FISH technique are also being used to produce **spectral karyotypes** in which individual chromosomes can be detected using probes labeled with dyes that will fluoresce at different wavelengths (see Chapter 8 opening photograph and Figure 19–1). Spectral karyotyping has proven to be extremely valuable for detecting deletions, translocations, duplications, and other anomalies in chromosome structure, such as the chromosomal rearrangements (discussed in Chapter 8), and for detecting chromosomal abnormalities in cancer cells (discussed in Chapter 19).

FIGURE 20–13 Northern blot analysis of *dfmr1* gene expression in *Drosophila* ovaries and embryos. A *dfmr1* transcript of approximately 2.8 kb is present in ovaries and 0- to 3-hr-old embryos. The *dfmr1* transcript peaks in abundance between 9 and 12 hr of embryonic development, when it measures 4.0 kb. These data suggest that *dfmr1* gene expression may be regulated at the levels of transcription or transcript processing during embryogenesis. The *dfmr1* gene is a homolog of the human *FMR1* gene. Loss-of-function mutations in *FMR1* result in human fragile-X mental retardation.

FIGURE 20–14 *In situ* hybridization of a zebrafish embryo 48 hours after fertilization showing expression of *atp2a1* mRNA, which encodes muscle-specific calcium pump. The probe revealing *atp2a1* expression produces dark blue staining. Notice that this staining is restricted to muscle cells surrounding the developing spinal cord of the embryo.

20.5 DNA Sequencing Is the Ultimate Way to Characterize DNA Structure at the Molecular Level

In a sense, cloned DNA, from a single gene to an entire genome, is completely characterized at the molecular level only when its nucleotide sequence is known. The ability to sequence DNA has greatly enhanced our understanding of genome organization and increased our knowledge of gene structure, function, and mechanisms of regulation.

Historically, the most commonly used method of DNA sequencing was developed by Fred Sanger and his colleagues and is known as **dideoxynucleotide chain-termination sequencing** or simply **Sanger sequencing**. In this technique, a double-stranded DNA molecule whose sequence is to be determined is converted to single strands that are used as a template for synthesizing a series of complementary strands. The DNA to be sequenced is mixed with a primer that is complementary to the target DNA or vector, along with DNA polymerase, and the four deoxyribonucleotide triphosphates (dATP, dCTP, dGTP, and dTTP) are added to each tube.

The key to the Sanger technique is the addition of a small amount of one modified deoxyribonucleotide (**Figure 20–15**), called a **dideoxynucleotide** (abbreviated ddNTP). Notice that dideoxynucleotides have a 3′ hydrogen instead of a 3′ hydroxyl group. Dideoxynucleotides are called chain-termination nucleotides because they lack the 3′ oxygen required to form a phosphodiester bond with another nucleotide. Thus when ddNTPs are included in a reaction as DNA synthesis takes place, the polymerase occasionally inserts a dideoxynucleotide instead of a deoxyribonucleotide into a growing DNA strand. Since the dideoxynucleotide has no 3′-OH group, it cannot form a 3′ bond with another nucleotide, and DNA synthesis terminates because DNA polymerase cannot add new nucleotides to a ddNTP. The Sanger reaction takes advantage of this key modification.

For example, in **Figure 20–16**, notice that the shortest fragment generated is a sequence that has added ddCTP to the 3′ end of the primer and the chain has terminated. Over time as the reaction proceeds, eventually a ddNTP will be inserted at every location in the newly synthesized DNA so that each strand synthesized differs in length by one nucleotide and is terminated by a ddNTP. This allows for separation of these DNA fragments by gel electrophoresis, which can then be used to determine the sequence.

When the Sanger technique was first developed, four separate reaction tubes, each with a different single ddNTP (e.g., ddATP, ddCTP, ddGTP, and ddTTP), were used. These reactions typically used either a radioactively labeled primer or a radioactively labeled ddNTP for analysis of the

FIGURE 20–15 Deoxynucleotides (top) have an OH group at the 3′ position in the deoxyribose molecule. Dideoxynucleotides (bottom) lack an OH group and have only hydrogen (H) at this position. Dideoxynucleotides can be incorporated into a growing DNA strand, but the lack of a 3′-OH group prevents formation of a phosphodiester bond with another nucleotide, terminating further elongation of the template strand.

sequence following polyacrylamide gel electrophoresis and autoradiography. Historically, this approach involved large polyacrylamide gels in which each reaction was loaded on a separate lane of the gel and ladder-like banding patterns revealed by autoradiography were read to determine the sequence. This original approach could typically read about 800 bases of 100 DNA molecules simultaneously. *Read length*—that is, the amount of sequence that can be generated in a single individual reaction and the total amount of DNA sequence generated in a sequence *run*, which is effectively read length times the number of reactions an instrument can run during a given period of time—has become a hot area for innovation in sequencing technology.

In the past 20 years, modifications of the Sanger technique led to technologies that allowed sequencing reactions to occur in a single tube. As shown in Figure 20–16, each of the four ddNTPs is labeled with a different-colored fluorescent dye. These reactions were carried out in PCR-like fashion using cycling reactions that permit greater read and run capabilities. The reaction products were separated through a single, ultrathin-diameter polyacrylamide tube gel called a capillary gel (capillary gel electrophoresis). As DNA fragments move through the gel, they are scanned with a laser. The laser stimulates fluorescent dyes on each DNA fragment, which then emit different wavelengths of light for each ddNTP. Emitted light is captured by a detector that amplifies and feeds this information into a computer to convert the light patterns into a DNA sequence that is

1. Reaction components
- DNA template
- Primer
- DNA polymerase
- dNTPs (dATP, dCTP, dGTP, dTTP)
- small amount of ddNTPs with fluorochromes

ddNTPs
ddATP—●
ddCTP—●
ddGTP—●
ddTTP—●

2. Primer extension and chain termination

3. Separate DNA fragments by capillary gel electrophoresis

Direction of movement of strands — Capillary gel

Laser — Detector

4. Laser and detector detect fluorescence of each ddNTP and provide input to a computer for sequence analysis

Chromatograph

FIGURE 20–16 Computer-automated DNA sequencing using the chain-termination (Sanger) method. (1) A primer is annealed to a sequence adjacent to the DNA being sequenced (usually near the multiple cloning site of a cloning vector). (2) A reaction mixture is added to the primer–template combination. This includes DNA polymerase, the four dNTPs, and small molar amounts of dideoxynucleotides (ddNTPs) labeled with fluorescent dyes. All four ddNTPs are added to the same tube, and during primer extension, all possible lengths of chains are produced. During primer extension, the polymerase occasionally (randomly) inserts a ddNTP instead of a dNTP, terminating the synthesis of the chain because the ddNTP does not have the OH group needed to attach the next nucleotide. Over the course of the reaction, all possible termination sites will have a ddNTP inserted. The products of the reaction are added to a single lane on a capillary gel, and the bands are read by a detector and imaging system. This process is computer automated, and robotic machines sequence several hundred thousand nucleotides in a 24-hour period and then store and analyze the data automatically. The sequence is obtained by extension of the primer and is read from the newly synthesized strand. Thus in this case, the sequence obtained begins with 5′-CTAGACATG-3′.

technically called an electropherogram or chromatograph. The data are represented as a series of colored peaks, each corresponding to one nucleotide in the sequence.

Since the early 1990s, DNA sequencing has largely been performed through computer-automated Sanger-reaction-based technology and is referred to as **computer-automated high-throughput DNA sequencing**. Such systems generate relatively large amounts of sequence DNA. Computer-automated sequences can achieve read

lengths of approximately 1000 bp with about 99.999 percent accuracy for about $0.50 per kb. Automated DNA sequencers often contain multiple capillary gels (as many as 96) that are several feet long and can process several thousand bases of sequences so that many of these instruments make it possible to generate over 2 million bp of sequences in a day! These systems became essential for the rapidly accelerating progress of the Human Genome Project.

Sequencing Technologies Have Progressed Rapidly

Nearly three decades since Fred Sanger was awarded part of the 1980 Nobel Prize in Chemistry (which he shared with Walter Gilbert and Paul Berg) for sequencing technology, DNA sequencing technologies have undergone an incredible evolution to dramatically improve sequencing capabilities. New innovations in sequencing technology are developing quickly. Sanger sequencing approaches (particularly those involving computer-automated instruments such as capillary electrophoresis) still have their place in everyday routine applications that require sequencing, such as sequencing a relatively short piece of DNA amplified by PCR.

When it comes to sequencing entire genomes, however, Sanger sequencing technologies are outdated. The costs of Sanger sequencing are relatively high compared to newer technologies, and Sanger sequencing output, even with computer-automated DNA sequencing, is simply not high enough to support the growing demand for genomic data. This demand is being driven in large part by personalized genomics (see Chapter 21) and the desire to reveal the genetic basis of human diseases, which will require tens of thousands of individual genome sequences. As we will discuss later in the text (see Chapter 21), the race is on to develop sequencing technologies that will allow the complete sequencing of an individual human genome for $1000. There is every indication that technology will allow this to happen relatively soon thanks to the development of **next-generation sequencing (NGS) technologies**.

Next-Generation and Third-Generation Sequencing Technologies

The development of genomics has spurred a demand for sequencers that are faster and capable of generating millions of bases of DNA sequences in a relatively short time, leading to the development of NGS approaches. Such sequencing technologies dispense with the Sanger technique and capillary electrophoresis methods (*First-Generation Sequencing*) in favor of sophisticated, parallel formats (simultaneous reaction formats) that synthesize DNA from tens of thousands of identical strands simultaneously and then use state-of-the art fluorescence imaging techniques to detect new synthesized strands and average sequence data across many molecules being sequenced. NGS technologies are providing an unprecedented capacity for generating massive amounts of DNA sequence data rapidly and at dramatically reduced costs per base.

The desire for next-generation sequencing within the research community and challenges such as the $1000

genome have led to an intense race among many companies eager to produce NGS methods. As a result, there are at least five NGS technologies. Next-generation sequencing started around 2005. Some of the first instruments were capable of producing as much data as 50 capillary electrophoresis systems and are up to 200 times faster and cheaper than conventional Sanger approaches. Companies such as Applied Biosystems (ABI, now merged with Life Technologies), Roche 454 Life Sciences, and Illumina led this effort. NGS instruments generally produce short read lengths of ~200–400 bp, and then these snippets of sequence are stitched together using software to produce a coherent, complete genome.

In 2005, Roche 454 Life Sciences was the first company to commercialize NGS technology. This approach uses a solid-phase method in which beads are attached to fragmented genomic DNA, which is then PCR amplified in separate water droplets in oil for each bead and loaded into multiwell plates and mixed with DNA polymerase. Multiwell plates often contain more than one million wells with one bead per well—each serving as a reaction tube for sequencing. Next, a sequencing technology called **pyrosequencing** is used to sequence DNA on the beads in each well. In pyrosequencing, a single, labeled nucleotide (e.g., dATP) is flowed over the wells. Each well contains a single bead along with primers annealed to the DNA on the bead. When a complementary nucleotide crosses a template strand adjacent to the primer, it is added to the 3' end of the primer by DNA polymerase.

Incorporation of a nucleotide results in the release of pyrophosphate, which initiates a series of chemiluminescent (light-releasing) reactions that ultimately produce light using the firefly enzyme luciferase. Emitted light from the reaction is captured and recorded to determine when a single nucleotide has been incorporated into a strand. By rapidly repeating the nucleotide flow step with each of the four nucleotides to determine which base is next in the sequence, this approach can generate read lengths of about 400 bases and on the order of 400 million bases (Mbp) of data per 10-hour run. NGS sequencing technologies are also creating major data management challenges for saving and storing such large image data files.

The Life Technologies Ion Torrent Personal Genome Machine and the Illumina HiSeq are two of the most common NGS platforms currently used in cutting-edge sequencing laboratories. Each instrument has unique features, but they work in similar ways using a *sequencing by synthesis* approach. This method involves using DNA fragments as templates for synthesizing new strands, incorporating nucleotides labeled with different dyes, washing away unincorporated nucleotides, imaging incorporated nucleotides, and repeating this cycle.

For example, the method developed by Illumina attaches DNA fragments to a solid support and then using reactions similar to the Sanger method, fluorescently tagged terminator nucleotides are added and detected. Then the fluorescent tags and terminator portions of the nucleotide are removed to allow another cycle of extension. This approach can now generate about 600 Gb of data in 10 days—enough to sequence four complete human genomes, with each base sequenced an average of 30 times for accuracy! The instrumentation needed to run these platforms is expensive. For example, the Illumina HiSeq instrument costs about $700,000. But given the massive amounts of sequence data the NGS methods can generate, the average cost per base is much lower than Sanger sequencing.

Shortly after NGS methods were commercialized, companies were announcing progress on **Third-Generation Sequencing (TGS)**. TGS methods are based on strategies that sequence a *single molecule* of single-stranded DNA, and at least four different approaches are being explored.

Pacific Biosciences' PacBio technology is generally considered the current leader in TGS. The PacBio instrument works by attaching single-stranded molecules of the DNA to be sequenced to a single molecule of DNA polymerase anchored to a substrate and then visualizing, in real time, the polymerase as it synthesizes a strand of DNA (see **Figure 20–17**). The DNA polymerase is confined within a hole, a nanopore of about 10 nm in diameter located within a thin layer of metal on a glass substrate. This configuration allows for the illumination necessary to detect individual nucleotides as they are added to single strands synthesized in the nanopore. The

polymerase adds fluorescent dye-labeled nucleotides to a newly synthesized growing strand of DNA. Because the dye is attached to a terminal phosphate chain of the nucleotide, it is cleaved when incorporated into the newly synthesized strand. The fluorescent dye flashes as the base is incorporated into the DNA strand. Each base flashes with a characteristic color that is detected and recorded.

The PacBio was one of the first "long-read" instruments to reach the market. It generates read lengths of over 1500 bp. Recently, the PacBio was used to sequence the genomes of five strains of *Vibrio cholera* involved in a cholera outbreak in Haiti in less than an hour. This genetic determination of the *Vibrio* strains resulted in rapid action to successfully treat the outbreak with antibiotics to which these bacteria were not resistant. Most TGS technologies still have somewhat high error rates for sequencing accuracy—about 15 percent errors in sequence generated. At around $750,000, these technologies also remain very expensive.

In other TGS approaches being developed, the single-stranded DNA molecule is captured in a nanopore, and individual bases from a single strand of DNA are cleaved off by an exonuclease to produce a signal that can be interpreted. Yet another TGS method being developed by IBM involves passing single-stranded DNA through a transistor to read individual bases based on electronic signals unique to each nucleotide. Which approach will emerge as the leader in TGS remains unclear, but there is no doubt that the development of TGS technologies represents another significant sequencing milestone for genomic studies.

1. DNA polymerase located in a nanopore anchored to a solid substrate binds a single-stranded DNA molecule to be sequenced.

2. DNA polymerase adds fluorescently tagged nucleotides to synthesize DNA.

3. Fluorescent tag is cleaved off each base as it is added to the DNA strand.

FIGURE 20–17 Third-Generation Sequencing. A simplified version of one approach to TGS is shown here. In this example, a DNA polymerase molecule anchored within a nanopore binds to a single strand of DNA. As the polymerase incorporates fluorescently labeled nucleotides into a newly synthesized strand (shown in orange), each base emits a characteristic color that can be detected.

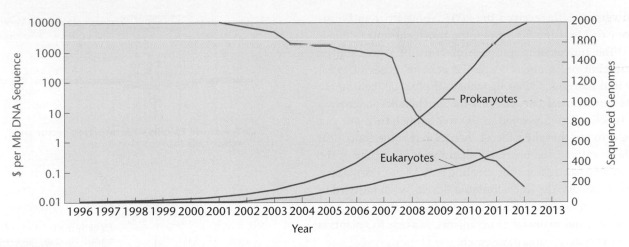

FIGURE 20–18 Rapidly decreasing sequence costs have enabled the rapid expansion of eukaryotic and prokaryotic genome sequencing. The number of eukaryotic and prokaryotic genomes sequenced has increased dramatically during the past decade due to significant improvements in high-throughput sequencing technologies and sharply decreasing costs (green line) of sequencing large numbers of base pairs.

The genomics research community has embraced NGS and third-generation sequencing technologies. Which approaches will eventually emerge as the sequencing methods of choice for the long-term is unclear, but what is clear is that the landscape of sequencing capabilities has dramatically changed for the better and never before have scientists had the ability to generate so much sequence data so quickly. Through 2006, new sequencing technologies were cutting sequencing costs in half about every two years (**Figure 20–18**). And keep an eye on the $1000 genome: there is every reason to believe sequencing technology will get us there soon, perhaps in 2015.

DNA Sequencing and Genomics

Our overview of DNA sequencing in this chapter is a great introduction to a detailed discussion of genomics and many related topics found later in the text (see Chapter 21). The principal techniques of recombinant DNA technology, particularly DNA cloning, were essential for making genome projects possible, but no technology has had a greater influence on our ability to study genomes than DNA sequencing. Rapid advances in sequencing technology that pushed the capabilities of computer-automated sequencing were driven by the demands of genome scientists (particularly those working on the Human Genome Project) to rapidly generate more sequence with greater accuracy and at lower cost. As a result of these technologies, you will learn about innovative approaches to genome sequencing that are providing data for a range of new research and clinical applications.

20.6 Creating Knockout and Transgenic Organisms for Studying Gene Function

Recombinant DNA technology has also made it possible to directly manipulate genes in organisms in ways that allow scientists to learn about gene function *in vivo*. These approaches also enable scientists to create genetically engineered plants and animals for research and for commercial applications. We conclude this chapter by briefly discussing gene knockout technology and creating transgenic animals as examples of *gene-targeting* methods that have revolutionized research in genetics. Throughout the book, the Modern Approaches to Understanding Gene Function boxes have highlighted examples of specific research projects involving gene-targeting approaches.

Gene Targeting and Knockout Animal Models

The concept behind *gene targeting* is to manipulate a specific allele, locus, or base sequence to learn about the functions of a gene of interest. Gene targeting focuses on manipulating a specific gene in the genome. In the 1980s, scientists devised a gene-targeting technique for creating **gene knockout** (often abbreviated as KO) organisms, specifically mice. The pioneers of knockout technology, Dr. Mario Capecchi of the University of Utah and colleagues Oliver Smithies of the University of North Carolina, Chapel Hill, and Sir Martin Evans of Cardiff

University, UK, received the 2007 Nobel Prize in Physiology or Medicine for developing this technique.

The fundamental purpose of creating a knockout is to disrupt or eliminate a specific gene or genes of interest and then ask, "what happens?" If physical, behavioral, and biochemical changes or other metabolic phenotypes or functions are observed in the KO animal, then one can begin to see that the gene of interest has some functional role or roles in the observed phenotypes. Thus one of the most valuable reasons for creating a KO is to learn about gene function. The KO techniques developed in mice led to similar technologies for making KOs in zebrafish, rats, pigs, fruit flies, and many other organisms. Making KO plants is also a very active area of research.

Knockout mice have revolutionized research in genetics, molecular biology, and biomedical research in many ways. Scientists have used knockout methods to create thousands of knockout organisms that have advanced our understanding of gene function, created animal models for many human diseases, and enabled scientists to make transgenic animals (which we will discuss below). Applications of KO technology have also provided the foundation for gene-targeting approaches in gene therapy that we discuss later in the text (see Special Topic Chapter 6—Gene Therapy).

Generally, generating a KO mouse or a transgenic mouse is a very labor-intensive project that can take several years of experiments and crosses and a significant budget to complete. However, once a KO mouse is made, assuming it is fertile, a colony of mice can be maintained; often KO mice are shared around the world so that other researchers can work with them. Many companies will produce KO mice for researchers. It is also possible to make *double-knockout animals (DKOs)* and even *triple-knockout animals (TKOs)*. This approach is typically used when scientists want to study the functional effects of disrupting two or three genes thought to be involved in a related mechanism or pathway.

A KO animal can be made in several ways (**Figure 20–19**). Here we outline a strategy for making KO mice, but the same basic methods apply when making most KO animals. The DNA sequence for the gene of interest to be targeted for KO must be known. Scientists also need to know some sequence information about noncoding sequences that flank the gene at its location in the genome. A *targeting vector* is then constructed. The purpose of the targeting vector is to create a segment of DNA that can be introduced into cells. It then undergoes homologous recombination with the gene of interest (the target gene) to disrupt or replace the gene of interest, thereby rendering it nonfunctional. The targeting vector contains a copy of the gene of interest that has been mutated by inserting a large segment of foreign DNA, essentially a large insertion

1. Designing the targeting vector

2. Transform ES cells with targeting vector and select cells for recombination

ES cells from agouti mouse

3. Microinject ES cells into blastocyst from black-colored mouse

Inner cell mass

4. Transfer into pseudo-pregnant foster mother, birth of chimeras

Normal   Chimeras

5. Chimeric mouse bred to black mouse to create mice heterozygous (+/−) for gene knockout

(+/−)   (+/+)

(+/−)   (+/+)

6. Breed heterozygous mice to produce mice homozygous (−/−) for gene knockout

FIGURE 20–19 A basic strategy for producing a knockout mouse.

mutation. This foreign DNA will disrupt the reading frame of the target gene so that if the gene is transcribed into mRNA and translated into protein, it will produce a nonfunctional protein.

To help scientists determine whether the targeting vector has been properly introduced into the genome, the insertion sequence typically contains a marker gene. The example shown in Figure 20–19 uses a marker sequence for neomycin resistance (*neoR*). Neomycin is an antibiotic that blocks protein synthesis in both prokaryotic and eukaryotic cells, and its role will become apparent momentarily. The gene for green fluorescent protein (GFP), the *lacZ* gene that we discussed earlier in this chapter, and other marker genes are also sometimes used as marker genes. These markers allow for very visual examples of KO or transgenic organisms and you will see an example of a GFP transgenic animal later in this section.

There are several ways to introduce the targeting vector into cells. One popular approach involves using electroporation to deliver the vector into **embryonic stem (ES) cells** grown in culture. The ES cells are harvested from the inner cell mass of a mouse embryo at the blastocyst stage. Alternatively, the targeting vector is directly injected into the blastocyst with the hopes that it will enter ES cells in the inner cell mass. Sometimes it is possible to make KOs by isolating newly fertilized eggs from a female mouse (or female of the desired animal species) and microinjecting the targeting vector DNA directly into the nucleus of the egg or into one of the pronuclei of a fertilized egg [**Figure 20–20(a)**].

Randomly, in a very small percentage of ES cells that have taken in the targeting vector, the actions of the endogenous enzyme recombinase will catalyze homologous recombination between the targeting vector and the sequence for the gene of interest. In the few recombinant ES cells that will be created, the targeting vector will usually replace the original gene on only one of two chromosomes.

Recombinant ES cells can be selected for by treating cultured ES cells with a reagent that will kill cells that lack the targeting vector. For the example shown in Figure 20–19, neomycin is added to cultured ES cells. Cells containing the targeting vector are resistant to neomycin, but ES cells that are not nonrecombinant die. Recombinant ES cells are then injected into a mouse embryo at the blastocyst stage where they will be incorporated into the inner cell mass of the blastocyst. The blastocyst is then placed into the uterus of a surrogate mother mouse, sometimes called a *pseudopregnant mouse*—a mouse previously impregnated by mating with a male mouse. The pseudopregnant mouse offers a uterus that is receptive to implantation of the blastocyst containing the targeting vector.

Of course, the surrogate will give birth to mice that arose from the original mating, but the surrogate will also give birth to mice that are *chimeras*: some cells in their body arise from KO stem cells, and others arise from stem cells of the donor blastocyst. Researchers screen for mice that contain the targeting vector by obtaining DNA from a sample of tail tissue, purifying the DNA, and performing PCR (and sometimes Southern blots) to verify that the targeting

(a)   **(b)**

FIGURE 20–20 (a) Microinjecting DNA into a fertilized egg to create a knockout or a transgenic mouse. A fertilized egg is held by a suction or holding pipette (seen below the egg), and a microinjection needle delivers cloned DNA into the nucleus of the egg. (b) On the left is a null mouse ($-/-$) for both copies of the obese (*ob*) gene, which produces a peptide hormone called leptin. The mouse on the right is wild type ($+/+$) for the *ob* gene. The *ob* knockout mouse weighs almost five times as much as its wild-type sibling. Naturally occurring mutations in the human *Ob* gene create weight disorders for affected individuals.

vector sequence is present in the animal's genome. As long as the targeting vector DNA is present in germ cells, the sequence will be inherited in all of the offspring generated by these mice, but typically most F1 generation KO mice produced this way are heterozygous (+/−) for the gene of interest and the targeting vector and not homozygous for the KO. Sibling matings of F1 animals can then be used to generate homozygous KO animals, referred to as *null mice* and given a −/− designation because they lack wild-type copies of the targeted gene of interest. As mentioned at the beginning of this section, KO animal models serve invaluable roles for learning about gene function, and they continue to be essential for biomedical research on disease genes [see **Figure 20–20(b)**].

Despite all of the work that goes into trying to produce a KO organism, sometimes viable offspring are never born. The KO results in *embryonic lethality*. Knocking out a gene that is important during embryonic development may kill the mouse before researchers have a chance to study it. Typically, researchers will examine embryos from the pseudopregnant mouse to see if they can determine at what stage of embryonic development the embryo is dying. This examination often reveals specific organ defects that can also be informative about the function of the KO gene.

If null mice for a particular gene of interest cannot be derived by traditional KO approaches, a **conditional knockout** can often provide a way to study such a gene. Conditional knockouts allow one to control when a target gene is disrupted. This study can be done at a particular time in the animal's development. For example, if a target gene displays embryonic lethality, one can use a conditional KO to allow an animal to progress through development and be born before disrupting. Another advantage of conditional KOs is that target genes can also be turned off in a particular tissue or organ instead of the entire animal.

One common approach for making conditional KOs is called the *Cre-Lox system* (**Figure 20–21**). With this method, conditional KOs are made by inserting sequences called *loxP* sites into the targeting vector on either side of the target gene sequence. These sequences will be introduced into the germ line via the same mechanism as a knockout. These mice can then be crossed to other mice with a germ line containing the Cre-recombinase gene (*Cre*), which encodes a viral enzyme that can recognize the *loxP* sequences, recombine them, and delete the gene between the *loxP* sequences.

A key to the Cre-Lox system is that the promoter for the *Cre* mouse strain can be designed as a tissue-specific promoter that will only be active in certain tissues. This example is shown in Figure 20–21. To prevent embryonic lethality, the promoter chosen for the *Cre* strain can be under the control of a particular hormone, dietary nutrients, or other conditions, and thus the promoter responsible for

© 2007 Nature Publishing Group

FIGURE 20–21 The Cre-Lox system for creating conditional knockouts.

expressing *Cre* can be turned on or off at different stages in the development of the animal to produce the KO under the desired specific conditions, depending on the research being carried out.

In 2006 a worldwide collaboration involving more than $100 million in funding was initiated to disable the ~20,000 genes in the mouse genome. The purpose was to create a KO mouse resource for the genetics research community that would help advance human disease research using these model organisms. Rather than a gene-by-gene approach to make KO, researchers are using a high-throughput technique that involves knocking out thousands of genes in embryonic stem cells and then creating offspring in which specific genes of interest can then be turned off.

Later in the text (see Special Topic Chapter 6—Gene Therapy), we discuss how gene-targeting methods with *transcription activator-like effector nucleases (TALENs)* and *zinc finger nucleases (ZFNs)* can be used for gene therapy. These

(a)

(b)

FIGURE 20–22 Examples of transgenic animals. (a) Transgenic mice incorporating the GFP gene from jellyfish enable scientists to tag particular genes with GFP to track gene activity, including activity in subsequent generations of mice generated from these transgenics. This procedure can be very valuable for examining the transgenerational effects on gene expression, including epigenetic changes. (b) The mouse on the left is transgenic for a rat growth hormone gene, cloned downstream from a mouse metallothionein promoter. When the transgenic mouse was fed zinc, the metallothionein promoter induced the transcription of the growth hormone gene, stimulating the growth of the transgenic mouse.

approaches have been used for the *in vivo* genetic engineering of mice, rats, and other species for targeted modifications of specific genes. Later in the text (see Special Topic Chapter 6) we also briefly mention *CRISPRs* (Clustered Regularly Interspaced Palindromic Repeats) as a powerful new tool for gene-targeting experiments, including engineering primates (which can be difficult to do with traditional KO methods).

Making a Transgenic Animal: The Basics

Transgenic animals (Figure 20–22), also sometimes called **knock-in animals**, express or often overexpress a particular gene of interest (the transgene). The method of creating transgenic animals is conceptually simple, and many of the steps are similar to the steps involved in making a KO. Moreover, as is true when making KOs, there are species-specific challenges associated with creating transgenics. Many of the prevailing techniques used to make transgenics were also developed in mice.

Conceptually, introducing a transgene into an organism involves steps similar to making a KO. But instead of trying to disrupt a target gene, a vector with the transgene is created to undergo homologous recombination into the host-cell genome. In some applications, tissue-specific promoter sequences can be used so that the transgene is expressed only in specific tissues. For example, tissue-specific promoters are used in the biotechnology industry to express specific recombinant products in milk for subsequent purification. It

is often much easier to make a transgenic than a KO because the vector just needs to be incorporated into the host genome somewhere (hopefully in a noncoding region) but often not at a particular locus as is necessary when making a KO.

The vector with the transgene can be put into ES cells or injected directly into embryos. Then, in a relatively small percentage of embryos or eggs, the transgenic DNA becomes inserted into the egg cell genome by recombination due to the action of naturally occurring DNA recombinases. After this stage, the rest of the process is similar to making a KO: embryos are placed into pseudopregnant females, and resulting crosses are used to derive mice that are homozygous for the transgene.

In a transgenic, the transgene is often overexpressed in order to study its effects on the appearance and functions of mice. There are many variations and purposes for making transgenics. Transgenic animals overexpressing certain genes, expressing human genes or genes from a different species, and expressing mutant genes are among examples of transgenics that are valuable models for basic and applied research to understand gene function.

As we will consider later in the text (see Chapter 22), transgenic animals and plants are also created in order to produce commercially valuable biotechnology products. Later in the text (see Special Topic Chapter 5—Genetically Modified Foods), you will learn about examples of transgenic food crops.

CTGACNCAC TA TAGGGCGAA T TCGAGCTCG G T ACCCGGNGG A TCC T C T AG A
10   20   30   40   50

Manipulating Recombinant DNA: Restriction Mapping and Designing PCR Primers

As you learned in this chapter, restriction enzymes are sophisticated "scissors" that molecular biologists use to cut DNA, and they are routinely used in genetics and molecular biology laboratories for recombinant DNA experiments. A wide variety of online tools assist scientists working with restriction enzymes and manipulating recombinant DNA for different applications. Here we explore **Webcutter** and **Primer3**, two sites that make recombinant DNA experiments much easier.

Exercise I – Creating a Restriction Map in Webcutter

Suppose you had cloned and sequenced a gene and you wanted to design a probe approximately 600 bp long that could be used to analyze expression of this gene in different human tissues by Northern blot analysis. Not too long ago, you had primarily two ways to approach this task. You could digest the cloned DNA with whatever restriction enzymes were in your freezer, then run agarose gels and develop restriction maps in the hope of identifying cutting sites that would give you the size fragment you wanted. Or you could scan the sequence with your eyes, looking for restriction sites of interest—a very time-consuming and eye-straining effort! Internet sites such as **Webcutter** take the guesswork out of developing restriction maps and make it relatively easy to design experiments for manipulating recombinant DNA. In this exercise, you will use Webcutter to create a restriction map of human DNA with the enzymes *Eco*RI, *Bam*HI, and *Pst*I.

1. Access **Webcutter** at http://bioinfo .ut.ee/primer3/. Go to the Companion Web site for *Concepts of Genetics* and open the Exploring Genomics exercise for this chapter. Copy the

sequence of cloned human DNA found there and paste it into the text box in Webcutter.

2. Scroll down to "Please indicate which enzymes to include in the analysis." Click the button indicating "Use only the following enzymes." Select the restriction enzymes *Eco*RI, *Bam*HI, and *Pst*I from the list provided, then click "Analyze sequence." (*Note*: Use the command, control, or shift key to select multiple restriction enzymes.)

3. After examining the results provided by Webcutter, create a table showing the number of cutting sites for each enzyme and the fragment sizes that would be generated by digesting with each enzyme. Draw a restriction map indicating cutting sites for each enzyme with distances between each site and the total size of this piece of human DNA.

Exercise II – Designing a Recombinant DNA Experiment

Now that you have created a restriction map of your piece of human DNA, you need to ligate the DNA into a plasmid DNA vector that you can use to make your probe (molecular biologists often refer to this as subcloning). To do this, you will need to determine which restriction enzymes would best be suited for cutting both the plasmid and the human DNA.

1. Referring back to the Companion Web site and the Exploring Genomics exercise for this chapter, copy the plasmid DNA sequence from Exercise II into the text box in Webcutter and identify cutting sites for the same enzymes you used in Exercise I. Then answer the following questions:

   a. What is the total size of the plasmid DNA analyzed in Webcutter?

   b. Which enzyme(s) could be used in a recombinant DNA experiment to ligate the plasmid to the *largest* DNA fragment from the human gene? Briefly explain your answer.

   c. What size recombinant DNA molecule will be created by ligating these fragments?

   d. Draw a simple diagram showing the cloned DNA inserted into the plasmid and indicate the restriction-enzyme cutting site(s) used to create this recombinant plasmid.

2. As you prepare to carry out this subcloning experiment, you find that the expiration dates on most of your restriction enzymes have long since passed. Rather than run an experiment with old enzymes, you decide to purchase new enzymes. Fortunately, a site called **REBASE®: The Restriction Enzyme Database** can help you. Over 300 restriction enzymes are commercially available rather inexpensively, but scientists are always looking for ways to stretch their research budgets as far as possible. REBASE is excellent for locating enzyme suppliers and enzyme specifics, particularly if you need to work with an enzyme that you are unfamiliar with. Visit **REBASE®** at http://rebase.neb.com/rebase/ rebase.html to identify companies that sell the restriction enzyme(s) you need for this experiment.

Exercise III – Designing PCR Primers

Giving this experiment more thought, you decide to try reverse transcriptase PCR (RT-PCR) first instead of Northern blotting because RT-PCR is a faster and more sensitive way to detect gene expression. Picking correct primers for a PCR experiment is not a trivial process. You have to be sure the primers can amplify the gene of interest, and you need to avoid primer self-annealing—or having primers bind to each other—among many other considerations. Fortunately, primer design is another task made much easier by the Internet. In this exercise, you will use **Primer3**, a PCR primer design site from the Whitehead Institute for Biomedical Research.

1. Access **Primer3** at http://bioinfo.ut.ee /primer3/. Copy the human DNA sequence from Exercise I into the text box, then click "Pick Primers."

2. On the next page, the sequences for the best recommended primers will appear at the top of the screen. Answer the following:

   a. What is the length, in base pairs, of the left (forward) primer and right (reverse) primer? Where does each of these primers bind in the gene sequence?

   b. The hybridization temperature for a PCR reaction is often set around 5 degrees below the melting temperature, or T_m (refer to Chapter 10 for a discussion of melting temperature). Based on the T_m for these primers, what might be the optimal hybridization temperature for this experiment?

   c. What size PCR product would you expect these primers to generate if you ran the DNA amplified by this PCR reaction on an agarose gel?

CASE STUDY | Should we worry about recombinant DNA technology?

Early in the 1970s, when recombinant DNA research was first developed, scientists realized that there may be unforeseen dangers, and after a self-imposed moratorium on all such research, they developed and implemented a detailed set of safety protocols for the construction, storage, and use of genetically modified organisms. These guidelines then formed the basis of regulations adopted by the federal government. Over time, safer methods were developed, and these stringent guidelines were gradually relaxed or, in many cases, eliminated altogether. Now, however, the specter of bioterrorism has re-focused attention on the potential misuses of recombinant DNA technology. For example, individuals or small groups might use the information in genome databases coupled with recombinant DNA technology to construct or reconstruct agents of disease, such as the smallpox virus or the deadly influenza virus.

1. Do you think that the question of recombinant DNA research regulation by university and corporations should be revisited to monitor possible bioterrorist activity?

2. Should freely available access to genetic databases, including genomes, and gene or protein sequences be continued, or should it be restricted to individuals who have been screened and approved for such access?

3. Forty years after its development, the use of recombinant DNA technology is widespread and is found even in many middle school and high school biology courses. Are there some aspects of gene splicing that might be dangerous in the hands of an amateur?

Summary Points

MasteringGenetics™ For activities, animations, and review quizzes, go to the Study Area.

1. Recombinant DNA technology was made possible by the discovery of specific proteins called restriction enzymes, which cut DNA at specific recognition sequences, producing fragments that can be joined together with other DNA fragments to form recombinant DNA molecules.

2. Recombinant DNA molecules can be transferred into any of several types of host cells where cloned copies of the DNA are produced during host-cell replication. Many kinds of host cells may be used for replication, including bacteria, yeast, and mammalian cells.

3. The polymerase chain reaction (PCR) allows DNA to be amplified without host cells and is a rapid, sensitive method with wide-ranging applications.

4. Historically, DNA libraries have been important for producing collections of cloned genes to identify genes and gene-regulatory regions of interest.

5. Once cloned, DNA sequences are analyzed through a variety of molecular techniques that allow scientists to study gene structure, expression, and function.

6. By determining the nucleotide sequence of a DNA segment, DNA sequencing is the ultimate way to characterize DNA at the molecular level.

7. Rapid advances in sequencing technologies have led to greatly increased sequencing capacities at reduced costs over historically used sequencing methods, providing scientists with unprecedented access to sequence data.

8. Gene knockout methods and transgenic animals are widely used to study gene function *in vivo*.

INSIGHTS AND SOLUTIONS

The recognition sequence for the restriction enzyme *Sau*3AI is GATC (see Figure 20–1); in the recognition sequence for the enzyme *Bam*HI—GGATCC—the four internal bases are identical to the *Sau*3AI sequence. The single-stranded ends produced by the two enzymes are identical. Suppose you have a cloning vector that contains a *Bam*HI recognition sequence and you also have foreign DNA that was cut with *Sau*3AI.

(a) Can this DNA be ligated into the *Bam*HI site of the vector, and if so, why?
(b) Can the DNA segment cloned into this sequence be cut from the vector with *Sau*3AI? With *Bam*HI? What potential problems do you see with the use of *Bam*HI?

Solution: (a) DNA cut with *Sau*3AI can be ligated into the vector's *Bam*HI cutting site because the single-stranded ends generated by the two enzymes are identical.
(b) The DNA can be cut from the vector with *Sau*3AI because the recognition sequence for this enzyme (GATC) is

maintained on each side of the insert. Recovering the cloned insert with *Bam*HI is more problematic. In the ligated vector, the conserved sequences are GGATC (left) and GATCC (right). The correct base for recognition by *Bam*HI will *follow* the conserved sequence (to produce GGATCC on the left) only about 25 percent of the time, and the correct base will *precede* the conserved sequence (and produce GGATCC on the right) about 25 percent of the time as well. Thus, *Bam*HI will be able to cut the insert from the vector (0.25 × 0.25 = 0.0625), or only about 6 percent, of the time.

Problems and Discussion Questions

MasteringGenetics™ Visit for instructor-assigned tutorials and problems.

HOW DO WE KNOW?

1. In this chapter we focused on how specific DNA sequences can be copied, identified, characterized, and sequenced. At the same time, we found many opportunities to consider the methods and reasoning underlying these techniques. From the explanations given in the chapter, what answers would you propose to the following fundamental questions?
   (a) In a recombinant DNA cloning experiment, how can we determine whether DNA fragments of interest have been incorporated into plasmids and, once host cells are transformed, which cells contain recombinant DNA?
   (b) When using DNA libraries to clone genes, what combination of techniques are used to identify a particular gene of interest?
   (c) What steps make PCR a chain reaction that can produce millions of copies of a specific DNA molecule in a matter of hours without using host cells?
   (d) How has DNA sequencing technology evolved in response to the emerging needs of genome scientists?

CONCEPT QUESTION

2. Review the Chapter Concepts list on page 489. All of these refer to recombinant DNA methods and applications. Write a short essay or sketch a diagram that provides an overview of how recombinant DNA techniques help geneticists study genes.
3. What roles do restriction enzymes, vectors, and host cells play in recombinant DNA studies? What role does DNA ligase perform in a DNA cloning experiment? How does the action of DNA ligase differ from the function of restriction enzymes?
4. The human insulin gene contains a number of sequences that are removed in the processing of the mRNA transcript. In spite

of the fact that bacterial cells cannot excise these sequences from mRNA transcripts, explain how a gene like this can be cloned into a bacterial cell and produce insulin.

5. Although many cloning applications involve introducing recombinant DNA into bacterial host cells, many other cell types are also used as hosts for recombinant DNA. Why?
6. Using DNA sequencing on a cloned DNA segment, you recover the nucleotide sequence shown below. Does this segment contain a palindromic recognition sequence for a restriction enzyme? If so, what is the double-stranded sequence of the palindrome, and what enzyme would cut at this sequence? (Consult Figure 20–1 for a list of restriction sites.)

   CAGTATGGATCCCAT

7. Restriction sites are palindromic; that is, they read the same in the 5′ to 3′ direction on each strand of DNA. What is the advantage of having restriction sites organized this way?
8. List the advantages and disadvantages of using plasmids as cloning vectors. What advantages do BACs and YACs provide over plasmids as cloning vectors?
9. What are the advantages of using a restriction enzyme whose recognition site is relatively rare? When would you use such enzymes?
10. The introduction of genes into plants is a common practice that has generated not only a host of genetically modified foodstuffs, but also significant worldwide controversy. Interestingly, a tumor-inducing plasmid is often used to produce genetically modified plants. Is the use of a tumor-inducing plasmid the source of such controversy?

11. In the context of recombinant DNA technology, of what use is a probe?

12. If you performed a PCR experiment starting with only one copy of double-stranded DNA, approximately how many DNA molecules would be present in the reaction tube after 15 cycles of amplification?

13. In a control experiment, a plasmid containing a *Hin*dIII recognition sequence within a kanamycin resistance gene is cut with *Hin*dIII, re-ligated, and used to transform *E. coli* K12 cells. Kanamycin-resistant colonies are selected, and plasmid DNA from these colonies is subjected to electrophoresis. Most of the colonies contain plasmids that produce single bands that migrate at the same rate as the original intact plasmid. A few colonies, however, produce two bands, one of original size and one that migrates much higher in the gel. Diagram the origin of this slow band as a product of ligation.

14. What advantages do cDNA libraries provide over genomic DNA libraries? Describe cloning applications where the use of a genomic library is necessary to provide information that a cDNA library cannot.

15. You have recovered a cloned DNA segment from a vector and determine that the insert is 1300 bp in length. To characterize this cloned segment, you isolate the insert and decide to construct a restriction map. Using enzyme I and enzyme II, followed by gel electrophoresis, you determine the number and size of the fragments produced by enzymes I and II alone and in combination, as recorded in the following table. Construct a restriction map from these data, showing the positions of the restriction-enzyme cutting sites relative to one another and the distance between them in units of base pairs.

Enzyme	Restriction Fragment Sizes (bp)
I	350, 950
II	200, 1100
I and II	150, 200, 950

16. To create a cDNA library, cDNA can be inserted into vectors and cloned. In the analysis of cDNA clones, it is often difficult to find clones that are full length—that is, many clones are shorter than the mature mRNA molecules from which they are derived. Why is this so?

17. Although the capture and trading of great apes has been banned in 112 countries since 1973, it is estimated that about 1000 chimpanzees are removed annually from Africa and smuggled into Europe, the United States, and Japan. This illegal trade is often disguised by simulating births in captivity. Until recently, genetic identity tests to uncover these illegal activities were not used because of the lack of highly polymorphic markers (markers that vary from one individual to the next) and the difficulties of obtaining chimpanzee blood samples. A study was reported in which DNA samples were extracted from freshly plucked chimpanzee hair roots and used as templates for PCR. The primers used in these studies flank highly polymorphic sites in human DNA that result from variable numbers of tandem nucleotide repeats. Several offspring and their putative parents were tested to determine whether the offspring were "legitimate" or the product of illegal trading. The data are shown in the following Southern blot.

Lane 1: father chimpanzee
Lane 2: mother chimpanzee
Lanes 3–5: putative offspring A, B, C

Examine the data carefully and choose the best conclusion.

(a) None of the offspring is legitimate.

(b) Offspring B and C are not the products of these parents and were probably purchased on the illegal market. The data are consistent with offspring A being legitimate.

(c) Offspring A and B are products of the parents shown, but C is not and was therefore probably purchased on the illegal market.

(d) There are not enough data to draw any conclusions. Additional polymorphic sites should be examined.

(e) No conclusion can be drawn because "human" primers were used.

18. List the steps involved in screening a genomic library. What must be known before starting such a procedure? What are the potential problems with such a procedure, and how can they be overcome or minimized?

19. To estimate the number of cleavage sites in a particular piece of DNA with a known size, you can apply the formula $N/4^n$ where N is the number of base pairs in the target DNA and n is the number of bases in the recognition sequence of the restriction enzyme. If the recognition sequence for *Bam*III is GGATCC and the λ phage DNA contains approximately 48,500 bp, how many cleavage sites would you expect?

20. In a typical PCR reaction, describe what is happening in stages occurring at temperature ranges (a) 90–95°C, (b) 50–70°C, and (c) 70–75°C.

21. We usually think of enzymes as being most active at around 37°C, yet in PCR the DNA polymerase is subjected to multiple exposures of relatively high temperatures and seems to function appropriately at 70–75°C. What is special about the DNA polymerizing enzymes typically used in PCR?

22. How are dideoxynucleotides (ddNTPs) structurally different from deoxynucleotides (dNTPs), and how does this structural difference make ddNTPs valuable in chain-termination methods of DNA sequencing?

23. Assume you have conducted a DNA sequencing reaction using the chain-termination (Sanger) method. You performed all the steps correctly and electrophoresced the resulting DNA fragments correctly, but when you looked at the sequencing gel, many of the bands were duplicated (in terms of length) in other lanes. What might have happened?

24. How is fluorescent *in situ* hybridization (FISH) used to produce a spectral karyotype?

25. What is the difference between a knockout animal and a transgenic animal?

26. One complication of making a transgenic animal is that the transgene may integrate at random into the coding region, or the regulatory region, of an endogenous gene. What might be the consequences of such random integrations? How might this complicate genetic analysis of the transgene?

27. When disrupting a mouse gene by knockout, why is it desirable to breed mice until offspring homozygous (−/−) for the knockout target gene are obtained?

28. What techniques can scientists use to determine if a particular transgene has been integrated into the genome of an organism?

Extra-Spicy Problems

29. The gel presented here shows the pattern of bands of fragments produced with several restriction enzymes. The enzymes used are identified above and below the gel and six possible restriction maps are shown in the column to the right.

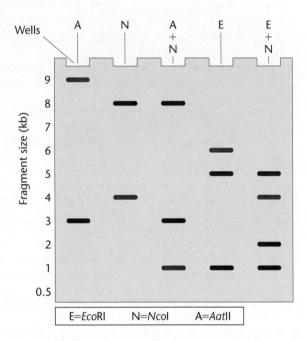

E=EcoRI   N=NcoI   A=AatII

One of the six restriction maps shown is consistent with the pattern of bands shown in the gel.
(a) From your analysis of the pattern of bands on the gel, select the correct map and explain your reasoning.
(b) In a Southern blot prepared from this gel, the highlighted bands (pink) hybridized with the gene *pep*. Where is the *pep* gene located?

30. A widely used method for calculating the annealing temperature for a primer used in PCR is 5 degrees below the T_m (°C), which is computed by the equation 81.5 + 0.41 × (%GC) − (675/N), where %GC is the percentage of GC nucleotides in the oligonucleotide and N is the length of the oligonucleotide. Notice from the formula that both the GC content *and* the length of the oligonucleotide are variables. Assuming you have the following oligonucleotide as a primer, compute the annealing temperature for PCR. What is the relationship between T_m (°C) and %GC? Why? (*Note:* In reality, this computation provides only a starting point for empirical determination of the most useful annealing temperature.)

$$5'-TTGAAAATATTTCCCATTGCC-3'$$

31. Most of the techniques described in this chapter (blotting, cloning, PCR, etc.) are dependent on intermolecular attractions (annealing) between different populations of nucleic acids. Length of the strands, temperature, and percentage of GC nucleotides weigh considerably on intermolecular associations. Two other components commonly used in hybridization protocols are monovalent ions and formamide. A formula that takes monovalent ion (Na⁺) and formamide concentrations into consideration to compute a T_m (temperature of melting) is as follows:

$$T_m = 81.5 + 16.6(\log M[Na^+]) + 0.41(\%GC) - 0.72(\%formamide)$$

(a) For the following concentrations of Na⁺ and formamide, calculate the T_m. Assume 45% GC content.

Na⁺	% Formamide
0.825	20
0.825	40
0.165	20
0.165	40

(b) Given that formamide competes for hydrogen bond locations of nucleic acid bases and monovalent cations are attracted to the negative charges of nucleic acids, explain why the T_m varies as described in part (a).

32. In humans, congenital heart disease is a common birth defect that affects approximately 1 out of 125 live births. Using reverse transcription PCR (RT-PCR), Zaidi et al. (2013) determined that approximately 10 percent of the cases resulted from point mutations, often involving histone function. To capture products of gene expression in developing hearts, they used oligo(dT) in their reverse transcription protocol.
(a) How would such a high %T in a primer influence annealing temperature?
(b) Compared with oligo(dT) primers, a pool of random sequence primers requires a trickier assessment of annealing temperature. Why?
(c) If one were interested in comparing the quantitative distribution of gene expression in say, the right and left side of a developing heart, how might one proceed using RT-PCR?

33. The U.S. Department of Justice has established a database that catalogs PCR amplification products from short tandem repeats of the Y (Y-STRs) chromosome in humans. The database contains polymorphisms of five U.S. ethnic groups (African Americans, European Americans, Hispanics, Native Americans, and Asian Americans) as well as worldwide population.

(a) Given that STRs are repeats of varying lengths, for example $(TCTG)_{9-17}$ or $(TAT)_{6-14}$, explain how PCR could reveal differences (polymorphisms) among individuals. How could the Department of Justice make use of those differences?
(b) Y-STRs from the nonrecombining region of the Y chromosome (NRY) have special relevance for forensic purposes. Why?
(c) What would be the value of knowing the ethnic population differences for Y-STR polymorphisms?
(d) For forensic applications, the probability of a "match" for a crime scene DNA sample and a suspect's DNA often culminates in a guilty or innocent verdict. How is a "match" determined, and what are the uses and limitations of such probabilities?

34. There are a variety of circumstances under which rapid results using multiple markers in PCR amplifications are highly desired, such as in forensics, pathogen analysis, or detection of genetically modified organisms. In multiplex PCR, multiple sets of primers are used, often with less success than when applied to PCR as individual sets. Numerous studies have been conducted to optimize procedures, but each has described the process as time consuming and often unsuccessful. Considering the information given in Problem 31, why should multiplex PCR be any different than single primer set PCR in terms of dependability and ease of optimization?

TGGCTTGGCCCTATCTGTCCTGTGTTGAAGCTGTGCCAATCCGAAAAGTCCAG
||||||||||||||||||| | || ||| ||||||||| |||| |||||||||
TGGCTTTGGCCCCTATCTTTTCTATGTCCAAGCTGTGCCCATCCAAAAAGTCCAA

ACCAAAACCCTCATCAAGACGATTGTCGCCAGGATCAATGACATTTCACACACG
|||||||||||||||||||||||| |||||| |||||||||||||||||||||||
ACCAAAACCCTCATCAAGACAATTGTCACCAGGATCAATGACATTTCACACACG

GTCTCCTCCAAACAGAGGGTCGCTGGTCTGGACTTCATTCCTGGGCTCCAACCA
||||||||||||||||| ||| | ||| |||||||||||||||||||||||||||
GTCTCCTCCAAACAGAAAGTCACCGGTTTGGACTTCATTCCTGGGCTCCACCCC

AGTTTGTCCAGGATGGACCAGACGTTGGCCATCTACCAACAGATCCTCAACAGT
| || |||| |||||||||| |||| |||||||||||||||||||| ||||||
ACCTTATCCAAGATGGACCAGACACTGGCAGTCTACCAACAGATCCTCACCAGT

TCCAGAAATGTGGTCCAAATATCTAATGACCTGGAGAACCTCCGGGACCTTCTC
|||||||| ||| |||||||||||| || ||||||||||||||||||| |||||
TCCAGAAACGTGATCCAAATATCCAACGACCTGGAGAACCTCCGGGATCTTCTT

CTGGCCTCCTCCAAGAGCTGCCCCTTGCCCCGGGCCAGGGGCCTGGAGACCTTT
|||||| ||| |||||||||||| ||||||| |||||| ||||| |||||||||||
CTGGCCTTCTCTAAGAGCTGCCACTTGCCCTGGGCCAGTGGCCTGGAGACCTTG

Alignment comparing DNA sequence for the leptin gene from dogs (top) and humans (bottom). Vertical lines and shaded boxes indicate identical bases. *LEP* encodes a hormone that functions to suppress appetite. This type of analysis is a common application of bioinformatics and a good demonstration of comparative genomics.

21

Genomics, Bioinformatics, and Proteomics

CHAPTER CONCEPTS

- Genomics applies recombinant DNA, DNA sequencing methods, and bioinformatics to sequence, assemble, and analyze genomes.

- Disciplines in genomics encompass several areas of study, including structural and functional genomics, comparative genomics, and metagenomics, and have led to an "omics" revolution in modern biology.

- Bioinformatics merges information technology with biology and mathematics to store, share, compare, and analyze nucleic acid and protein sequence data.

- The Human Genome Project has greatly advanced our understanding of the organization, size, and function of the human genome.

- Ten years after completion of the Human Genome Project, a new era of genomics studies is providing deeper insights into the human genome.

- Comparative genomics analysis has revealed similarities and differences in genome size and organization.

- Metagenomics is the study of genomes from environmental samples and is valuable for identifying microbial genomes.

- Transcriptome analysis provides insight into patterns of gene expression and gene-regulatory activity of a genome.

- Proteomics focuses on the protein content of cells and on the structures, functions, and interactions of proteins.

- Systems biology approaches attempt to uncover complex interactions among genes, proteins, and other cellular components.

The term **genome**, meaning the complete set of DNA in a single cell of an organism, was coined at a time when geneticists began to turn from the study of individual genes to a focus on the larger picture. To begin to characterize all of the genes in an organism's genome, geneticists typically followed a two-part classical genetics approach: (1) identify spontaneous mutations or collect mutants produced by chemical or physical agents, and (2) generate linkage maps using mutant strains as discussed earlier in the text (see Chapter 5).

These effective strategies were used to identify genes in many of the classic model organisms discussed in this book, such as *Drosophila*, maize, mice, bacteria, and yeast, as well as in viruses, such as bacteriophages. These approaches formed the technical backbone of genetic analysis and still have their applications today; however, they have several major limitations. For instance, conventional mutational analysis and linkage requires that at least one mutation for each gene be available before all the genes in a genome can be identified. Obtaining mutants and carrying out linkage studies are very time consuming processes, and when mutations are lethal or have no clear phenotype, they can be difficult or impossible to map. In addition, although researchers can generate mutations in animal models in a laboratory, they cannot do the same with humans; thus, identifying human genes by mutational analysis is largely limited to linkage mapping of inherited or spontaneously acquired mutant genes with clear phenotypes. Another fundamental limitation of these approaches is that, although they can be used for identifying and characterizing gene loci, they do not lead to a determination of DNA sequence. Nor are they particularly useful for studying noncoding areas of the genome such as DNA regulatory sequences.

In 1977, as recombinant DNA-based techniques were developed, Fred Sanger and colleagues began the field of **genomics**, the study of genomes, by using a newly developed method of DNA sequencing to sequence the 5400-nucleotide genome of the virus ϕX174. Other viral genomes were sequenced in short order, but even this technology was slow and labor-intensive, limiting its use to small genomes. In the 1980s, geneticists interested in mapping human genes began using recombinant DNA technology to map DNA sequences to specific chromosomes. Initially, most of these sequences were not actually full-length genes but marker sequences such as restriction fragment length polymorphisms (RFLPs). Once assigned to chromosomes, these markers were used in pedigree analysis to establish linkage between the markers and disease phenotypes for genetic disorders. This approach, called **positional cloning**, was used to map, isolate, clone, and sequence the genes for cystic fibrosis, neurofibromatosis, and dozens of other disorders. Positional cloning identified one gene at a time, and yet by the mid-1980s, it had been used to assign more than 3500 genes and markers to human chromosomes.

At this time it was estimated that there were approximately 100,000 genes in the human genome, and it was readily apparent that mapping by using existing methods would be a laborious, time-consuming, and nearly insurmountable task. As you will soon learn, this estimate for gene number turned out to be inaccurate. During the next three decades, the development of computer-automated DNA sequencing methods made it possible to consider sequencing the larger and more complex genomes of eukaryotes, including the 3.1 billion nucleotides that comprise the human genome. The development of recombinant DNA technologies coupled with the advent of new, powerful DNA sequencing methods and bioinformatics is responsible for rapidly accelerating the field of genomics.

Genomic technologies have developed so quickly that modern biological research is currently experiencing a genomics revolution. In this chapter, we will examine basic technologies used in genomics and then discuss examples of genome data and different disciplines of genomics. We will also discuss *transcriptome analysis,* the study of genes expressed in a cell or tissue (the "transcriptome"), and *proteomics,* the study of proteins present in a cell or tissue.

The chapter concludes with a brief look at *systems biology,* a new area of contemporary biology that incorporates and integrates genomics, transcriptome analysis, and proteomics data. Later in the text (see Chapter 22) we will continue our discussion of genomics by describing many modern applications of recombinant DNA and genomic technologies. Please note that some of the topics discussed in this chapter are explored in greater depth in later chapters (see Special Topic Chapter 1—Epigenetics, Special Topic Chapter 2—Emerging Roles of RNA, and Special Topic Chapter 4—Genomics and Personalized Medicine).

21.1 Whole-Genome Sequencing Is a Widely Used Method for Sequencing and Assembling Entire Genomes

As discussed earlier in the text (see Chapter 20), recombinant DNA technology made it possible to generate DNA libraries that could be used to identify, clone, and sequence specific genes of interest. But a primary limitation of library screening and even of most polymerase chain reaction (PCR) approaches is that they typically can identify only relatively small numbers of genes at a time. Genomics allows the sequencing of entire genomes. **Structural genomics** focuses on sequencing genomes and analyzing nucleotide sequences to identify genes and other important sequences such as gene-regulatory regions.

The most widely used strategy for sequencing and assembling an entire genome involves variations of a method called **whole-genome sequencing (WGS)**, also known as **shotgun cloning** or shotgun sequencing. In simple terms, this technique is analogous to you and a friend taking your respective copies of this genetics textbook and randomly ripping the pages into strips about 5 to 7 inches long. Each chapter represents a chromosome, and all of the letters in the entire book are the "genome." Then you and your friend would go through the painstaking task of comparing the pieces of paper to find places that match, overlapping sentences—areas where there are similar sentences on different pieces of paper. Eventually, in theory, many of the strips containing matching sentences would overlap in ways that you could use to reconstruct the pages and assemble the order of the entire text.

Figure 21–1 shows a basic overview of WGS. First, an entire chromosome is cut into short, overlapping fragments, either by mechanically shearing the DNA in various ways (such as excessive heat treatment or sonication in which sonic energy is used to break DNA) or by using restriction enzymes to cleave the DNA at different locations. For

1. **Genomic DNA cut into multiple overlapping fragments by digestion with different restriction enzymes to create a series of contiguous fragments, or "contigs"**

2. **Overlapping sequenced fragments aligned using computer programs to assemble an entire chromosome**

3. **Fragments aligned based on identical DNA sequences**

FIGURE 21-1 An overview of whole-genome sequencing (WGS) and assembly. This approach shows one strategy that involves using restriction enzymes to digest genomic DNA into contigs, which are then sequenced and aligned using bioinformatics to identify overlapping fragments based on sequence identity. Notice that *Eco*RI digestion of the portion of DNA depicted here produces two fragments (contigs 1, 2–4), whereas digestion with *Bam*HI produces three fragments (contigs 1–2, 3, 4).

use of algorithm-based software programs for creating a DNA-sequence **alignment**, in which similar sequences of bases, such as contigs, are lined up for comparison. Alignment identifies overlapping sequences, allowing scientists to reconstruct their order in a chromosome. **Figure 21–2** shows an example of contig alignment and assembly for a portion of human chromosome 2. For simplicity, this figure shows relatively short sequences for each contig, which in actuality would be much longer. The figure is also simplified in that, in actual alignments, assembled sequences do not always overlap only at their ends.

The whole-genome shotgun sequencing method was developed by J. Craig Venter and colleagues at The Institute for Genome Research (TIGR). In 1995, TIGR scientists used this approach to sequence the 1.83-million-bp genome of the bacterium *Haemophilus influenzae*. This was the first completed genome sequence from a free-living organism, and it demonstrated "proof of concept" that shotgun sequencing could be used to sequence an entire genome. Even after the genome for *H. influenzae* was sequenced, many scientists were skeptical that a shotgun approach would work on the larger genomes of eukaryotes. But improvement to shotgun approaches using next-generation sequencing technologies are now the predominant methods for sequencing genomes from nearly all species, including humans.

High-Throughput Sequencing and Its Impact on Genomics

Cutting a genome into contigs is not particularly difficult; however, a primary hurdle that had to be overcome to advance whole-genome sequencing was the question of how to sequence millions or billions of base pairs in a timely and cost-effective way. This was a major challenge for scientists working on the Human Genome Project (Section 21.4). The Sanger sequencing method discussed earlier in the text (see Chapter 20), was the predominant sequencing technique for a long time. However, a major limitation

simplicity, here we present a basic example of DNA shearing using restriction enzymes. Increasingly, nonenzymatic approaches for shearing DNA are being used. Different restriction enzymes can be used so that chromosomes are cut at different sites; or sometimes, *partial digests* of DNA using the same restriction enzyme are used. With partial digests, DNA is incubated with restriction enzymes for only a short period of time, so that not every site in a particular sequence is cut to completion by an individual enzyme. Restriction digests of whole chromosomes generate thousands to millions of overlapping DNA fragments. For example, a 6-bp cutter such as *Eco*RI creates about 700,000 fragments when used to digest the human genome! Because these overlapping fragments are adjoining segments that collectively form one continuous DNA molecule within a chromosome, they are called **contiguous fragments**, or "**contigs**."

In the next section, we will discuss the importance of bioinformatics to genomics. One of the earliest bioinformatics applications to be developed for genomic purposes was the

FIGURE 21-2 DNA-sequence alignment of contigs on human chromosome 2. Single-stranded DNA for three different contigs from human chromosome 2 is shown in blue, red, or green. The actual sequence from chromosome 2 is shown, but in reality, contig alignment involves fragments that are several thousand bases in length. Alignment of the three contigs allows a portion of chromosome 2 to be assembled. Alignment of all contigs for a particular chromosome would result in assembly of a completely sequenced chromosome.

of this technique was that even the best sequencing gels would typically yield only several hundred base pairs in each run and relatively few runs could be completed in a day. As a result, the overall production of sequence data was quite slow compared with modern techniques. Obviously, it would be very time consuming to manually sequence an entire genome by the Sanger method. The major technological breakthrough that made genomics possible was the development of computer-automated sequencers.

Many of the early computer-automated sequencers, designed for so-called **high-throughput sequencing**, could process millions of base pairs in a day. These sequencers contained multiple capillary gels that are several feet long. Some ran as many as 96 capillary gels at a time, each producing around 900 bases of sequence. Because these sequencers were computer automated, they could work around the clock, generating over 2 million bases of sequence in a day. In the past 15 years, high-throughput sequencing has increased the productivity of DNA-sequencing technology over 500-fold. The total number of bases that could be sequenced in a single reaction was doubling about every 24 months. At the same time, this increase in efficiency brought about a dramatic decrease in cost, from about $1.00 to less than $0.001 per base pair. As we will discuss in Section 21.4, without question the development of high-throughput sequencing was essential for the Human Genome Project. And as you know from earlier in the text (see Chapter 20), next- and third-generation sequencers now enable genome scientists to produce sequence nearly 50,000 times faster than sequencers in 2000 with greater output, improved accuracy, and reduced cost.

The Clone-by-Clone Approach

Prior to the widespread use of whole-genome sequencing approaches, genomes were being assembled using a **clone-by-clone** approach, also called **map-based cloning** (**Figure 21–3**). Initial progress on the Human Genome Project was based on this methodology, in which individual DNA fragments from restriction digests of chromosomes are aligned to create the restriction maps of a chromosome. These restriction fragments are then ligated into vectors such as bacterial artificial chromosomes (BACs) or yeast artificial chromosomes (YACs) to create libraries of contigs. Recall from earlier in the text (see Chapter 20) that BACs and YACs are good cloning vectors for replicating large fragments of DNA.

Prior to the development of high-throughput sequencing approaches, DNA fragments in BACs and YACs would often be further digested into smaller, more easily manipulated pieces that were then subcloned into cosmids or plasmids so that they could be sequenced in their entirety (Figure 21–3). After each sequenced fragment was analyzed for alignment overlaps, a chromosome could be assembled. The bioinformatics approaches we will discuss in the next section would then be used to identify possible protein-coding genes and assign them a location on the chromosome. For example, Figure 21–3 shows the use of map-based cloning to sequence part of chromosome 11, including part of the human β-globin gene.

Compared to whole-genome sequencing, the clone-by-clone approach is cumbersome and time consuming because of the time required to clone DNA fragments into different vectors, transform bacteria or yeast, select

Digest chromosomal DNA into many
small pieces with restriction enzymes

Human
chromosome

Average 400,000-bp fragment
cloned into yeast artificial
chromosome (YAC) or
bacterial artificial
chromosome (BAC)

Yeast artificial chromosome

Cosmid

Average 40,000-bp
fragment cloned into
cosmid

Restriction map

Overlapping clones

Average 4000-bp fragment
cloned into plasmid or
sequencing vector

Plasmid

Partial Nucleotide Sequence
(from human β-globin gene)
GGCACTGACTCTCTCTGCCTATGGTCTATTTTCCCACCCTAGGCTGCTGGTGGTCTACCC
TGGACCCAGAGGTTCTTTGAGTCCTTTGGGGATCTGTCCACTCCTGATGCTGTTATGG

Chromosome 11
144 million bases

Beckwith-Wiedemann syndrome	Freeman-Sheldon syndrome variant
Dopamine receptor	Jansky-Bielschowsky disease
Autonomic nervous system dysfunction	Diabetes mellitus, insulin-dependent
Thalassemia	Sickle-cell anemia
Diabetes mellitus, rare form	Thalassemias, beta
Hyperproinsulinemia, familial	Erythremias, beta
Breast cancer	Heinz body anemias, beta
Rhabdomyosarcoma	Bladder cancer
Lung cancer	Wilms tumor, type 2
Segawa syndrome, recessive	Adrenocortical carcinoma, hereditary
Hypoparathyroidism	Sjogren syndrome antigen
Tumor susceptibility gene	Osteoporosis
Breast cancer	Deafness, autosomal recessive
Usher syndrome	Leukemia, T-cell acute lymphoblastic
Atrophia areata	Hepatitis B virus integration site
Fanconi anemia	Lacticacidemia
Leukemia, myeloid and lymphocytic	T-cell leukemia/lymphoma
Acatalasemia	Diabetes mellitus, noninsulin-dependent
Peters anomaly	Cardiomyopathy, familial hypertrophic
Cataracts, congenital	Prostate cancer overexpressed gene
Keratitis	Coagulation factor II (thrombin)
Severe combined immunodeficiency,	Hypoprothrombinemia
B cell-negative	Dysprothrombinemia
Omenn syndrome	Complement component inhibitor
Wilms tumor, type I	Angioedema, hereditary
Denys-Drash syndrome	Smith-Lemli-Opitz syndrome, types I and II
	IgE responsiveness, atopic
	Bardet-Biedl syndrome

FIGURE 21–3 A clone-by-clone, or map-based, approach to genome sequencing involves cloning overlapping DNA fragments (contigs) into vectors. Different vectors, such as BACs, YACs, cosmids, and plasmids, are used depending on the size of each DNA fragment being analyzed. Overlapping clones are then sequenced and aligned to assemble an entire chromosome. Depicted here is a partial map of genes on chromosome 21 that are involved in human genetic disease conditions.

individual clones from the library for sequencing, and then carry out sequence analysis and assembly on relatively short sequences. Essentially, the clone-by-clone approach is the organized sequencing of contigs from a restriction map instead of random sequencing and assembly. As whole-genome sequencing approaches have become a routine method for assembling genomes, map-based cloning approaches are rarely used, and only then to resolve the problems encountered during whole-genome sequencing. For example, highly repetitive sequences in a chromosome may be difficult to align correctly in order to identify overlaps because with such sequences one cannot know for sure whether portions that are nearly identical are overlapping fragments or belong to different parts of a highly repetitive region. Frequently, there are also gaps between aligned contigs. In the textbook-ripping analogy, after you compare all your pieces of paper, you may be left with some very small ones that contain too few words to be matched with certainty to any others and with some pieces for which you just could not find matches. In these instances, a clone-by-clone approach may enable you to assemble the necessary contigs and complete the chromosome.

Draft Sequences and Checking for Errors

It is common for a draft sequence of a genome to be announced before a final sequence is eventually released. Draft sequences often contain gaps in areas that, for any number of reasons, may have been difficult to analyze. The decision to designate a sequence as "final" is dictated by the amount of error genome scientists are willing to accept as a cutoff.

Chromosome segments are typically sequenced more than once to ensure a high level of accuracy. The assembly of a final genomic sequence from multiple sequencing runs is known as **compiling**. One way to compile and error check is to sequence complementary strands of a DNA molecule separately and then use base-pairing rules to check for errors. Researchers using the shotgun method on the genome of the bacterium *Pseudomonas aeruginosa* sequenced the 6.3 million nucleotides seven times to ensure that the final sequence would be accurate. Yet even with this level of redundancy, the assembler software recognized 1604 regions that required further clarification. These regions were then reanalyzed and re-sequenced. Finally, relevant parts of the shotgun sequence were compared with the sequences of two widely separated genomic regions obtained by conventional cloning. The 81,843 nucleotides cloned and sequenced by the clone-by-clone method were in perfect agreement with the sequence obtained by the shotgun method. This level of care in checking for accuracy is not unusual; similar precautions are taken in almost every genome project.

Once compiled, a genome is analyzed to identify gene sequences, regulatory elements, and other features that reveal important information. In the next section we discuss the central role of bioinformatics in this process.

21.2 DNA Sequence Analysis Relies on Bioinformatics Applications and Genome Databases

Genomics necessitated the rapid development of **bioinformatics**, the use of computer hardware and software and mathematics applications to organize, share, and analyze data related to gene structure, gene sequence and expression, and protein structure and function. However, even before whole-genome sequencing projects had been initiated, a large amount of sequence information from a range of different organisms was accumulating as a result of gene cloning by recombinant DNA techniques. Scientists around the world needed databases that could be used to store, share, and obtain the maximum amount of information from protein and DNA sequences. Thus, bioinformatics software was already being used to compare and analyze DNA sequences and to create private and public databases. Once genomics emerged as a new approach for analyzing DNA, however, bioinformatics became even more important than before. Today, it is a dynamic area of biological research, providing new career opportunities for anyone interested in merging an understanding of biological data with information technology, mathematics, and statistical analysis.

Among the most common applications of bioinformatics are to compare DNA sequences, as in contig alignment; to identify genes in a genomic DNA sequence; to find gene-regulatory regions, such as promoters and enhancers; to identify structural sequences, such as telomeric sequences, in chromosomes; to predict the amino acid sequence of a putative polypeptide encoded by a cloned gene sequence; to analyze protein structure and predict protein functions on the basis of identified domains and motifs; and to deduce evolutionary relationships between genes and organisms on the basis of sequence information.

High-throughput DNA sequencing techniques were developed nearly simultaneously with the expansion of the Internet. As genome data accumulated, many DNA-sequence databases became freely available online. Databases are essential for archiving and sharing data with other researchers and with the public. One of the largest genomic databases, called **GenBank**, is maintained by the National Center for Biotechnology Information (NCBI) in Washington, D.C., and is the largest publicly available database of DNA sequences. GenBank shares and acquires data from databases in Japan and Europe; it contains more than 150 billion bases of sequence data from over 100,000 species; and it doubles in size roughly every 14–18 months! The Human Genome Nomenclature Committee, supported by the NIH, establishes rules for assigning names and symbols to newly cloned human genes. As sequences are identified and genes are named, each sequence deposited into Gen-Bank is provided with an **accession number** that scientists can use to access and retrieve that sequence for analysis.

The NCBI is an invaluable source of public access databases and bioinformatics tools for analyzing genome data. You have already been introduced to NCBI and GenBank through several Exploring Genomics exercises. In Exploring Genomics for this chapter, you will use NCBI and GenBank to compare and align contigs in order to assemble a chromosome segment.

Annotation to Identify Gene Sequences

One of the fundamental challenges of genomics is that, although genome projects generate tremendous amounts of DNA sequence information, these data are of little use until they have been analyzed and interpreted. Genome projects accumulate nucleotide sequences, and then scientists have to make sense of those sequences. Thus, after a genome has been sequenced and compiled, scientists are faced with the task of identifying gene-regulatory sequences and other sequences of interest in the genome so that gene maps can be developed. This process, called **annotation**, relies heavily on bioinformatics, and a wealth of different software tools are available to carry it out.

One initial approach to annotating a sequence is to compare the newly sequenced genomic DNA to the known sequences already stored in various databases. The NCBI provides access to **BLAST (Basic Local Alignment Search Tool)**, a very popular software application for searching through banks of DNA and protein sequence data. Using BLAST, we can compare a segment of genomic DNA to sequences throughout major databases such as Gen-Bank to identify portions that align with or are the same as existing sequences. **Figure 21–4** shows a representative example of a sequence alignment based on a BLAST search. Here a 280-bp chromosome 12 contig from the rat was used to search a mouse database to determine whether a sequence in the rat contig matched a known gene in mice. Notice that the rat contig (the query sequence in the

ref | NT_039455.6 | Mm8_39495_36
Mus musculus chromosome 8 genomic contig, strain C57BL/6J
Features in this part of subject sequence: insulin receptor
Score = 418 bits (226), Expect = 2e-114
Identities = 262/280 (93%), Gaps = 0/280 (0%)

```
Query   1       CAGGCCATCCCGAAAGCGAAGATCCCTTGAAGAGGTGGGCAATGTGACAGCCACTACACC   60
                ||||||||||||||||||||||||||||||||||||||||| ||||||||||||| ||||
Sbjct   174891  CAGGCCATCCCGAAAGCGAAGATCCCTTGAAGAGGTGGGGAATGTGACAGCCACCACACT   174832

Query   61      CACACTTCCAGATTTTCCCAACATCTCCTCCACCATCGCGCCCACAAGCCACGAAGAGCA   120
                |||||||||||||| |||||| |||||||| |||||| | ||||||||| || || |||||
Sbjct   174831  CACACTTCCAGATTTCCCCAACGTCTCCTCTACCATTGTGCCCACAAGTCAGGAGGAGCA   174772

Query   121     CAGACCATTTGAGAAAGTAGTAAACAAGGAGTCACTTGTCATCTCTGGCCTGAGCACTT   180
                |||| |||||||||||||| || |||||||||||||||||||||||||||||||||||||
Sbjct   174771  CAGGCCATTTGAGAAAGTGGTGAACAAGGAGTCACTTGTCATCTCTGGCCTGAGCACTT   174712

Query   181     CACTGGGTACCGCATTGAGCTGCAGGCATGCAATCAGGACTCCCCAGAAGAGAGGTGCAG   240
                ||||||||||||||||||||||||||||||||||||| || ||||||| |||||||||||
Sbjct   174711  CACTGGGTACCGCATTGAGCTGCAGGCATGCAATCAAGATTCCCCAGATGAGAGGTGCAG   174652

Query   241     CGTGGCTGCCTACGTCAGTGCCCGGACCATGCCTGAAGGT   280
                |||||||||||||||||||||||||||||||||||||||||
Sbjct   174651  TGTGGCTGCCTACGTCAGTGCCCGGACCATGCCTGAAGGT   174612
```

FIGURE 21–4 BLAST results showing a 280-base sequence of a chromosome 12 contig from rats (*Rattus norvegicus*, the "query") aligned with a portion of chromosome 8 from mice (*Mus musculus*, the "subject") that contains a partial sequence for the insulin receptor gene. Vertical lines indicate exact matches. The rat contig sequence was used as a query sequence to search a mouse database in GenBank. Notice that the two sequences show 93 percent identity, strong evidence that this rat contig sequence contains a gene for the insulin receptor.

FIGURE 21–5 Characteristics of a protein-coding gene that can be used during annotation to identify a gene in an unknown sequence of genomic DNA. Most eukaryotic genes are organized into coding segments (exons) and noncoding segments (introns). When annotating a genome sequence to determine whether it contains a gene, it is necessary to distinguish between introns and exons, gene-regulatory sequences, such as promoters and enhancers, untranslated regions (UTRs), and gene termination sequences.

BLAST search) aligned with base pairs 174,612 to 174,891 of mouse chromosome 8. The accession number for the mouse chromosome sequence, NT_039455.6, is indicated at the top of the figure. BLAST searches calculate a **similarity score**—also called the **identity** value—determined by the sum of identical matches between aligned sequences divided by the total number of bases aligned. Gaps, indicating missing bases in the two sequences, are usually ignored in calculating similarity scores. The aligned rat and mouse sequences were 93 percent similar and showed no gaps in the alignment. Notice that the BLAST report also provides an "Expect" value, or **E-value**, based on the number of matching sequences in the database that would be expected by chance. E-values take into account the length of the query sequence. By chance, shorter sequences have a much greater likelihood of being present in the database than longer sequences. The lower the E-value (the closer it is to 0), the higher the significance of the match. Significant alignments, indicating that DNA sequences are significantly similar, have E-values less than 1.0.

Because this mouse sequence on chromosome 8 is known to contain an insulin receptor gene (encoding a protein that binds the hormone insulin), it is highly likely that the rat contig sequence also contains an insulin receptor gene. We will return to the topic of similarity in Sections 21.3 and 21.6, where we consider how similarity between gene sequences can be used to infer function and to identify evolutionarily related genes through comparative genomics.

Hallmark Characteristics of a Gene Sequence Can Be Recognized during Annotation

A major limitation of this approach to annotation is that it only works if similar gene sequences are already in a database. Fortunately, it is not the only way to identify genes. Whether the genome under study is from a eukaryote or a prokaryote, several hallmark characteristics of genes can be searched for using bioinformatics software (**Figure 21–5**). We discussed many of these characteristics of a

"typical" gene earlier in the text (see Chapters 13 and 17). For instance, gene-regulatory sequences found upstream of genes are marked by identifiable sequences such as promoters, enhancers, and silencers. Recall from earlier in the text (see Chapter 17) that TATA box, GC box, and CAAT box sequences are often present in the promoter region of eukaryotic genes. Recall also that splice sites between **exons** and **introns** contain a predictable sequence (most introns begin with CT and end with AG) and such splice-site sequences are important for determining intron and exon boundaries. Interestingly, current estimates indicate that only 6 percent of human genes are transcribed from a single, linear stretch of DNA that does not contain any introns.

Downstream elements, such as termination sequences and well-defined sequences at the end of a gene, where a polyadenylation sequence signals the addition of a poly-A tail to the 3′ end of a mRNA transcript, are also important for annotation (Figure 21–5). Annotation can sometimes be a little bit easier for prokaryotic genes than for eukaryotic genes because there are no introns in prokaryotic genes. Gene-prediction programs are used to annotate sequences. These programs incorporate search elements for many of the criteria mentioned above and have become invaluable applications of bioinformatics.

Yet even with bioinformatics, identifying a gene in a particular sequence of DNA is not always straightforward, particularly when one is studying genes that do not code for proteins. In fact, a reasonable question whenever one sequences a genome is "where are the genes?" In other words, how does one know what sequences of a genome are genes and which sequences are not genes or parts of a gene? Consider the sequence presented in **Figure 21–6(a)**, which shows a portion of the human genome. From a casual inspection, it is not clear whether this sequence contains any genes and, if so, how many. Analysis of the sequence, however, reveals identifiable features that provide clues to the presence of a protein-coding gene. In addition, protein-coding genes contain one or more **open reading frames (ORFs)**, sequences of triplet nucleotides

(a)

```
gagccacacc  ctagggttgg  ccaatctact  cccaggagca  gggagggcag  gagccagggc
tgggcataaa  agtcagggca  gagccatcta  ttgcttacat  ttgcttctga  cacaactgtg
ttcactagca  acctcaaaca  gacaccatgg  tgcacctgac  tcctgaggag  aagtctgccg
ttactgccct  gtggggcaag  gtgaacgtgg  atgaagttgg  tggtgaggcc  ctgggcaggt
tggtatcaag  gttacaagac  aggtttaagg  agaccaatag  aaactgggca  tgtggagaca
gagaagactc  ttgggtttct  gataggcact  gactctctct  gcctattggt  ctattttccc
acccttaggc  tgctggtggt  ctaccccttg  acccagaagt  tctttgagtc  ctttggggat
ctgtccactc  ctgatgctgt  tatgggcaac  cctaaggtga  aggctcatgg  caagaaagtg
ctcggtgcct  ttagtgatgg  cctggctcac  ctggacaacc  tcaagggcac  ctttgccaca
ctgagtgagc  tgcactgtga  caagctgcac  gtggatcctg  agaacttcag  ggtgagtcta
tgggacccttt  gatgttttct  ttccccttct  tttctatggt  taagttcatg  tcataggaag
gggagaagta  acagggtaca  gtttagaatg  ggaaacagac  gaatgattgc  atcagtgtgg
aagtctcagg  atcgtttttag  tttctttttat  ttgctgttca  taacaattgt  tttctttttgt
ttaattcttg  ctttcttttt  ttttcttctc  cgcaatttttt actattatac  ttaatgcctt
aacattgtgt  ataacaaaag  gaaatatctc  tgagatacat  taagtaactt  aaaaaaaaac
tttacacagt  ctgcctagta  cattactatt  tggaatatat  gtgtgcttat  ttgcatattc
ataatctccc  tactttatttt tctttttattt ttaattgata  cataatcatt  atacatattt
atgggttaaa  gtgtaatgtt  ttaatatgtg  tacacatatt  gaccaaatca  gggtaatttt
gcatttgtaa  ttttaaaaaa  tgctttcttc  ttttaatata  cttttttgtt  tatcttatttt
ctaatacttt  ccctaatctc  tttctttcag  ggcaataatg  atacaatgta  tcatgcctct
ttgcaccatt  ctaaagaata  acagtgataa  tttctggggtt aaggcaatag  caatatttct
gcatataaat  atttctgcat  ataaattgta  actgatgtaa  gaggtttcat  attgctaata
gcagctacaa  tccagctacc  attctgcttt  tatttttatgg ttgggataag  gctggattat
tctgagtcca  agctaggccc  ttttgctaat  catgttcata  cctcttatct  tcctcccaca
gctcctgggc  aacgtgctgg  tctgtgtgct  ggcccatcac  tttggcaaag  aattcacccc
accagtgcag  gctgcctatc  agaaagtggt  ggctggtgtg  gctaatgccc  tggcccacaa
gtatcactaa  gctcgctttc  ttgctgtcca  atttctatta  aaggttcctt  tgttccctaa
gtccaactac  taaactgggg  gatattatga  agggccttga  gcatctggat  tctgcctaat
aaaaaacatt  tattttcatt  gcaatgatgt  atttaaatta  tttctgaata  ttttactaaa
```

(b)

```
gagccacacc  ctagggttgg  ccaatctact  cccaggagca  gggagggcag  gagccagggc
tgggcataaa  agtcagggca  gagccatcta  ttgcttacat  ttgcttctga  cacaactgtg
ttcactagca  acctcaaaca  gacaccatgg  tgcacctgac  tcctgaggag  aagtctgccg  ┐
ttactgccct  gtggggcaag  gtgaacgtgg  atgaagttgg  tggtgaggcc  ctgggcaggt  ├ Exon 1
tggtatcaag  gttacaagac  aggtttaagg  agaccaatag  aaactgggca  tgtggagaca
gagaagactc  ttgggtttct  gataggcact  gactctctct  gcctattggt  ctattttccc
acccttaggc  tgctggtggt  ctaccccttg  acccagaagt  tctttgagtc  ctttggggat  ┐
ctgtccactc  ctgatgctgt  tatgggcaac  cctaaggtga  aggctcatgg  caagaaagtg  ├ Exon 2
ctcggtgcct  ttagtgatgg  cctggctcac  ctggacaacc  tcaagggcac  ctttgccaca  │
ctgagtgagc  tgcactgtga  caagctgcac  gtggatcctg  agaacttcag  ggtgagtcta  ┘
tgggacccttt  gatgttttct  ttccccttct  tttctatggt  taagttcatg  tcataggaag
gggagaagta  acagggtaca  gtttagaatg  ggaaacagac  gaatgattgc  atcagtgtgg
aagtctcagg  atcgtttttag  tttctttttat  ttgctgttca  taacaattgt  tttctttttgt
ttaattcttg  ctttcttttt  ttttcttctc  cgcaatttttt actattatac  ttaatgcctt
aacattgtgt  ataacaaaag  gaaatatctc  tgagatacat  taagtaactt  aaaaaaaaac
tttacacagt  ctgcctagta  cattactatt  tggaatatat  gtgtgcttat  ttgcatattc
ataatctccc  tactttatttt tctttttattt ttaattgata  cataatcatt  atacatattt
atgggttaaa  gtgtaatgtt  ttaatatgtg  tacacatatt  gaccaaatca  gggtaatttt
gcatttgtaa  ttttaaaaaa  tgctttcttc  ttttaatata  cttttttgtt  tatcttatttt
ctaatacttt  ccctaatctc  tttctttcag  ggcaataatg  atacaatgta  tcatgcctct
ttgcaccatt  ctaaagaata  acagtgataa  tttctggggtt aaggcaatag  caatatttct
gcatataaat  atttctgcat  ataaattgta  actgatgtaa  gaggtttcat  attgctaata
gcagctacaa  tccagctacc  attctgcttt  tatttttatgg ttgggataag  gctggattat
tctgagtcca  agctaggccc  ttttgctaat  catgttcata  cctcttatct  tcctcccaca
gctcctgggc  aacgtgctgg  tctgtgtgct  ggcccatcac  tttggcaaag  aattcacccc  ┐
accagtgcag  gctgcctatc  agaaagtggt  ggctggtgtg  gctaatgccc  tggcccacaa  ├ Exon 3
gtatcactaa  gctcgctttc  ttgctgtcca  atttctatta  aaggttcctt  tgttccctaa  ┘
gtccaactac  taaactgggg  gatattatga  agggccttga  gcatctggat  tctgcctaat
aaaaaacatt  tattttcatt  gcaatgatgt  atttaaatta  tttctgaata  ttttactaaa
```

(c)

EXON 1   EXON 2   EXON 3

0.0   0.5   1.0   1.5   kb

FIGURE 21–6 Annotation of a DNA sequence containing part of the human β-globin gene. By convention, the sequence is presented in groups of ten nucleotides, although in reality the sequence is continuous. (a) The location of genes, if any, in this sequence is not readily apparent from a cursory glance. (b) The analyzed sequence, showing the location of an upstream regulatory sequence (green). The red box indicates a start triplet representing a start codon in mRNA. Open reading frames for three exons of the human β-globin gene are shown in blue. (c) Diagrammatic representation of three exons for the human β-globin gene encoded by the sequence shown in (a) and (b).

that, after transcription and mRNA splicing, are translated into the amino acid sequence of a protein. ORFs typically begin with an initiation sequence, usually ATG, which transcribes into the AUG start codon of an mRNA molecule, and end with a termination sequence, TAA, TAG, or TGA, which corresponds to the stop codons of UAA, UAG, and UGA in mRNA. Genetic information is encoded in groups of three nucleotides (triplets), but it is not always clear whether to begin the analysis of a sequence at the first nucleotide, the second, or the third. Typically, the sequence adjacent to a promoter is examined for a

start (initiation) triplet; however, ORFs can be used to identify a gene even when a promoter sequence is not apparent. Software programs can then analyze the ORFs three nucleotides at a time. The discovery of an ORF starting with an ATG followed at some distance by a termination sequence is usually a good indication that the coding region of a gene has been identified.

The way genes are organized in eukaryotic genomes (including the human genome) makes direct searching for ORFs more difficult in them than in prokaryotic genomes. First, many eukaryotic genes have introns. As a result, many, if not most, eukaryotic genes are not organized as continuous ORFs; instead, the gene sequences consist of ORFs (exons) interspersed with introns. Second, genes in humans and other eukaryotes are often widely spaced, increasing the chances of finding false ORFs in the regions between gene clusters.

Annotation of the sequence shown in Figure 21–6(a) reveals several identifiable indicators that the sequence contains a protein-coding gene: it includes a promoter sequence, an initiation codon, and three *exons* [**Figure 21–6(b)**]. The two unshaded regions between the exons represent introns that would be spliced out following transcription when the mRNA is processed [**Figure 21–6**(b) and (c)]. Using this sequence as the query in a search of genomic databases would reveal that it is the sequence of a single gene, the human β-globin gene.

Software designed for ORF analysis of eukaryotic genomes is highly valuable. Often such programs are used to make computational predictions of all ORFs (the ORFeome!) in a sequenced genome as a way to estimate the number of potential protein-coding genes in a genome. In addition to the features already mentioned, such software can be used to "translate" ORFs into possible polypeptide sequences as a way to predict the polypeptide encoded by a gene. Shown in **Figure 21–7** is a partial sequence for the first exon of the human tubulin alpha 3c gene (*TUBA3C*). Prediction programs scan potential ORFs in the 5′ to 3′ direction on both strands of a section of genomic DNA to predict possible reading frames in each direction. Figure 21–7 shows the results for the six possible reading frames in the sequence of interest. Amino acids are shown using the single-letter code for each residue. Notice the very different results obtained for each of the six frames. For instance, the 5′ to 3′ ORF 1 contains several stop codons interspersed among amino acids but no methionine residues that are evidence of a start codon. Other ORFs would contain too many methionines to produce a functional polypeptide. For this exon of *TUBA3C*, the 5′ to 3′ ORF 2 is correct.

Prediction programs can also search for **codon bias**, the more frequent use of one or two codons to encode an amino acid that can be specified by a number of different codons. For example, alanine can be encoded by GCA, GCT, GCC, and GCG. If the codons were used randomly, each would be used about 25 percent of the time. Yet in the human genome, GCC is used 41 percent of the time, and GCG only 11 percent of the time. Codon bias is present in exons but should not be present in introns or intergenic spacers.

NOW SOLVE THIS

21–1 In a sequence encompassing 99.4 percent of the euchromatic regions of human chromosome 1, Gregory et al. (Gregory, S.G. et al., *Nature*, 441:315–321, 2006) identified 3141 genes.

(a) How does one identify a gene within a raw sequence of bases in DNA?

(b) What features of a genome are used to verify likely gene assignments?

(c) Given that chromosome 1 contains approximately 8 percent of the human genome, and assuming that there are approximately 20,000 genes, would you consider chromosome 1 to be "gene rich"?

■ **HINT:** *This problem involves a basic understanding of bioinformatics and gene annotation approaches to determine how potential gene sequences can be identified in a stretch of sequenced DNA.*

(a) *Homo sapiens TUBA3C* (bp 1-300)

```
  1 ggttgaggtcaagtagtagcgttgggctgcggcagcggaggagctcaacatgcgtgagtg
 61 tatctctatccacgtggggcaggcaggagtccagatcggcaatgcctgctgggaactgta
121 ctgcctggaacatggaattcagcccgatggtcagatgccaagtgataaaaccattggtgg
181 tggggacgactccttcaacacgttcttcagtgagactggagctggcaagcacgtgcccag
241 agcagtgtttgtggacctggagcccactgtggtcgatgaagtgcgcacaggaacctatag (300)
```

(b) Predicted polypeptides

5′ to 3′ Frame 1
G **Stop** G Q V V A L G C G S G G A Q H A **Stop** V Y L Y P R G A G R S P D R Q C L L G
T V L P G T W N S A R W S D A K **Stop Stop** N H W W W G R L L Q H V L Q **Stop** D W
S W Q A R A Q S S V C G P G A H C G R **Stop** S A H R N L **Stop**

5′ to 3′ Frame 2
V E V K **Stop Stop** R W A A A A L L N **Met** R E C I S I H V G Q A G V Q I G N A C W
E L Y C L E H G I Q P D G Q **Met** P S D K T I G G G D D S F N T F F S E T G A G K H V
P R A V F V D L E P T V V D E V R T G T Y

5′ to 3′ Frame 3
L R S S S S V G L R Q R R S S T C V S V S L S T W G R Q E S R S A **Met** P A G N C T A
W N **Met** E F S P **Met** V R C Q V I K P L V V G T T P S T R S S V R L E L A S T C P E Q C
L W T W S P L W S **Met** K C A Q E P I

3′ to 5′ Frame 1
L **Stop** V P V R T S S T T V G S R S T N T A L G T C L P A P V S L K N V L K E S S P P P
Met V L S L G I **Stop** P S G **Stop** I P C S R Q Y S S Q Q A L P I W T P A C P T W I E I H
S R **Met** L S S S A A A A Q R Y Y L T S T

3′ to 5′ Frame 2
Y R F L C A L H R P Q W A P G P Q T L L W A R A C Q L Q S H **Stop** R T C **Stop** R S R P
H H Q W F Y H L A S D H R A E F H V P G S T V P S R H C R S G L L P A P R G **Stop** R Y
T H A C **Stop** A P P L P Q P N A T T **Stop** P Q

3′ to 5′ Frame 3
I G S C A H F I D H S G L Q V H K H C S G H V L A S S S L T E E R V E G V V P T T N G
F I T W H L T I G L N S **Met** F Q A V Q F P A G I A D L D S C L P H V D R D T L T H V E
L L R C R S P T L L L D L N

FIGURE 21–7 Predicted polypeptide sequences translated from potential ORFs in the human *TUBA3C* gene. (a) Nucleotides 1–300 of the first exon in the human *TUBA3C* gene. (b) A translation program predicts six possible polypeptide sequences from this exon. Which predicted sequence is correct?

Note: Methionine is highlighted using the three letter amino acid code (Met).

21.3 Genomics Attempts to Identify Potential Functions of Genes and Other Elements in a Genome

Reading a genome sequence is a surefire cure for insomnia. What is exciting is not the sequence of the nucleotides but the information that the sequence contains. After a genome has been annotated and ORFs have been identified, the next analytical task is to assign putative functions to all possible genes in the sequence. As the term suggests, **functional genomics** is the study of gene functions, based on the resulting RNAs or possible proteins they encode, and the functions of other components of the genome, such as gene-regulatory elements. Functional genomics can involve experimental approaches to confirm or refute computational predictions about genome functions (such as the number of protein-coding genes), and it also considers how genes are expressed and the regulation of gene expression.

Predicting Gene and Protein Functions by Sequence Analysis

One approach to assigning functions to genes is to use sequence similarity searches, as described in the previous section. Programs such as BLAST are used to search through databases to find alignments between the newly sequenced genome and genes that have already been identified, either in the same or in different species. You were introduced to this approach for predicting gene function in Figure 21–4, when we demonstrated how sequence similarity to the mouse gene was used to identify a gene in a rat contig as the insulin receptor gene. Inferring gene function from similarity searches is based on a relatively simple idea. If a genome sequence shows statistically significant similarity to the sequence of a gene whose function is known, then it is likely that the genome sequence encodes a protein with a similar or related function.

Another major benefit of similarity searches is that they are often able to identify **homologous genes**, genes that are evolutionarily related. After the human genome was sequenced, many ORFs in it were identified as protein-coding genes based on their alignment with related genes of known function in other species. As an example, **Figure 21–8** compares portions of the human leptin gene (*LEP*) with its homolog in mice (*ob/Lep*). These two genes are over 85 percent identical in sequence. The leptin gene was first discovered in mice. The match between the *LEP*-containing DNA sequence in humans and the mouse homolog sequence confirms the identity and leptin-coding function of this gene in human genomic DNA.

As an interesting aside, the leptin gene (also called *ob*, for obesity, in mice) is highly expressed in fat cells (adipocytes). This gene produces the protein hormone leptin, which targets cells in the brain to suppress appetite. Knockout mice lacking a functional *ob* gene grow dramatically overweight. A similar phenotype has been observed in small numbers of humans with particular mutations in *LEP*. Although it is important to note that weight control is not regulated by a single gene, the discovery of leptin has provided significant insight into lipid metabolism and weight disorders in humans. Further studies on leptin will

be important for understanding more about the genetics of weight disorders.

If homologous genes in different species are thought to have descended from a gene in a common ancestor, the genes are known as **orthologs**. In Section 21.6 we will consider the globin gene family. Mouse and human α-globin genes are orthologs evolved from a common ancestor. Homologous genes in the same species are called **paralogs**. The α- and β-globin subunits in humans are paralogs resulting from a gene-duplication event. Paralogs often have similar or identical functions.

Predicting Function from Structural Analysis of Protein Domains and Motifs

When a gene sequence is used to predict a polypeptide sequence, the polypeptide can be analyzed for specific structural domains and motifs. Identification of **protein domains**, such as ion channels, membrane-spanning regions, DNA-binding regions, secretion and export signals, and other structural aspects of a polypeptide that are encoded by a DNA sequence, can in turn be used to predict protein function. Recall from earlier in the text (see Chapter 17), for example, that the structures of many DNA-binding proteins have characteristic patterns, or **motifs**, such as the helix-turn-helix, leucine zipper, or zinc-finger motifs. These motifs can often easily be searched for using bioinformatics software, and their identification in a sequence is a common strategy for inferring the possible functions of a protein.

Investigators Are Using Genomics Techniques Such as Chromatin Immunoprecipitation to Investigate Aspects of Genome Function and Regulation

In this chapter and later in the text (see Chapter 22), we will consider a range of different genomic techniques that investigators are using that are valuable for functional genomics studies. One example is a technique called **chromatin immunoprecipitation (ChIP)**. Various techniques involving ChIP are designed to map protein–DNA interactions and are useful for identifying genes that are regulated by DNA-binding transcription factors.

To perform these techniques, researchers treat tissues or cultured cells with formaldehyde (**Figure 21–9**). Any proteins that are tightly bound to DNA will be crosslinked to the DNA by the formaldehyde. The researchers then extract DNA from the cells and shear it into small fragments. To isolate those DNA fragments that are bound to a specific protein, they add an antibody that recognizes (attaches to) the protein. These antibodies are usually attached to a bead or resin that enables the antibody to then be precipitated (by

Human *LEP* gene
```
GTCACCAGGATCAATGACATTTCACACACG- - -TCAGTCTCCTCCAAACAGAAAGTCACC
||||||||||||||||||||||||||||||   || || ||| |||| |||| |||||
GTCACCAGGATCAATGACATTTCACACACGCAGTCGGTATCCGCCAAGCAGAGGGTCACT
```
Mouse *ob/Lep* gene

```
GGTTTGGACTTCATTCCTGGGCTCCACCCCATCCTGACCTTATCCAAGATGGACCAGACA
|| |||||||||||||| |||||||| |||||| |||| || ||||||||||||||||||
GGCTTGGACTTCATTCCTGGGCTTCACCCCATTCTGAGTTTGTCCAAGATGGACCAGACT
```

```
CTGGCAGTCTACCAACAGATCCTCACCAGTATGCCTTCCAGAAACGTGATCCAAATATCC
|||||||||| |||||| |||||||||| |||||||| ||| ||| | || ||| ||
CTGGCAGTCTATCAACAGGTCCTCACCAGCCTGCCTTCCCAAAATGTGCTGCAGATAGCC
```

FIGURE 21–8 Comparison of the human *LEP* and mouse *ob/Lep* genes. Partial sequences for these homologs are shown with the human *LEP* gene on top and the mouse *ob/Lep* gene sequence below it. Notice from the number of identical nucleotides, indicated by vertical lines, that the nucleotide sequence for these two genes is very similar. Gaps are indicated by horizontal dashes.

Cell

Nucleus

Crosslink proteins to
DNA and lyse cells

Protein

DNA

Isolate chromatin and fragment it

Antibody

Add a protein-specific antibody
and purify protein–DNA complexes

Reverse crosslinks and isolate DNA

CAGACAAC
Sequence DNA

Chromosomal DNA

Each red box
denotes a
sequence read

Map sequence to genome

© 2007 AAAS

FIGURE 21–9 The ChIPSeq method screens for specific transcription factor binding sites across a whole genome. In this method, formaldehyde is added to tissues or cultured cells to crosslink DNA-binding proteins currently attached to chromatin when formaldehyde was added. Then the chromatin is extracted from cells and sheared into small fragments. An antibody or antibodies that recognize specific DNA-binding proteins of interest (POI), such as a transcription factor, are added to the mixture and the antibodies attach to the POI. Then the antibody, together with its protein–DNA fragment, is pulled out of the mixture (immunoprecipitated). The immunoprecipitated DNA fragments are released from crosslinked proteins and attached antibodies and are then sequenced. Sequence data reveal the DNA-binding site for the POI and these sequences can be mapped to specific locations in the genome.

DNA complexes to the bottom of the centrifuge tube. The investigators can then purify the immunoprecipitated DNA fragments by removing them from the antibody/protein.

At this stage, there are several options for analyzing precipitated DNA fragments. **Figure 21–9** demonstrates an approach called *ChIPSeq*. Here precipitated DNA fragments are directly sequenced by high-throughput approaches. This allows researchers to study an entire genome to locate binding sites for proteins such as transcription factors, histone-related proteins, and other proteins involved in chromatin structure.

In another approach called *ChIP-chip*, the captured DNA fragments can be labeled with a fluorescent tag and hybridized to a DNA microarray (described in Section 21.9) containing synthetic oligonucleotides or cloned DNAs representing the organism's entire genome. Any spot on the microarray that hybridizes to the labeled DNA represents a DNA sequence that bound the protein. Because each spot on the DNA microarray is known, the identity of each positive signal can be determined. DNA isolated by ChIP can also be sequenced to identify DNA sequences that are bound by DNA-binding proteins.

21.4 The Human Genome Project Revealed Many Important Aspects of Genome Organization in Humans

Now that you have a general idea of the basic strategies used for analyzing a genome, let's look at the largest genomics project completed to date. The **Human Genome Project (HGP)** was a coordinated international effort to determine the sequence of the human genome and to identify all the genes it contains. It has produced a plethora of information, much of which is still being analyzed and interpreted. What is clear from all the different kinds of genomes sequenced is that humans and all other species share a common set of genes

immunoprecipitation) from the mixture, along with the protein to which it binds and any DNA fragments that are crosslinked to the protein. Immunoprecipitation is usually accomplished by centrifugation of the antibody/protein/DNA complexes. Because the antibody has a bead attached to it, the mass of the bead is used to centrifuge the antibody/protein/

essential for cellular function and reproduction, confirming that all living organisms arose from a common ancestor.

Origins of the Project

The publicly funded Human Genome Project began in 1990 under the direction of James Watson, the co-discoverer of the double-helix structure of DNA. Eventually the public project was led by Dr. Francis Collins, who had previously led a research team involved in identifying the *CFTR* gene as the cause of cystic fibrosis. In the United States, the Collins-led HGP was coordinated by the Department of Energy and the National Center of Human Genome Research, a division of the National Institutes of Health. It established a 15-year plan with a proposed budget of $3 billion to identify all human genes, originally thought to number between 80,000 and 100,000, to sequence and map them all, and to sequence the approximately 3 billion base pairs thought to comprise the 24 chromosomes (22 autosomes, plus X and Y) in humans. Other primary goals of the HGP included the following:

- To establish functional categories for all human genes

- To analyze genetic variations between humans, including the identification of **single-nucleotide polymorphisms (SNPs)**

- To map and sequence the genomes of several model organisms used in experimental genetics, including *E. coli, S. cerevisiae, C. elegans, D. melanogaster,* and *M. musculus* (mouse)

- To develop new sequencing technologies, such as high-throughput computer-automated sequencers, in order to facilitate genome analysis

- To disseminate genome information among both scientists and the general public

Lastly, to deal with the impact that genetic information would have on society, the HGP set up the **ELSI program** (standing for Ethical, Legal, and Social Implications) to consider ethical, legal, and social issues arising from the HGP and to ensure that personal genetic information would be safeguarded and not used in discriminatory ways.

As the HGP grew into an international effort, scientists in 18 countries were involved in the project. Much of the work was carried out by the International Human Genome Sequence Consortium, involving nearly 3000 scientists working at 20 centers in six countries (China, France, Germany, Great Britain, Japan, and the United States).

In 1999, a privately funded human genome project led by J. Craig Venter at **Celera Genomics** (aptly named from a word meaning "swiftness") was announced. Celera's goal was to use whole-genome shotgun sequencing and computer-automated high-throughput DNA sequencers

to sequence the human genome more rapidly than HGP. The public project had proposed using a clone-by-clone approach to sequence the genome. Recall that Venter and colleagues had proven the potential of shotgun sequencing in 1995 when they completed the genome for *H. influenzae*. Celera's announcement set off an intense competition between the two teams, which both aspired to be first with the human genome sequence. This contest eventually led to the HGP finishing ahead of schedule and under budget after scientists from the public project began to use high-throughput sequencers and whole-genome sequencing strategies as well.

Major Features of the Human Genome

In June 2000, the leaders of the public and private genome projects met at the White House with President Clinton and jointly announced the completion of a draft sequence of the human genome. In February 2001, they each published an analysis covering about 96 percent of the euchromatic region of the genome. The public project sequenced euchromatic portions of the genome 12 times and set a quality control standard of a 0.01 percent error rate for their sequence. Although this error rate may seem very low, it still allows about 600,000 errors in the human genome sequence. Celera sequenced certain areas of the genome more than 35 times when compiling the genome.

The remaining work of completing the sequence by filling in gaps clustered around centromeres, telomeres, and repetitive sequences (regions rich in GC base pairs can be particularly tough to sequence and interpret), correcting misaligned segments, and re-sequencing portions of the genome to ensure accuracy. In 2003 genome sequencing and error fixing were deemed sufficient to pass the international project's definition of completion—that it contained fewer than 1 error per 10,000 nucleotides and that it covered 95 percent of the gene-containing portions of the genome. Yet even at the time of "completion" there were still some 350 gaps in the sequence that continued to be worked on.

And of course the HGP did not sequence the genome of every person on Earth. The assembled genomes largely consist of haploid genomes pooled from different individuals so that they provide a *reference genome* representative of major, common elements of a human genome widely shared among populations of humans. Examples of major features of the human genome are summarized in **Table 21.1**. As you can see in this table, many unexpected observations have provided us with major new insights. The genome is not static! Genome variations, including the abundance of repetitive sequences scattered throughout the genome, verify that the genome is indeed dynamic, revealing many evolutionary examples of sequences that have changed in

TABLE 21.1 Major Features of the Human Genome

- The human genome contains 3.1 billion nucleotides, but protein-coding sequences make up only about 2 percent of the genome.
- The genome sequence is ~99.9 percent similar in individuals of all nationalities. SNPs and copy number variations (CNVs) account for genome diversity from person to person.
- The genome is dynamic. At least 50 percent of the genome is derived from transposable elements, such as LINE and *Alu* sequences, and other repetitive DNA sequences.
- The human genome contains approximately 20,000 protein-coding genes, far fewer than the originally predicted number of 80,000–100,000 genes.
- The average size of a human gene is ~25 kb, including gene-regulatory regions, introns, and exons. On average, mRNAs produced by human genes are ~3000 nt long.
- Many human genes produce more than one protein through alternative splicing, thus enabling human cells to produce a much larger number of proteins (perhaps as many as 200,000) from only ~20,000 genes.
- More than 50 percent of human genes show a high degree of sequence similarity to genes in other organisms; however, more than 40 percent of the genes identified have no known molecular function.
- Genes are not uniformly distributed on the 24 human chromosomes. Gene-rich clusters are separated by gene-poor "deserts" that account for 20 percent of the genome. These deserts correlate with G bands seen in stained chromosomes. Chromosome 19 has the highest gene density, and chromosome 13 and the Y chromosome have the lowest gene densities.
- Chromosome 1 contains the largest number of genes, and the Y chromosome contains the smallest number.
- Human genes are larger and contain more and larger introns than genes in the genomes of invertebrates, such as *Drosophila*. The largest known human gene encodes dystrophin, a muscle protein. This gene, associated in mutant form with muscular dystrophy, is 2.5 Mb in length (Chapter 14), larger than many bacterial chromosomes. Most of this gene is composed of introns.
- The number of introns in human genes ranges from 0 (in histone genes) to 234 (in the gene for *titin*, which encodes a muscle protein).

that human cells produce about 100,000 proteins. At least half of the genes show sequence similarity to genes shared by many other organisms, and as you will learn in Section 21.7, a majority of human genes are similar in sequence to genes from closely related species such as chimpanzees. There is still no consensus among scientists worldwide about the exact number of human genes. One reason is that it is unclear whether or not many of the presumed genes produce functional proteins. Genome scientists continue to annotate the genome, and as mentioned earlier, functional genomics studies have important roles in determining whether or not computational predictions about the number of protein-coding and non–protein-coding genes are accurate.

The number of genes is much lower than the number of predicted proteins in part because many genes code for multiple proteins through **alternative splicing**. Recall from earlier in the text (see Chapter 13), that alternative splicing patterns can generate multiple mRNA molecules, and thus multiple proteins, from a single gene, through different combinations of intron–exon splicing arrangements. Initial estimates suggested that over 50 percent of human genes undergo alternative splicing to produce multiple transcripts and multiple proteins. Recent studies suggest that ~94–95 percent of human pre-mRNAs contain multiple exons that are processed to produce multiple transcripts and potentially multiple different protein products. Clearly, alternative splicing produces an incredible diversity of proteins beyond simple predictions based on the number of genes in the human genome.

Functional categories have been assigned for human genes, primarily on the basis of (1) functions determined previously (for example, from recombinant DNA cloning of human genes and known mutations involved in human diseases), (2) comparison to known genes and predicted protein sequences from other species, and (3) predictions based on annotation and analysis of protein functional domains and motifs (**Figure 21–10**). Although functional categories and assignments continue to be revised, the functions of over 40 percent of human genes remain unknown. Determining human gene functions, deciphering complexities of gene-expression regulation and gene interaction, and uncovering the relationships between human genes and phenotypes are among the many challenges for genome scientists.

Individual Variations in the Human Genome

The HGP has also shown us that in all humans, regardless of racial and ethnic origins, the genomic sequence is approximately 99.9 percent the same. As we discuss in other chapters, most genetic differences between humans result from **single-nucleotide polymorphisms (SNPs)** and **copy number variations (CNVs)**. Recall that SNPs are single-base changes in the genome and variations of many

structure and location. In many ways, the HGP has revealed just how little we know about our genome.

Two of the biggest surprises discovered by the HGP were that less than 2 percent of the genome codes for proteins and that there are only around 20,000 protein-coding genes. Recall that the number of genes had originally been estimated to be about 100,000, based in part on a prediction

Cell adhesion (577, 1.9%)
Miscellaneous (1318, 4.3%)
Viral protein (100, 0.3%)
Transfer/carrier protein (203, 0.7%)
Transcription factor (1850, 6.0%)
Nucleic acid enzyme (2308, 7.5%)
Signaling molecule (376, 1.2%)
Receptor (1543, 5.0%)
Kinase (868, 2.8%)
Select regulatory molecule (988, 3.2%)
Transferase (610, 2.0%)
Synthase and synthetase (313, 1.0%)
Oxidoreductase (656, 2.1%)
Lyase (117, 0.4%)
Ligase (56, 0.2%)
Isomerase (163, 0.5%)
Hydrolase (1227, 4.0%)

Chaperone (159, 0.5%)
Cytoskeletal structural protein (876, 2.8%)
Extracellular matrix (437, 1.4%)
Immunoglobulin (264, 0.9%)
Ion channel (406, 1.3%)
Motor (376, 1.2%)
Structural protein of muscle (296, 1.0%)
Proto-oncogene (902, 2.9%)
Select calcium-binding protein (34, 0.1%)
Intracellular transporter (350, 1.1%)
Transporter (533, 1.7%)

nucleic acid binding

signal transaction

enzyme

Molecular function unknown (12809, 41.7%)

FIGURE 21–10 A representation of the functional categories to which genes in the human genome have been assigned on the basis of similarity to proteins of known function. Among the most common genes are those involved in nucleic acid metabolism (7.5 percent of all genes identified), transcription factors (6.0 percent), receptors (5 percent), hydrolases (4 percent), protein kinases (2.8 percent), and cytoskeletal structural proteins (2.8 percent). A total of 12,809 predicted proteins (41 percent) have unknown functions, indicative of the work that is still needed to fully decipher our genome.

SNPs are associated with disease conditions. For example, SNPs cause sickle-cell anemia and cystic fibrosis. Later in the text (see Chapter 22), we will examine how SNPs can be detected and used for diagnosis and treatment of disease.

After the draft sequence of the human genome was completed, it initially appeared that most genetic variations between individuals (the 0.1 percent differences) were due to SNPs. While SNPs are important contributing factors to genome variation, structural differences that we discussed earlier in the text (see Chapter 12) such as deletions, duplications, inversions, and CNVs, which can span millions of bp of DNA, play much more important roles in genome variation than previously thought. As we discussed earlier in the text (see Chapters 8 and 12), recall that CNVs are duplications or deletions of relatively large sections of DNA on the order of several hundred or several thousand base pairs. Many of the CNVs that vary the most among genomes appear to be at least 1 kilobase.

Although most human DNA is present in two copies per cell, one from each parent, CNVs are segments of DNA that are duplicated or deleted, resulting in variations in the number of copies of a DNA segment inherited by individuals. In some cases CNVs are major deletions removing entire genes; other deletions affect gene function by frameshifts in the reading code. CNV sequences that are duplicated can result in overexpression of a particular gene, yet many deleted and duplicated CNVs do not present clearly identifiable phenotypes.

Current estimates of the number of CNVs in an individual genome range from about 12 CNVs to perhaps 4–5 dozen per person. Some studies estimate that there may be as many as 1500 CNVs greater than 1 kb among the human genome. Other studies claim there are more than 1.5 million deletions of less than 100 bp that contribute to genome variation between individuals.

Accessing the Human Genome Project on the Internet

It is now possible to access databases and other sites on the Internet that display maps for all human chromosomes. You will visit a number of these databases in Exploring Genomics exercises. **Figure 21–11(a)** displays a partial gene map for chromosome 12 that was taken from an NCBI database called Map Viewer. You may already have used Map Viewer for the Exploring Genomics exercises ealier in the text (see Chapters 5 and 12). This image shows an ideogram, or cytogenetic map, of chromosome 12. To the right of the ideogram is a column showing the contigs (arranged lying vertically) that were aligned to sequence this chromosome. The Hs UniG column displays a histogram representation of gene density on chromosome 12. Notice that relatively few genes are located near the centromere. Gene symbols, loci, and gene names (by description) are provided for selected genes; in this figure only 20 genes are shown. When accessing these maps on the Internet, one can magnify, or zoom in on, each region of the chromosome, revealing all genes mapped to a particular area.

FIGURE 21–11 (a) A gene map for chromosome 12 from the NCBI database Map Viewer. (b) Partial map of disease genes on human chromosome 21. Maps such as this depict genes thought to be involved in human genetic disease conditions.

You can see that most of the genes listed here have been assigned descriptions based on the functions of their products, some of which are transmembrane proteins, some enzymes such as kinases, some receptors, including several involved in olfaction, and so on. Other genes are described in terms of hypothetical products; they are presumed to be genes based on the presence of ORFs, but their function remains unknown [Figure 21–11(a)].

The HGP's most valuable contribution will perhaps be the identification of disease genes and the development of new treatment strategies as a result. Thus, extensive maps have been developed for genes implicated in human disease conditions. The disease gene map of chromosome 21 shown in **Figure 21–11(b)** indicates genes involved in amyotrophic lateral sclerosis (ALS), Alzheimer disease, cataracts, deafness, and several different cancers. Later in the text (see Chapter 22) we discuss implications of the HGP for the identification of genes involved in human genetic diseases, and for disease diagnosis, detection, and gene therapy applications.

21.5 The "Omics" Revolution Has Created a New Era of Biological Research

The Human Genome Project and the development of genomics techniques have been largely responsible for launching a new era of biological research—the era of "omics." It seems that every year, more areas of biological research are being described as having an omics connection. Some examples of "omics" are

- proteomics—the analysis of all the proteins in a cell or tissue

- metabolomics—the analysis of proteins and enzymatic pathways involved in cell metabolism

- glycomics—the analysis of the carbohydrates of a cell or tissue

- toxicogenomics—the analysis of the effects of toxic chemicals on genes, including mutations created by toxins and changes in gene expression caused by toxins

- metagenomics—the analysis of genomes of organisms collected from the environment

- pharmacogenomics—the development of customized medicine based on a person's genetic profile for a particular condition

- transcriptomics—the analysis of all expressed genes in a cell or tissue

We will consider several of these genomics disciplines in other parts of this chapter.

As evidence of the impact of genomics, a new field of nutritional science called nutritional genomics, or **nutrigenomics**, has emerged. Nutrigenomics focuses on understanding the interactions between diet and genes. We have all had routine medical tests for blood pressure, blood sugar levels, and heart rate. Based on these tests, your physician may recommend that you change your diet and exercise more to lose weight, or that you reduce your intake of sodium to help lower your blood pressure. Now several companies claim to provide nutrigenomics tests that analyze your genomes for genes thought to be associated with different medical conditions or aspects of nutrient metabolism. The companies then provide a customized nutrition report, recommending diet changes for improving your health and preventing illness, based on your genes! It is important to know that these tests have not been validated as accurate and they have not been approved by the U.S. Food and Drug Administration. It remains to be seen whether this approach as currently practiced is of valid scientific or nutritional value.

Stone-Age Genomics

In yet another example of how genomics has taken over areas of DNA analysis, a number of labs around the world are involved in analyzing "ancient" DNA. These so-called **stone-age genomics** studies are generating fascinating data from miniscule amounts of ancient DNA obtained from bone and other tissues such as hair that are tens of thousands to about 700,000 years old, and often involve samples from extinct species. Analysis of DNA from a 2400-year-old Egyptian mummy, bison, mosses, platypus, mammoths, Pleistocene-age cave bears and polar bears, coelacanths and Neanderthals are some of the most prominent examples of stone-age genomics. In 2013, scientists reported the oldest complete genome sequence generated to date. It came from a 700,000-year-old bone fragment from an ancient horse uncovered from the frozen ground in the Yukon Territory of Canada. This result is interesting in part because evolutionary biologists have used genomic data to estimate that ancient ancestors of modern horses branched off from other animal lineages around 4 million years ago— about twice as long ago as prior estimates.

In 2005, researchers from McMaster University in Canada and Pennsylvania State University published about 13 million bp from a 27,000-year-old woolly mammoth. This study revealed a ~98.5 percent sequence identity between mammoths and African elephants. Subsequent studies by other scientists have used whole-genome shotgun sequencing of mitochondrial and nuclear DNA from Siberian mammoths to provide data on the mammoth genome. These studies suggest that the mammoth genome differs from the African elephant by as little as 0.6 percent. These studies are also great demonstrations of how stable DNA can be under

FIGURE 21–12 Plot showing the number of genes on each human chromosome (blue), the average fraction of protein-coding bases that align to Roche 454 reads from James D. Watson's genome (green), and the fraction of coding bases that align to one or more mammoth reads (orange), using predicted elephant genes that map to the human chromosome based on sequence similarity—approximately 50 percent for each autosome, but only 31 percent for the X chromosome because the mammoth used for this study was male.

the right conditions, particularly when frozen. In the future, it may be possible to produce complete genome sequences from samples that are several million years old.

Perhaps even more intriguing are similarities that have been revealed between the mammoth and human genomes. For example, as shown in **Figure 21–12**, when the gene sequences from human chromosomes were aligned with sequences from the mammoth genome, approximately 50 percent of mammoth genes showed sequence alignment with human genes on autosomes. Incidentally, notice that this figure also shows the relative number of genes from James Watson's genome (which we will discuss in the next section) compared to the human genome reference sequence.

In Section 21.6 we will discuss recent work on the Neanderthal genome. Obtaining the genome of a human ancestor this old was previously unimaginable. This work is providing new insights into our understanding of human evolution.

After the HGP: What Is Next?

Since completion of a reference sequence of the human genome, studies have continued at a very rapid pace. For example, as a result of the HGP, many other major theme areas for human genome research have emerged, including cancer genome projects, analysis of the epigenome (including a Human Epigenome Project that is creating hundreds of maps of epigenetic changes in different cell and tissue types and evaluating potential roles of epigenetics in complex diseases), characterization of SNPs (the International HapMap Project) and CNVs for their role in genome variation, disease, and pharmacogenomics applications.

We have discussed aspects of a cancer genome project (Cancer Genome Atlas Project) earlier in the text (see Chapter 19). The epigenome is covered in depth later in the text (see Special Topic Chapter 1—Epigenetics). SNPs and pharmacogenomics are discussed later as well (see Special Topic Chapter 4—Genomics and Personalized Medicine). Here we consider four examples of human genome research that are extensions of the HGP: (1) the analysis of personal genomes, (2) the ENCODE Project, (3) the Human Microbiome Project, and (4) the Genome 10K Plan.

Personal Genome Projects and Personal Genomics

As we discussed earlier in this chapter and earlier in the text (see Chapter 20), new sequencing technologies, capable of generating longer sequence reads at higher speeds with greater accuracy, have greatly reduced the cost of DNA sequencing, and expectations for continued cost reductions along with continued technological advances are high (see **Figure 21–13**). These expectations led several companies to propose WGS for individual people—a personal genomics approach. In 2006, the X Prize Foundation announced the Archon Genomics X Prize, an award of $10 million to the first private group that develops technology capable of sequencing 100 human genomes with a high degree of accuracy in 10 days for under $10,000 per genome. There were eight competitors for this prize, but none could meet the 10-day requirement. Archon subsequently canceled the X Prize in part because sequencing technology was improving in speed and decreasing in cost without the need for a

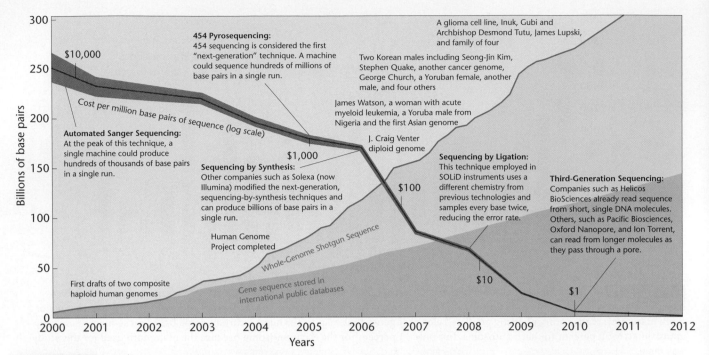

FIGURE 21-13 Human genome sequence explosion. Sequencing costs have steadily declined since 2000 due to innovations in sequencing technology. As a result, notice that the amount of whole-genome shotgun sequencing data stored in public databases—which include data on several individual genomes—has dramatically increased.

competition. Other groups are working on sequencing a personalized genome for a mere $1000! Two programs funded by the National Institutes of Health challenged scientists to develop sequencing technologies to complete a human genome for $1000 by 2014 (see the "Genetics, Technology, and Society" essay in Chapter 22).

In 2012, Life Technologies announced that their Ion Proton technology was used to sequence a genome for $1000. Whether the $1000 mark represents the costs of reagents to sequence a genome or actual costs when sequence preparation, labor, and analysis of the genome are taken into account can be debated. Whether the accuracy and completeness of the sequence coverage reported by Life Technologies is sufficient to definitively state that the $1000 genome threshold has been achieved has been challenged by other scientists.

As you will learn later in the text (see Chapter 22), having somebody such as a geneticist analyze genome data and consider how genome variations may affect a person's health takes a lot of time and money. So even if the cost of sequencing a person's genome is less than $1000, interpreting genome data to make sense for medical treatment may cost hundreds of thousands of dollars. Regardless of how the actual cost of sequencing a genome is calculated, the modern cost is substantially lower than the $3 billion cost of the HGP.

Pursuit of the $1000 genome was an indicator that DNA sequencing may eventually be affordable enough for individuals to consider acquiring a readout of their

own genetic blueprint. The genome of James D. Watson, who together with Francis Crick discovered the structure of DNA, was the focus of "Project Jim" by the Connecticut company 454 Life Sciences, which wanted to sequence the genome of a high-profile person and decided that the co-discoverer of DNA structure and the first director of the U.S. Human Genome Project should be that person. This company used their next-generation pyrosequencing approach (see Figure 21–13) for Project Jim, and within two years it was announced that six-fold coverage of Watson's genome was complete at a rough cost of just under $1 million. James Watson was then presented with two DVDs containing his genome sequence.

Human genome pioneer J. Craig Venter, whose accomplishments we have discussed in several chapters, had his genome completed by the J. Craig Venter Institute and deposited into GenBank in May 2007. George Church of Harvard and his colleagues started a **Personal Genome Project (PGP)** and recruited volunteers to provide DNA for individual genome sequencing on the understanding that the genome data will be made publicly available. Church's genome has been completed and is available online. The concept of a personal genome project raises the obvious question: would you have your genome sequenced for $10,000, $1000, or even for free?

Since the Watson and Venter genomes were completed, in 2008 the first complete genome sequence was provided for an individual "ancient" human, a Palaeo-Eskimo, obtained from ~4000-year-old permafrost-preserved hair. This work recovered about 78 percent of the diploid genome and revealed many interesting SNPs (of which about 7 percent have not been previously reported). As of 2013, more than 30,000 individual human genomes have been sequenced.

One especially intriguing example of personal genomics involves a genetics researcher who examined his own genome for insight about a medical condition. Dr. Richard Gibbs of Baylor College of Medicine in Texas led a group that sequenced the whole genome of his colleague Dr. James Lupski, a medical geneticist who has **Charcot-Marie-Tooth (CMT) disease**. This disease is a neurological condition that causes muscle weakness. Interestingly, mutations in over 30 genes, many of which were identified by Dr. Lupski, are involved in CMT, although Lupski did not carry any of these mutations. A comparison of Lupski's genome to the HGP reference sequence revealed many SNPs and other variations, but it was unclear how many of these were simply sequencing errors or variations that were not involved in CMT.

Focusing on genes previously linked to CMT and other neurological conditions, researchers found that Lupski's genome had two different mutations in the gene *SH3TC2*, which is expressed in Schwann cells that wrap around certain neurons to form the myelin sheath essential for impulse conductions in nerves. In one *SH3TC2* allele a nonsense mutation was revealed, and in Lupski's second allele for *SH3TC2* a new missense mutation was found. When genetic tests for these alleles were carried out on Lupski's parents and seven siblings, the nonsense mutation was found in one parent and two siblings who did not have the disease. The missense mutation was found in another parent and one grandparent, neither of whom had the disorder. Only siblings who inherited both mutated alleles had CMT disease. Many consider this the first clinically relevant success for personal genome sequencing—at least for identifying disease genes.

Exome Sequencing

The focus of personal genome projects has shifted toward **exome sequencing**, sequencing the 180,000 exons in a person's genome. This can be done at a cost of less than $1000 with <100× coverage. Exome sequencing reveals mutations involved in disease by focusing only on exons as protein-coding segments of the genome. Of course, a limitation of this approach is its failure to identify mutations in gene-regulatory regions that influence gene expression. As an example, a group of scientists called the 1000 Genomes Project Consortium reported on the genomes of 1092 individuals from 14 populations representing Europe, East Asia, sub-Saharan Africa, and the Americas. Whole-genome and exome-sequencing data revealed more than 38

million SNPs and many other structural variations (CNVs). One interpretation of this work is that it reveals clear variations in individuals and associates particular diseases with geographic or ancestral background. Thus sequencing genomes of individuals from diverse populations can help us better understand the spectrum of human genetic variation and to learn the causes of genetic diseases across diverse groups. We will come back to the topic of exome sequencing later in the text (see Chapter 22), when we discuss genetic testing.

Another particularly beneficial aspect of personal genome projects is the insight they are providing into genome variation. The HGP combined samples from different individuals to create a reference genome for a *haploid genome*. Personal genome projects sequence a diploid genome; consequently, such projects indicate that haploid genome comparisons may underestimate the extent of genome variation between individuals by five-fold or more. For example, when Venter's genome was analyzed, over 4 million variations were found between his maternal and paternal chromosomes alone. From what we are learning about personal genomes, genome variation between individuals may be closer to 0.5 percent than 0.1 percent, and in a 3-billion-bp genome this is a significant difference in sequence variation. Integrating genome data from several complete individual genomes of individuals from different ethnic groups will also be of great value in evolutionary genetics to address fundamental questions about human diversity, ancestry, and migration patterns.

In a related matter, PGPs are revealing that there can be significant *mosaicism* in human somatic cells. Thus, cells in an individual person do not all contain identical genomes. Because of the sophistication of WGS methods, mosaicisms for SNPs and CNVs have been found in skin, brain, blood, and stem cells from the same individual. We are only beginning to understand the frequency and effects of genetic mosaicism on health and disease.

Later in the text (see Chapter 22), we will consider how various approaches to personal genomics can be used for genetic testing.

Encyclopedia of DNA Elements (ENCODE) Project

In 2003, a few months after the announcement that the human genome had been sequenced, a group of about three dozen research teams around the world began the **Encyclopedia of DNA Elements (ENCODE) Project**. A main goal of ENCODE was to use both experimental approaches, including ChIP-based methods as we discussed in Section 21.3, and bioinformatics to identify and analyze functional elements of the genome, such as transcriptional start sites, promoters, and enhancers, which regulate the expression of human genes.

Recall from our previous discussions that only a relatively small percentage (2 percent) of the human genome codes for proteins. ENCODE focused not on genes but on all of the sequences, commonly referred to as "junk" DNA. So what are all of the other bases in the genome doing? The term *junk DNA* has always been a misnomer. We know that such sequences are important for chromosome structure, the regulation of gene expression, and other roles. Just because these sequences themselves do not code for protein does not mean that they are unimportant. Non–protein-coding sequences are discussed in greater detail later in the text (see Special Topic Chapter 2—Emerging Roles of RNA).

ENCODE studied gene expression in 147 different cell types because genome activity differs from cell to cell. After about a decade of research and a cost of $288 million, in 2012 a group of 30 research papers were published revealing the major findings of the ENCODE project. Highlights of what ENCODE revealed include the following.

- The majority, ~80 percent, of the human genome is considered functional. This is partly because large segments of the genome are transcribed into RNA. Most of these RNAs do not encode proteins. These various RNAs include tRNA, rRNAs, and miRNAs. For example, at least 13,000 sequences specify long noncoding RNAs (lncRNAs). Other reports suggest there may be over 17,000 lncRNAs. It may turn out that the number of noncoding RNA sequences will outnumber protein-coding genes.

- The functional sequences also include gene-regulatory regions: ~70,000 promoter regions and nearly 400,000 enhancer regions.

- There are 20,687 protein-coding genes in the human genome.

- A total of 11,224 sequences are characterized as pseudogenes, previously thought to be inactive in all individuals. Some of these are inactive in most individuals but occasionally active in certain cell types of some individuals, which may eventually warrant their reclassification as active, transcribed genes and not pseudogenes.

- SNPs associated with disease are enriched within noncoding functional elements of the genome, often residing near protein-coding genes.

Clearly, it is not accurate to dismiss non–protein-coding DNA as junk. These sequences are critically important as regulatory regions. Thus one important conclusion of ENCODE is that nearly 80 percent of the genome has some functional significance. The ENCODE findings have broadly defined the functional roles of the genome to include encoding proteins or noncoding RNAs and displaying biochemical properties such as binding regulatory proteins that influence transcription or chromatin structure. Consequently, regulation of gene expression is far more complex than previously thought, with gene expression being influenced by regulatory sequences that are near and far to the gene being transcribed.

Not all scientists agree with ENCODE's definition of sequence function. And within the scientific community there has been significant debate about ENCODE and its value given the cost of the project. But research teams are already using information from ENCODE to identify risk factors for certain diseases, with the hopes of developing appropriate cures and treatments.

EVOLVING CONCEPT OF A GENE

Based on the work of the ENCODE project, we now know that DNA sequences that have previously been thought of as "junk DNA," which do not encode proteins, are nonetheless often transcribed into what we call noncoding RNA (ncRNA). Since the function of some these RNAs is now being determined, we must consider whether the concept of the gene should be expanded to include DNA sequences that encode ncRNAs. At this writing, there is no consensus, but it is important for you to be aware of these current findings as you develop your final interpretation of a gene. ∎

The Human Microbiome Project

In 2007 the National Institutes of Health announced plans for the **Human Microbiome Project (HMP),** a $170 million project to complete the genomes of an estimated 600–1000 microorganisms, bacteria, viruses, and yeast that live on and inside humans. Microorganisms comprise ~1–2 percent of the human body, outnumbering human cells by about 10 to 1. Many microbes, such as *E. coli* in the digestive tract, have important roles in human health, and of course other microbes make us ill. The HMP has several major goals, including:

- Determining if individuals share a core human microbiome.

- Understanding whether changes in the microbiome can be correlated with changes in human health.

- Developing new methods, including bioinformatics tools, to support analysis of the microbiome.

- Addressing ethical, legal, and social implications raised by human microbiome research. Does this sound familiar? Recall that addressing ethical, legal, and social issues was a goal of the HGP.

The HMP has involved about 200 scientists at 80 institutions. In 2012 a series of papers were published summarizing recent findings from the HMP. The HMP analyzed 15 body sites from males and 18 sites from females from 242 healthy individuals in the United States and applied WGS of genomes for the microbes and viruses present at these sites. Each person was sampled up to three times over nearly two years. Researchers used bioinformatics to compare microbial and viral genome sequences obtained to sequences in publicly available databases. In addition to WGS analysis, sequences for 16S rRNA gene sequences in particular were used to compare bacterial samples. More than 2000 microbial sequences isolated from the human body have been sequenced to date.

The HMP has amassed more than 1000 times the sequencing data generated by the Human Genome Project. What concepts have we formulated about the human microbiome so far?

- Sequence data from the HMP have identified an estimated 81 to 99 percent of the microbes and viruses distributed among body areas in human males and females.

- As many as 1000 bacterial strains may be present in each person.

- An estimated 10,000 bacterial species may be part of the human microbiome.

- The microbiome starts at birth. Babies pick up bacteria from their mothers' microbiome.

- A surprise to HMP scientists is that the microbiome can be substantially different from person to person. Also, sequences for disease-causing bacteria are present in everyone's microbiome.

- In the human gut, for example, although the microbiome differs from person to person, it remains relatively stable over time in individuals.

There is no single "reference" human microbiome to which people can be compared. Microbial diversity varies greatly from individual to individual, and a personalization of the microbiome occurs in individuals. For instance, comparing sequences of the microbiomes from two healthy people of equivalent age reveals microbiomes that can be quite different. There are, however, similarities in certain parts of the body, with signature bacteria and characteristic genes associated with a particular location in the body.

Knowledge about the personalized nature of the microbiome will be valuable for improving human health and medicine, which in the future may include microbiome-specific therapeutic drugs. Scientists are trying to establish criteria for a healthy microbiome, which is expected to help

determine, for example, how bacteria help maintain normal health, how antibiotics can disturb a person's microbiome, and why certain individuals are susceptible to certain diseases, especially chronic conditions such as psoriasis, irritable bowel syndrome, and potentially even obesity.

Related to this project, a team of researchers at the University of California, Los Angeles, analyzed DNA sequences from 101 college students, 49 of whom had acne and 52 of whom did not. Over 1000 strains of *Propionibacterium acnes* (*P. acnes*) were isolated. Using WGS and bioinformatics, researchers clustered these strains into ten strain types (related strains). Six of these types were more common among acne-prone students, and one type appeared repeatedly in skin samples from students without acne. Sequence analysis of types associated with acne indicated gene clusters that may contribute to the skin disease. Further analysis of these strain types may help dermatologists develop new drugs targeted at killing acne-causing strains of *P. acnes*.

No Genome Left Behind and the Genome 10K Plan

Without question new sequencing technologies that have been developed as a result of the HGP are an important part of the transformational effect the HGP has had on modern biology. In the late 1990s, a room full of sequencers and several million dollars were required to sequence the 97-Mb genome of *C. elegans*. As a sign of modern times in the world of genomics, recently two sequencers and $500,000 produced a reasonably complete draft of the 750-Mb cod genome—in a month!

Recent headline-grabbing genomes that have been completed include:

- the tomato, which has 31,760 genes, more genes than humans!

- the potato, a vegetable that shares 92 percent of its DNA with tomatoes, a fruit

- chickpea, the second most widely grown legume after the soybean

- the red-spotted new, which has a genome of almost 10 billion base pairs!

Modern sequencing technologies are asking some to consider the question, "What would you do if you could sequence everything?" Partners around the world, including genome scientists and museum curators, have proposed sequencing 10,000 vertebrate genomes, the **Genome 10K** plan. Shortly after the HGP finished, the National Human Genome Research Institute (NHGRI) assembled a list of mammals and other vertebrates as priorities for genome sequencing in part because of their potential benefit for learning about the human genome through comparative genomics. Genome 10K will also provide insight into genome evolution and speciation.

21.6 Comparative Genomics Analyzes and Compares Genomes from Different Organisms

As of 2013, over 4300 whole genomes have been sequenced—including many model organisms and a number of viruses. About 200 of the completed genomes are from eukaryotes. This is quite extraordinary progress in a relatively short time span! Among these organisms are yeast (*Saccharomyces cerevisiae*)—the first eukaryotic genome to be sequenced to bacteria such as *E. coli,* the nematode roundworm (*Caenorhabditis elegans),* the thale cress plant (*Arabidopsis thaliana),* mice (*Mus musculus),* zebrafish (*Danio rerio),* and of course *Drosophila*. In the past few years, genomes for chimpanzees, dogs, chickens, gorillas, sea urchins, honey bees, pigs, pufferfish, rice, and wheat have all been sequenced.

These studies have demonstrated not only significant differences in genome organization between prokaryotes and eukaryotes but also many similarities between genomes of nearly all species. In this section we discuss interesting aspects of genomes in selected organisms. Analysis of the growing number of genome sequences confirms that all living organisms are related and descended from a common ancestor. Similar gene sets are used by organisms for basic cellular functions, such as DNA replication, transcription, and translation. These genetic relationships are the rationale for using model organisms to study inherited human disorders, the effects of the environment on genes, and interactions of genes in complex diseases, such as cardiovascular disease, diabetes, neurodegenerative conditions, and behavioral disorders.

Comparative genomics compares the genomes of different organisms to answer questions about genetics and other aspects of biology. It is a field with many research and practical applications, including gene discovery and the development of model organisms to study human diseases. It also incorporates the study of gene and genome evolution and the relationship between organisms and their environment. Comparative genomics uses a wide range of techniques and resources, such as the construction and use of nucleotide and protein databases containing nucleic acid and amino acid sequences, fluorescent *in situ* hybridization (FISH), and the creation of gene knockout animals. Comparative genomics can reveal genetic differences and similarities between organisms to provide insight into how those differences contribute to differences in phenotype, life cycle, or other attributes, and to ascertain the evolutionary history of those genetic differences.

Prokaryotic and Eukaryotic Genomes Display Common Structural and Functional Features and Important Differences

Since most prokaryotes have small genomes amenable to shotgun cloning and sequencing, many early genome projects have focused on prokaryotes, and more than 900 additional projects to sequence prokaryotic genomes are now under way. Many of the prokaryotic genomes already sequenced are from organisms that cause human diseases, such as cholera, tuberculosis, and leprosy. Traditionally, the bacterial genome has been thought of as relatively small (less than 5 Mb) and contained within a single circular DNA molecule. *E. coli,* used as the prototypical bacterial model organism in genetics, has a genome with these characteristics. However, the flood of genomic information now available has challenged the validity of this viewpoint for bacteria in general. Although most prokaryotic genomes are small, their sizes vary across a surprisingly wide range. In fact, there is some overlap in size between larger bacterial genomes (30 Mb in *Bacillus megaterium*) and smaller eukaryotic genomes (12.1 Mb in yeast). Gene number in bacterial genomes also demonstrates a wide range, from less than 500 to more than 5000 genes, a ten-fold difference.

In addition, although many bacteria have a single, circular chromosome, there is substantial variation in chromosome organization and number among bacterial species. An increasing number of genomes composed of linear DNA molecules are being identified, including the genome of *Borrelia burgdorferi,* the organism that causes Lyme disease. Sequencing of the *Vibrio cholerae* genome (the organism responsible for cholera) revealed the presence of two circular chromosomes. Other bacteria that have genomes with two or more chromosomes include *Rhizobium radiobacter* (formerly *Agrobacterium tumefaciens*), *Deinococcus radiodurans,* and *Rhodobacter sphaeroides.* The finding that some bacterial species have multiple chromosomes raises questions both about how replication and segregation of their chromosomes are coordinated during cell division and about what undiscovered mechanisms of gene regulation may exist in bacteria. The answers may provide clues about the evolution of multichromosome eukaryotic genomes.

We can make two generalizations about the organization of protein-coding genes in bacteria. First, gene density is very high, averaging about one gene per kilobase of DNA. For example, the genome of *E. coli* strain K12, which was sequenced in 1997 as the second prokaryotic genome to be sequenced, is 4.6 Mb in size, and it contains 4289

TABLE 21.2 Comparison of Selected Genomes

Organism (Scientific Name)	Approximate Size of Genome (in million [megabase, Mb] or billion [gigabase, Gb] bases) (Date Completed)	Number of Genes	Approximate Percentage of Genes Shared with Humans
Bacterium (*Escherichia coli*)	4.6 Mb (1997)	4403	not determined
Chicken (*Gallus gallus*)	1 Gb (2004)	~20,000–23,000	60%
Dog (*Canis familiaris*)	2.5 Gb (2003)	~18,400	75%
Chimpanzee (*Pan troglodytes*)	~3 Gb (2005)	~20,000–24,000	98%
Fruit fly (*Drosophila melanogaster*)	165 Mb (2000)	~13,600	50%
Human (*Homo sapiens*)	3.1 Gb (2004)	~20,000	100%
Mouse (*Mus musculus*)	~2.5 Gb (2002)	~30,000	80%
Pig (*Sus scrofa*)	~3 Gb (2012)	21,640	84%
Rat (*Rattus norvegicus*)	~2.75 Gb (2004)	~22,000	80%
Rhesus macaque (*Macaca mulatta*)	2.87 Gb (2007)	~20,000	93%
Rice (*Oryza sativa*)	389 Mb (2005)	~41,000	not determined
Roundworm (*Caenorhabditis elegans*)	97 Mb (1998)	19,099	40%
Sea urchin (*Strongylocentrotus purpuratus*)	814 Mb (2006)	~23,500	60%
Thale cress (plant) (*Arabidopsis thaliana*)	140 Mb (2000)	~27,500	not determined
Yeast (*Saccharomyces cerevisiae*)	12 Mb (1996)	~5700	30%

Adapted from Palladino, M. A. *Understanding the Human Genome Project*, 2nd ed. Benjamin Cummings, 2006.
Note: Billion bp (gigabase, Gb).

protein-coding genes in its single, circular chromosome. This close packing of genes in prokaryotic genomes means that a very high proportion of the DNA (approximately 85 to 90 percent) serves as coding DNA. Typically, only a small amount of a bacterial genome is noncoding DNA, often in the form of regulatory sequences or of transposable elements that can move from one place to another in the genome.

The second generalization we can make is that bacterial genomes contain operons. Recall from an earlier chapter (see Chapter 16), that operons contain multiple genes functioning as a transcriptional unit whose protein products are part of a common biochemical pathway). In *E. coli*, 27 percent of all genes are contained in operons (almost 600 operons). In other bacterial genomes, the organization of genes into transcriptional units is challenging our ideas about the nature of operons. For example, in *Aquifex aeolicus*, one polygenic transcription unit contains six genes involved in several different cellular processes with no apparent common relationships: two genes for DNA recombination, one for lipid synthesis, one for nucleic acid synthesis, one for protein synthesis, and one that encodes a protein for cell motility. Other polygenic transcription units in this species also contain genes with widely different functions. This finding, combined with similar results from other genome projects, raises interesting questions about the consensus that operons encode products that control a single metabolic pathway in bacterial cells.

The basic features of eukaryotic genomes are similar in different species, although genome size in eukaryotes is highly variable (Table 21.2). Genome sizes range from about 10 Mb in fungi to over 100,000 Mb in some flowering plants (a ten thousand-fold range); the number of chromosomes per genome ranges from two to the hundreds (about a hundred-fold range), but the number of genes varies much less dramatically than either genome size or chromosome number.

Eukaryotic genomes have several features not found in prokaryotes:

- **Gene density**. In prokaryotes, gene density is close to 1 gene per kilobase. In eukaryotic genomes, there is a wide range of gene density. In yeast, there is about 1 gene/2 kb, in Drosophila, about 1 gene/13 kb, and in humans, gene density varies greatly from chromosome to chromosome. Human chromosome 22 has about 1 gene/64 kb, while chromosome 13 has 1 gene/155 kb of DNA.

- **Introns**. Most eukaryotic genes contain introns. There is wide variation among genomes in the number of introns they contain and also wide variation from gene to gene. The entire yeast genome has only 239 introns, whereas just a single gene in the human genome can contain more than 100 introns. Regarding intron size, generally the size in eukaryotes is correlated with genome size. Smaller genomes have smaller average introns, and larger genomes have larger average intron sizes. But there are exceptions. For example, the genome of the pufferfish (*Fugu rubripes*) has relatively few introns.

- **Repetitive sequences**. The presence of introns and the existence of repetitive sequences are two major reasons for the wide range of genome sizes in eukaryotes. In some plants, such as maize, repetitive sequences are the dominant feature of the genome. The maize genome has about 2500 Mb of DNA, and more than two-thirds of that genome is composed of repetitive DNA. In the human, as discussed previously, about half of the genome is repetitive DNA.

Comparative Genomics Provides Novel Information about the Genomes of Model Organisms and the Human Genome

As mentioned earlier, the Human Genome Project sequenced genomes from a number of model nonhuman organisms too, including *E. coli, Arabidopsis thaliana, Saccharomyces cerevisiae, Drosophila melanogaster,* the nematode roundworm *Caenorhabditis elegans,* and the mouse *Mus musculus.* Complete genome sequences of such organisms have been invaluable for comparative genomics studies of gene function in these organisms and in humans. As shown in Table 21.2, the number of genes humans share with other species is very high, ranging from about 30 percent of the genes in yeast to ~80 percent in mice and ~98 percent in chimpanzees. The human genome even contains around 100 genes that are also present in many bacteria. Comparative genomics has shown us that many mutated genes involved in human disease are also present in model organisms. For instance, approximately 60 percent of genes mutated in nearly 300 human diseases are also found in *Drosophila.* These include genes involved in prostate, colon, and pancreatic cancers; cardiovascular disease; cystic fibrosis; and several other conditions. Here we consider how comparative genomics studies of several model organisms (sea urchins, dogs, chimpanzees, and Rhesus monkeys) and the Neanderthal genome have revealed interesting elements of the human genome.

The Sea Urchin Genome

In 2006, researchers from the Sea Urchin Genome Sequencing Consortium completed the 814 million bp genome of the sea urchin *Strongylocentrotus purpuratus* [pictured in Figure 21–20(a)]. Sea urchins are shallow-water marine invertebrates that have served as important model organisms, particularly for developmental biologists. One reason is that the sea urchin is a nonchordate deuterostome, and humans, with their spinal cord, are chordate deuterostomes. Fossil records indicate that sea urchins appeared during the Early Cambrian period, around 520 mya.

A combination of whole-genome shotgun sequencing and map-based cloning in BACs was used to complete the genome. Sea urchins have an estimated 23,500 genes, including representative genes for just about all major vertebrate gene families. Sequence alignment and homology searches demonstrate that the sea urchin contains many genes with important functions in humans, yet interestingly, important genes in flies and worms, such as certain cytochrome P-450 genes that play a role in the breakdown of toxic compounds, are missing from sea urchins. The sea urchin genome also has an abundance (~25 to 30 percent) of **pseudogenes**—nonfunctional relatives of protein-coding genes (we meet pseudogenes again in the next subsection). Sea urchins have a smaller average intron size than humans, supporting the general trend revealed by comparative genomics that intron size is correlated with overall genome size.

Another genome trend that urchins share with other eukaryotes is the presence of genes involved in innate immunity, the inborn defense mechanisms that provide broad-spectrum protection against many pathogens. Sea urchins have an extraordinarily rich number of genes providing innate immunity. For example, one very important category of innate immunity genes, the Toll-like receptors (TLRs), produce transmembrane proteins that are essential for pathogen recognition in nearly every cell type of vertebrates. Sea urchins have over 200 *Tlr* genes compared to 11 in humans. The abundance of these and other important innate immunity genes in sea urchins has led to categorizing these genes as the urchin "defensome." This characteristic of sea urchins may help explain how these organisms have adapted so well to the pathogen-loaded environments of seabeds.

Urchins have nearly 1000 genes for sensing light and odor, indicative of great sensory abilities. In this respect, their genome is more typical of vertebrates than invertebrates. A number of orthologs of human genes involved in hearing and balance are present in the sea urchin, as are many human-disease-associated orthologs, including protein kinases, GTPases, transcription factors, TLRs, transporters, and low-density lipoprotein receptors. Sea urchins and humans share approximately 7000 orthologs.

Another interesting aspect of the sea urchin genome project is that it has identified genes previously thought to be vertebrate-specific. One example, the *WntA* gene, important for patterning during embryonic development, as discussed earlier in the text (see Chapter 18), was thought to be absent from nonvertebrate deuterostomes. The sea urchin genome also contains genes that are not present in chordates. Further analysis of the urchin genome is expected to make important contributions to our understanding of evolutionary transitions between invertebrates and vertebrates.

The Dog Genome

In 2005 the genome for "man's best friend" was completed, and it revealed that we share about 75 percent of our genes with dogs (*Canis familiaris*), providing a useful model with which to study our own genome. Dogs have a genome that is similar in size to the human genome: about 2.5 billion base pairs with an estimated 18,400 genes. The dog offers several advantages for studying heritable human diseases. Dogs share many genetic disorders with humans, including over 400 single-gene disorders, sex-chromosome aneuploidies, multifactorial diseases (such as epilepsy), behavioral conditions (such as obsessive-compulsive disorder), and genetic predispositions to cancer, blindness, heart disease, and deafness. The molecular causes of at least 60 percent of inherited diseases in dogs, such as point mutations and deletions, are similar or identical to those found in humans. In addition, at least 50 percent of the genetic diseases in dogs are breed-specific, so that the mutant allele segregates in relatively homogeneous genetic backgrounds. Dog breeds resemble isolated human populations in having a small number of founders and a long period of relative genetic isolation. These properties make individual dog breeds useful as models of human genetic disorders.

In addition, differences in biology and behavior among dog breeds are well documented. Domestic dogs show greater variation in body size than all other living terrestrial vertebrates. The size difference between a Chihuahua and a Great Dane is an excellent example. Mapping and comparing DNA sequence differences (polymorphisms) among breeds may help identify genes that contribute to both physiological and behavioral differences. For instance, in 2007, genome-wide analysis of different large and small dog breeds revealed a locus on chromosome 15 where a single-nucleotide polymorphism in the insulin-like growth factor 1 gene (*Igf1*) is common in all small breeds of dogs but virtually absent from large dogs. It is well known that *Igf1* plays important roles in growth-hormone-regulated increases in muscle mass and bone growth during adolescence in humans. This study provides very strong evidence that mutation of *Igf1* is a primary determinant of body size in small dogs.

Dog breeders are now using genetic tests to screen dogs for inherited disease conditions, for coat color in Labrador retrievers and poodles, and for fur length in Mastiffs. Undoubtedly, we can expect many more genetic tests for dogs in the near future, including DNA analysis for size, type of tail, speed, sense of smell, and other traits deemed important by breeders and owners.

Finally, scientists have been using genomic data to determine the origin of domestic dogs. An analysis of 48,000 markers across the whole genomes of hundreds of dogs and gray wolves from different regions around the world showed that modern dogs shared more sequences in common with Middle Eastern wolves than with Asian wolves. Recent research based on sequence analysis of mitochondrial DNA (mtDNA) from the fossils of ancient dogs and wolves suggests that dogs originated in Europe from gray wolves that are now extinct. In this work, researchers compared mtDNA from samples 1000 to 36,000 years old from 77 dogs of different breeds, 49 wolves, and 4 coyotes. Based on mtDNA sequences, dogs appear to be more closely related to ancient wolves than to modern wolves. A similar conclusion was made by a team studying whole genomes. In addition, mtDNA sequences from ancient remains that most closely matched modern dogs were all from European gray wolf samples. Aging of the samples suggests that dog domestication began between 18,800 and 32,100 years ago among hunter-gatherers several thousand years before humans farmed in earnest. Scientists who believe that the domestication of dogs began in Asia have noted that the recent mtDNA study may be flawed because the researchers were unable to get DNA samples from ancient specimens from the Middle East and from East Asia. Ongoing research in this area will continue, and it will be interesting to see whether genomics can settle the debate about the origins of man's best friend.

The Chimpanzee Genome

Although the chimpanzee (*Pan troglodytes*) genome was not part of the HGP, its nucleotide sequence was completed in 2004. Overall, the chimp and human genome sequences differ by less than 2 percent, and 98 percent of the genes are the same. Comparisons between these genomes offer some interesting insights into what makes some primates humans and others chimpanzees.

The speciation events that separated humans and chimpanzees occurred less than 6.3 million years ago (mya). Genomic analysis indicates that these species initially diverged but then exchanged genes again before separating completely. Their separate evolution after this point is exhibited in such differences as that seen between the sequence of chimpanzee chromosome 22 and its human ortholog, chromosome 21 (**Table 21.3**; chimps have 48 chromosomes and humans have 46, so the numbering is different). These chromosomes have accumulated nucleotide substitutions that total 1.44 percent of the sequence. The most surprising difference is the discovery of 68,000 nucleotide insertions or deletions, collectively called **indels**, in the chimp and human chromosomes, a frequency of 1 indel every 470 bases. Many of these are *Alu* insertions in human chromosome 21. Although the overall difference in the nucleotide sequence is small, there are significant differences in the encoded genes. Only 17 percent of the genes analyzed encode identical proteins in both chromosomes;

TABLE 21.3 Comparisons between Human Chromosome 21 and Chimpanzee Chromosome 22

	Human 21	Chimpanzee 22
Size (bp)	33,127,944	32,799,845
%G + C Content	40.94	41.01
CpG Islands	950	885
SINEs (*Alu* elements)	15,137	15,048
Genes	284	272
Pseudogenes	98	89

the other 83 percent encode genes with one or more amino acid differences.

Differences in the time and place of gene expression also play a major role in differentiating the two primates. Using DNA microarrays (discussed in Section 21.9), researchers compared expression patterns of 202 genes in human and chimp cells from brain and liver. They found more species-specific differences in expression of brain genes than liver genes. To further examine these differences, Svante Pääbo and colleagues compared expression of 10,000 genes in human and chimpanzee brains and found that 10 percent of genes examined differ in expression in one or more regions of the brain. More importantly, these differences are associated with genes in regions of the human genome that have been duplicated subsequent to the divergence of chimps and humans. This finding indicates that genome evolution, speciation, and gene expression are interconnected. Further work on these segmental duplications and the genes they contain may identify genes that help make us human.

The Rhesus Monkey Genome

The Rhesus macaque monkey (*Macaca mulatta*), another primate, has served as one of the most important model organisms in biomedical research. Macaques have played central roles in our understanding of cardiovascular disease, aging, diabetes, cancer, depression, osteoporosis, and many other aspects of human health. They have been essential for research on AIDS vaccines and for the development of polio vaccines. The macaque's genome is the first monkey genome to have been sequenced. A main reason geneticists are so excited about the completion of this sequencing project is that macaques provide a more distant evolutionary window that is ideally suited for comparing and analyzing human and chimpanzee genomes. As we discussed in the preceding section, humans and chimpanzees shared a common ancestor approximately 6 mya. But macaques split from the ape lineage that led to chimpanzees and humans about 25 mya. The macaque and human genome

have thus diverged farther from one another, as evidenced by the ~93 percent sequence identity between humans and macaques compared to the ~98 percent sequence identity shared by humans and chimpanzees.

The macaque genome was published in 2007, and it was no surprise to learn that it consists of 2.87 billion bp (similar to the size of the human genome) contained in 22 chromosomes (20 autosomes, an X, and a Y) with ~20,000 protein-coding genes. Although comparative analyses of this genome are ongoing, a number of interesting features have been revealed so far. As in humans, about 50 percent of the genome consists of repeat elements (transposons, LINEs, SINEs). Gene duplications and gene families are abundant, including cancer gene families found in humans.

A number of interesting surprises have also been observed. For instance, recall from earlier in the text (see Chapter 4) and elsewhere our discussion about the genetic disorder phenylketonuria (PKU), an autosomal recessive inherited condition in which individuals cannot metabolize the amino acid phenylalanine due to mutation of the phenylalanine hydroxylase (*PAH*) gene. The histidine substitution encoded by a mutation in the *PAH* gene of humans with PKU appears as the wild-type amino acid in the protein from healthy macaques. Further analysis of the macaque genome and comparison to the human and chimpanzee genome will be invaluable for geneticists studying genetic variations that played a role in primate evolution.

The Neanderthal Genome and Modern Humans

In early 2009, a team of scientists led by Svante Pääbo at the Max Planck Institute for Evolutionary Anthropology in Germany and 454 Life Sciences reported completion of a rough draft of the Neanderthal (*Homo neanderthalensis*) genome encompassing more than 3 billion bp of Neanderthal DNA and about two-thirds of the genome. Previously, in 1997, Pääbo's lab sequenced portions of Neanderthal mitochondrial DNA from a fossil. In late 2006, Pääbo's group along with a number of scientists in the United States reported the first sequence of ~65,000 bp of nuclear DNA isolated from Neanderthal bone samples from Croatia. Bones from three females who lived in Vindija Cave in Croatia about 38,000 to 44,000 years ago were used to produce the draft sequence of the Neanderthal nuclear genome.

Because Neanderthals are members of the human family, and closer relatives to humans than chimpanzees, the Neanderthal genome is expected to provide an unprecedented opportunity to use comparative genomics to advance our understanding of evolutionary relationships between modern humans and our predecessors. In particular, scientists are interested in identifying areas in the genome where humans have undergone rapid evolution since splitting (diverging) from Neanderthals. Much of this analysis involves a comparative genomics approach to compare the Neanderthal genome to the human and chimpanzee genomes.

The human and Neanderthal genomes are 99 percent identical. Comparative genomics has identified 78 protein-coding sequences in humans that seem to have arisen since the divergence from Neanderthals and that may have helped modern humans adapt. Some of these sequences are involved in cognitive development and sperm motility. Of the many genes shared by these species, *FOXP2* is a gene that has been linked to speech and language ability. There are many genes that influence speech, so this finding does not mean that Neanderthals spoke as we do. But because Neanderthals had the same modern human *FOXP2* gene scientists have speculated that Neanderthals possessed linguistic abilities.

A 2008 study of the Neanderthal mitochondrial genome by Pääbo's team obtained 39 million sequence reads averaging 69 bp in length. Of 16,568 nucleotides present in mtDNA of modern humans, on average 206 differed from those of Neanderthals. These differences fall outside the variation among modern humans and led the research team to estimate that the most common point of ancestry, the divergence date between the two mtDNA lineages, was 660,000 years ago (±140,000). This study also provided interesting observations about rates of amino acid substitutions in key enzymes in the mitochondrial electron transport chain.

The realization that modern humans and Neanderthals lived in overlapping ranges as recently as 30,000 years ago has led to speculation about the interactions between modern humans and Neanderthals. Genome studies suggest that interbreeding took place between Neanderthals and modern humans an estimated 45,000 to 80,000 years ago in the eastern Mediterranean. In fact, the genome of non-African *H. sapiens* contains approximately 1–4 percent

of sequence inherited from Neanderthals. These exciting studies, previously thought to be impossible, are having ramifications in many areas of human evolution, and it will be interesting indeed to follow the progress of this work.

21.7 Comparative Genomics Is Useful for Studying the Evolution and Function of Multigene Families

Comparative genomics has also proven to be valuable for identifying members of **multigene families**, groups of genes that share similar but not identical DNA sequences through duplication and descent from a single ancestral gene. Their gene products frequently have similar functions, and the genes are often, but not always, found at a single chromosomal locus. A group of related multigene families is called a **superfamily**. Sequence data from genome projects are providing evidence that multigene families are present in many, if not all, genomes. One of the best-studied examples of gene family evolution is the **globin gene superfamily**, whose members encode very similar but not identical polypeptide chains with closely related functions (**Figure 21–14**). Other well-characterized

FIGURE 21–14 The evolutionary history of the globin gene superfamily. A duplication event in an ancestral gene gave rise to two lineages about 700 to 800 million years ago (mya). One line led to the myoglobin gene, which is located on chromosome 22 in humans; the other underwent a second duplication event about 500 mya, giving rise to the ancestors of the α-globin and β-globin gene subfamilies. Duplications beginning about 200 mya formed the β-globin gene subfamilies. In humans, the α-globin genes are located on chromosome 16, and the β-globin genes are on chromosome 11.

gene superfamilies include the histone, tubulin, actin, and immunoglobulin (antibody) gene superfamilies.

Recall that paralogs, which we defined in Section 21.3, are homologous genes present in the same single organism, believed to have evolved by gene duplication. The globin genes that encode the polypeptides in hemoglobin molecules are a paralogous multigene superfamily that arose by duplication and dispersal to occupy different chromosomal sites. In this family, an ancestral gene encoding an oxygen transport protein was duplicated about 800 mya, producing two sister genes, one of which evolved into the modern-day myoglobin gene. **Myoglobin** is an oxygen-carrying protein found in muscle. The other gene underwent further duplication and divergence about 500 mya and formed prototypes of the α-globin and β-globin genes. These genes encode proteins found in **hemoglobin**, the oxygen-carrying molecule in red blood cells. Additional duplications within these genes occurred within the last 200 million years. Events subsequent to each duplication dispersed these gene subfamilies to different chromosomes, and in the human genome, each now resides on a separate chromosome. Similar patterns of evolution are observed in other gene families, including the trypsin–chymotrypsin family of proteases, the homeotic selector genes of animals, and the rhodopsin family of visual pigments.

Adult hemoglobin is a tetramer containing two α- and two β-polypeptides (refer to Figure 14–20 for the structure of hemoglobin). Each polypeptide incorporates a heme group that reversibly binds oxygen. The α-globin gene cluster on chromosome 16 and the β-globin gene cluster on chromosome 11 share nucleotide- and amino acid–sequence similarity but the highest degree of sequence similarity is found within subfamilies.

The **α-globin** gene subfamily [**Figure 21–15(a)**] contains three genes: the ζ (zeta) gene, expressed only in early embryogenesis, and two copies of the α gene, expressed during the fetal (α_1) and adult stages (α_2). In addition, the cluster contains two pseudogenes (similar to ζ and α_1), which in this family are designated by the prefix Ψ (psi) followed by the symbol of the gene they most resemble. Thus, the designation $\Psi\alpha_1$ indicates a pseudogene of the fetal α_1 gene.

The organization of the α-globin subfamily members and the locations of their introns and exons demonstrate several characteristic features [Figure 21–15(a)]. First, the DNA encoding the three functional α genes occupies only

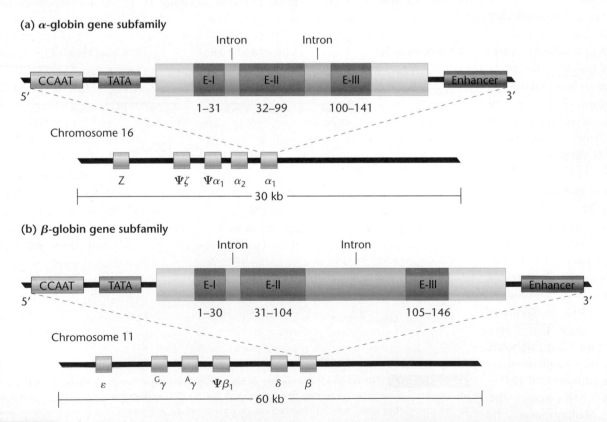

FIGURE 21–15 Organization of (a) the α-globin gene subfamily on chromosome 16 and (b) the β-globin gene subfamily on chromosome 11. Also shown in each case is the internal organization of the α_1 gene and the β gene, respectively. Both genes contain three exons (E-I, E-II, E-III) and two introns. The numbers below the exons indicate the location of amino acids in the gene product encoded by each exon.

a small portion of the 30-kb region containing the subfamily. Second, each functional gene in this subfamily contains two introns at precisely the same positions. Third, the nucleotide sequences within corresponding exons are nearly identical in the ζ and α genes. Each of these genes encodes a polypeptide chain of 141 amino acids. However, their intron sequences are highly divergent, even though the introns are about the same size. Note that much of the nucleotide sequence of each gene is contained in these noncoding introns.

The human β-globin gene cluster contains five genes spaced over 60 kb of DNA [**Figure 21–15(b)**]. In this and the α-globin gene subfamily, the order of genes on the chromosome parallels their order of expression during development. Three of the five genes are expressed before birth. The ε (epsilon) gene is expressed only during embryogenesis, while the two nearly identical γ genes ($^G\gamma$ and $^A\gamma$) are expressed only during fetal development. The polypeptide products of the two γ genes differ only by a single amino acid. The two remaining genes, δ and β, are expressed after birth and throughout life. A single pseudogene, $\Psi\beta_1$, is present in this subfamily. All five functional genes in this cluster encode proteins with 146 amino acids and have two similar-sized introns at exactly the same positions. The second intron in the β-globin subfamily is significantly larger than its counterpart in the functional α-globin subfamily. These features reflect the evolutionary history of each subfamily and the events such as gene duplication, nucleotide substitution, and chromosome translocations that produced the present-day globin superfamily.

21.8 Metagenomics Applies Genomics Techniques to Environmental Samples

Metagenomics, also called **environmental genomics**, is the use of whole-genome shotgun approaches to sequence genomes from entire communities of microbes in environmental samples of water, air, and soil. Oceans, glaciers, deserts, and virtually every other environment on Earth are being sampled for metagenomics projects. Human genome pioneer J. Craig Venter left Celera to form the J. Craig Venter Institute, and his group has played a central role in developing metagenomics as an emerging area of genomics research.

One of the institute's major initiatives has been a global expedition to sample marine and terrestrial microorganisms from around the world and to sequence their genomes. Through this project, called the *Sorcerer II Global Ocean Sampling* (GOS) Expedition, Venter and his

researchers traveled the globe by yacht, in a sailing voyage described as a modern-day version of Charles Darwin's famous voyage on the *H.M.S. Beagle*.

A key benefit of metagenomics is its potential for teaching us more about millions of species of bacteria, of which only a few thousand have been well characterized. Many new viruses, particularly bacteriophages, are also identified through metagenomics studies of water samples. Metagenomics is providing important new information about genetic diversity in microbes that is key to understanding complex interactions between microbial communities and their environment, as well as allowing phylogenetic classification of newly identified microbes. Metagenomics also has great potential for identifying genes with novel functions, some of which may have valuable applications in medicine and biotechnology.

The general method used in metagenomics to sequence genomes for all microbes in a given environment involves isolating DNA directly from an environmental sample without requiring cultures of the microbes or viruses. Such an approach is necessary because often it is difficult to replicate the complex array of growth conditions the microbes need to survive in culture.

For the *Sorcerer II* GOS project, samples of water from different layers in the water column were passed through high-density filters of various sizes to capture the microbes. DNA was then isolated from the microbes and subjected to shotgun sequencing and genome assembly. High-throughput sequencers on board the yacht operated nearly around the clock. One of the earliest expeditions by this group sequenced bacterial genomes from the Sargasso Sea off Bermuda. This project yielded over 1.2 million novel DNA sequences from 1800 microbial species, including 148 previously unknown bacterial species, and identified hundreds of photoreceptor genes. Many aquatic microorganisms rely on photoreceptors for capturing light energy to power photosynthesis. Scientists are interested in learning more about photoreceptors to help develop ways in which photosynthesis may be used to produce hydrogen as a fuel source. Medical researchers are also very interested in photoreceptors because in humans and many other species, photoreceptors in the retina of the eye are key proteins that detect light energy and transduce electrical signals that the brain eventually interprets to create visual images.

By early 2007, the GOS database contained approximately 6 billion bp of DNA from more than 400 uncharacterized microbial species! These sequences included 7.7 million previously uncharacterized sequences, encoding more than 6 million different potential proteins. This is almost twice the total number of previously characterized proteins in all other known databases worldwide (such

FIGURE 21-16   (a) Kingdom identifications for predicted proteins in NCBInr, NCBI Prokaryotic Genomes, the Institute for Genomics Research Gene Indices, and Ensembl databases. Notice that the publicly available databases of sequenced genomes and the predicted proteins they encode are dominated by eukaryotic sequences. (b) Kingdom identifications for novel predicted proteins in the Global Ocean Sampling (GOS) database. Bacterial sequences dominate this database, demonstrating the value of metagenomics for revealing new information about microbial genomes and microbial communities.

as the Swiss-Prot database discussed in the Exploring Genomics exercise for Chapter 14). **Figure 21–16(a)** shows the kingdom assignments for predicted protein sequences in publicly available databases worldwide, such as the

NCBI-nonredundant protein database (NCBInr), which accesses GenBank, Ensembl, and other well-known databases. Eukaryotic sequences comprise the majority (63 percent) of predicted proteins in these databases. Reviewing the kingdom assignments of approximately 6 million predicted proteins in the Global Ocean Sampling (GOS) dataset shows that, in contrast, the largest majority (90.8 percent) of sequences in this database are from the bacterial kingdom [**Figure 21–16(b)**].

The GOS Expedition also examined protein families corresponding to the predicted proteins encoded by the genome sequences in the GOS database: 17,067 families were medium (between 20 and 200 proteins) and large-sized (>200 proteins) clusters. A **Venn diagram**, like the image shown in **Figure 21–17**, is a common way to represent overlapping data in genomics datasets. In this figure, overlapping ovals indicate numbers of protein families belonging to certain sets of categories. Each area of the diagram is labeled with the number and percentage of families out of the 17,067 GOS medium- and large-sized clusters in each category or area of overlap. Of the 17,067 clusters in the GOS database, 3995 did not show significant homology to known protein families in prokaryotes, viruses, or eukaryotes (Figure 21–17). The results summarized in Figures 21–16 and 21–17 demonstrate the value of the GOS Expedition and of metagenomics for identifying novel microbial genes and potential proteins.

In Section 21.5 you learned about the Human Microbiome Project. This project represents an example of a metagenomics project in that it is intended to sequence the genomes of microbes and viruses present in and on humans as the "environment" being sampled. In fact, many of the techniques used in this project were based on metagenomics techniques used to sequence bacterial and viral genomes from marine water samples. Many other high-profile metagenomics applications have emerged recently, including the use of metagenomics to identify viruses and fungi thought to be involved in colony collapse disorder. One such malady has resulted in the loss of 50–90 percent of the honey bee population in beekeeping operations throughout the United States.

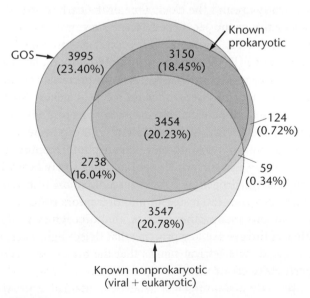

FIGURE 21–17   Venn diagram representation of 17,067 medium and large clusters of protein families grouped according to three categories: GOS, known prokaryotic sequences, and known nonprokaryotic sequences. Notice that the GOS project identified 3995 medium and large clusters of gene families that are unique to the GOS database and do not show significant homology to known protein families in prokaryotes or nonprokaryotes (viral and eukaryotes).

21.9 Transcriptome Analysis Reveals Profiles of Expressed Genes in Cells and Tissues

Once any genome has been sequenced and annotated, a formidable challenge still remains: that of understanding genome function by analyzing the genes it contains and the ways the genes expressed by the genome are regulated. **Transcriptome analysis**, also called **transcriptomics** or **global analysis of gene expression**, studies the expression of genes by a genome both qualitatively—by identifying which genes are expressed and which genes are not expressed—and quantitatively—by measuring varying levels of expression for different genes.

Even though in theory all cells of an organism possess the same gene in any cell or tissue type, certain genes will be highly expressed, others expressed at low levels, and some not expressed at all. Transcriptome analysis reveals gene-expression profiles that for the same genome may vary from cell to cell or from tissue type to tissue type. Identifying genes expressed by a genome is essential for understanding how the genome functions. Transcriptome analysis provides insights into (1) normal patterns of gene expression that are important for understanding how a cell or tissue type differentiates during development, (2) how gene expression dictates and controls the physiology of differentiated cells, and (3) mechanisms of disease development that result from or cause gene-expression changes in cells. Later in the text (see Chapter 22), we will consider why gene-expression analysis is gradually becoming an important diagnostic tool in certain areas of medicine. For example, examining gene-expression profiles in a cancerous tumor can help diagnose tumor type, determine the likelihood of tumor metastasis (spreading), and develop the most effective treatment strategy.

Microarray Analysis

A number of different techniques can be used for transcriptome analysis. PCR-based methods are useful because of their ability to detect genes that are expressed at low levels. **DNA microarray analysis** is widely used because it enables researchers to analyze all of a sample's expressed genes simultaneously.

Most microarrays, also known as **gene chips**, consist of a glass microscope slide onto which single-stranded DNA molecules are attached, or "spotted," using a computer-controlled high-speed robotic arm called an arrayer. Arrayers are fitted with a number of tiny pins. Each pin is immersed in a small amount of solution containing millions of copies of a different single-stranded DNA molecule. For example, many microarrays are made with single-stranded sequences of complementary DNA (cDNA) or expressed sequenced

tags (ESTs)—short fragments of cloned DNA from expressed genes. The arrayer fixes the DNA onto the slide at specific locations (points, or spots) that are recorded by a computer. A single microarray can have over 20,000 different spots of DNA (and over 1 million for exon-specific microarrays), each containing a unique sequence for a different gene. Entire genomes are available on microarrays, including the human genome. As you will learn later in the text (see Chapter 22), researchers are also using microarrays to compare patterns of gene expression in tissues in response to different conditions, to compare gene-expression patterns in normal and diseased tissues, and to identify pathogens.

To prepare a microarray for use in transcriptome analysis, scientists typically begin by extracting mRNA from cells or tissues (**Figure 21–18**). The mRNA is usually then reverse transcribed to synthesize cDNA tagged with fluorescently labeled nucleotides. The mRNA or cDNA can be labeled in a number of ways, but most methods involve the use of fluorescent dyes. Historically, microarray studies often involve comparing gene expression in different cell or tissue samples. cDNA prepared from one tissue is usually labeled with one color dye, red for example, and cDNA from another tissue is labeled with a different-colored dye, such as green. Labeled cDNAs are then denatured and incubated overnight with the microarray so that they will hybridize to spots on the microarray that contain complementary DNA sequences. Next, the microarray is washed, and then it is scanned by a laser that causes the cDNA hybridized to the microarray to fluoresce. The patterns of fluorescent spots reveal which genes are expressed in the tissue of interest, and the intensity of spot fluorescence indicates the relative level of expression. The brighter the spot, the more the particular mRNA is expressed in that tissue.

Microarrays have dramatically changed the way gene-expression patterns are analyzed. As discussed earlier in the text (see Chapter 20), Northern blot analysis was one of the earliest methods used for analyzing gene expression. Then PCR techniques proved to be rapid and more sensitive approaches. The biggest advantage of microarrays is that they enable thousands of genes to be studied simultaneously. As a result, however, they can generate an overwhelming amount of gene-expression data. Over 1 million gene-expression datasets are now available in publicly accessible databases. Most of these datasets have been generated in the past decade largely through microarray analysis. In addition, even when properly controlled, microarrays often yield variable results. For example, one experiment under certain conditions may not always yield similar patterns of gene expression as another identical experiment. Some of these differences can be due to real differences in gene expression, but others can be the result of variability in chip preparation, cDNA synthesis, probe hybridization, or washing conditions, all of which must be carefully

FIGURE 21–18 Microarray analysis for analyzing gene-expression patterns in a tissue.

controlled to limit such variability. Commercially available microarrays can reduce the variability that can result when individual researchers make their own arrays. You should also be aware that new methods for directly sequencing RNA (RNA-Seq, also called whole-transcriptome shotgun sequencing) will soon render microarrays obsolete!

Computerized microarray data analysis programs are essential for organizing gene-expression profile data from microarrays. For instance, **cluster algorithm** programs can be used to retrieve spot-intensity data from different locations on a microarray and to group gene-expression data from one or multiple microarrays into cluster images incorporating results from many experiments. Cluster analysis groups genes according to whether they show increased (upregulated) or decreased (downregulated) expression under the experimental conditions examined.

Figure 21–19(a) shows hierarchical clusters of upregulated and downregulated gene-expression patterns for the yeast *Saccharomyces cerevisiae* grown under different experimental culture conditions. Notice that different culture times reveal different patterns of downregulation

(a)

Experiments 1–15

10min 30min 50min 70min 90min 110min 130min 150min 170min 190min 210min 230min 250min 270min 290min

Genes

	unknown
SCW11	cell wall biogenesis glucanase (putative)
CLB6	cell cycle B-type cyclin; S phase
KCC4	bud growth protein kinase
MCD1	mitosis, sister chromatid cohesion
POL30	DNA replication DNA polymerase processivity factor
	unknown
RFA1	DNA replication replication factor A, 69 kD subunit
	unknown
STP3	tRNA splicing
TOS6	unknown; similar to Mid2p
ISR1	staurosporine resistance protein kinase
SRO4	bud site selection, plasma membrane protein
CSI2	cell wall biogenesis chitin synthase 3 subunit
SVS1	vanadate resistance
CLN2	cell cycle G1/S cyclin

Cluster of down-
regulated genes

Cluster of up-
regulated genes

(b)

Time (h) ⟶

FIGURE 21–19 (a) Hierarchical clusters in a microarray experiment using RNA samples from *Saccharomyces cerevisiae* grown for varying times in culture (experiments 1–15). Gene identities are labeled to the right of the array image. Red color in the array indicates upregulation in the experimental sample, and green indicates downregulation in the sample, as compared to a control culture. The intensity of the color indicates the magnitude of up- or downregulation. Brighter spots represent higher levels of expression than dimmer or black spots. The yellow oval highlights a cluster of downregulated genes, and the white oval highlights a cluster of upregulated genes. (b) High (red), intermediate (black), and low (green) levels of gene expression for *Drosophila* genes that exhibit a circadian rhythm. RNA samples from *Drosophila* were collected every four hours for six days and then used for microarray analysis. Each row shows all 36 responses of a single gene. Each column shows the gene-expression pattern for each time point sampled. Genes were arranged from top to bottom according to the time of peak activity.

(yellow oval) and upregulation (white oval). The identities of the genes in these regulated clusters indicate that many of the genes affected by the growth conditions of this experiment are genes involved in cell division.

Figure 21–19(b) reveals an interesting gene-expression profile for genes in *Drosophila* in which they display repeating patterns of expression as part of a **circadian rhythm** response. Circadian rhythms are oscillations in biological activity that occur on a regular cycle of time, such as 24 hours. Reductions in brain wave electrical activity that occur when you sleep, followed by the increased brain wave activity that occurs to wake you up, just before your alarm clock sounds in the morning, are examples of circadian responses. In the *Drosophila* microarray, each horizontal row shows expression results for a different gene. Notice how every several hours the expression for most genes is upregulated (red) and then downregulated (green) several hours later in a rhythmic pattern that repeats over the time course of this experiment (6 days). Results such as these are representative of the types of gene-expression profiles that can be revealed by microarrays. You will see similar representations of microarray data later in the text (see Chapter 24).

In Section 21.6 we briefly discussed the sea urchin genome and the importance of the sea urchin as a key model organism. Sea urchins have a relatively simple body

plan [**Figure 21–20(a)**]. They contain approximately 1500 cells with only a dozen cell types. Yet sea urchin development progresses through complex changes in gene expression that resemble vertebrate patterns of gene-expression changes during development. This is one reason urchins are a valuable model organism for developmental biology.

Scientists at NASA's Ames Genome Research Facility in Moffett, California, used microarrays to carry out a transcriptome study on sea urchin gene expression during the first two days of development (to the mid-late gastrula stage, about 48 hours postfertilization). This work revealed that approximately 52 percent of all genes in the sea urchin are active during this period of development: 11,500 of the sea urchin's 23,500 known genes were expressed in the embryo. The functional categories of genes expressed in the embryo were diverse, including genes for about 70 percent of the nearly 300 transcription factors in the sea urchin genome, along with genes involved in cell signaling, immunity, fertilization, and metabolism [**Figure 21–20(b)**]. Incredibly, 51,000 RNAs of unknown function were also expressed. Studies are underway to explain the differences between gene number and transcripts expressed, although it is already known that many sea urchin genes are extensively processed through alternative splicing. Further analysis of

(a)

(b)

FIGURE 21-20 (a) The sea urchin *Strongylocentrotus purpuratus*. (b) Transcriptome analysis of genes expressed in the sea urchin embryo. The *y*-axis of the histogram displays the percentage of annotated genes in different functional categories expressed in the embryo. The number at the top of each bar represents the total number of annotated genes in the corresponding functional category. Trans., transcription factors; Signal, signaling genes; Process, basic cellular processes, such as metabolism; Cytoskelet., cytoskeletal genes; Fertiliz., fertilization; and Biominer., biomineralization.

the sea urchin genome will undoubtedly reveal interesting aspects of gene function during sea urchin development and advance our understanding of the genetics of embryonic development in both invertebrates and vertebrates.

Now that we have considered genomes and transcriptomes, we turn our attention to the ultimate end products of most genes, the proteins encoded by a genome.

21.10 Proteomics Identifies and Analyzes the Protein Composition of Cells

As more genomes have been sequenced and studied, biologists have focused increasingly on understanding the complex structures and functions of the proteins the genomes encode. This interest is not surprising given that in most of the genomes sequenced to date, many newly discovered genes and their putative proteins have no known function. Keep in mind, in the ensuing discussion, that although every cell in the body contains an equivalent set of genes, not all cells express the same genes and proteins. **Proteome** is a term that represents the complete set of proteins encoded by a genome, but it is also often used to mean the entire complement of proteins in a cell. This definition would then include proteins that a cell acquired from another cell type.

Proteomics—the complete identification, characterization, and quantitative analysis of the proteome of a cell, tissue, or organism—can be used to reconcile differences between the number of genes in a genome and the number of different proteins produced. But equally important, proteomics also provides information about a protein's struc-

ture and function; posttranslational modifications; protein–protein, protein–nucleic acid, and protein–metabolite interactions; cellular localization of proteins; protein stability and aspects of translational and posttranslational levels of gene-expression regulation; and relationships (shared domains, evolutionary history) to other proteins. Proteomics projects have been used to characterize major families of proteins for some species. For example, about two-thirds of the *Drosophila* proteome has been well catalogued using proteomics.

Proteomics is also of clinical interest because it allows comparison of proteins in normal and diseased tissues, which can lead to the identification of proteins as biomarkers for disease conditions. Proteomic analysis of mitochondrial proteins during aging, proteomic maps of atherosclerotic plaques from human coronary arteries, and protein profiles in saliva as a way to detect and diagnose diseases are examples of such work.

Reconciling the Number of Genes and the Number of Proteins Expressed by a Cell or Tissue

Recall the one-gene:one-polypeptide hypothesis of George Beadle and Edward Tatum (see Chapter 14). Genomics has revealed that the link between gene and gene product is often much more complex. Genes can have multiple transcription start sites that produce several different types of transcripts. Alternative splicing and editing of pre-mRNA molecules can generate dozens of different proteins from a single gene. Remember the current estimate that over 50 percent of human genes produce more than one protein by alternative splicing.

As a result, proteomes are substantially larger than genomes. For instance, the ~20,000 genes in the human genome encode ~100,000 proteins, although some estimates suggest that the human proteome may be as large as 150,000–200,000 proteins.

Proteomes undergo dynamic changes that are coordinated in part by regulation of gene-expression patterns—the transcriptome. However, a number of other factors affect the proteome profile of a cell, further complicating the analysis of protein function. For instance, many proteins are modified by co-translational or posttranslational events, such as cleavage of signal sequences that target a protein for an organelle pathway, propeptides, or initiator methionine residues; by linkage to carbohydrates and lipids; or by the addition of chemical groups through methylation, acetylation, and phosphorylation and other modifications. Over a hundred different mechanisms of posttranslational modification are known. In addition, many proteins work via elaborate protein–protein interactions or as part of a large molecular complex.

Well before a draft sequence of the human genome was available, scientists were already discussing the possibility of a "Human Proteome Project." One reason such a project never came to pass is that there is no single human proteome: different tissues produce different sets of proteins. But the idea of such a project led to the **Protein Structure Initiative (PSI)** by the National Institute of General Medical Sciences (NIGMS), a division of the National Institutes of Health, involving over a dozen research centers. PSI is a multiphase project designed to analyze the three-dimensional structures of more than 4000 protein families. Proteins with interesting potential therapeutic properties are a top priority for the PSI, and to date the structures of over 6,000 proteins have been determined. Developing computation protein structural prediction methods, solving unique protein structures, disseminating PSI information, and focusing on the biological relevance of the work are major goals. There also are a number of other ongoing projects dedicated to identifying proteome profiles that correlate with diseases such as cancer and diabetes.

Proteomics Technologies: Two-Dimensional Gel Electrophoresis for Separating Proteins

With proteomics technologies, scientists have the ability to study thousands of proteins simultaneously, generating enormous amounts of data quickly and dramatically changing ways of analyzing the protein content of a cell.

The early history of proteomics dates back to 1975 and the development of **two-dimensional gel electrophoresis (2DGE)** as a technique for separating hundreds to thousands of proteins with high resolution. In this technique, proteins isolated from cells or tissues of interest are loaded onto a polyacrylamide tube gel and first separated by **isoelectric focusing**, which causes proteins to migrate according to their electrical charge in a pH gradient. During isoelectric focusing, proteins migrate until they reach the location in the gel where their net charge is zero compared to the pH of the gel (**Figure 21–21**). Then in a second migration, perpendicular to the first, the proteins are separated by their molecular mass using **sodium dodecyl sulfate polyacrylamide gel electrophoresis (SDS-PAGE)**. In this step, the tube gel is rotated 90° and placed on top of an SDS polyacrylamide gel; an electrical current is applied to the gel to separate the proteins by mass.

Proteins in the 2D gel are visualized by staining with Coomassie blue, silver stain, or other dyes that reveal the separated proteins as a series of spots in the gel (Figure 21–21). It is not uncommon for a 2D gel loaded with a complex mixture of proteins to show several thousand spots in the gel, as in Figure 21–21, which displays the complex mixture of proteins in human platelets (thrombocytes). Particularly abundant protein spots in this gel have been labeled with the names of identified proteins. With thousands of different spots on the gel, how are the identities of the proteins ascertained?

NOW SOLVE THIS

21–2 Annotation of a proteome attempts to relate each protein to a function in time and space. Traditionally, protein annotation depended on an amino acid sequence comparison between a query protein and a protein with known function. If the two proteins shared a considerable portion of their sequence, the query would be assumed to share the function of the annotated protein. Following is a representation of this method of protein annotation involving a query sequence and three different human proteins. Note that the query sequence aligns to common domains within the three other proteins. What argument might you present to suggest that the function of the query is not related to the function of the other three proteins?

—— Query amino acid sequence

Region of amino acid sequence match to query

■ **HINT:** *This problem asks you to think about sequence similarities between four proteins and predict functional relationships. The key to its solution is to remember that although protein domains may have related functions, proteins can contain several different interacting domains that determine protein function.*

For more practice, see Problems 24 and 26.

1st Dimension: Load protein sample onto an isoelectric focusing tube gel. Electrophoresis separates proteins according to their isoelectric point, where their net charge is zero compared to the pH of the gel

pH 4.0

pH 10.0

pH 4.0

Proteins

pH 10.0

2nd Dimension: Rotate tube gel 90° and place onto an SDS-polyacrylamide gel (SDS-PAGE). Electrophoresis separates proteins according to mass (molecular weight in kilodaltons, kDa)

Stained gel shows proteins as a series of spots separated by isoelectric point and molecular mass

SDS-PAGE

FIGURE 21–21 Two-dimensional gel electrophoresis (2DGE) is a useful method for separating proteins in a protein extract from cells or tissues that contains a complex mixture of proteins with different biochemical properties. The two-dimensional gel photo shows separations of human platelet proteins. Each spot represents a different polypeptide separated by molecular weight (*y*-axis) and isoelectric point, pH (*x*-axis). Known protein spots are labeled by name based on identification by comparison to a reference gel or by determination of protein sequence using mass spectrometry techniques. Notice that many spots on the gel are unlabeled, indicating proteins of unknown identity.

In some cases, 2D gel patterns from experimental samples can be compared to gels run with reference standards containing known proteins with well-characterized migration patterns. Many reference gels for different biological samples such as human plasma are available, and computer software programs can be used to align and compare the spots from different gels. In the early days of 2DGE, proteins were often identified by cutting spots out of a gel and sequencing the amino acids the spots contained. Only relatively small sequences of amino acids can typically be generated this way; rarely can an entire polypeptide be sequenced using this technique. BLAST and similar programs can be used to search protein databases containing amino acid sequences of known proteins. However, because of alternative splicing or posttranslational modifications, peptide sequences may not always match easily with the final product, and the identity of the protein may have to be confirmed by another approach. As you will learn in the next section, proteomics has incorporated other techniques to aid in protein identification, and one of these techniques is mass spectrometry.

Proteomics Technologies: Mass Spectrometry for Protein Identification

As important as 2DGE has been for protein analysis, **mass spectrometry (MS)** has been instrumental to the development of proteomics. Mass spectrometry techniques analyze ionized samples in gaseous form and measure the **mass-to-charge (*m/z*) ratio** of the different ions in a sample. Proteins analyzed by mass spectra generate *m/z* spectra that can be correlated with an *m/z* database containing known protein sequences to discover the protein's identity. Certain MS applications can provide peptide sequences directly from spectra. Some of the most valuable proteomics applications of this technology are to identify an unknown protein or proteins in a complex mix of proteins, to sequence peptides, to identify posttranslational modifications of proteins, and to characterize multiprotein complexes.

One commonly used mass spectrometry approach is **matrix-assisted laser desorption ionization (MALDI).** This approach is ideally suited for identifying proteins and is widely used for proteomic analysis of tissue samples

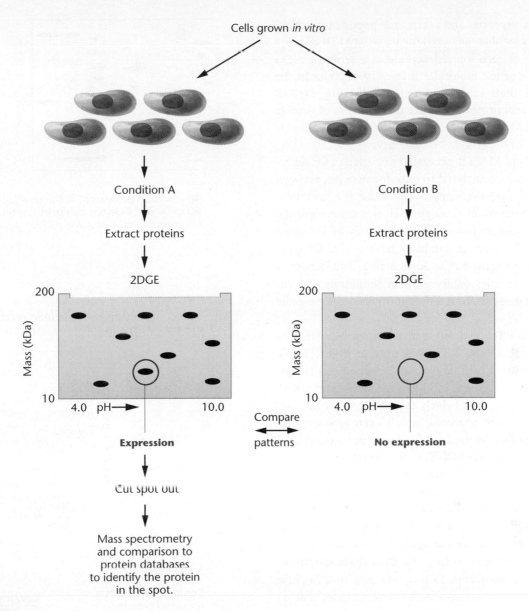

FIGURE 21–22 In a typical proteomic analysis, cells are exposed to different conditions (such as different growth conditions, drugs, or hormones). Then proteins are extracted from these cells and separated by 2DGE, and the resulting patterns of spots are compared for evidence of differential protein expression. Spots of interest are cut out from the gel, digested into peptide fragments, and analyzed by mass spectrometry to identify the protein they contain.

treated under different conditions. The proteins are first extracted from cells or tissues of interest and separated by 2DGE, after which MALDI (described below) is used to identify the proteins in the different spots. **Figure 21–22** shows an example in which two different sets of cells grown in culture are analyzed for protein differences. Just about any source providing a sufficient number of cells can be used: blood, whole tissues, and organs; tumor samples; microbes; and many other substances. Many proteins involved in cancer have been identified by the use of MALDI to compare protein profiles in normal tissue and tumor samples.

Protein spots are cut out of the 2D gel, and proteins are purified out of each gel spot. Computer-automated high-throughput instruments are available that can pick

all of the spots out of a 2D gel. Isolated proteins are then enzymatically digested with a protease (a protein-digesting enzyme) such as trypsin to create a series of peptides. This proteolysis produces a complex mixture of peptides determined by the cleavage sites for the protease in the original protein. Each type of protein produces a characteristic set of peptide fragments, and these are identified by MALDI as follows.

In MALDI, peptides are mixed with a low molecular weight and ultraviolet (UV) light-absorbing acidic matrix material (such as dihydroxybenzoic acid) and the mixture is then applied to a metal plate. A UV laser, often a nitrogen laser at a wavelength of 337 nm, is fired at the sample. As the matrix absorbs energy from the laser, heat accumulating on the matrix vaporizes and ionizes the peptide fragments. Released ions are then analyzed for mass; MALDI displays the *m/z* ratio of each ionized peptide as a series of peaks representative of the molecular masses of peptides in the mixture and their relative abundance (**Figure 21–23**). Because different proteins produce different sets of peptide fragments, MALDI produces a peptide "fingerprint" that is characteristic of the protein being analyzed.

Databases of MALDI-generated *m/z* spectra for different peptides can be analyzed to look for matches between *m/z* spectra of unknown samples and those of known proteins. One limitation of this approach is database quality. An unknown protein from a 2D gel can only be identified by MALDI if proteomics databases have a MALDI spectrum for that protein. But as is occurring with genomics databases, proteomics databases with thousands of well-characterized proteins from different organisms are rapidly developing.

MALDI is often coupled with a protein biochemistry technique for mass analysis called **time of flight (TOF)**. TOF moves ionized peptide fragments through an electrical field in a vacuum. Each ion has a speed that varies with its mass. The speed with which each ion crosses the vacuum chamber can be measured, and differences in the ions' kinetic energy can be used to develop a mass-dependent velocity profile—a MALDI-TOF spectrum—that shows each ion's "time of flight." MALDI-TOF spectra can then be compared to databases of spectra for known proteins, as described above for MALDI spectra.

Many other methods involve mass spectrometry. Some incorporate liquid chromatography (LC) to separate proteins by mass and then employ **tandem mass spectrometry (MS/MS)** approaches to generate *m/z* spectra. Also emerging are new mass spectrometry techniques that do not involve the running of gels. As we mentioned when discussing genomics, high-throughput 2DGE instruments and mass spectrometers can process thousands of samples in a single day. Instruments with faster sample-processing times and increased sensitivity are under development. These instruments may soon make "shotgun proteomics" a viable approach for characterizing entire proteomes.

An unknown protein cut out from a spot on a 2D gel is first digested into small peptide fragments using a protease such as trypsin.

Subject peptide fragments to mass spectrometry to produce mass-to-charge (*m/z*) spectra

Compare *m/z* spectra for unknown protein to a proteomics database of *m/z* spectra for known peptides. A spectrum match would identify the peptide sequence of the unknown protein.

FIGURE 21–23 Mass spectrometry for identifying an unknown protein isolated from a 2D gel. The mass-to-charge spectrum (*m/z*) (determined, for example, by MALDI) for trypsin-digested peptides from the unknown protein can be compared to a proteomics database for a spectrum match to identify the unknown protein. The peptide in this example was revealed to have the amino acid sequence serine (S)-glutamine (Q)-alanine (A)-alanine (A)-glutamic acid (E)-leucine (L)-leucine (L), shown in single-letter amino acid code.

FIGURE 21-24 (a) Mass spectrometry (MS) patterns for a trypsin-digested peptide sequence—GVQPP(OH)GPQGPR—from *T. rex*. The peptide sequence, shown here in single-letter amino acid code, contains a charged hydroxyl group characteristic of collagen. (b) Mass spectrometry of a synthetic version of collagen peptide shows good alignment with the *m/z* spectra for fragmented ions from the *T. rex* peptide, thus confirming the *T. rex* sequence as collagen and demonstrating the value of MS techniques.

Protein microarrays are also becoming valuable tools for proteomics research. These are designed around the same basic concept as microarrays (gene chips) and are often constructed with antibodies that specifically recognize and bind to different proteins. These microarrays are used, among other applications, for examining protein–protein interactions, for detecting protein markers for disease diagnosis, and for studying in biosensors designed to detect pathogenic microbes and potentially infectious bioweapons.

Identification of Collagen in *Tyrannosaurus rex* and *Mammut americanum* Fossils

As mentioned earlier, DNA has been recovered from fossils, but the general assumption has been that proteins degrade in fossilized materials and cannot be recovered. Mass spectrometry analysis of bone tissue from a *Tyrannosaurus rex* skeleton excavated from the Hell Creek Formation in eastern Montana and estimated to be 68 million years old is a good demonstration that fossilization does not fully destroy all proteins in well-preserved fossils under certain conditions. This research also demonstrates the power and sensitivity of mass spectrometry as a proteomics tool.

In this work, medullary tissue was removed from the inside of the left and right femoral bones. Medullary tissue is porous, spongy bone that contains bone marrow cells, blood vessels, and nerves. *T. rex* proteins extracted from the tissue showed cross-reactivity with antibodies to chicken collagen and were digested by the collagen-specific protease collagenase. These results suggested that the *T. rex* protein samples contained collagen, a major matrix component of bone, ligaments, tendons, and skin. To definitively identify the presence of collagen, tryptic peptides from the *T. rex* samples were analyzed by liquid chromatography and mass spectrometry (LC/MS; Figure 21–23). The *m/z* spectra for one of the *T. rex* peptides was identified from a database of *m/z* spectra as corresponding to collagen. Compare the spectrum for a collagen peptide in **Figure 21–24(a)** to that of a synthetic version of a collagen peptide [**Figure 21–24(b)**], and you will notice that the m/z ratios for all major ions align almost identically, confirming that the *T. rex* sequence is collagen. The *T. rex* peptide also contained a hydroxyl group attached to a proline residue. Proline hydroxylation is a characteristic feature of collagen. Furthermore, the amino acid sequence of *T. rex* collagen peptide aligned with an isoform of chicken collagen, demonstrating sequence similarity. Such work has provided excellent experimental evidence to support the widely accepted theory that birds and dinosaurs are close relatives.

Similar results were obtained for 160,000- to 600,000-year-old mastodon (*Mammut americanum*) peptides that showed matches to collagen from extant species, including collagen isoforms from humans, chimps, dogs, cows, chickens, elephants, and mice.

NOW SOLVE THIS

21–3 Because of its accessibility and biological significance, the proteome of human plasma has been intensively studied and used to provide biomarkers for such conditions as myocardial infarction (troponin) and congestive heart failure (B-type natriuretic peptide). Polanski and Anderson (Polanski, M., and Anderson, N. L., *Biomarker Insights*, 2: 1–48, 2006) have compiled a list of 1261 proteins, some occurring in plasma, that appear to be differentially expressed in human cancers. Of these 1261 proteins, only 9 have been recognized by the FDA as tumor-associated proteins. First, what advantage should there be in using plasma as a diagnostic screen for cancer? Second, what criteria should be used to validate that a cancerous state can be assessed through the plasma proteome?

■ **HINT**: *This problem asks you to consider criteria that are valuable for using plasma proteomics as a diagnostic screen for cancer. The key to its solution is to consider proteomics data that you would want to evaluate to determine whether a particular protein is involved in cancer.*

21.11 Systems Biology Is an Integrated Approach to Studying Interactions of All Components of an Organism's Cells

We conclude this chapter by discussing **systems biology**, an emerging discipline that incorporates data from genomics, transcriptomics, proteomics, and other areas of biology, as well as engineering applications and problem-solving approaches. Identifying genes and proteins by mutational analysis of genomes has been a very important and successful approach for characterizing genes when mutants showing visible phenotypes are found to be part of similar biochemical pathways. However, even extensive mutational analysis and screening will not provide a full understanding of complex cellular processes such as signal transduction pathways, metabolic pathways, and regulation of cell division, DNA replication, and gene expression. A more comprehensive, more integrated approach is needed.

As we mentioned earlier in this chapter, until relatively recently, much of what has been learned about gene and protein functions at the cellular, molecular, and biochemical levels has been acquired primarily through decades of work by scientists studying the functions of individual genes or relatively small numbers of genes and proteins. Many researchers have spent entire careers studying one gene or protein. However, just when it seems as if we know all there is to know about even the most well-characterized protein, another study reveals that it possesses novel functions. Such revelations demonstrate our incomplete understanding of the extreme complexity of genes and proteins in a cell. As a simple analogy, you could study the individual components of your cell phone, but until you focused on how the many components interact, you would not truly understand how a cell phone works.

Linking genomic studies to gene function and the physiology of different disease states is essential. For example, genome-wide association studies have uncovered many loci associated with diseases, but translating such information to make valuable and reliable diagnostic predictions and to develop drug targets of key proteins involved in disease is necessary. A major challenge in modern biology is to unravel the interactions of genes and proteins that enable complex processes such as cell division; this is what systems biology is all about. Proteins occasionally function alone, but more typically they work in complex interconnected networks under the regulation and control of other proteins or metabolites. Networks of interacting proteins form the regulatory framework controlling how cells respond to environmental signals, metabolize nutrients, move organelles, divide, and carry out many other processes. As genomics and proteomics have advanced, the discipline of systems biology has emerged as a more holistic approach to studying cell function by analyzing interactions among all of the molecular components of a biological system. Systems biology considers genes, proteins, metabolites, and other interacting molecules of a cell in order to understand molecular interactions and to integrate such information into models that can be used to better understand the biological functions of an organism.

In many ways, systems biology is interpreting genomic information in the context of the structure, function, and regulation of biological pathways. As is well known, biological systems are very complex. By studying relationships between all components in an organism, biologists are trying to build a "systems"-level understanding of how organisms function. Systems biologists typically combine recently acquired genomics and proteomics data with years of more traditional studies of gene and protein structure and function. Much of this data is retrieved from databases such as PubMed, GenBank, and other newly emerging genomics, transcriptomics, and proteomics resources. Systems models are used to diagram interactions within a cell or an entire organism, such as protein–protein interactions, protein–nucleic acid interactions, and protein–metabolite interactions (e.g., enzyme-substrate binding). These models help systems biologists understand the components of interacting pathways and the interrelationships of molecules in an interacting pathway. In recent years, the term **interactome** has arisen to describe the interacting components of a cell. Systems biologists use several different types of models to diagram protein interaction pathways. One of the most common model types is a **network map**—a sketch showing interacting proteins, genes, and other molecules. These diagrams are essentially the equivalent of an electrical wiring diagram. One disadvantage of network maps is that they are static diagrams that typically lack information about

when and where each interaction occurs. Even so, they are a useful foundation for generating computational models that allow the running of simulations to determine how signaling events occur. For example, major groups of kinases, enzymes that phosphorylate other proteins to affect their activity, have been network mapped to show their interactions with each other. Because kinases play such important roles in the regulation of most critical cellular processes, such information about the "kinome" has been very valuable for companies developing drug treatments targeted to certain metabolic pathways.

Network maps are helping scientists model intricate potential interactions of molecules involved in normal and disease processes. **Figure 21–25** shows an example of a network map. This map depicts a human disease network

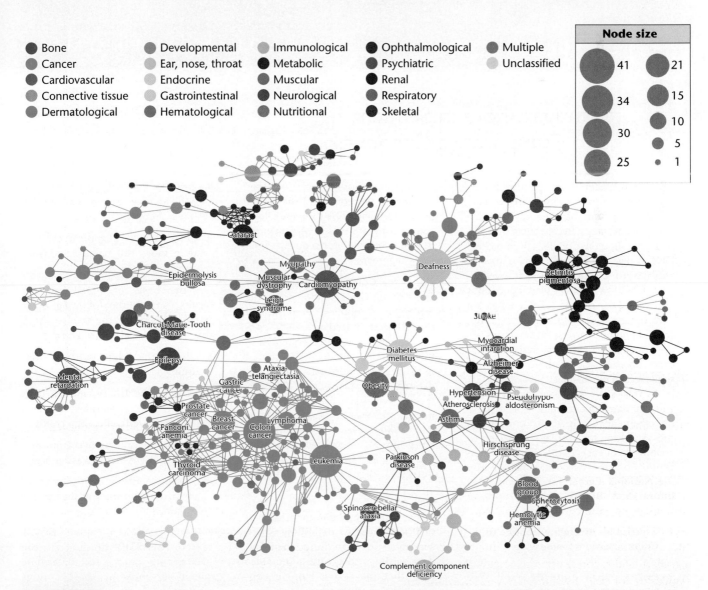

FIGURE 21–25 A systems biology model of human disease gene interactions. The model shows nodes corresponding to 22 specific disorders colored by class. Node size is proportional to the number of genes contributing to the disorder.

model illustrating the complexity of interactions between genes involved in 22 different human diseases. Look at the cluster of turquoise-colored nodes corresponding to genes involved in several different cancers. One aspect of the map that should be immediately obvious is that a number of cancers share interacting genes even though the cancers affect different organs. Knowing the genes involved and the protein interaction networks for different cancers is a major breakthrough for informing scientists about target genes and proteins to consider for therapeutic purposes.

Systems biology is becoming increasingly important in the drug discovery and development process, where its approaches can help scientists and physicians develop a

conceptual framework of gene and protein interactions in human disease that can then serve as the rationale for effective drug design. Understanding disease development and progression by defining interaction networks of molecules in normal and diseased tissue will be important for detecting and treating complex diseases such as cancer. Many databases are now being developed to model interactomes for human diseases, including breast and prostate cancer, diabetes, asthma, and cardiovascular disease. Systems biology is also being used to create biofuels and to design genetically modified organisms for cleaning up the environment, among a range of other exciting applications.

EXPLORING GENOMICS

Contigs, Shotgun Sequencing, and Comparative Genomics

MasteringGenetics™ Visit the Study Area: Exploring Genomics

In this chapter, we discussed how whole-genome shotgun sequencing methods can be used to assemble chromosome maps. Recall that in the technique of shotgun cloning, chromosomal DNA is digested with different restriction enzymes to create a series of overlapping DNA fragments called contiguous sequences, or "contigs." The contigs are then subjected to DNA sequencing, after which bioinformatics-based programs are used to arrange the contigs in their correct order on the basis of short overlapping sequences of nucleotides.

In this Exploring Genomics exercise you will carry out a simulation of contig alignment to help you to understand the underlying logic of this approach to creating sequence maps of a chromosome. For this purpose, you will use the **National Center for Biotechnology Information BLAST** site and apply a DNA alignment program called bl2seq.

■ **Exercise I – Arranging Contigs to Create a Chromosome Map**

1. Access BLAST from the NCBI Web site at http://blast.ncbi.nlm.nih.gov/ Blast.cgi. Locate and select the "Align

two sequences using BLAST (bl2seq)" category at the bottom of the BLAST homepage. The bl2seq feature allows you to compare two DNA sequences at a time to check for sequence similarity alignments.

2. Go to the Companion Web site for *Essentials of Genetics* and open the Exploring Genomics exercise for this chapter. Listed are eight contig sequences, called Sequences A through H, taken from an actual human chromosome sequence deposited in GenBank. For this exercise we have used short fragments; however, in reality contigs are usually several thousand base pairs long. To complete this exercise, copy and paste two sequences into the Align feature of BLAST and then run an alignment (by clicking on "Align"). Repeat these steps with other combinations of two sequences to determine which sequences overlap, and then use your findings to create a sequence map that places overlapping contigs in their proper order. Here are a few tips to consider:

■ Develop a strategy to be sure that you analyze alignments for all pairs of contigs.

■ Only consider alignment overlaps that show 100 percent sequence similarity.

3. On the basis of your alignment results, answer the following questions, referring to the sequences by their letter codes (A through H):

   a. What is the correct order of overlapping contigs?

   b. What is the length, measured in number of nucleotides, of each sequence overlap between contigs?

   c. What is the total size of the chromosome segment that you assembled?

   d. Did you find any contigs that do not overlap with any of the others? Explain.

4. Run a nucleotide-nucleotide BLAST search (BLASTn) on any of the overlapping contigs to determine which chromosome these contigs were taken from, and report your answer.

CASE STUDY | Your microbiome may be a risk factor for disease

A number of genes involved in susceptibility to inflammatory bowel disorders (IBDs), including Crohn disease and ulcerative colitis, have been identified. However, it is clear that other risk factors, both genetic and nongenetic, are important in triggering the onset of these diseases. Recent research has centered on understanding the role of the gut microbiome and its interactions with the host genome in IBD. It is known that the microbiome of those with IBD is different from that of those whose IBD is in remission, and it is also different from that of people who do not have IBD. These observations suggest that transfer of microbiota from unaffected individuals via fecal microbial transplantation (FMT) might be a successful treatment for IBD. This idea is supported by the use of FMT as an effective treatment in IBD individuals for a potentially life threatening infection caused by the bacterium *Clostridium difficile*. Currently, four clinical trials are underway to evaluate the use of FMT as a treatment for IBD.

1. If you had IBD, how would you react if your physician recommended that you enroll in one of these clinical studies to evaluate fecal transplants as a treatment?

2. Current treatment of IBD involves the use of anti-inflammatory drugs, but these drugs achieve remission only in some cases. If genetic analysis reveals that you carry susceptibility alleles for IBD that respond to periodic FMT as a therapy, would you agree to try this method?

3. Before agreeing to FMT, what would you want to know about the microbiomes of individuals who do not have IBD?

Summary Points

MasteringGenetics™ For activities, animations, and review quizzes, go to the Study Area.

1. High-throughput computer-automated DNA sequencing methods coupled with bioinformatics enable scientists to assemble sequence maps of entire genomes.

2. Bioinformatics is essential for the analysis of genomes and proteomes. Bioinformatics applies computer hardware and software together with statistical approaches to analyze biological sequence data.

3. Annotation is used to identify protein-coding DNA sequencing and noncoding sequences such as regulatory elements, while bioinformatics programs are used to identify open reading frames that predict possible polypeptides coded for by a particular sequence.

4. Functional genomics predicts gene function based on sequence analysis.

5. The Human Genome Project revealed many surprises about human genetics, including gene number, the high degree of DNA sequence similarity between individuals and between humans and other species, and showed that many genes encode multiple proteins.

6. Genomics has led to other related "omics" disciplines that are rapidly changing how modern biologists study DNA, RNA, and proteins and many aspects of cell function.

7. The genomes for many important model organisms have been completed. Genomic analysis of model prokaryotes and eukaryotes has revealed similarities and important fundamental differences in genome size, gene number, and genome organization.

8. Studies in comparative genomics are revealing fascinating similarities and differences in genomes from different organisms, including the identification and analysis of gene families.

9. Metagenomics, or environmental genomics, sequences genomes of microorganisms from environmental samples, often identifying new sequences that encode proteins with novel functions.

10. DNA chips or microarrays are valuable for transcriptome analysis in studying expression patterns for thousands of genes simultaneously.

11. Methods such as two-dimensional gel electrophoresis and mass spectrometry are valuable for analyzing proteomes—the protein content of a cell.

12. Systems biology approaches are designed to provide an integrated understanding of the interactions between genes, proteins, and other molecules that govern complex biological processes.

INSIGHTS AND SOLUTIONS

1. One of the main problems in annotation is deciding how long a putative ORF must be before it is accepted as a gene. Shown at the right are three different ORF scans of the same *E. coli* genome region—the region containing the *lacY* gene. Regions shaded in brown indicate ORFs. The top scan was set to accept ORFs of 50 nucleotides as genes. The middle and bottom scans accepted ORFs of 100 and 300 nucleotides as genes, respectively. How many putative genes are detected in each scan? The longest ORF covers 1254 bp; the next longest, 234 bp; and the shortest, 54 bp. How can we decide the actual number of genes in this region? In this type of ORF scan, is it more likely that the number of genes in the genome will be overestimated or underestimated? Why?

Solution: Generally one can examine conserved sequences in other organisms to indicate that an ORF is likely a coding region. One can also match a sequence to previously described sequences that are known to code for proteins. The problem is not easily solved—that is, deciding which ORF is actually a gene. The shorter the ORFs scan, the more likely the overestimate of genes because ORFs longer than 200 are less likely to occur by chance. For these scans, notice that the 50-bp scans produce the highest number of possible genes, whereas the 300-bp scan produces the lowest number (1) of possible genes.

2. Sequencing of the heterochromatic regions (repeat-rich sequences concentrated in centromeric and telomeric areas) of the *Drosophila* genome indicates that within 20.7 Mb, there are 297 protein-coding genes (Bergman et al. 2002. http://genomebiology.com/2002/3/12/research/0086). Given that the euchromatic regions of the genome contain 13,379 protein-coding genes in 116.8 Mb, what general conclusion is apparent?

Solution: Gene density in euchromatic regions of the *Drosophila* genome is about one gene per 8730 base pairs, while gene density in heterochromatic regions is one gene per 70,000 bases (20.7 Mb/297). Clearly, a given region of heterochromatin is much less likely to contain a gene than the same-sized region in euchromatin.

50
Sequenced strand

Complementary strand

100
Sequenced strand

Complementary strand

300
Sequenced strand

Complementary strand

Problems and Discussion Questions

MasteringGenetics™ Visit for instructor-assigned tutorials and problems.

HOW DO WE KNOW?

1. In this chapter, we focused on the analysis of genomes, transcriptomes, and proteomes and considered important applications and findings from these endeavors. At the same time, we found many opportunities to consider the methods and reasoning by which much of this information was acquired. From the explanations given in the chapter, what answers would you propose to the following fundamental questions:
   (a) How do we know which contigs are part of the same chromosome?
   (b) How do we know if a genomic DNA sequence contains a protein-coding gene?
   (c) What evidence supports the concept that humans share substantial sequence similarities and gene functional similarities with model organisms?

   (d) How can proteomics identify differences between the number of protein-coding genes predicted for a genome and the number of proteins expressed by a genome?
   (e) What evidence indicates that gene families result from gene duplication events?
   (f) How have microarrays demonstrated that, although all cells of an organism have the same genome, some genes are expressed in almost all cells, whereas other genes show cell- and tissue-specific expression?

CONCEPT QUESTION

2. Review the Chapter Concepts list on page 522. All of these pertain to how genomics, bioinformatics, and proteomics approaches have changed how scientists study genes and proteins. Write a short essay that explains how recombinant DNA techniques were used to identify and study genes compared

to how modern genomic techniques have revolutionized the cloning and analysis of genes.

3. What is functional genomics? How does it differ from comparative genomics?

4. Compare and contrast whole-genome shotgun sequencing to a map-based cloning approach.

5. What is bioinformatics, and why is this discipline essential for studying genomes? Provide two examples of bioinformatics applications.

6. List and describe three major goals of the Human Genome Project.

7. How do high-throughput techniques such as computer-automated and next-generation sequencing and mass spectrometry facilitate research in genomics and proteomics? Explain.

8. BLAST searches and related applications are essential for analyzing gene and protein sequences. Define BLAST, describe basic features of this bioinformatics tool, and provide an example of information provided by a BLAST search.

9. What are pseudogenes, and how are they produced?

10. Describe the human genome in terms of genome size, the percentage of the genome that codes for proteins, how much is composed of repetitive sequences, and how many genes it contains. Describe two other features of the human genome.

11. What functional information about a genome can be determined through applications of chromatin immunoprecipitation (ChIP)?

12. The Human Genome Project has demonstrated that in humans of all races and nationalities approximately 99.9 percent of the sequence is the same, yet different individuals can be identified by DNA fingerprinting techniques. What is one primary variation in the human genome that can be used to distinguish different individuals? Briefly explain your answer.

13. Annotation involves identifying genes and gene-regulatory sequences in a genome. List and describe characteristics of a genome that are hallmarks for identifying genes in an unknown sequence. What characteristics would you look for in a prokaryotic genome? A eukaryotic genome?

14. Through the Human Genome Project (HGP), a relatively accurate human genome sequence was published in 2003 from combined samples from different individuals. It serves as a reference for a haploid genome. Recently, genomes of a number of individuals have been sequenced under the auspices of

the Personal Genome Project (PGP). How do results from the PGP differ from those of the HGP?

15. Describe the significance of the Genome 10K plan.

16. It can be said that modern biology is experiencing an "omics" revolution. What does this mean? Explain your answer.

17. Metagenomics studies generate very large amounts of sequence data. Provide examples of genetic insight that can be learned from metagenomics.

18. What are gene microarrays? How are microarrays used?

19. In a draft annotation and overview of the human genome sequence, F.A. Wright et al. (*Genome Biol.* 2001: 2(7): Research0025) presented a graph similar to the one shown here. The graph details the approximate number of genes from each chromosome that are expressed only in embryos. Review earlier information in the text on human chromosomal aneuploids and correlate that information with the graph. Does this graph provide insight as to why some aneuploids occur and others do not?

20. Annotation of the human genome sequence reveals a discrepancy between the number of protein-coding genes and the number of predicted proteins actually expressed by the genome. Proteomic analysis indicates that human cells are capable of synthesizing more than 100,000 different proteins and perhaps three times this number. What is the discrepancy, and how can it be reconciled?

Extra-Spicy Problems

21. Genomic sequencing has opened the door to numerous studies that help us understand the evolutionary forces shaping the genetic makeup of organisms. Using databases containing the sequences of 25 genomes, scientists (Kreil, D.P. and Ouzounis, C.A., *Nucl. Acids Res.* 29: 1608–1615, 2001) examined the relationship between GC content and global amino acid composition. They found that it is possible to identify thermophilic species on the basis of their amino acid composition alone, which suggests that evolution in a hot environment selects for a certain whole organism amino acid composition. In what way might evolution in extreme environments influence genome and amino acid composition? How might evolution in

extreme environments influence the interpretation of genome sequence data?

22. The β-globin gene family consists of 60 kb of DNA, yet only 5 percent of the DNA encodes gene products. Account for as much of the remaining 95 percent of the DNA as you can.

23. M. Stoll and colleagues have compared candidate loci in humans and rats in search of loci in the human genome that are likely to contribute to the constellation of factors leading to hypertension. Through this research, they identified 26 chromosomal regions that they consider likely to contain hypertension genes. How can comparative genomics aid in the identification of genes responsible for such a complex human

disease? The researchers state that comparisons of rat and human candidate loci to those in the mouse may help validate their studies. Why might this be so?

24. Homology can be defined as the presence of common structures because of shared ancestry. Homology can involve genes, proteins, or anatomical structures. As a result of "descent with modification," many homologous structures have adapted different purposes.

(a) List three anatomical structures in vertebrates that are homologous but have different functions.

(b) Is it likely that homologous proteins from different species have the same or similar functions? Explain.

(c) Under what circumstances might one expect proteins of similar function to not share homology? Would you expect such proteins to be homologous at the level of DNA sequences?

25. Comparisons between human and chimpanzee genomes indicate that a gene that may function as a wild type or normal gene in one primate may function as a disease-causing gene in another (The Chimpanzee Sequence and Analysis Consortium, *Nature*, 437: 69–87, 2005). For instance, the *PPARG* locus (regulator of adipocyte differentiation) is associated with type 2 diabetes in humans but functions as a wild-type gene in chimps. What factors might cause this apparent contradiction? Would you consider such apparent contradictions to be rare or common? What impact might such findings have on the use of comparative genomics to identify and design therapies for disease-causing genes in humans?

26. Traditionally, gene sequence homology implied functional similarity. Even though two proteins may contain over 60 percent sequence identity, only about 38 percent have identical functions (Roy et al., 2008). In some cases, closely related homologs may engender completely different classes of proteins (enzymes). Consider the 3D structure of two proteins with 60 percent homology with entirely different functions. Explain how different functions may evolve by discussing the position of the homologous amino acid track, its relation to nonhomologous tracks, and the role that chaperones (Chapter 14) may play in determining protein function.

27. The discovery that *M. genitalium* has a genome of 0.58 Mb and only 470 protein-coding genes has sparked interest in determining the minimum number of genes needed for a living cell. In the search for organisms with smaller and smaller genomes, a new species of Archaea, *Nanoarchaeum equitans*, was discovered in a high-temperature vent on the ocean floor. This prokaryote has one of the smallest cell sizes ever discovered, and its genome is only about 0.5 Mb. However, organisms such as *M. genitalium*, *N. equitans*, and other microbes with very small genomes are either parasites or symbionts. How does this affect the search for a minimum genome? Should the definition of the minimum genome size for a living cell be redefined?

28. Whole Exome Sequencing (WES) is becoming a procedure to help physicians identify the cause of a genetic condition that has defied diagnosis by traditional means. The implication here is that exons in the nuclear genome are sequenced in the hopes that, by comparison with the genomes of nonaffected individuals, a diagnosis might be revealed.

(a) What are the strengths and weaknesses of this approach?

(b) If you were ordering WES for a patient, would you also include an analysis of the patient's mitochondrial genome?

E. coli have been genetically engineered to produce lycopene, the antioxidant found in tomatoes, which also gives the fruit its characteristic color.

22 Applications and Ethics of Genetic Engineering and Biotechnology

CHAPTER CONCEPTS

- Recombinant DNA technology, genetic engineering, and biotechnology have revolutionized medicine and agriculture.

- Genetically modified plants and animals can serve as bioreactors to produce therapeutic proteins and other valuable protein products.

- Genetic modifications of plants have resulted in herbicide and pest resistant crops, and crops with improved nutritional value; similarly, transgenic animals are being created to produce therapeutic proteins and to protect animals from disease.

- A synthetic genome has been assembled and transplanted into a donor bacterial strain, elevating interest in potential applications of synthetic biology.

- Applications of recombinant DNA technology and genomics have become essential for diagnosing genetic disorders, determining genotypes, and scanning the human genome to detect diseases.

- Genome-wide association studies (GWAS) scan for hundreds or thousands of genetic differences in an attempt to link genome variations to particular traits and diseases.

- Medical clinics are adopting whole genome sequencing of an individual's DNA for disease diagnosis and treatment.

- Computational services for predicting offspring based on a couple's genetics are being advertised to consumers.

- Almost all applications of genetic engineering and biotechnology present unresolved ethical dilemmas that involve important moral, social, and legal issues.

Since the dawn of recombinant DNA technology in the 1970s, scientists have harnessed **genetic engineering** not only for biological research, but also for applications in medicine, agriculture, and biotechnology. Genetic engineering refers to the alteration of an organism's genome and typically involves the use of recombinant DNA technologies to add a gene or genes to a genome, but it can also involve gene removal. The ability to manipulate DNA *in vitro* and to introduce genes into living cells has allowed scientists to generate new varieties of plants, animals, and other organisms with specific traits. These organisms are called **genetically modified organisms (GMOs)**. Industry analysts estimate that genetic engineering will lead to U.S. commercial products worth over $60 billion in the near future. Many of these products will be developed by the **biotechnology** industry.

Biotechnology is the use of living organisms to create a product or a process that helps improve the quality of life for humans or other organisms. Biotechnology as a modern industry began in earnest shortly after recombinant DNA technology developed. But biotechnology is actually a science dating back to ancient civilization and the use of microbes to make many important products, including beverages such as wine and beer, vinegar, breads, and cheeses. Modern biotechnology relies heavily on recombinant DNA technology, genetic engineering, and genomics applications, and these areas will be highlighted in this chapter. Existing products and new developments that occur seemingly every day make the biotechnology industry one of the most rapidly developing branches of the workforce worldwide, encompassing nearly 5000 companies in 54 countries.

The development of the biotechnology industry and the rapid growth in the number of applications for DNA technologies have raised serious concerns about using our power to manipulate genes and to apply gene technologies. Genetic engineering and biotechnology have the potential to provide solutions to major problems globally and to significantly alter how humans deal with the natural world; hence, they raise ethical, social, and economic questions that are unprecedented in human experience. These complex issues cannot be fully explored in the context of an introductory genetics textbook.

This chapter will therefore present only a selection of applications that illustrate the power of genetic engineering and biotechnology and the complexity of the dilemmas they engender. We will begin by explaining how genetic engineering occurs in animals. We briefly describe how genetic engineering has affected the production of pharmaceutical products, and we examine the impact of genetic technologies on the diagnosis and treatment of human diseases, including gene therapy approaches. Finally, we explore some of the social, ethical, and legal implications of genetic engineering and biotechnology.

Please note that many of the topics discussed in this chapter are covered in more detail later in the text (see Special Topic Chapter 3—DNA Forensics, Special Topic Chapter 4—Genomics and Personalized Medicine, Special Topic Chapter 5—Genetically Modified Foods, and Special Topic Chapter 6—Gene Therapy).

22.1 Genetically Engineered Organisms Synthesize a Wide Range of Biological and Pharmaceutical Products

The most successful and widespread application of recombinant DNA technology has been production by the biotechnology industry of recombinant proteins as **biopharmaceutical** products—particularly, therapeutic proteins to treat diseases. Prior to the recombinant DNA era, biopharmaceutical proteins such as insulin, clotting factors, or growth hormones were purified from tissues such as the pancreas, blood, or pituitary glands. Clearly, these sources were in limited supply, and the purification processes were expensive. In addition, products derived from these natural sources could be contaminated by disease agents such as viruses. Now that human genes encoding important therapeutic proteins can be cloned and expressed in a number of host-cell types, we have more abundant, safer, and less expensive sources of biopharmaceuticals. **Biopharming** is a commonly used term to describe the production of valuable proteins in genetically modified (GM) animals and plants.

In this section, we outline several examples of therapeutic products that are produced by expression of cloned genes in transgenic host cells and organisms. It should not surprise you that cancers, arthritis, diabetes, heart disease, and infectious diseases such as AIDS are among the major diseases that biotechnology companies are targeting for treatment by recombinant therapeutic products. Table 22.1 provides a short list of important recombinant products currently synthesized in transgenic bacteria, plants, yeast, and animals.

Insulin Production in Bacteria

Many therapeutic proteins have been produced by introducing human genes into bacteria. In most cases, the human gene is cloned into a plasmid, and the recombinant vector is introduced into the bacterial host. Large quantities of the transformed bacteria are grown, and the recombinant human protein is recovered and purified from bacterial extracts.

The first human gene product manufactured by recombinant DNA technology was human insulin, called Humulin, which was licensed for therapeutic use in 1982 by the **U.S. Food and Drug Administration (FDA)**, the government agency responsible for regulating the safety of food and drug products and medical devices. In 1977, scientists at Genentech, the San Francisco biotechnology company cofounded in 1976 by Herbert Boyer (one of the pioneers of using plasmids for recombinant DNA technology) and Robert Swanson isolated and cloned the gene for insulin and expressed it in bacterial cells. Genentech, short for "genetic engineering technology," is also generally regarded as the world's first biotechnology company.

Previously, insulin was chemically extracted from the pancreas of cows and pigs obtained from slaughterhouses. **Insulin** is a protein hormone that regulates glucose metabolism. Individuals who cannot produce insulin have diabetes, a disease that, in its more severe form (type I), affects more than 2 million individuals in the United States. Although synthetic human insulin can now be produced by another process, a look at the original genetic engineering

TABLE 22.1 Examples of Genetically Engineered Biopharmaceutical Products Available or Under Development

Gene Product	Condition Treated	Host Type
Erythropoitin	Anemia	*E. coli*; cultured mammalian cells
Interferons	Multiple sclerosis, cancer	*E. coli*; cultured mammalian cells
Tissue plasminogen activator tPA	Heart attack, stroke	Cultured mammalian cells
Human growth hormone	Dwarfism	Cultured mammalian cells
Monoclonal antibodies against vascular endothelial growth factor (VEGF)	Cancers	Cultured mammalian cells
Human clotting factor VIII	Hemophilia A	Transgenic sheep, pigs
C1 inhibitor	Hereditary angioedema	Transgenic rabbits
Recombinant human antithrombin	Hereditary antithrombin deficiency	Transgenic goats
Hepatitis B surface protein vaccine	Hepatitis B infections	Cultured yeast cells, bananas
Immunoglobulin IgG1 to HSV-2	Herpesvirus infections	Transgenic soybeans glycoprotein B
Recombinant monoclonal antibodies	Passive immunization against rabies (also used in diagnosing rabies), cancer, rheumatoid arthritis	Transgenic tobacco, soybeans, cultured mammalian cells
Norwalk virus capsid protein	Norwalk virus infections	Potato (edible vaccine)
E. coli heat-labile enterotoxin	*E. coli* infections	Potato (edible vaccine)

method is instructive, as it shows both the promise and the difficulty of applying recombinant DNA technology.

Clusters of cells embedded in the pancreas synthesize a precursor polypeptide known as preproinsulin. As this polypeptide is secreted from the cell, amino acids are cleaved from the end and the middle of the chain. These cleavages produce the mature insulin molecule, which contains two polypeptide chains (the *A* and *B* chains) joined by disulfide bonds. The *A* subunit contains 21 amino acids, and the *B* subunit contains 30.

In the original bioengineering process, synthetic genes that encode the *A* and *B* subunits were constructed by oligonucleotide synthesis (63 nucleotides for the *A* polypeptide and 90 nucleotides for the *B* polypeptide). Each synthetic oligonucleotide was inserted into a separate vector, adjacent to the *lacZ* gene encoding the bacterial form of the enzyme β-galactosidase. When transferred to a bacterial host, the *lacZ* gene and the adjacent synthetic oligonucleotide were transcribed and translated as a unit. The product is a **fusion protein**—that is, a hybrid protein consisting of the amino acid sequence for β-galactosidase attached to the amino acid sequence for one of the insulin subunits (**Figure 22–1**). The fusion proteins were purified from bacterial extracts and treated with cyanogen bromide, a chemical that cleaves the fusion protein from the β-galactosidase. When the fusion products were mixed, the two insulin subunits spontaneously united, forming an intact, active insulin molecule. The purified injectable insulin was then packaged for use by diabetics.

Shortly after insulin became available, growth hormone—used to treat children who suffer from a form of dwarfism—was cloned. Soon, recombinant DNA technology made that product readily available too, as well as a wide variety of other medically important proteins that were once difficult to obtain in adequate amounts. Since recombinant insulin ushered in the biotechnology era, well over 200 recombinant products have entered the market worldwide. In recent years, the development of many other, nonbiopharmaceutical products has been a very active area of research. One example includes the production in *E. coli* of the antioxidant lycopene found in tomatoes (see the opening photograph at the beginning of this chapter). Lycopene produced by *E. coli* is not yet available for human consumption.

Transgenic Animal Hosts and Pharmaceutical Products

Although bacteria have been widely used to produce therapeutic proteins, there are some disadvantages in using prokaryotic hosts to synthesize eukaryotic proteins. One problem is that bacterial cells often cannot process and modify eukaryotic proteins. As a result, they frequently cannot add the carbohydrates and phosphate groups to proteins that are needed for full biological activity. In addition, eukaryotic proteins produced in prokaryotic cells often do not fold into the proper three-dimensional conformation and are therefore inactive. To overcome these difficulties and increase yields, many biopharmaceuticals are now produced in eukaryotic hosts. As seen in Table 22.1, eukaryotic hosts may include cultured eukaryotic cells (plant or animal) or transgenic farm animals. For example, a herd of goats or cows can serve as very effective **bioreactors** or

(a)

(b)

FIGURE 22–1 (a) Humulin, a recombinant form of human insulin, was the first therapeutic protein produced by recombinant DNA technology to be approved for use in humans. (b) To synthesize recombinant human insulin, synthetic oligonucleotides encoding the insulin A and B chains were inserted (in separate vectors) at the tail end of a cloned *E. coli lacZ* gene. The recombinant plasmids were transformed into *E. coli* host cells, where the β-gal/insulin fusion protein was synthesized and accumulated in the cells. Fusion proteins were then extracted from the host cells and purified. Insulin chains were released from β-galactosidase by treatment with cyanogen bromide. The insulin subunits were purified and mixed to produce a functional insulin molecule.

biofactories—living factories—that could continuously make milk containing the desired therapeutic protein that can then be isolated in a noninvasive way.

Yeast are also valuable hosts for expressing recombinant proteins. Even insect cells are valuable for this purpose, through the use of a gene delivery system (virus) called **baculovirus**. Recombinant baculovirus containing a gene of interest is used to infect insect cell lines, which then express the protein at high levels. Baculovirus-insect cell expression is particularly useful for producing human recombinant proteins that are heavily glycosylated. Regardless of the host, therapeutic proteins may then be purified from the host cells—or when **transgenic animals** are used, isolated from animal products such as milk.

Refer to our discussion earlier in the text (see Chapter 20) on how transgenic animals can be created to allow for expression of a transgene of interest. Biotechnology companies are working on expressing many different genes in transgenic animals for the purpose of expressing, isolating, and purifying commercially valuable proteins.

An example of a biopharmaceutical product synthesized in transgenic animals is the human protein α1-antitrypsin. A deficiency of the enzyme α1-antitrypsin is associated with the heritable form of emphysema, a progressive and fatal respiratory disorder common among people of European ancestry. To produce α1-antitrypsin for use in treating this disease, the human gene was cloned into a vector at a site adjacent to a sheep promoter sequence that specifically activates transcription in milk-producing cells of the sheep mammary glands. Genes placed next to this promoter are expressed only in mammary tissue. This fusion gene was microinjected into sheep zygotes fertilized *in vitro*. The fertilized zygotes were transferred to surrogate mothers. The resulting transgenic sheep developed normally and produced milk containing high concentrations of functional human α1-antitrypsin. This human protein is present in concentrations of up to 35 grams per liter of milk and can be easily extracted and purified. A small herd of lactating transgenic sheep can provide an abundant supply of this protein.

In 2006, recombinant human **antithrombin**, an anticlotting protein, became the world's first drug extracted from the milk of farm animals to be approved for use in humans. Scientists at GTC Biotherapeutics introduced the human antithrombin gene into goats. By placing the gene adjacent to a promoter for beta casein, a common protein in milk, GTC scientists were able to target antithrombin expression in the mammary gland. As a result, antithrombin protein is highly expressed in the milk. In one year, a single goat will produce the equivalent amount of antithrombin that in the past would have been isolated from ~90,000 blood collections.

Recombinant DNA Approaches for Vaccine Production

Another successful application of recombinant DNA technology for therapeutic purposes is the production of vaccines. Vaccines stimulate the immune system to produce antibodies against disease-causing organisms and thereby confer immunity against specific diseases. Traditionally, two types of vaccines have been used: **inactivated vaccines**, which are prepared from killed samples of the infectious virus or bacteria; and **attenuated vaccines**, which are live viruses or bacteria that can no longer reproduce but can cause a mild form of the disease. Inactivated vaccines include the vaccines for rabies and influenza; vaccines for tuberculosis, cholera, and chickenpox are examples of attenuated vaccines.

Genetic engineering is being used to produce **subunit vaccines**, which consist of one or more surface proteins from the virus or bacterium but not the entire virus or bacterium. Often the surface protein is produced through recombinant DNA technology by cloning and expressing the genes encoding the protein to be used for the vaccine. This surface protein acts as an antigen that stimulates the immune system to make antibodies that act against the organism from which it was derived. One of the first subunit vaccines was made against the **hepatitis B virus**, which causes liver damage and cancer. The gene that encodes the hepatitis B surface protein was cloned into a yeast expression vector, and the cloned gene was expressed in yeast host cells. The protein was then extracted and purified from the host cells and packaged for use as a vaccine.

In 2005, the FDA approved **Gardasil**, a subunit vaccine produced by the pharmaceutical company Merck and the first cancer vaccine to receive FDA approval. Gardasil targets four strains of **human papillomavirus (HPV)** that cause ~70 percent of cervical cancers. Approximately 70 percent of sexually active women will be infected by an HPV strain during their lifetime. Gardasil is designed to provide immune protection against HPV prior to infection but is not effective against existing infections. You may have heard of Gardasil through media coverage of the legislation proposed in several states that would require all adolescent school girls to receive a Gardasil vaccination regardless of whether or not they are sexually active.

Vaccine Proteins Can Be Produced by Plants

Plants offer several other advantages for expressing recombinant proteins. For instance, once a transgenic plant is made, it can easily be grown and replicated in a greenhouse or field, and it will provide a constant source of recombinant protein. In addition, the cost of expressing a recombinant protein in a transgenic plant is typically much lower than making the same protein in bacteria, yeast, or mammalian cells.

No recombinant proteins expressed in transgenic plants have yet been approved for use by the FDA as therapeutic proteins for humans, although about a dozen products are close to making it through final clinical trials. Some edible vaccines are now in clinical trials. For example, a vaccine against a bacterium that causes cholera has been produced in genetically engineered potatoes and used to successfully vaccinate human volunteers.

Developing countries face serious difficulties in manufacturing, transporting, and storing vaccines. Most vaccines need refrigeration and must be injected under sterile conditions. In many rural areas, refrigeration and sterilization facilities are not available. In addition, in many cultures people are fearful of being injected with needles. To overcome these problems, scientists are attempting to develop vaccines that can be synthesized in edible food plants. These vaccines would need to be inexpensive to produce, would not require refrigeration, and would not have to be given under sterile conditions by trained medical personnel.

Tests using vaccine-producing bananas are currently under way. Bananas are considered to be perhaps the best edible vaccine candidate for a hepatitis B vaccine. Genetically engineered edible plants are being used for trials to vaccinate infants, children, and adults against many infectious diseases. But a number of technical questions about vaccine delivery in plants need to be answered if edible plant vaccines are to become more widely used. For example, how can vaccine dose be carefully controlled when fruits and vegetables grow to different sizes and express different amounts of the vaccine? Will vaccine proteins pass through the digestive tract unaltered so that they maintain their ability to provide immune protection? Nevertheless, these are exciting prospects.

DNA-Based Vaccines

Lastly, it warrants mentioning that **DNA-based vaccines** have been attempted for many years, and recently there has been renewed interest in using these vaccines to protect against viral pathogens. In this approach, DNA encoding proteins from a particular pathogen are inserted into plasmid vectors, which are then injected directly into an individual or delivered via a viral vector similar to the way certain viruses are used for gene therapy. The idea here is that pathogen proteins encoded by the delivered DNA would be produced and trigger an immune response that could provide protection should an immunized person be exposed to the pathogen in the future.

For example, trials are underway using plasmid DNA encoding protein antigens from HIV as an attempt to vaccinate individuals against HIV. Thus far a major limitation of DNA-based vectors has been that they typically result in very low production of protein encoded by delivered genes, and thus the immune response in vaccinated persons is insufficient to provide the desired protection. Work on DNA-based vaccines continues to be an active area of exploration, but whether they will ever have significant roles in the vaccine market remains to be seen.

NOW SOLVE THIS

22–1 In order to vaccinate people against diseases by having them eat antigens (such as the cholera toxin) or antibodies expressed in an edible vaccine, the antigen must reach the cells of the small intestine. What are some potential problems of this method?

■ **HINT:** *This problem asks you to consider why edible vaccines may not be effective. The key to its solution is to consider the molecular structure of the antigen or antibody and its recognition by the immune system.*

22.2 Genetic Engineering of Plants Has Revolutionized Agriculture

For millennia, farmers have manipulated the genetic makeup of plants and animals to enhance food production. Until the advent of genetic engineering 30 years ago, these genetic manipulations were primarily restricted to **selective breeding**—the selection and breeding of naturally occurring or mutagen-induced variants. In the last 50 to 100 years, genetic improvement of crop plants through the traditional methods of artificial selection and genetic crosses has resulted in dramatic increases in productivity and nutritional enhancement. For example, maize yields have increased fourfold over the last 60 years, and more than half of this increase is due to genetic improvement by artificial selection and selective breeding (**Figure 22–2**). Modern maize has substantially larger ears and kernels than the predecessor crops, including hybrids from which it was bred.

Recombinant DNA technology provides powerful new tools for altering the genetic constitution of agriculturally important organisms. Scientists can now identify, isolate, and clone genes that confer desired traits, then specifically and efficiently introduce these into organisms. As a result, it is possible to quickly introduce insect resistance, herbicide resistance, or nutritional characteristics into farm plants and animals, a primary purpose of **agricultural biotechnology**.

There are many examples of applications of recombinant DNA and genomics involving the use of plants; we will defer those discussions in detail. Genetic modifications of plant crops are discussed in greater detail

later in the text (see Special Topic Chapter 5—Genetically Modified Foods). In this section we primarily consider genetic manipulations to produce transgenic crop plants of agricultural value. In Section 22.3, we will discuss examples of genetic manipulations of agriculturally important animals.

Worldwide, millions of acres of genetically engineered crops have been planted, particularly herbicide- and pest-resistant soybeans, corn, cotton, and canola; over 50 different transgenic crop varieties are available, including alfalfa, corn, rice, potatoes, tomatoes, tobacco, wheat, and cranberries.

Several of the main reasons for generating transgenic crops include:

■ Improving the growth characteristics and yield of agriculturally valuable crops

■ Increasing the nutritional value of crops

■ Providing crop resistance against insect and viral pests, drought, and herbicides

In addition, many new GM crops that will soon be on the market will be designed for ethanol production and for making biodiesel fuel—that is, for providing sustainable sources of energy.

Insights from plant genome sequencing projects will undoubtedly be the catalyst for analysis of genetic diversity in crop plants, identification of genes involved in

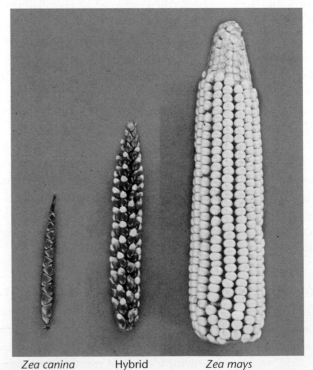

Zea canina   Hybrid   *Zea mays*

FIGURE 22–2 Selective breeding is one of the oldest methods of genetic alteration of plants. Shown here is teosinte (*Zea canina*, left), a selectively bred hybrid (center), and modern corn (*Zea mays*).

crop domestication and breeding traits, and subsequent enhancement of a variety of desirable traits through genetic engineering. In the past several years genome projects have been completed for many major food and industrial crops, including the three crops that account for most of the world's caloric intake: maize, rice, wheat. We will now examine other, more successful examples of genetically engineered plants used in agriculture. Some of the ethical and social concerns associated with these practices will be examined in Section 22.7.

22.3 Transgenic Animals Serve Important Roles in Biotechnology

Although genetically engineered plants are major players in modern agriculture, commercial applications of transgenic animals are less widespread. Most transgenic animals are created for research purposes to study gene function. Nonetheless, some high-profile examples of genetically engineered farm animals have aroused public interest and controversy. It is expected that in the future transgenic animals may increasingly be available for commercial purposes.

Examples of Transgenic Animals

Oversize mice containing a human growth hormone transgene were some of the first transgenic animals created. Attempts to create farm animals containing transgenic growth hormone genes have not been particularly successful, probably because growth is a complex, multigene trait. One notable exception is the transgenic Atlantic salmon, bearing copies of a Chinook salmon growth hormone gene adjacent to a constitutive promoter (see Special Topic Chapter 5—Genetically Modified Foods).

As discussed in Section 22.1, currently, the major uses for transgenic farm animals are as bioreactors to produce useful pharmaceutical products, but a number of other interesting transgenic applications are under development. Several of these applications are designed to increase milk production or increase nutritional value of milk. Significant research efforts are also being made to protect farm animals against common pathogens that cause disease and animal loss (including potential bioweapons that could be used in a terrorist attack on food animals) and put the food supply at risk. For instance, controlling mastitis in cattle by creating transgenic cows has shown promise (**Figure 22–3**). **Mastitis** is an infection of the mammary glands. It is the most costly disease affecting the dairy industry, leading to over $2 billion in losses in the United States. Mastitis can block milk ducts, reducing milk output, and can also contaminate the

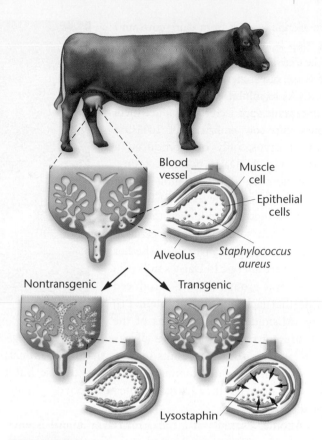

FIGURE 22–3 Transgenic cows for battling mastitis. The mammary glands of nontransgenic cows are highly susceptible to infection by the skin microbe *Staphylococcus aureus*. Transgenic cows express the lysostaphin transgene in milk, where it can kill *S. aureus* before they can multiply in sufficient numbers to cause inflammation and damage mammary tissue.

milk with pathogenic microbes. Infection by the bacterium *Staphylococcus aureus* is the most common cause of mastitis, and most cattle with mastitis typically do not respond well to conventional treatments with antibiotics. As a result, mastitis is a significant cause of herd reduction.

In an attempt to create cattle resistant to mastitis, transgenic cows were generated that possessed the lysostaphin gene from *Staphylococus simulana*. Lysostaphin is an enzyme that specifically cleaves components of the *S. aureus* cell wall. Transgenic cows expressing this protein in milk produce a natural antibiotic that wards off *S. aureus* infections. These transgenic cows do not completely solve the mastitis problem because lysostaphin is not effective against other microbes such as *E. coli* and *S. uberis* that occasionally cause mastitis; moreover, there is also the potential that *S. aureus* may develop resistance to lysostaphin. Nonetheless, scientists are cautiously optimistic that transgenic approaches have a strong future for providing farm animals with a level of protection against major pathogens.

Researchers in New Zealand have engineered a cow to produce hypoallergenic milk. This research effort has been spurred by the fact that an estimated 2–3 percent of babies are allergic to milk from dairy cows and develop a reaction to a protein called β-lactoglobulin (BLG). The approach of these researchers involved designing miRNAs to inhibit BLG and then using a transgenic approach to introduce these genes into cow embryos. Of 100 GM cow embryos, only one produced a calf, Daisy. As Daisy began lactating, researchers found that her milk did not have any detectable levels of BLG. Currently, studies are underway to determine if Daisy's milk is less allergenic to mice, with future plans to test whether humans are allergic to Daisy's milk.

Several groups recently produced cattle that lack the prion protein *PrP* gene. Misfolded configurations of the PrP protein result in **mad cow disease**, or *bovine spongiform encephalitis*. Early results indicate that these animals are resistant to the development of mad cow disease, but it is not yet known if they are fully protected from developing the disease.

Another example of a transgenic farm animal is **enviroPig**, a pig with salivary glands that express the gene encoding the enzyme phytase. These pigs are able to break down dietary phosphorus, thereby reducing excretion of phosphorus, which is a major pollutant in pig farms. The initial line of EnviroPigs had genes that were found to be unstable during reproduction, and often these genes were bred out of the pigs in subsequent generations. A modified version of these transgenic pigs, called the Cassie line, was subsequently produced. Although no studies report a food safety risk from eating meat from these pigs, research on the Cassie line has stopped because transgenic food animals have not been embraced by either consumers or food suppliers.

Scientists at Yorktown Industries of Austin, Texas, created the **GloFish**, a transgenic strain of zebrafish (*Danio rerio*) containing a red fluorescent protein gene from sea anemones. Marketed as the first GM pet in the United States, GloFish fluoresce bright pink when illuminated by ultraviolet light (**Figure 22–4**). GM critics describe these fish as an abuse of genetic technology. However, GloFish may not be as frivolous a use of genetic engineering as some believe. A variation of this transgenic model, incorporating a heavy-metal-inducible promoter adjacent to the red fluorescent protein gene, has shown promise in a bioassay for heavy metal contamination of water. When these transgenic zebrafish are in water contaminated by mercury and other heavy metals, the promoter becomes activated, inducing transcription of the red fluorescent protein gene. In this way, zebrafish fluorescence can be used as a bioassay to measure heavy metal contamination and uptake by living organisms.

FIGURE 22–4 GloFish, marketed as the world's first GM pet, are a controversial product of genetic engineering.

22.4 Synthetic Genomes and the Emergence of Synthetic Biology

Studying genomes has led to a fundamental question: "what is the minimum number of genes necessary to support life?" Scientists are interested in this question in part because the answers are expected to provide ways to create artificial cells or designer organisms based on genes encoded by a **synthetic genome** constructed in the laboratory. To create cells with a synthetic genome, we need a better understanding of the minimum number of genes required to maintain life. Of course, viruses are not included in this discussion because they cannot replicate on their own.

How Simple Can a Genome Be?

To help advance synthetic genome work, we can use the small genomes of obligate parasites to address this question. For example, the bacterium *Mycoplasma genitalium*, a human parasitic pathogen, is among the simplest self-replicating prokaryotes known and has served as a model for understanding the minimal elements of a genome necessary for a self-replicating cell. *M. genitalium* has a genome of 580 kb. *M. genitalium* can cause diseases in a wide range of hosts, including insects, plants, and humans. In humans, it causes genital infections.

In 1995, a team involving J. Craig Venter, Hamilton Smith, and Clyde Hutchison III sequenced the *M. genitalium* genome. With 485 protein-coding genes, it is one of the smallest bacterial genomes to be sequenced. In contrast, the 1.8-Mb genome of *Haemophilus influenzae* (the first bacterial genome sequenced) has 1783 genes. Which of the 482 protein-encoding genes carried by *M. genitalium* are close to the minimum gene set needed for life? Can we define life in terms of a number of specific genes? A combination of bioinformatics and experimental methods can be used to answer these questions including comparative genomics approaches to compare the *M. genitalium* genome to the genomes of other relatives such as *M. pneumoniae* and *H. influenzae.* By comparing the nucleotide sequences of the *M. genitalium* genes with the *H. influenzae* genes, researchers identified 240 genes that are orthologous for these species. In addition to these shared genes, 16 genes with different sequences but identical functions were identified. These represent essential functions performed by nonorthologous genes. Thus, comparative genomics estimates that 256 genes may represent the minimum gene set needed for life.

J. Craig Venter and his colleagues used an experimental approach to determine how many of the *M. genitalium* genes are essential for life. They used transposon-based methods to selectively mutate genes in *M. genitalium.* Mutations in essential genes would produce a lethal phenotype, but mutation of nonessential genes would not affect viability or show any obvious negative impacts. They found that about 100 of the 480 genes were nonessential and that the minimum gene set for *M. genitalium* is about 381 genes.

Recently, *M. genitalium* lost its title for having the smallest genome. A microbe called *Tremblaya princeps* has been sequenced which contains only 120 protein-coding genes. But is it ultimately misleading to think about a minimal genome? *T. princeps* lives only on a type of insect called a mealybug. The organisms live in a symbiotic relationship. Mealybugs drink tree sap, and *T. princeps* metabolizes the sap into vitamins and amino acids that the bugs need to survive. But this story is much more complicated. A bacterium called *Moranella endobia,* with a small genome of 406 genes, lives with *T. princeps.* The mealybugs rely on both microbes to survive, and similarly both microbes cannot live without each other. This is a great reminder that life can exist because of the relationships that organisms have with each other, and thus life does not exist in a vacuum by programming the genome to its minimal size. The context of what constitutes a minimal genome is essential.

Transplantation of a Synthetic Genome

In 2008 scientists from the J. Craig Venter Institute (JCVI) reported a complete chemical synthesis of the 580-kb *M. genitalium* genome. They could not yet demonstrate the functionality of the synthetic genome they produced because it could not be transplanted into another bacterium. **Genome transplantation** is effectively the true test of the functionality of a synthetic genome. From an earlier chapter (see Chapter 20), recall that if a plasmid containing a gene of interest were introduced into bacteria, the expression of genes in the plasmid, whether they were antibiotic resistance genes or a human gene such as insulin, would demonstrate successful transformation of bacteria. Transplanting an entire synthetic genome with the expectation that genes in the synthetic genome would completely transform the phenotype of the cell is essential.

In 2010 JCVI scientists published the first report of a functional synthetic genome. In this approach they designed and had chemically synthesized more than one thousand 1080-bp segments called cassettes covering the entire 1.08-Mb *M. mycoides* genome [**Figure 22–5(a)**]. To assemble these segments correctly, the sequences had 80-bp sequences at each end which overlapped with their neighbor sequences. These sequences were cloned in *E. coli.* Then, using the yeast *Saccharomyces cerevisiae,* a homologous recombination approach was used to assemble the sequences into 11 separate 100-kb assemblies that were eventually combined to completely span the entire 1.08-Mb *M. mycoides* genome [**Figure 22–5(b)**].

The entire assembled genome, called JCVI-syn1.0, was then transplanted into a close relative, *M. capricolum,* as recipient cells. This resulted in cells with the JCVI-syn1.0 genotype and phenotype of a new strain of *M. mycoides.* JCVI-syn1.0 was forced into the existing natural genome of *M. capricolum* (although many of the mechanistic details about genome transplantation are unclear). As shown in **Figure 22–5(c)**, JCVI determined that the recipient cells were taken over to become JCVI-syn.1.0 *M. mycoides* in part because they were shown to express the *lacZ* gene which was incorporated into the synthetic genome [Figure 22–5(c)]. Selection for tetracycline resistance and a determination that recipient cells also made proteins characteristic of *M. mycoides* and not *M. capricolum* were also used to verify strain conversion.

One particularly impressive accomplishment of these experiments was that the synthetic DNA was "naked" DNA, because it did not contain any proteins from *M. mycoides.* Therefore it was capable of transcribing all of the appropriate genes and translating all of the protein products necessary for life as *M. mycoides*! This is not a trivial accomplishment. The synthetic genome effectively rebooted the *M. capricolum* recipient cells to change them from one form to another. When this work was announced, J. Craig Venter claimed: "This is equivalent to changing a Macintosh computer into a PC by inserting a new piece of PC software." This is tedious work. Ninety-nine percent of the experiments involved failed! A single base error among a million bp would derail the project for several months.

Venter and others have used recombinant DNA technology to construct synthetic copies of viral genomes. This approach has demonstrated that a minimal genome can be created and assembled for nonliving entities such as viruses. For example, the genome for polio virus and the 1918 influenza strain responsible for the pandemic flu have

FIGURE 22–5 Building a synthetic version of the 1.08-Mb *Mycoplasma mycoides* genome JCVI-syn1.0. (a) Overview of the approach used to produce *M. mycoides* JCVI-syn1.0. (b) Assembly of the synthetic *M. mycoides* genome in yeast occurred in three steps. (1) 1080-bp segments (cassettes) were produced from overlapping synthetic oligonucleotides (orange arrows), (2) segments were recombined in sets of 10 to produce 109 ~10-kb assemblies (blue arrows), then (3) these were combined in sets of 10 to produce 11 ~100-kb assemblies (green arrows). Assemblies were carried out in yeast to create the entire synthetic genome called JCVI-syn1.0. (c) Images of *M. mycoides* JCVI-syn1.0 (top) and wild-type *M. mycoides* (bottom). Cells with the synthetic genome express the *lacZ* gene and are thus blue in color, wild-type cells do not express the *lacZ* gene and are white in color.

been assembled this way. But Venter's recent work with *M. mycoides* JCVIsyn1.0, a decade-long project that cost about $40 million, is being hailed as a defining moment in the emerging field of **synthetic biology**. Synthetic biology applies engineering principles and designs to biological systems.

This work did not create life from an inanimate object since it was based on converting one living strain into another. Also the *Mycoplasma* strains used lack a cell wall typically found in other bacteria, which could be a barrier to genome transplantation in other bacterial species. There are many fundamental questions about synthetic genomes and genome transplantation that need to be answered. But clearly these studies provided key "proof of concept" that synthetic genomes could be produced, assembled, and successfully transplanted to create a microbial strain encoded by a synthetic genome and bring scientists closer to producing novel synthetic genomes incorporating genes for specific traits of interest.

What are other potential applications of synthetic genomes and synthetic biology? One of JCVI's goals is to create microorganisms that can be used to synthesize biofuels. Other possibilities exist such as creating synthetic microbes with genomes engineered to express gene products to degrade pollutants (bioremediation), the synthesis of new biopharmaceutical products, synthesizing chemicals and fuels from sunlight and carbon dioxide, genetically programmed bacteria to help us heal, "semisynthetic" crops that contain synthetic chromosomes encoding genes for beneficial traits such as drought resistance or improved photosynthetic efficiency, and the ability to make "prosthetic genomes." Work on synthetic genomes and synthetic biology has led to speculation of a future world in which new bacteria, and perhaps new animal and plant cells, can be designed and even programmed to be controlled as we want them to! In the future, could synthetic genomes be used to create life from inanimate components? Stay tuned!

Synthetic Biology for Bioengineering Applications

Because of the complexity of creating an entire genome, synthetic biologists are using *bioengineering* approaches to put together parts of genes in different ways. Consider the components of a gene such as protein-coding sequences, start and stop triplets and promoters and other regulatory sequences. Can these gene parts be interchanged and combined in unique ways, essentially reconstituting biological functions, for novel and valuable bioengineering applications?

In many ways this approach is borrowed from computer science. The parts of a circuit board and board design transformed computing. In synthetic biology, cells are DNA-driven machines where DNA sequences provide the software code that directs proteins to do work for cells. The Massachusetts Institute of Technology now maintains a Registry of Standard Biological Parts (see http://partsregistry.org) with thousands of working parts or interchangeable "components" for synthetic biology. Some believe that synthetic biology will transform applications of biology in the future. Even if novel applications develop slowly, synthetic biology will help us develop a deeper understanding of how the parts of a biological system work, such as component

segments of a gene (regulatory sequences including promoters enhancers, coding and noncoding sequences and termination sequences).

George Church of Harvard University is one of the leaders in this field. His team has created a synthetic gene circuit in *E. coli* by coupling a series of three genes in a row. This system uses recombinase enzymes to cut stretches of DNA that flip the pieces and insert them back into the genome. Each flip of a DNA piece is essentially an on or off switch, like a string of 0s and 1s in the binary code in a computer program. If this system is connected to a promoter sequence for a gene, each time the gene is turned on, the recombinases flip a section of DNA. Because the DNA of bacterial cells is altered, this creates a memory of the number of times a gene was turned on that can be determined by sequence analysis of flipped regions. Thus a DNA circuit has a memory for counting events. These gene circuits have also been coupled to genes producing bioluminescent proteins as a way to report gene circuit activity (see **Figure 22–6**).

For example, Church's team has connected this recombinase system to target sequences around the promoter for a gene controlling the production of green fluorescent protein (GFP). Each time this system is turned on, recombinases flip DNA sequences that turn on the promoter for GFP, cells express GFP, and they glow. The team can measure the number of inputs (turning on gene expression) by either sequencing the DNA or by monitoring GFP fluorescence from the cells. Computer scientists refer to these

FIGURE 22–6 Gene circuits. In response to stimuli, bacteria engineered by synthetic biology produce flashes of fluorescence under the control of three genes in a circuit.

properties as logic functions and memory, in which specific inputs cause a program to respond (logic) and the program retains a memory.

As another interesting example of synthetic biology, geneticists are reengineering the genetic code by creating new codon combinations and thus *genetically recoded organisms* (GROs). This approach may be used to incorporate novel amino acids into proteins to change the chemical properties of particular proteins to make them resistant to degradation or provide stability under harsh conditions of temperature or pH, which can be valuable for novel commercial applications of recombinant proteins.

22.5 Genetic Engineering and Genomics Are Transforming Medical Diagnosis

Geneticists are applying knowledge about the human genome and the genetic basis of many diseases to a wide range of medical applications. Gene-based technologies have already had a major impact on the diagnosis of disease and are revolutionizing medical treatments and the development of specific and effective pharmaceuticals. In large part as a result of the Human Genome Project, researchers are identifying genes involved in both single-gene diseases and complex genetic traits. Methods based on recombinant DNA and genomics technologies are making this possible. In this section, we provide an overview of representative examples that demonstrate how gene-based technologies are being used to diagnose genetic diseases.

Using DNA-based tests, scientists can directly examine a patient's DNA for mutations associated with disease. Gene testing was one of the first successful applications of recombinant DNA technology, and currently more than 900 gene tests are in use. These tests usually detect DNA mutations associated with single-gene disorders that are inherited in a Mendelian fashion. Examples of such genetic tests are those that detect sickle-cell anemia, cystic fibrosis, Huntington disease, hemophilias, and muscular dystrophies. Other genetic tests have been developed for complex disorders such as breast and colon cancers.

Gene tests are used to perform prenatal diagnosis of genetic diseases, to identify carriers, to predict the future development of disease in adults, to confirm the diagnosis of a disease detected by other methods, and to identify genetic diseases in embryos created by *in vitro* fertilization. For genetic testing of adults, DNA from white blood cells is commonly used. Alternatively, many genetic tests can be carried out on cheek cells collected by swabbing the inside of the mouth, or hair cells. Some genetic testing can be carried out on gametes.

Prenatal Genetic Testing

The genetic testing of adults is increasing, as is the screening of newborns for genetic disorders (an ethically controversial issue that we will discuss in Section 22.8). In newborns, a simple prick of the heel of a baby produces a few drops of blood that are used to check the newborn for genetic disorders. Over the past two decades more genetic tests have been used to detect genetic conditions in babies than in adults.

All states now require newborn screening for certain medical conditions. And there are about 60 conditions that can be screened for. In the U.S., newborn screening identifies about 12,500 children with medical disorders out of approximately 4 million babies born each year.

For prenatal diagnosis, fetal cells are obtained by **amniocentesis** or **chorionic villus sampling**. **Figure 22–7** shows the procedure for amniocentesis, in which a small volume of the amniotic fluid surrounding the fetus is removed. Amniotic fluid contains fetal cells that can be used for karyotyping, genetic testing, and other procedures. For chorionic villus sampling, cells from the fetal portion of the placental wall (the chorionic villi) are sampled through a vacuum tube, and analyses can be carried out on this tissue. Captured fetal cells can then be subjected to genetic analysis, usually involving techniques that involve PCR (such as allele-specific oligonucleotide testing, described later in this section).

Noninvasive procedures are being developed for prenatal genetic testing of fetal DNA. These procedures are making prenatal testing easier with little to no risk to the fetus. Circulating in each person's bloodstream is cell-free DNA that is released from dead and dying cells. This DNA is cut up into small fragments by enzymes in the blood. The blood of a pregnant woman contains snippets of DNA from cells of the fetus. It is estimated that ~3 to 10 percent of the DNA in a pregnant mother's blood belong to her baby. It is now possible to analyze these traces of fetal DNA to determine if the baby has certain types of genetic conditions such as Down syndrome. Such tests require about a tablespoon of blood.

DNA in the blood is sequenced to analyze **haplotypes**, contiguous segments of DNA that do not undergo recombination during gamete formation, that distinguish which DNA segments are maternal and which are from the fetus (see **Figure 22–8**). If a fetal haplotype contained a specific mutation, this would also be revealed by sequence analysis. In addition, nearly complete fetal genome sequences have been assembled from maternal blood. These are developed by sequencing DNA fragments from maternal blood and

FIGURE 22–7 For amniocentesis, the position of the fetus is first determined by ultrasound, and then a needle is inserted through the abdominal and uterine walls to recover amniotic fluid and fetal cells for genetic or biochemical analysis.

comparing those fragments to sequenced genomes from the mother and father. Bioinformatics software is then used to organize the genetic sequences from the fetus in an effort to assemble the fetal genome. Currently, this technology results in an assembled genome sequence with segments missing, so it does not capture the entire fetal genome. It has been shown, however, that whole genome shotgun sequencing

FIGURE 22–8 Deducing fetal genome sequences from maternal blood. For any given chromosome, a fetus inherits one copy of a haplotype from the mother (maternal copies, M1 or M2) and another from the father (paternal copies, P1 or P2). For simplicity, a single-stranded sequence of DNA from each haplotype is shown. Here the fetus inherited haplotypes are M2 and P2 from the mother and father, respectively. DNA from the blood of a pregnant woman would contain paternal haplotypes inherited by the fetus (P2, blue), maternal haplotypes that are not passed to the fetus (M1, orange), and maternal haplotypes that are inherited by the fetus (M2, yellow). The maternal haplotype inherited by the fetus (M2) would be present in excess amounts relative to the haplotype that is not inherited (M1). These haplotype sequences can be detected by whole genome shotgun sequencing.

of maternal plasma DNA can be used to accurately sequence the entire exome of a fetus.

Tests for fetal genetic analysis based on maternal blood samples started to arrive on the market in 2011. Sequenom of San Diego, California was one of the first companies to launch such a test—**Materni21,** a Down syndrome test that can also be used to test for trisomy 13 (Patau syndrome) and trisomy 18 (Edward syndrome). The Materni21 test analyzes 36-bp fragments of DNA to identify chromosome 21 from the fetus. Sequenom claims that this test is highly accurate with a false positive rate of just 0.2 percent. The Materni21 test can be done as early as week 10 (about the same time at which CVS sampling can be done, which is about 4 to 6 weeks earlier than amniocentesis can be performed). While not intended to replace amniocentesis, it can help prevent some women from having amniocentesis after a false positive report from ultrasound or protein marker tests.

Several companies have followed the Sequenom approach. Nationwide, it has been estimated that the future market for these tests could be greater than $1 billion. As we will discuss later in this chapter, there are many ethical issues associated with prenatal genetic testing. Most insurance companies are not yet paying for these new tests, which can cost around $2000. Recently, California agreed to subsidize noninvasive prenatal testing for women through the state's genetic diseases program, which screens ~400,000 women each year.

In Section 22.9 we will discuss preconception testing and recent patents for computing technologies designed to predict the genetic potential of offspring (destiny tests).

Genetic Tests Based on Restriction Enzyme Analysis

A classic method of genetic testing is **restriction fragment length polymorphism (RFLP) analysis**. As we will discuss in the next section, PCR-based methods have largely replaced RFLP analysis; however, applications of this approach are still used occasionally, and for historical purposes it is also helpful to compare RFLP analysis to new approaches, which were largely not widespread prior to completion of the HGP. To illustrate this method, we examine the prenatal diagnosis of **sickle-cell anemia**. As we have discussed before, this disease is an autosomal recessive condition common in people with family origins in areas of West Africa, the Mediterranean basin, and parts of the Middle East and India. It is caused by a single amino acid substitution in the β-globin protein, as a consequence of a single-nucleotide substitution in the β-globin gene. The single-nucleotide substitution also eliminates a cutting site in the β-globin gene for the restriction enzymes MstII and CvnI. As a result, the mutation alters the pattern of restriction fragments seen on Southern blots. These differences in restriction cutting sites are used to prenatally diagnose sickle-cell anemia and to establish the parental genotypes and the genotypes of other family members who may be heterozygous carriers of this condition.

DNA is extracted from tissue samples and digested with MstII. This enzyme cuts three times within a region of the normal β-globin gene, producing two small DNA fragments. In the mutant sickle-cell allele, the middle MstII site is destroyed by the mutation, and one large restriction fragment is produced by MstII digestion (**Figure 22–9**). The restriction-enzyme-digested DNA fragments are separated by gel electrophoresis, transferred to a nylon membrane, and visualized by Southern blot hybridization, using a probe from this region. Figure 22–9 shows the results of RFLP analysis for sickle-cell anemia in one family. Both parents (I-1 and I-2) are heterozygous carriers of the mutation. MstII digestion of the parents' DNA produces a large band (because of the mutant allele) and two smaller bands (from the normal allele) in each case. The parents' first child (II-1) is homozygous normal because she has only the two smaller bands. The second child (II-2) has sickle-cell anemia; he has only one large band and is homozygous for

FIGURE 22–9 RFLP diagnosis of sickle-cell anemia. In the mutant β-globin allele (β^S), a point mutation (GAG → GTG) has destroyed a cutting site for the restriction enzyme MstII, resulting in a single large fragment on a Southern blot. In the pedigree, the family has one unaffected homozygous normal daughter (II-1), an affected son (II-2), and an unaffected carrier fetus (II-3). The genotype of each family member can be read directly from the blot and is shown below each lane.

the mutant allele. The fetus (II-3) has a large band and two small bands and is therefore heterozygous for sickle-cell anemia. He or she will be unaffected but will be a carrier.

22–2 You are asked to assist with a prenatal genetic test for a couple, each of whom is found to be a carrier for a deletion in the β-globin gene that produces β-thalassemia when homozygous. The couple already has one child who is unaffected and is not a carrier. The woman is pregnant, and the couple wants to know the status of the fetus. You receive DNA samples obtained from the fetus by amniocentesis and from the rest of the family by extraction from white blood cells. Using a probe that binds to the mutant allele, you obtain the following blot. Is the fetus affected? What is its genotype for the β-globin gene?

■ **HINT:** *This problem is concerned with interpreting results of RFLP analysis of a fetus. The key to its solution is to remember that differences in the number and location of restriction sites create RFLPs that can be used to determine genotype.*

22.5 GENETIC ENGINEERING AND GENOMICS ARE TRANSFORMING MEDICAL DIAGNOSIS | **583**

Only about 5 to 10 percent of all point mutations can be detected by restriction enzyme analysis because most mutations occur in regions of the genome that do not contain restriction enzyme cutting sites. However, now that the HGP has been completed and many disease-associated mutations are known, geneticists can employ synthetic oligonucleotides to detect these mutations, as described next.

Genetic Testing Using Allele-Specific Oligonucleotides

A common method of genetic testing involves the use of synthetic DNA probes known as **allele-specific oligonucleotides (ASOs)**. Scientists use these short, single-stranded fragments of DNA to identify alleles that differ by as little as a single nucleotide. In contrast to restriction enzyme analysis, which is limited to cases for which a mutation changes a restriction site, ASOs detect single-nucleotide changes (**single-nucleotide polymorphisms** or **SNPs**), including those that do not affect restriction enzyme cutting sites. As a result, this method offers increased resolution and wider application. Under proper conditions, an ASO will hybridize only with its complementary DNA sequence and not with other sequences, even those that vary by as little as a single nucleotide.

Genetic testing using ASOs and PCR analysis is now available to screen for many disorders, such as sickle-cell anemia. In the case of sickle-cell screening, DNA is extracted, and a region of the β-globin gene is amplified by PCR. A small amount of the amplified DNA is spotted onto strips of a DNA-binding membrane, and each strip is hybridized to an ASO synthesized to resemble the relevant sequence from either a normal or mutant β-globin gene (**Figure 22–10**). The ASO is tagged with a molecule that is either radioactive or fluorescent, to allow for visualization of the ASO hybridized to DNA on the membrane. This rapid, inexpensive, and accurate technique is used to diagnose a wide range of genetic disorders caused by point mutations. Although highly effective, SNPs can affect probe binding leading to false positive or false negative results that may not reflect a genetic disorder, particularly if precise hybridization conditions are not used. Sometimes DNA sequencing is carried out on amplified gene segments to confirm identification of a mutation.

Because ASO testing makes use of PCR, small amounts of DNA can be analyzed. As a result, ASO testing is ideal for **preimplantation genetic diagnosis (PGD)**. PGD is the genetic analysis of single cells from embryos created by *in vitro* fertilization (**Figure 22–11**). When sperm and eggs are mixed to create zygotes, the early-stage embryos are grown in culture. A single cell can be removed from an early-stage embryo using a vacuum pipette to gently aspirate one cell

Region of β-globin gene amplified by PCR

DNA is spotted onto binding filters and hybridized with ASO probe

(a) Genotypes   *AA*   *AS*   *SS*

Normal (β^A) ASO: 5′ – CTCCTGAGGAGAAGTCTGC – 3′

(b) Genotypes   *AA*   *AS*   *SS*

Mutant (β^S) ASO: 5′ – CTCCTGTGGAGAAGTCTGC – 3′

FIGURE 22–10 Allele-specific oligonucleotide (ASO) testing for the β-globin gene and sickle-cell anemia. The β-globin gene is amplified by PCR, using DNA extracted from white blood cells or cells obtained by amniocentesis. The amplified DNA is then denatured and spotted onto strips of DNA-binding membranes. Each strip is hybridized to a specific ASO and visualized on X-ray film after hybridization and exposure. (a) Results observed when the three possible genotypes are hybridized to an ASO from the normal β-globin allele: *AA*-homozygous individuals have normal hemoglobin that has two copies of the normal β-globin gene and will show heavy hybridization; *AS*-heterozygous individuals carry one normal β-globin allele and one mutant allele and will show weaker hybridization; *SS*-homozygous sickle-cell individuals carry no normal copy of the β-globin gene and will show no hybridization to the ASO probe for the normal β-globin allele. (b) Results observed when DNA for the three genotypes are hybridized to the probe for the sickle-cell β-globin allele: no hybridization by the *AA* genotype, weak hybridization by the heterozygote (*AS*), and strong hybridization by the homozygous sickle-cell genotype (*SS*).

away from the embryo (Figure 22–11). This could possibly kill the embryo, but if it is done correctly the embryo will often continue to divide normally. DNA from the removed cell is then typically analyzed by FISH (for chromosome analysis) or by ASO testing (Figure 22–11). The genotypes for each cell can then be used to decide which embryos will be implanted into the uterus.

Any alleles that can be detected by ASO testing can be used for PGD. Sickle-cell anemia, cystic fibrosis, and dwarfism are often tested for by PGD, but alleles for many other conditions are often analyzed. As you will learn in Section 22.6, it is now becoming possible to carry out whole genome sequencing on individual cells. This method is now being applied for PGD of single cells from an embryo created by IVF.

At the 8- to 16-cell stage, one cell from an embryo is gently removed with a suction pipette. The remaining cells continue to grow in culture.

DNA from an isolated cell is amplified by PCR with primers for the β-globin gene. Small volumes of denatured PCR products are spotted onto two separate DNA-binding membranes.

One membrane is hybridized to a probe for the normal β-globin allele (β^A) and the other membrane is hybridized to a probe for the mutant β-globin allele (β^S).

Membrane hybridized to a probe for the normal β-globin allele (β^A)   Membrane hybridized to a probe for the mutant β-globin allele (β^S)

In this example, hybridization of the PCR products to the probes for both the β^A and β^S alleles reveals that the cell analyzed by PGD has a carrier genotype ($\beta^A\beta^S$) for sickle-cell anemia.

FIGURE 22–11 A single cell from an early-stage human embryo created by *in vitro* fertilization can be removed and subjected to preimplantation genetic diagnosis (PGD) by ASO testing. DNA from each cell is isolated, amplified by PCR with primers specific for the gene of interest, then subjected to ASO analysis as shown in Figure 22–10. In this example, a region of the β-globin gene was amplified and analyzed by ASO testing to determine the sickle-cell genotype for this cell.

ASOs can also be used to screen for disorders that involve deletions instead of single-nucleotide mutations. An example is the use of ASOs to diagnose **cystic fibrosis (CF)**. CF is an autosomal recessive disorder associated with a defect in a protein called the **cystic fibrosis transmembrane conductance regulator (CFTR)**, which regulates chloride ion transport across the plasma membrane. A small deletion called Δ*508* is found in 70 percent of all mutant copies of the *CFTR* gene. To detect carriers of the Δ*508* mutation, ASOs are made by PCR from cloned samples of the normal and mutant alleles. DNA extracted from

individuals to be tested is amplified by PCR and then hybridized to each ASO (**Figure 22–12**). In affected individuals, only the ASO from the mutant allele hybridizes. In heterozygotes, both ASOs hybridize, and in normal homozygotes, only the ASO from the normal allele hybridizes.

CF affects approximately 1 in 2000 individuals of northern European descent. Screening in these populations can detect carriers who can be counseled about their genetic status with respect to CF. However, geneticists have evidence of more than 1000 different mutations for this gene. Not all of these alleles can be screened for because ASO tests have not been generated for all of these variants. Keep in mind also that an ASO test can only screen for specific alleles targeted by the test. Thus, a negative result does not necessarily eliminate someone from having other mutant alleles for a particular condition. Furthermore, it is likely that still more CF mutations remain to be identified. Consequently, CF screening is not widespread but will no doubt become commonplace when tests can detect a majority of all possible mutations.

NOW SOLVE THIS

22–3 The DNA sequence surrounding the site of the sickle-cell mutation in the β-globin gene, for normal and mutant genes, is as follows.

Each type of DNA is denatured into single strands and applied to a DNA-binding membrane. The membrane containing the two spots is hybridized to an ASO of the sequence

5′-GACTCCTGAGGAGAAGT-3′

Which spot, if either, will hybridize to this probe?

5′-GACTCCTGAGGAGAAGT-3′

3′-CTGAGGACTCCTCTTCA-5′

Normal DNA

5′-GACTCCTGTGGAGAAGT-3′

3′-CTGAGGACACCTCTTCA-5′

Sickle-cell DNA

HINT: *This problem asks you to analyze results of an ASO test. The key to its solution is to understand that ASO analysis is done under conditions that allow only identical nucleotide sequences to hybridize to the ASO on the membrane.*

For more practice see Problems 8, 10, and 24.

Genetic Testing Using DNA Microarrays and Genome Scans

Both RFLP and ASO analyses are efficient methods of screening for gene mutations; however, they can only detect the presence of one or a few specific mutations whose identity and locations in the gene are known. There is also a need for genetic tests that detect complex

ASO for normal DNA sequence in region of Δ508 mutation in cystic fibrosis

5'–CACCAAAGATGATATTTTC–3'

Region deleted in Δ508

ASO for mutant DNA sequence in region around Δ508 deletion

5'–CACCAATGATATTTTC–3'

FIGURE 22–12 Detecting a deletion in the *CFTR* gene by ASO testing. ASOs for the region spanning the most common mutation in CF (the Δ508 allele) are prepared from cloned copies of the normal allele and the Δ508 allele, which contains a small deletion, and spotted onto DNA-binding membranes. In screening, the CF alleles carried by an individual are amplified by PCR, labeled, and hybridized to the ASOs on the membranes. The genotype of each family member can then be read directly from the membranes. DNA from the parents (I-1 and I-2) hybridizes to both ASOs, indicating that they each carry one normal allele and one mutant allele and are therefore heterozygous. DNA from II-1 hybridizes only to the Δ508 ASO, indicating that this family member is homozygous for the mutation and has cystic fibrosis. DNA from II-2 hybridizes only to the ASO from the normal CF allele, indicating that this individual carries two normal alleles. DNA from II-3 shows two hybridization spots, so the person is heterozygous and a carrier for CF.

mutation patterns or previously unknown mutations in genes associated with genetic diseases and cancers. For example, the gene that is responsible for cystic fibrosis (the *CFTR* gene) contains 27 exons and encompasses

250 kilobases of genomic DNA. As mentioned earlier, of the 1000 known mutations of the *CFTR* gene, about half of these are point mutations, insertions, and deletions—and they are widely distributed throughout the gene. Similarly, over 500 different mutations are known to occur within the tumor suppressor *p53* gene, and any of these mutations may be associated with, or predispose a patient to, a variety of cancers. In order to screen for mutations in these genes, comprehensive, high-throughput methods are required.

From an earlier chapter (see Chapter 21) recall that one emerging high-throughput screening technique is based on the use of **DNA microarrays (Figure 22–13)**. DNA microarrays (also called DNA chips or gene chips) are small, solid supports, usually glass or polished quartz-based, on which known fragments of DNA are deposited in a precise pattern. Each spot on a DNA microarray is called a **field** (sometimes also called a feature). The DNA fragments that are deposited in a DNA microarray field—called probes—are single-stranded and may be oligonucleotides synthesized *in vitro* or longer fragments of DNA created from cloning or PCR amplification. There are typically over a million identical molecules of DNA in each field. The numbers and types of DNA sequences on a microarray are dictated by the type of analysis that is required. For example, each field on a microarray might contain a DNA sequence derived from each member of a gene family, or sequence variants from one or several genes of interest, or a sequence derived from each gene in an organism's genome. Some microarrays use identical sequences as probes in each field for a particular gene; other microarrays use many different probes for the same gene. What makes DNA microarrays so amazing is the immense amount of information that can be simultaneously generated from a single array. DNA microarrays the size of postage stamps (just over 1 cm square) can contain up to 500,000 different fields, each representing a different DNA sequence. Earlier in the text (see Chapter 21), you learned about the use of microarrays for transcriptome analysis. Scientists are using DNA microarrays in a wide range of applications, including the detection of mutations in genomic DNA and the detection of gene-expression patterns in diseased tissues.

Human genome microarrays containing probes for most human genes are available. Geneticists can use a type of DNA microarray known as a **genotyping microarray** to detect mutations in specific genes. Probes on a genotyping microarray consist of short oligonucleotides, about 20 nucleotides long. These probes are designed to methodically scan through the gene of interest, one nucleotide at a time, checking for the presence of a mutation at each position in the gene. Each position in the gene is tested by a set of five oligonucleotides (and hence five fields, arranged in a column) that are identical in sequence except for one

FIGURE 22–13 A commercially available DNA microarray, called a GeneChip, marketed by Affymetrix, Inc. This microarray can be used to analyze expression for approximately 50,000 RNA transcripts. It contains 22 different probes for each transcript and allows scientists to simultaneously assess the expression levels of most of the genes in the human genome.

nucleotide that differs in each of them, being either A, C, G, T, or a deletion (**Figure 22–14**).

The genomic DNA sample to be tested on such a microarray is cleaved into small fragments, and the DNA regions of interest are amplified by PCR, labeled with a fluorescent dye, and then hybridized to the microarray. DNA molecules with a sequence that exactly matches the probe sequence present in a microarray field will hybridize to that field. DNA molecules that differ by one or more nucleotides will hybridize less efficiently or not at all, depending on the hybridization conditions. After washing off DNA that does not hybridize to the microarray, scientists analyze the microarray with a fluorescence scanner to determine which fields hybridized to the test DNA sample and which fields did not.

Under stringent hybridization conditions, the PCR-amplified DNA fragment will hybridize most efficiently to its exact complement but less efficiently to the other possible sequence variants. Hence, the strongest hybridization among the five fields will be to the oligonucleotide probe that contains the correct nucleotide at the tested position. The sequence of the test DNA can therefore be determined by reading through the columns and noting the fields to which the hybridization is most intense (**Figure 22–15**). DNA microarrays have been designed to scan for mutations in many disease-related genes, including the *p53* gene, which is mutated in a majority of human cancers, and the *BRCA1* gene, which, when mutated, predisposes women to breast cancer. Figure 22–15 shows results for a genotypic microarray for the *p53* gene. In this example, hybridization of PCR-amplified DNA fragments from a patient appears as green or blue-green spots on the microarray [**Figure 22–15(b)**]. Interpreting the hybridization pattern reveals the *p53* gene sequence from the patient ("target").

In addition to testing for mutations in single genes, DNA microarrays can contain probes that detect SNPs. SNPs occur randomly about every 100 to 300 nucleotides throughout the human genome, both inside and outside of genes. SNPs crop up in an estimated 15 million positions in the genome where these single-based changes reveal differences from one person to the next. Certain SNP sequences at a specific locus are shared by certain segments of the population. In addition, certain SNPs cosegregate with genes associated with some disease conditions. By correlating the presence or absence of a particular SNP with a genetic disease, scientists are able to use the SNP as a genetic testing marker.

The presence of SNPs as probes on a DNA microarray allows scientists to simultaneously screen thousands of genes that might be involved in single-gene diseases as well as those involved in disorders exhibiting multifactorial inheritance. This technique, known as **genome scanning**,

Region of wild-type ***p53* gene to be tested:**		5′ – acttgtcatg gcgactgtcc acctttgtgc – 3′
Set 1	Probe 1	3′ – tgaacagtaa cgctgacagg – 5′
	Probe 2	3′ – tgaacagtac cgctgacagg – 5′
	Probe 3	3′ – tgaacagtat cgctgacagg – 5′
	Probe 4	3′ – tgaacagtag cgctgacagg – 5′
	Probe 5	3′ – tgaacagta– cgctgacagg – 5′
Set 2	Probe 1	3′ – gaacagtac agctgacagg t – 5′
	Probe 2	3′ – gaacagtac cgctgacagg t – 5′
	Probe 3	3′ – gaacagtac tgctgacagg t – 5′
	Probe 4	3′ – gaacagtac ggctgacagg t – 5′
	Probe 5	3′ – gaacagtac –gctgacagg t – 5′
Set 3	Probe 1	3′ – aacagtac cactgacagg tg – 5′
	Probe 2	3′ – aacagtac ccctgacagg tg – 5′
	Probe 3	3′ – aacagtac ctctgacagg tg – 5′
	Probe 4	3′ – aacagtac cgctgacagg tg – 5′
	Probe 5	3′ – aacagtac c–ctgacagg tg – 5′

FIGURE 22–14 Example of the oligonucleotide probe design for use on a genotyping DNA microarray. Each probe would occupy a different field on the microarray. Each set of five probes is aligned under the nucleotide position to be tested (highlighted in blue). Each of the otherwise identical probes in a set contains either an A, C, T, G or a deletion at the test position. One probe in each set is complementary to the wild-type DNA sequence; all other probes are complementary to potential mutations at the same position. Each nucleotide in the gene is tested with a set of five probes, and each probe set is offset from the previous set by one nucleotide. The pattern is repeated throughout the gene until every nucleotide has been tested. These particular probes are designed to test for mutations in the human *p53* gene.

(a)

(b)

FIGURE 22–15 A *p53* GeneChip (Affymetrix, Inc.) after hybridization to *p53* PCR products. (a) This DNA microarray contains over 65,000 fields, each about 50 micrometers square. The microarray tests for mutations within the entire 1.2-kb coding sequence of the human *p53* gene. The dotted vertical lines are generated by control fields and allow for alignment of the DNA chip during scanner analysis. (b) An enlarged portion of the *p53* microarray. Each square is a field to which the test DNA has or has not hybridized. Each row represents one of the four nucleotides or a deletion in the test position of the probe. Each column represents the nucleotide position being tested. The column outlined in white shows that the test DNA sample has a C at this position in the *p53* sequence based on its hybridization to the G in this field. The column marked with an asterisk (*) is the alignment control. The sequence of the *p53* gene is shown under the photo.

makes it possible to analyze a person's DNA for dozens or hundreds of disease alleles, including those that might predispose the person to heart attacks, asthma, diabetes, Alzheimer disease, and other genetically defined disease subtypes. Genome scans are now occasionally used when physicians encounter patients with chronic illnesses where the underlying cause cannot be diagnosed.

Finally, **array comparative genomic hybridization (CGH)** is a microarray-based technique that is used to identify copy number variants (CNVs) throughout the genome which may be involved in genetic disease conditions. Recall from earlier in the text (see Chapter 21), that CNVs are relatively large (~500 bp to several Mb) insertions or deletions, which together with SNPs comprise a majority of genome variations between individuals.

Originally developed to identify chromosomal changes in tumor sample, a CGH array uses oligonucleotides that span the entire genome of a species based on the reference sequence for that species.

Human genome CGH arrays are made using bacterial artificial chromosomes (BACs) that contain reference sequences spanning the entire genome. Test genomic DNA from an individual with a particular disorder and control DNA from a healthy individual are labeled differentially with fluorescent tags and then hybridized to the CGH array. Once scanned, fluorescent ratios on the array are analyzed and used to indicate the relative presence or absence of hybridization in the samples. Low or no binding of a DNA sample to a particular field on the array can be one indication of the presence of a CNV, such as a duplication or deletion in the genome. Array CGH is a rapid way of examining an individual genome for CNVs, but these do not reveal very small variations in the genome; nor do they recognize translocations or inversions that can contribute to genetic diseases.

Genetic Analysis Using Gene-Expression Microarrays

The arrays that we just discussed analyze genomic DNA to test for the presence or absence of a specific sequence such as a mutant allele for a particular disease. **Gene-expression microarrays** are a widely used technique in both basic research and genetic testing for detecting gene-expression patterns for specific genes.

Gene-expression microarrays are effective for analyzing gene-expression patterns in genetic diseases because the progression of a tissue from a healthy to a diseased state is almost always accompanied by changes in expression of hundreds to thousands of genes. Because mRNA expression is being detected through gene expression microarrays, these arrays provide a powerful tool for diagnosing genetic disorders and gene-expression changes. Expression microarrays may contain probes for only a few specific genes thought to be expressed differently in cell types or may contain probes representing each gene in the genome. Although microarray techniques provide novel information about gene expression, keep in mind that DNA microarrays do not directly provide us with information about protein levels in a cell or tissue. We often infer what predicted protein levels may be based on mRNA expression patterns, but this may not always be accurate.

In one type of expression microarray analysis, mRNA is isolated from two different cell or tissue types—for example, normal cells and cancer cells arising from the same cell type (**Figure 22–16**). The mRNA samples contain transcripts from each gene that is expressed in that cell type. Some genes are expressed more efficiently than others;

Normal   Tumor

Isolate RNA. Use RT-PCR
to produce cDNA labeled
with fluorescent dyes.

Combine
equal
amounts

Hybridize denatured cDNA
to microarray

Scan microarray
and analyze to reveal
hybridization pattern

mRNA present in
relatively equal
amounts in normal
and cancer cells

mRNA present only   mRNA present only
in normal cells   in cancer cells

FIGURE 22–16 Microarray procedure for analyzing gene expression in normal and cancer cells. The method shown here is based on a two-channel microarray in which cDNA samples from the two different tissues are competing for binding to the same probe sets. Colors of dots on an expression microarray represent levels of gene expression. In this example, green dots represent genes expressed only in one cell type (e.g., normal cells), and red dots represent genes expressed only in another cell type (e.g., cancer cells). Intermediate colors represent different levels of expression of the same gene in the two cell types. Only a small portion of the DNA microarray is shown.

therefore, each type of mRNA is present at a different level. The level of each mRNA can be used to develop a gene-expression profile that is characteristic of the cell type. Isolated mRNA molecules are converted into cDNA molecules, using reverse transcriptase. The cDNAs from the normal cells are tagged with fluorescent dye-labeled nucleotides (for example, green), and the cDNAs from the cancer cells are tagged with a different fluorescent dye-labeled nucleotide (for example, red).

The labeled cDNAs are mixed together and applied to a DNA microarray. The cDNA molecules bind to complementary single-stranded probes on the microarray but not to other probes. Keep in mind that each field or feature does not consist of just one probe, but rather they contain thousands of copies of the probe. After washing off the nonbinding cDNAs, scientists scan the microarray with a laser, and a computer captures the fluorescent image pattern for analysis. The pattern of hybridization appears as a series of colored dots, with each dot corresponding to one field of the microarray (Figure 22–16).

The color patterns revealed on the microarray provide a sensitive measure of the relative levels of each cDNA in the mixture. In the example shown in Figure 22–16, if an mRNA is present only in normal cells, the probe representing the gene encoding that mRNA will appear as a green dot because only "green" cDNAs have hybridized to it. Similarly, if an mRNA is present only in the cancer cells, the microarray probe for that gene will appear as a red dot. If both samples contain the same cDNA, in the same relative amounts, both cDNAs will hybridize to the same field, which will appear yellow (Figure 22–16). Intermediate colors indicate that the cDNAs are present at different levels in the two samples.

Expression microarray profiling has revealed that certain cancers have distinct patterns of gene expression and that these patterns correlate with factors such as the cancer's stage, clinical course, or response to treatment. In one such experiment, scientists examined gene expression in both normal white blood cells and in cells from a white blood cell cancer known as **diffuse large B-cell lymphoma (DLBCL)**. About 40 percent of patients with DLBCL respond well to chemotherapy and have long survival times. The other 60 percent respond poorly to therapy and have short survival. The investigators assayed the expression profiles of 18,000 genes and discovered that there were two types of DLBCL, with almost inverse patterns of gene expression (**Figure 22–17**). One type of DLBCL, called GC B-like, had an expression pattern dramatically different from that of a second type, called activated B-like. Patients with the activated B-like pattern of gene expression had much lower survival rates than patients with the GC B-like pattern. The researchers concluded that DLBCL is actually two different

(a)

(b)

FIGURE 22–17 (a) Gene-expression analysis generated from expression DNA microarrays that analyzed 18,000 genes expressed in normal and cancerous lymphocytes. Each row represents a summary of the gene expression from one particular gene; each column represents data from one cancer patient's sample. The colors represent ratios of relative gene expression compared to normal control cells. Red represents expression greater than the mean level in controls, green represents expression lower than in the controls, and the intensity of the color represents the magnitude of difference from the mean. In this summary analysis, the cancer patients' samples are grouped by how closely their gene-expression profiles resemble each other. The cluster of cancer patients' samples marked with orange at the top of the figure are GC B-like DLBCL cells. The blue cluster contains samples from cancer patients within the activated B-like DLBCL group. (b) Gene-expression profiling and survival probability. Patients with activated B-like profiles have a poorer chance of survival (16 in 21) than those with GC B-like profiles (6 in 19). Data such as these demonstrate the value of microarray analysis for diagnosing disease conditions.

diseases with different outcomes. Once this type of analysis is introduced into routine clinical use, it may be possible to adjust therapies for each group of cancer patients and to identify new specific treatments based on gene-expression profiles. Similar gene-expression profiles have been generated for many other cancers, including breast, prostate, ovarian, and colon cancer. Gene-expression microarrays are providing tremendous insight into both substantial and subtle variations in genetic diseases.

Several companies are now promoting **nutrigenomics** services in which they claim to use genotyping and gene-expression microarrays to identify allele polymorphisms and gene-expression patterns for genes involved in nutri-

ent metabolism. For example, polymorphisms in genes such as that for apolipoprotein A (*APOA1*), involved in lipid metabolism, and that for *MTHFR* (methylenetetrahydrofolate reductase), involved in metabolism of folic acid, have been implicated in cardiovascular disease. Nutrigenomics companies claim that microarray analysis of a patient's DNA sample for genes such as these and others enables them to judge whether a patient's allele variations or gene-expression profiles warrant dietary changes to potentially improve health and reduce the risk of diet-related diseases.

Application of Microarrays for Gene Expression and Genotype Analysis of Pathogens

Among their many applications, microarrays are also providing infectious disease researchers with powerful new tools for studying pathogens. Genotyping microarrays are being used to identify strains of emergent viruses, such as the virus that causes the highly contagious condition called Severe Acute Respiratory Syndrome (SARS) as well as the H5N1 avian influenza virus, the cause of bird flu, which has killed people in Asia, leading to the slaughter of over 80 million chickens and causing concern about possible pandemic outbreaks.

Whole-genome transcriptome analysis of pathogens is being used to inform researchers about genes that are important for pathogen infection and replication (**Figure 22–18**). In this approach, bacteria, yeast, protists, or viral pathogens are used to infect host cells *in vitro*, and then expression microarrays are used to analyze pathogen gene-expression profiles. Patterns of gene activity during pathogen infection of host cells and replication are useful for identifying pathogens and understanding mechanisms of infection. But of course a primary goal of infectious disease research is to prevent infection. Gene-expression profiling is also a valuable approach for identifying important pathogen genes and the proteins they encode that may prove to be useful targets for subunit vaccine development or for drug treatment strategies to prevent or control infectious disease. This strategy primarily informs researchers about how a pathogen responds to its host.

Similarly, researchers are evaluating host responses to pathogens (**Figure 22–19**). This type of detection has been accelerated in part by the need to develop pathogen-detection strategies for military and civilian use both for detecting outbreaks of naturally emerging pathogens such as SARS and avian influenza and for potential detection of outbreaks such as anthrax (caused by the bacterium *Bacillus anthracis*) that could be the result of a bioterrorism event. Host-response gene-expression profiles are

FIGURE 22–18 Whole genome expression profiling enables researchers to identify genes that are actively expressed when pathogens infect host cells and replicate. Knowing which genes are critical for pathogen infection and replication can help scientists target proteins as vaccine and drug-treatment candidates for preventing or treating infectious diseases.

developed by exposing a host to a pathogen and then using expression microarrays to analyze host gene-expression patterns.

Figure 22–19 shows the different gene-expression profiles for mice following exposure to *Neisseria meningitidis,* the SARS virus, or *E. coli.* In this example, although there are several genes that are upregulated or downregulated by each pathogen, notice how each pathogen strongly induces different prominent clusters of genes that reveal a host gene-expression response to the pathogen and provide a signature of pathogen infection. Comparing such host gene-expression profiles following exposure to different pathogens provides researchers with a way to quickly diagnose and classify infectious diseases. Scientists are developing databases of both pathogen and host-response expression profile data that can be used to identify pathogens efficiently.

FIGURE 22–19 Gene-expression microarrays can reveal host-response signatures for pathogen identification. In this example, mice were infected with different pathogens: *Neisseria meningitidis,* the virus that causes Severe Acute Respiratory Syndrome (SARS), and *E. coli.* Mouse tissues were then used as the source of mRNA for gene-expression microarray analysis. Increased expression compared to uninfected control mice is shown in shades of yellow. Decreased expression compared to uninfected controls is indicated in shades of blue. Notice that each pathogen elicits a somewhat different response in terms of which major clusters of host genes are activated by pathogen infection (circles).

22.6 Genetic Analysis by Individual Genome Sequencing

The ability to sequence and analyze individual genomes is rapidly changing the ways that scientists and physicians evaluate a person's genetic information. Genome sequencing is being utilized in medical clinics at an accelerated rate. Many major hospitals around the world are setting up clinical sequencing facilities for use in identifying the causes of rare diseases.

Recently, whole genome sequencing has provided new insights into the genetics of anorexia, Alzheimer disease, autism, Proteus syndrome, and other diseases. Proteus syndrome, a rare congenital disorder that causes atypical bone development, tumors, and other conditions, was the subject of the acclaimed movie *Elephant Man*. Already there have been some very exciting success stories whereby whole genome sequencing of an individual's DNA has led to improved treatment of diseases in children and adults.

For example, through individual genome sequencing, researchers in Newfoundland identified a mutation in a gene called *AVRD5*. Newfoundlanders have one of the highest incidences in the world of a rare condition called *arrhythmogenic right ventricular cardiomyopathy* (*ARVC*), a condition in which affected individuals often have no symptoms but then die suddenly from irregular electrical impulses within the heart. Mutations of the *AVRD5* gene lead to such cases of premature death through ARVC. Approximately 50 percent of males and 5 percent of females die by age 40, and 80 percent of males and 20 percent of females die by age 50. Individuals carrying this mutation are now being implanted with internal cardiac defibrillators that can be used to restart their hearts if electrical impulses stop or become irregular.

Diseases that are caused by multiple genes are much harder to diagnose and treat based on sequencing data. For example, whole genome sequencing of individuals affected by **autism spectrum disorder (ASD)** has revealed the involvement of more than 100 different genes. The genetics of ASD is particularly complex because of the broad range of phenotypes associated with this disorder. While whole genome sequencing of individuals affected by ASD has revealed inherited mutations, it has also identified sporadic *de novo* mutations. In the future, sequence-based knowledge of these mutations may help physicians develop patient-specific treatment strategies.

Recall our introduction of the concept of **exome sequencing** (see Chapter 21). In early 2014, sequencing an entire genome costs about $3000, and sequencing an exome costs less than $1000. Exome sequencing in clinical settings is now producing some promising results. For example, from the time he was born, Nicholas Volmer had to live with unimaginable discomfort from an undiagnosed condition that was causing intestinal fistulas (holes from his gut to outside of his body) that were leaking body fluids and feces and requiring constant surgery. By 3 years of age, Nicholas had been to the operating room more than 100 times. A team at the Medical College of Wisconsin decided to have Nicholas's exome sequenced. Applying bioinformatics to compare his sequence to that of the general population, they identified a mutation in a gene on the X chromosome called *X-linked inhibitor of apoptosis* (*XIAP*). *XIAP* is known to be linked to another condition that can often be corrected by a bone marrow transplant. In 2010 a bone marrow transplant saved Nicholas's life and largely restored his health. Shortly thereafter the popular press was describing Nicholas as the first child saved by DNA sequencing.

The National Institutes of Health began an initiative in 2008 called the Undiagnosed Diseases Program. Its goal is to use exome sequencing to help diagnose rare and mysterious disease conditions of unknown genetic basis. In this program, exome sequences from an individual with a disorder can be compared to exome sequences from healthy family members and reference sequences to identify mutations that may be involved in the disease. To date, the program has diagnosed over 40 cases. Unfortunately, however, even though the mutations responsible for these rare conditions have been identified, few cures or drug treatments have been developed for them.

We now have the ability to sequence the genome from a *single cell*! Single-cell sequencing typically involves isolating DNA from a single cell and then executing *whole genome amplification (WGA)* to produce sufficient DNA to be sequenced. Reliable amplification of the genome to produce enough DNA for sequencing without introducing errors remains a major challenge.

Single-cell sequencing allows scientists to explore how the genome varies from cell to cell. These studies are revealing that different mutant genes can vary greatly between individual cells. As another example, a team of researchers sequenced the genomes of individual spermatozoa. This approach may lead to evaluating the gametes of a particular individual to learn about recombination "hot spots" (areas of the sperm genome that are most prone to undergo recombination), to determine how abnormalities in recombination may lead to birth defects, and to detect and diagnose potential reproductive problems. Such research will also help scientists better understand how factors such as diet and age affect mutation rates in gametes.

Genome sequencing is quickly becoming standard practice in medical clinics, and there is every reason to expect genome-based diagnosis to become an essential part of mainstream medicine in the future.

22.7 Genome-Wide Association Studies Identify Genome Variations That Contribute to Disease

Microarray-based genomic analysis has led geneticists to employ powerful new strategies called **genome-wide association studies (GWAS)** in their quest to identify genes that may influence disease risk. During the past 8 years there has been a dramatic expansion in the number of GWAS being reported. For example, GWAS for height differences, autism, obesity, diabetes, macular degeneration, myocardial infarction, arthritis, hypertension, several cancers, bipolar disease, autoimmune diseases, Crohn disease, schizophrenia, amyotrophic lateral sclerosis, multiple sclerosis, and behavioral traits (such as intelligence) are among the many GWAS that have been widely publicized in the scientific literature and popular press. GWAS have resulted in approximately 1000 scientific publications linking nearly 3000 genetic variations to about 150 traits.

How are GWAS carried out? In a GWAS, the genomes of thousands of unrelated individuals with a particular disease are analyzed, typically by microarray analysis, and results are compared with genomes of individuals without the disease as an attempt to identify genetic variations that may confer risk of developing the disease. Many GWAS involve large-scale use of SNP microarrays that can probe on the order of 500,000 SNPs to evaluate results from different individuals. Other GWAS approaches can look for specific gene differences or evaluate CNVs or changes in the epigenome, such as methylation patterns in particular regions of a chromosome. By determining which SNPs, CNVs, or epigenome changes co-occur in individuals with the disease, scientists can calculate the disease risk associated with each variation. Analysis of GWAS results requires statistical analysis to predict the relative potential impact (association or risk) of a particular genetic variation on development of a disease phenotype.

Figure 22–20 shows a typical representation of one way that results from GWAS are commonly reported. Called

FIGURE 22-20 A GWAS study for Type 2 diabetes revealed 386,371 genetic markers, clustered here by chromosome number. Markers above the black line appeared to be significantly associated with the disease.

a Manhattan plot, such representations are "scatterplots" that are used to display data with a large number of data points. The x-axis typically plots a particular position in the genome; in this case loci on each chromosome are plotted in a different color code. The y-axis plots results of a genotypic association test. There are several ways that association can be calculated. Shown here is a negative log of p values that shows loci determined to be significantly associated with a particular condition. The top line of this plot establishes a threshold value for significance. Marker sequences with significance levels exceeding 10^{-5}, corresponding to 5.0 on the y-axis, are likely disease-related sequences (Figure 22–20).

One prominent study that brought the potential of GWAS to light involved research in the United States and Iceland on 4500 patients with a history of heart attack, technically a myocardial infarction (MI), and 12,767 control patients. This work was done with microarrays containing 305,953 SNPs. Among the most notable results, the study revealed variations in tumor-suppressor genes on chromosome 9 (*CDKN2A* and *CDKN2B*). Twenty-one percent of MI individuals were homozygous for deleterious mutations in the *CDKN2A* and *CDKN2B* genes, and these individuals showed a 1.63 enhanced risk of MI compared with noncarriers, including individuals homozygous for wild-type alleles. These variations were correlated with those in people of European descent, but interestingly, these same mutant alleles are not prominent in African-Americans. Does this mean that these genetic markers are not MI risk factors among this ethnicity?

Examples such as this lead to many questions and ethical concerns about patients involved in GWAS and their emotional responses to knowing about genetic risk data. For example,

- What does it mean if an individual has 3, 5, 9, or 30 risk alleles for a particular condition?

- How do we categorize rare, common, and low-frequency risk alleles to determine the overall risk for developing a disease?

- GWAS often reveal dozens of DNA variations, but many variations have only a modest effect on risk. How does one explain to a person that he or she has a gene variation that changes a risk difference for a particular disease from 12 to 16 percent over an individual's lifetime? What does this information mean?

- If the sum total of GWAS for a particular condition reveals about 50 percent of the risk alleles, what are the other missing elements of heritability that may contribute to developing a complex disease?

In some cases, risk data revealed by GWAS may help patients and physicians develop diet and exercise plans designed to minimize the potential for developing a particular disease. But the number of risk genes identified by most GWAS is showing us that, unlike single-gene disorders, complex genetic disease conditions involve a multitude of genetic factors contributing to the total risk for developing a condition. We need such information to make meaningful progress in disease diagnosis and treatment, which is ultimately a major purpose of what GWAS are all about.

22.8 Genomics Leads to New, More Targeted Medical Treatment Including Personalized Medicine

Genomic technologies are changing medical diagnosis and allowing scientists to manufacture abundant and effective therapeutic proteins. The examples already available today are a strong indication that in the near future, we will see even more transformative medical treatments based on genomics and advanced DNA-based technologies. In this section, we provide a brief introduction to pharmacogenomics and rational drug design, topics that will be considered in greater detail later in the text (see Special Topic Chapter 4—Genomics and Personalized Medicine).

Pharmacogenomics and Rational Drug Design

Every year, more than 2 million Americans experience serious side effects of medications, and more than 100,000 die from adverse drug reactions. Until recently, the selection of effective medications for each individual has been a random, trial-and-error process. The new field of **pharmacogenomics** promises to lead to more specific, effective, and personally customized drugs that are designed to complement each person's individual genetic makeup.

In the 1950s, scientists discovered that individual reactions to drugs had a hereditary component. We now know that many genes affect how different individuals react to drugs. Some of these genes encode products such as cell-surface receptors that bind a drug and allow it to enter a cell, as well as enzymes that metabolize drugs. For example, liver enzymes encoded by the cytochrome *P450* gene family affect the metabolism of many modern drugs, including those used to treat cardiovascular and neurological conditions. DNA sequence variations in these genes result in enzymes with different abilities to metabolize and utilize these drugs. Thus, gene variants that encode inactive forms of the cytochrome P450 enzymes are associated with a patient's inability to break down drugs in the body, leading to drug overdoses. A genetic test that recognizes some of these variants is currently being used to screen patients who are recruited into clinical trials for new drugs.

Another example is the reaction of certain people to the thiopurine drugs used to treat childhood leukemias (**Figure 22–21**). Some individuals have sequence variations in the gene encoding the enzyme thiopurine methyltransferase (TPMT), which breaks down thiopurines. Anticancer drugs such as 6-mercaptopurine (6-MP) that are commonly used to treat leukemia have a thiopurine structure. In individuals with mutations in the *TPMT* gene, thiopurine cancer drugs can build up to toxic levels. As a result, although some patients, such as those who are homozygous for the wild-type *TPMT* gene, respond well to 6-MP treatment, others who are heterozygotes or homozygous for mutations in *TPMT* can have severe or even fatal reactions to 6-MP. At first a genetic test was developed to detect *TPMT* gene variants, but now a simple blood test is enough to enable clinicians to tailor the drug dosage to the individual. As a result of this new technology, toxic effects of 6-MP have decreased, and survival rates for childhood leukemia patients treated with 6-MP have increased—a great example of pharmacogenomics in action.

Several methods are being developed for expanding the uses of pharmacogenomics. One promising method involves the detection of SNPs. Perhaps researchers will be able to identify a shared SNP sequence in the DNA of people who also share a heritable reaction to a drug. If the SNP segregates with a part of the genome containing the gene responsible for the drug reaction, it may be possible to devise gene tests based on the SNP, without even knowing the identity of the gene responsible for the drug reaction. In the future, DNA microarrays may be used to screen a patient's genome for multiple drug reactions.

Knowledge from genetics and molecular biology is also contributing to the development of new drugs targeted at specific disease-associated molecules. Most drug development is currently based on trial-and-error testing of chemicals in lab animals, in the hope of finding a chemical that has a useful effect. In contrast, **rational drug design** involves the synthesis of specific chemical substances that affect specific gene products. An example of a rational drug design product is the new drug imatinib, trade name **Gleevec**, used to treat chronic myelogenous leukemia (CML). Geneticists had discovered that CML cells contain the Philadelphia chromosome, which results from a reciprocal translocation between chromosomes 9 and 22. Gene cloning revealed that the t(9;22) translocation creates a fusion of the *C-ABL* proto-oncogene with the *BCR* gene. This *BCR-ABL* fusion gene encodes a powerful fusion protein that causes cells to escape cell-cycle control. The fusion protein, which acts as a tyrosine kinase, is not present in noncancer cells from CML patients.

To develop Gleevec, chemists used high-throughput screens of chemical libraries to find a molecule that bound

Individuals respond differently to the anti-leukemia drug 6-mercaptopurine.	The diversity in responses is due to mutations in a gene called thiopurine methyltransferase (*TPMT*).	After a simple blood test, individuals can be given doses of medication that are tailored to their genetic profile.
Most people metabolize the drug quickly. Doses need to be high enough to treat leukemia and prevent relapses.	Normal TPMT enzyme	High dose for TPMT homozygote
Others metabolize the drug slowly and need lower doses to avoid toxic side effects of the drug.	Normal and mutant TPMT (✹) enzyme	Moderate dose for TPMT heterozygote
A small portion of people metabolize the drug so poorly that its effects can be fatal.	Mutant TPMT enzyme	Low dose for an extra slow metabolizer (TPMT-deficient homozygote)

FIGURE 22–21 Pharmacogenomics approaches to drug development are saving lives. Different individuals with the same disease, in this case childhood leukemia, often respond differently to a drug treatment because of subtle differences in gene expression. The dose of an anticancer drug such as 6-MP that works for one person may be toxic for another person. A simple gene or enzyme test to identify genetic variations can enable physicians to prescribe a drug treatment and dosage based on a person's genetic profile.

to the BCR-ABL enzyme. After chemical modifications to make the inhibitory molecule bind more tightly, tests showed that it specifically inhibited BCR-ABL activity. Clinical trials revealed that Gleevec was effective against CML, with minimal side effects and a higher remission rate than that seen with conventional therapies. Gleevec is now used to treat CML and several other cancers. With scientists discovering more genes and gene products associated with diseases, rational drug design promises to become a powerful technology within the next decade.

Gene Therapy

Although drug treatments are often effective in controlling symptoms of genetic disorders, the ideal outcome of medical treatment is to cure these diseases. In an effort to cure genetic diseases, scientists are actively investigating **gene therapy**—a therapeutic technique that aims to transfer normal genes into a patient's cells. In theory, the normal genes will be transcribed and translated into functional gene products, which, in turn, will bring about a normal phenotype.

In many ways, gene therapy is the ultimate application of recombinant technology and genomics. Although there have been some successful applications of gene therapy, it has proven to be technically challenging for many reasons. We will discuss gene therapy in detail later in the text (see Special Topic Chapter 6—Gene Therapy).

22.9 Genetic Engineering, Genomics, and Biotechnology Create Ethical, Social, and Legal Questions

Geneticists use recombinant DNA and genomic technologies to identify genes, diagnose and treat genetic disorders, produce commercial and pharmaceutical products, and solve crimes. However, the applications that arise from these technologies raise important ethical, social, and legal issues that must be identified, debated, and resolved. Here we present a brief overview of some current ethical debates concerning the uses of genetic technologies.

Genetic Testing and Ethical Dilemmas

When the Human Genome Project was first discussed, scientists and the general public raised concerns about how genome information would be used and how the interests of both individuals and society can be protected. To address these concerns, the **Ethical, Legal, and Social Implications (ELSI) Program** was established. The ELSI Program considers a range of issues, including the impact of genetic information on individuals, the privacy and confidentiality of genetic information, and implications for medical practice, genetic counseling, and reproductive decision making. Through research grants, workshops, and public forums, ELSI is formulating policy options to address these issues.

ELSI focuses on four areas in its deliberations concerning these various issues: (1) privacy and fairness in the use and interpretation of genetic information, (2) ways to transfer genetic knowledge from the research laboratory to clinical practice, (3) ways to ensure that participants in genetic research know and understand the potential risks and benefits of their participation and give informed consent, and (4) public and professional education.

A majority of the most widely applied genetic tests that have been used to date have provided patients and physicians with information that improve quality of life. One example involves prenatal testing for phenylketonuria (PKU) and implementing dietary restrictions to diminish the effects of the disease. But many of the potential benefits and consequences of genetic testing are not always clear. For example,

- We have the technologies to test for genetic diseases for which there are no effective treatments. *Should we test people for these disorders?*

- With current genetic tests, a negative result does not necessarily rule out future development of a disease; nor does a positive result always mean that an individual will get the disease. *How can we effectively communicate the results of testing and the actual risks to those being tested?*

- *What information should people have before deciding to have a genome scan or a genetic test for a single disorder or have their whole genome sequenced?*

- Sequencing fetal genomes from the maternal bloodstream has revealed examples of mutations in the fetal genome (for example, a gene involved in Parkinson disease). *How might parents and physicians use this information?*

- *How can we protect the information revealed by such tests?*

- Since sharing patient data through electronic medical records is a significant concern, *what issues of consent need to be considered?*

- *How can we define and prevent genetic discrimination?*

Let's explore a specific case. In 2011, a case in Boston revealed the dangers of misleading results based on genetic testing. A prenatal ultrasound of a pregnant woman revealed a potentially debilitating problem (Noonan syndrome) involving the spinal cord of the woman's developing fetus. Physicians ordered a DNA test, which came back positive gene variant in a database that listed the gene as implicated in Noonan syndrome. The parents chose to terminate the pregnancy. Months later it was learned that the locus linked to Noonan was not involved in the disease, yet there was no effective way to inform the research community.

To minimize these kinds of problems in the future, the National Institutes of Health (NIH) National Center for Biotechnology Information (NCBI) has developed a database called ClinVar (see www.ncbi.nlm.nih.gov/clinvar/) which integrates data from clinical genetic testing labs and research literature to provide an updated resource for researchers and physicians.

Disclosure of incidental results is another ethically challenging issue. When someone has his or her genome sequenced or has a test done for a particular locus thought to be involved in a disease condition, the analysis sometimes reveals other mutations that could be of significance to the patient. Researchers and clinicians are divided on whether such information should be disclosed to the patient. What do you think?

Earlier in this chapter we discussed preimplantation genetic diagnosis (PGD), which provides couples with the ability to screen embryos created by *in vitro* fertilization for genetic disorders. As we learn more about genes involved in human traits, will other, nondisease-related genes be screened for by PGD? Will couples be able to select embryos with certain genes encoding desirable traits for height, weight, intellect, and other physical or mental characteristics? What do you think of using genetic testing to purposely select for an embryo with a genetic disorder? There have been several well-publicized cases of couples seeking to use prenatal diagnosis or PGD to select for embryos with dwarfism and deafness.

As identification of genetic traits becomes more routine in clinical settings, physicians will need to ensure genetic privacy for their patients. There are significant concerns about how genetic information could be used in negative ways by employers, insurance companies, governmental agencies, or the general public. Genetic privacy and prevention of genetic discrimination will be increasingly important in the coming years. In 2008, the **Genetic Information Nondiscrimination Act** was signed into law in the United States. This legislation is designed to prohibit the improper use of genetic information in health insurance and employment.

Direct-to-Consumer Genetic Testing and Regulating the Genetic Test Providers

The past decade has seen dramatic developments in **direct-to-consumer (DTC) genetic tests**. A simple Web search will reveal many companies offering DTC genetic tests. As of 2014, there are approximately 1900 diseases for which such tests are now available (in 1993 there were about 100 such tests). Most DTC tests require that a person mail a saliva sample, hair sample, or cheek cell swab to the company. For a range of pricing options, DTC companies largely use SNP-based tests such as ASO tests to screen for different mutations. For example, in 2007 Myriad Genetics, Inc. began a major DTC marketing campaign of its tests for *BRCA1* and *BRCA2*. Mutations in these genes increase risk of developing breast and ovarian cancer. DTC testing companies report absolute risk, the probability that an individual will develop a disease, but how such risks results are calculated is highly variable and subject to certain assumptions.

Such tests are controversial for many reasons. For example, the test is purchased online by individual consumers and requires no involvement of a physician or other health-care professionals such as a nurse or genetic counselor to administer or to interpret results. There are significant questions about the quality, effectiveness, and accuracy of such products because currently the DTC industry is largely self-regulated. The FDA does not regulate DTC genetic tests. There is at present no comprehensive way for patients to make comparisons and evaluations about the range of tests available and their relative quality.

Most companies make it clear that they are not trying to diagnose or prevent disease, nor that they are offering health advice, so what is the purpose of the information that test results provide to the consumer?

Web sites and online programs from DTC companies provide information on what advice a person should pursue if positive results are obtained. But is this enough? If results are not understood, might negative tests not provide a false sense of security? Just because a woman is negative for *BRCA1* and *BRCA2* mutations *does not* mean that one cannot develop breast or ovarian cancer. Refer to Problem 17 for an example of a personal decision that actress Angelina Jolie made based on the results of a genetic test.

In June 2010, the FDA announced that five genetic test manufacturers (Illumina, Pathway Genomics, NaviGenics, 23andMe, and deCODEme Genetics) would need FDA approval before their tests could be sold to consumers. This action was prompted when Pathway Genomics announced plans to market a DTC kit for "comprehensive genotyping" in the pharmacy chain Walgreens. Pathway Genomics and the other companies had been selling their DTCs through company Web sites for several years. Pathway and others claimed that because their DTC kits are Clinical Laboratory Improvement Amendments (CLIA) approved that no further regulation was required. CLIA regulates certain laboratory tests but is not part of the FDA. Pathway and deCODEme dropped out of the DTC market.

Whether the FDA will oversee DTC genetic tests in the future is unclear. However, at the time of publication of this edition, the FDA has not revealed any definitive plans to regulate or oversee DTC genetic tests. But because some DTC genetic testing companies, such as 23andMe, offer health-related analyses or health reports, they do fall under FDA regulations. The FDA continues to issue warnings to DTC companies to provide what the FDA considers to be appropriate health-related interpretations of genetic tests. There are varying opinions on the regulatory issue. Some believe that the FDA has no business regulating DTC tests and that consumers should be free to purchase products according to their own needs or interests. Others insist that the FDA must regulate DTCs in the interest of protecting consumers.

In 2010, the National Institutes of Health announced it will create the **Genetic Testing Registry (GTR)** designed to increase transparency by publicly sharing information about the utility of their tests, research for the general public, patients, health-care workers, genetic counselors, insurance companies, and others. The GTR is intended to allow individuals and families access to key resources to make more well-informed decisions about their health and genetic tests. But participation in the GTR by DTC companies has not been made mandatory yet, so will companies involved in genetic testing participate?

DNA and Gene Patents

Intellectual property (IP) rights are also being debated as an aspect of the ethical implications of genetic engineering, genomics, and biotechnology. Patents on intellectual property (isolated genes, new gene constructs, recombinant cell types, GMOs) can be potentially lucrative for the patent-holders but may also pose ethical and scientific problems. Why is protecting IP important for companies? Consider this issue. If a company is willing to spend millions or billions of dollars and several years doing research and development (R&D) to produce a valuable product, then shouldn't it be afforded a period of time to protect its discovery so that it can recover R&D costs and made a profit on its product?

Genes in their natural state as products of nature cannot be patented. Consider the possibilities for a human gene that has been cloned and then patented by the scientists who did the cloning. The person or company holding the patent could require that anyone attempting to do research with the patented gene pay a licensing fee for its use. Should a diagnostic test or therapy result from the research, more fees and royalties may be demanded, and as a result the costs of a genetic test may be too high for many patients to afford. But limiting or preventing the holding of patents for genes or genetic tools could reduce the incentive for pursuing the research that produces such genes and tools, especially for companies that need to profit from their research. Should scientists and companies be allowed to patent DNA sequences from naturally living organisms? And should there be a lower or an upper limit to the size of those sequences? For example, should patents be awarded for small pieces of genes, such as expressed sequence tags

(ESTs), just because some individual or company wants to claim a stake in having cloned a piece of DNA first, even if no one knows whether the DNA sequence has a use? Can or should investigators be allowed to patent the entire genome of any organism they have sequenced?

As of 2014, the U.S. Patent and Trademark Office has granted patents for more than 35,000 genes or gene sequences, including an estimated 20 percent of human genes. Incidentally the patenting of human genes has led some to use the term *patentome*! Some scientists are concerned that to award a patent for simply cloning a piece of DNA is awarding a patent for too little work. Given that computers do most of the routine work of genome sequencing, who should get the patent? What about individuals who figure out *what* to do with the gene? What if a gene sequence has a role in a disease for which a genetic therapy may be developed? Many scientists believe that it is more appropriate to patent novel technology and applications that make use of gene sequences than to patent the gene sequences themselves.

In recent years Congress has been considering legislation that would ban the patenting of human genes and any sequences, functions, or correlations to naturally occurring products from a gene. The patenting of genetic tests is also under increased scrutiny in part because of concerns that a patented test can create monopolies in which patients cannot get a second opinion if only one company holds the rights to conduct a particular genetic test. Recent analysis has estimated that as many as 64 percent of patented tests for disease genes make it very difficult or impossible for other groups to propose a different way to test for the same disease.

In 2010 a landmark case brought by the American Civil Liberties Union against Myriad Genetics contended that Myriad could not patent the *BRCA1* and *BRCA2* sequences used to diagnose breast cancer. Myriad's BRACAnalysis product has been used to screen over a million women for *BRCA* 1 and 2 during its period of patent exclusivity. A U.S. District Court judge ruled Myriad's patents invalid on the basis that DNA in an isolated form is not fundamentally different from how it exists in the body. Myriad was essentially accused of having a monopoly on its tests, which have existed for a little over a decade based on its exclusive licenses in the United States.

This case went to the Supreme Court in 2013, which rendered a 9–0 ruling against Myriad, stripping it of five of its patent claims for the *BRCA1* and *BRCA2* genes, largely based on the view that natural genes are a product of nature and just because they are isolated does not mean they can be patented. The Court ruled that cDNA sequences produced in a lab can continue to be patentable. Myriad still holds about 500 valid claims related to *BRCA* gene testing.

...e Genome Sequence Analysis Presents ...ny Questions of Ethics

To date, the majority of genetic testing applications have involved approaches such as amniocentesis and chorionic villus sampling for identifying chromosomal defects and testing for individual genes through methods such as ASO analysis. Even microarray analysis has not been widely used for genetic testing. But in the next decade and beyond, it is expected that whole genome sequencing of adults and babies will increasingly become common in clinical settings. A Genomic Sequencing and Newborn Screening Disorders Program is underway to sequence the exomes of more than 1500 babies. Both infants with illnesses and babies who are healthy will be part of this screening program. This will allow scientists to carry out comparative genomic analyses of specific sequences to help identify genes involved in disease conditions.

Screening of newborns is important to help prevent or minimize the impacts of certain disorders. Earlier in this section we mentioned the positive impact of early screening for PKU. Each year routine blood tests from a heel prick of newborn babies reveal rare genetic conditions in several thousand infants in the United States alone. A small number of states allow parents to opt out of newborn testing. In the future, should DNA sequencing at the time of birth be required? Do we really know enough about which human genes are involved in disease to help prevent disease in children? Estimates suggest that sequencing can identify approximately 15 to 50 percent of children with diseases that currently cannot be diagnosed by other methods. What is the value of having sequencing data for healthy children?

As exciting as this period of human genetics and medicine is becoming, many of the whole genome sequencing studies of individuals are happening in a largely unregulated environment, especially with respect to DNA collection, the variability and quality control of DNA handling protocols, sequence analysis, storage, and confidentiality of genetic information (see the Genetics, Technology, and Society box on the next page), which is raising significant ethical concerns.

Preconception Testing, Destiny Predictions, and Baby-Predicting Patents

Companies are now promoting the ability to do *preconception* testing and thus make "destiny predictions" about the potential phenotypes of hypothetical offspring based on computation methods for analyzing sequence data of parental DNA samples. The company 23andMe has been awarded a U.S. patent for a computational method called the *Family Traits Inheritance Calculator* to use parental DNA samples to predict a baby's traits, including eye color and the risk of certain diseases. This patent includes applications of technologies to screen sperm and ova for *in vitro fertilization* (IVF).

Currently, gender selection of embryos generated by IVF is very common. But could preconception testing lead to the selection of "designer babies"? Fear of *eugenics* surrounds these conversations, particularly as genetic analysis starts moving away from disease conditions to nonmedical traits such as hair color, eye color, other physical traits, and potentially behavioral traits. The patent has been awarded for a process that will compare the genotypic data of an egg provider and a sperm provider to suggest gamete donors that might result in a baby or hypothetical offspring with particular phenotypes of interest to a prospective parent. What do you think about this?

A company called GenePeeks claims to have a patent-pending technology for reducing the risk of inherited disorders by "digitally weaving" together the DNA of prospective parents. GenePeeks plans to sequence the DNA of sperm donors and women who want to get pregnant to inform women about donors who are most genetically compatible for the traits they seek in offspring. Their proprietary computing technology is intended to use sequence data to examine virtual progeny from donor-client pairings to estimate the likelihood of particular diseases from prospective parents. Initially the company claims that it plans to focus on looking at around 100,000 loci involved in rare disease. Will technologies such as this become widespread and attract consumer demand in the future? What do you think? Would you want this analysis done before deciding whether to have a child with a particular person?

Patents and Synthetic Biology

The J. Craig Venter Institute (JCVI) has filed two patent applications for what is being called "the world's first-ever human-made life form." The patents are intended to cover the minimal genome of *M. genitalium,* which JCVI believes are the genes essential for self-replication. One of these patent applications is designed to claim the rights to synthetically constructed organisms. Another U.S. patent issued to a different group of researchers covers application of a minimal genome for *E. coli,* which has generated even more concern given its relative importance compared with *M. genitalium.* What do you think? Should it be possible to patent a minimal genome or a synthetic organism?

Consider these other ethical issues about synthetic biology. Synthetic biology has the potential to be used for harmful purposes (such as bioterrorism). What regulatory policies and restrictions should be placed on applications of synthetic biology and on patents of these applications? The ability to modify life forms offends some people. How will this issue be addressed by the synthetic biology research community?

GENETICS, TECHNOLOGY, AND SOCIETY

Privacy and Anonymity in the Era of Genomic Big Data

Our lives are surrounded by Big Data. Enormous quantities of personal information are stored on private and public databases, revealing our purchasing preferences, search engine histories, social contacts, and even GPS locations. We allow this information to be collected in exchange for services that we perceive as valuable, or at least innocuous. But often we do not know how this information may be used in the future, and we do not consider how its distribution may affect us, our families, and our relationships.

Perhaps the most personal of all Big Data entries are those obtained from personal genome sequences and genomic analyses. Tens of thousands of individuals are now donating DNA for whole genome sequencing—to be carried out by both private gene-sequencing companies and public research projects. Most people who donate their DNA for sequence analysis do so with the assumption, or promise, that this data will remain anonymous and private. Even when we are informed that many DNA sequence databases, especially those used in large genomic research projects, will be available to others, we express little concern. After all, what consequences could possibly come from access to gigabytes of anonymous A's, C's, T's, and G's? Surprisingly, the answer is—quite a lot.

One of the first inklings of genetic privacy problems arose in 2005, when a 15-year-old boy named Ryan Kramer tracked down his anonymous sperm-donor father using his own Y chromosome sequence data and the Internet (Motluk, A., *New Scientist* 2524: November 3, 2005). Ryan submitted a DNA sample to a genealogy company that generates Y chromosome profiles, matches them against entries in their database, and puts people into contact with others who share similar genetic profiles, indicating relatedness. Two men contacted Ryan, and both had the same last name, with different spellings. Ryan combined the last names with the only information that he had about his sperm-donor father—date of birth, birth place, and college degree. Using an Internet people-search service, he obtained the names of everyone born on that date in that place. On the list, there was one man with the same last name as his two Y chromosome relatives. Through another Internet search, Ryan confirmed that the man also had the appropriate college degree. He then contacted his sperm-donor father. Since this report, other children of sperm donors have used DNA genealogy searching to find their paternal parent. In these cases, the sperm donors had not submitted their DNA to genealogy companies, but their identities could be determined indirectly. The implications for sperm donors have been unsettling, as most are promised anonymity. In some cases, donors are troubled to learn that they have fathered dozens of offspring.

More recently, several published reports reveal the ease with which anyone's identity can be traced using whole genome DNA sequences. For example, a research team led by Dr. Yaniv Erlich of the Whitehead Institute described how anonymous entries in the *1000 Genomes Project* database could be traced and identified (Gymrek, M. et al. 2013. *Science* 339:321–324). The searches took only a few hours and used free, publicly available Internet sources. To begin, they converted a number of randomly chosen Y chromosome sequences from the database into STR profiles, and then they used the profiles to search two free public genealogy databases. These searches yielded family surnames and other information such as geographical location and pedigrees. Internet searches of obituaries, other genealogy Web sites, and demographic data revealed the names and locations of 50 people in three different families—starting from the whole genome sequences of only five individuals.

Studies similar to Erlich's show that a person's identity and other personal information such as age, sex, body mass index, glucose, insulin, lipid levels, and disease susceptibilities can be revealed, starting with anonymous RNA expression-level data or data from SNP genotyping microarrays. In addition, in certain circumstances, an individual's DNA profile—even one obtained from a complex DNA mixture—can be queried against national and international forensic DNA databases, as described later in the text (see Special Topic Chapter 3—DNA Forensics). Some of these databases contain entries from persons only accused, but not convicted, of crimes, as well as entries obtained from crime scene evidence.

To many people, the implications of "genomic de-identifications" are disturbing. Genomic information leaks could reveal personal medical information, physical appearance, and racial origins. They could also be used to synthesize DNA to plant at a crime scene or could be used in unforeseen ways in the future as we gain more information that resides in our genome. The consequences of genomic information leaks are not limited to the person whose genome was sequenced, but encompass family members from many generations, who share the person's genetic heritage.

It may be time to address questions revolving around genome data privacy and anonymity before it is too late to put the genome-genie back into the bottle.

Your Turn

1. Would you donate your DNA to a research project designed to discover the genetic links to certain cancers? If not, why not? If so, what privacy assurances would you need to make you comfortable about your donation?

Some of the consequences of genome data leaks as they pertain to research projects are outlined in Brenner, S.E. 2013. Be prepared for the big genome leak. *Nature* 498: 139.

(continued)

Genetics, Technology, and Society, continued

2. Genome data privacy issues are being debated by scientists and regulatory agencies. What are some of their concerns about privacy, and what ideas are being proposed to deal with these concerns?

To begin a discussion about privacy, informed consent, and regulations, see Hayden, E.C. 2012.

Informed consent: a broken contract. *Nature* 486:312–314.

3. One way to deal with issues of genome data leaks is to make all personal genome data open and accessible. What are the advantages and disadvantages of this approach?

This approach is being taken by the Personal Genome Project. Read about their nonanonymous approach to DNA data at http://www.personalgenomes.org/non-anonymous.

CASE STUDY | Cancer-killing bacteria

Ralph, a 57-year-old man, was diagnosed with colon cancer. His oncologist discussed the use of radiation and chemotherapy as treatments for this cancer and explained that each of these therapies kills actively dividing normal and cancer cells, causing debilitating side effects. Ralph decided to carefully review his options and went for a second opinion to a cancer clinic at a major teaching hospital. There he learned that researchers in a synthetic biology program were testing the use of genetically modified *E. coli* cells that selectively invade and kill cancer cells, with no effects on normal cells. Ralph decided to participate in this trial, and at an appointment to learn about the details, he was informed that he would be part of a Phase III trial, comparing the effects of the modified bacterial cells against conventional chemotherapy. As part of the trial, he would be randomly assigned to receive one or the other treatment. He was disappointed to learn this, because he assumed that he would receive the bacterial therapy.

1. What are Ralph's options at this point?

2. Should he reconsider and try radiation and chemotherapy instead?

3. Or should he enroll on the chance that he would receive therapy using the genetically modified bacteria and that it would be more effective than conventional therapy?

Summary Points

MasteringGenetics™ For activities, animations, and review quizzes, go to the Study Area.

1. Recombinant DNA technology can be used to produce valuable biopharmaceutical protein products such as therapeutic proteins for treating disease.

2. Transgenic animals with improved growth characteristics or desirable phenotypes are being genetically engineered for a number of different applications.

3. Interest in synthetic biology and its potential applications has been spurred by the creation of a synthetic genome successfully used in a genome transplantation experiment in bacteria.

4. A variety of different molecular techniques, including restriction fragment length polymorphism analysis, allele-specific oligonucleotides tests, and DNA microarrays, can be used to identify genotypes associated with both normal and disease phenotypes.

5. Preimplantation genetic diagnosis and noninvasive methods for deducing a fetal genome from maternal blood allow for genetic analysis of a developing fetus.

6. Whole genome sequencing of individual genomes is entering medical clinics and becoming valuable for diagnosis and treating genetic conditions.

7. Genome-wide association studies can reveal genetic variations linked with disease conditions within populations.

8. Pharmacogenomics provides the basis for customized medical intervention based on an individual's genotype.

9. Applications of genetic engineering and biotechnology involve a range of ethical, social, and legal dilemmas with important scientific and societal implications.

INSIGHTS AND SOLUTIONS

1. Research by Petukhova et al. (*Nature* 466:113–117, 2010) involved a GWAS study to analyze 1054 cases of patients with alopecia areata (AA) and 3278 controls. Alopecia areata is a condition that leads to major hair loss and affects approximately 5.3 million people in the United States alone.

(a) A Manhattan plot from this work is shown on the top of the following page:

Based on your interpretation of this plot, which chromosomes were associated with loci that may contribute to AA?

(b) Of the 139 SNPs significantly associated with AA, several genes are involved in controlling the activation and proliferation of regulatory T lymphocytes (Treg cells) and cytotoxic T lymphocytes, genes involved in antigen presentation to immune cells, immune regulatory molecules such as the interleukins, and genes expressed in the hair follicle itself. Speculate how these candidate genes may help scientists understand how AA progresses as a disease.

Solution: (a) Investigators identified eight genomic regions with SNPs that exceed the genome-wide significance value of 5×10^{-7} (red line). These regions were clustered on chromosomes 2, 4, 6, 9, 10, 11, and 12.

(b) AA is an autoimmune disease in which the immune system attacks hair follicles, resulting in hair loss that can permeate across the entire scalp and even the whole body. AA hair follicles are attacked by T cells. The identification of candidate genes involved in T-cell proliferation, immune system regulation, and follicular development may potentially help investigators develop cures for AA.

2. Infection by HIV-1 (human immunodeficiency virus) weakens the immune system and results in the symptoms of AIDS (acquired immunodeficiency syndrome). Specifically, HIV infects and kills cells of the immune system that carry a cell-surface receptor known as CD4. An HIV surface protein known as gp120 binds to the CD4 receptor and allows the virus to enter the cell. The gene encoding the CD4 protein has been cloned. How might this clone be used along with recombinant DNA techniques to combat HIV infection?

Solution: Researchers hope that clones of the *CD4* gene can be used in the design of systems for the targeted delivery of drugs and toxins to combat the infection. For example, because infection depends on an interaction between the viral gp120 protein and the CD4 protein, the cloned *CD4* gene has been modified to produce a soluble form of the protein (sCD4) that, because of its solubility, would circulate freely in the body. The idea is that HIV might be prevented from infecting cells if the gp120 protein of the virus first encounters and binds to extra molecules of the soluble form of the CD4 protein. Once bound to the extra molecules, the virus would be unable to bind to CD4 proteins on the surface of immune system cells. Studies in cell-culture systems indicate that the presence of sCD4 effectively prevents HIV infection of tissue culture cells. However, studies in HIV-positive humans have been somewhat disappointing, mainly because the strains of HIV used in the laboratory are different from those found in infected individuals. In another strategy, the *CD4* gene has been fused with genes encoding bacterial toxins. The resulting fusion protein contains CD4 regions that should bind to gp120 on the surface of HIV-infected cells and toxin regions that should then kill the infected cell. In tissue culture experiments, cells infected with HIV are killed by this fusion protein, whereas uninfected cells survive.

Problems and Discussion Questions

MasteringGenetics™ Visit for instructor-assigned tutorials and problems.

HOW DO WE KNOW?

1. In this chapter, we focused on a number of interesting applications of genetic engineering, genomics, and biotechnology. At the same time, we found many opportunities to consider the methods and reasoning by which much of this information was acquired. From the explanations given in the chapter, what answers would you propose to the following fundamental questions:

(a) What experimental evidence confirms that we have introduced a useful gene into a transgenic organism and that it performs as we anticipate?

(b) How can we use DNA analysis to determine that a human fetus has sickle-cell anemia?

(c) How can DNA microarray analysis be used to identify specific genes that are being expressed in a specific tissue?

(d) How are GWAS carried out, and what information do they provide?

(e) What are some of the technical reasons why gene therapy is difficult to carry out effectively?

CONCEPT QUESTION

2. Review the Chapter Concepts list on page 569. Most of these center on applications of genetic technology that are becoming

widespread. Write a short essay that summarizes the impacts that genomic applications are having on society and the ethical issues presented by these applications.

3. One of the main safety issues associated with genetically modified crops is the potential for allergenicity caused by introducing an allergen or by changing the level of expression of a host allergen. Based on the observation that common allergenic proteins often contain identical stretches of a few (six or seven) amino acids, researchers developed a method for screening transgenic crops to evaluate potential allergenic properties (Kleter & Peijnenburg, 2002. *BMC Struct. Biol.* 2: 8). How do you think they accomplished this?

4. Why are most recombinant human proteins produced in animal or plant hosts instead of bacterial host cells?

5. There are more than 1000 cloned farm animals in the United States. In the near future, milk from cloned cows and their offspring (born naturally) may be available in supermarkets. These cloned animals have not been transgenically modified, and they are no different than identical twins. Should milk from such animals and their natural-born offspring be labeled as coming from cloned cows or their descendants? Why?

6. One of the major causes of sickness, death, and economic loss in the cattle industry is *Mannheimia haemolytica*, which causes bovine pasteurellosis, or shipping fever. Noninvasive delivery of a vaccine using transgenic plants expressing immunogens would reduce labor costs and trauma to livestock. An early step toward developing an edible vaccine is to determine whether an injected version of an antigen (usually a derivative of the pathogen) is capable of stimulating the development of antibodies in a test organism. The following table assesses the ability of a transgenic portion of a toxin (Lkt) of *M. haemolytica* to stimulate development of specific antibodies in rabbits.

Immunogen Injected	Antibody Production in Serum
Lkt50*—saline extract	+
Lkt50—column extract	+
Mock injection	−
Pre-injection	−

*Lkt50 is a smaller derivative of Lkt that lacks all hydrophobic regions. + indicates at least 50 percent neutralization of toxicity of Lkt; − indicates no neutralization activity.
Source: Modified from Lee et al. 2001. *Infect. and Immunity* 69: 5786–5793.

(a) What general conclusion can you draw from the data?
(b) With regards to development of a usable edible vaccine, what work remains to be done?

7. Describe how the team from the J. Craig Venter Institute created a synthetic genome. How did they demonstrate that the genome converted the recipient strain of bacteria into a different strain?

8. Suppose you develop a screening method for cystic fibrosis that allows you to identify the predominant mutation Δ*508* and the next six most prevalent mutations. What must you consider before using this method to screen a population for this disorder?

9. Sequencing the human genome and the development of microarray technology promise to improve our understanding of normal and abnormal cell behavior. How are microarrays dramatically changing our understanding of complex diseases such as cancer?

10. A couple with European ancestry seeks genetic counseling before having children because of a history of cystic fibrosis

(CF) in the husband's family. ASO testing for CF reveals that the husband is heterozygous for the Δ*508* mutation and that the wife is heterozygous for the *R117* mutation. You are the couple's genetic counselor. When consulting with you, they express their conviction that they are not at risk for having an affected child because they each carry different mutations and cannot have a child who is homozygous for either mutation. What would you say to them?

11. When genome scanning technologies become widespread, medical records will contain the results of such testing. Who should have access to this information? Should employers, potential employers, or insurance companies be allowed to have this information? Would you favor or oppose having the government establish and maintain a central database containing the results of individuals' genome scans?

12. What limits the use of differences in restriction enzyme sites as a way of detecting point mutations in human genes?

13. Might it make sense someday to sequence every newborn's genome at the time of birth? What are the potential advantages and concerns of this approach?

14. What is the main purpose of genome-wide association studies (GWAS)? How can information from GWAS be used to inform scientists and physicians about genetic diseases?

15. The family of a sixth-grade boy in Palo Alto, California, was informed by school administrators that he would have to transfer out of his middle school because they believed his mutation of the *CFTR*, which does not produce any symptoms associated with cystic fibrosis, posed a risk to other students at the school who have cystic fibrosis. After missing 11 days of school, a settlement was reached to have the boy return to school. Based on what you know about GINA, the Genetic Information Nondiscrimination Act, what ethical problems might you associate with this example?

16. Dominant mutations can be categorized according to whether they increase or decrease the overall activity of a gene or gene product. Although a loss-of-function mutation (a mutation that inactivates the gene product) is usually recessive, for some genes, one dose of the normal gene product, encoded by the normal allele, is not sufficient to produce a normal phenotype. In this case, a loss-of-function mutation in the gene will be dominant, and the gene is said to be *haploinsufficient*. A second category of dominant mutation is the gain-of-function mutation, which results in a new activity or increased activity or expression of a gene or gene product. The gene therapy technique currently used in clinical trials involves the "addition" to somatic cells of a normal copy of a gene. In other words, a normal copy of the gene is inserted into the genome of the mutant somatic cell, but the mutated copy of the gene is not removed or replaced. Will this strategy work for either of the two aforementioned types of dominant mutations?

17. In 2013 the actress Angelina Jolie elected to have prophylactic double-mastectomy surgery to prevent breast cancer based on a positive test for mutation of the *BRCA1* gene. What are some potential positive and negative consequences of this high-profile example of acting on the results of a genetic test?

18. The Genetic Testing Registry is intended to provide better information to patients, but companies involved in genetic testing are not required to participate. Should company participation be mandatory? Why or why not? Explain your answers.

19. Should the FDA regulate direct-to-consumer genetic tests, or should these tests be available as a "buyer beware" product?

Extra-Spicy Problems

20. Would you have your genome sequenced, if the price was affordable? Why or why not? If you answered yes, would you make your genome sequence publicly available? How might such information be misused?

21. Following the tragic shooting of 20 children at a school in Newtown, Connecticut, in 2012, Connecticut's state medical examiner requested a full genetic analysis of the killer's genome. What do you think investigators might be looking for? What might they expect to find? Might this analysis lead to oversimplified analysis of the cause of the tragedy?

22. Private companies are now offering personal DNA sequencing along with interpretation. What services do they offer? Do you think that these services should be regulated, and if so, in what way? Investigate one such company, 23andMe, at http://www.23andMe.com.

23. Host transgenic mammals are often made by injecting transgenic DNA into a pronucleus, a process that is laborious, technically demanding, and typified by yields of less than 1 percent. Lately, the engineered lentivirus, a retrovirus, has been used to generate transgenic pigs, rats, mice, and cattle with greater than 10 percent efficiency (Whitelaw, 2004). Lentivectors have reverse transcriptase activity, can infect both dividing and nondividing cells, and are replication-defective. Present, in a labeled diagram, a strategy for producing a transgenic mammal carrying a pharmaceutically important gene using a lentivector.

24. Yeager, M., et al. (*Nature Genetics* 39: 645–649, 2007) and Sladek, R. et al. (*Nature* 445: 881–885, 2007) have used single-nucleotide polymorphisms (SNPs) in genome-wide association studies (GWAS) to identify novel risk loci for prostate cancer and Type 2 diabetes mellitus, respectively. Each study suggests that disease-risk genes can be identified that significantly contribute to the disease state. Given your understanding of such complex diseases, what would you consider as reasonable factors to consider when interpreting the results of GWAS studies?

25. In March, 2010 Judge R. Sweet ruled to invalidate Myriad Genetics' patents on the *BRCA1* and *BRCA2* genes. Sweet wrote that since the genes are part of the natural world, they are not patentable. Myriad Genetics also holds patents on the development of a direct-to-consumer test for the *BRCA1* and *BRCA2* genes.

    (a) Would you agree with Judge Sweet's ruling to invalidate the patenting of the *BRCA1* and *BRCA2* genes? If you were asked to judge the patenting of the direct-to-consumer test for the *BRCA1* and *BRCA2* genes, how would you rule?

    (b) J. Craig Venter has filed a patent application for his "first-ever human made life form." This patent is designed to cover the genome of *M. genitalium*. Would your ruling for Venter's "organism" be different from Judge Sweet's ruling on patenting of the *BRCA1* and *BRCA2* genes?

26. A number of mouse models for human cystic fibrosis (CF) exist. Each of these mouse strains is transgenic and bears a different specific *CFTR* gene mutation. The mutations are the same as those seen in the varieties of human CF. These transgenic CF mice are being used to study the range of different phenotypes that characterize CF in humans. They are also used as models to test potential CF drugs. Unfortunately, most transgenic mouse CF strains do not show one of the most characteristic symptoms of human CF, that of lung congestion. Can you think of a reason why mouse CF strains do not display this symptom of human CF?

A field of pumpkins, where size is under the influence of additive alleles.

23

Quantitative Genetics and Multifactorial Traits

CHAPTER CONCEPTS

- Quantitative inheritance results in a range of measurable phenotypes for a polygenic trait.

- With some exceptions, polygenic traits tend to demonstrate continuous variation.

- Quantitative traits can be explained in Mendelian terms whereby certain alleles have an additive effect on the traits under study.

- The study of polygenic traits relies on statistical analysis.

- Heritability values estimate the genetic contribution to phenotypic variability under specific environmental conditions.

- Twin studies allow an estimation of heritability in humans.

- Quantitative trait loci (QTLs) can be mapped and identified.

Up to this point in the text, most of our examples of phenotypic variation have been those that have been assigned to distinct and separate categories; for example, human blood type was A, B, AB, or O; squash fruit shape was spherical, disc shaped, or elongated; and fruit fly eye color was red or white (see Chapter 4). Typically in these traits, a genotype will produce a single identifiable phenotype, although phenomena such as variable penetrance and expressivity, pleiotropy, and epistasis can obscure the relationship between genotype and phenotype.

In this chapter, we will look at traits that are not as clear cut, including many that are of medical or agricultural importance. The traits on which we focus show much more variation, often falling into a continuous range of phenotypes that are more difficult to classify into distinct categories. Most of these traits show *continuous variation,* including, for example, height in humans, milk and meat production in cattle, yield and seed protein content in various crops. Continuous variation across a range of phenotypes is measured and described in quantitative terms, so this genetic phenomenon is known as **quantitative inheritance**. And because the varying phenotypes result from the input of genes at more than one, and often many, loci, they are also said to be **polygenic** (literally "of many genes").

To further complicate the link between the genotype and phenotype, the genotype generated at fertilization establishes a quantitative range within which a particular individual can fall. However, the final phenotype is often also influenced by environmental factors to which that individual is exposed. Human height, for example, is genetically influenced, but is also affected by environmental factors such as nutrition. Quantitative (polygenic) traits whose phenotypes result from both gene action and environmental influences are often termed **multifactorial,** or **complex** traits. Often these terms are used interchangeably. For consistency throughout the chapter, we will utilize the term *multifactorial* in our discussions.

In this chapter, we will examine examples of quantitative inheritance, multifactorial traits, and some of the statistical techniques used to study them. We will also consider how geneticists assess the relative importance of genetic versus environmental factors contributing to continuous phenotypic variation, and we will discuss approaches to identifying and mapping genes that influence quantitative traits.

Please note that some of the topics discussed in this chapter are explored later in the text (see Special Topic Chapter 1—Epigenetics).

FIGURE 23–1 A graphic depiction of predisposing alleles characteristic of a threshold trait within a population, illustrated by Type II diabetes.

23.1 Not All Polygenic Traits Show Continuous Variation

In addition to quantitative traits that display continuous variation, there are two other classes of polygenic traits. **Meristic traits** are those in which the phenotypes are described by whole numbers. Examples of meristic traits include the number of seeds in a pod or the number of eggs laid by a chicken in a year. These are quantitative traits, but they do not have an infinite range of phenotypes: for example, a pod may contain 2, 4, or 6 seeds, but not 5.75. **Threshold traits** are polygenic (and frequently multifactorial), but they are distinguished from continuous and meristic traits by having a small number of discrete phenotypic classes. Threshold traits are currently of heightened interest to human geneticists because an increasing number of diseases are now thought to show this pattern of polygenic inheritance. One example is **Type II diabetes**, also known as adult-onset diabetes because it typically affects individuals who are middle aged or older. A population can be divided into just two phenotypic classes for this trait—individuals who have Type II diabetes and those who do not—so at first glance, it may appear to more closely resemble a simple monogenic trait. However, no single adult-onset diabetes gene has been identified. Instead, the combination of alleles present at multiple contributing loci gives an individual a greater or lesser likelihood of developing the disease. These varying levels of liability form a continuous range: at one extreme are those at very low risk for Type II diabetes, while at the other end of the distribution are those whose genotypes make it highly likely they will develop the disease (**Figure 23–1**). As with many threshold traits, environmental factors also play a role in determining the final phenotype, with diet and lifestyle having significant impact on whether an individual with moderate to high genetic liability will actually develop Type II diabetes.

23.2 Quantitative Traits Can Be Explained in Mendelian Terms

The question of whether continuous phenotypic variation could be explained in Mendelian terms caused considerable controversy in the early 1900s. Some scientists argued that, although Mendel's unit factors, or genes, explained patterns of discontinuous segregation with discrete phenotypic classes, they could not also account for the range of phenotypes seen in quantitative patterns of inheritance. However, geneticists William Bateson and G. Udny Yule, adhering to a Mendelian explanation, proposed the **multiple-factor** or **multiple-gene hypothesis**, in which many genes, each individually behaving in a Mendelian fashion, contribute to the phenotype in a *cumulative* or *quantitative* way.

The Multiple-Gene Hypothesis for Quantitative Inheritance

The **multiple-gene hypothesis** was initially based on a key set of experimental results published by Herman Nilsson-Ehle in 1909. Nilsson-Ehle used grain color in wheat to test the concept that the cumulative effects of alleles at multiple loci produce the range of phenotypes seen in quantitative traits. In one set of experiments, wheat with red grain was crossed to wheat with white grain (**Figure 23–2**). The F_1 generation demonstrated an intermediate pink color, which at first sight suggested incomplete dominance of two alleles at a single locus. However, in the F_2 generation, Nilsson-Ehle did not observe the typical segregation of a monohybrid cross. Instead, approximately 15/16 of the plants showed some degree of red grain color, while 1/16 of the plants showed white grain color. Careful examination of the F_2 revealed that grain with color could be classified into four different shades of red. Because the F_2 ratio occurred in sixteenths, it appears that two genes, each with

FIGURE 23–2 How the multiple-factor hypothesis accounts for the 1:4:6:4:1 phenotypic ratio of grain color when all alleles designated by an uppercase letter are additive and contribute an equal amount of pigment to the phenotype.

two alleles, control the phenotype and that they segregate independently from one another in a Mendelian fashion.

If each gene has one potential **additive allele** that contributes approximately equally to the red grain color and one potential **nonadditive allele** that fails to produce any red pigment, we can see how the multiple-factor hypothesis could account for the various grain color phenotypes. In the P_1 both parents are homozygous; the red parent contains only additive alleles (*AABB* in Figure 23–2), while

the white parent contains only nonadditive alleles (*aabb*). The F_1 plants are heterozygous (*AaBb*), contain two additive (*A* and *B*) and two nonadditive (*a* and *b*) alleles, and express the intermediate pink phenotype. Each of the F_2 plants has 4, 3, 2, 1, or 0 additive alleles. F_2 plants with no additive alleles are white (*aabb*) like one of the P_1 parents, while F_2 plants with 4 additive alleles are red (*AABB*) like the other P_1 parent. Plants with 3, 2, or 1 additive alleles constitute the other three categories of red color observed in the F_2 generation. The greater the number of additive alleles in the genotype, the more intense the red color expressed in the phenotype, as each additive allele present contributes equally to the cumulative amount of pigment produced in the grain.

Nilsson-Ehle's results showed how continuous variation could still be explained in a Mendelian fashion, with additive alleles at multiple loci influencing the phenotype in a quantitative manner, but each individual allele segregating according to Mendelian rules. As we saw in Nilsson-Ehle's initial cross, if two loci, each with two alleles, were involved, then five F_2 phenotypic categories in a 1:4:6:4:1 ratio would be expected. However, there is no reason why three, four, or more loci cannot function in a similar fashion in controlling various quantitative phenotypes. As more quantitative loci become involved, greater and greater numbers of classes appear in the F_2 generation in more complex ratios. The number of phenotypes and the expected F_2 ratios for crosses involving up to five gene pairs are illustrated in **Figure 23–3**.

Additive Alleles: The Basis of Continuous Variation

The multiple-gene hypothesis consists of the following major points:

1. Phenotypic traits showing continuous variation can be quantified by measuring, weighing, counting, and so on.

2. Two or more gene loci, often scattered throughout the genome, account for the hereditary influence on the phenotype in an *additive way*. Because many genes may be involved, inheritance of this type is called *polygenic*.

3. Each gene locus may be occupied by either an *additive* allele, which contributes a constant amount to the phenotype, or a *nonadditive* allele, which does not contribute quantitatively to the phenotype.

1 Gene pair $Aa \times Aa$

2 Gene pairs $AaBb \times AaBb$

3 Gene pairs $AaBbCc \times AaBbCc$

4 Gene pairs $AaBbCcDd \times AaBbCcDd$

5 Gene pairs $AaBbCcDdEe \times AaBbCcDdEe$

FIGURE 23–3 The genetic ratios (on the *x*-axis) resulting from crossing two heterozygotes when polygenic inheritance is in operation with 1–5 gene pairs. The histogram bars indicate the distinct F₂ phenotypic classes, ranging from one extreme (left end) to the other extreme (right end). Each phenotype results from a different number of additive alleles.

4. The contribution to the phenotype of each additive allele, though often small, is approximately equal. While we now know this is not always true, we have made this assumption in the above discussion.

5. Together, the additive alleles contributing to a single quantitative character produce substantial phenotypic variation.

Calculating the Number of Polygenes

Various formulas have been developed for estimating the number of **polygenes**, the genes contributing to a quantitative trait. For example, if the ratio of F₂ individuals resembling *either* of the two extreme P₁ phenotypes can be determined, the number of polygenes involved (*n*) may be calculated as follows:

$$1/4^n = \text{ratio of F}_2 \text{ individuals expressing either extreme phenotype}$$

In the example of the red and white wheat grain color summarized in Figure 23–2, 1/16 of the progeny are either red *or* white like the P₁ phenotypes. This ratio can be substituted on the right side of the equation to solve for *n*:

$$\frac{1}{4^n} = \frac{1}{16}$$

$$\frac{1}{4^2} = \frac{1}{16}$$

$$n = 2$$

Table 23.1 lists the ratio and the number of F₂ phenotypic classes produced in crosses involving up to five gene pairs.

For low numbers of polygenes (*n*), it is sometimes easier to use the equation

$$(2n + 1) = \text{the number of distinct phenotypic categories observed}$$

For example, when there are two polygenes involved (*n* = 2), then (2*n* + 1) = 5 and each phenotype is the result of 4, 3, 2, 1, or 0 additive alleles. If *n* = 3, 2*n* + 1 = 7 and each phenotype is the result of 6, 5, 4, 3, 2, 1, or 0 additive alleles. Thus, working backwards with this rule and knowing the number of phenotypes, we can calculate the number of polygenes controlling them.

It should be noted, however, that both of these simple methods for estimating the number of polygenes involved in a quantitative trait assume not only that all the relevant alleles contribute equally and additively, but also that phenotypic expression in the F₂ is not affected significantly by environmental factors. As we will see later, for many quantitative traits, these assumptions may not be true.

TABLE 23.1 Determination of the Number of Polygenes (*n*) Involved in a Quantitative Trait

n	Individuals Expressing Either Extreme Phenotype	Distinct Phenotypic Classes
1	1/4	3
2	1/16	5
3	1/64	7
4	1/256	9
5	1/1024	11

NOW SOLVE THIS

23–1 A homozygous plant with 20-cm-diameter flowers is crossed with a homozygous plant of the same species that has 40-cm-diameter flowers. The F_1 plants all have flowers 30 cm in diameter. In the F_2 generation of 512 plants, 2 plants have flowers 20 cm in diameter, 2 plants have flowers 40 cm in diameter, and the remaining 508 plants have flowers of a range of sizes in between.

(a) Assuming that all alleles involved act additively, how many genes control flower size in this plant?

(b) What frequency distribution of flower diameter would you expect to see in the progeny of a backcross between an F_1 plant and the large-flowered parent?

■ **HINT:** *This problem provides F_1 and F_2 data for a cross involving a quantitative trait and asks you to calculate the number of genes controlling the trait. The key to its solution is to remember that unless you know the total number of distinct F_2 phenotypes involved, then the ratio (not the number) of parental phenotypes reappearing in the F_2 must be used in your determination of the number of genes involved.*

For more practice, see Problems 4, 5, 6, and 7.

23.3 The Study of Polygenic Traits Relies on Statistical Analysis

Before considering the approaches that geneticists use to dissect how much of the phenotypic variation observed in a population is due to genotypic differences among individuals and how much is due to environmental factors, we need to consider the basic statistical tools they use for the task. It is not usually feasible to measure expression of a polygenic trait in every individual in a population, so a random subset of individuals is usually selected for measurement to provide a *sample*. It is important to remember that the accuracy of the final results of the measurements depends on whether the sample is truly random and representative of the population from which it was drawn. Suppose, for example, that a student wants to determine the average height of the 100 students in his genetics class, and for his sample he measures the two students sitting next to him, both of whom happen to be centers on the college basketball team. It is unlikely that this sample will provide a good estimate of the average height of the class, for two reasons: First, it is too small; second, it is not a representative subset of the class (unless all 100 students are centers on the basketball team).

If the sample measured for expression of a quantitative trait is sufficiently large and also representative of the population from which it is drawn, we often find that the data form a **normal distribution**; that is, they produce a characteristic

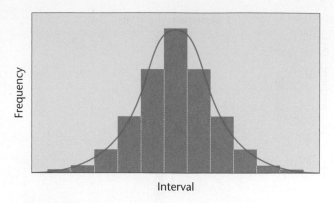

FIGURE 23–4 Normal frequency distribution, characterized by a bell-shaped curve.

bell-shaped curve when plotted as a frequency histogram (**Figure 23–4**). Several statistical concepts are useful in the analysis of traits that exhibit a normal distribution, including the mean, variance, standard deviation, standard error of the mean, and covariance.

The Mean

The mean provides information about where the central point lies along a range of measurements for a quantitative trait. **Figure 23–5** shows the distribution curves for two different sets of phenotypic measurements. Each of these sets of measurements clusters around a central value (as it happens, they both cluster around the same value). This clustering is called a central tendency, and the central point is the mean.

Specifically, the **mean** ($\overline{X}$) is the arithmetic average of a set of measurements and is calculated as

$$\overline{X} = \frac{\Sigma X_i}{n}$$

where $\overline{X}$ is the mean, ΣX_i represents the sum of all individual values in the sample, and n is the number of individual values.

The mean provides a useful descriptive summary of the sample, but it tells us nothing about the range or spread of the data. As illustrated in Figure 23–5, a symmetrical distribution

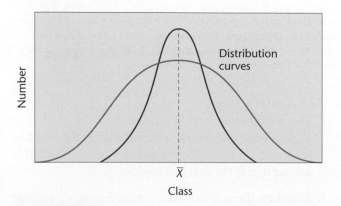

FIGURE 23–5 Two normal frequency distributions with the same mean but different amounts of variation.

of values in the sample may, in one case, be clustered near the mean. Or a set of measurements may have the same mean but be distributed more widely around it. A second statistic, the variance, provides information about the spread of data around the mean.

Variance

The **variance** (s^2) for a sample is the average squared distance of all measurements from the mean. It is calculated as

$$s^2 = \frac{\Sigma(X_i - \overline{X})^2}{n - 1}$$

where the sum (Σ) of the squared differences between each measured value (X_i) and the mean ($\overline{X}$) is divided by one less than the total sample size $n - 1$.

As Figure 23–5 shows, it is possible for two sets of sample measurements for a quantitative trait to have the same mean but a different distribution of values around it. This range will be reflected in different variances. Estimation of variance can be useful in determining the degree of genetic control of traits when the immediate environment also influences the phenotype.

Standard Deviation

Because the variance is a squared value, its unit of measurement is also squared (m^2, g^2, etc.). To express variation around the mean in the original units of measurement, we can use the square root of the variance, a term called the **standard deviation** (s):

$$s = \sqrt{s^2}$$

Table 23.2 shows the percentage of individual values within a normal distribution that fall within different multiples of the standard deviation. The values that fall within one standard deviation to either side of the mean represent 68 percent of all values in the sample. More than 95 percent of all values are found within two standard deviations to either side of the mean. This means that the standard deviation s can also be interpreted in the form of a probability. For example, a sample measurement picked at random has a 68 percent probability of falling within the range of one standard deviation.

TABLE 23.2	Sample Inclusion for Various s Values
Multiples of s	Sample Included (%)
$\overline{X} \pm 1s$	68.3
$\overline{X} \pm 1.96s$	95.0
$\overline{X} \pm 2s$	95.5
$\overline{X} \pm 3s$	99.7

Standard Error of the Mean

If multiple samples are taken from a population and measured for the same quantitative trait, we might find that their means vary. Theoretically, larger, truly random samples will represent the population more accurately, and their means will be closer to each other. To measure the accuracy of the sample mean we use the **standard error of the mean** ($S_{\overline{X}}$), calculated as

$$S_{\overline{X}} = \frac{s}{\sqrt{n}}$$

where s is the standard deviation and $\sqrt{n}$ is the square root of the sample size. Because the standard error of the mean is computed by dividing s by $\sqrt{n}$, it is always a smaller value than the standard deviation.

Covariance and Correlation Coefficient

Often geneticists working with quantitative traits find they have to consider two phenotypic characters simultaneously. For example, a poultry breeder might investigate the correlation between body weight and egg production in hens: Do heavier birds tend to lay more eggs? The **covariance** statistic measures how much variation is common to both quantitative traits. It is calculated by taking the deviations from the mean for each trait (just as we did for estimating variance) for each individual in the sample. This gives a pair of values for each individual. The two values are multiplied together, and the sum of all these individual products is then divided by one fewer than the number in the sample. Thus the covariance **cov$_{XY}$** of two sets of trait measurements, X and Y, is calculated as

$$\text{cov}_{XY} = \frac{\Sigma\left[(X_i - \overline{X})(Y_i - \overline{Y})\right]}{n - 1}$$

The covariance can then be standardized as yet another statistic, the **correlation coefficient** (r). The calculation of r is

$$r = \text{cov}_{XY}/S_X S_Y$$

where S_X is the standard deviation of the first set of quantitative measurements X, and S_Y is the standard deviation of the second set of quantitative measurements Y. Values for the correlation coefficient r can range from -1 to $+1$. Positive r values mean that an increase in measurement for one trait tends to be associated with an increase in measurement for the other, while negative r values mean that increases in one trait are associated with decreases in the other. Therefore, if heavier hens do tend to lay more eggs, a positive r value can be expected. A negative r value, on the other hand, suggests that greater egg production is more likely from less heavy birds. One important point to note about correlation coefficients is that even significant r

values—close to +1 or −1—do not prove that a cause-and-effect relationship exists between two traits. Correlation analysis simply tells us the extent to which variation in one quantitative trait is associated with variation in another, not what causes that variation.

Analysis of a Quantitative Character

To apply these statistical concepts, let's consider a genetic experiment that crossed two different homozygous varieties of tomato. One of the tomato varieties produces fruit averaging 18 oz in weight, whereas fruit from the other averages 6 oz. The F_1 obtained by crossing these two varieties has fruit weights ranging from 10 to 14 oz. The F_2 population contains individuals that produce fruit ranging from 6 to 18 oz. The results characterizing both generations are shown in **Table 23.3**.

The mean value for the fruit weight in the F_1 generation can be calculated as

$$\overline{X} = \frac{\Sigma X_i}{n} = \frac{626}{52} = 12.04$$

The mean value for fruit weight in the F_2 generation is calculated as

$$\overline{X} = \frac{\Sigma X_i}{n} = \frac{872}{72} = 12.11$$

Although these mean values are similar, the frequency distributions in Table 23.3 show more variation in the F_2 generation. The range of variation can be quantified as the sample variance s^2, calculated, as we saw above, as the sum of the squared differences between each value and the mean, divided by one less than the total number of observations.

$$s^2 = \frac{\Sigma(X_i - \overline{X})^2}{n - 1}$$

When the above calculation is made, the variance is found to be 1.29 for the F_1 generation and 4.27 for the F_2 generation. When converted to the standard deviation ($s = \sqrt{s^2}$), the values become 1.13 and 2.06, respectively. Therefore, the distribution of tomato weight in the F_1 generation can be

23–2 The following table shows measurements for fiber lengths and fleece weight in a small flock of eight sheep.

	Sheep Fiber Length (cm)	Fleece Weight (kg)
1	9.7	7.9
2	5.6	4.5
3	10.7	8.3
4	6.8	5.4
5	11.0	9.1
6	4.5	4.9
7	7.4	6.0
8	5.9	5.1

(a) What are the mean, variance, and standard deviation for each trait in this flock?

(b) What is the covariance of the two traits?

(c) What is the correlation coefficient for fiber length and fleece weight?

(d) Do you think greater fleece weight is correlated with an increase in fiber length? Why or why not?

This problem provides data for two quantitative traits in a flock of sheep. After making numerous statistical calculations, you are asked in part (d) to determine if the traits are correlated.

■ **HINT:** *This problem provides data for two quantitative traits and asks you to make numerous statistical calculations, ultimately determining if the traits are correlated. The key to its solution is that once the calculation of the correlation coefficient (r) is completed, you must interpret that value—whether it is positive or negative, and how close to zero it is.*

described as 12.04 ± 1.13, and in the F_2 generation it can be described as 12.11 ± 2.06.

Assuming that both tomato varieties are homozygous at the loci of interest and that the alleles controlling fruit weight act additively, we can estimate the number of polygenes involved in this trait. Since 1/72 of the F_2 offspring have a phenotype that overlaps one of the parental strains (72 total F_2 offspring; one weighs 6 oz, one weighs 18 oz;

TABLE 23.3 Distribution of F_1 and F_2 Progeny Derived from a Theoretical Cross Involving Tomatoes

		Weight (oz)												
		6	7	8	9	10	11	12	13	14	15	16	17	18
Number of	F_1					4	14	16	12	6				
Individuals	F_2	1	1	2	0	9	13	17	14	7	4	3	0	1

see Table 23.3), the use of the formula $1/4^n = 1/72$ indicates that n is between 3 and 4, providing evidence of the number of genes that control fruit weight in these tomato strains.

23.4 Heritability Values Estimate the Genetic Contribution to Phenotypic Variability

The question most often asked by geneticists working with multifactorial traits and diseases is how much of the observed phenotypic variation in a population is due to genotypic differences among individuals and how much is due to environment. The term **heritability** is used to describe *what proportion of total phenotypic variation in a population is due to genetic factors*. For a multifactorial trait in a given population, a high heritability estimate indicates that much of the variation can be attributed to genetic factors, with the environment having less impact on expression of the trait. With a low heritability estimate, environmental factors are likely to have a greater impact on phenotypic variation within the population.

The concept of heritability is frequently misunderstood and misused. It should be emphasized that heritability indicates neither how much of a trait is genetically determined nor the extent to which an individual's phenotype is due to genotype. In recent years, such misinterpretations of heritability for human quantitative traits have led to controversy, notably in relation to measurements such as intelligence quotients, or IQs. Variation in heritability estimates for IQ among different racial groups tested led to incorrect suggestions that unalterable genetic factors control differences in intelligence levels among humans of different ancestries. Such suggestions misrepresented the meaning of heritability and ignored the contribution of genotype-by-environment interaction variance to phenotypic variation in a population. Moreover, heritability is not fixed for a trait. For example, a heritability estimate for egg production in a flock of chickens kept in individual cages might be high, indicating that differences in egg output among individual birds are largely due to genetic differences, as they all have very similar environments. For a different flock kept outdoors, heritability for egg production might be much lower, as variation among different birds may also reflect differences in their individual environments. Such differences could include how much food each bird manages to find and whether it competes successfully for a good roosting spot at night. Thus a heritability estimate tells us the proportion of phenotypic variation that can be attributed to genetic variation *within a certain population in a particular environment*. If we measure heritability for the same trait among different populations in a range of environments, we frequently find that the calculated heritability values have large standard errors. This is an important point to remember when considering heritability estimates for traits in human populations. A mean heritability estimate of 0.65 for human height does not mean that your height is 65 percent due to your genes, but rather that in the populations sampled, on average, *65 percent of the overall variation in height could be explained by genotypic differences among individuals*.

With this subtle but important distinction in mind, we will now consider how geneticists divide the phenotypic variation observed in a population into genetic and environmental components. As we saw in the previous section, variation can be quantified as a sample variance: taking measurements of the trait in question from a representative sample of the population and determining the extent of the spread of those measurements around the sample mean. This gives us an estimate of the total **phenotypic variance** in the population (V_P). Heritability estimates are obtained by using different experimental and statistical techniques to partition V_P into **genotypic variance** (V_G) and **environmental variance** (V_E) components.

An important factor contributing to overall levels of phenotypic variation is the extent to which individual genotypes affect the phenotype differently depending on the environment. For example, wheat variety A may yield an average of 20 bushels an acre on poor soil, while variety B yields an average of 17 bushels. On good soil, variety A yields 22 bushels, while variety B averages 25 bushels an acre. There are differences in yield between the two genotypically distinct varieties, so variation in wheat yield has a genetic component. Both varieties yield more on good soil, so yield is also affected by environment. However, we also see that the two varieties do not respond to better soil conditions equally: The genotype of wheat variety B achieves a greater increase in yield on good soil than does variety A. Thus, we have differences in the interaction of genotype, with environment contributing to variation for yield in populations of wheat plants. This third component of phenotypic variation is **genotype-by-environment interaction variance** ($V_{G \times E}$) (**Figure 23–6**).

We can now summarize all the components of total phenotypic variance V_P using the following equation:

$$V_P = V_G + V_E + V_{G \times E}$$

In other words, total phenotypic variance can be subdivided into genotypic variance, environmental variance, and genotype-by-environment interaction variance. When obtaining heritability estimates for a multifactorial trait, researchers often assume that the genotype-by-environment interaction variance is small enough that it can be ignored or combined

(a)

(b)

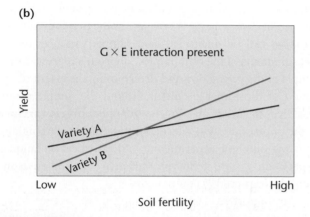

FIGURE 23–6 Differences in yield between two wheat varieties at different soil fertility levels. (a) No genotype-by-environment, or G × E, interaction: The varieties show genetic differences in yield but respond equally to increasing soil fertility. (b) G × E interaction present: Variety A outyields B at low soil fertility, but B yields more than A at high fertility levels.

with the environmental variance. However, it is worth remembering that this kind of approximation is another reason heritability values are *estimates* for a given population in a particular context, not a *fixed attribute* for a trait.

Animal and plant breeders use a range of experimental techniques to estimate heritabilities by partitioning measurements of phenotypic variance into genotypic and environmental components. One approach uses inbred strains containing genetically homogeneous individuals with highly homozygous genotypes. Experiments are then designed to test the effects of a range of environmental conditions on phenotypic variability. Variation *between* different inbred strains reared in a constant environment is due predominantly to genetic factors. Variation *among* members of the same inbred strain reared under different conditions is more likely to be due to environmental factors. Other approaches involve analysis of variance for a quantitative trait among offspring from different crosses, or

comparing expression of a trait among offspring and parents reared in the same environment.

Broad-Sense Heritability

Broad-sense heritability (represented by the term H^2) measures the contribution of the genotypic variance to the total phenotypic variance. It is estimated as a proportion:

$$H^2 = \frac{V_G}{V_P}$$

Heritability values for a trait in a population range from 0.0 to 1.0. A value approaching 1.0 indicates that the environmental conditions have little impact on phenotypic variance, which is therefore largely due to genotypic differences among individuals in the population. Low values close to 0.0 indicate that environmental factors, not genotypic differences, are largely responsible for the observed phenotypic variation within the population studied. Few quantitative traits have very high or very low heritability estimates, suggesting that both genetics and environment play a part in the expression of most phenotypes for the trait.

The genotypic variance component V_G used in broad-sense heritability estimates includes all types of genetic variation in the population. It does not distinguish between quantitative trait loci with alleles acting additively as opposed to those with epistatic or dominance effects. Broad-sense heritability estimates also assume that the genotype-by-environment variance component is negligible. While broad-sense heritability estimates for a trait are of general genetic interest, these limitations mean this kind of heritability is not very useful in breeding programs. Animal or plant breeders wishing to develop improved strains of livestock or higher-yielding crop varieties need more precise heritability estimates for the traits they wish to manipulate in a population. Therefore, another type of estimate, narrow-sense heritability, has been devised that is of more practical use.

Narrow-Sense Heritability

Narrow-sense heritability (h^2) is the proportion of phenotypic variance due to additive genotypic variance alone. Genotypic variance can be divided into subcomponents representing the different modes of action of alleles at quantitative trait loci. As not all the genes involved in a quantitative trait affect the phenotype in the same way, this partitioning distinguishes among three different kinds of gene action contributing to genotypic variance. **Additive variance, V_A**, is the genotypic variance due to the additive action of alleles at quantitative trait loci. **Dominance variance, V_D**, is the deviation from the additive components that results when phenotypic expression in heterozygotes is not precisely intermediate between the two homozygotes. **Interactive variance, V_I,** is the deviation from the additive components that occurs when two or more loci behave epistatically. The amount of interactive variance is often negligible, and so this component is often excluded from calculations of total genotypic variance.

The partitioning of the total genotypic variance V_G is summarized in the equation

$$V_G = V_A + V_D + V_I$$

and a narrow-sense heritability estimate based only on that portion of the genotypic variance due to additive gene action becomes

$$h^2 = \frac{V_A}{V_P}$$

Omitting V_I and separating V_P into genotypic and environmental variance components, we obtain

$$h^2 = \frac{V_A}{V_E + V_A + V_D}$$

Heritability estimates are used in animal and plant breeding to indicate the potential response of a population to artificial selection for a quantitative trait. Narrow-sense heritability, h^2, provides a more accurate prediction of selection response than broad-sense heritability, H^2, and therefore h^2 is more widely used by breeders.

Artificial Selection

Artificial selection is the process of choosing specific individuals with preferred phenotypes from an initially heterogeneous population for future breeding purposes. Theoretically, if artificial selection based on the same trait preferences is repeated over multiple generations, a population can be developed containing a high frequency of individuals with the desired characteristics. If selection is for a simple trait controlled by just one or two genes subject to little environmental influence, generating the desired population of plants or animals is relatively fast and easy. However, many traits of economic importance in crops and livestock, such as grain yield in plants, weight gain or milk yield in cattle, and speed or stamina in horses, are polygenic and frequently multifactorial. Artificial selection for such traits is slower and more complex. Narrow-sense heritability estimates are valuable to the plant or animal breeder because, as we have just seen, they estimate the proportion of total phenotypic variance for the trait that is due to additive genetic variance. Quantitative trait alleles with additive impact are those most easily manipulated by the breeder. Alleles at quantitative trait loci that generate dominance effects or interact epistatically (and therefore contribute

to V_D or V_I) are less responsive to artificial selection. Thus narrow-sense heritability, h^2, can be used to predict the impact of selection. The higher the estimated value for h^2 in a population, the more likely the breeder will observe a change in phenotypic range for the trait in the next generation after artificial selection.

Partitioning the genetic variance components to calculate h^2 and predict response to selection is a complex task requiring careful experimental design and analysis. The simplest approach is to select individuals with superior phenotypes for the desired quantitative trait from a heterogeneous population and breed offspring from those individuals. The mean score for the trait of those offspring ($M2$) can then be compared to that of: (1) the original population's mean score (M) and (2) the selected individuals used as parents ($M1$). The relationship between these means and h^2 is

$$h^2 = \frac{M2 - M}{M1 - M}$$

This equation can be further simplified by defining $M2 - M$ as the **selection response (R)**—the degree of response to mating the selected parents—and $M1 - M$ as the **selection differential (S)**—the difference between the mean for the whole population and the mean for the selected population—so h^2 reflects the ratio of the response observed to the total response possible. Thus,

$$h^2 = \frac{R}{S}$$

A narrow-sense heritability value obtained in this way by selective breeding and measuring the response in the offspring is referred to as an estimate of **realized heritability**.

As an example of a realized heritability estimate, suppose that we measure the diameter of corn kernels in a population where the mean diameter M is 20 mm. From this population, we select a group with the smallest diameters, for which the mean $M1$ equals 10 mm. The selected plants are interbred, and the mean diameter $M2$ of the progeny kernels is 13 mm. We can calculate the realized heritability h^2 to estimate the potential for artificial selection on kernel size:

$$h^2 = \frac{M2 - M}{M1 - M}$$
$$h^2 = \frac{13 - 20}{10 - 20}$$
$$= \frac{-7}{-10}$$
$$= 0.70$$

This value for narrow-sense heritability indicates that the selection potential for kernel size is relatively high.

The longest running artificial selection experiment known is still being conducted at the State Agricultural Laboratory in Illinois. Since 1896, corn has been selected for both high and low oil content. After 76 generations, selection continues to result in increased oil content (**Figure 23–7**). With each cycle of successful selection, more of the corn plants accumulate a higher percentage of additive alleles involved in oil production. Consequently, the narrow-sense heritability h^2 of increased oil content in succeeding generations has declined (see parenthetical values at generations 9, 25, 52, and 76 in Figure 23–7) as artificial selection comes closer and closer to optimizing the genetic potential for oil production. Theoretically, the process will continue until all individuals in the population possess a uniform genotype that includes all the additive alleles responsible for high oil content. At that point, h^2 will be reduced to zero, and response to artificial selection will cease. The decrease in response to selection for low oil content shows that heritability for low oil content is approaching this point.

Table 23.4 lists narrow-sense heritability estimates expressed as percentage values for a variety of quantitative traits in different organisms. As you can see, these h^2 values vary, but heritability tends to be low for quantitative traits that are essential to an organism's survival. Remember, this does not indicate the absence of a genetic contribution to the observed phenotypes for such traits. Instead, the low h^2

TABLE 23.4 Estimates of Heritability for Traits in Different Organisms

Trait	Heritability (h^2)
Mice	
Tail length	60%
Body weight	37
Litter size	15
Chickens	
Body weight	50
Egg production	20
Egg hatchability	15
Cattle	
Birth weight	45
Milk yield	44
Conception rate	3

values show that natural selection has already largely optimized the genetic component of these traits during evolution. Egg production, litter size, and conception rate are examples of how such physiological limitations on selection have already been reached. Traits that are less critical to survival, such as body weight, tail length, and wing length, have higher heritabilities because more genotypic variation for such traits is still present in the population. Remember also that any single heritability estimate can only provide information about one population in a specific environment. Therefore, narrow-sense heritability is a more valuable predictor of response to selection when estimates are calculated for many populations and environments and show the presence of a clear trend.

23.5 Twin Studies Allow an Estimation of Heritability in Humans

Human twins are useful subjects for examining how much phenotypic variance for a multifactorial trait is due to the genotype as opposed to the environment. In these studies, the underlying principle has been that **monozygotic (MZ)**, or **identical, twins** are derived from a single zygote that divides mitotically and then spontaneously splits into two separate cells. Both cells give rise to a genotypically identical embryo. **Dizygotic (DZ)**, or **fraternal, twins,** on the other hand, originate from two separate fertilization events and are only as genetically similar as any two siblings, with an average of 50 percent of their alleles in common. For a given trait, therefore, phenotypic differences between pairs of MZ twins will be equivalent to the environmental variance (V_E) (because the genotypic variance is zero).

FIGURE 23–7 Response of corn selected for high and low oil content over 76 generations. The numbers in parentheses at generations 9, 25, 52, and 76 for the "high oil" line indicate the calculation of heritability at these points in the continuing experiment.

Phenotypic differences between DZ twins, however, display both environmental variance (V_E) and approximately half the genotypic variance (V_G). Comparing the extent of phenotypic variance for the same trait in MZ and DZ sets of twins provides an estimate of broad-sense heritability for the trait.

Twins are said to be **concordant** for a given trait if both express it or neither expresses it. If one expresses the trait and the other does not, the pair is said to be **discordant**. Comparison of concordance values of MZ versus DZ twins reared together illustrates the potential value for heritability assessment. (See the Now Solve This feature on the next page, for example.)

Before any conclusions can be drawn from twin studies, the data must be examined carefully. For example, if concordance values approach 90 to 100 percent in MZ twins, we might be inclined to interpret that as a large genetic contribution to the phenotype of the trait. In some cases—for example, blood types and eye color—we know that this is indeed true. In the case of contracting measles, however, a high concordance value merely indicates that the trait is almost always induced by a factor in the environment—in this case, a virus.

It is more meaningful to compare the *difference* between the concordance values of MZ and DZ twins. If concordance values are significantly higher in MZ twins, we suspect a strong genetic component in the determination of the trait. In the case of measles, where concordance is high in both types of twins, the environment is assumed to be the major contributing factor. Such an analysis is useful because phenotypic characteristics that remain similar in different environments are likely to have a strong genetic component.

Twin Studies Have Several Limitations

Interesting as they are, human twin studies contain some unavoidable sources of error. For example, MZ twins are often treated more similarly by parents and teachers than are DZ twins, especially when the DZ siblings are of different sex. This circumstance may inflate the environmental variance for DZ twins. Another possible error source is interactions between the genotype and the environment that produce variability in the phenotype. These interactions can increase the total phenotypic variance for DZ twins compared to MZ twins raised in the same environment, influencing heritability calculations. Overall, heritability estimates for human traits based on twin studies should therefore be considered approximations and examined very carefully before any conclusions are drawn.

Although they must often be viewed with caution, classical twin studies, based on the assumption that MZ twins share the same genome, have been valuable for estimating heritability over a wide range of traits including multifactorial disorders such as cardiovascular disease, diabetes, and mental illness, for example. These disorders clearly have genetic components, and twin studies provide a foundation for studying interactions between genes and environmental factors. However, results from genomics research have challenged the view that MZ twins are truly identical and have forced a reevaluation of both the methodology and the results of twin studies. Such research has also opened the way to new approaches to the study of interactions between the genotype and environmental factors.

The most relevant genomic discoveries about twins include the following:

- By the time they are born, MZ twins do not necessarily have identical genomes.

- Gene-expression patterns in MZ twins change with age, leading to phenotypic differences.

We will address these points in order. First, MZ twins develop from a single fertilized egg, where sometime early in development the resulting cell mass separates into two distinct populations creating two independent embryos. Until that time, MZ twins have identical genotypes. Subsequently, however, the genotypes can diverge slightly. For example, differences in *copy number variation* (*CNV*)—variation in the number of copies of numerous large DNA sequences (usually 1000 bp or more)—may arise, differentially producing genetically distinct populations of cells in each embryo (see Chapter 8 for a discussion of CNV). This creates a condition called *somatic mosaicism,* which may result in a milder disease phenotype in some disorders and may play a similar role in phenotypic discordance observed in some pairs of MZ twins.

At this point, it is difficult to know for certain how often CNV arises after MZ twinning, but one estimate suggests that such differences are believed to occur in 10 percent of all twin pairs. In those pairs where it does occur, one estimate is that such divergence takes place in 15 to 70 percent of the somatic cells. In one case, a CNV difference between MZ twins has been associated with chronic lymphocytic leukemia in one twin, but not the other.

The second genomic difference between MZ twins involves **epigenetics**—the chemical modification of their DNA and associated histones. An international study of epigenetic modifications in adult European MZ twins showed that MZ twin pairs are epigenetically identical at birth, but adult MZ twins show significant differences in the *methylation patterns* of both DNA and histones. Such epigenetic changes in turn affect patterns of gene expression. The accumulation of epigenetic changes and gene-expression profiles may explain some of the observed phenotypic discordance and susceptibility to diseases in adult MZ twins.

For example, a clear difference in DNA methylation patterns is observed in MZ twins discordant for Beckwith–Wiedemann syndrome, a genetic disorder associated with variable developmental overgrowth of certain tissues and organs and an increased risk of developing cancerous and noncancerous tumors. Affected infants are often larger than normal, and one in five die early in life.

Other complex disorders displaying a genetic component are similarly being investigated using epigenetic analysis in twin studies. These include susceptibility to several neurobiological disorders, including schizophrenia and autism, as well as to the development of Type 1 diabetes, breast cancer, and autoimmune disease.

Progressive, age-related genomic modifications may be the result of MZ twins being exposed to different environmental factors, or from failure of epigenetic marking following DNA replication. These findings also indicate that concordance studies in DZ twins must take into account genetic as well as *epigenetic differences* that contribute to discordance in these twin pairs.

NOW SOLVE THIS

23–3 The following table gives the percentage of twin pairs studied in which both twins expressed the same phenotype for a trait (concordance). Percentages listed are for concordance for each trait in monozygotic (MZ) and dizygotic (DZ) twins. Assuming that both twins in each pair were raised together in the same environment, what do you conclude about the relative importance of genetic versus environmental factors for each trait?

Trait	MZ %	DZ %
Blood types	100	66
Eye color	99	28
Mental retardation	97	37
Measles	95	87
Hair color	89	22
Handedness	79	77
Idiopathic epilepsy	72	15
Schizophrenia	69	10
Diabetes	65	18
Identical allergy	59	5
Cleft lip	42	5
Club foot	32	3
Mammary cancer	6	3

■ **HINT:** *This problem asks you to evaluate the relative importance of genetic versus environmental contributions to specific traits by examining concordance values in MZ versus DZ twins. The key to its solution is to examine the difference in concordance values and to factor in what you have learned about the genetic differences between MZ and DZ twins.*

The realization that epigenetics may play an important role in the development of phenotypes promises to make twin studies an especially valuable tool in dissecting the interactions among genes and the role of environmental factors in the production of phenotypes. Once the degree of epigenetic differences between MZ and DZ twin pairs has been defined, molecular studies on DNA and histone modification can link changes in gene expression with differences in the concordance rates between MZ and DZ twins.

We will discuss the most recent findings involving epigenetics and summarize its many forms and functions later in the text (see Special Topic Chapter 1—Epigenetics).

23.6 Quantitative Trait Loci Are Useful in Studying Multifactorial Phenotypes

Environmental effects, interaction among segregating alleles, and the large number of genes that may contribute to a polygenic phenotype make it difficult to: (1) identify all genes that are involved; and (2) determine the effect of each gene on the phenotype. However, because many quantitative traits are of economic or medical relevance, it is often desirable to obtain this information. In such studies, a chromosome region is identified as containing one or more genes contributing to a quantitative trait known as a **quantitative trait locus (QTL)**.* When possible, the relevant gene or genes contained within a QTL are isolated and studied.

The modern approach used to find and map QTLs involves looking for associations between DNA markers and phenotypes. One way to do this is to begin with individuals from two lines created by artificial selection that are highly divergent for a phenotype (fruit weight, oil content, bristle number, etc.). For example, **Figure 23–8** illustrates a generic case of QTL mapping. Over many generations of artificial selection, two divergent lines become highly homozygous, which facilitates their use in QTL mapping. Individuals from each of the lines with divergent phenotypes [generation 25 in **Figure 23–8(a)**] are used as parents to create an F_1 generation whose members will be heterozygous at most of the loci contributing to the trait. Additional crosses, either among F_1 individuals or between the F_1 and the inbred parent lines, result in F_2 generations that carry different portions of the parental genomes [**Figure 23–8(b)**] with different QTL genotypes and associated phenotypes. This segregating F_2 is known as the **QTL mapping population**.

Researchers then measure phenotypic expression of the trait among individuals in the mapping population and

---

*We utilize QTLs to designate the plural form, quantitative trait loci.

(a)

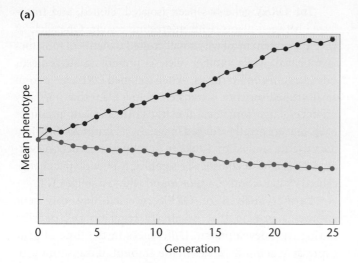

FIGURE 23–8 (a) Individuals from highly divergent lines created by artificial selection are chosen from generation 25 as parents. (b) The thick bars represent the genomes of individuals selected from the divergent lines as parents. These individuals are crossed to produce an F_1 generation (not shown). An F_2 generation is produced by crossing members of the F_1. As a result of crossing over, individual members of the F_2 generation carry different portions of the P_1 genome, as shown by the colored segments of the thick bars. DNA markers and phenotypes in individuals of the F_2 generation are analyzed. (c) Statistical methods are used to determine the probability that a DNA marker is associated with a QTL that affects the phenotype. The results are plotted as the likelihood of association against chromosomal location. Units on genetic maps are measured in centimorgans (cM), determined by crossover frequencies. Peaks above the horizontal line represent significant results. The data show five possible QTLs, with the most significant findings at about 10 cM and 60 cM.

(b)

(c)

not vary among individuals with different genotypes at that marker locus. However, if a DNA marker *is* linked to a QTL, then different genotypes at that marker locus will also differ in their phenotypic expression of the trait. When this occurs, the marker locus and the QTL are said to *cosegregate*. Consistent cosegregation establishes the presence of a QTL at or near the DNA marker along the chromosome—in other words, the marker and QTL are linked. When numerous QTLs for a given trait have been located, a genetic map is created, showing the probability that specific chromosomal regions are associated with the phenotype of interest [**Figure 23–8(c)**]. Further research using genomic techniques identifies genes in these regions that contribute to the phenotype.

QTL mapping has been used extensively in agriculture, including plants such as corn, rice, wheat, and tomatoes (**Table 23.5**), and livestock such as cattle, pigs, sheep,

TABLE 23.5 QTLs for Quantitative Phenotypes

Organism	Quantitative Phenotype	QTLs Identified
Tomato	Soluble solids	7
	Fruit mass	13
	Fruit pH	9
	Growth	5
	Leaflet shape	9
	Height	9
Maize	Height	11
	Leaf length	7
	Grain yield	18
	Number of ears	10

Source: Used with permission of Annual Reviews of Genetics, from "Mapping Polygenes" by S.D. Tanksley, *Annual Review of Genetics*, Vol. 27:205–233, Table 1, December 1993. © Annual Reviews, Inc.

identify genomic differences among individuals by using chromosome-specific DNA markers such as restriction *fragment length polymorphisms (RFLPs)*, *microsatellites*, and *single-nucleotide polymorphisms (SNPs)* (see Chapter 21). Computer-based statistical analysis is used to search for linkage between the markers and a component of phenotypic variation associated with the trait. If a DNA marker (such as those markers described above) *is not* linked to a QTL, then the phenotypic mean score for the trait will and chickens. For example, hundreds of QTLs have been located in the tomato, and its genome has been sequenced. Many chromosome regions responsible for quantitative traits such as fruit size, shape, soluble solid content, and acidity have been identified. These QTLs are distributed on all 12 chromosomes representing the haploid genome of this plant.

A research program conducted by Steven Tanksley and his colleagues at Cornell University has focused on mapping and characterizing quantitative traits in the tomato, including fruit shape and weight. We will describe one aspect of this research, which represents a model approach in the study of QTLs. While the cultivated tomato can weigh up to 1000 grams, fruit from the related wild species thought to be the ancestor of the modern tomato weighs only a few grams [**Figure 23–9(a)**]. QTL mapping has identified more than 28 QTLs related to this thousand-fold variation in fruit weight. More than ten years of work was required to localize, identify, and clone one of these QTLs, called *fw2.2* (on chromosome 2). Within this QTL, a specific gene, *ORFX,* has been identified, and alleles at this locus are responsible for about 30 percent of the variation in fruit weight.

FIGURE 23–9 (a) The ancestral and modern-day tomato. (b) Phenotypic effect of the *fw2.2* transgene in the tomato. When the allele causing small fruit is transferred to a plant that normally produces large fruit, the fruit is reduced in size (+). A control fruit (−) that has not been transformed is shown for comparison.

The *ORFX* gene has been isolated, cloned, and transferred between plants, with interesting results. One allele of *ORFX* is present in all wild small-fruited varieties of tomatoes investigated, while another allele is present in all domesticated large-fruited varieties. When a cloned *ORFX* gene from small-fruited varieties is transferred to a plant that normally produces large tomatoes, the transformed plant produces fruits that are greatly reduced in weight [(**Figure 23–8(b)**]. In the varieties studied by Tanksley's group, the reduction averaged 17 grams, a statistically significant phenotypic change caused by the action of a gene found within a single QTL.

Further analysis of *ORFX* revealed that this gene encodes a protein that negatively regulates cell division during fruit development. Differences in the time of gene expression and differences in the amount of transcript produced lead to small or large fruit. Higher levels of expression mediated by transferred *ORFX* alleles exert a negative control over cell division, resulting in smaller tomatoes.

Yet *ORFX* and other related genes cannot account for all the observed variation in tomato size. Analysis of another QTL, *fas* (located on chromosome 11), indicates that the development of extreme differences in fruit size resulting from artificial selection also involves an increase in the number of compartments in the mature fruit. The small, ancestral stocks produce fruit with two to four seed compartments, but the large-fruited present-day strains have eight or more compartments. Thus, the QTLs that affect fruit size in tomatoes work by controlling at least two developmental processes: cell division early in development and the determination of the number of ovarian compartments.

The discovery that QTLs can control levels of gene expression has led to new, molecular definitions of phenotypes associated with quantitative traits. For example, the phenotype investigated may be the amount of an RNA transcript produced by a gene (**expression QTLs, or eQTLs**), or the amount of protein produced (**protein QTLs, or pQTLs**). These molecular phenotypes are polygenically controlled in the same way as more conventional phenotypes, such as fruit weight. Gene expression, for example, is controlled by *cis* factors, including promoters, and by *trans*-acting transcription factors (see Chapter 17 for a discussion of gene regulation in eukaryotes).

Expression QTLs (eQTLs) and Genetic Disorders

eQTLs are rapidly becoming an important tool in identifying genes responsible for complex diseases such as asthma, cleft lip, Type 2 diabetes, and coronary artery disease. For example, across the globe, asthma cases have risen dramatically over the last three decades, and this disease is now a major public health concern. Genome-wide association studies (GWAS) have identified loci that confer susceptibility to asthma and other pulmonary diseases. However, the functions of many of these genes are unknown, and GWAS alone are unable to establish which alleles of these loci are responsible for susceptibility or the mechanism of their action.

To identify genes directly involved in asthma susceptibility, researchers collected lung specimens from over 1000 individuals and used lung-specific gene expression as a phenotype to study how genetic variants (DNA polymorphisms) are linked to both gene expression (eQTLs) and the asthma phenotype. Integration of the GWAS and the eQTL data identified a network of 34 genes that constitute the most likely gene set that causes asthma. Six of these genes were identified as drivers that control the other genes in the network. These genes are candidates for drug discovery studies to develop therapies for this chronic and sometimes fatal disease. Similar approaches are likely to reveal the genetic networks that underlie other complex genetic disorders.

GENETICS, TECHNOLOGY, AND SOCIETY

The Green Revolution Revisited: Genetic Research with Rice

Of the 7 billion people now living on Earth, over 800 million do not have enough to eat. That number is expected to grow by an additional 1 million people each year for the next several decades. How will we be able to feed the estimated 8 billion people on Earth by 2025?

The past gives us some reasons to be optimistic. In the 1950s and 1960s, in the face of looming population increases, plant scientists around the world set about to increase the production of crop plants, including the three most important grains—rice, wheat, and maize. These efforts became known as the *Green Revolution*. The approach was three-fold: (1) to increase the use of fertilizers, pesticides, and irrigation; (2) to bring more land under cultivation; and (3) to develop improved varieties of crop plants by intensive plant breeding.

The results were dramatic. Developing nations more than doubled their production of rice, wheat, and maize between 1961 and 1985. Nations that were facing widespread famine in the 1960s were able to feed themselves and became major exporters of grain.

The Green Revolution saved millions of people from starvation and improved the quality of life for millions more; however, its effects may be diminishing. The rate of increase in grain yields has slowed since the 1980s, due to slower growth in irrigation development and fertilizer use. If food production is to keep pace with the projected increase in the world's population, we will have to depend more and more on the genetic improvement of crop plants to provide higher yields. But are we approaching the theoretical limits of yield in important crop plants? Recent work with rice suggests that the answer to this question may be a resounding no.

About half of the Earth's population depends on rice for basic nourishment. The Green Revolution for rice began in 1960, aided by the establishment of the International Rice Research Institute (IRRI). One of their major developments was the breeding of a rice variety with improved disease resistance and higher yield. The IRRI research team crossed a Chinese rice variety (*Dee-geo-woo-gen*) and an Indonesian variety (*Peta*) to create a new cultivar known as IR8. IR8 produced a greater number of rice kernels per plant, when grown in the presence of fertilizers and irrigation. Under these cultural practices, IR8 plants were so top-heavy with grain that they tended to fall over—a trait called "lodging." To reduce lodging, IRRI breeders crossed IR8 with a dwarf native variety to create semi-dwarf lines. Due in part to the adoption of the semi-dwarf IR8 lines, the world production of rice doubled in 25 years.

Predictions suggest that a 40 percent increase in the annual rice harvest may be necessary to keep pace with anticipated population growth during the next 30 years. As land and water resources become more scarce and the prices of fertilizers and pesticides grow, more emphasis will be placed on creating new rice varieties that have even higher yields and greater disease resistance.

Geneticists are now using several strategies to develop more productive rice. Conventional hybridization and selection techniques, such as those used to create the IR8 strain, continue to produce varieties that contribute to a productivity increase of between 1 and 10 percent a year. Dozens of quantitative trait loci (QTLs) from wild rice appear to contribute to increased yields, and scientists are attempting to introduce these traits into current dwarf varieties of domestic rice. Genomics and genetic engineering are also contributing to the new Green Revolution for rice. In 2002, the rice genome was the first cereal crop genome to be sequenced. Research is now concentrated on assigning a function to all the genes in the rice genome. Once identified and characterized, these genes may be transferred into crop plants, speeding the creation of rice varieties with desirable traits, such as disease resistance, tolerance to drought and salinity, and improved nutritional content.

Your Turn

Take time, individually or in groups, to answer the following questions. Investigate the references and links to help you understand some of the technologies and issues surrounding the new Green Revolution.

1. Almost half of the world's rice is grown in soils that are poor in nutrients, subject to flooding or drought, or farmed by people unable to afford fertilizers. Can genetic research address these limitations?

(continued)

Genetics, Technology, and Society, continued

One recent study indicates that a QLT locus in a wild rice variety may confer tolerance to several of these factors. Read about the promising research on the PSTOL1 gene in Gamuyao, R. et al. 2012. The protein kinase Pstol1 from traditional rice confers tolerance of phosphorus deficiency. *Nature* 488: 535–539.

2. A serious complication in our efforts to feed the Earth's population is global climate change. Given your assessment of current climate change predictions, what traits should we introduce into rice plants, and what methods can we use to do this?

To learn more about the effects of global climate change on agriculture, read Battisti, D. S. and Naylor, R. L. 2009. Historical warnings of future food insecurity with unprecedented seasonal heat. *Science* 323: 240–244.

3. Despite its benefits, the Green Revolution has been the subject of controversy. What are the main criticisms of the Green Revolution, and how can we mitigate some of the Green Revolution's negative aspects?

A discussion of this topic can be found in Pingali, P.L. 2012. Green Revolution: Impacts, limits, and the path ahead. *Proc. Natl. Acad. Sci. USA* 109 (31): 12302–12308.

CASE STUDY | A genetic flip of the coin

On July 11, 2008, twin sons were born to Stephan Gerth from Germany and Addo Gerth from Ghana. Stephan is very fair-skinned with blue eyes and straight hair; Addo is dark-skinned, with brown eyes and curly hair. The first born of the twins, Ryan, is fair-skinned, with blue eyes and straight hair; his brother, Leo, has light brown skin, brown eyes, and curly hair. Although the twins' hair texture and eye color were the same as those of one or the other parent, the twins had different skin colors, intermediate to that of their parents. Experts explained that the blending effect of skin color in the twins resulted from quantitative inheritance involving at least three different gene pairs, whereas hair texture and eye color are not quantitatively inherited. Using this as an example of quantitative genetics, we can ask the following questions:

1. What approach is used in estimating how many gene pairs are involved in a quantitative trait? Why would this be extremely difficult in the case of skin color in humans?

2. Would either parent need to have mixed-race ancestry for the twins to be so different?

3. Would twins showing some parental traits (hair texture, eye color) but a blending of other traits (skin color in this case) seem to be a commonplace event, or are we looking at a "one in a million" event?

Summary Points

MasteringGenetics™ For activities, animations, and review quizzes, go to the Study Area.

1. Quantitative inheritance results in a range of phenotypes due to the action of additive alleles from two or more genes, as influenced by environmental factors.
2. Numerous statistical methods are essential during the analysis of quantitative traits, including the mean, variance, standard deviation, standard error, covariance, and the correlation coefficient.
3. Heritability is an estimate of the relative contribution of genetic versus environmental factors to the range of phenotypic variation seen in a quantitative trait in a particular population and environment.
4. Twin studies are used to estimate the heritability of multifactorial traits in humans.
5. Quantitative trait loci, or QTLs, may be identified and mapped using DNA markers.

INSIGHTS AND SOLUTIONS

1. In a certain plant, height varies from 6 to 36 cm. When 6-cm and 36-cm plants were crossed, all F_1 plants were 21 cm. In the F_2 generation, a continuous range of heights was observed. Most were around 21 cm, and 3 of 200 were as short as the 6-cm P_1 parent.

   (a) What mode of inheritance does this illustrate, and how many gene pairs are involved?

   (b) How much does each additive allele contribute to height?

   (c) List all genotypes that give rise to plants that are 31 cm.

Solution:

(a) Polygenic inheritance is illustrated when a trait is continuous and when alleles contribute additively to the phenotype. The 3/200 ratio of F_2 plants is the key to determining the number of gene pairs. This reduces to a ratio of 1/66.7, very close to 1/64. Using the formula $1/4^n = 1/64$ (where 1/64 is equal to the proportion of F_2 phenotypes as extreme as either P_1 parent), $n = 3$. Therefore, three gene pairs are involved.

(b) The variation between the two extreme phenotypes is

$$36 - 6 = 30 \text{ cm}$$

Because there are six potential additive alleles (*AABBCC*), each contributes

$$30/6 = 5 \text{ cm}$$

to the base height of 6 cm, which results when no additive alleles (*aabbcc*) are part of the genotype.

(c) All genotypes that include five additive alleles will be 31 cm (5 alleles × 5 cm/allele + 6 cm base height = 31 cm). Therefore, *AABBCc*, *AABbCC*, and *AaBBCC* are the genotypes that will result in plants that are 31 cm.

2. In a cross separate from the above-mentioned F_1 crosses, a plant of unknown phenotype and genotype was testcrossed, with the following results:

1/4   11 cm
2/4   16 cm
1/4   21 cm

An astute genetics student realized that the unknown plant could be only one phenotype but could be any of three genotypes. What were they?

Solution: When testcrossed (with *aabbcc*), the unknown plant must be able to contribute either one, two, or three additive alleles in its gametes in order to yield the three phenotypes in the offspring. Since no 6-cm offspring are observed, the unknown plant never contributes all nonadditive alleles (*abc*). Only plants that are homozygous at one locus and heterozygous at the other two loci will meet these criteria. Therefore, the unknown parent can be any of three genotypes, all of which have a phenotype of 26 cm:

AABbCc

AaBbCC

AaBBCc

For example, in the first genotype (*AABbCc*),

AABbCc × *aabbcc*

yields

1/4   *AaBbCc*   21 cm
1/4   *AaBbcc*   16 cm
1/4   *AabbCc*   16 cm
1/4   *Aabbcc*   11 cm

which is the ratio of phenotypes observed.

3. The mean and variance of corolla length in two highly inbred strains of *Nicotiana* and their progeny are shown in the following table. One parent (P_1) has a short corolla, and the other parent (P_2) has a long corolla. Calculate the broad-sense heritability (H^2) of corolla length in this plant.

Strain	Mean (mm)	Variance (mm)
P_1 short	40.47	3.12
P_2 long	93.75	3.87
F_1 ($P_1 \times P_2$)	63.90	4.74
F_2 ($F_1 \times F_1$)	68.72	47.70

Solution: The formula for estimating heritability is $H^2 = V_G/V_P$, where V_G and V_P are the genetic and phenotypic components of variation, respectively. The main issue in this problem is obtaining some estimate of two components of phenotypic variation: genetic and environmental factors. V_P is the combination of genetic and environmental variance. Because the two parental strains are true breeding, they are assumed to be homozygous, and the variance of 3.12 and 3.87 is considered to be the result of environmental influences. The average of these two values is 3.50. The F_1 is also genetically homogeneous and gives us an additional estimate of the impact of environmental factors. By averaging this value along with that of the parents,

$$\frac{4.74 + 3.50}{2} = 4.12$$

we obtain a relatively good idea of environmental impact on the phenotype. The phenotypic variance in the F_2 is the sum of the genetic (V_G) and environmental (V_E) components. We have estimated the environmental input as 4.12, so 47.70 minus 4.12 gives us an estimate of V_G of 43.58. Heritability then becomes 43.58/47.70, or 0.91. This value, when interpreted as a percentage, indicates that about 91 percent of the variation in corolla length is due to genetic influences.

Problems and Discussion Questions

MasteringGenetics™ Visit for instructor-assigned tutorials and problems.

HOW DO WE KNOW?

1. In this chapter, we focused on a mode of inheritance referred to as quantitative genetics, as well as many of the statistical parameters utilized to study quantitative traits. Along the way, we found opportunities to consider the methods and reasoning by which geneticists acquired much of their understanding of quantitative genetics. From the explanations given in the chapter, what answers would you propose to the following fundamental questions:

(a) How do we know that threshold traits are actually polygenic even though they may have as few as two discrete phenotypic classes?

(b) How can we ascertain the number of polygenes involved in the inheritance of a quantitative trait?

(c) What findings led geneticists to postulate the multiple-factor hypothesis that invoked the idea of additive alleles to explain inheritance patterns?

(d) How do we assess environmental factors to determine if they impact the phenotype of a quantitatively inherited trait?

(e) How do we know that monozygotic twins are not identical genotypically as adults?

2. Review the Chapter Concepts list on page 604. These all center around quantitative inheritance and the study and analysis of polygenic traits. Write a short essay that discusses the difference between the more traditional Mendelian and neo-Mendelian modes of inheritance (qualitative inheritance) and quantitative inheritance.

3. Define the following: (a) polygenic, (b) additive alleles, (c) correlation, (d) monozygotic and dizygotic twins, (e) heritability, (f) QTL, and (g) continuous variation.

4. A dark-red strain and a white strain of wheat are crossed and produce an intermediate, medium-red F_1. When the F_1 plants are interbred, an F_2 generation is produced in a ratio of 1 dark-red: 4 medium-dark-red: 6 medium-red: 4 light-red: 1 white. Further crosses reveal that the dark-red and white F_2 plants are true breeding.

(a) Based on the ratios in the F_2 population, how many genes are involved in the production of color?

(b) How many additive alleles are needed to produce each possible phenotype?

(c) Assign symbols to these alleles and list possible genotypes that give rise to the medium-red and light-red phenotypes.

(d) Predict the outcome of the F_1 and F_2 generations in a cross between a true-breeding medium-red plant and a white plant.

5. Height in humans depends on the additive action of genes. Assume that this trait is controlled by the four loci R, S, T, and U and that environmental effects are negligible. Instead of additive versus nonadditive alleles, assume that additive and partially additive alleles exist. Additive alleles contribute two units, and partially additive alleles contribute one unit to height.

(a) Can two individuals of moderate height produce offspring that are much taller or shorter than either parent? If so, how?

(b) If an individual with the minimum height specified by these genes marries an individual of intermediate or moderate height, will any of their children be taller than the tall parent? Why or why not?

6. An inbred strain of plants has a mean height of 24 cm. A second strain of the same species from a different geographical region also has a mean height of 24 cm. When plants from the two strains are crossed together, the F_1 plants are the same height as the parent plants. However, the F_2 generation shows a wide range of heights; the majority are like the P_1 and F_1 plants, but approximately 4 of 1000 are only 12 cm high and about 4 of 1000 are 36 cm high.

(a) What mode of inheritance is occurring here?

(b) How many gene pairs are involved?

(c) How much does each gene contribute to plant height?

(d) Indicate one possible set of genotypes for the original P_1 parents and the F_1 plants that could account for these results.

(e) Indicate three possible genotypes that could account for F_2 plants that are 18 cm high and three that account for F_2 plants that are 33 cm high.

7. Erma and Harvey were a compatible barnyard pair, but a curious sight. Harvey's tail was only 6 cm long, while Erma's was 30 cm. Their F_1 piglet offspring all grew tails that were 18 cm. When inbred, an F_2 generation resulted in many piglets (Erma and Harvey's grandpigs), whose tails ranged in 4-cm intervals from 6 to 30 cm (6, 10, 14, 18, 22, 26, and 30). Most had 18-cm tails, while 1/64 had 6-cm tails and 1/64 had 30-cm tails.

(a) Explain how these tail lengths were inherited by describing the mode of inheritance, indicating how many gene pairs were at work, and designating the genotypes of Harvey, Erma, and their 18-cm-tail offspring.

(b) If one of the 18-cm F_1 pigs is mated with one of the 6-cm F_2 pigs, what phenotypic ratio will be predicted if many offspring resulted? Diagram the cross.

8. In the following table, average differences of height, weight, and fingerprint ridge count between monozygotic twins (reared together and apart), dizygotic twins, and nontwin siblings are compared:

Trait	MZ Reared Together	MZ Reared Apart	DZ Reared Together	Sibs Reared Together
Height (cm)	1.7	1.8	4.4	4.5
Weight (kg)	1.9	4.5	4.5	4.7
Ridge count	0.7	0.6	2.4	2.7

Based on the data in this table, which of these quantitative traits has the highest heritability values?

9. What kind of heritability estimates (broad sense or narrow sense) are obtained from human twin studies?

10. List as many human traits as you can that are likely to be under the control of a polygenic mode of inheritance.

11. Corn plants from a test plot are measured, and the distribution of heights at 10-cm intervals is recorded in the following table:

Height (cm)	Plants (no.)
100	20
110	60
120	90
130	130
140	180
150	120
160	70
170	50
180	40

Calculate (a) the mean height, (b) the variance, (c) the standard deviation, and (d) the standard error of the mean. Plot a rough graph of plant height against frequency. Do the values represent a normal distribution? Based on your calculations, how would you assess the variation within this population?

12. The following variances were calculated for two traits in a herd of hogs.

Trait	V_P	V_G	V_A
Back fat	30.6	12.2	8.44
Body length	52.4	26.4	11.70

(a) Calculate broad-sense (H^2) and narrow-sense (h^2) heritabilities for each trait in this herd.

(b) Which of the two traits will respond best to selection by a breeder? Why?

13. The mean and variance of plant height of two highly inbred strains (P_1 and P_2) and their progeny (F_1 and F_2) are shown here.

Strain	Mean (cm)	Variance
P_1	34.2	4.2
P_2	55.3	3.8
F_1	44.2	5.6
F_2	46.3	10.3

Calculate the broad-sense heritability (H^2) of plant height in this species.

14. A hypothetical study investigated the vitamin A content and the cholesterol content of eggs from a large population of chickens. The variances (V) were calculated, as shown here:

	Trait	
Variance	Vitamin A	Cholesterol
V_P	123.5	862.0
V_E	96.2	484.6
V_A	12.0	192.1
V_D	15.3	185.3

(a) Calculate the narrow-sense heritability (h^2) for both traits.

(b) Which trait, if either, is likely to respond to selection?

15. In a herd of dairy cows the narrow-sense heritability for milk protein content is 0.76, and for milk butterfat it is 0.82. The correlation coefficient between milk protein content and butterfat is 0.91. If the farmer selects for cows producing more butterfat in their milk, what will be the most likely effect on milk protein content in the next generation?

16. In an assessment of learning in *Drosophila*, flies were trained to avoid certain olfactory cues. In one population, a mean of 8.5 trials was required. A subgroup of this parental population that was trained most quickly (mean = 6.0) was interbred, and their progeny were examined. These flies demonstrated a mean training value of 7.5. Calculate realized heritability for olfactory learning in *Drosophila*.

17. Suppose you want to develop a population of *Drosophila* that would rapidly learn to avoid certain substances the flies could detect by smell. Based on the heritability estimate you obtained in Problem 16, do you think it would be worth doing this by artificial selection? Why or why not?

18. In a population of tomato plants, mean fruit weight is 60 g and h^2 is 0.3. Predict the mean weight of the progeny if tomato plants whose fruit averaged 80 g were selected from the original population and interbred.

19. In a population of 100 inbred, genotypically identical rice plants, variance for grain yield is 4.67. What is the heritability for yield? Would you advise a rice breeder to improve yield in this strain of rice plants by selection?

20. Many traits of economic or medical significance are determined by quantitative trait loci (QTLs) in which many genes, usually scattered throughout the genome, contribute to expression.

(a) What general procedures are used to identify such loci?

(b) What is meant by the term *cosegregate* in the context of QTL mapping? Why are markers such as RFLPs, SNPs, and microsatellites often used in QTL mapping?

Extra-Spicy Problems

MasteringGenetics™ Visit for instructor-assigned tutorials and problems.

21. A 3-inch plant was crossed with a 15-inch plant, and all F_1 plants were 9 inches. The F_2 plants exhibited a "normal distribution," with heights of 3, 4, 5, 6, 7, 8, 9, 10, 11, 12, 13, 14, and 15 inches.

(a) What ratio will constitute the "normal distribution" in the F_2?

(b) What will be the outcome if the F_1 plants are testcrossed with plants that are homozygous for all nonadditive alleles?

22. In a cross between a strain of large guinea pigs and a strain of small guinea pigs, the F_1 are phenotypically uniform, with an average size about intermediate between that of the two parental strains. Among 1014 F_2 individuals, 3 are about the same size as the small parental strain and 5 are about the same size as the large parental strain. How many gene pairs are involved in the inheritance of size in these strains of guinea pigs?

23. Type A1B brachydactyly (short middle phalanges) is a genetically determined trait that maps to the short arm of chromosome 5 in humans. If you classify individuals as either having or not having brachydactyly, the trait appears to follow a single-locus, incompletely dominant pattern of inheritance. However, if one examines the fingers and toes of affected individuals, one sees a range of expression from extremely short to only slightly short. What might cause such variation in the expression of brachydactyly?

24. In a series of crosses between two true-breeding strains of peaches, the F_1 generation was uniform, producing 30-g peaches. The F_2 fruit mass ranges from 38 to 22 g at intervals of 2 g.

(a) Using these data, determine the number of polygenic loci involved in the inheritance of peach mass.

(b) Using gene symbols of your choice, give the genotypes of the parents and the F_1.

25. Students in a genetics laboratory began an experiment in an attempt to increase heat tolerance in two strains of *Drosophila melanogaster*. One strain was trapped from the wild six weeks before the experiment was to begin; the other was obtained from a *Drosophila* repository at a university laboratory. In which strain would you expect to see the most rapid and extensive response to heat-tolerance selection, and why?

26. Consider a true-breeding plant, *AABBCC*, crossed with another true-breeding plant, *aabbcc*, whose resulting offspring are *AaBbCc*. If you cross the F_1 generation, and independent assortment is operational, the expected fraction of offspring in each phenotypic class is given by the expression $N!/M!(N - M)!$ where N is the total number of alleles (six in this example) and M is the number of uppercase alleles. In a cross of

AaBbCc × AaBbCc, what proportion of the offspring would be expected to contain two uppercase alleles?

27. Canine hip dysplasia is a quantitative trait that continues to affect most large breeds of dogs in spite of approximately 40 years of effort to reduce the impact of this condition. Breeders and veterinarians rely on radiographic and universal registries to facilitate the development of breeding schemes for reducing its incidence. Data (Wood and Lakhani. 2003. *Vet. Rec.* 152: 69–72) indicate that there is a "month-of-birth" effect on hip dysplasia in Labrador retrievers and Gordon setters, whereby the frequency and extent of expression of this disorder vary depending on the time of year dogs are born. Speculate on how breeders attempt to "select" out this disorder and what the month-of-birth phenomenon indicates about the expression of polygenic traits.

28. Floral traits in plants often play key roles in diversification, in that slight modifications of those traits, if genetically determined, may quickly lead to reproductive restrictions and evolution. Insight into genetic involvement in flower formation is often acquired through selection experiments that expose realized heritability. Lendvai and Levin (2003) conducted a series of artificial selection experiments on flower size (diameter) in *Phlox drummondii.* Data from their selection experiments are presented in the following table in modified form and content.

Year	Treatment	Mean (mm)
1997	Control	30.04
	Selected parents	34.13
	Offspring	32.21
1998	Control	28.11
	Selected parents	31.98
	Offspring	31.90
1999	Control	29.68
	Selected parents	31.81
	Offspring	33.74

(a) Considering that differences in control values represent year-to-year differences in greenhouse conditions, calculate (in mm) the average response to selection over the three-year period.
(b) Calculate the realized heritability for each year and the overall realized heritability.
(c) Assuming that the realized heritability in phlox is relatively high, what factors might account for such a high response?
(d) In terms of evolutionary potential, is a population with high heritability likely to be favored compared to one with a low realized heritability?

29. In 1988, Horst Wilkens investigated blind cavefish, comparing them with members of a sibling species with normal vision that are found in a lake [Wilkens, H. (1988). *Ecol. Biol.* 23: 271–367]. We will call them cavefish and lakefish. Wilkens found that cavefish eyes are about seven times smaller than lakefish eyes. F_1 hybrids have eyes of intermediate size. These data, as well as the $F_1 \times F_1$ cross and those from backcrosses ($F_1 \times$ cavefish and $F_1 \times$ lakefish), are depicted below. Examine Wilkens's results and respond to the following questions:

(a) Based strictly on the F_1 and F_2 results of Wilkens's initial crosses, what possible explanation concerning the inheritance of eye size seems most feasible?
(b) Based on the results of the F_1 backcross with cavefish, is your explanation supported? Explain.
(c) Based on the results of the F_1 backcross with lakefish, is your explanation supported? Explain.
(d) Wilkens examined about 1000 F_2 progeny and estimated that 6–7 genes are involved in determining eye size. Is the sample size adequate to justify this conclusion? Propose an experimental protocol to test the hypothesis.
(e) A comparison of the embryonic eye in cavefish and lakefish revealed that both reach approximately 4 mm in diameter. However, lakefish eyes continue to grow, while cavefish eye size is greatly reduced. Speculate on the role of the genes involved in this problem.

A colorized cross section of the human brain. The average brain contains about 86 billion neurons, each of which is connected to many other neurons by synapses.

24 Neurogenetics

CHAPTER CONCEPTS

- Behavior is a complex response to stimuli that is mediated both by genes and by the environment.

- Lines of evidence including observations on species-specific behaviors and the use of artificial selection have established the role of genetics in behavior. In humans, studies of families, twins, and adoptions confirm that many forms of behavior in our species have a genetic basis.

- Genetic and molecular studies of behavior in model organisms and in humans are centered on understanding the role of genes and environment in shaping the development, structure, and function of the nervous system, and its components, especially the synapse.

- Genetic and genomic approaches to the study of behavior have been successfully used in *Drosophila* and the mouse, making them useful model organisms for the study of nervous system function and the mechanisms that underlie human behavioral disorders.

- Many human behavioral disorders are complex responses to stimuli. These responses are mediated by genes, environmental factors, and interactions among genes and the environment. More recently, newly developed genomic techniques are being used to study the role of genes in human behavior.

Behavior is generally defined as a reaction to stimuli, whether internal or external, that alter an organism's response to its environment. Animals run, remain still, or counterattack in the presence of a predator; birds build complex and distinctive nests in response to a combination of internal and external signals; plants bend toward light; and humans behave in both simple and complex ways guided by their intellect, emotions, and culture.

The role of heredity in behavior was first examined in the nineteenth century by Francis Galton, who systematically studied behavior and heredity. In one of his early studies, he examined his own family (he was a cousin of Charles Darwin) trying to find a pattern of inheritance associated with intelligence. By the early 1900s, clear-cut cases of genetic influence on behavior had been identified, but at the time, behavior was primarily of interest to psychologists, who categorized behavior as either innate or conditioned. Innate behavior is present at birth (reflexes, for example), while conditioned behavior is learned through experience. At this time, psychologists thought that conditioned behaviors were produced by environmental factors to the exclusion of genetic influences. The difference between a genetic and an environmental approach to behavior was the starting point for the nature versus nurture debate. In this simplistic (and false) dichotomy, behavior is controlled entirely either by genes or by the environment.

This controversy presented a distorted view of the nature of behavioral responses. After all, any behavior must rely on the expression of an individual's genotype, which takes place within a hierarchy of environmental settings (that is, gene expression depends on interactions within the cell, the tissue, the organ, the organism, and finally the population and surrounding environment). Without genes and their environments, there could be no behavior. Nevertheless, the nature–nurture controversy flourished well into the 1950s, when it became clear that behavioral patterns were the result of the interaction of genetic and environmental factors. The prevailing view today is that most behaviors are complex traits involving a number of genes, as well as interactions between the products of these genes and environmental influences. In this scenario, the genotype provides the biological underpinnings or mental ability (or both) required to execute a behavior and further determines the limitations of environmental influences.

The definition of behavior based on observable changes in the relationship of a cell or an organism to its environment as the result of some stimulus broadly identifies the phenotype that geneticists use as a starting point for investigating the biological basis of behavior. Evidence that some behaviors have a genetic basis comes from several lines of evidence: observable species-specific behaviors, such as courtship rituals, and artificial selection, which draws upon individual variations in behavior among organisms in populations that can be used to establish strains with heritable differences in behavior. In humans, twin studies have provided evidence for the role of heredity in behavioral responses.

Because the nervous system senses the environment, processes the information, and initiates the response that we perceive as behavior, much of the study of behavior in genetics focuses on the development, structure, and function of the nervous system and its components. In this chapter, we will examine several approaches to studying the genetic basis of behavior, and consider what we have learned about the genetic and molecular basis of human behavior from research and the use of model organisms. Please note that some of the topics discussed in this chapter are explored in greater depth later in the text (see Special Topic Chapter 1—Epigenetics).

24.1 The Central Nervous System Receives Sensory Input and Generates Behavioral Responses

Behavior is an innate or a learned response to environmental stimuli. These stimuli are received and processed by the nervous system, which generates a response in the

Central Nervous System (CNS)

Brain

Spinal cord

FIGURE 24–1 The central nervous system is composed of the brain and the spinal cord.

form of behavior and stores this and other experiences as memories. For these reasons, the nervous system is the central focus of behavior genetics. In humans and other vertebrates, the brain and the spinal cord (**Figure 24–1**) form the central nervous system (CNS), while the peripheral nervous system includes the nerves that radiate from the CNS.

Organization of Cells in the Central Nervous System

At the cellular level, the central nervous system contains several cell types, including nerve cells, or neurons (**Figure 24–2**). The nucleus of a neuron is contained in the cell body, and there are two types of cytoplasmic extensions, which allow the cell to receive and send signals. These signals, in the form of electrical impulses, are received by cytoplasmic extensions called dendrites located at one end of the cell. These electrical impulses move across the cell to cytoplasmic extensions called axons at the other end of the cell. From the axon, the signal may be transferred to adjacent neurons. During this process, the impulse is propagated by the transport of sodium and potassium ions across the plasma membrane of the neuron (Figure 24–2). The movement of these charged ions depolarizes the membrane and can be monitored by measuring changes in the electrical potential of the membrane.

Although the human nervous system is composed of billions of neurons, they do not work individually, but instead are tightly integrated into functional groups. The patterns of synaptic connections between and among neurons form circuits (**Figure 24–3**) that determine the capacities of each functional group. Diverging circuits [**Figure 24–3(a)**]

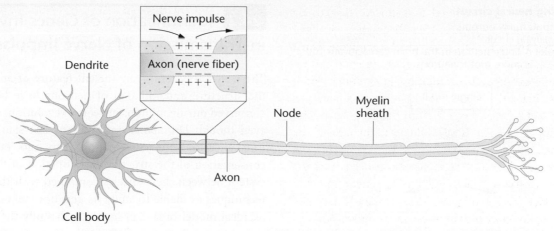

FIGURE 24–2 A nerve cell (neuron) has extensions called dendrites that carry impulses toward the cell body and also has one or more axons that carry impulses away from the cell body. The axon is encased in a sheath of myelin, except at nodes spaced at intervals along the axon. The movement of nerve impulses is accelerated by jumping from node to node. Electrodes placed on either side of the neuron's plasma membrane can record the electric potential across the membrane. When the neuron is at rest, there is more sodium outside the cell and more potassium inside the cell. When a nerve impulse is generated, sodium moves into the cell, and potassium moves out, altering the electric potential. As the impulse moves away, sodium and potassium ions are pumped in opposite directions to restore the original electric potential.

receive input from one neuron and distribute this signal to many other neurons. This typically occurs when external stimuli are received by the sensory system and distributed to many different parts of the brain. In converging circuits [**Figure 24–3(b)**], a variable number of neurons may input signals to a single neuron. This concentrates input from several sources and generates a single response.

Synapses Transfer Information between Neurons

Information flow through the chains of neurons that make up the nervous system depends on junctions that functionally connect neurons to each other. **Synapses** are junctions between the axon of one neuron and the dendrite of another neuron (**Figure 24–4**). The gap separating two neurons at a synapse is called the **synaptic cleft**, a fluid-filled space approximately 30–50 nm wide. Neurons sending impulses toward the synapse are called presynaptic neurons, while those that transmit impulses away from the synapse are known as postsynaptic neurons (Figure 24–4).

The tips of axons contain vesicles, each of which is filled with neurotransmitter molecules. When a nerve impulse arrives at the end of the axon, it triggers the release of neurotransmitters into the synaptic cleft. These chemical signals diffuse across the cleft and bind to receptor molecules on the membrane of the postsynaptic neuron. Neurotransmitter binding produces a change in the shape of the receptor, which in turn generates a nerve impulse in the postsynaptic cell. In other words, the nerve impulse arrives as an electrical signal at the axon, where it causes the release, diffusion, and binding of a chemical signal, which

in turn generates a new electrical impulse in the dendrite on the other side of the synapse.

As long as a neurotransmitter remains bound to its receptor, nerve impulses continue to be generated by the postsynaptic neuron. Generally, the effects of the neurotransmitter are terminated in a few milliseconds. This occurs by reuptake or enzymatic degradation of the neurotransmitter, or by its diffusion out of the synapse (Figure 24–4). Several different classes of chemicals can act as neurotransmitters (Table 24.1), and each is associated with a specific type of receptor.

TABLE 24.1 Some Neurotransmitters in the Central Nervous System

Acetylcholine (Ach) amines
Norepinephrine
Dopamine
Serotonin

Amino acids
GABA (γ-aminobutryic acid)
Glutamate
Glycine

Peptides
Endorphins
Tachykinins
Somatostatin
Cholecystokinin

Gases and lipids
Nitric oxide (NO)
Carbon monoxide (CO)
Endocannabinoids

(a) Diverging neural circuit:
- One input, many outputs
- An *amplifying* circuit
- **Example:** A single neuron in the brain can acitvate 100 or more motor neurons

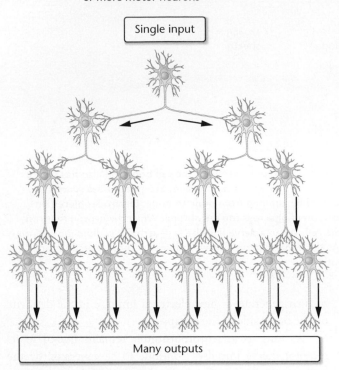

Single input

Many outputs

(b) Converging neural circuit:
- Many inputs, one output
- A *concentrating* circuit
- **Example:** Different sensory stimuli can all elicit the same memory

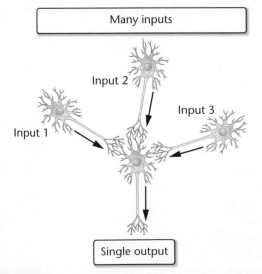

Many inputs

Input 1

Input 2

Input 3

Single output

FIGURE 24–3 Two major types of nerve circuits in the brain. (a) Diverging circuits take a single impulse and distribute it to many motor neurons. (b) Converging circuits consolidate multiple impulses and generate a single output response.

24.2 Identification of Genes Involved in Transmission of Nerve Impulses

The nervous system is an ancient feature of animals, and the structure and function of neurons have been highly conserved during millions of years of evolution. As a result, even though *Drosophila* and humans last shared a common ancestor some 800 million years ago, evolutionary conservation of the structure and function of the nervous system between these species combined with the genomic techniques available to study its genetics make *Drosophila* an ideal model organism in which to study the molecular genetics of behavior and the nervous system. The wide-ranging and sophisticated array of genetic tools available to study *Drosophila* include marker chromosomes, strains with duplicated and deleted chromosome regions, and an extensive collection of mutant strains displaying aberrant behavioral traits. These genetic resources along with the information gained from its genome sequence make it possible to use *Drosophila* as a model organism to identify and isolate genes involved in behavior. In turn, these *Drosophila* genes may be used to probe the human genome for related human genes.

As a case in point, Barry Ganetzky and his colleagues screened behavioral mutants of *Drosophila* to identify those with electrophysiological abnormalities in the generation and propagation of nerve impulses. Two general classes of such mutants have been isolated: those with defects in the movement of sodium and those with defects in potassium transport (**Table 24.2**). One mutant identified in the screening procedure is a temperature-sensitive allele of the *paralytic* gene. Flies homozygous for this mutant allele become paralyzed when exposed to temperatures at or above 29°C, but recover rapidly when the temperature is lowered to 25°C. Electrophysiological studies showed that mutant flies have defective sodium transport associated with the conduction of nerve impulses.

Subsequently, Ganetzky and his colleagues mapped, isolated, and cloned the *paralytic* gene. This locus encodes a sodium channel protein, which controls the movement of sodium across the membrane of nerve cells in many different organisms, from flies to humans. The human version of the *para* gene is called *SCN1A*, which encodes part of the human sodium channel gene. Mutations in this gene produce fever-induced epileptic seizures and generalized epilepsy. These same researchers found that another mutant allele, called *Shaker* (originally isolated over 40 years ago as a behavioral mutant), encodes a potassium channel protein. This gene has also been cloned and characterized. Because the mechanism of nerve impulse conduction has been highly conserved during animal evolution, the cloned

FIGURE 24–4 The stages in transmission of a nerve impulse across the synapse.

TABLE 24.2 Behavioral Mutants of *Drosophila* in Which Nerve Impulse Transmission Is Affected

Mutation	Map Location	Ion Channel Affected	Phenotype
nap^{ts}	2-56.2	Sodium	Adults and larvae paralyzed at 37.5°C; reversible at 25°C
$para^{ts}$	1-53.9	Sodium	Adults paralyzed at 29°C, larvae at 37°C; reversible at 25°C
Tip-E	3-13.5	Sodium	Adults and larvae paralyzed at 39–40°C; reversible at 25°C
sei^{ts}	2-10.6	Sodium	Adults paralyzed at 38°C, larvae unaffected; adults recover at 25°C
Sh	1-57.7	Potassium	Aberrant leg shaking in adults exposed to ether
eag	1-50.0	Potassium	Aberrant leg shaking in adults exposed to ether
Hk	1-30.0	Potassium	Ether-induced leg shaking
sio	3-85.0	Potassium	At 22°C, adults are weak fliers; at 38°C, adults are weak, uncoordinated

Drosophila genes were used as probes to isolate the equivalent human potassium ion channel gene, *KCN1A*, which maps to chromosome 12. Mutations in this gene cause involuntary muscle tremors and postural changes, a condition called episodic ataxia Type 1.

Ganetzky's group used *eag*, another *Drosophila* behavioral mutant allele, as a probe to identify the equivalent gene in humans, which is called *KCNH2*. This gene encodes a protein component of the potassium channel. In humans, loss-of-function mutations in this gene produce a genetic disorder associated with potentially fatal cardiac arrhythmias. The isolation and cloning of this gene have made it possible to screen and identify family members at risk for this fatal disorder. Mutations in ion channel genes, collectively called channelopathies, are being used to study the molecular basis of nerve impulse transmission in humans.

NOW SOLVE THIS

24–1 Assume that you discovered a fruit fly that walked with a limp and was continually off balance as it moved. Describe how you would determine whether this behavior was due to an injury (induced in the environment) or to an inherited trait. Assuming that it was inherited, what are the various ways a gene might lead to this trait? Describe how you would determine the mechanism of gene expression experimentally if the gene were X-linked.

■ **HINT:** *This problem involves an understanding of how traits are inherited and transmitted to offspring in Mendelian crosses and the expected outcome of crosses involving recessive, dominant, and X-linked genes. The key to its solution is to first determine whether your analysis will begin by first identifying and isolating the gene, or by using the behavior as a phenotypic marker.*

24.3 Synapses Are Involved in Many Human Behavioral Disorders

The development, structure, function, and maintenance of synapses are essential for normal brain function and normal patterns of behavior. Each neuron in the human brain contains, on average, 1000 synapses, connecting it to a multitude of other neurons, resulting in a total of about 100 trillion synapses in the brain.

A research team using proteomics (see Chapter 21) isolated and identified 1461 proteins associated with synapses. Screening the human genome with the proteomic data matched each protein to a different gene. These 1461 genes constitute about 7.5 percent of the human genome's 20,000 genes, illustrating both the complexity of the syn-

TABLE 24.3 Some Behavioral Disorders with Synaptic Defects	
Alzheimer disease	Huntington disease
Angelman syndrome	MAOA deficiency
Autism	Major depressive disorder
Bipolar disorder	Phelan–McDermid syndrome
Charcot–Marie–Tooth syndrome	Rett syndrome
Down syndrome	Schizophrenia
Epilepsy	Tuberous sclerosis syndrome
Fragile-X syndrome	

apse and its importance in brain function. Matching the cataloged synapse genes with known genetic disorders revealed that mutations in 169 of these genes are associated with 269 different heritable diseases, many of which have behavioral components (Table 24.3). These disorders, which affect millions of people, include epilepsy, Alzheimer disease, Huntington disease, some forms of autism and learning disabilities, as well as addiction and drug abuse and many rare behavioral disorders.

At the cellular level, the phenotypes of these disorders involve changes in neuron structure, neurodegeneration, and dysfunctional synaptic transmission. As we will see later in this chapter, different behavioral disorders often involve the same genes and encoded protein sets, raising the possibility that treatments developed for one disorder may be effective in treating other, genetically related disorders. Some examples of single-gene human behavioral disorders involving synaptic genes will be presented before we consider disorders with more complex causes.

A Defect in Neurotransmitter Breakdown

In 1993, researchers identified a family with a new form of mild intellectual disability and behavioral changes. All affected males in this family engaged in aggressive and frequently violent behavior (**Figure 24–5**). This characteristic pattern of behavior was often triggered by fear, frustration, or anger, and included arson, attempted rape, and stabbings. Pedigree analysis indicated that this trait is X-linked. The gene was mapped to a location near another gene that encodes the enzyme monoamine oxidase type A (MAOA). In the nervous system, this enzyme acts in the synapse to break down several types of neurotransmitters. Recall that once neurotransmitters have generated a nerve impulse in the postsynaptic neuron, they must be cleared from the synapse. The mutant *MAOA* allele present in affected family members encodes a nonfunctional form of this enzyme.

FIGURE 24–5 Mutations in the *MAOA* gene cosegregate with aggressive behavior. Affected males are shown by filled symbols. Symbols with dots inside represent females known to be heterozygous carriers of the mutant allele.

Failure to clear neurotransmitters from the synapse disrupts the normal function of the nervous system, which is reflected in the behavioral phenotype and the presence of elevated levels of neurotransmitter-related chemicals in the urine of affected individuals.

Additional research in children and young adults with behavioral problems has revealed that another allele of the *MAOA* gene is associated with a predisposition to criminal and delinquent behavior, but this behavior is manifested only after exposure to certain environmental factors. While there is some question as to whether the effects of MAOA metabolism are primary or secondary effects in these behaviors, the association suggests that pharmacological treatment of these conditions may be possible.

Fragile-X Syndrome and Synapses

Fragile-X syndrome is one of the most common causes of heritable intellectual deficits and affects about 1 in 4000 males and 1 in 8000 females. This disorder also causes autism in about 15–30 percent of all cases. Fragile-X (or Martin–Bell syndrome) is caused by a dominantly inherited mutant allele on the X chromosome (see Chapter 8 for a discussion of the genetic aspects of fragile-X syndrome).

The normal allele in fragile-X syndrome encodes a protein called FMRP (Fragile-X Mental Retardation Protein). At the cellular level, FMRP is an RNA-binding protein that represses translation. In normal cells, FMRP regulates the translation of a number of synaptic proteins. Most of these proteins are required to maintain synaptic strength, which is the level of response generated by increases or decreases in synaptic activity.

When the neurotransmitter glutamine is released and crosses the synapse, it binds to mGluR5 receptors, a class of receptors involved in learning and memory. Binding of glutamine activates mGluR5 signaling pathways which stimulate protein synthesis in the regions near the synapse. The normal FMRP protein modulates mGLuR5-stimulated synaptic protein synthesis [**Figure 24–6(a)**], by binding to ribosomes and reducing translation of these proteins during a critical phase of brain development.

In those affected with fragile-X syndrome, the mutant allele is inactive, and no FMRP is produced [**Figure 24–6(b)**]. As a result, mGluR5-stimulated protein synthesis is unchecked, resulting in overproduction of certain synaptic proteins, causing alterations in the structure and function of affected neurons. One result is reduction in the interconnection of brain neurons, leading to the intellectual deficits and other problems that define fragile-X syndrome. Once it was established that many of the symptoms of this syndrome are caused by the failure to regulate the mGluR5 pathway, sequencing studies on autistic children with fragile-X syndrome identified a number of mutations in the mGuR5 pathway, linking autism to fragile X.

The central role of the mGluR5 receptor in fragile-X syndrome and some forms of autism has focused attention on the development of drugs for use in the treatment of mGluR5-mediated neurodevelopmental disorders. Several mGluR5 inhibitors are now in clinical trials for the treatment of fragile-X syndrome (Table 24.4). If these trials are successful, fragile-X syndrome will be the first neurodevelopmental syndrome with an available treatment, lessening the burden on children with fragile X and their families. If these drugs are approved for fragile-X syndrome, researchers expect that clinical trials using these same drugs for fragile-X associated autism will follow shortly after.

TABLE 24.4 Drugs in Clinical Trials for Treatment of Fragile-X Syndrome

Pharmaceutical Firm	Drug
Neuren Pharmaceuticals	NNZ-2266
Novartis	AFQ056
Roche	RO4917523
Seaside Therapeutics	STX107

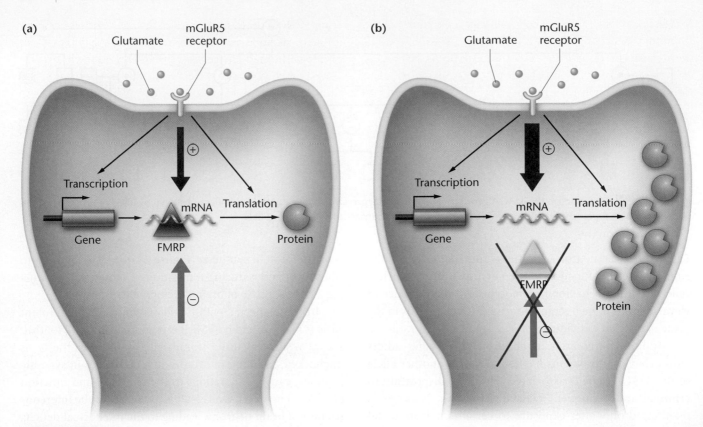

FIGURE 24–6 Action of FMRP protein in normal and fragile-X cells. (a) In normal cells, binding of the neurotransmitter glutamine to mGluR5 receptors initiates the synthesis of synaptic proteins. FMRP binds to mRNA and prevents overproduction of these proteins. (b) In fragile-X syndrome, no FMRP is produced. As a result, when glutamate binding stimulates production of synaptic proteins, this process is unregulated, and proteins are overproduced. The accumulation of these proteins and their action on synapses produce the intellectual deficits and intellectual disabilities association with this disorder.

24.4 Animal Models Play an Important Role in the Study of Huntington Disease and Learning Behavior

In many cases, studying the genetics of behavior has proven more difficult to characterize in humans than in other organisms. In part, this is because some forms of behavior, including aspects of *intelligence*, *language*, *personality*, and *emotion*, present two problems when they are studied. First, these traits are difficult to define objectively and to measure quantitatively. Second, even behavioral abnormalities controlled primarily by single genes are affected by environmental factors, and there is a wide range of variation in the individual responses to these factors as the boundaries between normal and abnormal behavior are defined.

The use of animal models of human behavioral disorders presents an opportunity to separate behavioral phenotypes into their components. This makes it possible to study the developmental, structural, and functional neuronal mechanisms related to these behaviors individually and at times and in ways that are difficult or impossible to do with humans. In addition, behavior in animal models can be studied in controlled conditions that limit the impact of environmental factors on specific forms of behavior. The mouse is a widely used model organism for these studies partly because humans and mice have about 90 percent of their genes in common, and a wide range of strains with specific behavioral phenotypes are available. In addition, genomic techniques make it possible to create transgenic strains by transferring human genes into mice. Here we will consider two ways in which model organisms are used to study the genetic basis of specific human behaviors: analysis of single genes associated with behavioral disorders, and the study of learning and memory.

Huntington Disease Is a Neurodegenerative Behavioral Disorder

Huntington disease (HD) is inherited as an autosomal dominant late-onset disorder that affects about 1 in 10,000 people, causing death in selected brain cells that produces associated behavioral changes. In most cases, symptoms appear between the ages of 30 and 50 as a gradual loss of motor function and coordination. As structural degeneration of the brain progresses, personality changes occur. The symptoms are caused by brain-cell death in specific brain regions, including the cerebral cortex and the striatum, which receives signals from the cerebral cortex and generates responses related to body movements. Most victims die within 10 to 15 years after the onset of the disease.

The *HD* gene, on chromosome 4, encodes a large protein (350 kDa) called huntingtin (HTT) that is essential for the survival of certain neurons in adult brains. Mutant HD alleles have an expanded number of cytosine-adenine-guanine (CAG) trinucleotide repeats in exon 1 (see Chapter 15 for a discussion of trinucleotide repeats). Normal alleles of the *HD* gene carry 7 to 34 CAG repeats, which specify insertion of multiple copies of the amino acid glutamine near the HTT amino terminus. In mutant alleles, expansion of the CAG repeats places additional glutamine residues into the encoded protein. The addition of more than 40 CAG repeats and the additional glutamine residues cause HTT to become toxic and cause cell death in certain regions of the brain, leading to behavioral abnormalities.

HD is one of several behavioral disorders associated with the progressive accumulation of misfolded proteins that cause cell death in specific regions of the brain, leading to behavioral consequences. Some of these disorders include Alzheimer disease (AD), amyotrophic lateral sclerosis (ALS), and Parkinson disease. Transgenic animal models of HD and these other neurodegenerative diseases have been developed and are being used to study the molecular events of synthesis, processing, and aggregation of mutant proteins, and the links between protein accumulation, cell death, and behavioral changes.

A Transgenic Mouse Model of Huntington Disease

Several animal models of HD are being used to study the normal function of huntingtin, to analyze the disease process, and to study its effects at the molecular level. The ultimate goal of these studies is the development of drugs to slow or stop the degeneration and death of human brain cells and halt or reverse the clinical symptoms of the disorder. To study whether there is a relationship between CAG repeat length and disease progression, researchers constructed transgenic mice carrying human *HD* genes with 16, 48, or 89 copies of the CAG repeat. In the vector used for gene transfer, the *HD* gene was placed adjacent to a promoter and an enhancer to ensure high levels of expression (see Chapter 22 for a discussion of transgenic organisms). Mice carrying the human transgene were monitored

from birth to death to determine the age of onset and progression of abnormal behavior. Animals carrying 48- or 89-repeat human *HD* genes showed behavioral abnormalities as early as 8 weeks, and by 20 weeks, these mice also showed motor-coordination abnormalities compared with the control animals and mice carrying human *HD* genes with 16 CAG repeats.

At various ages, brains of wild-type mice and of transgenic animals carrying mutant alleles with 16, 48, and 89 copies of the CAG repeat were examined for changes in structure. Degenerating neurons and cell loss were evident in mice carrying 48 and 89 repeats, but no changes were seen in brains of wild-type mice or of those carrying a 16-repeat transgene (**Figure 24–7**).

The behavioral changes and the degeneration in specific brain regions in the transgenic mice parallel the progression of HD in humans. Researchers using these mice are examining changes in brain structure that occur before the onset of early symptoms and developing experimental treatments to slow or reverse cell loss. Having a mouse model for the disease allows researchers to administer treatment at specific times in disease progression and to evaluate the outcome of treatments in the presymptomatic stages of HD.

Mechanism of Huntington Disease

Although the *HD* gene was mapped, isolated, and characterized some 30 years ago, the *mechanism* by which mutant forms of the HTT protein (mHTT) cause HD is

FIGURE 24–7 Relative levels of neuronal loss in HD transgenic mice. Cell counts show a significant reduction of certain neurons (small-medium neurons) in the striatum in the brains of *HD* 48 mutants (middle column) and *HD* 89 mutants (right column) compared to wild-type mice (left column). Cell loss in this brain region is also found in humans with HD, making these transgenic mice valuable models to study the course of this disease.

still unknown. HTT is expressed in all cells of the body, with the highest levels in the brain and testes. mHTT causes cell death initially in striatal cells of the brain. Several mechanisms have been proposed to explain this region-specific pattern of cell death, including abnormal mitochondrial metabolism, and increased activity of proteases associated with nuclear inclusions containing HTT fragments. The discovery that mHTT binds to Rhes, a small protein localized to cells in the brain's striatal region, may explain the cell-specific toxicity of the mHTT protein. Experiments show that when bound to Rhes, mHTT is chemically modified and converted to a form that causes cell death. Low levels of Rhes are also found in cells of the cerebral cortex, another region of the brain in which mHTT causes cell death. In a mouse model of HD, deletion of the Rhes gene reduces damage to the striatum and diminishes loss of motor function. All these data suggest that the interaction of Rhes with mHTT is important in the pathology of HD.

However, HTT is a multifunctional protein that interacts with more than 100 different proteins, including those involved with synaptic function, transcription, cell signaling, and intracellular transport, offering other avenues for the role of this protein in selective cell death. Recent work has focused on the role of mHTT in the disruption of transcriptional regulation. In affected individuals, onset of HD is associated with decreases in mRNA levels for genes encoding certain neurotransmitter receptors. In a transgenic HD mouse model, researchers used cDNA arrays to screen nearly 6000 mRNAs from striatal cells. They found lower levels of mRNA from a small set of genes involved in signaling pathways that are critical to striatal cell function. Similar results were found in another transgenic HD mouse model and are consistent with findings from HD patients, implicating aberrant gene expression and synaptic dysfunction as one of the underlying causes of HD.

Treatment Strategies for Huntington Disease

The symptoms of HD are caused by the toxic effects of mHTT accumulation in certain regions of the brain, which result in cell death and behavioral symptoms. Although the effects of this abnormal protein have been known for over 15 years, there are no treatments available to slow or halt the onset or progress of this neurodegenerative disorder. It is clear that therapies that reduce levels of mHTT are a possible way of treating this disorder. Based on this idea, researchers used *Drosophila* to conduct a genome-wide RNAi-based screen to identify genes that modify levels of mHTT. Results identified 13 such genes. Testing in a *Drosophila* HD model confirmed

FIGURE 24–8 Possible mechanism for NUB1 degradation of mHTT. Increased expression of NUB1 by β-interferon facilitates marking of mHTT molecules for degradation by intracellular pathways. Reducing mHTT levels lowers the toxic effects of this mutant protein.

that expression of one of these genes, *NUB1*, significantly lowered levels of mHTT and reduced cell death. At the cellular level, binding of NUB1 targets mHTT for degradation, and effective therapy would depend on finding a way to raise levels of this protein. As it turns out, cellular levels of NUB1 can be upregulated (**Figure 24–8**) by using β-interferon, a drug approved by the U.S. Food and Drug Administration (FDA) for the treatment of other neurodegenerative disorders. Testing this therapy in mouse models of HD is the next step in assessing the potential of manipulating levels of NUB1 in the brain as a treatment for HD.

NOW SOLVE THIS

24–2 Transgenic mice carrying mutant alleles of the human *HD* gene are created by transferring cloned human *HD* genes into the mice. This process adds copies of the mutant human *HD* gene to the mouse genome, but does not replace or inactivate the normal mouse alleles of the *HD* gene. Based on what you have learned about the structure and function of the normal and mutant *HD* alleles, is it likely that the presence of the normal mouse *HD* gene and mouse HTT poses a problem in these experiments by elevated levels of HTT caused by the additive effects of mouse and human HTT?

■ **HINT:** *This problem involves an understanding of the structure and action of the normal and mutant versions of the HTT molecule.*

Drosophila as an Animal Model for Learning and Memory

Researchers gain a great advantage when they can study the genetics of a complex behavior in a model organism, such as learning or memory in *Drosophila*. In this case, researchers used an olfactory-based shock-avoidance learning system in fruit flies to identify genes that control learning and memory. In this system, flies are presented with a pair of odors, one of which is associated with an electric shock. They quickly learn to avoid the odor associated with the shock.

The demonstration that *Drosophila* can learn opened the way to selecting mutants that are defective in learning and memory (**Table 24.5**). To accomplish this, males from an inbred wild-type strain were treated with mutagens and mated to females from the same strain. Their progeny were

recovered and mated to produce strains that carried a mutagenized X chromosome. Mutations that affected learning were selected by testing for responses in the olfactory shock apparatus. A number of learning-deficient mutants, including *dunce*, *turnip*, *rutabaga*, and *cabbage*, were isolated in this way. In addition, a memory-deficient mutant, *amnesia*, which learns normally but forgets about four times faster than normal, was also recovered. Each of these mutations represents a single gene defect that affects a specific form of behavior. Because of the method used to recover them, most of the first mutants identified were X-linked genes. By using other methods, autosomal genes that control learning and memory have been identified.

Dissecting the Mechanisms and Neural Pathways in Learning

Analysis of these mutants identified both the biochemical pathways and the neural mechanisms involved in learning and memory. One group of *Drosophila* learning mutations is defective in a signal transduction pathway that plays an important role in learning. In cells of the nervous system and many other cell types, cyclic adenosine monophosphate (cAMP) is produced from adenosine triphosphate (ATP) in the cytoplasm in response to signals received at the cell surface (see **Figure 24–9**). Once produced, cyclic AMP (cAMP) activates protein kinases, which, in turn, phosphorylate proteins, transfer the signal to the nucleus, and initiate a cascade of changes in transcriptional patterns of gene expression. Behavioral mutants of *Drosophila* were among the first to show the link between cAMP metabolism and learning. The *rutabaga* (*rut*) locus encodes adenyl cyclase, the enzyme that synthesizes cAMP from ATP.

TABLE 24.5   Some *Drosophila* Mutations That Affect Learning and Memory

Behavior Genes	Molecular Function	Behavior Phenotype, Function
dunce (dnc)	cAMP-specific phosphodiesterase	Locomotor rhythms, ethanol tolerance
rutabaga (rut)	Adenyl cyclase	Courtship learning, ethanol tolerance, grooming
amnesiac (amn); cheapdate (chpd)	Neuropeptide	Ethanol tolerance
latheo (lat)	DNA-replication factor	Larval feeding
Shaker (Sh)	Voltage-sensitive potassium channel	Courtship suppression, gestation defect, ether sensitivity
G proteins 60 A	Heterotrimeric G protein	Visual behavior, cocaine sensitivity
DCO; cAMP-dependent protein kinase I (Pka-C1)	Protein Ser/Thr kinase	Locomotor rhythms, ethanol tolerance
cAMP-response-element-binding protein B at 17A	Transcription factor	Locomotor rhythms (CrebB17A); dCREB
Calcium/calmodulin-dependent protein kinase II (CaMKII)	Protein Ser/Thr kinase	Courtship suppression
Neurofibromatosis 1 (Nf1)	Ras GTPase activator	Embryonic, nervous system defects

Source: Adapted by permission from Macmillan Publishers Ltd: *Nature Reviews Genetics*, "Drosophila: Genetics Meets Behavior," by M.B. Sokolowski. *Nature Reviews Genetics* 2:879–890, table 1, p. 882. Copyright 2001, www.nature.com/nrg.

FIGURE 24–9 The pathway for cyclic AMP (cAMP) synthesis and degradation. ATP is converted into cAMP by the enzyme adenyl cyclase; cAMP affects short-term memory via the potassium channel in the plasma membrane and affects long-term memory by regulating the transcription factor CREB. In *Drosophila*, the *rutabaga* gene encodes adenyl cyclase. When produced, the enzyme is inactive; it is converted to an active form by a protein encoded by the *turnip* gene. The active form of adenyl cyclase is inactivated by the protein encoded by the *dunce* gene. Mutations in any of these genes affect learning and memory in *Drosophila*.

Homozygous mutant *rutabaga* flies do not have short-term or long-term memories, and do not learn the association between specific odors and electric shocks. The *dunce* (*dnc*) locus encodes the structural gene for the enzyme cAMP phosphodiesterase, which degrades adenyl cyclase. Mutant alleles of *dunce* cause an increase in cAMP levels, and learning and memory deficits in homozygous flies. The *turnip* (*tur*) mutation occurs in a gene encoding a G protein, which indirectly activates adenyl cyclase.

Analysis of these mutations also identified parts of the fly's nervous system where sensory information is processed and where both short-term and long-term memory are formed. Cells in the *Drosophila* brain, called *mushroom body neurons* (**Figure 24–10**), integrate and process sensory input and form short-term and long-term memories. When olfactory stimuli and electric shock stimuli arrive at a mushroom body simultaneously, *rutabaga*-encoded adenyl cyclase is stimulated, increasing cAMP levels, which activates other genes whose activity is critical for learning and memory. The increase in cAMP also leads to changes in the excitability of mushroom body neurons. Elevated levels of cAMP upregulate expression of a protein kinase, which enhances both short-term and long-term memory. These results confirm that these two types of memory involve different populations of neurons. Short-term memory is mediated by changes in potassium channels. Long-term memory is associated with changes in gene expression within mushroom body neurons, which is controlled by

FIGURE 24–10 Green fluorescent protein (GFP) labeling of the neurons in the mushroom body region of the *Drosophila* brain. Cells in this region are important in learning and memory.

a transcriptional activator, CREB (cAMP response element binding protein). CREB binds to elements upstream of cAMP inducible genes and changes the pattern of gene expression, encoding long-term memories.

Drosophila Is an Effective Model for Learning and Memory in Humans

The biochemical pathways that control learning and memory in *Drosophila* are similar to those in other organisms, including mice and humans. The mammalian homologs of the *Drosophila* genes are active in parts of the mouse brain involved in learning and memory. Identification of these genes in *Drosophila* has provided insight into the mechanisms of learning and memory in humans. Drugs that act on the *rutabaga* pathway have been developed and are being used to treat memory deficits in humans. Studies on the human version of the *dunce* gene (called *PDE4B*) have shown that mutant alleles of this gene are part of the spectrum of symptoms associated with schizophrenia. Other genes activated by CREB during learning and memory formation in *Drosophila* are being evaluated for their role in learning and in behavioral disorders in humans.

24.5 Behavioral Disorders Have Environmental Components

Geneticists, psychologists, and social scientists have a long history of interest in the social and environmental context of human behavior. Most human behavior involves interactions between two individuals or among individuals

MODERN APPROACHES TO UNDERSTANDING GENE FUNCTION

RbAp48 and a Potential Molecular Mechanism for Age-Related Memory Loss

You have likely heard someone (perhaps one of your professors) make the exclamation "I forgot what I wanted to say—it must be my age!" or a similar statement. In this last "Modern Approaches to Understanding Gene Function" entry, we focus on an exciting recent finding that links a specific gene in the brain to age-related memory loss or dementia. The experimental basis of this work provides an elegant example of how scientists are using molecular approaches to gradually develop an understanding of the genetic basis of cognitive behaviors. As of 2010, an estimated 36 million people ages 65 and older were living with some form of dementia, and many of these individuals do not have Alzheimer disease (AD).

By examining human brains from young and old adults who died without signs of neurological diseases, neuroscientists identified a specific region of the hippocampus, called the dentate gyrus (DG), as a primary memory center affected by aging. Because this region of the brain is different from the region where AD is typically manifested, researchers speculated that the cellular and molecular basis for age-related memory loss is distinctly different from AD.

A research team at Columbia University Medical Center led by Nobel laureate Dr. Eric Kandler carried out microarray analysis to study gene-expression patterns in the DG. This team identified 17 candidate age-related genes. Because expression of the gene RbAp48 showed a decline that correlated with aging of the DG, they hypothesized that this gene may play a key role in age-related memory loss. RbAp48 encodes a histone-binding protein that modifies histone acetylation. Kandler and colleagues then turned to mouse models to study the roles of RbAp48 in age-related memory loss.

They created transgenic mice expressing a mutant (dominant-negative) version of the RbAp48 gene called RbAp48DN. By overexpressing the RbAp48DN transgene, researchers could essentially override the functions of the wild-type protein. The transgene vector restricted expression of RbAp48DN to the forebrain, and expression was under the control of a promoter inhibited by the antibiotic doxycycline (dox). By supplementing mouse food with dox, researchers could turn expression of the transgene off in mice at different times and ages as desired (see figure panel a).

Results:

Prematurely inhibiting RbAp48 in young mice (2.4 months old) caused them to lose their way through mazes and perform poorly on memory-related tasks just like older mice (figure panel b). Overexpression of RbAp48 in forgetful older mice (15 months) made them as sharp as young mice when cognitive behaviors associated with memory were tested (see figure panel c). Of the many interesting results reported in the paper, investigators also noted that:

- They could not induce AD by manipulating levels of RbAP48.
- Functional magnetic resonance imaging (MRI) showed that the DG was affected in impaired young mice expressing RbAp48DN.
- Abnormal histone acetylation patterns were detected in regions of the brain where RbAp48 was inhibited.

Conclusions:

The body of work presented in this paper reinforced evidence suggesting

(a) In situ *hybridization results showing* RbAp48DN *transgene expression in mice with no dox treatment (Transgene ON). Treating mice with dox (DT) turns the transgene off (Transgene OFF). (b) Results of novel object recognition tests, essentially the time it takes for mice to discriminate between familiar and new objects. The higher the score on the discrimination index, the more rapidly animals are demonstrating discrimination based on memory of familiar objects. Notice that young mice (2.5 months) expressing the* RbAp48DN *transgene score significantly worse on this test than wild-type control mice. (c) Novel object recognition test comparing wild-type aged mice (15 months) receiving DG injections of lentiviral vectors expressing* RbAp48 *or green-fluorescent protein (GFP) as a negative control. Notice that* RbAp48-*injected mice do substantially better on this memory test. Researchers observed similar results with a memory test involving a maze. *, indicates statistically significant difference in results* that age-related memory loss is not the same as AD. *RbAp48* appears to be a key gene involved in the development of age-related memory loss. Its role in histone acetylation points clearly to an epigenetic cause. The authors also provided evidence connecting *RbAp48* to a protein kinase A (PKA)–cyclic adenosine monophosphate (cAMP) response element binding protein 1 (CREB1)–CREB-binding protein (CBP). Clinically, it has been shown that drugs enhancing the PKA-CREB-CBP pathway are known to improve

age-related functions in mice. Might it be possible to test the effects of these drugs for treating age-related memory problems in humans?

Reference:

Pavlopoulos, E., et al. 2013. Molecular mechanism for age-related memory loss: the histone-binding protein RbAp48. *Sci. Transl. Med.* 5:1–12.

Questions to Consider:

1. Based on what you now know about using knockout and transgenic

animals to study gene function, speculate about why the researchers did not create *RbAp48* knockout mice to test their hypothesis.

2. The results of this paper are compelling. What other information might be important to determine if *RbAp48* should be a target for developing drugs designed to treat memory loss?

---

in groups. Evidence from family studies and twin studies provides clear evidence for the role of genetics, especially multifactorial inheritance in human behavioral traits and disorders. **Figure 24–11** shows the results from twin studies for some disorders. Behavior has both genetic and nongenetic components. Heritability studies provide the best evidence for the role of nongenetic factors in behavior. In the following sections we will discuss several disorders associated with social behavior.

In contrast to behavioral disorders that are controlled by single genes, such as Huntington disease, many behavioral traits are polygenic with strong environmental components, making it difficult to associate them with specific genes.

Schizophrenia Is a Complex Behavioral Disorder

Schizophrenia is a term that describes a collection of mental disorders affecting 1 percent of the U.S. population, with

symptoms appearing in late adolescence or early adulthood. Affected individuals have delusions, thought disorders, psychotic symptoms, and often exhibit antisocial behavior.

Schizophrenia is clearly a familial disorder, with relatives of schizophrenics having a much higher incidence of the condition than the general population (**Figure 24–12**). Furthermore, the closer the genetic or biological relationship to an affected individual, the greater a person's likelihood of developing the disorder. Twin studies have helped establish a genetic link to schizophrenia. If both twins express a trait, they are *concordant* for that trait; if one expresses the trait, but the other does not, they are *discordant* for that trait. In studies of schizophrenia in monozygotic and dizygotic twins, concordance is higher in monozygotic twins than in dizygotic twins.

The genetic contributions to schizophrenia have been difficult to identify. Simple monohybrid inheritance and dihybrid inheritance have been discounted as causes of schizophrenia. Schizophrenia is now considered to be a multifactorial and quantitative trait, influenced by genes, by the environment, and by interactions between the genotype and environmental factors.

The search for genes causing schizophrenia parallels the development of technologies for identifying genes associated with complex traits. Beginning in the late 1980s, linkage studies using restriction fragment length polymorphism (RFLP) markers identified chromosome regions that segregated in families with affected members. By 2000, a small number of candidate genes had been identified on chromosomes 6, 8, and 13. The role of some of the encoded proteins in brain development and synaptic impulse

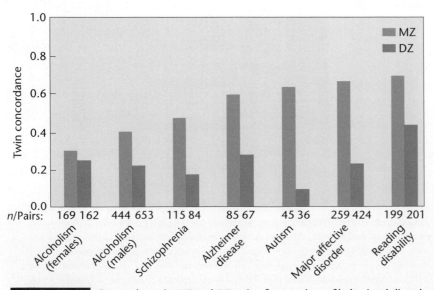

FIGURE 24–11 Concordance in MZ and DZ twins for a variety of behavioral disorders.

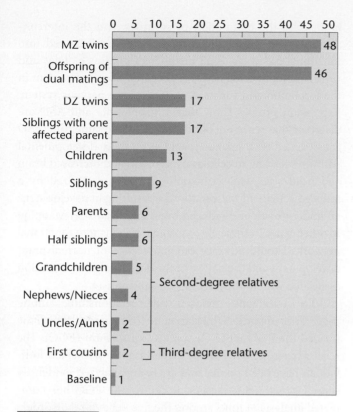

FIGURE 24–12 Relative lifetime risk of schizophrenia for non-related individuals and for relatives of schizophrenics.

FIGURE 24–13 Results of a genome-wide association study (GWAS) to detect SNPs on the short arm of chromosome 6 (6p) that are associated with schizophrenia. SNPs above the statistical threshold for association (red line) are shown as red diamonds. Seven SNPs spanning 209 kb of DNA show significance. Red circles represent SNPs at the threshold of statistical significance; green circles indicate SNPs with no association. The x-axis marks the location of the SNPs in million base pairs within the 6p22.1 region.

transmission supports the idea that these genes may play a role in schizophrenia. New experimental methods developed during and after the Human Genome Project have used haplotype mapping and high-throughput sequencing approaches to study schizophrenia. Foremost among these are genome-wide association studies (GWAS) that utilize some of the more than 10 million single-nucleotide polymorphisms (SNPs) present in the human genome (SNPs are discussed in Chapter 21). Subsets of closely linked SNPs called **haplotypes** (that are inherited in blocks) serve as markers for specific chromosome regions. In GWAS, researchers scan thousands of genomes looking for an association between specific haplotypes and a trait, in this case, schizophrenia (**Figure 24–13**). The haplotypes are markers that identify chromosome regions that may contain genes associated with schizophrenia.

The evidence from GWAS regarding schizophrenia indicates that no single gene or allele makes a significant contribution to this disorder. Instead, the results point to the involvement of hundreds of genes, each of which contributes only a small amount to schizophrenia. GWAS are based on the assumption that common gene variants (present in more than 5 percent of the population) contribute to disease risk (the common disease/common variant hypothesis, abbreviated as CDCV). In this case, common variants identified by GWAS contribute only about 4 to 30 percent

of the risk for schizophrenia. Large-scale whole genome resequencing to identify allelic variants associated with gene–phenotype associations are proposed as a means of identifying these variants.

GWAS have also implicated copy number variants (CNVs) as important factors in the development of schizophrenia and other psychiatric disorders. Copy number variants (see Chapter 8 for a discussion) can alter the dosage of genes and the number of regulatory regions that control these genes. Deletion CNVs and large duplication CNVs are generally associated with more severe phenotypes than small duplication CNVs.

Studies on CNVs have shown that newly arising (*de novo*) CNVs representing both deletions and duplications are three to four times more frequent in cases of schizophrenia than in normal individuals. Many genes in these *de novo* CNVs are involved in brain development and function, providing clues to the cellular basis of schizophrenia. Some of these genes will be discussed in the next section.

Several Behavioral Disorders Share a Genetic Relationship

Historically, the diagnosis of psychiatric disorders has been based on specific clinical behavioral symptoms, first defined in the nineteenth century. Now, however, the distinction among many such disorders is beginning to blur as researchers identify genes, SNP haplotypes, and CNVs shared by affected individuals. Recent evidence suggests that at least five psychiatric disorders—schizophrenia, autism spectrum disorders (ASD), bipolar disorder, major depressive disorder, and attention-deficit/hyperactivity disorder (ADHD)—all share common genetic components.

The first indication of this shared relationship came from work on schizophrenia and ASD.

Like schizophrenia, family studies and twin studies show that **autism spectrum disorders (ASD)** are complex, multifactorial diseases with genetic components. It is estimated that ASD affects about 3.4 per 1000 children between the ages of 3 and 10 years. These disorders are characterized by severe and pervasive deficits in (1) thinking, (2) language skills, (3) feelings, and (4) social interaction. These disorders range from a severe form called autism through several intermediates to a mild form with no intellectual disability or language deficit. Some rare mutations and chromosomal rearrangements are associated with ASD but, taken together, account for only about 5 to 15 percent of all cases. GWAS results have identified SNPs associated with susceptibility to ASD. Some of these SNPs are also risk factors for schizophrenia, indicating that these disorders may be related. Other studies reveal the existence of rare CNVs associated with the development of both disorders. CNVs covering seven genomic regions have been linked to both schizophrenia and ASD (Table 24.6). In two of these regions, deletions are associated with an increased risk of autism, and duplications are associated with an increased risk of schizophrenia (16p11.2, 22q13.3). In two others (1q21.1, 22.q11.21), deletions increase the risk of schizophrenia, and duplications are associated with ASD. The region at 16p13.1 supports a model of overlap between the two conditions.

Further work has shown that genes in these chromosomal regions play important roles in the development of brain cells, the maturation of synapses, and the interconnection of neurons. These genes have been mapped into functional pathways using methods of systems biology, and reveal interconnected nodes of gene interaction important in the formation and function of parts of the nervous system. Expression profiles show that schizophrenia and ASD are disorders that represent opposite sides of the same coin. ASD is associated with increased activity in these developmental pathways leading to cellular overgrowth and increased brain and head size, while schizophrenia is characterized by a reduced activity in these pathways, resulting in developmental undergrowth and reduced brain and head size. Mapping of other genes in these chromosomal regions into functional networks should advance our knowledge of normal brain development and the nature of the defects in gene regulation associated with both schizophrenia and autism.

To investigate genome-wide relationships among psychiatric disorders, researchers from across the globe formed the Psychiatric Genomics Consortium (PGC). The results from genetic studies on thousands of affected individuals have been pooled and are being analyzed to identify shared genetic risk factors. Recently, the PGC has completed analysis of links among the five behavioral disorders listed above. SNP data from over 33,000 affected individuals were used to estimate heritability explained by SNPs shared across these disorders. SNPs at four loci show significance above the 0.05 level (**Figure 24–14**) demonstrating cross-disorder associations.

SNPs in regions on the short arm of chromosome 3 and the long arm of chromosome 10, as well as SNPs within calcium channel subunits encoded by genes on the short arm of chromosome 10 and the long arm of chromosome 12, are involved. The pairs of disorders showing the highest SNP heritabilities were schizophrenia-bipolar disorder, bipolar disorder-major depressive disorder, major depressive disorder-attention-deficit/hyperactivity disorder, and schizophrenia-autism spectrum disorders. These results, coupled with the results of other analyses, point to the role of neuronal calcium channel defects as a common risk factor in all five disorders, and are an example of *pleiotropy*, a condition in which a single gene may have multiple effects. If the results of the PGC study are confirmed, it will mark an important turning point in the diagnosis and treatment of mental illness; behavioral disorders will be defined by their underlying biological causes instead of clinical symptoms. In addition, new and more effective drug therapies can be developed from an understanding of the molecular pathways that define these disorders.

TABLE 24.6 Frequencies of CNV Deletions or Duplications Dssociated with Autism or Schizophrenia

CNV Locus	Condition	Deletion Cases	Duplication Cases
1q21.1	Autism	2	**10**
	Schizophrenia	**15**	4
15q13.3	Autism	3	2
	Schizophrenia	**10**	4
16p11.2	Autism	**14**	5
	Schizophrenia	5	**24**
16p13.1	Autism	0	**3**
	Schizophrenia	8	**23**
17p12	Autism	4	1
	Schizophrenia	**8**	0
22q11.21	Autism	1	**8**
	Schizophrenia	**16**	1
22q13.3	Autism	**5**	0
	Schizophrenia	0	**4**

Entries in bold indicate that the CNV is statistically documented as a risk factor for the condition specified.

From: Crespi, B, et al., 2010. Comparative genomics of autism and schizophrenia. Proc. Nat. Acad. Sci. 107: 1736–1741; their Table 1, page 1737.
Contact: crespi@sfu.ca

Epigenetics and Mental Illness

Exposure to environmental factors in prenatal stages or early in life can have profound effects on behavior, and these effects can be transmitted to offspring. These effects

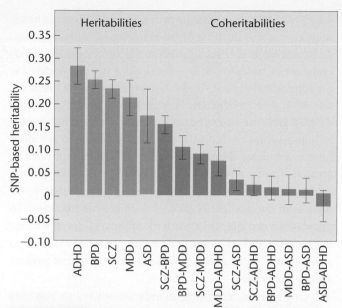

FIGURE 24–14 Genome-wide SNP-based heritability for individual behavioral disorders (blue columns) and cross-disorder heritability for pairs of behavioral disorders (green columns). Degrees of heritability are indicated on the *y*-axis. Four pairs of disorders (SCZ-BPD, BPD-MDD, SCZ-MDD, and MDD-ADHD) show strong correlation. The existence of pleiotropic effects between several pairs of disorders indicates that they may share underlying genes. ADHD = attention-deficit/hyperactivity disorder; SCZ = schizophrenia; BPD = bipolar disorder; MDD = major depressive disorder; ASD = autism spectrum disorders.

are mediated by epigenetic changes to DNA and/or histones that do not change the sequence of nucleotides. Some epigenetic modifications involve addition or removal of methyl groups to DNA sequences in or near promoter regions. Normally, addition of methyl groups to DNA silences genes, and removal activates genes.

Twin studies offer an opportunity to study the relationship of genomic epigenetic changes to mental illness. Monozygotic (MZ) twins share the same genome, and cases of discordance, in which one twin has a disorder such as schizophrenia, bipolar disorder, or autism, and the other does not, offer opportunities to explore whether or not epigenetic changes may be involved. In one large study, researchers studied methylation patterns at 27,000 different sites in the genome using DNA from 22 pairs of MZ twins discordant for schizophrenia or bipolar disorder. There were significant differences in methylation patterns, many of which were in or near genes previously shown to be risk factors for both disorders. One gene, *ST6GALNAC1*, had up to a 20 percent difference in promoter methylation in twins affected with either disorder, compared to the unaffected twin. This result confirms a previous study using postmortem brain tissue that showed a 25 percent methylation pattern difference in the same gene.

The twin study also showed increased methylation of the *ZNF659* gene in twins with schizophrenia and undermethylation in twins with bipolar disorder, suggesting that opposite levels of gene activity might partially define differences between these disorders.

While these epigenetic studies do not establish a causal relationship between epigenetic changes and specific forms of mental illness, they do suggest how environmental factors may affect the development and severity of these disorders. Please note that some of the topics discussed in this section are explored in greater depth later in the text (see Special Topic Chapter 1—Epigenetics).

Addiction and Alcoholism Are Behaviors with Genetic and Environmental Causes

Addiction results from multistep physiological processes that follow exposure to an environmental agent. The brain undergoes adaptation to the agent, leading to changes in brain function. Research has established that addictions are related to other psychiatric conditions by common genes and neural pathways. Although research into the genetic and molecular basis of addictions has lagged behind work on disorders of mental function such as schizophrenia, bipolar disorder, depression, and others, the cost of addictions and substance use disorders in the United States is more than $480 billion/year, more than the combined costs of diabetes and cancer.

Family, adoption, and especially twin studies all show that addictions of many different types are heritable (**Figure 24–15**). Most addictions are inherited as complex traits with no clear-cut signs of simple Mendelian inheritance. Polygenic inheritance with a substantial

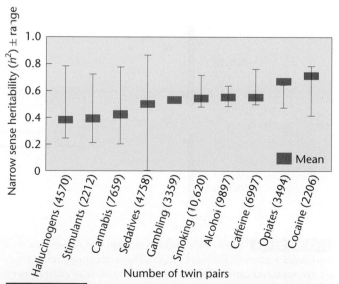

FIGURE 24–15 The heritability of several addictive behavioral disorders derived from twin studies. Higher heritabilities are associated with higher risks.

environmental input may be involved, but the complexity of neural pathways and the variations in the genes that control those pathways can lead to enough heterogeneity in the phenotypes so that identification of the genes responsible may be difficult. Genome scans have identified relevant chromosome regions and genes that encode synaptic receptors, neurotransmitters, and other proteins involved in synapse function and maintenance. In the following section, we will consider the use of alcohol (ethanol), the most widely used addictive drug, and one of the most studied and best known addictions.

Excessive use of alcohol to the point of addiction has two major consequences: (1) damage to the brain, nervous system, and other organ systems, including the liver; and (2) an individual's loss of ability to function in the workplace, the home, and social settings. About 75 percent of the U.S. population consumes alcohol, and of these individuals, 25 percent engage in binge drinking and 10 percent are classified as alcoholics. Evidence for the involvement of genetics in alcoholism can be derived from animal models; in mice, alcohol preference is a selectable trait. In humans, pedigree analysis show a 25 to 50 percent risk of alcoholism in sons of alcoholics. Twin studies show 50 percent concordance for alcoholism in MZ twins, and a 28 percent rate in same-sex DZ twins.

Two genes encode enzymes that catalyze linked steps in alcohol metabolism (**Figure 24–16**). Alcohol dehydrogenase (ADH1B) is an enzyme that converts alcohol to acetaldehyde, which in turn is converted to acetate by aldehyde dehydroge-

nase 2 (ALDH2). Accumulation of acetaldehyde causes histamine release and flushing of the skin, headache, and nausea. Acetaldehyde is also recognized as a potent mutagen; accumulation of this metabolic intermediate is a risk factor for gastrointestinal cancer. Allelic variants of each gene affect the rate of alcohol metabolism. A high activity SNP allele of the *ADH1B* gene increases the catalytic efficiency of the enzyme in homozygotes by 100-fold, converting alcohol to acetaldehyde much faster than the enzyme ALDH2 can convert the acetaldehyde to acetate. An allele of the *ALDH2* gene lowers the activity of ALDH2, also raising acetaldehyde levels because of the slow conversion of acetaldehyde to acetate. In populations carrying either or both of these alleles, the flushing reaction and its associated symptoms cause aversion to alcohol, and these alleles represent genotypes that protect against alcoholism.

Other genes, encoding neurotransmitters or proteins that affect synapse function, have been proposed to be involved in alcoholism. Work in animal models (mouse and rat) has identified over 100 genes that may be involved in alcoholism. This finding indicates that multifactorial inheritance, perhaps with each gene making a small contribution to the phenotype, may be involved, along with a diverse array of environmental factors.

At the cellular level, what is known is that all addictive drugs, including alcohol—in spite of differences in chemical structure and actions—eventually enhance the synaptic release of dopamine in a region of the brain called the striatum. Repeated use of these substances causes long-lasting

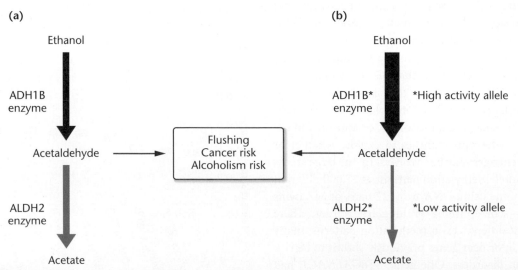

FIGURE 24–16 Allelic differences in alcohol metabolism. (a) In this pathway, normal-activity alleles convert ethanol into acetaldehyde and acetate at constant rates. Acetaldehyde accumulation leads to facial flushing and more serious risks, including alcoholism and gastrointestinal cancer. (b) The high-activity allele of *ADH1B* converts ethanol to acetaldehyde about 100 times faster than the normal allele. The low-activity allele of *ALDH2* converts acetaldehyde to acetate much more slowly than the normal allele. Individuals carrying one or the other or both alleles have increased rates of flushing, headache, and nausea. This reaction reduces alcohol consumption or causes an aversion to alcohol, reducing the risk of alcoholism.

changes in synaptic function and connections among neurons in brain circuits. These circuit dysfunctions in addiction are shared with disorders such as schizophrenia, depression, and anxiety disorders. What remains is to fill in the gaps between the action of drugs on the synapse and their associated behaviors.

CASE STUDY | Primate models for human disorders

Huntington disease (HD) is a dominantly inherited, adult-onset neurodegenerative disorder that affects about 1 in 10,000 people. Onset is around 50 years of age, there is no treatment, and the disorder inevitably causes dementia and loss of motor control, and is fatal. To study the cellular and molecular mechanisms associated with HD, animal models, including mice and *Drosophila*, have been created by transferring mutant human *HD* genes into these organisms. However, some of the behavioral changes seen in HD mice and fruit flies are difficult to correlate with those seen in affected humans. To more closely replicate the cognitive and motor changes in HD, researchers have created a primate model using rhesus macaques, which are one of our closest relatives and share many similarities with humans, including life span, cellular metabolism, as well as endocrine and reproductive functions. However, their use raises several important questions.

1. What are the ethical concerns related to research with primate models of human disease?

2. Does it seem likely that results from using rhesus macaques will translate directly to an understanding of the disease process in humans and lead to treatment?

3. If the primate HD model is successful, should it be used for other human behavioral disorders such as Alzheimer or Parkinson disease?

EXPLORING GENOMICS

HomoloGene: Searching for Behavioral Genes

This chapter discussed some of the complexities of understanding behavior—in humans and other species—as a product of both genes and environment. In this exercise, we will explore the NCBI database **HomoloGene** to search for genes implicated in behavioral conditions. HomoloGene is a database of homologs from several eukaryotic species, and it contains genes that have been implicated in behavioral conditions both in animal models and in humans. Some of these are mutant genes, which, on the basis of single-nucleotide polymorphisms or linkage mapping, are thought to contribute to a behavioral phenotype. Keep in mind that correlation of a gene with a particular behavioral condition does not necessarily mean that the gene is the cause of the condition. Nor does it mean that the gene is the only one involved in the behavioral condition or that the condition is entirely due to genetics.

Nonetheless, exploring HomoloGene is an interesting way to search for putative behavioral genes and learn more about them.

■ **Exercise I – HomoloGene**

1. Access **HomoloGene** from the ENTREZ site at http://www.ncbi.nlm.nih.gov/homologene/

2. Search HomoloGene using the following list of terms related to behavioral conditions in humans. What human genes are listed in the top two categories of gene homologs that result from the HomoloGene search for each condition? Name these genes and identify their chromosomal loci. Notice the list of other species thought to share homologs of each gene.

   a. alcoholism

   b. depression

   c. nicotine addiction

   d. seasonal affective disorder

   e. intelligence

3. For each of the top two categories of homologs, click on the category title to open a report on those genes. Then use the links for individual genes to learn more about the functions of those genes. In addition to other good resources, the "Additional Links" category at the bottom of each gene report page will provide you with access to the Online Mendelian Inheritance in Man (OMIM) site that we have used for other exercises.

4. Search HomoloGene for any behavioral conditions you are interested in to see if the database contains genes that may be implicated in those conditions.

Summary Points

1. Behavior is a multifactorial trait controlled by genes, environmental factors, and interactions among these genes and the environment.
2. Several lines of evidence, including family and twin studies, confirm that many human behaviors have genetic components.
3. The structure and function of synapses and other components of the nervous are the focus of current research on behavior.
4. Because of the large number of genes in common, *Drosophila* and other organisms are useful for the study of behavioral disorders in humans.
5. Genomic technology has opened new avenues of investigation into the development of the human nervous system and the mechanisms of behavioral disorders.

INSIGHTS AND SOLUTIONS

Bipolar disorder is a mental illness associated with pervasive and wide mood swings. It is estimated that 1 in 100 individuals has or will suffer from this disorder at least once in his or her lifetime. Genetic studies indicate that bipolar disorder is familial and that mutations in several genes are involved. In an attempt to identify genes associated with bipolar disorder (this condition was formerly called manic depression), researchers began by using conventional genetic analysis. In 1987, two separate studies using pedigree analysis, RFLP analysis, and a variety of other genetic markers reported a linkage between manic depression and, in one report, markers on the X chromosome and, in the other report, markers on the short arm of chromosome 11. At the time, these reports were hailed as landmark discoveries. It was thought that genes controlling this behavioral disorder could be identified, mapped, and sequenced in much the same way as genes for cystic fibrosis, neurofibromatosis, and other disorders. It was hoped that this discovery would open the way to the development of therapeutic strategies based on knowledge of the nature of the gene product and its mechanism of action. One of the challenges of human genetics results from the fact that some disorders show variable times of onset, and the bipolar studies provide an example of this. Following the original analysis identifying markers, some of the controls (unaffected individuals) who did not carry the markers subsequently developed bipolar disorder. This outcome weakened the evidence for linkage. These findings do not exclude the role of major genes on the X chromosome and chromosome 11 in bipolar disorder, but they do exclude linkage to the markers used in the original reports. This setback not only caused embarrassment and confusion, but also forced a reex-amination of the validity of the newly developed recombinant DNA-based methods used in mapping other human genes and of the analysis of data from linkage studies involving complex behavioral traits. Several factors have been proposed to explain the flawed conclusions reported in the original studies. What do you suppose some of these factors were?

Solution: Although some of the criticisms were directed at the choice of markers, most of the factors at work in this situation appear to be related to the phenotype of manic depression. At least three confounding factors have been identified. One factor relates to the diagnosis of bipolar disorder itself. The phenotype is complex and not as easily quantified as height or weight. In addition, mood swings are a universal part of everyday life, and it is not always easy to distinguish transient mood alterations and the role of environmental factors from disorders having a biological or genetic basis (or both). A second confounding factor is that, in the populations studied, there may in fact be more than one major X-linked gene and more than one major autosomal gene that trigger bipolar disorder. A third factor is age of onset. There is a positive correlation between age and the appearance of the symptoms of bipolar disorder. Therefore, at the time of a pedigree study, younger individuals who will be affected later in life may not show any signs of bipolar disorder. Taken together, these factors illustrate the difficulty in researching the genetic basis of complex behavioral traits. Individually or in combinations, the factors described might skew the results enough so that the guidelines for proof that are adequate for other traits are not stringent enough for behavioral traits with complex phenotypes and complex underlying causes.

Problems and Discussion Questions

HOW DO WE KNOW?

1. In this chapter we focused on how genes that control the development, structure, and function of the nervous system and interactions with environmental factors produce behavior. At the same time, we found many opportunities to consider the methods and reasoning by which much of this information was acquired. From the explanations given in the chapter, what answers would you propose to the following fundamental questions:
(a) How do we know there is genetic variation for a specific behavior that is present in strains of a species?
(b) How do we know that *Drosophila* can learn and remember?

(c) How do we know how the mutant gene product in Huntington disease functions?

(d) How do we know that schizophrenia has genetic components?

CONCEPT QUESTION

2. Review the Chapter Concepts list on page 625. One of these concepts describes the focus of genetics and molecular biology on the structure and function of the nervous system. Write a short essay on the role of the synapse, neurotransmitters, and receptors in human behavioral disorders.

3. In humans, the chemical phenylthiocarbamide (PTC) is either tasted or not. When the offspring of various combinations of taster and nontaster parents are examined, the following data are obtained:

Parents	Offspring
Both tasters	All tasters
Both tasters	1/2 tasters
	1/2 nontasters
Both tasters	3/4 tasters
	1/4 nontasters
One taster and One nontaster	All tasters
One taster	1/2 tasters
One nontaster	1/2 nontasters
Both nontasters	All nontasters

Based on these data, how is PTC tasting behavior inherited?

4. Various approaches have been applied to study the genetics of problem and pathological gambling (PG), and within-family vulnerability has been well documented. However, family studies, while showing clusters within blood relatives, cannot separate genetic from environmental influences. Eisen (2001) applied "twin studies" using 3359 twin pairs from the Vietnam-era Twin Registry and found that a substantial portion of the variance associated with PG can be attributed to inherited factors. How might twin studies be used to distinguish environmental from genetic factors in complex behavioral traits such as PG?

5. *Caenorhabditis elegans* has become a valuable model organism for the study of development and genetics for a variety of reasons. The developmental fate of each cell (1031 in males and 959 in hermaphrodites) has been mapped. *C. elegans* has only 302 neurons whose pattern of connectivity is known, and it displays a variety of interesting behaviors including chemotaxis, thermotaxis, and mating behavior, to name a few. In addition, isogenic lines have been established. What advantage would the use of *C. elegans* have over other model organisms in the study of animal behavior? What are likely disadvantages?

6. Using the behavioral phenotypes of a series of 18 mutants falling into five phenotypic classes, Thomas (1990) described the genetic program that controls the cyclic defecation motor program in *Caenorhabditis elegans*. The first step in each cycle is contraction of the posterior body muscles, followed by contraction of the anterior body muscles. Finally, anal muscles open and expel the intestinal contents. Below is a list of selected mutants (simplified) that cause defects in defecation.

Gene	Phenotype
exp	failure to open the anus and expel intestinal contents
unc	failure to contract anterior body muscles
pbo	failure to contract posterior body muscles
aex	failure to open the anus and expel intestinal contents and failure to contract anterior body muscles
cha	alteration of cycle periodicity, all other components being completely functional

Present a simple schematic that illustrates genetic involvement in *C. elegans* defecation. Account for the action of the *aex* gene and speculate on the involvement and placement of the *cha* gene.

7. Discuss why the study of human behavior genetics has lagged behind that of other organisms.

8. J. P. Scott and J. L. Fuller studied 50 traits in five pure breeds of dogs. Almost all the traits varied significantly in the five breeds, but very few bred true in crosses. What can you conclude with respect to the genetic control of these behavioral traits?

Extra-Spicy Problems

MasteringGenetics™ Visit for instructor-assigned tutorials and problems.

9. Although not discussed in this chapter, *C. elegans* is a model system whose life cycle makes it an excellent choice for the genetic dissection of many biological processes. *C. elegans* has two natural sexes: hermaphrodite and male. The hermaphrodite is essentially a female that can generate sperm as well as oocytes, so reproduction can occur by hermaphrodite self-fertilization or hermaphrodite–male mating. In the context of studying mutations in the nervous system, what is the advantage of hermaphrodite self-fertilization with respect to the identification of recessive mutations and the propagation of mutant strains?

10. In July 2006, a population of flies, *Drosophila melanogaster*, rode the space shuttle *Discovery* to the International Space Station

(ISS) where a number of graviperception experiments and observations were conducted over a nine-generation period. Frozen specimens were collected by astronauts and returned to Earth. Researchers correlated behavioral and physiological responses to microgravity with changes in gene activity by analyzing RNA and protein profiles. The title of the project is "*Drosophila* Behavior and Gene Expression in Microgravity." If you were in a position to conduct three experiments on the behavioral aspects of these flies, what would they be? How would you go about assaying changes in gene expression in response to microgravity? Given that humans share over half of the genome and proteins of *Drosophila*, how would you justify the expense of such a project in terms of improving human health?

11. Of a variety of investigational approaches that have been applied to the study of schizophrenia, two separate approaches, twin studies and genomic analysis, have provided strong support for a genetic component.
    (a) Provide a summary of the contribution that each has played in understanding schizophrenia.
    (b) Speculate on the value that genomic analysis using samples from monozygotic and dizygotic twins might have for enhancing research on schizophrenia.
12. Describe the use of single-nucleotide polymorphisms (SNPs) in the study of genetic causes of schizophrenia.
13. Autism, a relatively common complex of human disorders, can range from severe to mild. What evidence indicates a possible link between genetics and autism?
14. An interesting and controversial finding by Wedekind and colleagues (1995) suggested that a sense of smell, flavored with various HLA (human leukocyte antigen) haplotypes, plays a role in mate selection in humans. Women preferred T-shirts from men with HLA haplotypes unlike their own. The HLA haplotypes are components of the major histocompatibility complex (MHC) and are known to have significant immunological functions. In addition to humans, mice and fish also condition mate preference on MHC constitution. The three-spined stickleback (*Gasterosteus aculeatus*) has recently been studied to determine whether females use an MHC odor-based system to select males as mates. Examine the following data (modified from Milinski et al., 2005) and provide a summary conclusion. Why might organisms evolve a mate selection scheme for assessing and optimizing MHC diversity?

	Male with Optimal MHC	Male with Nonoptimal MHC
Gravid female time spent (seconds)	350	250
Number spawning females	11	3

The table compares odor-based choices made by gravid females for males with optimal MHC alleles and males with nonoptimal MHC alleles. Gravid females chose different amounts of time (seconds) for exposure to males with optimal MHC alleles versus those with nonoptimal MHC alleles. The number of females spawning when exposed to different males with different MHC complements is also presented in the table.

15. Describe studies indicating that the degree of DNA methylation (removal or addition), coupled with changes in trinucleotide repeats, can play a role in mental illness. How have twin studies aided our understanding of the role of DNA methylation in the study of mental illness?
16. Fragile-X syndrome is characterized by intellectual deficits, some dysmorphia, and hyperactivity. It is caused by abnormal expansion of a $(CGG)_n$ repeat in the 5'-untranslated region of the *FMR1* gene and as such results in hypermethylation of CpGs. Considering the role of the *FMR1* gene in expression of fragile-X syndrome, what is the relationship between hypermethylation and *FMR1* gene expression?
17. There are at least eight known progressive neuronal dysfunction diseases in humans that are caused by abnormal numbers of CAG repeats within the coding regions of specific genes. Genes carrying such mutations are typically of the gain-of-function class and often share a common mechanism of progressive pathogenesis. Why are such genes "gain-of-function"? Speculate on why such diseases are probably caused by a common mechanism of pathogenesis.

These ladybird beetles, from the Chiricahua Mountains in Arizona, show considerable phenotypic variation.

25 Population and Evolutionary Genetics

CHAPTER CONCEPTS

- Most populations and species harbor considerable genetic variation.

- This variation is reflected in the alleles distributed among populations of a species.

- The relationship between allele frequencies and genotype frequencies in an ideal population is described by the Hardy–Weinberg law.

- Selection, migration, and genetic drift can cause changes in allele frequency.

- Mutation creates new alleles and changes allele frequencies only in very small populations.

- Nonrandom mating changes population genotype frequency but does not change allele frequency.

- A reduction in gene flow between populations, accompanied by selection or genetic drift, can lead to reproductive isolation and speciation.

- Genetic differences between populations or species are used to reconstruct evolutionary history.

In the mid-nineteenth century, Alfred Russel Wallace and Charles Darwin identified natural selection as the mechanism of evolution. In his book, *On the Origin of Species,* published in 1859, Darwin provided evidence that populations and species are not fixed, but change, or evolve, over time as a result of natural selection. However, Wallace and Darwin could not explain either the origin of the variations that provide the raw material for evolution or the mechanisms by which such variations are passed from parents to offspring. Gregor Mendel published his work on the inheritance of traits in 1866, but it received little notice at the time. The rediscovery of Mendel's work in 1900 began a 30-year effort to reconcile Mendel's concept of genes and alleles with the theory of evolution by natural selection. As twentieth-century biologists applied the principles of Mendelian genetics to populations, both the source of variation (mutation and recombination) and the mechanism of inheritance (segregation of alleles) were explained. We now view evolution as a consequence of changes in genetic material through mutation and changes in allele frequencies in populations over time. This union of population genetics with the theory of natural selection generated a new view of the evolutionary process, called *neo-Darwinism.*

In addition to natural selection, other forces including mutation, migration, and drift, individually and collectively, alter allele frequencies and bring about evolutionary divergence that eventually may result in **speciation,** the formation of new species. Speciation is facilitated by environmental diversity. If a population is spread over a geographic range encompassing a number of ecologically distinct subenvironments

647

with different selection pressures, the populations occupying these areas may gradually adapt and become genetically distinct from one another. Genetically differentiated populations may remain in existence, become extinct, reunite with each other, or continue to diverge until they become reproductively isolated. Populations that are reproductively isolated are regarded as separate species. Genetic changes within populations can modify a species over time, transform it into another species, or cause it to split into two or more species.

Population geneticists investigate patterns of genetic variation within and among groups of interbreeding individuals. As changes in genetic structure form the basis for evolution of a population, population genetics has become an important subdiscipline of evolutionary biology. In this chapter, we examine the population genetics processes of **microevolution**—defined as evolutionary change within populations of a species—and then consider how molecular aspects of these processes can be extended to **macroevolution**—defined as evolutionary events leading to the emergence of new species and other taxonomic groups.

25.1 Genetic Variation Is Present in Most Populations and Species

A **population** is a group of individuals belonging to the same species that live in a defined geographic area and actually or potentially interbreed. In thinking about the human population, we can define it as everyone who lives in the United States, or in Sri Lanka, or we can specify a population as all the residents of a particular small town or village.

The genetic information carried by members of a population constitutes that population's **gene pool.** At first glance, it might seem that a population that is well adapted to its environment must be highly homozygous because it is assumed that the most favorable allele at each locus is present at a high frequency. In addition, a look at most populations of plants and animals reveals many phenotypic similarities among individuals. However, a large body of evidence indicates that, in reality, most populations contain a high degree of heterozygosity. This built-in genetic diversity is not necessarily apparent in the phenotype; hence, detecting it is not a simple task. Nevertheless, the diversity within a population can be revealed by several methods.

Detecting Genetic Variation by Artificial Selection

One way to determine whether genetic variation exists in a population is to use artificial selection. If there is little or no variation present in the genes controlling a particular phenotype, selection will have little or no effect on the phenotype. If genetic variation is present, the phenotype will change over a few generations. A dramatic example of this test is the domestic dog. The broad array of sizes, shapes, colors, and behaviors seen in different breeds of dogs all arose from the effects of selection on the genetic variation present in wolves, from which all domestic dogs are descended. Genetic and archaeological evidence indicates that the domestication of wolves took place at least 10,000 years ago and possibly much earlier. On a shorter time scale, laboratory selection experiments on the fruit fly *Drosophila melanogaster* can cause significant changes over a few generations in almost every phenotype imaginable, including size, shape, developmental rate, fecundity, and behavior.

Variations in Nucleotide Sequence

The most direct way to estimate genetic variation is to compare the nucleotide sequences of genes carried by individuals in a population. In one study, Martin Kreitman examined the *alcohol dehydrogenase* locus (*Adh*) in *Drosophila melanogaster* (**Figure 25–1**). This locus has two alleles, the *Adh-f* and the *Adh-s* alleles. The encoded proteins differ by only a single amino acid (thr versus lys at codon 192). To determine whether the amount of genetic variation detectable at the protein level (one amino acid difference) corresponds to the amount of variation at the nucleotide level, Kreitman cloned and sequenced *Adh* genes from individuals representing five natural populations of *Drosophila* (**Figure 25–2**).

The 11 cloned genes from these five populations contained a total of 43 nucleotide variations in the *Adh* sequence of 2721 base pairs. These variations are distributed throughout the gene: 14 in exon-coding regions, 18 in introns, and 11 in the untranslated flanking regions. Of the 14 variations in coding regions, only one leads to an amino acid replacement—the one in codon 192, producing the two alleles. The other 13 coding-region nucleotide substitutions do not lead to amino acid replacements and are silent variations in this gene.

Among the most intensively studied human genes is the locus encoding the cystic fibrosis transmembrane conductance regulator (CFTR). Recessive loss-of-function

FIGURE 25–1 Organization of the *Adh* locus of *Drosophila melanogaster.*

	Exon 3	Intron 3	Exon 4
Consensus Adh sequence:	C C C C	G G A A T	C T C C A* C T A G
Strain			
Wa-S	T T • A	C A • T A	A C • • • • • •
Fl1-S	T T • A	C A • T A	A C • • • • • •
Ja-S	• • • •	• • • • •	• • • T • T • C A
Fl-F	• • • •	• • • • •	• • G T C T C C •
Ja-F	• • A •	• • G • •	• • G T C T C C •

FIGURE 25–2 DNA sequence variation in parts of the *Drosophila Adh* gene in a sample of the laboratory strains derived from the five natural populations. The dots represent nucleotides that are the same as the consensus sequence; letters represent nucleotide polymorphisms. An A/C polymorphism (A*) in codon 192 creates the two *Adh* alleles (F and S). All other polymorphisms are silent or noncoding.

mutations in the *CFTR* locus cause **cystic fibrosis,** a disease that affects secretory glands and lungs, leading to susceptibility to bacterial infections. More than 1900 different mutations in the *CFTR* gene have been identified. Among these are missense mutations, amino acid deletions, nonsense mutations, frameshifts, and splice defects. **Figure 25–3** shows a map of the 27 exons in the *CFTR* gene, with many exons identified by function. The histogram above the map shows the locations of some of the disease-causing mutations and the number of copies of each mutation that have been identified. One mutation, a 3-bp deletion in exon 10 called ΔF508, accounts for 67 percent of all mutant cystic fibrosis alleles, but several other mutations were present in

at least 100 of the chromosomes surveyed. In populations of European ancestry, between 1 in 44 and 1 in 20 individuals are heterozygous carriers of mutant alleles. Note that Figure 25–3 includes only the sequence variants that alter the function of the CFTR protein. There are undoubtedly many more *CFTR* alleles with silent sequence variants that do not change the amino acid sequence of the protein and do not affect its function.

Studies of other organisms, including the rat, the mouse, and the mustard plant *Arabidopsis thaliana,* have produced similar estimates of nucleotide diversity in various genes. These studies indicate that there is an enormous reservoir of genetic variability within most populations. At the DNA level most, and perhaps all, genes exhibit diversity from individual to individual. Alleles representing these variations are distributed among members of a population.

Explaining the High Level of Genetic Variation in Populations

The finding that populations harbor considerable genetic variation at the amino acid and nucleotide levels came as a surprise to many evolutionary biologists. The early consensus had been that selection would favor a single optimal (wild-type) allele at each locus and that, as a result, populations would have high levels of homozygosity. This expectation was shown conclusively to be wrong, and considerable research and argument have ensued concerning the forces that maintain such high levels of genetic variation.

The **neutral theory** of molecular evolution, proposed by Motoo Kimura in 1968, proposes that mutations leading to amino acid substitutions are usually detrimental, with only a very small fraction being favorable. Some mutations are neutral; that is, they are functionally equivalent to the allele they replace. Mutations that are favorable or detrimental are preserved or removed from the population, respectively, by natural selection. However, the frequency of the neutral alleles in a population will be determined by mutation rates and random genetic drift, and not by selection. Some neutral mutations will drift to fixation in the population; other neutral mutations will be lost. At any given time, a population may contain several neutral alleles at any particular locus. The diversity of alleles at most

FIGURE 25–3 The locations of disease-causing mutations in the cystic fibrosis gene. The histogram shows the number of copies of each identified mutation. (The vertical axis is a logarithmic scale.) The genetic map below the histogram shows the location and relative sizes of the 27 exons of the *CFTR* locus. The boxes at the bottom indicate the functions of different domains of the CFTR protein.

loci does not, therefore, reflect the action of natural selection, but instead is a function of population size (larger populations have more variation) and the fraction of mutations that are neutral. The alternative explanation for the surprisingly high genetic variation in populations is natural selection. There are several examples in which enzyme or protein variations are maintained by adaptation to certain environmental conditions. The well-known advantage of sickle-cell anemia heterozygotes when infected by malarial parasites is such an example.

Fitness differences of a fraction of a percent would be sufficient to maintain such a variation, but at that level their presence would be difficult to measure. Current data are therefore insufficient to determine what fraction of molecular genetic variation is neutral and what fraction is subject to selection. The neutral theory nonetheless serves a crucial function: It points out that some genetic variation is expected simply as a result of mutation and drift. In addition, the neutral theory provides a working hypothesis for studies of molecular evolution. In other words, biologists must find positive evidence that selection is acting on allele frequencies at a particular locus before they can reject the simpler assumption that only mutation and drift are at work.

25.2 The Hardy–Weinberg Law Describes Allele Frequencies and Genotype Frequencies in Populations

Often when we examine a single gene in a population, we find that distribution of the alleles of this gene results in individuals with different genotypes. Key elements of population genetics are the calculation of allele frequencies and genotype frequencies in the population, and the determination of how these frequencies change from one generation to the next. Population geneticists use these calculations to answer questions such as: How much genetic variation is present in a population? Are genotypes randomly distributed in time and space, or do discernible patterns exist? What processes affect the composition of a population's gene pool? Do these processes produce genetic divergence among populations that may lead to the formation of new species? Changes in allele frequencies in a population that do not result in reproductive isolation are examples of microevolution. In the following sections, we will discuss microevolutionary changes in population gene pools, and in later sections, we will consider macroevolution and the process of speciation.

The relationship between the relative proportions of alleles in the gene pool and the frequencies of different genotypes in the population was elegantly described in a mathematical model developed independently by the British mathematician Godfrey H. Hardy and the German physician Wilhelm Weinberg. This model, called the **Hardy–Weinberg law,** describes what happens to allele and genotype frequencies in an "ideal" population that is infinitely large and randomly mating, and that is not subject to any evolutionary forces such as mutation, migration, or selection. Under these conditions, the Hardy–Weinberg model makes two predictions:

1. The frequencies of alleles in the gene pool do not change over time.

2. If two alleles at a locus, *A* and *a*, are considered, then as we will show later in this chapter, after one generation of random mating, the frequencies of the genotypes *AA:Aa:aa* in the population can be calculated as $p^2 + 2pq + q^2 = 1$, where p = frequency of allele *A* and q = frequency of allele a.

A population that meets these criteria, and in which the frequencies of p and q, two alleles at a given locus, result in the predicted genotypic frequencies, is said to be in Hardy–Weinberg equilibrium. It is rare for a real population to conform totally to the Hardy–Weinberg model and for all allele and genotype frequencies to remain unchanged for generation after generation.

The Hardy–Weinberg model uses Mendelian principles of segregation and simple probability to explain the relationship between allele and genotype frequencies in a population. We can demonstrate how this works by considering the example of a single autosomal gene with two alleles, *A* and *a,* in a population where the frequency of *A* is 0.7 and the frequency of *a* is 0.3. Note that 0.7 + 0.3 = 1, indicating that all the alleles of gene *A* present in the population are accounted for. This means that the probability that any female gamete will contain *A* is 0.7, and the probability that a male gamete will contain *A* is also 0.7. The probability that *both* gametes will contain *A* is 0.7 × 0.7 = 0.49. Thus we predict that in the offspring, the genotype *AA* will occur 49 percent of the time. The probability that a zygote will be formed from a female gamete carrying *A* and a male gamete carrying *a* is 0.7 × 0.3 = 0.21, and the probability of a female gamete carrying *a* being fertilized by a male gamete carrying *A* is 0.3 × 0.7 = 0.21, so the frequency of genotype *Aa* in the offspring is 0.21 + 0.21 = 0.42 = 42 percent. Finally, the probability that a zygote will be formed from two gametes carrying *a* is 0.3 × 0.3 = 0.09, so the frequency of genotype *aa* is 9 percent. As a check on our calculations, note that 0.49 + 0.42 + 0.09 = 1.0, confirming that we have accounted for all possible genotypic combinations in the zygotes. These calculations are summarized in **Figure 25–4**.

Now that we know the frequencies of genotypes in the next generation, what will be the frequency distribution of

Sperm

	fr(A) = 0.7	fr(a) = 0.3
fr(A) = 0.7	fr(AA) = 0.7 × 0.7 = 0.49	fr(Aa) = 0.7 × 0.3 = 0.21
Eggs		
fr(a) = 0.3	fr(aA) = 0.3 × 0.7 = 0.21	fr(aa) = 0.3 × 0.3 = 0.09

FIGURE 25–4 Calculating genotype frequencies from allele frequencies. Gametes represent samples drawn from the gene pool to form the genotypes of the next generation. In this population, the frequency of the *A* allele is 0.7, and the frequency of the *a* allele is 0.3. The frequencies of the genotypes in the next generation are calculated as 0.49 for *AA*, 0.42 for *Aa*, and 0.09 for *aa*. Under the Hardy–Weinberg law, the frequencies of *A* and *a* remain constant from generation to generation.

Sperm

	fr(A) = p	fr(a) = q
fr(A) = p	fr(AA) = p^2	fr(Aa) = pq
Eggs		
fr(a) = q	fr(aA) = qp	fr(aa) = q^2

FIGURE 25–5 The general description of allele and genotype frequencies under Hardy–Weinberg assumptions. The frequency of allele *A* is *p*, and the frequency of allele *a* is *q*. After mating, the three genotypes *AA*, *Aa*, and *aa* have the frequencies p^2, $2pq$, and q^2, respectively.

alleles in this new generation? Under the Hardy–Weinberg law, we assume that all genotypes have equal rates of survival and reproduction. This means that in the next generation, all genotypes contribute equally to the new gene pool. The *AA* individuals constitute 49 percent of the population, and we can predict that the gametes they produce will constitute 49 percent of the gene pool. These gametes all carry allele *A*. Similarly, *Aa* individuals constitute 42 percent of the population, so we predict that their gametes will constitute 42 percent of the new gene pool. Half (0.5) of these gametes will carry allele *A*. Thus, the frequency of allele *A* in the gene pool is 0.49 + (0.5)0.42 = 0.7. The other half of the gametes produced by *Aa* individuals will carry allele *a*. The *aa* individuals constitute 9 percent of the population, so their gametes will constitute 9 percent of the new gene pool. All these gametes carry allele *a*. Thus, we can predict that the allele *a* in the new gene pool is (0.5)0.42 + 0.09 = 0.3. As a check on our calculation, note that 0.7 + 0.3 = 1.0, accounting for all of the gametes in the gene pool of the new generation.

For the general case, we use variables instead of numerical values for the allele frequencies in the Hardy–Weinberg model. Imagine a gene pool in which the frequency of allele *A* is *p* and the frequency of allele *a* is *q*, such that *p* + *q* = 1. If we randomly draw male and female gametes from the gene pool and pair them to make a zygote, the probability that both will carry allele *A* is *p* × *p*. Thus, the frequency of genotype *AA* among the zygotes is p^2. The probability that the female gamete carries *A* and the male gamete carries *a* is *p* × *q*, and the probability that the female gamete carries *a* and the male gamete carries *A* is *q* × *p*. Thus, the frequency of genotype *Aa* among the zygotes is $2pq$. Finally, the probability that both gametes carry *a* is *q* × *q*, making

the frequency of genotype *aa* among the zygotes q^2. Therefore, the distribution of genotypes among the zygotes is

$$p^2 + 2pq + q^2 = 1$$

These calculations are summarized in **Figure 25–5**.

In other words, this population does not change or evolve with respect to the locus being examined. Remember, however, the assumptions about the theoretical population described by the Hardy–Weinberg model:

1. Individuals of all genotypes have equal rates of survival and equal reproductive success—that is, there is no selection.

2. No new alleles are created or converted from one allele into another by mutation.

3. Individuals do not migrate into or out of the population.

4. The population is infinitely large, which in practical terms means that the population is large enough that sampling errors and other random effects are negligible.

5. Individuals in the population mate randomly.

These assumptions are what make the Hardy–Weinberg model so useful in population genetics research. By specifying the conditions under which the population does not evolve, the Hardy–Weinberg model can be used to identify the real-world forces that cause allele frequencies to change. Application of this model can also reveal "neutral genes" in a population gene pool—those not being operated on by the forces of evolution.

The Hardy–Weinberg model has three additional important consequences. First, it shows that dominant traits do not necessarily increase from one generation to the next. Second, it demonstrates that **genetic variability** can be maintained in a population since, once established in an ideal population, allele frequencies remain unchanged.

Third, if we invoke Hardy–Weinberg assumptions, then knowing the frequency of just one genotype enables us to calculate the frequencies of all other genotypes at that locus. This is particularly useful in human genetics because we can calculate the frequency of heterozygous carriers for recessive genetic disorders even when all we know is the frequency of affected individuals.

NOW SOLVE THIS

25–1 Calculate the frequency of the *AA*, *Aa*, and *aa* genotypes after one generation if the initial population consists of 0.2 *AA*, 0.6 *Aa*, and 0.2 *aa* genotypes and meets the requirements of the Hardy–Weinberg relationship. What genotype frequencies will occur after a second generation?

■ **HINT:** *This problem involves an understanding of how to use the Hardy–Weinberg law. The key to its solution is to use allele frequencies to calculate genotype frequencies for all genotypes in the second generation.*

25.3 The Hardy–Weinberg Law Can Be Applied to Human Populations

To show how allele frequencies are measured in a real population, let's consider a gene that influences an individual's susceptibility to infection by HIV-1, the virus responsible for AIDS (acquired immunodeficiency syndrome). A small number of individuals who make high-risk choices (such as unprotected sex with HIV-positive partners) remain uninfected. Some of these individuals are homozygous for a mutant allele of a gene called *CCR5*.

The *CCR5* gene **(Figure 25–6)** encodes a protein called the C-C chemokine receptor-5, often abbreviated CCR5. Chemokines are signaling molecules associated with the immune system. The CCR5 protein is also a receptor for strains of HIV-1, allowing it to gain entry into cells. The mutant allele of the *CCR5* gene contains a 32-bp deletion, making the encoded protein shorter and nonfunctional. The normal allele is called *CCR51* (also called *1*), and the mutant allele is called *CCR5-Δ32* (also called *Δ32*).

TABLE 25.1	*CCR5* Genotypes and Phenotypes
Genotype	**Phenotype**
1/1	Susceptible to sexually transmitted strains of HIV-1
1/Δ32	Susceptible but may progress to AIDS slowly
Δ32/Δ32	Resistant to most sexually transmitted strains of HIV-1

Δ32/Δ32 individuals are resistant to HIV-1 infection. Heterozygous *1/Δ32* individuals are susceptible to HIV-1 infection but progress more slowly to AIDS. **Table 25.1** summarizes the genotypes possible at the *CCR5* locus and the phenotypes associated with each.

The discovery of the *CCR5-Δ32* allele generates two important questions: Which human populations carry the *Δ32* allele, and how common is it? To address these questions, teams of researchers surveyed members of several populations. Genotypes were determined by direct analysis of DNA **(Figure 25–7)**. In one population, 79 individuals had genotype *1/1*, 20 were (*1/Δ32*), and 1 was *Δ32/Δ32*. This population has 158 *1* alleles carried by the *1/1* individuals plus 20 *1* alleles carried by *1/Δ32* individuals, for a total of 178. The frequency of the *CCR51* allele in the sample population is thus 178/200 = 0.89 = 89 percent. Copies of the *CCR5-Δ32* allele were carried by 20 *1/Δ32* individuals, plus 2 carried by the *Δ32/Δ32* individual, for a total of 22. The frequency of the *CCR5-Δ32* allele is thus 22/200 = 0.11 = 11 percent. Notice that $p + q = 1$, confirming that we have accounted for all the alleles of this gene in the population. **Table 25.2** shows two methods for computing the frequencies of the *1* and *Δ32* alleles in the population surveyed.

Can we expect the *CCR5-Δ32* allele to increase in human populations because it offers resistance to infection by HIV? This specific question is difficult to answer directly, but as we have seen earlier in this chapter, when factors such as natural selection, mutation, migration, or genetic drift are present, the allele frequencies in a population may change from one generation to the next.

By determining allele frequencies over more than one generation, it is possible to determine whether the frequencies remain in equilibrium because the Hardy–Weinberg

FIGURE 25–6 Organization of the *CCR5* gene in region 3p21.3. The gene contains 4 exons and 2 introns (there is no intron between exons 2 and 3). The arrow shows the location of the 32-bp deletion in exon 4 that confers resistance to HIV-1 infection.

FIGURE 25-7 Allelic variation in the *CCR5* gene. Michel Samson and colleagues used PCR to amplify a part of the *CCR5* gene containing the site of the 32-bp deletion, cut the resulting DNA fragments with a restriction enzyme, and ran the fragments on an electrophoresis gel. Each lane reveals the genotype of a single individual. The *1* allele produces a 332-bp fragment and a 403-bp fragment; the *Δ32* allele produces a 332-bp fragment and a 371-bp fragment. Heterozygotes produce three bands.

assumptions are operating, or whether allele frequencies or genotype frequencies are changing because one or more of these assumptions is not operating.

Testing for Hardy–Weinberg Equilibrium in a Population

One way to see whether one (or more) of the Hardy–Weinberg assumptions does not hold in a given population is to determine whether the population's genotypes are in equilibrium. To do this, we first determine the genotype frequencies either directly from the phenotypes (if heterozygotes are recognizable) or by analyzing proteins or DNA sequences. We then calculate the allele frequencies from the genotype frequencies, as demonstrated earlier. Finally,

we use the allele frequencies in the parental generation to predict the offspring's genotype frequencies. According to the Hardy–Weinberg law, genotype frequencies are predicted to fit the $p^2 + 2pq + q^2 = 1$ relationship. If they do not, then one or more of the assumptions are invalid for the population in question.

To demonstrate, let's examine *CCR5* genotypes in a population. Our population includes 283 individuals; of these, 223 have genotype *1/1*; 57 have genotype *1/Δ32*; and 3 have genotype *Δ32/Δ32*. These numbers represent the following genotype frequencies: *1/1* = 223/283 = 0.788, *1/Δ32* = 57/283 = 0.201, and *Δ32/Δ32* = 3/283 = 0.011, respectively. From the genotype frequencies, we can compute the *CCR51* allele frequency as 0.89 and the frequency of the *CCR5-Δ32* allele as 0.11. Once we know the allele frequencies, we can use the Hardy–Weinberg law to determine whether this population is in equilibrium. The allele frequencies predict the genotype frequencies in the next generation as follows:

Expected frequency of genotype

$$1/1 = p^2 = (0.89)^2 = 0.792$$

Expected frequency of genotype

$$1/\Delta 32 = 2pq = 2(0.89)(0.11) = 0.196$$

Expected frequency of genotype

$$\Delta 32/\Delta 32 = q^2 = (0.11)^2 = 0.012$$

These expected frequencies are nearly identical to the frequencies observed in the parental generation. Our test of this population has failed to provide evidence that Hardy–Weinberg assumptions are being violated. The conclusion can be confirmed by using the whole numbers utilized in

TABLE 25.2 Methods of Determining Allele Frequencies from Data on Genotypes

(a) Counting Alleles	Genotype			
	1/1	*1/Δ32*	*Δ32/Δ32*	Total
Number of individuals	79	20	1	100
Number of 1 alleles	158	20	0	178
Number of Δ32 alleles	0	20	2	22
Total number of alleles	158	40	2	200

Frequency of *CCR51* in sample: 178/200 = 0.89 = 89%
Frequency of *CCR5-Δ32* in sample: 22/200 = 0.11 = 11%

(b) From Genotype Frequencies	Genotype			
	1/1	*1/Δ32*	*Δ32/Δ32*	Total
Number of individuals	79	20	1	100
Genotype frequency	79/100 = 0.79	20/100 = 0.20	1/100 = 0.01	1.00

Frequency of *CCR51* in sample: 0.79 + (0.5)0.20 = 0.89 = 89%
Frequency of *CCR5-Δ32* in sample: (0.5)0.20 + 0.01 = 0.11 = 11%

calculating the genotype frequencies to perform a χ^2 analysis (see Chapter 3). In this case, neither the genotype frequencies nor the allele frequencies are changing in this population, meaning that the population is in equilibrium, and that selection, drift, migration, mutation, and nonrandom mating are not operating in this population.

25–2 Suppose you are monitoring the allelic and genotypic frequencies of the MN blood group (see Chapter 4 for a description of the MN blood group) in a small human population. You find that for 1-year-old children, the genotype frequencies are MM = 0.25, MN = 0.5, and NN = 0.25. The genotypic frequencies for adults are MM = 0.3, MN = 0.4, and NN = 0.3.

(a) Calculate the M and N allele frequencies for 1-year-old children and for adults.
(b) Are the allele frequencies in equilibrium in this population?
(c) Are the genotype frequencies in equilibrium?

■ **HINT:** *This problem involves an understanding of how to use the Hardy–Weinberg Law to calculate allele and genotype frequencies, and the factors that cause these to change from generation to generation.*

Calculating Frequencies for Multiple Alleles in Populations

Although we have used one-gene two-allele systems as examples, many genes have several alleles, all of which can be found in a single population. The ABO blood group in humans (discussed in Chapter 4) is such an example. The locus *I* (isoagglutinin) has three alleles, I^A, I^B, and i, yielding six possible genotypic combinations (I^AI^A, I^BI^B, ii, I^AI^B, I^Ai, I^Bi). Remember that in this case I^A and I^B are codominant alleles and that both of these are dominant to i. The result is that homozygous I^AI^A and heterozygous I^Ai individuals are phenotypically identical, as are I^BI^B and I^Bi individuals, so we can distinguish only four phenotypic combinations.

By adding another variable to the Hardy–Weinberg equation, we can calculate both the genotype and allele frequencies for the situation involving three alleles. Let *p*, *q*, and *r* represent the frequencies of alleles I^A, I^B, and *i*, respectively. Note that because there are three alleles,

$$p + q + r = 1$$

Under Hardy–Weinberg assumptions, the frequencies of the genotypes are given by

$$(p + q + r)^2 = p^2 + q^2 + r^2 + 2pq + 2pr + 2qr = 1$$

If we know the frequencies of blood types for a population, we can then estimate the frequencies for the three alleles of the ABO system. For example, in one population sampled, the following blood-type frequencies are observed: A = 0.53, B = 0.133, O = 0.26. Because the *i* allele is recessive, the population's frequency of type O blood equals the proportion of the recessive genotype r^2. Thus,

$$r^2 = 0.26$$
$$r = \sqrt{0.26}$$
$$r = 0.51$$

Using *r*, we can calculate the allele frequencies for the I^A and I^B alleles. The I^A allele is present in two genotypes, I^AI^A and I^Ai. The frequency of the I^AI^A genotype is represented by p^2 and the I^Ai genotype by $2pr$. Therefore, the combined frequency of type A blood and type O blood is given by

$$p^2 + 2pr + r^2 = 0.53 + 0.26$$

If we factor the left side of the equation and take the sum of the terms on the right,

$$(p + r)^2 = 0.79$$
$$p + r = \sqrt{0.79}$$
$$p = 0.89 - r$$
$$p = 0.89 - 0.51 = 0.38$$

Having calculated *p* and *r*, the frequencies of allele I^A and allele *i*, we can now calculate the frequency for the I^B allele:

$$p + q + r = 1$$
$$q = 1 - p - r$$
$$= 1 - 0.38 - 0.51$$
$$= 0.11$$

The phenotypic and genotypic frequencies for this population are summarized in Table 25.3.

TABLE 25.3 Calculating Genotype Frequencies for Multiple Alleles in a Hardy–Weinberg Population Where the Frequency of Allele I^A = 0.38, Allele I^B = 0.11, and Allele i = 0.51

Genotype	Genotype Frequency	Phenotype	Phenotype Frequency
I^AI^A	$p^2 = (0.38)^2 = 0.14$	A	0.53
I^Ai	$2pr = 2(0.38)(0.51) = 0.39$		
I^BI^B	$q^2 = (0.11)^2 = 0.01$	B	0.12
I^Bi	$2qr = 2(0.11)(0.51) = 0.11$		
I^AI^B	$2pq = 2(0.38)(0.11) = 0.084$	AB	0.08
ii	$r^2 = (0.51)^2 = 0.26$	O	0.26

Calculating Allele Frequencies for X-linked Traits

The Hardy–Weinberg law can be used to calculate allele and genotype frequencies for X-linked traits, as long as we remember that in an XY sex-determination system, the homogametic (XX) sex has two copies of an X-linked allele, whereas the heterogametic sex (XY) only has one copy. Thus, for mammals (including humans) where the female is XX and the male is XY, the frequency of the X-linked allele in the gene pool and the frequency of males expressing the X-linked trait will be the same. This is because each male only has one X chromosome, and the probability of any individual male receiving an X chromosome with the allele in question must be equal to the frequency of the allele. The probability of any individual female having the allele in question on both X chromosomes will be q^2, where q is the frequency of the allele.

To illustrate this for a recessive X-linked trait, let's consider the example of red-green color blindness, which affects 8 percent of human males. The frequency of the color blindness allele is therefore 0.08; in other words, 8 percent of X chromosomes carry it.

The other 92 percent of X chromosomes carry the dominant allele for normal red-green color vision. If we define p as the frequency of the normal allele and q as the frequency of the color blindness allele, then $p = 0.92$ and $q = 0.08$. The frequency of color-blind females (with two affected X chromosomes) is $q^2 = (0.08)^2 = 0.0064$, and the frequency of carrier females (having one normal and one affected X chromosome) is $2pq = 2(0.08)(0.92) = 0.147$. In other words, 14.7 percent of females carry the allele for red-green color blindness and can pass it to their children, although they themselves have normal color vision.

An important consequence of the difference in allele frequency for X-linked genes between male and female gametes is that for a rare recessive allele, the trait will be expressed at a much higher frequency among XY individuals than among those who are XX. So, for example, diseases such as hemophilia and Duchenne muscular dystrophy (DMD) in humans, both of which are caused by recessive mutations on the X chromosome, are much more common in boys, who need only to inherit a single copy of the mutated allele to suffer from the disease. Girls who inherit two affected X chromosomes will also have the disease; but with a rare allele, the probability of this occurrence is small.

Calculating Heterozygote Frequency

A useful application of the Hardy–Weinberg law, especially in human genetics, allows us to estimate the frequency of heterozygotes in a population. The frequency of a recessive trait can usually be determined by counting individuals with the homozygous recessive phenotype in a sample

of the population. With this information and the Hardy–Weinberg law, we can then calculate the allele and genotype frequencies for this gene.

Cystic fibrosis, an autosomal recessive trait, has an incidence of about $1/2500 = 0.0004$ in people of northern European ancestry. Individuals with cystic fibrosis are easily distinguished from the population at large by such symptoms as extra-salty sweat, excess amounts of thick mucus in the lungs, and susceptibility to bacterial infections. Because this is a recessive trait, individuals with cystic fibrosis must be homozygous. Their frequency in a population is represented by q^2 (provided that mating has been random in the previous generation). The frequency of the recessive allele is therefore

$$q = \sqrt{q^2} = \sqrt{0.0004} = 0.02$$

Because $p + q = 1$, the frequency of p is

$$p = 1 - q = 1 - 0.02 = 0.98$$

In the Hardy–Weinberg equation, the frequency of heterozygotes is $2pq$. Thus,

$$2pq = 2(0.98)(0.02)$$
$$= 0.04 \text{ or 4 percent, or } 1/25$$

Thus, heterozygotes for cystic fibrosis are rather common (about $1/25$ individuals, or 4 percent of the population), even though the incidence of homozygous recessives is only $1/2500$, or 0.04 percent. Calculations such as these are estimates because the population may not meet all Hardy–Weinberg assumptions.

NOW SOLVE THIS

25-3 If the albino phenotype occurs in $1/10,000$ individuals in a population at equilibrium and albinism is caused by an autosomal recessive allele a, calculate the frequency of (a) the recessive mutant allele; (b) the normal dominant allele; (c) heterozygotes in the population; (d) mating between heterozygotes.

■ **HINT:** *This problem involves an understanding of the method of calculating allele and genotype frequencies. The key to its solution is to first determine the frequency of the albinism allele in this population.*

25.4 Natural Selection Is a Major Force Driving Allele Frequency Change

To understand evolution, we must understand the forces that transform the gene pools of populations and can lead to the formation of new species. Chief among the mechanisms transforming populations is **natural selection,** discovered independently by Darwin and by Alfred Russel Wallace. The Wallace–Darwin concept of natural selection can be summarized as follows:

1. Individuals of a species exhibit variations in phenotype—for example, differences in size, agility, coloration, defenses against enemies, ability to obtain food, courtship behaviors, and flowering times.

2. Many of these variations, even small and seemingly insignificant ones, are heritable and passed on to offspring.

3. Organisms tend to reproduce in an exponential fashion. More offspring are produced than can survive. This causes members of a species to engage in a struggle for survival, competing with other members of the community for scarce resources. Offspring also must avoid predators, and in sexually reproducing species, adults must compete for mates.

4. In the struggle for survival, individuals with particular phenotypes will be more successful than others, allowing the former to survive and reproduce at higher rates.

As a consequence of natural selection, populations and species change. The phenotypes that confer improved ability to survive and reproduce become more common, and the phenotypes that confer poor prospects for survival and reproduction may eventually disappear. Under certain conditions, populations that at one time could interbreed may lose that capability, thus segregating their adaptations into particular niches. If selection continues, it may result in the appearance of new species.

Detecting Natural Selection in Populations

Recall that measuring allele frequencies and genotype frequencies using the Hardy–Weinberg law is based on certain assumptions about an ideal population: large population size, lack of migration, presence of random mating, absence of selection and mutation, and equal survival rates of offspring.

However, if all genotypes do not have equal rates of survival or do not leave equal numbers of offspring, then allele frequencies may change from one generation to the next. To see why, let's imagine a population of 100 individuals in which the frequency of allele A is 0.5 and that of allele a is 0.5. Assuming the previous generation mated randomly, we find that the genotype frequencies in the present generation are $(0.5)^2 = 0.25$ for AA, $2(0.5)(0.5) = 0.5$ for Aa, and $(0.5)^2 = 0.25$ for aa. Because our population contains 100 individuals, we have 25 AA individuals, 50 Aa individuals, and 25 aa individuals. Now suppose that individuals with different genotypes have different rates of survival: All 25 AA individuals survive to reproduce, 90 percent or 45 of the Aa individuals survive to reproduce, and 80 percent or 20 of

the aa individuals survive to reproduce. When the survivors reproduce, each contributes two gametes to the new gene pool, giving us $2(25) + 2(45) + 2(20) = 180$ gametes. What are the frequencies of the two alleles in the surviving population? We have 50 A gametes from AA individuals, plus 45 A gametes from Aa individuals, so the frequency of allele A is $(50 + 45)/180 = 0.53$. We have 45 a gametes from Aa individuals, plus 40 a gametes from aa individuals, so the frequency of allele a is $(45 + 40)/180 = 0.47$.

These differ from the frequencies we started with. The frequency of allele A has increased, whereas the frequency of allele a has declined. A difference among individuals in survival or reproduction rate (or both) is an example of natural selection. Natural selection is the principal force that shifts allele frequencies within large populations and is one of the most important factors in evolutionary change.

Fitness and Selection

Selection occurs whenever individuals with a particular genotype enjoy an advantage in survival or reproduction over other genotypes. However, selection may vary from less than 1 to 100 percent. In the previous hypothetical example, selection was strong. Weak selection might involve just a fraction of a percent difference in the survival rates of different genotypes. Advantages in survival and reproduction ultimately translate into increased genetic contribution to future generations. An individual organism's genetic contribution to future generations is called its **fitness.** Genotypes associated with high rates of reproductive success are said to have high fitness, whereas genotypes associated with low reproductive success are said to have low fitness.

Hardy–Weinberg analysis also allows us to examine fitness. By convention, population geneticists use the letter w to represent fitness. Thus, w_{AA} represents the relative fitness of genotype AA, w_{Aa} the relative fitness of genotype Aa, and w_{aa} the relative fitness of genotype aa. Assigning the values $w_{AA} = 1$, $w_{Aa} = 0.9$, and $w_{aa} = 0.8$ would mean, for example, that all AA individuals survive, 90 percent of the Aa individuals survive, and 80 percent of the aa individuals survive, as in the previous hypothetical case.

Let's consider selection against deleterious alleles. Fitness values, $w_{AA} = 1$, $w_{Aa} = 1$, and $w_{aa} = 0$ describe a situation in which a is a homozygous lethal allele. As homozygous recessive individuals die without leaving offspring, the frequency of allele a will decline. The decline in the frequency of allele a is described by the equation

$$q_g = \frac{q_0}{1 + gq_0}$$

where q_g is the frequency of allele a in generation g, q_o is the starting frequency of a (i.e., the frequency of a in generation zero), and g is the number of generations that have passed.

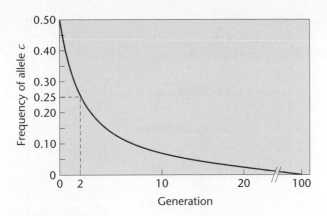

FIGURE 25–8 Change in the frequency of a lethal recessive allele, *a*. The frequency of *a* is halved in two generations and halved again by the sixth generation. Subsequent reductions occur slowly because the majority of *a* alleles are carried by heterozygotes.

Figure 25–8 shows what happens to a lethal recessive allele with an initial frequency of 0.5. At first, because of the high percentage of *aa* genotypes, the frequency of allele *a* declines rapidly. The frequency of *a* is halved in only two generations. By the sixth generation, the frequency is halved again. By now, however, the majority of *a* alleles are carried by heterozygotes. Because *a* is recessive, these heterozygotes are not selected against. Consequently, as more time passes, the frequency of allele *a* declines ever more slowly. As long as heterozygotes continue to mate, it is difficult for selection to completely eliminate a recessive allele from a population.

Figure 25–9 shows the outcome of different degrees of selection against a nonlethal recessive allele, *a*. In this case, the intensity of selection varies from strong (red curve) to weak (blue curve), as well as intermediate values (yellow, purple, and green curves). In each example, the frequency of the deleterious allele, *a*, starts at 0.99 and declines over time. However, the rate of decline depends heavily on the strength of selection. When selection is strong and only 90 percent of the heterozygotes and 80 percent of the *aa* homozygotes survive (red curve), the frequency of allele *a*

drops from 0.99 to less than 0.01 in about 85 generations. However, when selection is weak, and 99.8 percent of the heterozygotes and 99.6 percent of the *aa* homozygotes survive (blue curve), it takes 1000 generations for the frequency of allele *a* to drop from 0.99 to 0.93. Two important conclusions can be drawn from this example. First, over thousands of generations, even weak selection can cause substantial changes in allele frequencies; because evolution generally occurs over a large number of generations, selection is a powerful force in evolutionary change. Second, for selection to produce rapid changes in allele frequencies, the differences in fitness among genotypes must be large.

The manner in which selection affects allele frequencies allows us to make some inferences about the *CCR5-Δ32* allele that we discussed earlier. Because individuals with genotype *Δ32/Δ32* are resistant to most sexually transmitted strains of HIV-1, while individuals with genotypes *1/1* and *1/Δ32* are susceptible, we might expect AIDS to act as a selective force causing the frequency of the *Δ32* allele to increase over time. Indeed, it probably will, but the increase in frequency is likely to be slow in human terms. In fact, it will take about 100 generations (about 2000 years) for the frequency of the *Δ32* allele to reach just 0.11. In other words, the frequency of the *Δ32* allele will probably not change much over the next few generations in most populations that currently harbor it.

There Are Several Types of Selection

The phenotype is the result of the combined influence of the individual's genotype at many different loci and the effects of the environment. Selection for traits can be classified as (1) directional, (2) stabilizing, or (3) disruptive.

In **directional selection (Figure 25–10)** phenotypes at one end of the spectrum present in the population become selected for or against, usually as a result of changes in

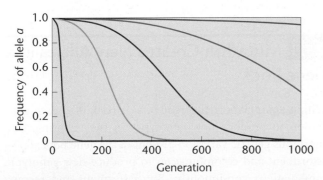

FIGURE 25–9 The effect of selection on allele frequency. The rate at which a deleterious allele is removed from a population depends heavily on the strength of selection.

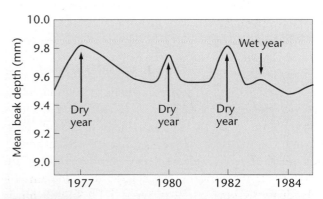

FIGURE 25–10 Beak size in finches during dry years increases because of strong selection. Between droughts, selection for large beak size is not as strong, and birds with smaller beak sizes survive and reproduce, increasing the number of birds with smaller beaks.

the environment. A carefully documented example comes from research by Peter and Rosemary Grant and their colleagues, who study the medium ground finches (*Geospiza fortis*) of Daphne Major Island in the Galapagos Islands. The beak size of these birds varies enormously. In 1976, for example, some birds in the population had beaks less than 7 mm deep, while others had beaks more than 12 mm deep. In 1977, a severe drought killed some 80 percent of the finches. Big-beaked birds survived at higher rates than small-beaked birds because when food became scarce, the big-beaked birds were able to eat a greater variety of seeds. When the drought ended in 1978, the offspring of the survivors inherited their parents' big beaks. Between 1976 and 1978, the beak depth of the average finch in the Daphne Major population increased by just over 0.5 mm, shifting the average beak size toward one phenotypic extreme.

Stabilizing selection, in contrast, tends to favor intermediate phenotypes, with those at both extremes being selected against. Over time, this will reduce the phenotypic variance in the population but without a significant shift in the mean. One of the clearest demonstrations of stabilizing selection is shown by a study of human birth weight and survival for 13,730 children born over an 11-year period. **Figure 25–11** shows the distribution of birth weight and the percentage of mortality at 4 weeks of age. Infant mortality increases on either side of the optimal birth weight of 7.5 pounds. Stabilizing selection acts to keep a population well adapted to its current environment.

Disruptive selection is selection against intermediates and for both phenotypic extremes. It can be viewed as the opposite of stabilizing selection because the intermediate types are selected against. This will result in a population with an increasingly bimodal distribution for the trait, as we can see in **Figure 25–12**. In one set of experiments using *Drosophila*, after several generations of disruptive artificial selection for bristle number, in which only flies with high

FIGURE 25–12 The effect of disruptive selection on bristle number in *Drosophila*. When individuals with the highest and lowest bristle number were selected, the population showed a nonoverlapping divergence in only 12 generations.

or low bristle numbers were allowed to breed, most flies could be easily placed in a low- or high-bristle category. In natural populations, such a situation might exist for a population in a heterogeneous environment.

25.5 Mutation Creates New Alleles in a Gene Pool

Within a population, the gene pool is reshuffled each generation to produce new genotypes in the offspring. The enormous genetic variation present in the gene pool allows assortment and recombination to produce new genotypic combinations continuously. But assortment and recombination do not produce new alleles. **Mutation** alone acts to create new alleles. It is important to keep in mind that

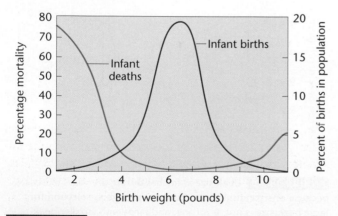

FIGURE 25–11 Relationship between birth weight and mortality in humans.

mutational events occur at random—that is, without regard for any possible benefit or disadvantage to the organism. In this section, we consider whether mutation, by itself, is a significant factor in changing allele frequencies.

To determine whether mutation is a significant force in changing allele frequencies, we measure the rate at which they are produced. As most mutations are recessive, it is difficult to observe mutation rates directly in diploid organisms. Indirect methods use probability and statistics or large-scale screening programs to estimate mutation rates. For certain dominant mutations, however, a direct method of measurement can be used. To ensure accuracy, several conditions must be met:

1. The allele must produce a distinctive phenotype that can be distinguished from similar phenotypes produced by recessive alleles.

2. The trait must be fully expressed or completely penetrant so that mutant individuals can be identified.

3. An identical phenotype must never be produced by nongenetic agents such as drugs or chemicals.

Mutation rates can be stated as the number of new mutant alleles per given number of gametes. Suppose that for a given gene that undergoes mutation to a dominant allele, 2 out of 100,000 births exhibit a mutant phenotype. In these two cases, the parents are phenotypically normal. Because the zygotes that produced these births each carry two copies of the gene, we have actually surveyed 200,000 copies of the gene (or 200,000 gametes). If we assume that the affected births are each heterozygous, we have uncovered two mutant alleles out of 200,000. Thus, the mutation rate is 2/200,000 or 1/100,000, which in scientific notation is written as 1×10^{-5}. In humans, a dominant form of dwarfism known as **achondroplasia** fulfills the requirements for measuring mutation rates. Individuals with this skeletal disorder have an enlarged skull, short arms and legs, and can be diagnosed by X-ray examination at birth. In a survey of almost 250,000 births, the mutation rate (μ) for achondroplasia has been calculated as

$$\mu = 1.4 \times 10^{-5} \pm 0.5 \times 10^{-5}$$

Knowing the rate of mutation, we can estimate the extent to which mutation can cause allele frequencies to change from one generation to the next. We represent the normal allele as d and the allele for achondroplasia as D.

Imagine a population of 500,000 individuals in which everyone has genotype dd. The initial frequency of d is 1.0, and the initial frequency of D is 0. If each individual contributes two gametes to the gene pool, the gene pool will contain 1,000,000 gametes, all carrying allele d. Although the gametes are in the gene pool, 1.4 of every 100,000 d

alleles mutate into a D allele. The frequency of allele d is now $(1,000,000 - 14)/1,000,000 = 0.999986$, and the frequency of allele D is $14/1,000,000 = 0.000014$. From these numbers, it will clearly be a long time before mutation, by itself, causes any appreciable change in the allele frequencies in this population. In other words, mutation generates new alleles but by itself does not alter allele frequencies at an appreciable rate in large populations. However, in very small populations, mutation can alter allele frequencies.

25.6 Migration and Gene Flow Can Alter Allele Frequencies

Occasionally, a species becomes divided into populations that are separated geographically. Various evolutionary forces, including selection, can establish different allele frequencies in such populations. **Migration** occurs when individuals move between the populations. Imagine a species in which a given locus has two alleles, A and a. There are two populations of this species, one on a mainland and one on an island. The frequency of A on the mainland is represented by p_m, and the frequency of A on the island is p_i. If there is migration from the mainland to the island, the frequency of A in the next generation on the island (p_i') is given by

$$p_i' = (1 - m)p_i + mp_m$$

where m represents migrants from the mainland to the island and migration is random with respect to genotype.

As an example of how migration might affect the frequency of A in the next generation on the island (p_i'), assume that $p_i = 0.4$ and $p_m = 0.6$ and that 10 percent of the parents of the next generation are migrants from the mainland ($m = 0.1$). In the next generation, the frequency of allele A on the island will therefore be

$$\begin{aligned} p_i' &= [(1 - 0.1) \times 0.4] + (0.1 \times 0.6) \\ &= 0.36 + 0.06 \\ &= 0.42 \end{aligned}$$

In this case, migration from the mainland has changed the frequency of A on the island from 0.40 to 0.42 in a single generation.

These calculations reveal that the change in allele frequency attributable to migration is proportional to the differences in allele frequency between the donor and recipient populations and to the rate of migration. If either m is large or p_m is very different from p_i, then a rather large change in the frequency of A can occur in a single generation. If migration is the only force acting to change the allele frequency

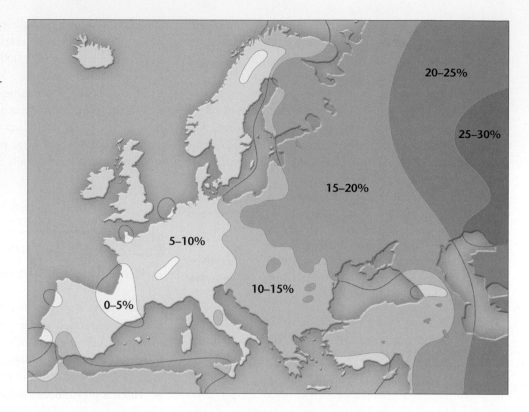

FIGURE 25-13 Migration as a force in evolution. The I^B allele of the *ABO* locus is present in a gradient from east to west. This allele shows the highest frequency in central Asia and the lowest in northeast Spain. The gradient parallels the waves of Mongol migration into Europe following the fall of the Roman Empire and is a genetic relic of human history.

20–25%

25–30%

15–20%

5–10%

10–15%

0–5%

on the island, then equilibrium will be attained only when $p_i = p_m$. These guidelines can often be used to estimate migration in cases where it is difficult to quantify. As m can have a wide range of values, the effect of migration can substantially alter allele frequencies in populations, as shown for the I^B allele of the ABO blood group in **Figure 25–13**.

25.7 Genetic Drift Causes Random Changes in Allele Frequency in Small Populations

In small populations, significant random fluctuations in allele frequencies are possible by chance alone, a situation known as **genetic drift.** The degree of fluctuation increases as the population size decreases. In addition to small population size, drift can arise through the **founder effect,** which occurs when a population originates from a small number of individuals. Although the population may later increase to a large size, the genes carried by all members are derived from those of the founders (assuming no mutation, migration, or selection, and the presence of random mating). Drift can also arise via a **genetic bottleneck.** Bottlenecks develop when a large population undergoes a drastic but temporary reduction in numbers. Even though the population recovers, its genetic diversity has been greatly reduced.

Founder Effects in Human Populations

Allele frequencies in certain human populations demonstrate the role of genetic drift in natural populations. Native Americans living in the southwestern United States have a high frequency of oculocutaneous albinism (OCA). In the Navajo, who live primarily in northeast Arizona, albinism occurs with a frequency of 1 in 1500–2000, compared with whites (1 in 36,000) and African-Americans (1 in 10,000). There are four different forms of OCA (OCA1–4), all with varying degrees of melanin deficiency in the skin, eyes, and hair. OCA2 is caused by mutations in the *P* gene, which encodes a plasma membrane protein. To investigate the genetic basis of albinism in the Navajo, researchers screened for mutations in the *P* gene. In their study, all Navajo with albinism were homozygous for a 122.5-kb deletion in the *P* gene, spanning exons 10–20 (**Figure 25–14**). This deletion allele was not present in 34 individuals belonging to other Native American populations.

Using a set of PCR primers, researchers were able to identify homozygous affected individuals and heterozygous carriers (**Figure 25–15**) and surveyed 134 normally pigmented Navajo and 42 members of the Apache, a tribe closely related to the Navajo. Based on this sample, the heterozygote frequency in the Navajo is estimated to be 4.5 percent. No carriers were found in the Apache population that was studied.

The 122.5-kb deletion allele causing OCA2 was found only in the Navajo population and not in members of other Native American tribes in the southwestern United States,

(a)

(b)

FIGURE 25–14 Genomic DNA digests from a Navajo affected with albinism (N5) and a normally pigmented individual (C). (a) Hybridization with a probe covering exons 11–15 of the *P* gene; there are no hybridizing fragments detected in N5. (b) Hybridization with a probe covering exons 15–20 of the *P* gene; there are no hybridizing fragments detected in N5. This confirms the presence of a deletion in affected individuals.

Courtesy of Murray Brilliant, "A 122.5 kilobase deletion of P gene underlies the high prevalence of oculocutaneous albinism type 2 in the Navajo population." From: American Journal Human Genetics *72:62–72, Figure 1, 65. Published by University of Chicago Press.*

suggesting that the mutant allele is specific to the Navajo and may have arisen in a single individual who was one of a small number of founders of the Navajo population. Using other methods, workers originally estimated the age of the mutation to be between 400 and 11,000 years. To narrow this range, they relied on tribal history. Navajo oral tradition indicates that the Navajo and Apache became separate populations between 600 and 1000 years ago. Because the deletion is not found in the Apaches, it probably arose in the Navajo population after the tribes split. On this basis, the deletion is estimated to be 400 to 1000 years old and probably arose as a founder mutation.

FIGURE 25–15 PCR screens of Navajo affected with albinism (N4 and N5) and the parents of N4 (N2 and N3). Affected individuals (N4 and N5), heterozygous carriers (N2 and N3), and a homozygous normal individual (C) each give a distinctive band pattern, allowing detection of heterozygous carriers in the population. Molecular size markers (M) are in the first lane.

Courtesy of Murray Brilliant, "A 122.5 kilobase deletion of P gene underlies the high prevalence of oculocutaneous albinism type 2 in the Navajo population." From: American Journal Human Genetics *72: 62–72, Figure 3, p. 67. Published by University of Chicago Press.*

25.8 Nonrandom Mating Changes Genotype Frequency but Not Allele Frequency

We have explored how violations of the first four assumptions of the Hardy–Weinberg law, in the form of selection, mutation, migration, and genetic drift, can cause allele frequencies to change. The fifth assumption is that the members of a population mate at random; in other words, any one genotype has an equal probability of mating with any other genotype in the population. Nonrandom mating can change the frequencies of genotypes in a population. Subsequent selection for or against certain genotypes has the potential to affect the overall frequencies of the alleles they contain, but it is important to note that nonrandom mating *does not itself directly change allele frequencies*.

Nonrandom mating can take one of several forms. In **positive assortive mating,** similar genotypes are more likely to mate than dissimilar ones. This often occurs in humans: A number of studies have indicated that many people are more attracted to individuals who physically resemble them (and are therefore more likely to be genetically similar as well). **Negative assortive mating** occurs when dissimilar genotypes are more likely to mate; some plant species have inbuilt pollen/stigma recognition systems that prevent fertilization between individuals with the same alleles at key loci. However, the form of nonrandom mating most commonly found to affect genotype frequencies in population genetics is **inbreeding.**

Inbreeding

Inbreeding occurs when mating individuals are more closely related than any two individuals drawn from the population at random; loosely defined, inbreeding is mating among relatives. For a given allele, inbreeding increases the proportion of homozygotes in the population. A completely inbred population will theoretically consist only of homozygous genotypes.

To describe the intensity of inbreeding in a population, geneticist Sewall Wright devised the **coefficient of inbreeding (F).** F quantifies the probability that the two alleles of a given gene in an individual are identical *because they are descended from the same single copy of the allele in an ancestor.* If $F = 1$, all individuals in the population are homozygous, and both alleles in every individual are derived from the same ancestral copy. If $F = 0$, no individual has two alleles derived from a common ancestral copy.

One method of estimating F for an individual is shown in **Figure 25–16.** The fourth-generation female (shaded pink) is the daughter of first cousins (yellow). Suppose her great-grandmother (green) was a carrier of a recessive lethal allele, a. What is the probability that the fourth-generation female will inherit two copies of her great-grandmother's lethal allele? For this to happen, (1) the great-grandmother had to pass a copy of the allele to her son, (2) her son had to pass it to his daughter, and (3) his daughter had to pass it to her daughter (the pink female). Also, (4) the great-grandmother had to pass a copy of the allele to her daughter, (5) her daughter had to pass it to her son, and (6) her son had to pass it to his daughter (the pink female). Each of the six necessary events has an individual probability of $1/2$, and they *all* have to happen, so the probability that the pink female will inherit two copies of her great-grandmother's

lethal allele is $(1/2)^6 = 1/64$. To calculate an overall value of F for the pink female as a child of a first-cousin marriage, remember that she could also inherit two copies of any of the other three alleles present in her great-grandparents. Because any of four possibilities would give the pink female two alleles identical by descent from an ancestral copy,

$$F = 4 \times (1/64) = 1/16$$

25–4 A prospective groom, who is normal, has a sister with cystic fibrosis (CF), an autosomal recessive disease. Their parents are normal. The brother plans to marry a woman who has no history of CF in her family. What is the probability that they will produce a CF child? They are both Caucasian, and the overall frequency of CF in the Caucasian population is 1/2500—that is, 1 affected child per 2500. (Assume the population meets the Hardy–Weinberg assumptions.)

■ **HINT:** *This problem involves an understanding of how recessive alleles are transmitted (see Chapter 3) and the probability of receiving a recessive allele from a heterozygous parent. The key to its solution is to first work out the probability that each parent carries the mutant allele.*

25.9 Reduced Gene Flow, Selection, and Genetic Drift Can Lead to Speciation

A **species** can be defined as a group of actually or potentially interbreeding organisms that is reproductively isolated in nature from all other such groups. In sexually reproducing organisms, speciation transforms the parental species into another species, or divides a single species into two or more separate species. Changes in morphology or physiology and adaptation to ecological niches may also occur but are not necessary components of the speciation event.

Populations within a species may carry considerable genetic variation, present as differences in alleles or allele frequencies at a variety of loci. Genetic divergence of these populations can reflect the action of natural selection, genetic drift, or both. In an earlier section, we saw that the migration of individuals between populations tends

The chance that this female will inherit two copies of her great-grandmother's a allele is

$$F = \frac{1}{2} \times \frac{1}{2} \times \frac{1}{2} \times \frac{1}{2} \times \frac{1}{2} \times \frac{1}{2} = \frac{1}{64}$$

Because the female's two alleles could be identical by descent from any of four different alleles,

$$F = 4 \times \frac{1}{64} = \frac{1}{16}$$

FIGURE 25–16 Calculating the coefficient of inbreeding (F) for the offspring of a first cousin marriage.

to homogenize allele frequencies among populations. In other words, migration counteracts the tendency of populations to diverge.

When gene flow between populations is reduced or absent, the populations may diverge to the point that members of one population are no longer able to interbreed successfully with members of the other. When populations reach the point where they are reproductively isolated from one another, they have become different species, according to the biological species concept. The genetic changes that result in reproductive isolation between or among populations and that lead to the formation of new species or higher taxonomic groups represent an example of macroevolution. We will restrict our discussion to the macroevolutionary changes that lead to the formation of new species.

The biological barriers that prevent or reduce interbreeding between populations are called **reproductive isolating mechanisms.** These mechanisms may be ecological, behavioral, seasonal, mechanical, or physiological.

Prezygotic isolating mechanisms prevent individuals from mating in the first place. Individuals from different populations may not find each other at the right time, may not recognize each other as suitable mates, or may try to mate but find that they are unable to do so.

Postzygotic isolating mechanisms create reproductive isolation even when the members of two populations are willing and able to mate with each other. For example, genetic divergence may have reached the stage where the viability or fertility of hybrids is reduced. Hybrid zygotes may be formed, but all or most may be inviable. Alternatively, the hybrids may be viable, but be sterile or suffer from reduced fertility. Yet again, the hybrids themselves may be fertile, but their progeny may have lowered viability or fertility. In all these situations, hybrids are genetic dead-ends. These postzygotic mechanisms act at or beyond the level of the zygote and are generated by genetic divergence.

Postzygotic isolating mechanisms waste gametes and zygotes and lower the reproductive fitness of hybrid survivors. Selection will therefore favor the spread of alleles that reduce the formation of hybrids, leading to the development of prezygotic isolating mechanisms, which in turn prevent interbreeding and the formation of hybrid zygotes and offspring. In animal evolution, one of the most effective prezygotic mechanisms is behavioral isolation, involving courtship behavior.

Changes Leading to Speciation

Formation of the Isthmus of Panama about 3 million years ago created a land bridge connecting North and South America and separated the Caribbean Sea from the Pacific Ocean. After identifying seven Caribbean species of snapping shrimp (**Figure 25–17**) and seven similar Pacific

FIGURE 25–17   A snapping shrimp (genus *Alpheus*).

species, researchers matched them in pairs. Members of each pair were closer to each other in structure and appearance than to any other species in its own ocean. Analysis of allele frequencies and mitochondrial DNA sequences confirmed that the members of each pair were one another's closest genetic relatives. In other words, the ancestors of each pair were members of a single species. When the isthmus closed, each of the seven ancestral species was divided into two separate populations, one in the Caribbean and the other in the Pacific. But after 3 million years of separation, were members of these populations different species?

Males and females were paired together, and successful matings between Caribbean–Pacific couples versus those of Caribbean–Caribbean or Pacific–Pacific pairs were calculated. In three of the seven species pairs, transoceanic couples refused to mate altogether. For the other four pairs, transoceanic couples were 33, 45, 67, and 86 percent as likely to mate with each other compared to the same-ocean pairs.

Of the transoceanic pairs that mated, only 1 percent produced viable offspring, while 60 percent of same-ocean pairs produced viable offspring. We can conclude that 3 million years of separation has resulted in complete or nearly complete speciation, involving strong pre- and postzygotic isolating mechanisms for all seven species pairs.

The Rate of Macroevolution and Speciation

How much time is required for speciation? As we saw in the example above, the time needed for genetic divergence and formation of new species can occur over a span of several million years. In fact, the average time for speciation ranges from 100,000 to 10,000,000 years. However, rapid speciation over much shorter time spans has been reported in a number of cases, including fishes in East African lakes, marine salmon, palm trees on isolated islands, polyploid plants, and brown algae in the Baltic Sea.

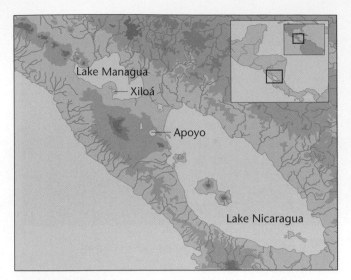

FIGURE 25–18 Lake Apoyo in Nicaragua occupies the crater of an inactive volcano. The lake formed about 23,000 years ago. Two species of cichlid fish in the lake share a close evolutionary relationship.

(a)

(b)

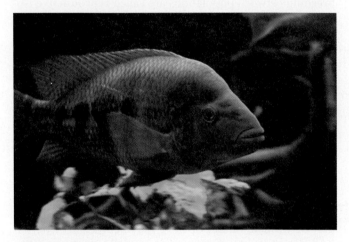

FIGURE 25–19 The two species of cichlids in Lake Apoyo exhibit distinctive morphologies: (a) *Amphilophus citrinellus*, (b) *Amphilophus zaliosus*.

In Nicaragua, Lake Apoyo was formed within the last 23,000 years in the crater of a volcano (**Figure 25–18**). This small lake is home to two species of cichlid fish: the Midas cichlid, *Amphilophus citrinellus*, and the Arrow cichlid, *A. zaliosus*. The Midas is the most common cichlid in the region and is found in nearby lakes; the Arrow cichlid is found only in Lake Apoyo.

To establish the evolutionary origin of the Arrow cichlid, researchers used a variety of approaches, including phylogenetic, morphological, and ecological analyses. Sequence analysis of mitochondrial DNA established that the two species form a monophyletic group, indicating that there was first a population expansion of the Midas cichlid, followed by an ongoing expansion of the Arrow cichlid. Further analysis using a PCR-based method strengthened the conclusion that these two species are monophyletic and that *A. zaliosus* evolved from *A. citrinellus*. Members of the two species have distinctive morphologies (**Figure 25–19**), including jaw specializations that reflect different food preferences, which were confirmed by analysis of stomach contents. In addition, the two species are reproductively isolated, a conclusion that was substantiated by laboratory experiments. Using a molecular clock calibrated for cichlid mtDNA, it is estimated that *A. zaliosus* evolved from *A. citrinellus* sometime within the last 10,000 years. This, and examples from other species, provide unambiguous evidence that depending on the strength of selection and that of other parameters of the Hardy–Weinberg law, species formation can occur over a much shorter time scale than the usual range of 100,000–10,000,000 years.

25.10 Phylogeny Can Be Used to Analyze Evolutionary History

Speciation is associated with changes in the genetic structure of populations and with genetic divergence of those populations. Therefore, we should be able to use genetic differences among present-day species to reconstruct their evolutionary histories, or phylogenies. These relationships are most often presented in the form of phylogenetic trees (**Figure 25–20**), which show the ancestral relationships among a group of organisms. These groups can be species, or larger groups. In a phylogenetic tree, branches represent lineages over time. The length of a branch can be arbitrary, or it can be derived from a time scale, showing the length of time between speciation events. Points at which lines diverge, called nodes, show when a species split into two or more species. Each node represents a common ancestor of

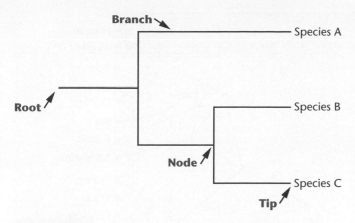

FIGURE 25–20 Elements of a phylogenetic tree showing the relationships among several species. The root represents a common ancestor to all species on the tree. Branches represent lineages through time. The points at which the branches separate are called nodes, and at the tips of the branches are the living or extinct species.

the species diverging at that node. The tips of the branches represent species (or a larger group) alive today (or those that ended in extinction). Groups that consist of an ancestral species and all its descendants are called monophyletic groups. The root of a phylogenetic tree represents the oldest common ancestor to all the groups shown in the tree.

Constructing Phylogenetic Trees from Amino Acid Sequences

In an important early example of phylogenetic analysis, W. M. Fitch and E. Margoliash used data on the amino acid sequence of cytochrome c in a variety of organisms to construct a phylogenetic tree. **Cytochrome c** is a eukaryotic mitochondrial protein whose amino acid sequence has changed very slowly over time. For example, the amino acid sequence in humans and chimpanzees is identical, and humans and rhesus monkeys show only one amino acid difference. This high degree of similarity is remarkable considering that the fossil record indicates that the lines leading to humans and monkeys diverged from a common ancestor approximately 20 million years ago. Using these data, Margoliash postulated the idea of **genetic equidistance,** meaning that the differences in amino acid sequence between species and major groups of organisms is proportional to their evolutionary distance. For example, fish were early vertebrates, and the number of amino acid differences between individual species of fish and individual species of mammals should be similar. In fact, the differences between the sequence from tuna and horse, pig, rabbit, and human falls in the range of 17–21 amino acid differences, and the distance between yeast and vertebrates ranges from 43 to 48.

However, more than one nucleotide change may be required to generate an amino acid substitution. When the nucleotide changes necessary for all amino acid differences

observed in a protein are totaled, the **minimal mutational distance** between the genes of any two species is established.

Fitch used data on the minimal mutational distances between the cytochrome c genes of 19 organisms to construct a phylogenetic tree showing their evolutionary history (**Figure 25–21**). The black dots on the tips of the branches represent existing species. Common ancestors are linked to them by green lines and red dots showing that ancestral species evolved and diverged to produce the modern species. The tree culminates in a single common ancestor for all the species on the tree, represented by the red dot on the extreme left. Numbers on the lines represent corrected minimal mutational differences.

Molecular Clocks Measure the Rate of Evolutionary Change

In many cases, we would like to estimate not only which members of a set of species are most closely related, but also when their common ancestors lived. The phylogenetic analysis of amino acid sequences and the concept of genetic equidistance led to the idea of constructing and using **molecular clocks** to measure the rate of change in amino acid or nucleotide sequences as a way to infer evolutionary relationships and estimate time of divergence from a common ancestor.

To be useful, molecular clocks must be carefully calibrated. Molecular clocks can only measure changes in amino acids or nucleotides; they are linear over certain time scales, and times and dates must be added to the clock using independent evidence such as the fossil record. **Figure 25–22** shows a molecular clock showing divergence times for humans and other vertebrates based on the fossil record [**Figure 22–22(a)**], and molecular data [**Figure 25–22(b)**]. In both cases, changes in amino acid sequence and nucleotide sequence increase linearly with time.

Genomics and Molecular Evolution

The development of genome projects, bioinformatics, and the emergence of comparative genomics has revolutionized the field of molecular evolution. Using these methods, researchers are studying the origin, evolution, and function of gene duplications (discussed in Chapters 8 and 21), the evolution of the human genome, and more recently, the role of natural selection in human adaptations. As we will see in the following section, comparative genomics can be used to provide a detailed picture of how our genome compares to those of our closest relatives and ancestors.

The Complex Origins of Our Genome

For most of the twentieth century, ideas about how and where our species arose were derived entirely from the study of fossils. In the mid-1980s, geneticists began to study levels of genetic diversity in mitochondrial DNA

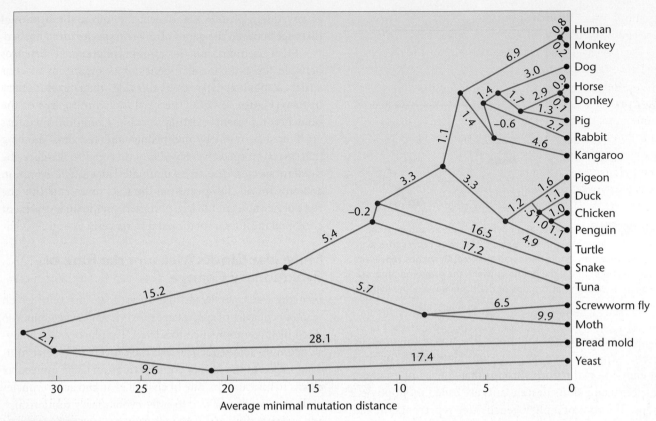

FIGURE 25-21 Phylogenetic tree constructed by comparing homologies in cytochrome c amino acid sequences.

(mtDNA) from present-day population groups as a way of inferring where *Homo sapiens* originated. Phylogenetic trees constructed from these results showed the highest levels of diversity in African populations, with much less diversity in populations of Europe, Asia, and the Americas.

Molecular clock estimates indicate that all non-African populations had their origins about 50,000 years ago. These and other studies of genetic variation in modern populations extrapolate backwards in time to conclude that *H. sapiens* originated in Africa from earlier species of *Homo*, and that

FIGURE 25-22 Relationship between the number of amino acid substitutions and the number of nucleotide substitutions for 4198 nuclear genes from 10 vertebrate species. Humans versus (1) chimpanzee, (2) orangutan, (3) macaque, (4) mouse, (5) cow, (6) opossum, (7) chicken, (8) western clawed frog, and (9) zebrafish. In (a) the data are calculated by divergence times based on the fossil record, and in (b), based on molecular data. Synonymous nucleotide substitutions do not result in the replacement of an amino acid; non-synonymous nucleotide substitutions result in a different amino acid in the protein.

migrations from Africa beginning about 50,000–60,000 years ago dispersed our species across Europe and Asia where we replaced other, preexisting human species, including *H. neanderthalensis.*

This relatively straightforward account of the origin and dispersal of our species and the history of our genome became more complicated with advances in DNA sequencing technology that allowed the recovery and genomic sequencing of DNA from fossil humans. This new field, called **paleogenomics,** along with the continuing discovery of fossils representing other human species, is revolutionizing the study of human evolution. We will begin by discussing what we know about the genome of the Neanderthals and the contributions they made to our genome. We will then describe the findings establishing that at least one other species has also added alleles to our genome.

Neanderthals, *Homo neanderthalensis,* lived in Europe and western Asia from some 300,000 years ago until they disappeared about 30,000 years ago. For at least 30,000 years, Neanderthals coexisted with anatomically modern humans (*Homo sapiens*) in several regions, raising several questions about the relationship between Neanderthals and modern humans: (1) Were Neanderthals direct ancestors of modern humans? (2) Did Neanderthals and *H. sapiens* interbreed, so that descendants of the Neanderthals are alive today? Or did the Neanderthals die off and become extinct? (3) What can we say about the similarities and differences between our genome and that of the Neanderthals?

To answer these and other questions, DNA from three Neanderthal skeletons recovered from a cave in Croatia was sequenced and assembled into a genome sequence. As part of this project, the genomes of five individuals from our species, all living in different parts of the world were also sequenced.

The Neanderthal genome is the same size as the genome of our species, and contains about 3.2 billion base pairs. Sequence comparison shows it is 99.7 percent identical to our genome. As a point of reference, both the Neanderthal genome and our genome are about 98.8 percent identical to that of the chimpanzee.

By comparing the Neanderthal genome sequence with the genomes of five present-day humans and with the chimpanzee genome, researchers were able to identify amino acid-coding differences in 90

genes that originated after the split between the Neanderthal and human lineages. These genes are involved in cognitive development, skin morphology, and skeletal development. In addition, there is evidence that several regions of the modern human genome have undergone positive selection in the interval since Neanderthals and modern humans last shared a common ancestor.

Perhaps the most unexpected finding in this analysis is that the genomes of present-day humans in Europe and Asia, but not Africa, are composed of 1–4 percent Neanderthal sequences. However, the recent discovery that the 1–4 percent figure actually represents different parts of the Neanderthal genome present in different individuals suggests that upwards of 20 percent of the Neanderthal genome may be present in our DNA. Interbreeding with Neanderthals may have occurred somewhere in the Middle East, before humans migrated into Europe and Asia. No Neanderthal contributions to African genomes were detected, but it is possible that a larger sampling of African populations will determine whether some Africans carry Neanderthal genes.

A phylogenetic tree showing the pattern and times of divergence of Neanderthals and our species is presented in **Figure 25–23**. The tree shows that Neanderthals and humans last shared a common ancestor about 706,000 years ago and that the isolating split between Neanderthals and human populations occurred about 370,000 years ago. From these studies, several conclusions can be drawn. First, Neanderthals are not direct ancestors of our species. Second, Neanderthals and members of our species interbred, and Neanderthals

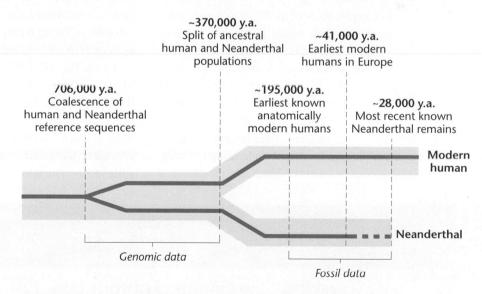

FIGURE 25–23 Estimated times of divergence of human and Neanderthal genomic sequences and, subsequently, of their populations, relative to landmark events in both human and Neanderthal evolution. These estimates are based on sequencing about 65,000 base pairs of Neanderthal DNA (y.a. = years ago). "Sequencing and analysis of Neanderthal genomic DNA," by J.P. Noonan et al., from SCIENCE, 314. Copyright © 2006 by AAAS. Reprinted with permission.

contributed to our genome. The extent of this contribution remains to be determined. As a species, Neanderthals are extinct, but some of their genes survive as part of our genome. Third, from what we know about the Neanderthal genome, we share most genes and other sequences with them.

Our Genome Is a Mosaic

When *H. sapiens* migrated out of Africa, parts of Europe and Asia were already occupied by members of other human species. The most well known of these is the Neanderthals, and their contribution to the genomes of non-African populations was described earlier in this chapter. However, the human family has been expanded by the discovery of fossils from other species. In 2004, human fossils were unearthed on the island of Flores, in Indonesia. Members of this species, called *H. floresiensis*, were only about 1 meter (39 inches) tall, and the fossil evidence suggests that this species was in existence at least 38,000 years ago, a time frame that overlaps with the presence of our species in the same area. Because of the tropical climate, no DNA for genomic sequencing has been recovered from the *H. floresiensis* fossils, so their contribution to our genome, if any, remains to be determined.

In 2008, human fossils were discovered in a cave near Denisova, Siberia. A complete mtDNA genome sequence from this fossil showed that the Denisovans belonged to a group separate from both Neanderthals and our species. A nuclear genome sequence obtained from the Denisovan fossils shows they are more closely related to Neanderthals than to our species. However, analysis of modern human populations shows that Denisovan DNA is part of the genome of some members of our species. For example, 4–6% of the DNA in the genomes of Melanesians, residents of an island group in the South Pacific, is derived from Denisovans. In addition, Denisovan alleles are found in the genomes of Australian aborigines, Polynesian, Fujian, and east Indonesian populations. There is no evidence that Denisovans contributed to the genomes of populations now living in south or east Asia, who probably migrated to these areas after the Denisovans became extinct.

As things stand now, we know that the genomes of some members of our species outside of Africa are mosaics that

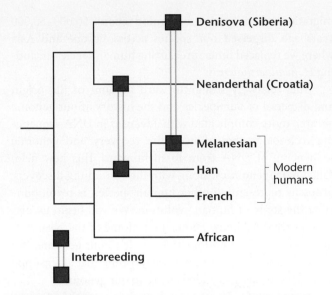

FIGURE 25–24 A phylogenetic tree showing the relationship between modern human populations and the Neanderthals and Denisovans. These two groups branched off from our last common ancestor before our species left Africa. Genomic analysis shows there was interbreeding between some members of our species with the Neanderthals and the Denisovans, making our genome a mosaic with contributions from two other human species.

contain DNA from one or two other sources (**Figure 25–24**). The Neanderthal and Denisovan genomes were assembled from fossils that are 40,000 to 80,000 years old. A recent analysis of the Denisovan genome shows evidence of interbreeding with an earlier, as yet unidentified, hominin population. The recent sequencing of a genome from a 700,000-year-old horse fossil opens the possibility that genome sequences can be recovered from fossil remains of much older human species such as *Homo erectus* (1.9 million to about 150,000 years ago), or *H. heidelbergensis*, a species that lived in Europe and Asia some 700,000 to 200,000 years ago and may have been the source of the unknown components of the Denisovan genome. If this is the case, we can expect exciting answers to questions about the similarities and differences between our genome and those of other human species. The information we derive will provide revolutionary insights into the evolution of our species and other human species that preceded us on this planet.

GENETICS, TECHNOLOGY, AND SOCIETY

Tracking Our Genetic Footprints out of Africa

Based on the physical traits and distribution of hominid fossils, most paleoanthropologists agree that a large-brained, tool-using hominid they call *Homo erectus* appeared in east Africa about 2 million years ago. This species used simple stone tools and hunted, but did not fish, build houses, or follow ritual burial practices. About 1.7 million years ago, *H. erectus* spread into Eurasia and south Asia. Most scientists also agree that *H. erectus* likely developed into *H. heidelbergensis*—a species that became the ancestor to our species (in Africa), Neanderthals (in Europe), and Denisovans (in Asia). These hominids were anatomically robust, with large, heavy skeletons and skulls. These groups disappeared 50,000 to 30,000 years ago—around the same time that anatomically modern humans (*H. sapiens*) appeared all over the world. The events that led to the appearance of *H. sapiens* throughout Europe and Asia are a source of controversy.

At present, two main hypotheses explain the origins of modern humans: the multiregional hypothesis and the out-of-Africa hypothesis. The multiregional hypothesis is based primarily on archaeological and fossil evidence. It proposes that *H. sapiens* developed gradually and simultaneously all over the world from existing *H. heidelbergensis* groups, including Neanderthals. Interbreeding between these groups eventually made *H. sapiens* a genetically homogeneous species. Natural selection then created the regional variants that we see today. In the multiregional view, our genetic makeup should include significant contributions from many *H. heidelbergensis* groups, including Neanderthals. In contrast, the out-of-Africa hypothesis, based primarily on genetic analyses of modern human populations, contends that *H. sapiens* evolved from the descendants of *H. heidelbergensis* in sub-Saharan Africa about 200,000 years ago. A small band of *H. sapiens* (probably fewer than 1000) then left Africa around 50,000 years ago. By 40,000 years ago, they had reached Europe, Asia, and Australia. In the out-of-Africa model, *H. sapiens* replaced all existing hominins, without interbreeding. In this way, *H. sapiens* became the only species in the genus by about 30,000 years ago.

Although the out-of-Africa hypothesis is still debated, most genetic evidence appears to support it. Humans all over the globe are remarkably similar genetically. DNA sequences from any two people chosen at random are 99.9 percent identical. More genetic identity exists between two persons chosen at random from a human population than between two chimpanzees chosen at random from a chimpanzee population. Interestingly, about 90 percent of the genetic differences that do exist occur between individuals rather than between populations. This unusually high degree of genetic relatedness in all humans around the world supports the idea that our species arose recently from a small founding group of humans.

Studies of mitochondrial DNA sequences from current human populations reveal that the highest levels of genetic variation occur within African populations. Africans show twice the mitochondrial DNA sequence diversity of non-Africans. This implies that the earliest branches of *H. sapiens* diverged in Africa and had a longer time to accumulate mitochondrial DNA mutations, which are thought to accumulate at a constant rate over time.

DNA sequences from mitochondrial, Y-chromosome, and chromosome-21 markers support the idea that human roots are in east Africa and that the migration out of Africa occurred through Ethiopia, along the coast of the Arabian Peninsula, and outward to Eurasia and Southeast Asia. Recent data based on nuclear microsatellite variants and whole genome single-nucleotide polymorphism (SNP) analysis further support the notion that humans migrated out of Africa and dispersed throughout the world from a small founding population.

As with any explanation of human origins, the out-of-Africa hypothesis is actively debated. As methods to sequence DNA from ancient fossils improve, it may be possible to fill the gaps in the genetic pathway leading out of Africa and to resolve those age-old questions about our origins.

Your Turn

1. When the sequence of Neanderthal DNA was reported, it was suggested that the Neanderthal genome is so different from ours that they came from two separate species that diverged about 600,000 years ago. However, recent data suggest that there was some interbreeding between *H. sapiens* and Neanderthals. Discuss evidence that supports, and refutes, the idea that Neanderthals and *H. sapiens* interbred in Europe and that Denisovans and *H. sapiens* interbred in Asia. How do these ideas affect the out-of-Africa hypothesis?

Start your investigations by reading Stoneking, M. and Krause, J. 2011. Learning about human population history from ancient and modern genomes. *Nat. Rev. Genet.* 12(9): 603–614.

2. If all people on Earth are very similar genetically, how did we come to have the range of physical differences, which some describe as racial differences? How has modern genomics contributed to the debate about the validity and definition of the term *race*?

For an interesting discussion of race, human variation, and genomic studies, see Lewontin, R.C. 2006. Confusion about human races, on the *Social Sciences Research Center website*—raceandgenomics.ssrc.org/Lewontin. *A study of the genetic differences between human population groups can be found in* Witherspoon, D.J. et al. 2007. Genetic similarities within and between human populations. *Genetics 176(1): 351–359.*

3. Geneticists study mitochondrial and Y-chromosome DNA to determine the ancestry of modern humans. Why are these two types of DNA used in lineage studies? What is meant by the terms *mitochondrial Eve* and *Y-chromosome Adam*?

To read the original paper hypothesizing a mitochondrial Eve, see Cann, R.L. et al. 1987. Mitochondrial DNA and human evolution. *Nature 325: 31–36. For a discussion of Y-chromosome Adam, see* Gibbons, A. 1997. Y Chromosome shows that Adam was an African. *Science 278: 804–805.*

CASE STUDY | An unexpected outcome

A newborn screening program identified a baby with a rare autosomal recessive disorder called arginosuccinic aciduria (AGA), which causes high levels of ammonia to accumulate in the blood. Symptoms usually appear in the first week after birth and can progress to include severe liver damage, developmental delay, and mental retardation. AGA occurs with a frequency of about 1 in 70,000 births. There is no history of this disorder in either the father's or mother's family. The above case raises several questions:

1. Since it appears that the unaffected parents are heterozygotes, would it be considered unusual that there would be no family history of the disorder? How would they be counseled about risks to future children?

2. If the disorder is so rare, what is the frequency of heterozygous carriers in the population?

3. What are the chances that two heterozygotes will meet and have an affected child?

Summary Points

MasteringGenetics™ For activities, animations, and review quizzes, go to the Study Area.

1. Genetic variation is a characteristic of most populations. In some cases, this can be observed at the phenotypic level, but analysis at the amino acid and nucleotide levels provides a more direct way to estimate genetic variation.

2. Using the assumptions of the Hardy–Weinberg law, it is possible to estimate allele and gene frequencies in populations.

3. The Hardy–Weinberg law can be applied to determining allele and genotype frequencies for multiple alleles and X-linked alleles, as well as calculating the frequency of heterozygotes for a given gene.

4. Natural selection changes allele frequency in populations leading to evolutionary change. Selection for quantitative traits can involve directional selection, stabilizing selection, or disruptive selection.

5. In addition to natural selection, other forces act on allele frequencies in populations. These include mutation, migration,

and genetic drift. Nonrandom mating changes genotype frequencies but does not change allele frequencies.

6. The formation of new species depends on the formation of subpopulations and the accumulation of enough genetic differences that, when reunited, members of the separated populations cannot interbreed.

7. Phylogenetic analysis using morphology, amino acid sequences, or nucleotide sequences can be used to construct phylogenetic trees showing the evolutionary relationships among a group of organisms. When calibrated with molecular clocks, the evolutionary changes on a phylogenetic tree can be calibrated with a time scale.

8. Phylogenetic analysis combined with genome sequence data from humans, Neanderthals, and other hominids has helped scientists reconstruct the relationship between Neanderthals and our species.

INSIGHTS AND SOLUTIONS

1. Tay–Sachs disease is caused by loss-of-function mutations in a gene on chromosome 15 that encodes a lysosomal enzyme. Tay–Sachs is inherited as an autosomal recessive condition. Among Ashkenazi Jews of Central European ancestry, about 1 in 3600 children are born with the disease. What fraction of the individuals in this population are carriers?

Solution: If we let p represent the frequency of the wild-type enzyme allele and q the total frequency of recessive loss-of-function alleles, and if we assume that the population is in Hardy–Weinberg equilibrium, then the frequencies of the genotypes are given by p^2 for homozygous normal, $2pq$ for carriers, and q^2 for individuals with Tay–Sachs. The frequency of Tay–Sachs alleles is thus

$$q = \sqrt{q^2} = \sqrt{\frac{1}{3600}} = 0.017$$

Since $p + q = 1$, we have

$$p = 1 - q = 1 - 0.017 = 0.983$$

Therefore, we can estimate that the frequency of carriers is

$$2pq = 2(0.983)(0.017) = 0.033 \text{ or about 1 in 30}$$

2. A single plant twice the size of others in the same population suddenly appears. Normally, plants of that species reproduce by self-fertilization and by cross-fertilization. Is this new giant plant simply a variant, or could it be a new species? How would you determine which it is?

Solution: One of the most widespread mechanisms of speciation in higher plants is polyploidy, the multiplication of entire sets of chromosomes. The result of polyploidy is usually a larger plant with larger flowers and seeds. There are two ways of testing the new variant to determine whether it is a new species. First, the giant plant should be crossed with a normal-sized plant to see whether the giant plant produces viable, fertile offspring. If it does not, then the two different types of plants would appear to be reproductively isolated. Second, the giant plant should be cytogenetically screened to examine its chromosome complement. If it has twice the number of its normal-sized neighbors, it is a tetraploid that may have arisen spontaneously. If the chromosome number differs by a factor of two and the new plant is reproductively isolated from its normal-sized neighbors, it is a new species.

Problems and Discussion Questions

HOW DO WE KNOW?

1. Population geneticists study changes in the nature and amount of genetic variation in populations, the distribution of different genotypes, and how forces such as selection and drift act on genetic variation to bring about evolutionary change in populations and the formation of new species. From the explanation given in the chapter, what answers would you propose to the following fundamental questions?
   (a) How do we know how much genetic variation is in a population?
   (b) How do geneticists detect the presence of genetic variation as different alleles in a population?
   (c) How do we know whether the genetic structure of a population is static or dynamic?
   (d) How do we know when populations have diverged to the point that they form two different species?
   (e) How do we know the age of the last common ancestor shared by two species?

CONCEPT QUESTION

2. Read the Chapter Concepts list on page 647. All these pertain to the principles of population genetics and the evolution of species. Write a short essay describing the roles of mutation, migration, and selection in bringing about speciation.

3. Price et al. (1999. *J. Bacteriol.* 181: 2358–2362) conducted a genetic study of the toxin transport protein (PA) of *Bacillus anthracis,* the bacterium that causes anthrax in humans. Within the 2294-nucleotide gene in 26 strains they identified five point mutations—two missense and three synonyms—among different isolates. Necropsy samples from an anthrax outbreak in 1979 revealed a novel missense mutation and five unique nucleotide changes among ten victims. The authors concluded that these data indicate little or no horizontal transfer between different *B. anthracis* strains.
   (a) Which types of nucleotide changes (missense or synonyms) cause amino acid changes?
   (b) What is meant by horizontal transfer?
   (c) On what basis did the authors conclude that evidence of horizontal transfer is absent from their data?

4. The genetic difference between two *Drosophila* species, *D. heteroneura* and *D. sylvestris,* as measured by nucleotide diversity, is about 1.8 percent. The difference between chimpanzees (*P. troglodytes*) and humans (*H. sapiens*) is about the same, yet the latter species are classified in different genera. In your opinion, is this valid? Explain why.

5. The use of nucleotide sequence data to measure genetic variability is complicated by the fact that the genes of higher eukaryotes are complex in organization and contain 5' and 3' flanking regions as well as introns. Researchers have compared the nucleotide sequence of two cloned alleles of the *γ globin* gene from a single individual and found a variation of 1 percent. Those differences include 13 substitutions of one nucleotide for another and 3 short DNA segments that have been inserted in one allele or deleted in the other. None of the changes takes place in the gene's exons (coding regions). Why do you think this is so, and should it change our concept of genetic variation?

6. The ability to taste the compound PTC is controlled by a dominant allele *T,* while individuals homozygous for the recessive allele *t* are unable to taste PTC. In a genetics class of 125 students, 88 can taste PTC and 37 cannot. Calculate the frequency of the *T* and *t* alleles and the frequency of the genotypes in this population.

7. Consider rare disorders in a population caused by an autosomal recessive mutation. From the frequencies of the disorder in the population given, calculate the percentage of heterozygous carriers:
   (a) 0.0064
   (b) 0.000081
   (c) 0.09
   (d) 0.01
   (e) 0.10

8. What must be assumed in order to validate the answers in Problem 7?

9. In a population where only the total number of individuals with the dominant phenotype is known, how can you calculate the percentage of carriers and homozygous recessives?

10. Determine whether the following two sets of data represent populations that are in Hardy–Weinberg equilibrium (use chi-square analysis if necessary):
    (a) CCR5 genotypes: $1/1$, 60 percent; $1/\Delta 32$, 35.1 percent; $\Delta 32/\Delta 32$, 4.9 percent
    (b) Sickle-cell hemoglobin: *AA,* 75.6 percent; *AS* 24.2 percent; *SS* 0.2 percent

11. If 4 percent of a population in equilibrium expresses a recessive trait, what is the probability that the offspring of two individuals who do not express the trait will express it?

12. Consider a population in which the frequency of allele A is $p = 0.7$ and the frequency of allele *a* is $q = 0.3$, and where the alleles are codominant. What will be the allele frequencies after one generation if the following occurs?
    (a) $w_{AA} = 1, w_{Aa} = 0.9, w_{aa} = 0.8$
    (b) $w_{AA} = 1, w_{Aa} = 0.95, w_{aa} = 0.9$
    (c) $w_{AA} = 1, w_{Aa} = 0.99, w_{aa} = 0.98$
    (d) $w_{AA} = 0.8, w_{Aa} = 1, w_{aa} = 0.8$

13. If the initial allele frequencies are $p = 0.5$ and $q = 0.5$ and allele *a* is a lethal recessive, what will be the frequencies after 1, 5, 10, 25, 100, and 1000 generations?

14. Under what circumstances might a lethal dominant allele persist in a population?

15. Assume that a recessive autosomal disorder occurs in 1 of 10,000 individuals (0.0001) in the general population and that in this population about 2 percent (0.02) of the individuals are carriers for the disorder. Estimate the probability of this disorder occurring in the offspring of a marriage between first cousins. Compare this probability to the population at large.

16. One of the first Mendelian traits identified in humans was a dominant condition known as *brachydactyly.* This gene causes an abnormal shortening of the fingers or toes (or both). At the time, some researchers thought that the dominant trait would spread until 75 percent of the population would be affected (because the phenotypic ratio of dominant to recessive is 3:1). Show that the reasoning was incorrect.

17. Describe how populations with substantial genetic differences can form. What is the role of natural selection?

18. Achondroplasia is a dominant trait that causes a characteristic form of dwarfism. In a survey of 50,000 births, five infants with achondroplasia were identified. Three of the affected infants

had affected parents, while two had normal parents. Calculate the mutation rate for achondroplasia and express the rate as the number of mutant genes per given number of gametes.

19. A recent study examining the mutation rates of 5669 mammalian genes (17,208 sequences) indicates that, contrary to popular belief, mutation rates among lineages with vastly different generation lengths and physiological attributes are remarkably constant (Kumar, S., and Subramanian, S. 2002. *Proc. Natl. Acad. Sci. [USA]* 99: 803–808). The average rate is estimated at 12.2×10^{-9} per bp per year. What is the significance of this finding in terms of mammalian evolution?

20. What are considered significant factors in maintaining the surprisingly high levels of genetic variation in natural populations?

21. A botanist studying water lilies in an isolated pond observed three leaf shapes in the population: round, arrowhead, and scalloped. Marker analysis of DNA from 125 individuals showed the round-leaf plants to be homozygous for allele *r1*, while the plants with arrowhead leaves were homozygous for a different allele at the same locus, *r2*. Plants with scalloped leaves showed DNA profiles with both the *r1* and *r2* alleles. Frequency of the *r1* allele was estimated at 0.81. If the botanist counted 20 plants with scalloped leaves in the pond, what is the inbreeding coefficient *F* for this population?

22. A farmer plants transgenic Bt corn that is genetically modified to produce its own insecticide. Of the corn borer larvae feeding on these Bt crop plants, only 10 percent survive unless they have at least one copy of the dominant resistance allele *B* that confers resistance to the Bt insecticide. When the farmer first plants Bt corn, the frequency of the *B* resistance allele in the corn borer population is 0.02. What will be the frequency of the resistance allele after one generation of corn borers fed on Bt corn?

23. In an isolated population of desert bighorn sheep, a mutant recessive allele *c* when homozygous causes curled coats in both males and females. The normal dominant allele *C* produces straight coats. A biologist studying these sheep counts four with curled coats. She also takes blood samples from the population for DNA analysis, which reveals that 17 of the sheep are heterozygous carriers of the *c* allele. What is the inbreeding coefficient *F* for this population?

24. To increase genetic diversity in the bighorn sheep population described in Problem 23, ten sheep are introduced from a population where the *c* allele is absent. Assuming that random mating occurs between the original and the introduced sheep, and that the *c* allele is selectively neutral, what will be the frequency of *c* in the next generation?

25. What genetic changes take place during speciation?

26. Some critics have warned that the use of gene therapy to correct genetic disorders will affect the course of human evolution. Evaluate this criticism in light of what you know about population genetics and evolution, distinguishing between somatic gene therapy and germ-line gene therapy.

Extra-Spicy Problems

MasteringGenetics™ Visit for instructor-assigned tutorials and problems.

27. A form of dwarfism known as Ellis–van Creveld syndrome was first discovered in the late 1930s, when Richard Ellis and Simon van Creveld shared a train compartment on the way to a pediatrics meeting. In the course of conversation, they discovered that they each had a patient with this syndrome. They published a description of the syndrome in 1940. Affected individuals have a short-limbed form of dwarfism and often have defects of the lips and teeth, and polydactyly (extra fingers). The largest pedigree for the condition was reported in an Old Order Amish population in eastern Pennsylvania by Victor McKusick and his colleagues (1964). In that community, about 5 per 1000 births are affected, and in the population of 8000, the observed frequency is 2 per 1000. All affected individuals have unaffected parents, and all affected cases can trace their ancestry to Samuel King and his wife, who arrived in the area in 1774. It is known that neither King nor his wife was affected with the disorder. There are no cases of the disorder in other Amish communities, such as those in Ohio or Indiana.

    (a) From the information provided, derive the most likely mode of inheritance of this disorder. Using the Hardy–Weinberg law, calculate the frequency of the mutant allele in the population and the frequency of heterozygotes, assuming Hardy–Weinberg conditions.

    (b) What is the most likely explanation for the high frequency of the disorder in the Pennsylvania Amish community and its absence in other Amish communities?

28. List the barriers that prevent interbreeding and give an example of each.

29. What are the two groups of reproductive isolating mechanisms? Which of these is regarded as more efficient, and why?

30. The original source of new alleles, upon which selection operates, is mutation, a random event that occurs without regard to selectional value in the organism. Although many model organisms have been used to study mutational events in populations, some investigators have developed abiotic molecular models. Soll (2006) examined one such model to study the relationship between both deleterious and advantageous mutations and population size in a ligase molecule composed of RNA (a ribozyme). Soll found that the smaller the population of molecules, the more likely it was that not only deleterious mutations but also advantageous mutations would disappear. Why would population size influence the survival of both types of mutations (deleterious and advantageous) in populations?

31. A number of comparisons of nucleotide sequences among hominids and rodents indicate that inbreeding may have occurred more in hominid than in rodent ancestry. When an ancient population bottleneck leaving approximately 10,000 individuals occurred in humans, Knight (2005) and Bakewell (2007) both suggested that this event may have left early humans with a greater chance of genetic disease. Why would a population bottleneck influence the frequency of genetic disease?

32. Shown below are two homologous lengths of the alpha and beta chains of human hemoglobin. Consult a genetic code dictionary (Figure 13.7) and determine how many amino acid substitutions may have occurred as a result of a single nucleotide substitution. For any that cannot occur as a result of a single change, determine the minimal mutational distance.

> alpha: ala val ala his val asp asp met pro
> beta: gly leu ala his leu asp asn leu lys

33. Recent reconstructions of evolutionary history are often dependent on assigning divergence in terms of changes in amino acid or nucleotide sequences. For example, a comparison of cytochrome c shows 10 amino acid differences between humans and dogs, 24 differences between humans and moths, and 38 differences between humans and yeast. Such data provide no information as to the absolute times of divergence for humans, dogs, moths, and yeast. How might one calibrate the molecular clock to an absolute time clock? What problems might one encounter in such a calibration?

34. Comparisons of Neanderthal mitochondrial DNA with that of modern humans indicate that they are not related to modern humans and did not contribute to our mitochondrial heritage. However, because Neanderthals and modern humans are separated by at least 25,000 years, this does not rule out some forms of interbreeding causing the modern European gene pool to be derived from both Neanderthals and early humans (called Cro-Magnons). To resolve this question, Caramelli et al. (2003. *Proc. Natl. Acad. Sci. [USA]* 100: 6593–6597) analyzed mitochondrial DNA sequences from 25,000-year-old Cro-Magnon remains and compared them to four Neanderthal specimens and a large dataset derived from modern humans. The results are shown in the graph

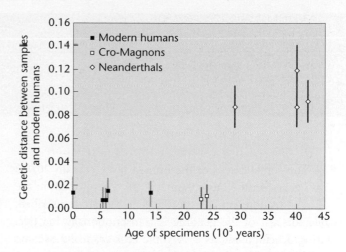

The *x*-axis represents the age of the specimens in thousands of years; the *y*-axis represents the average genetic distance. Modern humans are indicated by filled squares; Cro-Magnons, open squares; and Neanderthals, diamonds.

(a) What can you conclude about the relationship between Cro-Magnons and modern Europeans? What about the relationship between Cro-Magnons and Neanderthals?

(b) From these data, does it seem likely that Neanderthals made any mitochondrial DNA contributions to the Cro-Magnon gene pool or the modern European gene pool?

Epigenetics

The somatic cells of the human body contain 20,000 genes. In the more than 200 cell types present in the body, different cell-specific gene sets are transcribed, while the rest of the genome is transcriptionally inactive. During development, as embryonic cells gradually become specialized cells with adult phenotypes, programs of gene expression become more and more restricted. Until recently, it was thought that most regulation of gene expression is coordinated by *cis*-regulatory elements as well as DNA-binding proteins and transcription factors, and that this regulation can occur at any of the steps in gene expression (see Chapter 17). For example, transcriptional regulation, steps in mRNA processing, and other stages of posttranscriptional regulation control the amount of gene product synthesized from a DNA template. However, as we have learned more about genome organization and the regulation of gene expression, it is clear that classical regulatory mechanisms cannot fully explain how some phenotypes arise. For example, monozygotic twins have identical genotypes but often have different phenotypes. In addition, although one allele of each gene is inherited maternally and one is inherited paternally, in some cases, only the maternal or paternal allele is expressed, while the other is transcriptionally silent.

The newly emerging field of epigenetics is providing us with a molecular basis for understanding how heritable changes other than those in DNA sequence can influence phenotypic variation (**ST Figure 1–1**). These advances greatly extend our understanding of gene regulation and have application in wide-ranging areas including genetic disorders, cancer, and behavior.

An **epigenetic trait** is a stable, mitotically and meiotically heritable phenotype that results from changes in the pattern of gene expression without alterations of the DNA sequence. **Epigenetics** is the study of the ways in which chemical modifications to DNA and histones alter cell- and tissue-specific patterns of gene expression. These reversible modifications of DNA and chromatin structure mediate the interaction of the genome with a variety of environmental factors and generate changes in the patterns of gene expression in response to these factors. The **epigenome**

> **"The newly emerging field of epigenetics is providing us with a basis for understanding how heritable changes other than those in DNA sequence can influence phenotypic variation."**

refers to the pattern of epigenetic modifications present in a cell at a given time. During its life span, an organism has one genome, which can be modified in diverse cell types at different times to produce many epigenomes.

Current research efforts are focused on several aspects of epigenetics: how an epigenome arises in developing and differentiated cells and how these epigenomes are transmitted via mitosis and meiosis, making them heritable traits. In addition, because epigenetically controlled alterations to the genome are associated with common diseases such as cancer, diabetes, and asthma, efforts are also directed toward developing drugs that can modify or reverse disease-associated epigenetic changes in cells.

Here we will focus on how epigenetics is associated with some heritable genetic disorders, cancer, and environment–genome interactions. Because epigenetic changes are potentially reversible, we will also examine how knowledge of molecular mechanisms of epigenetics is being used to develop drugs and treatments for human diseases.

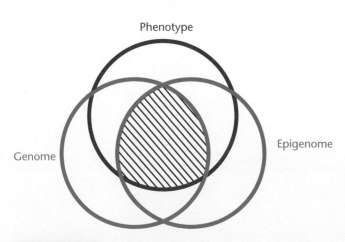

ST FIGURE 1–1 The phenotype of an organism is the product of interactions between the genome and the epigenome. The genome is constant from fertilization throughout life, but cells, tissues, and the organism develop different epigenomes as a result of epigenetic reprogramming of gene activity in response to environmental stimuli. These reprogramming events lead to phenotypic changes through the life cycle.

BOX 1
The Beginning of Epigenetics

C. H. Waddington coined the term *epigenetics* in the 1940s to describe how environmental influences on developmental events can affect the phenotype of the adult. He showed that by altering environmental conditions during development, organisms with identical genotypes can develop different phenotypes. Using *Drosophila melanogaster*, Waddington found that wing vein patterns could be altered by administering heat shocks during pupal development. Offspring of flies with these environmentally induced changes showed the alternative phenotype without the need for continued environmental stimulus. He called this phenomenon "genetic assimilation." In other words, interactions between the environment and the genome during certain stages of development produced heritable phenotypic changes.

In the 1970s, Holliday and Pugh extended the definition of epigenetics by proposing that changes in the program of gene expression during development depend on the methylation of specific bases in DNA, and that altering methylation patterns affects the resulting phenotype. Waddington's pioneering work, the methylation model of Holliday and Pugh, and the discovery that expression of genes from both the maternal and paternal genomes is required for normal development all helped set the stage for the birth of epigenetics and epigenomics as fields of scientific research.

Epigenetic Alterations to the Genome

Unlike the genome, which is identical in all cell types of an organism, the epigenome is cell-type specific and changes throughout the life cycle in response to environmental cues. Like the genome, the epigenome can be transmitted to daughter cells by mitosis and to future generations by meiosis. In the following sections, we will examine mechanisms of epigenetic changes and their role in imprinting, cancer, and environment–genome interactions, providing a snapshot of the many roles played by this recently discovered mechanism of gene regulation.

There are three major epigenetic mechanisms: (1) reversible modification of DNA by the addition or removal of methyl groups; (2) chromatin remodeling by the addition or removal of chemical groups to histone proteins; and (3) regulation of gene expression by noncoding RNA molecules.

DNA Methylation

In mammals, DNA methylation takes place after replication and during cell differentiation. This process involves the addition of a methyl group ($-CH_3$) to cytosine, a reaction catalyzed by a family of enzymes called DNA methyltransferases (DNMTs). Methylation takes place almost exclusively on cytosine bases located adjacent to a guanine base, a combination called a CpG dinucleotide. Many of these dinucleotides are clustered in regions called CpG islands, which are located in and near promoter sequences adjacent to genes (**ST Figure 1–2**). CpG islands and promoters adjacent to essential genes (housekeeping genes) and cell-specific genes are unmethylated, making them available for transcription. Genes with adjacent methylated CpG islands and methylated promoters are transcriptionally silenced. The methyl groups in CpG dinucleotides occupy the major groove of DNA and silence genes by blocking the binding of transcription factors necessary to form transcription complexes.

Methylation of CpG islands is a normal process during development. For example, inactivation of one of the X chromosomes in mammalian females is associated with DNA methylation of these groups (see Chapter 7 for a detailed explanation of X-inactivation). In addition, CpG methylation during development creates a parent-specific pattern of gene transcription called genomic imprinting. Abnormal patterns of DNA methylation are associated with specific human diseases, including cancer.

(a) Promoter is unmethylated and gene can be transcribed

CpG island in promoter   Gene

(b) Promoter is methylated and gene is silenced

CpG island in promoter   Gene

⚲ Unmethylated CpG island   ⚫ Methylated CpG island

ST FIGURE 1–2 Methylation patterns of CpG dinucleotides in promoters control activity of adjacent genes.

Histone Modification and Chromatin Remodeling

In addition to DNA methylation, histone modification is an important epigenetic mechanism of gene regulation. Recall that chromatin is a dynamic structure composed of DNA wound around a core of 8 histone proteins to form nucleosomes. The N-terminal region of each histone extends beyond the nucleosome, and the amino acids in these tails can be covalently modified in several ways, including the addition of acetyl, methyl, and phosphate groups (**ST Figure 1–3**). Several sets of proteins are involved in modifying histones. These include proteins that add chemical groups to histones ("writers"), proteins that interpret those modifications ("readers"), and proteins that remove those chemical groups ("erasers"). Some of the proteins involved in histone modification are shown in **ST Table 1.1**.

These modifications alter the structure of chromatin, making genes on nucleosomes accessible or inaccessible

ST TABLE 1.1 Epigenetic Chromatin Modifier Proteins

Type	Number Identified
Writers	78
Protein methyltransferases	
Histone acetyltransferases	
Readers	156
Tudor domain-containing proteins	
MBT domain-containing proteins	
Chromodomain-containing proteins	
Erasers	42
Histone deacetylases	
Lysine demethylases	

for transcription. Histone acetylation, for example, makes genes on these modified nucleosomes available for transcription [**ST Figure 1–4(a)**]. This modification is reversible, and removing (erasing) acetyl groups changes the chromatin configuration from an "open" to a "closed" configuration, silencing genes by making them unavailable for transcription [**ST Figure 1–4(b)**].

We are learning that specific combinations of histone modifications control the transcriptional status of a chromatin region. For example, whether or not lysine 9 on histone H3 will be methylated is controlled by modifications made elsewhere on this protein. On one hand, if serine 10 is phosphorylated, methylation of lysine 9 is inhibited. On the other hand, if lysine 14 is deacetylated, methylation of lysine 9 is facilitated. Many combinations of histone modifications are possible, and the sum of the complex patterns and interactions of histone modifications that alter chromatin organization and gene expression is called the **histone code.** Combinations of these changes allow differentiated cells to carry out cell-specific patterns of gene transcription and to respond to external signals that modify these patterns without any changes in DNA sequence.

MicroRNAs and Long Noncoding RNAs

In addition to messenger RNA (mRNA), genome transcription produces several classes of noncoding RNAs. Two of these, microRNAs (miRNAs) and long noncoding RNAs (lncRNAs), play important roles in epigenetic regulatory networks. miRNAs are involved in controlling pattern formation in developing embryos as well as cell signaling.

miRNAs are transcribed as precursor molecules about 70–100 nucleotides long, containing a double-stranded stem-loop and single-stranded regions. Processing removes the single-stranded regions, and the loops move to the cytoplasm where they are altered further. The resulting double-stranded RNA is incorporated into a protein complex where one RNA strand is removed and degraded, forming a mature RNA-induced silencing complex (RISC) containing the remaining

Histones

DNA

ST FIGURE 1–3 Clusters of histones in nucleosomes have their N-terminal tails covalently modified in epigenetic modifications that alter patterns of gene expression. Ac = acetyl groups, Me = methyl groups, P = phosphate groups.

"Open" configuration.
DNA is unmethylated and histones are acetylated.
Genes can be transcribed.

(a)

"Closed" configuration.
DNA is methylated at CpG islands (black circles) and histones are deacetylated.
Genes cannot be transcribed.

(b)

ST FIGURE 1–4 Epigenetic modifications to the genome alter the spacing of nucleosomes. In the open configuration, nucleosome positions are shifted, CpGs are unmethylated, and the genes on the DNA are available for transcription. In the closed configuration, DNA is tightly wound onto the nucleosomes, CpGs are methylated, and genes on the DNA are unavailable for transcription.

single miRNA strand. RISCs act as repressors of gene expression by binding to and destroying target mRNA molecules carrying sequences complementary to the RISC miRNA. mRNAs partially complementary to the RISC miRNA are modified, making these mRNAs less likely to be translated by ribosomes, resulting in downregulation of gene expression.

In addition to forming RISC complexes, miRNAs also associate with a different set of proteins to form RNA-induced transcriptional silencing (RITS) complexes. RITS complexes reversibly convert euchromatic chromosome regions into facultative heterochromatin, silencing the genes located within these newly created heterochromatic regions.

Long noncoding RNAs (lncRNAs) share many properties in common with mRNAs; they often have 5′ caps, 3′ poly-A tails, and are spliced. What distinguishes lncRNAs from coding (mRNA) transcripts is the lack of an extended open reading frame that codes for the insertion of amino acids into a polypeptide.

lncRNAs are found in the nucleus and the cytoplasm and through a variety of mechanisms are involved in regulating almost every stage of gene expression. As epigenetic modulators, lncRNAs bind to chromatin-modifying enzymes and direct their activity to specific regions of the genome. At these sites, the lncRNAs direct chromatin modification, altering the pattern of gene expression.

In summary, epigenetic modifications alter chromatin structure by several mechanisms including DNA methylation, histone acetylation, and action of RNAs, without changing the sequence of DNA. These epigenetic changes create an epigenome that, in turn, can regulate normal development and generate changes in gene expression as a response to environmental signals.

Epigenetics and Imprinting

Mammals inherit a maternal and a paternal copy of each autosomal gene, and usually both copies of these genes are expressed in the offspring. Imprinting is an epigenetically regulated process in which genes are expressed in a parent-of-origin pattern; that is, certain genes show expression of only the maternal allele or the paternal allele. Parent-specific patterns of allele expression are laid down in germ-line cells during gamete formation and are inherited via mitosis in somatic cells.

Differential methylation of CpG-rich regions and methylation of promoter sequences produce allele-specific imprinting and subsequent gene silencing. Once a gene has been imprinted, it remains transcriptionally silent during embryogenesis and development. Most imprinted genes direct aspects of growth during prenatal development. For example, in mice, genes on the maternal X chromosome are expressed in the placenta, while genes on the paternal X chromosome are silenced. Having only one functional allele makes imprinted genes highly susceptible to the deleterious effects of mutations. Because imprinted genes are clustered at a limited number of sites in the genome, mutation in one gene can have an impact on the function of adjacent imprinted genes, amplifying its impact on the phenotype.

ST TABLE 1.3 Some Cancer-Related Genes Inactivated by Hypermethylation in Human Cancers

Gene	Locus	Function	Related Cancers
BRCA1	17q21	DNA repair	Breast, ovarian
APC	5q21	Nucleocytoplasmic signaling	Colorectal, duodenal
MLH1	3p21	DNA repair	Colon, stomach
RB1	13q14	Cell-cycle control point	Retinoblastoma, osteosarcoma
AR	Xq11-12	Nuclear receptor for androgen; transcriptional activator	Prostate
ESR1	6q25	Nuclear receptor for estrogen; transcriptional activator	Breast, colorectal

hypomethylation of repetitive sequences leads to transcriptional activation of transposable DNA sequences such as LINEs and SINEs, further increasing genomic instability.

While widespread hypomethylation is a hallmark of cancer cells, hypermethylation at CpG islands and promoters silences tumor-suppressor genes (ST Table 1.3), often in a specific pattern. For example, the breast cancer gene BRCA1 is hypermethylated and inactivated in breast and ovarian cancer, and hypermethylation of the DNA repair gene MLH1 is a key step in the development of some forms of colon cancer. Epigenetic studies have revealed a unique pattern of abnormal DNA methylation that defines each type of cancer. Analysis of these patterns, called the CpG island methylator phenotype (CIMP), provides a way to identify tumor types and subtypes, and predict the sites to which the tumor will metastasize.

Epigenetic inactivation of tumor-suppressor genes plays a primary role in tumor formation as well as an important complementary role to mutational changes that accompany the transformation of normal cells into malignant cells. For example, in a bladder cancer cell line, one allele of the cell-cycle control gene CDKN2A is mutated, and the other, normal allele is inactivated by hypermethylation. Because both alleles are inactivated (although by different mechanisms), cells are able to escape control of the cell cycle and divide continuously. In many clinical cases, a combination of mutation and epigenetic hypermethylation occurs in familial forms of cancer.

However, the majority of hypermethylated genes in cancer cells are not tumor-suppressor genes, suggesting that the pattern of hypermethylation may result from a widespread deregulation of the methylation process rather than a targeted event.

In addition to altered patterns of methylation, many cancers also have disrupted histone modification profiles. In some cases, mutations in the genes of the histone-modifying proteins such as histone acetyltransferase (HAT) and histone deacetylase (HDAC) are linked to the development of cancer. For example, individuals with Rubinstein–Taybi syndrome inherit a germ-line mutation that produces a dysfunctional HAT and have a greater than 300-fold increased risk of cancer. In other cases, HDAC complexes are selectively recruited to tumor-suppressor genes by mutated, oncogenic DNA binding proteins. Action of the HDAC complexes at these genes converts the chromatin to a closed configuration and inhibits transcription, causing the cell to lose control of the cell cycle.

Mechanisms that cause epigenetic changes in cancer cells are not well understood, partly because they take place very early in the conversion of a normal cell to a cancerous one and partly because by the time the cancer is detected, alterations in the methylation pattern have already occurred. The MLH1 gene has an important role in genome stability, and silencing this gene by hypermethylation causes instability in repetitive microsatellite sequences, which, in turn, is an important step in the development of colon cancer and several other cancers. In some individuals with colon cancer, the MLH1 promoter in normal cells of the colon is already silenced by hypermethylation, indicating that this epigenetic event occurs very early in tumor formation, before the development of downstream genetic mutations.

The fact that such changes occur very early in the transformation process has led to the proposal that epigenetic changes leading to cancer may occur within adult stem cells in normal tissue. Three lines of evidence support this idea: (1) epigenetic mechanisms can replace mutations as a way of silencing individual tumor-suppressor genes or activating oncogenes; (2) global hypomethylation may cause genomic instability and the large-scale chromosomal changes that are a characteristic feature of cancer; and (3) epigenetic modifications can silence multiple genes, making them more effective in transforming normal cells into malignant cells than sequential mutations of single genes. A model of cancer based on epigenetic changes in colon stem cells as initial events in carcinogenesis followed by mutational events is shown in ST Figure 1–7.

Analysis of data from the Cancer Genome Atlas (TCGA) shows the importance of epigenetic events in cancer. In ovarian cancer, mutations in nine specific genes are predominant, but promoter hypermethylation is observed in 168 genes. These genes are epigenetically silenced, and their reduced expression is linked to the development and maintenance of this cancer. In addition to changing ideas about the origins of cancer, the fact that epigenetic changes are potentially reversible makes it possible to develop new classes of drugs for chemotherapy. The focus of epigenetic therapy is the reactivation of genes silenced by methylation or histone modification, essentially reprogramming the pattern of gene expression in cancer cells. Several epigenetic drugs have

(a)   (b)   (c)   (d)   (e)

■ Stem cells

■ Stem cells with epigenetic changes

■ Epigenetically altered stem cell with genetic mutations

■ Stem cell begins to divide

Uncontrolled growth / Metastasis

ST FIGURE 1-7 The epigenetic stem cell model proposes that both epigenetic changes and mutations are involved in the origins of cancer.

been approved by the U.S. Food and Drug Administration, and another 12–15 drugs are in clinical trials. One approved drug, Vidaza, is used in the treatment of myelodysplastic syndrome, a precursor to leukemia, and for treatment of acute myeloid leukemia. This drug is an analog of cytidine and is incorporated into DNA during replication during the S phase of the cell cycle. Methylation enzymes (methyltransferases) bind irreversibly to Vidaza, preventing methylation of DNA at many other sites, effectively reducing the amount of methylation in cancer cells. Other drugs that inhibit histone deacetylases (HDAC) have been approved by the FDA for use in epigenetic therapy. Experiments with cancer cell lines indicate that inhibiting HDAC activity results in the re-expression of tumor-suppressor genes. The HDAC inhibitor Zolinza is used to treat some forms of lymphoma.

The development of epigenetic drugs for cancer therapy is still in its infancy. The approved epigenetic drugs are only moderately effective on their own and are best used in combination with other anticancer drugs. To develop more effective drugs, several important questions remain to be answered: What causes cancer cells to respond to certain epigenetic drugs? What combination of epigenetic drugs and conventional anticancer drugs are most effective on specific cancers? Which epigenetic markers will be effective in predicting sensitivity or resistance to newly developed drugs? Further research into the mechanisms and locations of epigenetic genome modification in cancer cells will allow the design of more potent drugs to target epigenetic events as a form of cancer therapy.

Epigenetics and the Environment

Environmental agents including nutrition, exposure to chemicals, and physical factors, such as temperature, can alter gene expression by affecting the epigenome. In humans it is difficult to determine the relative contributions of environmental or learned behavior as factors in altering

---

BOX 2
What More We Need to Know about Epigenetics and Cancer

The discovery that epigenetic changes may be as important as genetic changes in the origin, maintenance, and metastasis of cancers has opened new avenues of cancer research. Key discoveries about epigenetic mechanisms include the finding of tumor-specific deregulation of genes by altered DNA methylation profiles and histone modifications, the discovery that epigenetic changes in histones or

DNA methylation are interconnected, and the recognition that epigenetic changes can affect hundreds of genes in a single cancer cell. These advances were made in the span of a few years, and while it is clear that epigenetics plays a key role in cancer, many questions remain to be answered before we can draw conclusions about the relative contributions of genetics and epigenetics to the development of cancer. Some of these questions are as follows:

• Is global hypomethylation in cancer cells a cause or an effect of the malignant condition?

• Do these changes arise primarily in stem cells or in differentiated cells?

• Once methylation alterations begin, what triggers hypermethylation in cancer cells?

• Is hypermethylation a process that targets certain gene classes, or is it a random event?

• Can we develop drugs that target cancer cells and reverse tumor-specific epigenetic changes?

• Can we target specific genes for reactivation, while leaving others inactive?

the epigenome, but there is indirect evidence that changes in nutrition and exposure to agents that affect the developing fetus can have detrimental effects during adulthood.

Women who were pregnant during the 1944–1945 famine in the Netherlands had children with increased risks for obesity, diabetes, and coronary heart disease. In addition, as adults, these individuals had significantly increased liability for schizophrenia and other neuropsychiatric disorders. Members of the F_2 generation also had abnormal patterns of weight gain and growth.

The most direct evidence for the role of environmental factors in modifying the epigenome comes from studies in experimental animals. A low-protein diet fed to pregnant rats results in permanent changes in the expression of several genes in both the F_1 and F_2 offspring. Increased expression of these genes is associated with hypomethylation of their promoters. Other evidence indicates that epigenetic changes triggered by this diet modification were gene-specific.

A dramatic example of how epigenome modifications affect the phenotype comes from the study of coat color in mice, where color is controlled by the dominant allele *Agouti* (*A*). In homozygous *AA* mice, the allele is active only during a specific time during hair development, resulting in a yellow band on an otherwise black hair shaft, producing the agouti phenotype. A nonlethal mutant allele (A^{vy}) causes yellow pigment formation along the entire hair shaft, resulting in yellow fur color. This allele is the result of the insertion of a transposable element near the transcription start site of the *Agouti* gene. A promoter element within the transposon is responsible for this change in gene expression. Researchers found that the degree of methylation in the transposon's promoter is related to the amount of yellow pigment deposited in the hair shaft and that the amount of methylation varies from individual to individual. The result is variation in coat color phenotypes even in genetically identical mice (**ST Figure 1–8**). In these mice, coat colors range from yellow (unmethylated promoter) to pseudoagouti (highly methylated promoter). In addition to a gradation in coat color, there is also a gradation in body weight. Yellow mice are more obese than the brown, pseudoagouti mice. Alleles such as A^{vy} that show variable expression from individual to individual in genetically identical strains caused by epigenetic modifications are called *metastable epialleles*. Metastable refers to the changeable nature of the epigenetic modifications, and epiallele refers to the heritability of the epigenetic status of the allele.

To evaluate the role of environmental factors in modifying the epigenome, the diet of pregnant A^{vy} mice was supplemented with methylation precursors, including folic acid, vitamin B_{12}, and choline. In the offspring, coat-color variation was reduced and shifted toward the pseudoagouti (highly methylated) phenotype. The shift in coat color was accompanied by increased methylation of the transposon's promoter. These findings have applications to epigenetic diseases in

| Yellow | Slightly mottled | Mottled | Heavily mottled | Pseudo-agouti |

ST FIGURE 1–8 Variable expression of yellow phenotype in mice caused by diet-related epigenetic changes in the genome.

humans. For example, the risk of colorectal cancer is linked directly to dietary folate deficiency and activity differences in enzymes leading to the synthesis of methyl donors.

In addition to foods that mediate epigenetic changes in gene expression via methylation, it has recently been discovered that some foods such as rice, cabbage, wheat, and potatoes are the source of miRNAs circulating in the blood and serum of humans. Studies on one target gene showed that plant miRNAs downregulate expression of this gene and that this effect is reversible by treatment with anti-miRNAs. This preliminary but highly significant work shows that miRNAs can act across species and even across kingdoms to regulate expression of target genes, and suggests that environmental factors may play a major role in epigenetic regulation of gene expression.

Epigenome Projects

As the role of the epigenome in disease has become increasingly clear, researchers across the globe have formed multidisciplinary projects to map all the epigenetic changes that occur in the normal genome and to study the role of the epigenome in specific diseases.

These include:

- NIH Roadmap Epigenomics Project
- Human Epigenome Project (HEP)
- International Human Epigenome Consortium (IHEC)
- International Cancer Genome Consortium (ICGC)

In conclusion, we will discuss some of these projects and their goals.

The NIH Roadmap Epigenomics Project is focused on how epigenetic mechanisms controlling stem cell differentiation and organ formation generate biological responses to external and internal stimuli that result in disease. One program of this project is the Human Epigenome Atlas, which catalogs normal human epigenomes to serve as reference standards. The Atlas provides detailed information about epigenomic modifications at specific loci, in different cell types and physiological states, as well as genotypes. These data allow researchers to perform comparative analysis of epigenomic data across genomic regions or entire genomes.

The Human Epigenome Project is a multinational, public/private consortium organized to identify, map, and establish the functional significance of all DNA methylation patterns in the human genome across all the major tissue types in the body. Analysis of these methylation patterns may show that genetic responses to environmental cues mediated by epigenetic changes are a pathway to disease.

The International Human Epigenome Consortium (IHEC) is global program established to determine how the epigenome has altered human populations in response to environmental factors. The consortium will begin by cataloging the epigenomes of 1000 individuals from different populations around the world. The catalog will also include the epigenomes of 250 different cell types.

Although these projects are in the early stages of development, the information already available strongly suggests that we are on the threshold of a new era in genetics, one in which we can study the development of disease at the genomic level, and understand impact of environmental factors on gene expression. The results of these projects may help explain how environmental settings in early life can affect predisposition to adulthood diseases.

Selected Readings and Resources

Journal Articles and Reviews

Burdge, G.C., and Lillicrop, K.A. 2010. Nutrition, epigenetics, and developmental plasticity: Implications for understanding human disease. *Annu. Rev. Nutr.* 30: 315–339.

Mercer, T.R., and Mattick, J.S. 2013. Structure and function of long noncoding RNAs in epigenetic regulation. *Nat Struct. Mol. Biol.* 20: 300–307.

Petronis, A. 2010. Epigenetics as a unifying principle in the aetiology of complex traits and diseases. *Nature* 465: 721–727.

Sandoval, J., and Esteller, M. 2012. Cancer epigenomics: Beyond genomics. *Curr. Opin. Genet. Develop.* 22: 50–55.

Soejima, H., and Higashimoto, K. 2013. Epigenetic and genetic alterations of the imprinting disorder Beckwith-Wiedemann syndrome and related disorders. *J. Hum. Genet.* 58: 402–409.

Weaver, I.C., Cervoni, N., Chanpagne, F.A., D'Allesio, A.C., Sharma, S., Seckl, J.R., Dymov, S., Szyf, M., and Meany, M.J. 2004. Epigenetic programming by maternal behavior. *Nat. Neurosci.* 7: 847–854.

Web Sites

Human Epigenome Project. www.epigenome.org

Human Epigenome Atlas. http://www.genboree.org/epigenomeatlas/index.rhtml

Computational Epigenetics Group. http://www.computational-epigenetics.de

Review Questions

1. What are the major mechanisms of epigenetic genome modification?
2. What parts of the genome are reversibly methylated? How does this affect gene expression?
3. What are the roles of proteins in histone modification?
4. Describe how reversible chemical changes to histones are linked to chromatin modification.
5. What is the histone code?
6. What is the difference between silencing genes by imprinting and silencing by epigenetic modifications?
7. Why are changes in nucleosome spacing important in changing gene expression?
8. How do microRNAs regulate epigenetic mechanisms during development?
9. What is the role of imprinting in human genetic disorders?

Discussion Questions

1. Imprinting disorders do not involve changes in DNA sequence, but only the methylated state of the DNA. Does it seem likely that imprinting disorders could be treated by controlling the maternal environment in some way, perhaps by dietary changes?
2. Should fertility clinics be required by law to disclose that some assisted reproductive technologies (ARTs) can result in epigenetic diseases? How would you and your partner balance the risks of ART with the desire to have a child?
3. How can the role of epigenetics in cancer be reconciled with the idea that cancer is caused by the accumulation of mutations in tumor-suppressor genes and proto-oncogenes?
4. Would the knowledge that plant miRNAs can affect gene expression in your body affect your food choices?

Emerging Roles of RNA

In 1958, Francis Crick proposed his theory for the central dogma of molecular biology, which described how genetic information flows from DNA to RNA to protein. Proteins, as the end products of the gene, were viewed as the functional units of the cell, while DNA was considered a stable molecule that stores genetic information. RNA was considered as the temporary message between DNA and protein. This insightful model was the basis for the emerging field of molecular biology and is still considered accurate today. However, this model did not anticipate many other types of **noncoding RNAs (ncRNAs)** that today are known to play important roles in genetic processes. Advancing rapidly in the early 1990s and continuing to this day, studies have revealed that ncRNAs are more abundant, more diverse, and more important than we could ever have imagined.

While it has been known for well over a decade that only ~1.5 percent of 3.2 billion base pairs making up the human genome encode proteins, we have recently learned that more than 75 percent of the human genome is in fact transcribed into RNA. Among these many transcripts are numerous examples of ncRNAs that have experimentally determined biological roles. Earlier in the text, we introduced several examples. You may recall from studying DNA replication that RNA serves as a primer for DNA synthesis and as a template molecule for reverse transcription of telomere sequences by telomerase (Chapter 11). And **small nuclear RNAs (snRNAs)** bound by several proteins (**snRNPs**) catalyze the splicing of pre-mRNAs as they are converted to mature transcripts (Chapter 13). Still another example is the relatively recent finding that the 23*S* prokaryotic and 28*S* eukaryotic rRNAs within the ribosome are responsible for catalyzing peptide bond formation during translation (Chapter 14).

The key to RNA's versatility lies in its structural diversity. While RNA is transcribed as a single strand that can serve as an informational molecule such as mRNA, it can also form complementary bonds with other nucleic acids, creating DNA/RNA duplexes and RNA/RNA duplexes (double-stranded RNA), or it can fold back on itself to form hairpin or stem-loop structures. As with proteins, such three-dimensional folding imparts enormous structural and thus

> **"Noncoding RNAs have myriad functions in the cell, including catalyzing reactions, modifying protein activity, defending the cell against foreign nucleic acids, and regulating gene expression."**

functional diversity to RNA molecules. Additionally, RNAs can associate with proteins and modify their activity or recruit them to other nucleic acids through complementary base pairing.

As our knowledge of the diversity of RNA structure and function has increased, it has shifted several paradigms for how we think about life at the molecular level. Whereas we once thought only proteins could be enzymes, we are now searching for ways to use catalytic RNAs as therapeutics to fight disease. Whereas we once thought that most of the human genome was "junk DNA," we are now discovering that most noncoding sequences can be transcribed and even display important anticancer functions. Whereas we never imagined that RNA could regulate gene expression, we now know that it does so at the level of both transcription and translation. As you will soon learn, RNA discoveries have even changed our views on how life began. In this Special Topics chapter we will examine the versatility of RNA and highlight some modern applications of RNAs as research tools and therapeutic agents. **ST Table 2.1** provides an overview of the many types of RNA molecules that we will discuss.

Catalytic Activity of RNAs: Ribozymes and the Origin of Life

In the 1960s, several scientists including Carl Woese, Francis Crick, and Leslie Orgel postulated that RNAs could be catalysts based on the fact that RNAs can form complex secondary structures. However, the first examples of RNAs acting as biological catalysts, or **ribozymes**, came many years later in the early 1980s from two different studies. Tom Cech's lab at the University of Colorado at Boulder discovered that introns (Group I introns) in some RNAs could be spliced out in the complete absence of any proteins. Such self-splicing introns demonstrated that RNAs could break and form phosphodiester bonds (see Chapter 13). Sidney Altman's lab at Yale University discovered that the M1 RNA moiety of RNase P is a ribozyme. RNase P cleaves the 5′ leader sequence of precursor

ST TABLE 2.1   Different Classes of RNAs

RNA type (abbreviation)	Function	Example(s)	Size
Messenger RNA (mRNA)	Determines the amino acid sequence of polypeptides and has untranslated regions (UTRs) that can influence stability, localization, and translation.	Human beta-actin mRNA encodes a 375 aa protein that is part of the cytoskeleton.	Variable
Noncoding RNA (ncRNA)	Any RNA that does not code for polypeptides.	tRNAs, rRNAs, and miRNAs are all examples of ncRNAs.	Variable
Transfer RNA (tRNA)	Transfers the amino acids to a growing polypeptide chain during translation.	tRNA^{Met}, tRNA^{Ala}	73–94 nt
Ribosomal RNA (rRNA)	Components of the ribosome.	The 23S rRNA is a component of the prokaryotic ribosomal large subunit and is a ribozyme.	120–5070 nt
Small nuclear RNA (snRNA)	Components of spliceosomes and participate in catalysis of pre-mRNA splicing.	The U2 and U6 snRNAs are involved in the catalysis of pre-mRNA splicing.	~120 nt
Small nucleolar RNA (snoRNA)	Guide the chemical modifications of other RNAs such as rRNAs, tRNAs, and snRNAs.	A complex of snoRNA and protein catalyzes the conversion of some uridines to pseudouridines in rRNAs.	~70–200 nt
Telomerase RNA component (TERC)	An RNA that associates with the telomerase and serves as a template for adding telomere repeats to the ends of chromosomes.	The TERC is complementary to the telomere sequence 5′-TTAGGG-3′.	438–541 nt
Small RNA (sRNA)	Small noncoding RNAs in prokaryotes that regulate gene expression by binding to mRNAs to influence translation or by binding proteins and modifying their function.	In low iron conditions an sRNA called *RyhB* is expressed to block translation of nonessential iron-containing proteins.	50–500 nt
Clusters of regularly interspersed short palindromic repeats RNA (CRISPR; crRNA)	Present in many bacteria and archaea. Following insertion of foreign DNA into CRISPR loci in the genome, crRNAs transcribed from these regions guide nucleases to invading complementary DNAs to destroy them.	Bacteriophage DNA sequences that are inserted into *E. coli* CRISPR loci are transcribed and processed into crRNAs that target endonucleases to destroy bacteriophage DNA.	24–72 nt
Small noncoding RNA (sncRNA)	This is a general term used to describe short eukaryotic RNAs that associate with RISC and regulate mRNA or transcription.	miRNAs, siRNAs, and piRNAs are examples of small noncoding RNAs.	20–31 nt; double-stranded; 2-nt 3′ overhang
Small interfering RNA (siRNA)	Short dsRNA sequences processed by Dicer that participate in transcriptional and/or posttranscriptional mechanisms of gene regulation.	Introduction of long dsRNAs in *C. elegans* leads to Dicer-mediated processing into siRNAs that associate with RISC and target complementary mRNAs for destruction.	20–25 nt; double-stranded; 2-nt 3′ overhang
Endogenous small interfering RNA (endo-siRNA)	siRNAs that are derived from endogenous sources such as bi-directional transcription of repetitive sequences such as centromeres and transposons that are processed by Dicer.	Endo-siRNAs expressed from LINE-1 retrotransposon sequences and processed by Dicer lead to DNA methylation and transcriptional silencing of LINE-1 loci.	20–25 nt; double-stranded; 2-nt 3′ overhang
Micro RNA (miRNA)	Short dsRNA sequences that participate in transcriptional and/or posttranscriptional mechanisms of gene regulation. Initially form hairpin structures prior to processing to the mature form.	*let-7* miRNAs negatively regulate proto-oncogene *RAS* mRNAs by sites in the 3′ UTR. This partly explains why cancer cells often have no or low expression of *let-7*.	21–24 nt; double-stranded; 2-nt 3′ overhang

(continued)

SPECIAL TOPIC 2

Piwi-interacting RNA (piRNA)	Short dsRNA sequences processed by a Dicer-independent mechanism and associated with Piwi proteins. Participate in transcriptional and/or posttranscriptional mechanisms to silence transposons and repetitive sequences in germ cells.	piRNAs and Piwi proteins form a specific type of RISC that functions to protect germ cells against the potential harm of transposons.	26–31 nt; double-stranded; 2-nt 3' overhang
Long noncoding RNA (lncRNA)	RNAs that are longer than 200 nt and do not encode for polypeptides. lncRNAs have various functions including epigenetic modifications of DNA and regulating the activity of transcription factors.	The lncRNA *Xist* is involved in the epigenetic modifications that lead to X chromosome inactivation in placental mammals.	> 200 nt
Circular RNA (circRNA)	A type of lncRNA. Act as "sponges" to soak up miRNAs and thus allow expression of miRNA targets.	The circRNA called CDR1as/ciRS-7 acts as a sponge to soak up *miR-7* and thus allow expression of *miR-7* targets.	Variable
Extracellular RNA (exRNA)	Various types of RNAs such as mRNAs and miRNAs that are secreted in association with proteins or in vesicles for protection and that serve to signal other cells.	exRNAs are found in many types of human bodily fluids, and their functions are currently being investigated.	Variable

tRNAs during the process of tRNA biogenesis. Cech and Altman were awarded the 1989 Nobel Prize in Chemistry "for their discovery of catalytic properties of RNA."

The discovery of ribozymes has had major implications for theories involving the molecular origins of life. Since DNA encodes proteins and proteins are required to replicate DNA, this presents a "chicken or the egg" paradox as to which may have preceded the other as life originated on Earth. However, since RNA can both encode information and catalyze reactions, it is attractive to hypothesize that RNA was the precursor to cellular life. At the center of this **RNA World Hypothesis**, coined by Walter Gilbert in 1986, is the possibility that RNAs can be self-replicating.

Can an RNA molecule catalyze the synthesis of an identical RNA molecule? If we examine the naturally occurring ribozymes, the repertoire of ribozyme-catalyzed reactions is fairly limited. Most ribozymes catalyze the cleavage or formation of phosphodiester bonds. One notable exception is the ribosome, as discussed earlier; the 23S prokaryotic and 28S eukaryotic large subunit rRNAs are ribozymes that catalyze peptide bond formation. However, naturally occurring ribozymes are limited in their catalytic activity in that they generally are only able to catalyze a reaction once. For example, self-splicing introns cut themselves out and ligate the exons together but can neither repeat this reaction on other molecules nor reverse it. Thus far, there are only three examples of naturally occurring ribozymes that are capable of "multiple turnover": the ribosome, snRNPs, and RNase P. So the naturally occurring ribozymes fall far short of the self-replicating molecules postulated in the RNA World Hypothesis. Nonetheless, one may predict that self-replicating RNAs did once exist but that during evolution, they were usurped by the more stable informational storage of DNA and the more efficient catalysis of enzymes.

Genetic Engineering of Ribozymes

To better understand the potential of ribozymes, scientists have turned toward genetically engineering them. By starting with a large collection of lab-synthesized RNA molecules of varying sequences, scientists have been able to identify and isolate molecules with specific catalytic activity. Using this process, dubbed *in vitro* **evolution**, lab-synthesized ribozymes with novel functions have been created. These functions include RNA and DNA phosphorylation, carbon–carbon bond formation, RNA aminoacylation, and other reactions. Importantly, ribozymes with RNA polymerase activity have also been isolated. Recently, the Holliger lab at the University of Cambridge reported a ribozyme polymerase called tC19Z, which can reliably copy RNA molecules up to 95 nucleotides long (**ST Figure 2–1**). One template RNA that tC19Z copied successfully was that of another ribozyme, which was subsequently shown to be functional. Such a finding lends further credibility to the RNA World Hypothesis, but it remains an open question as to how complex molecules such as the ribonucleotide building blocks of RNAs could be synthesized in a prebiotic world.

Genetically engineered ribozymes are also currently being investigated for therapeutic use. Angiozyme, designed to block angiogenesis, or the growth of new blood vessels, was the first ribozyme to be tested in clinical trials. Cancer cells often secrete a protein called vascular endothelial growth factor (VEGF), which signals through VEGF receptors on cells of blood vessels to induce vascularization of tumors. This provides the cancer cells a supply of oxygen and nutrients as well as a route for spreading to other parts of the body. To battle this problem, Angiozyme targets VEGF receptor mRNAs

ST FIGURE 2–1 A ribozyme polymerase. The lab-synthesized tC19Z ribozyme is capable of copying RNA templates up to 95 nucleotides long, with a sequence complementary to the ssC19 5′ end of the ribozyme.

for destruction to prevent formation of the receptor proteins, thus stopping angiogenesis. Angiozyme showed promising results in animal tests and progressed to phase II clinical trials on patients with metastatic breast cancer. Although analysis of patient blood serum showed a significant reduction in VEGF receptor levels, Angiozyme was not effective at fighting cancer and further development of the drug was halted. This study suggests that there is potential for ribozymes as drugs because there was specific target inhibition, but the study also demonstrates the complex nature of fighting cancer. There are ongoing clinical trials for ribozymes engineered for multiple targets associated with fighting HIV infection.

Small Noncoding RNAs Play Regulatory Roles in Prokaryotes

Prokaryotic small noncoding RNAs (**sRNAs**) were discovered decades ago, but their regulatory functions are still being elucidated and new sRNAs are still being discovered. It is thought that *E. coli* contains roughly 80–100 sRNAs, and other species are reported to have three times that number. sRNAs are generally between 50 and 500 nucleotides long and are involved in gene regulation and the modification of protein function. sRNAs involved in gene regulation

are often transcribed from loci that partially overlap the coding genes that they regulate. However, they are transcribed from the opposite strand of DNA and in the opposite direction, making them complementary to mRNAs transcribed from that locus In other cases, sRNAs are complementary to target mRNAs, but are transcribed from loci that do not overlap target genes. sRNAs regulate gene expression by binding to mRNAs (usually at the 5′ end) that are being transcribed. In some cases, sRNA binding to mRNAs blocks translation of the mRNA by blocking the ribosome binding site (RBS). In other cases, binding enhances translation by preventing secondary structures from forming in the mRNA that would block translation, often by masking the RBS (see **ST Figure 2–2**). Thus, sRNAs can be both negative and positive regulators of gene expression.

sRNAs have been shown to play important roles in gene regulation in response to changing environmental conditions or stress. For example, the sRNA *DsrA* of *E. coli* is upregulated in response to low temperature and promotes the expression of genes that enable the long-term survival of the cell under stressful conditions, or stationary phase (see Figure 6–1). *DsrA* binds to *rpoS* mRNA to promote the translation of the RpoS stress response sigma factor, which is the primary transcriptional regulator of genes that promote stationary phase. In contrast, *RyhB* sRNA from *E. coli* is a negative

ST FIGURE 2–2 Bacterial small noncoding RNAs regulate gene expression. Bacterial sRNAs can be negative regulators of gene expression by binding to mRNAs and preventing translation by masking the ribosome binding site (RBS), or they can be positive regulators of gene expression by binding to mRNAs and preventing secondary structures (that would otherwise mask an RBS) and enable translation.

regulator of gene expression. In response to low iron levels, *RyhB* is transcribed to inhibit the translation of several non-essential iron-containing enzymes so that the more critical iron-containing enzymes can utilize what little iron is present in the cytoplasm.

sRNAs also play a critical role in bacterial cell communication. Bacterial cells communicate to sense their population density and determine cellular behaviors that are appropriate for low-density or high-density populations. This bacterial cell communication is called **quorum sensing** (see the Genetics, Technology and Society essay in Chapter 16). For example, pathogenic bacteria are often harmless at low cell density because they do not express **virulence factors**, or the molecules that enable them to colonize the host, evade/suppress the immune system, and obtain nutrients from the host. At low cell density, virulence factors will not be at a high enough concentration to achieve their goals. However, pathogenic bacteria monitor their population size and change their gene expression to launch an attack of virulence factors in high concentrations that will be successful. The pathogen *Vibrio cholera* can infect the human small intestine and secrete virulence factors, including the cholera toxin, which causes vomiting and diarrhea. Production of virulence factors is dependent on the activity of the HapR transcription factor. HapR is not produced when the bacteria are at low density due to the activity of four sRNAs, *Qrr1–4*. These sRNAs bind to *hapR* mRNA and prevent its translation. However, when the population reaches a critical threshold, determined by increasing concentrations of an **autoinducer** molecule secreted by the cells, *Qrr1–4* transcription is down-regulated, thus allowing HapR to upregulate cholera toxin production. Current research is investigating ways in which the quorum sensing pathways of pathogenic bacteria can be exploited by drugs to prevent infections.

In addition to regulating mRNA translation, sRNAs can modulate protein activity. The *E. coli* 6S RNA is a 184-nucleotide sRNA that accumulates during stationary phase and functions to repress the transcription of genes that mediate vegetative growth. It accomplishes this by binding to RNA polymerases associated with the RpoD sigma factor that promotes the transcription of genes required for vegetative growth. 6S RNA has a hairpin structure that binds to the active site of the RNA polymerase and mimics double-stranded DNA, thus blocking the RNA polymerase from binding to promoter regions of target genes.

Prokaryotes Have an RNA-Guided Viral Defense Mechanism

Biological warfare between viruses (bacteriophages) and prokaryotes as a result of their coevolution has led to a diversity of defense mechanisms. For example, bacteria express endonucleases (restriction enzymes), which cleave specific DNA sequences. Such restriction enzymes destroy foreign bacteriophage DNA, while the host's genomic DNA is protected by DNA methylation. These same restriction enzymes have been adopted by molecular biologists for use in recombinant DNA technology (see Chapter 20). Bacteria can also defend against bacteriophage attack by blocking bacteriophage adsorption, blocking DNA insertion, and inducing suicide in infected cells. All of these defense mechanisms are **innate** because they are not tailored to a specific pathogen. In contrast, recent research has identified an **adaptive** viral defense strategy whereby previous infection by a pathogen provides immunity to that cell and its descendants. In 2007, researchers at a Danish food science company called Danisco sought to create a strain of *Streptococcus thermophilus* that was more resistant to bacteriophage attack, thus making it more efficient for use in the production of yogurt and cheese. The Danisco researchers found that when they exposed *S. thermophilus* to a particular bacteriophage, it essentially became immune to it. The Danisco research group and others identified an adaptive defense mechanism that uses RNA as a guide for destroying viral DNA.

The adaptive viral defense mechanism is dependent on a genomic feature called a **CRISPR**, so named because it contains clustered regularly interspaced short palindromic repeats (**ST Figure 2–3**). CRISPR sequences were first identified in 1987 in the *E. coli* genome based on a simple description of repeated DNA sequences with unique spacer sequences between them. These spacers remained a mystery until 2005 when three independent studies demonstrated that the spacer sequences of CRISPRS were identical to bacteriophage sequences. We now know that insertion of fragments of phage DNA into CRISPR loci is required for adaptive immunity. CRISPR-associated genes (*cas*) are found adjacent to CRISPR loci and are required for various aspects of adaptive immunity (ST Figure 2–3). There are many different types of Cas proteins, and they include proteins with DNase, RNase, and helicase domains, as well as proteins of unknown function.

The **CRISPR/Cas** mechanism for adaptive immunity has three discrete steps (ST Figure 2–3). The first step is the integration of invading phage DNA into CRISPR loci and is often referred to as **acquisition**. It is not completely clear how the host cell fragments phage DNA and inserts it into these specific CRISPR loci. However, one of the Cas proteins, Cas1 from *E. coli*, is a double-stranded DNase and is thought to be involved in this process. Certain sequences in phage genomes also appear to be targeted for CRISPR integration.

After acquisition, the second step is the transcription of CRISPR loci and the processing of CRISPR-derived RNAs (crRNAs). This step is referred to as **crRNA biogenesis**, which also requires assistance from Cas proteins. CasE from *E. coli* is an endoribonuclease that cleaves long precursor

ST FIGURE 2–3 The CRISPR/Cas system mediates an adaptive immune response in prokaryotes. CRISPR loci contain repeat sequences derived from foreign viral DNA separated by spacer sequences. *cas* genes, located nearby in the genome, are involved in CRISPR-mediated adaptive immunity. The CRISPR/Cas mechanism for adaptive immunity has three steps of acquisition (viral DNA is inserted into CRISPR loci), crRNA biogenesis (CRISPR loci are transcribed and processed into short crRNAs), and interference (crRNAs direct Cas proteins to viral DNA to destroy it).

species, has both helicase and DNase domains and is important for target DNA cleavage. Amazingly, this system is able to distinguish "self" DNA from foreign DNA; otherwise the CRISPR/Cas system would cleave CRISPR spacers in the genome since they contain bacteriophage sequences. "Self" identification is possible because the crRNAs contain CRISPR repeat sequences that are complementary to the "self" DNA and inhibit cleavage. Complementarity outside of the spacer region prevents DNA cleavage presumably because of conformational changes to the CRISPR-associated ribonucleoprotein complexes.

Although the details of the mechanism have been studied in just a select few species, it is already apparent that the CRISPR/Cas system is variable with respect to the number of CRISPR loci, the number of repeats, the length of the repeats, the length of the spacers, and the *cas* genes. It is also apparent, however, that some variation of the CRISPR/Cas adaptive defense system is present in roughly 48 percent of sequenced bacterial species and roughly 95 percent of sequenced Archaea, suggesting that it is an ancient and successful defense strategy. Furthermore, evidence suggests that this defense strategy is not just active against bacteriophages; this system is active against plasmid DNA as well.

CRISPR/Cas has been harnessed as an important tool for molecular biology. By expressing components of the CRISPR/Cas system in eukaryotic cells, scientists are able to specifically and efficiently target genes for

crRNAs (pre-crRNAs) into mature crRNAs. Each mature crRNA contains a spacer sequence (determined by the integrated phage DNA fragment) flanked by repeat sequences. In some species, CRISPR repeat sequences form secondary structures such as stem-loops that are required for processing. In other species, a short RNA called a transactivating CRISPR RNA (tracrRNA) is also required for processing. tracrRNAs are complementary to CRISPR repeat sequences in the pre-crRNA and bind to them to form secondary structures.

The third and final step is the targeting and cleavage of phage DNA sequences complementary to crRNAs. This step is referred to as **interference**. Mature crRNAs associate with one or more Cas proteins to form CRISPR-associated ribonucleoprotein complexes, which bind to foreign DNA through crRNA-DNA complementary interactions. When a complementary crRNA-DNA match is made, the complex catalyzes cleavage of both strands of the foreign DNA within the region of complementarity. Cas3, found in many

mutation. The CRISPR/Cas system of *Streptococcus pyrogenes* has been used most extensively for this purpose because only three things are needed to target a specific DNA sequence: the mature crRNA, the Cas9 endonuclease, and a tracrRNA (see above) required for crRNA interaction with Cas9. However, the crRNA and tracRNA can be genetically engineered and expressed as a hybrid small guide RNA (sgRNA), which provides the requisite secondary structure needed for activity. Thus, by inserting Cas9 and sgRNAs, one can target a specific gene for interruption. This can be done by inserting the genes encoding for Cas9 and the sgRNA or by injecting *in vitro* transcribed sgRNA and mRNA for Cas9. Since this technique was published in 2012, it has been successfully used to target genes for mutation in *Drosophila, C. elegans,* zebrafish, *Arabidopsis,* mice, and cultured human cells, demonstrating the broad applicability and the fast pace with which this is being adopted as a tool for science.

BOX 1

RNA-Guided Gene Therapy with CRISPR/Cas Technology

The CRISPR/Cas system has proved to be an efficient and specific genome-editing tool that has been exploited by scientists to induce mutations in target genes of interest. Based on this success, a company called Editas Medicine, based out of Cambridge, Massachusetts, aims "to translate its genome editing technology into a novel class of human therapeutics that enable precise and corrective molecular modification to treat the underlying cause of a broad range of diseases at the genetic level." Simply put, Editas Medicine hopes to develop CRISPR/Cas technology for gene therapy.

Current gene therapy approaches involve treating individuals with disease-causing mutations by inserting a functional copy of the gene, often using a viral vector (see Chapter 22). There are some concerns and limitations associated with this approach. For example, viral vectors may insert the replacement genes randomly into the genome, which may disrupt the function of other important genes. Indeed, the viral vectors themselves may cause dangerous immune responses. Significantly, traditional gene therapy approaches are limited to treating diseases caused by recessive, loss-of-function mutations. In contrast, adding a normal allele does not ameliorate diseases caused by dominant, gain-of-function alleles,

which result in toxic levels of gene expression and/or encode aberrant toxic proteins.

Founded by five academic scientists with expertise in CRISPR/Cas technology and supported by $43 million in venture capital investment, Editas Medicine thinks that CRISPR/Cas technology may offer a solution to some of the problems of traditional gene therapy strategies. Although we do not know their precise strategies or their intended target diseases, one can speculate on how CRISPR/Cas can be used for gene therapy. Since the CRISPR/Cas system uses RNA as a guide to direct the Cas9 endonuclease to complementary DNA sequences in the genome, small guide RNAs (sgRNAs) may be engineered to target disease-causing mutant alleles. For recessive genetic disorders, CRISPR/Cas can be used to induce a double-stranded break in the target gene, which activates the DNA repair machinery. If a normal copy of the gene is inserted into cells along with the CRISPR/Cas components, it can be used as a template for correcting the mutant allele by homologous recombination (see Chapter 15). This has a distinct advantage over traditional gene therapy methods because the gene is corrected in its native location in the genome rather than being randomly inserted or not integrated into a chromosome at all.

Although traditional gene therapy methods are not useful for treating dominant genetic diseases, CRISPR/Cas may be effective and thus extend the reach of gene therapy to a greater

range of diseases. Most of the individuals afflicted with dominant disorders are heterozygous; they have a dominant mutant allele and a normal allele. In theory, CRISPR/Cas may be used to specifically inactivate the dominant mutant allele, rendering it a recessive, loss-of-function allele. In many cases, the undisrupted allele would then be able to restore normal gene function.

Despite encouraging foundational studies on CRISPR/Cas genome editing, bright minds working on the problem, and financial backing, there are some important hurdles to overcome before Editas Medicine can achieve its goals. For example, how will sgRNAs and Cas9 (or genes encoding these components) be delivered to the appropriate target cells in the patient effectively and without causing damaging side-effects? Delivery is a difficult problem for all gene therapy strategies. However, a concern specific to CRISPR/Cas is that some studies found that the Cas9 endonuclease cleaves DNA at off-target loci in the genome. It will be important to achieve absolute target specificity before this strategy will be safe for therapeutic applications. There are reasons to be optimistic that this problem will be solved. Studies on the vast diversity of Cas proteins in prokaryotes may discover endonucleases more suitable than Cas9, and genetic engineering of Cas9 may improve its fidelity. CRISPR/Cas genome editing was first described in 2012, so we are only beginning to understand the ways in which this technology can be harnessed for application.

Small Noncoding RNAs Mediate the Regulation of Eukaryotic Gene Expression

As discussed above, small noncoding RNAs (sRNAs) regulate gene expression and modulate protein activity in prokaryotes. Indeed, small noncoding RNAs are present in eukaryotes as well. Despite the fact that they are both called small noncoding RNAs, the prokaryotic and eukaryotic varieties differ in terms of their length, biosynthesis,

mechanisms of action, and repertoire of regulatory activities. To help keep this distinction clear, scientists have applied the abbreviation sRNA to refer to the prokaryotic variety and refer to **small noncoding RNAs** in eukaryotes as **sncRNAs**. sncRNAs are short (20–31 nucleotides long) double-stranded RNAs with a 2-nucleotide 3′ overhang and are involved in silencing gene expression at the transcriptional or posttranscriptional levels through a process called **RNA-induced gene silencing**.

There are three different types of sncRNAs, which are classified according to their biogenesis and function. Small interfering RNAs (**siRNAs**) protect the cell from exogenous RNAs, such as from retroviral genomes. However, the exploitation of the siRNA mechanism for research and application has already proved indispensable and still has enormous potential. MicroRNAs (**miRNAs**) play important roles in regulating gene expression, and their malfunction is associated with human diseases (see Chapter 17 for additional coverage of siRNAs and miRNAs). The recently identified and poorly understood Piwi-interacting RNAs (**piRNAs**) protect the germ cells from the harmful effects of mobile DNA elements. We will consider the three types of sncRNAs separately.

siRNAs and RNA Interference

Nobel Prize-winning research from Andrew Fire and Craig Mello in 1998 demonstrated that when double-stranded RNA (dsRNA) is introduced into the cells of *C. elegans*, it leads to a "potent and specific" degradation of complementary mRNAs through a process we call **RNA interference (RNAi)**. We now know a great deal about the molecular basis of RNAi, that it functions broadly in eukaryotes, and how to harness it as a tool for research and as a therapeutic agent. When double-stranded RNAs (dsRNAs) are present in the cytoplasm of a eukaryotic cell, they are recognized and cleaved into ~22-nucleotide-long RNAs with a 2-nucleotide 3′ overhang by an RNAse III protein called **Dicer**. These **siRNAs** then associate with the **RNA-induced silencing complex (RISC)**, which contains an **Argonaute** family protein that binds RNA and has endonuclease or "slicer" activity. RISC cleaves and evicts one of the two strands of the siRNA and retains the other strand as a siRNA "guide" to recruit RISC to a complementary mRNA. RISC then cleaves the mRNA in the middle of the region of siRNA/mRNA complementarity (see **ST Figure 2–4**). Cleaved mRNA fragments lacking a methylated cap or a poly-A tail are then quickly degraded in the cell by nucleases.

The discovery of RNAi in 1998 led to an almost immediate revolution in the investigation of gene function. Traditionally, scientists elucidated the function of specific genes by studying mutants lacking that gene's function. This strategy, known as **forward genetics**, often involves random mutagenesis, screening for mutant phenotypes, mapping of the mutations, and identification of the gene bearing the mutation. Since this process is potentially labor-intensive and expensive, many scientists have turned to using **reverse genetics** approaches whereby a specific gene's function is inhibited to determine the phenotypic outcome. RNAi is an extremely powerful tool for reverse genetics because as long as a gene's sequence

ST FIGURE 2–4 RNA interference pathways. Double-stranded RNA is processed into short interfering RNAs (siRNAs) by Dicer. siRNAs then associate with the RNA induced silencing complex (RISC) containing an Argonaute (AGO) family protein. RISC unwinds the siRNAs into single-stranded siRNAs and cleaves mRNAs complementary to the siRNA. MicroRNA (miRNA) genes are transcribed as primary-miRNAs (pri-miRNAs), which are trimmed at the 5′ and 3′ ends by Drosha to form pre-miRNAs. Pre-miRNAs are exported to the cytoplasm and processed by Dicer. These miRNAs then associate with RISC, and single-stranded miRNAs target RISC to mRNAs. If the miRNA and mRNA are perfectly complementary, the mRNA is destroyed; however, if there is a partial match, translation is inhibited.

is known, one can quickly synthesize dsRNA corresponding to that sequence to inhibit or "knock down" that gene's function. As an example of how quickly RNAi became a tool for research, five years after the discovery of RNAi, the Ahringer lab from the University of Cambridge used RNAi on a massive scale to determine the loss-of-function phenotypes for 86 percent of the genes in the *C. elegans* genome. Subsequently, many genome-wide RNAi screens have been performed to test genes, one at a time, for roles in molecular, cellular, and developmental biology pathways.

siRNAs are also important tools for biomedical research and have great potential as therapeutic agents (see Chapter 17). Thus far, there have been over 30 clinical trials for siRNA drugs to treat diseases, such as asthma, cancer, and vision impairment. Despite substantial evidence that siRNAs are effective against a broad range of gene targets, siRNA delivery to target cells remains difficult. siRNAs are rapidly degraded when injected into the bloodstream, and they cannot passively cross the plasma membrane. Due to these siRNA delivery problems, several pharmaceutical companies, such as Novartis, Pfizer, and Roche, abandoned research and clinical trials involving siRNA drugs.

Since 2011, there has been a recent resurgence of siRNA drug development due to reports of successful delivery of siRNAs using either nanoparticles or cell-penetrating peptides. Clearly, an effective delivery solution will need to be identified before siRNAs will gain widespread use as therapeutic agents. As a promising start, Alnylam Pharmaceuticals recently reported successful phase I clinical trials with an siRNA drug and nanoparticle delivery system that treats transthyretin amyloidosis, a disorder characterized by nervous system and cardiac problems due to buildup of a mutant form of the transthyretin (TTR) protein.

Although the initial studies of RNAi involved the introduction of lab-synthesized dsRNAs, naturally occurring dsRNAs have been described as well, such as bi-directional transcription of genomic loci and retroviral genomes. siRNAs produced without insertion of lab-synthesized RNAs are called **endogenous siRNAs (endo-siRNAs)**. In fact, it is thought that the RNAi pathway evolved as a defense strategy against retroviruses, which often have dsRNA genomes. In that model, retroviral dsRNA would be chopped into siRNAs, which then guide RISC to retroviral transcripts to destroy them.

miRNAs Regulate Posttranscriptional Gene Expression

Another type of sncRNA present in eukaryotes is the miRNA (see Chapter 17). Unlike siRNAs, miRNAs are derived from the self-complementary transcripts of miRNA genes. These initial transcripts called **primary miRNAs (pri-miRNAs)** are "capped and tailed," and some contain introns like messenger RNAs. However, due to their self-complementary sequences, pri-miRNAs form hairpin structures. A nuclear enzyme called **Drosha** removes the non–self-complementary 5′ and 3′ ends to produce **pre-miRNAs**. These hairpins, which are single-stranded, are then exported to the cytoplasm and cleaved by **Dicer** to produce mature double-stranded miRNAs. miRNAs are very similar to siRNAs and associate with RISC to target complementary mRNAs. If the miRNA/mRNA match is perfect (common in plants), the target mRNA is cleaved by RISC, but if the miRNA/mRNA match is partial (common in animals) it blocks translation by the ribosome (ST Figure 2–4).

miRNAs are found in animals, plants, viruses, and possibly fungi, and have been shown to regulate genes involved in diverse cellular processes such as stress responses in plants, development in *C. elegans*, and cell-cycle control in mammalian cells. Why is miRNA-mediated posttranscriptional regulation so widespread? Wouldn't it be more efficient for the cell to repress a gene's transcription rather than transcribe a second gene to destroy/inhibit the mRNA of the first gene? The answer to these questions partly comes from the fact that mRNAs may be translated many times after transcription is stopped. To achieve an efficient and rapid change in gene expression, a cell can turn off transcription and employ an miRNA to target the existing mRNAs in the cytoplasm. For example, miRNAs are key regulators of mammalian embryonic stem cells (ES cells), the cells of the embryo that give rise to all differentiated cell types of the organism. ES cells express the "stemness genes" *Oct4*, *Sox2*, *KLF4*, *Lin28*, and *Myc*, which suppress differentiation and promote stem cell maintenance or self-renewal. Loss of these genes results in premature differentiation of ES cells while persistent activity results in an inability to produce specialized cells—both scenarios are lethal. To enable daughter cells of ES cells to differentiate, they express *miR-145* and *let-7* miRNAs, which target and downregulate stemness mRNAs (**ST Figure 2–5**). A better understanding of miRNA regulation of cellular differentiation is likely to improve stem cell therapy by ensuring that patients receive cells that properly differentiate into the desired cell types rather than fail to differentiate and pose a risk for tumor formation.

piRNAs Protect the Genome for Future Generations

Transposons are mobile DNA sequences that can change their position in the eukaryotic genome. This mobility is dependent on the activity of enzymes called transposases that are often encoded by genes within transposons (see Chapter 15). When transposons "jump" in the genome, they can cause mutations by inserting into genes and disrupting gene function. Therefore, it is important to silence transposons and prevent their transposition, especially in the germ cells that carry the genome forward to future generations. Piwi-interacting RNAs (piRNAs) are sncRNAs that are important for transposon silencing in germ cells and embryonic cells in animals. Animals lacking piRNAs show defects in gametogenesis and are sterile, or pass along mutations to offspring. piRNAs are named for their association with Piwi proteins, which are a subclass of the Argonaute family of proteins in RISC. piRNAs with Piwi-containing RISCs are able to target transposon-derived

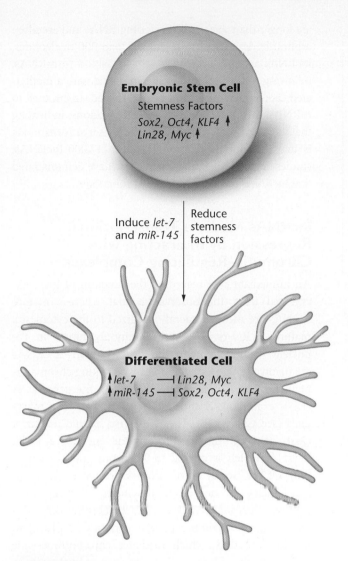

ST FIGURE 2–5 miRNAs regulate embryonic stem cell differentiation. Several genes associated with embryonic stem cell identity (*Sox2, Oct4, KLF4, Lin28,* and *Myc*) are repressed in differentiating cells by *miR-145* and *let-7* to enable cells to acquire specialized functions and inhibit self-renewal.

RNA-Induced Transcriptional Silencing

Heterochromatic regions of the eukaryotic chromosome, characterized by tightly packaged and transcriptionally repressed DNA, play critical structural roles (see Chapter 12). For example, centromeres are heterochromatic and are important for attaching chromosomes to spindle microtubules during cell division. Heterochromatic sequences such as centromeres are characterized by the modification of histone proteins within nucleosomes that are important for packaging and transcriptional repression. For example, nucleosomes associated with heterochromatin are generally methylated at lysine 9 on histone 3 (H3K9Me). Proteins associated with chromatin condensation and transcriptional repression such as the heterochromatin protein 1 (HP1) bind to H3K9Me and mediate heterochromatin formation. H3K9 methylation is dependent on the activity of a **histone methyltransferase** (HMT); several studies have identified DNA binding proteins that complex with HMTs and direct this complex to specific sequences. Importantly, studies have also found that sncRNAs can also direct heterochromatin formation to specific sites in the genome.

In contrast to RNAi, which results in posttranscriptional inhibition of gene expression, sncRNAs involved in heterochromatin formation use a mechanism known as **RNA-induced transcriptional silencing (RITS)**. RITS was first described in the fission yeast *Schizosaccharomyces pombe* when the deletion of several genes involved in the RNAi pathway, such as Argonaute and Dicer, resulted in loss of H3K9 methylation at centromere nucleosomes and loss of centromere function. In 2004, the Moazed lab at Harvard University identified a complex including an Argonaute protein, a heterochromatin-associated protein, and siRNAs produced by Dicer. The siRNAs associated with this RITS complex are complementary to centromeric DNA and are required for recruiting the complex to the centromere and heterochromatin formation.

Paradoxically, transcription from heterochromatic regions such as centromeres is important for transcriptional silencing by RITS. The siRNAs that target the RITS complex to centromeres have siRNAs derived from centromeric transcription that occurs during S phase of the cell cycle. When centromeric transcription occurs, an **RNA-directed RNA polymerase (RdRP)** binds to nascent transcripts and catalyzes the formation of dsRNA from single-stranded transcripts. The dsRNA is then a substrate for Dicer and leads to the formation of siRNAs complementary to centromeric DNA. The RITS complex associates with these siRNAs and targets centromeric transcripts. Through an unknown mechanism, this complex at centromeric loci leads to recruitment of HMTs and H3K9 methylation, which triggers heterochromatin formation (**ST Figure 2–6**). In support of this model, tethering of the RNAi machinery

RNAs due to their complementary sequences and cause their transcriptional repression, presumably by promoting DNA methylation. Although piRNA biogenesis is poorly understood, they are transcribed from regions of the genome that contain transposon DNA sequences called piRNA clusters. It is thought that piRNA clusters may derive from damaged or nonfunctional transposons in the genome. The long piRNA transcripts are processed by a Dicer-independent mechanism and are often longer than other sncRNAs, with a range of 26–31 nucleotides. It is not yet clear how different the piRNA pathway is from other sncRNA pathways but it is evident that this pathway is important for protecting the genome from the damaging effects of transposon activity.

ST FIGURE 2–6 RNA-induced transcriptional silencing. Bi-directional transcription of centromeric DNA (or RdRP activity on single-stranded transcripts) produces dsRNA that is processed by Dicer into siRNAs. These siRNAs associate with the RITS complex and recruit it to nascent transcripts. Histone methyltransferase (HMT) associated with RITS mediates H3K9 methylation of nearby nucleosomes, which leads to heterochromatin assembly.

to other chromosomal loci leads to heterochromatin formation and transcriptional silencing of these loci.

While RITS was characterized in *S. pombe*, RNAi machinery is known to be involved in transcriptional silencing and heterochromatin formation in plants, *Drosophila*, *C. elegans*, and mammals. Further studies will help to elucidate how similar these mechanisms are in diverse species.

Long Noncoding RNAs Are Abundant and Have Diverse Functions

In addition to small noncoding RNAs discussed above, eukaryotic genomes also encode many **long noncoding RNAs (lncRNAs)**. One obvious distinction is that lncRNAs

are longer than the small noncoding RNAs and are often arbitrarily designated to be longer than 200 nucleotides. lncRNAs are produced in a similar fashion to mRNAs; following transcription they are modified with a methylated cap, a poly-A tail, and can be spliced. In contrast to mRNAs, they have **no** start and stop codons, indicating that they do not encode protein. The conservative estimate is that the human genome encodes ~17,000 lncRNAs; studies of just a small fraction of these have demonstrated that lncRNAs have diverse cellular functions.

lncRNAs Mediate Transcriptional Repression by Interacting with Chromatin-Regulating Complexes

An immediate clue regarding the function of lncRNAs emerged from the observation that whereas mature mRNAs are most frequently localized to the cytoplasm, mature lncRNAs are most commonly found in the nucleus. Consistent with this finding, many lncRNAs are involved in gene regulation by recruiting chromatin-regulating complexes to specific loci in the genome. A classic example is X chromosome inactivation in mammals (see Chapter 7). The *X-inactive specific transcript* (*Xist*) gene on the X chromosome encodes a 17-kb lncRNA, which is critical to X chromosome inactivation. Of the two X chromosomes present in mammalian females, the one randomly chosen for inactivation expresses *Xist* lncRNAs that coat the chromosome. *Xist* recruits the polycomb repressor complex 2 (PRC2) to the inactivated X, which mediates chromosome-wide trimethylation of lysine 27 on histone 3 of nucleosomes, leading to chromatin condensation and transcriptional silencing. It is unclear how *Xist* spreads across the inactivated X, but recent studies demonstrate that the first loci on the X chromosome to acquire *Xist* lncRNAs are located near the *Xist* gene in terms of the three-dimensional architecture of the chromosome. Surprisingly, it appears that proximity to the site of transcription is more important than a specific sequence required for *Xist* lncRNA localization.

Similar mechanisms of lncRNA-mediated transcriptional repression are found in diverse eukaryotes and include gene-specific as well as chromosome-wide transcriptional silencing. For example, *Hotair* is a 2.2-kb lncRNA expressed from human chromosome 12 that mediates transcriptional repression of several target genes on chromosome 2. Similar to *Xist*, *Hotair* recruits PRC2 to target genes, which causes H3K27 methylation and transcriptional silencing (**ST Figure 2–7**). While the normal role of *Hotair* is not specifically known, overexpression of *Hotair* in cancer cells is linked with a poor prognosis due to increased chances for metastasis. Hopefully, future studies will help to elucidate how *Hotair* overexpression affects specific genes to promote cancer metastasis.

ST FIGURE 2–7 The *Hotair* long noncoding RNA regulates chromatin. The lncRNA *Hotair* is expressed from human chromosome 12 and recruits the polycomb repressor complex 2 (PRC2) to several target genes on chromosome 2. PRC2 catalyzes methylation of nearby nucleosomes (H3K27me3), which mediates chromatin condensation. Overexpression of *Hotair* in cancer indicates poor prognosis and likelihood of metastasis, presumably due to repression of the target genes on chromosome 2.

lncRNAs Regulate Transcription Factor Activity

lncRNAs can also associate with and regulate the activity of transcription factors. For example, the androgen receptor (AR) both binds testosterone and serves as transcription factor to activate target genes important for male development. Recent studies have demonstrated that ARs function as a transcription factor is regulated by two lncRNAs: PRNCR1 and PCGEM1. AR binds to enhancer sequences called androgen response elements (AREs) that are located at a distance from the target genes they enhance. In order to activate transcription of the target genes, the DNA is looped to bring the enhancer and AR closer to the target gene's promoter and the transcriptional machinery. PRNCR1 and PCGEM1 play important roles as "liaisons" in making this DNA loop by physically bridging the gap between AR and the promoter (**ST Figure 2–8**). Without these lncRNAs, AR cannot activate transcription of target genes. This work has added significance because androgen signaling is known to promote the growth of prostate cancer. Even eliminating testosterone by castration only delays cancer progression since the cancer cells often evolve to have mutant forms of AR that do not require testosterone for activity. Preliminary studies show that inhibiting PRNCR1 and PCGEM1 blocks the growth of both androgen-dependent and androgen-independent prostate cancer cells, suggesting that blocking these lncRNAs may be a new strategy for fighting prostate cancer.

Circular RNAs Act as "Sponges" to Soak Up MicroRNAs

RNA molecules adopt diverse shapes such as the cloverleaf characteristic of tRNAs and the stem-loop structure of

ST FIGURE 2–8 Long noncoding RNAs mediate transcriptional activation. The lncRNAs PCGEM1 and PRNCR1 act as liaisons between the androgen receptor (AR) and the promoter to activate the transcription of target genes. PRNCR1 binds to AR and recruits DOT1L, an enzyme that methylates AR. PCGEM1 binds methylated AR and recruits Pygo2, a protein that binds methylated H3K4 at promoters.

microRNAs. RNA can also adopt a closed circular configuration with no free 5′-phosphate or 3′-OH ends. The genomes of some viruses, such as hepatitis D, are single-stranded circular RNA molecules, and self-splicing introns in rRNAs sometimes form circles. More recently, the roles of eukaryotic circular lncRNAs in gene regulation are being investigated.

Circular RNAs (circRNAs) were first described in the cytoplasm of eukaryotic cells in 1979 using electron microscopy; there were also several other reports of their existence, but none provided evidence of a biological function. Therefore, many scientists dismissed them as a rare genetic error or an artifact of the molecular biology methods used to identify them. However, recent studies have provided compelling evidence not only that circRNAs exist, but also that they do indeed have a biological function.

In a search for eukaryotic circRNAs, Patrick Brown's group at Stanford University used RNA-seq (next-generation sequencing of RNA) to identify transcripts from human cells that had scrambled exon sequences, such as the fourth exon being followed by the second exon. To provide evidence that

these scrambled exon transcripts are indeed circRNAs, the Stanford group showed that they are highly resistant to digestion by RNase R, a 3′ to 5′ exonuclease, providing strong evidence that these RNA molecules lack 3′ ends. This study clearly demonstrated that circRNAs exist in human cells and went on to establish that circRNAs account for a substantial proportion of the total transcripts for hundreds of genes.

Such abundance suggests that circRNAs must be functional. Two studies originating from the Max Delbruck Center for Molecular Medicine and from Aarhus University and the University of Southern Denmark demonstrated that they are indeed functional. These studies demonstrate that some circRNAs contain many sites that are complementary to specific microRNA sequences and thus serve to function as "sponges" to soak up or sequester miRNAs along with their RISC proteins (**ST Figure 2–9**). One circRNA in particular, interchangeably called CDR1as and ciRS-7 (circRNA naming has not been standardized), is a sponge for *miR-7*. Expression of CDR1as/ciRS-7 leads to sequestration of the *miR-7* miRNAs and thus allows the expression

ST FIGURE 2–9 Circular RNAs are microRNA sponges. (a) circRNAs are postulated to form from circular splicing and (b) function as miRNA "sponges" that bind and sequester miRNAs from their mRNA targets. circRNAs are also postulated to be miRNA or RNA binding protein (RBP) delivery vehicles, RBP sponges, or regulators of RBPs and mRNAs.

BOX 2
Do Extracellular RNAs Play Important Roles in Cellular Communication?

In addition to the abundance and diversity of RNAs within cells, RNAs are also found outside of cells. RNAs are prevalent in blood, sweat, tears, and other body fluids. These **extracellular RNAs (exRNAs)**, which include mRNAs, miRNAs, siRNAs, lncRNAs, and tRNAs, are often enclosed in vesicles to protect them from degradation by ubiquitous RNases. Since RNAs are secreted from cells, it raises the possibility that they are internalized by other cells and can serve as a form of cell–cell communication. Although there is not yet convincing evidence that this is true in mammals, studies from plants (*A. thaliana*) and *C. elegans* clearly show that RNAs passed from cell to cell are indeed functional.

Experiments in *A. thaliana* demonstrated that exRNAs influence cells at a long distance from the cells that secrete them. When roots expressing a transgene carrying an inverted repeat RNA to target green fluorescent protein (GFP) were grafted to a plant expressing GFP in leaves, GFP expression was silenced in the leaves and siRNAs derived from the inverted repeats were found in the vascular tissue of the plant's stem (**ST Figure 2–10**). This strongly suggests that siRNAs can be transported within plants and affect gene expression in distant cells. An attractive implication of this mechanism is that a plant's ability to sense environmental conditions (such as stress) in one part of the plant can lead to an adaptive response in another part of the plant.

Studies in *C. elegans* have demonstrated that the effects of RNAi are both systemic and, in some cases, transgenerational. When worms are fed dsRNA, a membrane protein called SID-2 mediates the endocytosis of dsRNA into intestinal cells, which in turn likely secrete the dsRNAs into the body cavity. A second dsRNA channel (transport) protein, called SID-1, mediates the uptake of dsRNAs from the body cavity into most of the other cells of the worm where Dicer cleaves the dsRNAs into siRNAs that target mRNAs for destruction. Even cells of the germ line receive dsRNAs through this mechanism, thus passing the effect on to offspring. It is thought that that this mechanism evolved as part of an immune response whereby a damaged viral particle that spills its

ST FIGURE 2–10 RNAs are transported between cells in plants. *A. thaliana* scion (stem and leaves) expressing the green fluorescent protein (GFP) was grafted onto a rootstock expressing an inverted repeat of a partial GFP sequence. Transcription of the inverted repeats in roots created hairpin RNAs that were processed by Dicer to generate siRNAs. siRNAs spread through the plant and, with RISC, inhibited GFP expression in the leaves, demonstrating that siRNAs can signal between cells. GFP-positive regions are green, while non-GFP (silenced) regions are red due to autofluorescence of chlorophyll. Note that silencing is more prominent along vascular tissue, through which the siRNAs are transported.

(continued)

of *miR-7* target mRNAs. Given that *miR-7* targets alpha synuclein mRNA, which encodes a protein that aggregates in Parkinson disease patients due to lower levels of *miR-7*, it is plausible that CDR1as/ciRS-7 plays an important role in the nervous system. Another circRNA is produced from transcripts for the male-determining gene *Sry* (see Chapter 7) in mouse testes. *Sry* circRNAs have 16 sites for *miR-138* binding and are postulated to act as sponges for *miR-138*. It is still unclear how this circRNA functions in the context of sex determination or testes differentiation. Since miRNAs are abundant in stem cells where they negatively regulate genes required for differentiation, it will be interesting to see if circRNAs are expressed when stem cells begin to differentiate in order to soak up miRNAs, thus allowing the expression of genes required for differentiation.

There are still many unanswered questions about circRNAs. How do circRNAs form? One hypothesis is that they originate during RNA splicing where a 3′ splice site for a downstream exon is spliced to a 5′ splice site of an upstream exon (ST Figure 2–9). Do circRNAs have other functions? This remains to be seen but postulated functions include acting as an miRNA or RNA-binding protein (RBP; see below) delivery vehicle, acting as an RBP sponge, and acting as regulators of RBPs or mRNAs (ST Figure 2–9). Finally, circRNAs were also shown to exist in *S. solfataricus* (and related species), which is a sulfur-metabolizing aerobic archaeon. Thus far, there are no known roles for circRNAs in prokaryotes.

mRNA Localization and Translational Regulation in Eukaryotes

In this final section we shift from noncoding RNAs to messenger RNAs (mRNAs). Although we have known since 1960 that mRNAs encode for proteins, we are still learning about how mRNAs are posttranscriptionally regulated in eukaryotes. It has become clear that mRNAs are not simply translated as soon as they reach the cytoplasm, but rather that mRNAs can be localized to discrete locations within the cell and then locally translated. mRNA localization and localized translational control create asymmetric protein distributions within the cell that define cellular regions with distinct functions. For example, different proteins localized to the highly branched dendrites of a neuron enable them to receive sensory information, while the proteins present in the axon of a neuron mediate the release of neurotransmitters that signal to other cells (see Figure 24–6).

Since mRNA localization and localized translational control are common and important in diverse cell types, it is important to understand how mRNAs are localized and translationally regulated. As soon as mRNAs are transcribed, they begin to associate with a class of proteins called **RNA-binding proteins (RBPs)**, which influence splicing, nuclear export, localization, stability, degradation, and translation. Much of the research on mRNA localization and translational regulation has focused on RBPs and their interactions with mRNAs. One of the best-described RBP/mRNA interactions is the localization and translational control of actin mRNAs in crawling cells.

Following injury, fibroblasts migrate to the site of the wound and assist in wound healing. Fibroblasts and many other types of migrating cells control their direction of movement by controlling where within the cell they polymerize new actin microfilaments. The "leading edge" of the cell where this actin polymerization occurs is called the lamellipodium. A series of elegant studies by the Singer lab at the Albert Einstein College of Medicine showed that actin mRNA is localized to lamellipodia and that localization is dependent on a 54-nucleotide element in the actin 3′ untranslated region of the mRNA transcript termed a **zip code**. The actin zip code sequence is a binding site for a RBP called **zip code binding protein 1 (ZBP1)**. ZBP1 binds actin mRNAs and prevents translation initiation as well as promotes the transport of the mRNA to the lamellipodia. Once the mRNAs arrive at the final destination, a kinase called **Src** phosphorylates ZBP1, which disrupts RNA binding and allows translation initiation (**ST Figure 2–11**). Since Src activity is limited to the cell periphery, this mechanism allows cells to transport mRNAs in a translationally repressed state to the cell periphery where they become translated at the site of actin polymerization. Consistent with this model, mouse fibroblasts lacking ZBP1 have reduced actin mRNA localization and reduced directional motility.

(a)

(b)

ST FIGURE 2–11 Localization and translational regulation of actin messenger RNA. (a) Actin mRNA (red) is localized to the leading edge of a fibroblast cell where it becomes translated into actin protein (green). The nucleus is stained blue. (b) The RNA binding protein ZBP1 associates with actin mRNA in the nucleus and escorts it to the cytoplasm. ZBP1 binds cytoskeleton motor proteins (MP), which transport ZBP1 and actin mRNA to the cell periphery. At the cell periphery ZBP1 is phosphorylated by Src and dissociates from actin mRNA, allowing it to be translated. Actin translation and polymerization at the leading edge direct cell movement.

There is some evidence suggesting that this actin mRNA localization mechanism is used in other cell types as well. Local translation of actin in the neurites (cellular projections) of neurons is required for neurite outgrowth and axon guidance decisions, and mouse neurons lacking ZBP1 have reduced neurite length and exhibit defects in axon guidance.

mRNA localization and translational control are likely to be widespread mechanisms in diverse species and cell types. For example, *Drosophila nanos* mRNA, which encodes a translational repressor, is localized to the posterior pole of *Drosophila* embryos and to the dendrites of some neurons. Loss of *nanos* mRNA localization results in embryos that develop with anterior/posterior patterning defects and

neurons with a reduced number of dendritic branches and a concomitant loss of sensory function. By tagging *nanos* mRNAs with a fluorescent molecule in living cells, the Gavis lab from Princeton University demonstrated that *nanos* mRNAs are transported in **ribonucleoprotein (RNP) particles** to dendrites where they are locally translated. This transport is dependent on the motor protein dynein, which "walks" along microtubules of the cytoskeleton. These studies and many others have demonstrated how mRNA localization and localized protein synthesis are critical for neuronal function. In fact, defects in mRNA localization in neurons have been implicated in human disorders such as fragile-X syndrome, spinal muscular atrophy, and spinocerebellar ataxia.

Selected Readings and Resources

Journal Articles

Bardil, P., and Hammer, B.K. (2012). Non-coding sRNAs regulate virulence in the bacterial pathogen *Vibrio cholerae*. *RNA Biology* 9: 392–401.

Cech, T.R. (2012). The RNA Worlds in Context. *Cold Spring Harbor Perspectives in Biology* 4.

Eliscovich, C., Buxbaum, A.R., Katz, Z.B., and Singer, R.H. (2013). mRNA on the move: The road to its biological destiny. *Journal of Biological Chemistry* 288: 28.

The ENCODE Project Consortium (2012). An integrated encyclopedia of DNA elements in the human genome. *Nature* 498: 57–74.

Hentze, M.W., and Priess, T. (2013). Circular RNAs: Splicing's enigma variations. *The EMBO Journal* 32: 923–925.

Kung, J.T.Y., Colognori, D., and Lee, J.T. (2013). Long noncoding RNAs: Past, present, and future. *Genetics* 193: 651–659.

Lejeune, E., Bayne, E.H., and Allshire, R.C. (2010). On the connection between RNAi and heterochromatin at centromeres. *Cold Spring Harbor Symposia on Quantitative Biology* 75: 275–283.

Leslie, M. (2013). NIH effort gambles on mysterious extracellular RNAs. *Science* 341: 947.

Lujambio, A., and Lowe, S.W. (2012). The microcosmos of cancer. *Nature* 482: 347–355.

Pennisi, E. (2013). The CRISPR craze. *Science* 341: 833–836.

Web Sites

Exploring Life's Origins: Understanding the RNA World. http://exploringorigins.org/rnaworld.html

microRNA.org. http://www.microrna.org

Nature Reviews Web Focus: RNA. http://www.nature.com/nrm/focus/rna/index.html

Nature Reviews Genetics: Video Animation: RNA Interference. http://www.nature.com/nrg/multimedia/rnai/animation/index.html

National Center for Advancing Translational Sciences—Extracellular RNA Communication. http://www.ncats.nih.gov/research/reengineering/exrna/exrna.html

Review Questions

1. What are some of the different roles that RNA plays in biological systems?
2. What arguments support the RNA World Hypothesis?
3. What types of reactions do ribozymes catalyze? What types of chemical bonds are formed or broken?
4. How is bacterial DNA methylation and expression of restriction enzymes an innate defense strategy, whereas the CRISPR/Cas system is an adaptive defense strategy?
5. What are the three types of small noncoding RNAs in eukaryotic cells, and how are they different from one another?
6. The mechanism for RNA-induced transcriptional silencing of heterochromatic DNA is paradoxical. For example, how does it make sense that centromeric DNA in fission yeast first needs to be transcribed before it can be transcriptionally silenced?
7. Circular RNAs have been referred to as molecular "sponges." What does this mean, and what do they "soak up"?
8. Although exRNAs are found in many fluids within plants and animals, why are they usually found within vesicles or bound by proteins?
9. How and why are eukaryotic mRNAs transported and localized to discrete regions of the cell?

Discussion Questions

1. The RNA World Hypothesis suggests that the earliest forms of life used RNA as a genome instead of DNA. Why then do we not see organisms alive today with RNA genomes?
2. Bacterial sRNAs can bind to mRNAs through complementary binding to regulate gene expression. What determines whether the sRNA/mRNA binding will promote or repress mRNA translation?
3. In many cases, ncRNAs serve as "guides" to direct proteins to other nucleic acids. What are some examples of ncRNAs acting as "guides," and what purposes do they serve?
4. Prokaryotes and eukaryotes have both evolved mechanisms to defend against viral/foreign nucleic acids. How are these mechanisms similar, and how are they different?
5. Extracellular RNAs are abundant in human bodily fluids, but there is currently very little evidence for their potential functions in the body. Speculate on the roles that exRNAs might play in human biology.
6. How is it possible that a given mRNA in a cell is found throughout the cytoplasm but the protein that it encodes is only found in a few specific regions of the cytoplasm? Cite a few different possibilities.

DNA Forensics

Genetics is arguably the most influential science today—dramatically affecting technologies in fields as diverse as agriculture, archaeology, medical diagnosis, and disease treatment.

One of the areas that has been the most profoundly altered by modern genetics is forensic science. **Forensic science** (or *forensics*) uses technological and scientific approaches to answer questions about the facts of criminal or civil cases. Prior to 1986, forensic scientists had a limited array of tools with which to link evidence to specific individuals or suspects. These included some reliable methods such as blood typing and fingerprint analysis, but also many unreliable methods such as bite mark comparisons and hair microscopy.

Since the first forensic use of **DNA profiling** in 1986 (Box 1), **DNA forensics** (also called **forensic DNA fingerprinting** or **DNA typing**) has become an important method for police to identify sources of biological materials. DNA profiles can now be obtained from saliva left on cigarette butts or postage stamps, pet hairs found at crime scenes, or bloodspots the size of pinheads. Even biological samples that are degraded by fire or time are yielding DNA profiles that help the legal system determine identity, innocence, or guilt. Investigators now scan large databases of stored DNA profiles in order to match profiles generated from crime scene evidence. DNA profiling has proven the innocence of hundreds of people who were convicted of serious crimes and even sentenced to death. Forensic scientists have used DNA profiling to identify victims of mass disasters such as the Asian Tsunami of 2004 and the September 11, 2001 terrorist attacks in New York. They have also used forensic DNA analysis to identify endangered species and animals trafficked in the illegal wildlife trade. The power of DNA forensic analysis has captured the public imagination, and DNA forensics is featured in several popular television series.

The applications of DNA profiling extend beyond forensic investigations. These include paternity and family relationship testing, identification of plant materials, verification of military casualties, and evolutionary studies.

It is important for all of us to understand the basics of forensic DNA analysis. As informed citizens, we need to monitor its uses and potential abuses. Although DNA profiling is well validated as a technique and is considered the gold standard of forensic identification, it is not without controversy and the need for legislative oversight.

In this Special Topic chapter, we will explore how DNA profiling works and how the results of profiles are interpreted. We will learn about DNA databases, the potential problems associated with DNA profiling, and the future of this powerful technology.

DNA Profiling Methods

VNTR-Based DNA Fingerprinting

The era of DNA-based human identification began in 1984, with Dr. Alec Jeffreys's publication on DNA loci known as **minisatellites**, or **variable number of tandem repeats (VNTRs)**. As described earlier in the text (see Chapter 12), VNTRs are located in noncoding regions of the genome and are made up of DNA sequences of between 15 and 100 bp long, with each unit repeated a number of times. The number of repeats found at each VNTR locus varies from person to person, and hence VNTRs can be from 1 to 20 kilobases (kb) in length, depending on the person. For example, the VNTR

5′- GACTGCCTGCTAAGAT**GACTGCCTGCTAAGAT GACTGCCTGCTAAGAT**-3′

is comprised of three tandem repeats of a 16-nucleotide sequence (highlighted in bold).

VNTRs are useful for DNA profiling because there are as many as 30 different possible alleles (repeat lengths) at any VNTR in a population. This creates a large number of possible genotypes. For example, if one examined four different VNTR loci within a population, and each locus had 20 possible alleles, there would be more than 2 billion (4^{20}) possible genotypes in this four-locus profile.

To create a VNTR profile (also known as a DNA fingerprint), scientists extract DNA from a tissue sample and digest it with a restriction enzyme that cleaves on either side of the VNTR repeat region (**ST Figure 3–1**). The digested

> "Even biological samples degraded by fire or time are yielding DNA profiles that help determine identity, innocence, or guilt."

is present in as many as 100 copies per cell. The presence of *HER-2* overexpression is associated with increased tumor invasiveness, metastasis, and cell proliferation, as well as a poorer patient prognosis.

Using recombinant DNA technology, Genentech Corporation in California developed a monoclonal antibody known as trastuzumab (or Herceptin) that is designed to bind specifically to the extracellular region of the HER-2 receptor. When bound to the receptor, Herceptin appears to inhibit the signaling capability of HER-2 and may also flag the HER-2-expressing cell for destruction by the patient's immune system. In cancer cells that overexpress HER-2, Herceptin treatment causes cell-cycle arrest, and in some cases, death of the cancer cells.

Because Herceptin will only act on breast cancer cells that have amplified *HER-2* genes, it is important to know the HER-2 phenotype of each cancer. In addition, Herceptin has potentially serious side-effects. Hence, its use must be limited to those who could benefit from the treatment. A number of molecular assays have been developed to determine the gene and protein status of breast cancer cells. Two types of tests are used routinely to determine the amount of *HER-2* overexpression in cancer cells: immunohistochemistry (IHC) and fluorescence *in situ* hybridization (FISH). In IHC assays, an antibody that binds to the HER-2 protein is added to fixed tissue on a slide. The presence of bound antibody is then detected with a stain and observed under the microscope [**ST Figure 4–2(a)**]. The FISH assay (which is described in Chapter 10) assesses the number of *HER-2* genes by comparing the fluorescence signal from a HER-2 probe with a control signal from another gene that is not amplified in the cancer cells [**ST Figure 4–2(b)**].

Herceptin has had a major effect on the treatment of HER-2 positive breast cancers. When Herceptin is used in combination with chemotherapy, there is a 25 to 50 percent increase in survival, compared with the use of chemotherapy alone. Herceptin is now one of the biggest selling biotechnology products in the world, generating more than $5 billion in annual sales.

There are now dozens of drugs whose prescription and use depend on the genetic status of the target cells. Approximately 10 percent of FDA-approved drugs have labels that include pharmacogenomic information (**ST Table 4.1**). For example, about 40 percent of colon cancer patients respond to the drugs **Erbitux**® (cetuximab) and **Vectibix**® (panitumumab). These two drugs are monoclonal antibodies that bind to **epidermal growth factor receptors (EGFRs)** on the surface of cells and inhibit the EGFR signal transduction pathway. In order to work, cancer cells must express EGFR on their surfaces and must also have a wild-type *K-RAS* gene. The presence of EGFR can be assayed using a staining test and observation of cancer cells under a microscope. Mutations in the *K-RAS* gene can be detected using assays based on the polymerase chain reaction (PCR) method, which is described earlier in the text (see Chapter 20).

Another example of treatment decisions being informed by genetic tests is that of the **Oncotype DX**® Assay (Genomic Health Inc.). This assay analyzes the expression (amount of mRNA) from 21 genes in breast cancer samples, in order to help physicians select appropriate treatments and predict the course of the disease. These genes were chosen because their levels of gene expression correlate with breast cancer recurrence after initial treatment. Based on the mRNA expression levels revealed in the assay results, scientists calculate a "Recurrence Score," estimating

ST FIGURE 4–2   HER-2 protein and gene-amplification assays. (a) Normal and breast cancer cells within a biopsy sample, stained by HER-2 immunohistochemistry. Cell nuclei are stained blue. Cancer cells that overexpress HER-2 protein stain brown at the cell membrane. (b) Cancer cells assayed for *HER-2* gene copy number by fluorescence *in situ* hybridization. Cell nuclei are stained blue. *HER-2* gene DNA appears bright red. Chromosome 17 centromeres stain green. The degree of *HER-2* gene amplification is expressed as the ratio of red staining foci to green staining foci.

ST TABLE 4.1 Examples of Personalized Medicine Drugs and Diagnostics

Therapy	Gene Test	Description
Herceptin® (trastuzumab)	*HER-2* amplification	Breast cancer test to accompany Herceptin use
Erbitux® (cetuximab)	*EGFR* expression, *K-RAS* mutations	Protein and mutation analysis prior to treatment
Gleevec® (imatinib)	*BCR/ABL* fusion	Gleevec used in treatment of Philadelphia chromosome-positive chronic myelogenous leukemia
Gleevec® (imatinib)	*C-KIT*	Gleevec used in stomach cancers expressing mutated *C-KIT*
Tarceva® (erlotinib)	*EGFR* expression	Lung cancer for EGFR-positive tumors
Drugs/surgery	*MLH1, MSH2, MSH6*	Gene mutations related to colon cancers
Hormone/chemotherapies	Oncotype DX® test	Selection of breast cancer patients for chemotherapy
Chemotherapies	Aviara Cancer TYPE ID®	Classifies 39 tumor types using gene-expression assays
Rituximab	PGx Predict®	Detects CD-20 variants that predict response to rituximab in non-Hodgkin lymphoma

© 2011 Personalized Medicine Coalition

the likelihood that the cancer will recur within a ten-year period. Those patients with a low-risk rating would likely not benefit by adding chemotherapy to their treatment regimens and so can be treated with hormones alone. Those with higher risk scores would likely benefit from more aggressive therapies.

Reducing Adverse Drug Reactions

Every year, about 2 million people in the United States have serious side-effects from pharmaceutical drugs, and approximately 100,000 people die. The costs associated with these **adverse drug reactions (ADRs)** are estimated to be $136 billion annually. Although some ADRs result from drug misuse, others result from a patient's inherent physiological reactions to a drug.

Sequence variations in a large number of genes can affect drug responsiveness (ST Table 4.2). Of particular significance are the genes that encode the cytochrome P450 families of enzymes. These family members are encoded by 57 different genes. People with some cytochrome P450 gene variants metabolize and eliminate drugs slowly, which can lead to accumulations of the drug and overdose side-effects. In contrast, other people have variants that cause drugs to be eliminated quickly, leading to reduced effectiveness. An example of gene variants that affect drug responses is that of *CYP2D6* gene. This member of the cytochrome P450 family encodes the debrisoquine hydroxylase enzyme, which is involved in the metabolism of approximately 25 percent of all pharmaceutical drugs, including diazepam, acetaminophen, clozapine, beta blockers, tamoxifen, and codeine. There are more than 70 variant alleles of this gene. Some mutations in this gene reduce the activity of the encoded enzyme, and others can increase it. Approximately 80 percent of

ST TABLE 4.2 Examples of Variant Gene Products That Affect Drug Responses

Gene Product	Variant Phenotype	Drugs Affected	Response
Acetyl transferase NAT2	Slow, rapid acetylators	Isoniazid, sulfamethazine, dapsone, paraminosalicylic acid, heterocyclic amines	Slow: toxic neuritis, lupus erythematosus, bladder cancer; Rapid: colorectal cancer
Thiopurine methyltransferase	Poor TPMT methylators	6-mercaptopurine, 6-thioguanine, azathioprine	Bone marrow toxicity, liver damage
Catechol O-methyl transferase	High, low methylators	Levodopa, methyldopa	Low or increased response
CYP2C19	Poor, extensive hydroxylators	Mephenytoin, hexobarbital, proguanil, etc.	Poor or increased toxicity, poor efficacy (proguanil)
β_2 Adrenoceptor	Enhanced receptor downregulation	Albuterol, ventolin	Poor asthma control
5-HT2A serotonergic receptor	Multiple polymorphisms	Clozapine	Variable drug efficiencies
Multiple drug resistance transporter	Overexpression in cancer	Vinblastine, doxorubicin, paclitaxel, etc.	Drug resistance

© 2000 Spring Science + Business Media.

ST FIGURE 4–3 *CYP2D6* pharmacogenetic profile in a Swedish population. Individuals were tested for their ability to metabolize debrisoquine to 4-hydroxydebrisoquine, as an indication of the efficiency of debrisoquine hydroxylase enzyme activity. The population sample was divided into the categories UMs (ultra-rapid metabolizers), EMs (extensive metabolizers), and PMs (poor metabolizers). The "cut-off" label indicates the cut-off between extensive and poor metabolizers.

people are homozygous or heterozygous for the wild-type *CYP2D6* gene and are known as extensive metabolizers (**ST Figure 4–3**). Approximately 10 to 15 percent of people are homozygous for alleles that decrease activity (poor metabolizers), and the remainder of the population have duplicated genes (ultra-rapid metabolizers). Poor metabolizers are at increased risk for ADRs, whereas ultra-rapid metabolizers may not receive sufficient dosages to have an effect on their conditions.

In 2005, the FDA approved a microarray gene test called the **AmpliChip® CYP450** assay (Roche Diagnostics) that detects 29 genetic variants of two cytochrome P450 genes—*CYP2D6* and *CYP2C19*. This test detects single-nucleotide polymorphisms (SNPs) as well as gene duplications and deletions. The AmpliChip CYP450 assay is an example of a genotyping microarray, such as those described earlier in the text (see Chapter 22). After scanning with an automated scanner, the data are analyzed by computer software, and the *CYP2D6/CYP2C19* genotype of the individual is generated.

Another example of pharmacogenomics in personalized medicine is that of the *CYP2C9* and *VKORC1* genes and the drug **warfarin.** Warfarin (also known as Coumadin) is an anticoagulant drug that is prescribed to prevent blood clots after surgery and to aid people with cardiovascular conditions who are prone to clots. Warfarin inhibits the vitamin K-dependent synthesis of several clotting factors. There is an approximately ten-fold variability between patients in the doses of warfarin that have a therapeutic response. In the past, physicians attempted to adjust the doses of warfarin through a trial-and-error process during the first year of treatment. If

the dosage of warfarin is too high, the patient may experience serious hemorrhaging; if it is too low, the patient may develop life-threatening blood clots. It is estimated that 20 percent of patients are hospitalized during their first six months of treatment due to warfarin side-effects.

Variations in warfarin activity are affected by polymorphisms in several genes, particularly *CYP2C9* and *VKORC1*. Two single-nucleotide polymorphisms in *CYP2C9* lead to reduced elimination of warfarin and increased risk of hemorrhage. About 25 percent of Caucasians are heterozygous for one of these polymorphisms and 5 percent appear to be homozygous. About 5 percent of patients of Asian and African descent carry these variants. Patients who are heterozygous or homozygous for some alleles of *CYP2C9* require a 10 to 90 percent lower dose of warfarin.

The FDA recommends the use of *CYP2C9* and *VKORC1* genetic tests to predict the likelihood that a patient may have an adverse reaction to warfarin. Several companies offer tests to detect polymorphisms in these genes, using methods based on PCR amplification and allele-specific primers. It is estimated that the use of warfarin genetic tests could prevent 17,000 strokes and 85,000 serious hemorrhages per year. The savings in health care could reach $1.1 billion per year.

Pharmacogenomic tests and treatments, and the genetic information on which they are based, are rapidly advancing. A source of updated information on all aspects of pharmacogenomics can be found on the Pharmacogenomics Knowledge Base, which is described in Box 2.

Personalized Medicine and Disease Diagnostics

The ultimate goal of personalized medicine is to apply information from a patient's full genome to help physicians diagnose disease and select treatments tailored to that particular patient. Not only will this information be gleaned from genome sequencing, but it will also be informed by gene-expression information derived from transcriptomic, proteomic, metabolomic, and epigenetic tests.

BOX 2
The Pharmacogenomics Knowledge Base (PharmGKB): Genes, Drugs, and Diseases on the Web

The Pharmacogenomics Knowledge Base (PharmGKB) is a publicly available Internet database and information source developed by Stanford University. It is funded by the National Institutes of Health (NIH) and forms part of the NIH Pharmacogenomics Research Network, a U.S. research consortium. The goal of PharmGKB is to provide researchers and the general public with information that will increase the understanding of how genetic variation contributes to an individual's reaction to drugs. On the PharmGKB Web site (see **ST Figure 4–4**), you may search for genes and variants that affect drug reactions, information on a large number of drugs, diseases and their genetic links, pharmacogenomic pathways, gene tests, and relevant publications. Visit the PharmGKB Web site at http://www.pharmgkb .org.

ST FIGURE 4–4 The PharmGKB Knowledge Pyramid. A visual representation of the types of information available at www.pharmgkb.org.

At the present time, the most prevalent use of genomic information for disease diagnostics is genetic testing that examines specific disease-related genes and gene variants. Most existing genetic tests detect the presence of mutations in single genes that are known to be linked to a disease (**ST Table 4.3**). Currently, more than 1600 such genetic tests are available. A comprehensive list of genetic tests can be viewed on the NIH Genetic Testing Registry at www.ncbi .nlm.nih.gov/gtr/. The technologies used in many of these genetic tests are presented earlier in the text (see Chapter 22).

Genetic tests are classified according to their uses, and they fall into one or more groups. *Diagnostic tests* are designed to detect the presence or absence of gene variants or mutations linked to a suspected genetic disorder in a symptomatic patient. *Predictive tests* detect mutations and variants in patients with a family history of a known genetic disorder—for example, Huntington disease or *BRCA*-linked breast cancer. *Carrier tests* help physicians identify patients who carry a gene mutation linked to a disorder that might be passed on to their offspring—such as Tay–Sachs or cystic fibrosis. *Preimplantation tests* are performed on early embryos in order to select embryos for implantation that do not carry a suspected disease. *Prenatal tests* detect potential genetic diseases in a fetus. The test for Down syndrome is a well-known example.

Over the last decade, genome sequencing methods have progressed rapidly in speed, accuracy, and cost-effectiveness. In addition, other "omics" technologies such as transcriptomics and proteomics are providing major insights into how DNA sequences lead to gene expression and, ultimately, to phenotype. (Refer to Chapter 21 for descriptions of techniques and data emerging from human "omics" technologies.) As these technologies become more rapid and cost-effective, they will begin to make important contributions to personalized medicine.

Although the application of "omics" to personalized medicine has not yet entered routine medical care, several proof-of-principle cases illustrate the way in which whole genome analysis may develop in the future. They also reveal some of the limitations that must be overcome before

ST TABLE 4.3 **Some Single-Gene Defects for Which Genetic Tests Are Available**

Disease	Gene Mutation	Description
Achondroplasia	*FGFR3* gene. 99% of patients have a G to A point mutation at nucleotide 1138 (G380R substitution)	Abnormal bone growth
Hereditary breast/ovarian cancer	*BRCA1* and *BRCA2* genes. Deletions, duplications, and point mutations	Predisposition to breast, ovarian, prostate, and other cancers
Duchenne muscular dystrophy	*DMD* gene. Point mutations, deletions, insertions, splicing mutations	Early-onset progressive muscular weakness, heart disease
Fragile-X syndrome	*FMR1* gene. Primarily expanded trinucleotide (CGG) repeats and loss of function	Mental retardation, developmental disorders
Friedrich ataxia	*FXN* gene. 98% of cases have expanded trinucleotide (GAA) repeats in intron 1	Ataxia, muscle weakness, spasticity, heart and other organ dysfunctions
Hemophilia A	*F8* gene. Point mutations, insertions, deletions, inversions	Factor VIII blood-clotting defects, bleeding
Huntington disease	*HTT* (*HD*) gene. Trinucleotide (CAG) repeat expansions	Midlife onset of progressive motor and cognitive disorders
Lesch-Nyhan syndrome	*HPRT1* gene. Point mutations, deletions, duplications	Developmental, motor, and cognitive disorders
Marfan syndrome	*FBN1* gene. Point mutations, splicing mutations, deletions	Connective tissue disorders affecting numerous organs
Polycystic kidney disease, dominant	*PKD1* and *PKD2* genes. Sequence variants, partial or whole-gene deletions and duplications	Cysts in kidney, liver, and other organs, vascular abnormalities
Sickle-cell disease	*HBB* gene. Point mutation leading to Glu to Val substitution at amino acid 6	Early-onset anemia

© Gene Reviews

genome-based medicine becomes commonplace and practical. In the next two sections, we will describe several of these studies as they pertain to the diagnosis of cancers and other diseases.

Personal Genomics and Cancer

As we learned earlier in the text (see Chapter 19), cancer is a genetic disease at the level of somatic cells. High-throughput sequencing of normal and cancer genomes, along with RNA sequencing and protein profiling of normal and cancer cells, has revealed more of the mutations and gene rearrangements associated with specific cancers. Studies such as the Cancer Genome Atlas project are amassing data equivalent to 20,000 genome projects on normal and tumor DNA from patients with more than 20 different types of cancer. Such studies are revealing that cancers once classified in general terms (such as "prostate cancer") are in fact many different diseases based on their genetic profiles. For example, in the past, blood cancers were categorized into two large groups: leukemias and lymphomas. Today, we know that each category can be broken down into more than 40 different types, based on gene mutation and expression characteristics. Similarly, breast cancer is now thought to be at least 10 separate diseases, based on genomic and gene-expression data. The recognition that tumors differ significantly in gene expres-

sion will likely be used in the future to tailor therapies to attack or modify specific gene-expression aberrations.

Another significant discovery from cancer genome research is that every tumor is genetically unique, even though common cellular pathways are involved. This realization indicates that each cancer may require a personalized treatment and that the genomic "net" that is cast to detect altered gene function must be wide enough to capture all relevant defects within each cancer. The potential for whole genome sequencing and gene-expression assays in cancer diagnosis and treatment is illustrated by a case described in Box 3. This story illustrates the enormous quantities of resources involved in genomic sequencing and gene-expression assays, as well as the interpretation of the resulting data. It also shows that genomic sequencing alone may not be sufficient to detect the most important defects in cancer cells, including those that would be suitable targets for therapy. The story points out that few gene-specific drugs are currently available and those that do exist are expensive and may not be covered by medical insurance. The patient in this story had been fortunate that a key defect in his cancer had been detectable using genomic techniques and could be targeted by an existing drug. As most cancers contain dozens to hundreds of genetic and gene-expression defects, and more than one gene product may drive the cells to form cancers, the goal of developing

BOX 3

Personalized Cancer Diagnostics and Treatments: The Lukas Wartman Story [1]

During his final year of medical school in 2002, Dr. Lukas Wartman began to experience symptoms of fatigue, fever, and bone pain. After months of tests, he was given a diagnosis of adult acute lymphoblastic leukemia (ALL). Following two years of chemotherapies, his cancer went into remission for five years. When the ALL recurred, his doctors treated him with intensive chemotherapy and a bone marrow transplant, which put him back into remission for another three years. After his second relapse, all attempts at treatment failed and he was rapidly deteriorating.

At the time of his second relapse, Dr. Wartman was working as a physician-scientist at Washington University, researching the genetics of leukemias. His colleagues, including Dr. Timothy Ley, associate director of the Washington University Genome Institute, decided to rush into a last-minute effort to save him. Making round-the-clock use of the university's sequencing facilities and supercomputers, the research team sequenced the entire genomes of his normal and cancer cells. They also analyzed his RNA types and expression levels using RNAseq technologies.

As they had expected, Dr. Wartman's cancer DNA contained many gene mutations. Unfortunately, no drugs were available that would attack the products of these mutated genes. The RNA sequence analysis, however, revealed unexpected results. It showed that the fms-related tyrosine kinase 3 (*FLT3*) gene, although having a normal DNA sequence, was overexpressed in his cancer cells—perhaps due to mutations in the gene's regulatory regions. The *FLT3* gene encodes a protein kinase that is involved in normal hematopoietic cell growth and differentiation, and its overexpression would be a potentially important contributor to Dr. Wartman's cancer. Equally interesting, and fortunate, was that the drug sunitinib, or Sutent, was known to inhibit the FLT3 kinase and had been approved for use in the treatment of advanced kidney cancers.

Dr. Wartman decided to try sunitinib. Unfortunately, the drug cost $330 per day, and Dr. Wartman's insurance company refused to pay for it. In addition, the drug company Pfizer refused to supply the drug to him under its compassionate use program. Despite these setbacks, he collected enough money to buy a week's worth of sunitinib. Within days of starting treatment, his blood counts were approaching normal. Within two weeks his bone marrow was free of cancer cells. At this point Pfizer reversed its decision and supplied Dr. Wartman with the drug. In addition, he underwent a second bone marrow transplant to help ensure that the cancer would not return. Although Dr. Wartman's long-term prognosis is still uncertain, his successful experience with personalized cancer treatment has given him hope and has spurred research into the regulation of the *FLT3* gene in other cancers.

[1] This story was reported in Kolata, G., In treatment for leukemia, glimpses of the future. *New York Times*, July 7, 2012.

drugs for each of these defects remains a challenging one. Despite these challenges, it is a story of future promise for the role of cancer diagnosis and gene-specific treatments in personalized medicine.

Personal Genomics and Disease Diagnosis: Analyzing One Genome

In 2010, the journal *Lancet* published a report illustrating the type of information that we can currently obtain from personal whole genome sequencing.[1] The personal genome sequence in this study was the first one to be sequenced using a method known as true single-molecule sequencing (tSMS™). Some high-throughput methods, such as those described earlier in the text (see Chapters 20 and 21), require cloning or PCR amplification of template DNA prior to sequencing. In contrast, the tSMS method directly sequences individual genomic DNA strands with minimum processing. The sequencing of this genome took about a week, was

performed with one machine, used the services of three people, and cost $48,000. The genome sequence was that of Dr. Stephen Quake, a Stanford University professor who developed the technology and headed the research group. He was a healthy 40-year-old male who had a family history of arthritis, aortic aneurysm, coronary artery disease, and sudden cardiac death.

By comparing the patient's sequence with other human genome sequences in databases, they discovered a total of 2.6 million SNPs and 752 copy number variations. The researchers then sorted through the genome sequence data to determine which of these variants might have an effect on phenotype. This was accomplished by searching known SNPs in several large databases, manually creating their own disease-associated SNP database, and calculating likelihood ratios for various disease risks. The analysis required the combined efforts of more than two dozen scientists and clinicians over a period of about a year, and information gleaned from more than a dozen sequence databases, new and existing sequence analysis tools, and hundreds of individually accessed research papers.

[1] Ashley, E.A., et al. 2010. Clinical assessment incorporating a personal genome. *Lancet* 375: 1525–1535.

To determine how this patient may respond to pharmaceutical drugs, the researchers searched the PharmGKB database (see Box 2) for the presence of known variants within pharmacogenomically important genes. The patient was found to have 63 clinically relevant SNPs within genes associated with drug reactions. In addition, his genome contained six previously unknown SNPs that could alter amino acid sequences in drug-response genes. For example, the genome sequence revealed that the patient was heterozygous for a null mutation in the *CYP2C19* gene. This mutation could make him sensitive to a range of drugs, including those used to treat aspects of heart disease. He would also be more sensitive than normal to warfarin, based on SNPs within his *VKORC1* and *CYP4F2* genes. In contrast, the patient's sequence contained gene variants associated with good responses to statins; however, other gene variants suggested that he might require higher-than-normal statin dosages.

The search for mutations within genes that directly affect disease conditions revealed several potentially damaging variants. The patient was heterozygous for a SNP within the *CFTR* gene that would change a glycine to arginine at position 458. This mutation could lead to cystic fibrosis if it was passed on to a son or daughter who also inherited a defective *CFTR* gene from the other parent. Similarly, the patient was heterozygous for a recessive mutation in the hereditary haemochromatosis protein precursor gene (*HFE*), which is associated with the development of haemochromatosis, a serious condition leading to toxic accumulations of iron. Also, the patient was heterozygous for a recessive mutation in the solute carrier family 3 (*SLC3A1*) gene. This mutation is linked to cystinuria, an inherited disorder characterized by inadequate excretion of cysteine and development of kidney stones. The scientists discovered a heterozygous SNP within the parafibromin (*CDC73*) gene that would create a prematurely terminated protein. This gene is a tumor-suppressor gene linked to the development of hyperparathyroidism and parathyroid tumors. The presence of this SNP increased the risk that the patient might develop these types of tumors, if any of the patient's cells experienced a loss-of-heterozygosity mutation in the other copy of the gene.

The analysis of this patient's genome sequence for the purpose of predicting future development of multifactorial disease was more challenging. Genome-wide association studies have revealed large numbers of sequence variants that are associated with complex diseases; however, each of these variants most often contributes only a small part of the susceptibility to disease. Because not all variants have been discovered or characterized, it is difficult to establish a numerical risk score for each of these diseases based on the presence of one or more SNPs. As an example, the researchers discovered SNPs within three genes (*TMEM43*,

DSP, and *MYBPC3*) that may be associated with sudden cardiac death. However, the exact effects of two of these SNPs are still unclear, and the other SNP had not previously been described. The patient had five SNPs in genes associated with an increased risk of developing myocardial infarction and two SNPs associated with a lower risk. Among the SNPs associated with increased risk, a variant in the apolipoprotein A precursor (*LPA*) gene is associated with a five-fold increased plasma lipoprotein(a) concentration and a two-fold increased risk of coronary artery disease. By taking into consideration the simultaneous potential effects of many different SNPs, as well as the patient's own environmental and personal lifestyle factors, the researchers concluded that the patient's genetics contributed to a significantly increased risk for eight conditions (such as Type 2 diabetes, obesity, and coronary artery disease) and a decreased risk for seven conditions (such as Alzheimer disease). The patient was offered the services of clinical geneticists, counselors, and clinical lab directors in order to help interpret the information generated from the genome sequence. Genetic counseling covered areas such as the psychological and reproductive implications of genetic disease risk, the possibilities of discrimination based on genetic test results, and the uncertainties in risk assessments.

In 2012, another study of personal genome analysis was reported (Box 4). This study combined data from whole genome sequencing, transcriptomics, proteomics, and metabolomics profiles from a single patient at multiple time points over a 14-month period. This in-depth multilevel personal profiling allowed the patient to be monitored through both healthy and diseased states, as he contracted two virus infections and a period of Type 2 diabetes. This research points out how complex changes in gene expression may affect phenotype and shows the importance of looking beyond the raw sequence of an individual DNA. It also indicates that gene-expression profiles can be monitored by current technologies and may be applied in the future as part of personalized medical testing.

Technical, Social, and Ethical Challenges

There are still many technical hurdles to overcome before personalized medicine will become a standard part of medical care. The technologies of genome sequencing, "omics" profiling, microarray analysis, and SNP detection need to be faster, more accurate, and cheaper. Scientists expect that these challenges will be overcome in the near future; however, genome analysis needs to be used with caution until the technology becomes highly accurate and reliable. Even

BOX 4
Beyond Genomics: Personal Omics Profiling

A study published by a research team led by Dr. Michael Snyder of Stanford University provides an example of how multiple "omics" technologies can be used to examine one person's healthy and diseased states.[1]

Blood samples were taken from a healthy individual (Dr. Snyder) at 20 time points over a 14-month study period. The patient's whole genome sequence was generated at each time point using two different methods and backed up by exome sequencing using three different methods. In addition, his genome sequence was compared to that of his mother. Concurrently, whole-transcriptome sequencing, proteomic profiling, and metabolomics assays were performed.

Dr. Snyder's genome sequence revealed a number of SNPs that are known to be associated with elevated risks for coronary artery disease, basal cell carcinoma, hypertriglyceridemia, and Type 2 diabetes. A mutation in the *TERT* gene, which is involved in telomere replication, gave an increased risk for aplastic anemia. These data were followed by a series of medical tests. Dr. Snyder had no signs of aplastic anemia, and his telomere lengths were close to normal. Similarly, his mother, who shared his mutation in the *TERT* gene, had no symptoms of aplastic anemia. Medical tests revealed he did have elevated triglyceride levels, which he subsequently controlled using medication. Blood glucose levels were initially normal but became abnormally high after he became infected with respiratory syncytial virus (RSV). In response to these data, Dr. Snyder modified his diet and exercise regime and later brought his blood glucose down to normal levels. An analysis of drug response gene variants revealed that he should have good responses to diabetic drugs.

Using RNAseq technologies, the researchers monitored the numbers and types of more than 19,000 mRNAs and miRNAs transcribed from more than 12,000 genes over 20 time points. The data showed that sets of genes were coordinately regulated in response to conditions such as RSV infection and glucose levels. The researchers also found that RNA species underwent differential splicing and editing during changes in physiological states. Editing events included changes of adenosine to inosine and cytidine to uridine, and many of these RNA edits altered the amino acid sequences of translated proteins.

The researchers also profiled the levels of more than 6000 proteins and metabolites over the time course of the study. Like the RNA data, the protein and metabolite data showed coordinated changes that occur through virus infections and glucose level changes. Some of these changes were shared between RNA, protein, and metabolites and others were unique to each category. The medical significance of these patterns will be addressed in future studies.

[1] Chen, R. et al. 2012. Personal omics profiling reveals dynamic molecular and medical phenotypes. *Cell* 148: 1293–1307.

a low rate of error in genetic sequences or test results could lead to misdiagnoses and inappropriate treatments. Perhaps an even greater challenge lies in the ability of scientists to store and interpret the vast amount of emerging sequence data. Each personal genome generates the letter-equivalent of 200 large phone books, which must be stored in databases, mined for relevant sequence variants, and meaning assigned to each sequence variant. To undertake these kinds of analyses, scientists need to gather data from large-scale population genotyping studies that will link sequence variants to phenotype, disease, or drug responses. Experts suggest that such studies will take the coordinated efforts of public and private research teams and more than a decade to complete. Scientists will also need to develop efficient automated systems and algorithms to deal with this massive amount of information. Moreover, these data analyses will have to consider that genetic variants contribute only partially to personal phenotype. Personalized medicine will also need to integrate information about environmental, personal, lifestyle, and epigenetic factors.

Another technical challenge for personalized medicine is the development of automated health information technologies. Health-care providers will need to use electronic health records to store, retrieve, and analyze each patient's genomic profile, as well as to compare this information with constantly advancing knowledge about genes and disease. Currently, fewer than 10 percent of hospitals and physicians in the United States have access to these types of information technologies.

Personalized medicine has a number of societal implications. To make personalized medicine available to everyone, the costs of genetic tests, as well as the genetic counseling that accompanies them, must be reimbursed by insurance companies, even in cases where there are no prior diseases or symptoms. Regulatory changes are required to ensure that genetic tests and genomic sequencing are accurate and that the data generated are reliably stored in databases that guarantee the patient's privacy. At the present time, less than 1 percent of genetic tests are regulated by agencies such as the FDA.

Personalized medicine also requires changes to medical education. In the future, physicians will be expected to use genomics information as part of their patient management. For this to be possible, medical schools will need to train future physicians to interpret and explain genetic data. In addition, more genetic counselors and genomics specialists will be required. These specialists will need to understand genomics and disease, as well as to manipulate bioinformatic data. As of 2010, there were only about 2500 genetic counselors and 1100 clinical geneticists in North America.

The ethical aspects of the new personalized medicine are also diverse and challenging. For example, it is sometimes argued that the costs involved in the development of genomics and personalized medicine are a misallocation of limited resources. Some argue that science should solve larger problems facing humanity, such as the distribution of food and clean water, before embarking on personalized medicine. Similarly, some critics argue that such highly specialized and expensive medical care will not be available to everyone and represents a worsening of economic inequality. There are also concerns about how we will protect the privacy of genome information that is contained in databases and private health-care records. In addition, there need to be effective ways to prevent discrimination in employment or insurance coverage, based on information derived from genomic analysis.

Most experts agree that we are at the beginning of a personalized medicine revolution. Information from genetics and genomics research is already increasing the effectiveness of drugs and enabling health-care providers to predict diseases prior to their occurrence. In the future, personalized medicine will touch almost every aspect of medical care. By addressing the upcoming challenges of the new personalized medicine, we can guide its use for the maximum benefit to the greatest number of people.

Selected Readings and Resources

Journal Articles

Ashley, E.A., et al. 2010. Clinical assessment incorporating a personal genome. *Lancet* 375: 1525–1535.

Collins, F. 2010. Has the revolution arrived? *Nature* 464: 674–675.

McLeod, H.L. 2013. Cancer pharmacogenomics: Early promise, but concerted effort needed. *Science* 339: 1563–1566.

Ormond, K.E., et al. 2010. Challenges in the clinical application of whole-genome sequencing. *Lancet* 375: 1749–1751.

Pushkarev, D., et al. 2009. Single-molecule sequencing of an individual human genome. *Nature Biotech* 27: 847–850.

Ross, J.S. 2009. The HER-2 receptor and breast cancer: Ten years of targeted anti-HER-2 therapy and personalized medicine. *The Oncologist* 14: 320–368.

Soon, W.W., et al. 2013. High-throughput sequencing for biology and medicine. *Mol. Systems Biol.* 9: 640; doi:10.1038/msb.2012.61.

Venter, J.C. 2010. Multiple personal genomes await. *Nature* 464: 676–677.

Web Sites

Personalized Medicine Coalition, 2011. The Case for Personalized Medicine. http://www.personalizedmedicinecoalition.org/Resources/The_Case_for_Personalized_Medicine

U.S. Food and Drug Administration, 2010. Table of Valid Genomic Biomarkers in the Context of Approved Drug Labels. http://www.fda.gov/Drugs/ScienceResearch/ResearchAreas/Pharmacogenetics/ucm083378.htm

U.S. National Institutes of Health, Genetics Home Reference. What is pharmacogenomics? http://ghr.nlm.nih.gov/handbook/genomicresearch/pharmacogenomics

Review Questions

1. What is pharmacogenomics, and how does it differ from pharmacogenetics?
2. Describe how the drug Herceptin works. What types of gene tests are ordered prior to treatment with Herceptin?
3. What is the Oncotype DX Assay, and how is it used?
4. How do the cytochrome P450 proteins affect drug responses? Give two examples.
5. What types of genetic tests are currently available, and how are they classified?
6. Give two examples of how genomic studies have altered our understanding of cancers.
7. Why is it necessary to examine gene-expression profiles, in addition to genome sequencing, for effective personalized medicine?
8. Using the PharmGKB database, explain the relationship between *CYP2D6* variants and the response of patients to the breast cancer drug, tamoxifen.

Discussion Questions

1. In this chapter, we present three case studies that use personalized genomics analysis to predict and treat diseases. Although these cases have shown how personalized medicine may evolve in the future, they have triggered controversy. What are some objections to these types of studies, and how can these objections be addressed?

2. What are the biggest challenges that must be overcome before personalized medicine becomes a routine component of medical care? What do you think is the most difficult of these challenges and why?

3. How can we ensure that a patient's privacy is maintained as genome information accumulates within medical records?

How would you feel about allowing your genome sequence to be available for use in research?

4. As gene tests and genomic sequences become more commonplace, how can we prevent the emergence of "genetic discrimination" in employment and medical insurance?

Genetically Modified Foods

Throughout the ages, humans have used selective breeding techniques to create plants and animals with desirable genetic traits. By selecting organisms with naturally occurring or mutagen-induced variations and breeding them to establish the phenotype, we have evolved varieties that now feed our growing populations and support our complex civilizations.

Although we have had tremendous success shuffling genes through selective breeding, the process is a slow one. When recombinant DNA technologies emerged in the 1970s and 1980s, scientists realized that they could modify agriculturally significant organisms in a more precise and rapid way—by identifying and cloning genes that confer desirable traits, then introducing these genes into organisms. Genetic engineering of animals and plants promised an exciting new phase in scientific agriculture, with increased productivity, reduced pesticide use, and enhanced flavor and nutrition.

Beginning in the 1990s, scientists created a large number of genetically modified (GM) food varieties. The first one, approved for sale in 1994, was the Flavr Savr tomato—a tomato that stayed firm and ripe longer than non-GM tomatoes. Soon afterward, other GM foods were developed: papaya and zucchini with resistance to virus infection, canola containing the tropical oil laurate, corn and cotton plants with resistance to insects, and soybeans and sugar beets with tolerance to agricultural herbicides. By 2012, more than 200 different GM crop varieties had been created. Worldwide, GM crops are planted on 170 million hectares of arable land, with a global value of $15 billion for GM seeds.

Although many people see great potential for GM foods—to help address malnutrition in a world with a growing human population and climate change—others question the technology, oppose GM food development, and sometimes resort to violence to stop the introduction of GM varieties (**ST Figure 5.1**). Even Golden Rice—a variety of rice that contains the vitamin A precursor and was developed on a humanitarian nonprofit basis to help alleviate vitamin A deficiencies in the developing world—has been the target

> **"Genetic engineering of animals and plants promised an exciting new phase in scientific agriculture, with increased productivity, reduced pesticide use, and enhanced flavor and nutrition."**

of opposition and violence. On August 8, 2013, 400 protesters broke through security fences surrounding a field trial of Golden Rice in the Bicol region of the Philippines. Within 15 minutes, they had uprooted and trampled most of the GM rice plants. The attackers argued that Golden Rice was a threat to human health and biodiversity and would lead to Western corporate control of local food crops.

Opposition to GM foods is not unique to Golden Rice. In 2013, approximately two million people marched against GM foods in rallies held in 52 countries. Some countries have outright bans on all GM foods, whereas others embrace the technologies. Opponents cite safety and environmental concerns, while some scientists and commercial interests extol the almost limitless virtues of GM foods. The topic of GM food attracts hyperbole and exaggerated rhetoric, information, and misinformation—on both sides of the debate.

So, what are the truths about GM foods? In this Special Topic chapter, we will introduce the science behind GM foods and examine the promises and problems

ST FIGURE 5-1 Anti-GM protesters attacking a field of genetically-modified maize in southwestern France. In July 2004, hundreds of activists opposed to GM crops destroyed plants being tested by the US biotech company Pioneer Hi-Bred International.

of the new technologies. We will look at some of the controversies and present information to help us evaluate the complex questions that surround this topic.

What Are GM Foods?

GM foods are derived from **genetically modified organisms (GMOs)**, specifically plants and animals of agricultural importance. GMOs are defined as organisms whose genomes have been altered in ways that do not occur naturally. Although the definition of GMOs includes organisms that have been genetically modified by selective breeding, the most commonly used definition refers to organisms modified through genetic engineering or recombinant DNA technologies. Genetic engineering allows one or more genes to be cloned and transferred from one organism to another—either between individuals of the same species or between those of unrelated species. It also allows an organism's endogenous genes to be altered in ways that lead to enhanced or reduced expression levels. When genes are transferred between unrelated species, the resulting organism is called **transgenic**. The term **cisgenic** is sometimes used to describe gene transfers within a species. In contrast, the term **biotechnology** is a more general one, encompassing a wide range of methods that manipulate organisms or their components—such as isolating enzymes or producing wine, cheese, or yogurt. Genetic modification of plants or animals is one aspect of biotechnology.

In 2012, it was estimated that GM crops were grown in approximately 30 countries on 11 percent of the arable land on Earth. The majority of these GM crops (almost 90 percent) are grown in five countries—the United States, Brazil, Argentina, Canada, and India. Of these five, the United States accounts for approximately half of the acreage devoted to GM crops. According to the U.S. Department of Agriculture, 93 percent of soybeans and 88 percent of maize grown in the United States are from GM crops. In the United States, more than 70 percent of processed foods contain ingredients derived from GM crops.

Soon after the release of the Flavr Savr tomato in the 1990s, agribusinesses devoted less energy to designing GM foods to appeal directly to consumers. Instead, the market shifted toward farmers, to provide crops that increased productivity. By 2012, approximately 200 different GM crop varieties were approved for use as food or livestock feed in the United States. However, only about two dozen are widely planted. These include varieties of soybeans, corn, sugar beets, cotton, canola, papaya, and squash. ST Table 5.1 lists some of the common GM food crops available for planting in the United States. Of these GM crops, by far the most widely planted are varieties that are herbicide tolerant or insect resistant. At the time of writing this chapter, no

ST TABLE 5.1   Some GM Crops Approved for Food, Feed, or Cultivation in the United States*

Crop	Number of Varieties	GM Characteristics
Soybeans	19	Tolerance to glyphosate herbicide Tolerance to glufosinate herbicide Reduced saturated fats Enhanced oleic acid Enhanced omega-3 fatty acid
Maize	68	Tolerance to glyphosate herbicide Tolerance to glufosinate herbicide Bt insect resistance Enhanced ethanol production
Cotton	30	Tolerance to glyphosate herbicide Bt insect resistance
Potatoes	28	Bt insect resistance
Canola	23	Tolerance to glyphosate herbicide Tolerance to glufosinate herbicide Enhanced lauric acid
Papaya	4	Resistance to papaya ringspot virus
Sugar beets	3	Tolerance to glyphosate herbicide
Rice	3	Tolerance to glufosinate herbicide
Zucchini squash	2	Resistance to zucchini, watermelon, and cucumber mosaic viruses
Alfalfa	2	Tolerance to glyphosate herbicide
Plum	1	Resistance to plum pox virus

* Information from the International Service for the Acquisition of Agri-Biotech Applications, www.isaaa.org.

GM food animal was approved for consumption, although a GM salmon variety was nearing market approval in the United States (Box 1). A number of agriculturally important animals such as goats and sheep have been genetically modified to produce pharmaceutical products in their milk. The use of transgenic animals as bioreactors is discussed earlier in the text (see Chapter 22).

Herbicide-Resistant GM Crops

Weed infestations destroy about 10 percent of crops worldwide. To combat weeds, farmers often apply herbicides before seeding a crop and between rows after the crops are growing. As the most efficient broad-spectrum herbicides also kill crop plants, herbicide use may be difficult and limited. Farmers also use tillage to control weeds; however, tillage damages soil structure and increases erosion.

Herbicide-tolerant varieties are the most widely planted of GM crops, making up approximately 70 percent of all GM crops. The majority of these varieties contain a bacterial gene that confers tolerance to the broad-spectrum herbicide **glyphosate**—the active ingredient in commercial herbicides such as Roundup®. Studies have shown that

BOX 1
The Tale of GM Salmon—Downstream Effects?

It took 18 years and about $60 million, but the first GM animal to be approved as human food—the AquAdvantage salmon—may soon hit the U.S. market.

The AquAdvantage salmon is an Atlantic salmon that is genetically modified to grow twice as fast as its non-GM cousins, reaching marketable size in one and a half years rather than the usual three years. Scientists at AquaBounty Technologies in Massachusetts created the variety by transforming an Atlantic salmon with a single gene encoding the Chinook salmon growth hormone. The gene was cloned downstream of the antifreeze protein gene promoter from an eel. This promoter stimulates growth hormone synthesis in the winter, a time when the fish's own growth hormone gene is not expressed. The rapid growth of the GM salmon allows fish farmers to double their productivity.

AquaBounty intends to sell GM fish eggs to two facilities—one in the United States and one in Panama—that will raise the salmon and market them. To ensure that the fish will not escape the facilities, the company promises to sell only fertilized eggs that are female, triploid, and sterile. The facilities are to be approved only if the tanks are located inland and have sufficient filters to ensure that eggs and small fish cannot escape.

Despite these assurances, environmental groups are planning to fight the sale of GM salmon. Some grocery chains in the United States have banned GM fish, and legislators in several western U.S. states are trying to block the approval of the AquAdvantage salmon based on fears that the accidental release of these fish could contaminate wild salmon populations with transgenes and disturb normal ecosystems.

Supporters of GM fish point out that the GM salmon are very unlikely to escape their facilities, and if any did escape, they would be poorly adapted to wild conditions. Critics of the new GM salmon point out that the technique used to create sterile triploids (pressure-shocking the fertilized eggs) still allows a small percentage of fertile diploids to remain in the stock. They state that even a few fertile fish, if they escaped into the wild, could have long-term effects on

wild populations. A study published in 2013 shows that it is possible for the AquAdvantage salmon to breed successfully with a close relative, the brown trout.[*] In laboratory conditions, the hybrids grew more quickly than either the GM or non-GM varieties, and in closed stream-like systems, the hybrids outcompeted both parental fish varieties for food supplies. The authors point out that these results should be taken into account during environmental assessments, although it is still not known whether the hybrid salmon–trout variety could successfully breed in the wild. If GM salmon could escape, breed, and introduce transgenes into wild populations, there could be unknown negative downstream effects on fish ecosystems.

[*]Oke, K.B., et al. 2013. Hybridization between genetically modified Atlantic salmon and wild brown trout reveals novel ecological interactions. *Proc. R. Soc. B.* **280** (1763): 20131047.

The AquAdvantage salmon grows twice as fast as a non-GM Atlantic salmon, reaching market size in half the time.

glyphosate is effective at low concentrations, is degraded rapidly in soil and water, and is not toxic to humans.

Farmers who plant glyphosate-tolerant crops can treat their fields with glyphosate, even while the GM crop is growing. This approach is more efficient and economical than mechanical weeding and reduces soil damage caused by repeated tillage. It is suggested that there is less environmental impact when using glyphosate, compared with having to apply higher levels of other, more toxic, herbicides.

Recently, evidence suggests that some weeds may be developing resistance to glyphosate, thereby reducing the

effectiveness of glyphosate-tolerant crops. (This and other concerns about herbicide-tolerant GM plants are described later in this chapter.) One method used to engineer a glyphosate-tolerant plant is described in the next section.

Insect-Resistant GM Crops

The second most prevalent GM modifications are those that make plants resistant to agricultural pests. Insect damage is one of the most serious threats to worldwide food production. Farmers combat insect pests using crop rotation and predatory organisms, as well as applying insecticides.

The most widely used GM insect-resistant crops are the **Bt crops**. *Bacillus thuringiensis* (Bt) is group of soil-dwelling bacterial strains that produce crystal (Cry) proteins that are toxic to certain species of insects. These Cry proteins are encoded by the bacterial *cry* genes and form crystal structures during sporulation. The Cry proteins are toxic to Lepidoptera (moths and butterflies), Diptera (mosquitoes and flies), Coleoptera (beetles), and Hymenoptera (wasps and ants). Insects must ingest the bacterial spores or Cry proteins in order for the toxins to act. Within the high pH of the insect gut, the crystals dissolve and are cleaved by insect protease enzymes. The Cry proteins bind to receptors on the gut wall, leading to breakdown of the gut membranes and death of the insect.

Each insect species has specific types of gut receptors that will match only a few types of Bt Cry toxins. As there are more than 200 different Cry proteins, it is possible to select a Bt strain that will be specific to one pest type.

Bt spores have been used for decades as insecticides in both conventional and organic gardening, usually applied in liquid sprays. Sunlight and soil rapidly break down the Bt insecticides, which have not shown any adverse effects on groundwater, mammals, fish, or birds. Toxicity tests on humans and animals have shown that Bt causes few negative effects.

To create Bt crops, scientists introduce one or more cloned *cry* genes into plant cells using methods described in the next section. The GM crop plants will then manufacture their own Bt Cry proteins, which will kill the target pest species when it eats the plant tissues.

Although Bt crops have been successful in reducing crop damage, increasing yields, and reducing the amounts of insecticidal sprays used in agriculture, they are also controversial. Early studies suggested that Bt crops harmed Monarch butterfly populations, although more recent studies have drawn opposite conclusions (Box 2). Other concerns still exist and these will be discussed in subsequent sections of this chapter.

GM Crops for Direct Consumption

To date, most GM crops have been designed to help farmers increase yields. Also, most GM food crops are not consumed directly by humans, but are used as animal feed or as sources of processed food ingredients such as oils, starches, syrups, and sugars. For example, 98 percent of the U.S. soybean crop is used as livestock feed. The remainder is processed into a variety of food ingredients, such as lecithin, textured soy proteins, soybean oil, and soy flours. However, a few GM foods have been developed for direct consumption. Examples are rice, squash, and papaya (Box 3).

One of the most famous and controversial examples of GM foods is **Golden Rice**—a rice variety designed to synthesize beta-carotene (the precursor to **vitamin A**) in the rice grain endosperm.

Vitamin A deficiency is a serious health problem in more than 60 countries, particularly countries in Asia and Africa. The World Health Organization estimates that 190 million of the world's children and 19 million pregnant women are vitamin A deficient. Between 250,000 and 500,000 children with vitamin A deficiencies become blind each year, and half of these will die within a year of losing their sight. As vitamin A is also necessary for immune system function, deficiencies lead to increases in many other conditions, including diarrhea and virus infections. The most seriously affected people live in the poorest countries and have a basic starch-centered diet, often mainly rice. Vitamin A is normally found in dairy products and can be synthesized in the body from beta-carotene found in orange-colored fruits and vegetables and in green leafy vegetables.

Several approaches are being taken to alleviate the vitamin A deficiency status of people in developing countries. These include supplying high-dose vitamin A supplements and growing fresh fruits and vegetables in home gardens. These initiatives have had partial success, but the expense of delivering education and supplementation has impeded the effectiveness of these programs.

In the 1990s, scientists began to apply recombinant DNA technology to help solve vitamin A deficiencies in people with rice-based diets. Although the rice plant naturally produces beta-carotene in its leaves, it does not produce it in the rice grain endosperm, which is the edible part of the rice. The beta-carotene precursor, geranylgeranyldiphosphate, is present in the endosperm, but the enzymes that convert it to beta-carotene are not synthesized (**ST Figure 5–2**).

In the first version of Golden Rice, scientists introduced the genes *phytoene synthase* (*psy*) cloned from the daffodil plant and *carotene desaturase* (*crtI*) cloned from the bacterium *Erwinia uredovora* into rice plants. The bacterial *crtI* gene was chosen because the enzyme encoded by this gene can perform the functions of two of the missing rice enzymes, thereby simplifying the transformation process. The resulting plant produced rice grains that were a yellow color due to the presence of beta-carotene (**ST Figure 5–3**). This strain synthesized modest levels of beta-carotene—but only enough to potentially supply 15–20 percent of the recommended daily allowance of vitamin A. In the second version of the GM plant, called Golden Rice 2, the daffodil *psy* gene was replaced with the *psy* gene from maize. Golden Rice 2 produced beta-carotene levels that were more than 20-fold greater than those in Golden Rice. In the next section we describe the methods used to create Golden Rice 2.

BOX 2
The Monarch Butterfly Story

In 1999, three years after the introduction of Bt corn in the United States, scientists published a report that ignited the anti-GM movement and triggered years of intensive research. The scientists had conducted a laboratory assay in which they fed milkweed leaves, coated with pollen from either non-GM or Bt corn, to Monarch butterfly larvae. They concluded that Bt corn pollen reduced larval survival by approximately 50 percent. Concerned about the possibility of unintended harm to nontarget organisms, the U.S. Department of Agriculture commissioned scientists from the United States and Canada to provide detailed follow-up research. In 2001, these studies culminated in a series of five published papers that examined Monarch butterfly biology and ecology and how these may be affected by different types of Bt corn and Bt proteins—in both laboratory and field conditions.

Data from these studies explained and contradicted the initial study. First, the authors of the original 1999 study had fed larvae on pollen contaminated with ground-up corn anthers, which contain 100-fold higher levels of the Cry1Ab protein than found in pollen. In the field, larvae do not eat anthers or other parts of corn plants, as larvae feed exclusively on milkweed leaves. Second, in laboratory tests, larvae were found to be sensitive to Cry1Ab and Cry1Ac proteins, but not to other Cry proteins. Third, the levels of Cry1Ab and Cry1Ac proteins present in Bt cornfields had little, if any, effects on Monarch butterfly larvae. The studies also examined the survival of larvae on Bt cornfields compared with non-Bt cornfields that are sprayed with a pyrethroid insecticide used to control cornfield pests. Larval survival on milkweed within pesticide-treated fields was between 0 and 10 percent,

whereas survival within Bt cornfields was 80 to 93 percent.

Although these studies established a low risk for Monarch butterflies, a new twist in the tale may be emerging. Since 1993, the numbers of Monarch butterflies wintering in Mexico has dropped dramatically. Numbers have dropped significantly each year since 2007—including a 30 percent drop in 2011–2012 and a 59 percent drop in 2012–2013. The reasons for these declines appear to be complex. In Mexico, butterfly reserves have suffered from logging, water diversion, and drought. In the United States and Canada, where Monarch butterflies lay their eggs each year, milkweed habitat has suffered from drought,

human development, and changes in agricultural practices. Tillage, mowing, and herbicide use have destroyed millions of acres of milkweed habitat. Along with the use of conventional herbicides that kill weeds, the growing of glyphosate-tolerant corn and soybean crops has resulted in efficient suppression of weeds in fields that used to contain small numbers of milkweed plants. By affecting milkweeds, herbicide-tolerant GM crops may be contributing to the serious decline in Monarch butterfly populations. Scientists are proposing a program to plant milkweed plants along north–south highways from Texas to Canada, to provide food for Monarch butterfly larvae.

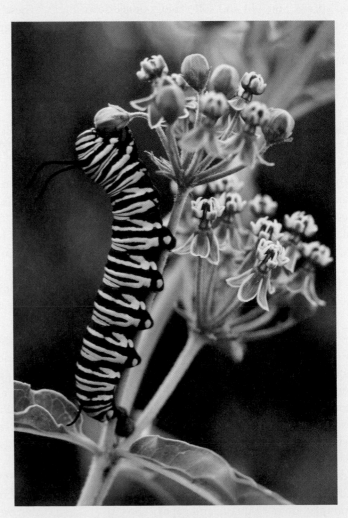

Monarch butterfly larvae feed exclusively on milkweed.

BOX 3
The Success of Hawaiian GM Papaya

n the mid-1990s, the papaya ringspot virus (PRSV) spread rapidly throughout Hawaii's papaya fields and threatened to destroy the industry within a few years. To try to stop the destruction of Hawaiian papaya, a team of scientists from the University of Hawaii, the USDA Agricultural Research Center in Hawaii, and the Upjohn Company cloned the coat protein gene of PRSV and introduced it into cultured papaya cells using biolistic transformation. The goal was to create PRSV resistance using a mechanism known as pathogen-derived resistance. The presence of virus coat proteins within the plant is thought to interfere with the disassembly and movement of an infecting virus, slowing or preventing infection. Researchers tested resistance to PRSV in the transformed papaya plants and developed two GM varieties—SunUp and Rainbow. SunUp was homozygous for the PRSV coat protein gene, and Rainbow was an F_1 hybrid of SunUp and a non-GM variety Kapoho. After three years of field testing and two years of moving through federal regulatory processes, GM papaya was approved for use. Seeds were given for free to farmers who immediately planted them to replace their virus-devastated fields.

Within three years, papaya harvests in Hawaii doubled and consumer acceptance was positive. Virus-resistant GM papaya is credited with saving the Hawaiian papaya industry.

An interesting side-effect of the presence of GM papaya in Hawaii was the recovery of non-GM and organically grown papaya. Because PRSV levels declined due to the presence of virus-resistant fields and the abandoning of infected fields, some growers can now produce non-GM papaya, albeit on a smaller scale than before the virus spread throughout Hawaii. At the present time, more than 70 percent of Hawaiian papaya

down and destroyed by anonymous attackers. Efforts to introduce GM papaya in Thailand have failed, and the government recently banned GM foods. Japan has approved the sale of GM papaya, but only if it is labeled as genetically modified.

(a)   (b)

A test field of GM papaya. The "Rainbow" variety, growing in the center of the field, is unaffected by PRSV. The "Sunrise" non-GM variety surrounds the GM papaya and is severely infected.

Clinical trials have shown that the beta-carotene in Golden Rice 2 is efficiently converted into vitamin A in humans and that about 150 grams of uncooked Golden Rice 2 (which is close to the normal daily rice consumption of children aged 4–8 years) would supply all of the childhood daily requirement for vitamin A.

At the present time, Golden Rice 2 is undergoing field, biosafety, and efficacy testing in preparation for approval by government regulators in Bangladesh and the Philippines. If Golden Rice 2 proves useful in alleviating vitamin A deficiencies and is approved for use, seed will be made available at the same price as non-GM seed and farmers will be allowed to keep and replant seed from their own crops.

Despite the promise of Golden Rice 2, controversies remain. Critics of GM foods suggest that Golden Rice could make farmers too dependent on one type of food or might have long-term health or environmental effects. These and other controversies surrounding GM foods are discussed in subsequent sections of this chapter.

Methods Used to Create GM Plants

Most GM plants are created using one of two approaches: the **biolistic method** or *Agrobacterium tumefaciens-mediated transformation* technology. Both methods

ST FIGURE 5–2 Beta-carotene pathway in Golden Rice 2. Rice plant enzymes and genes involved in beta-carotene synthesis are shown on the right. The enzymes that are not expressed in rice endosperm are indicated with an "X." The genes inserted into Golden Rice 2 are shown on the left.

ST FIGURE 5–3 Non-GM and Golden Rice 2. Golden Rice 2 contains high levels of beta-carotene, giving the rice endosperm a yellow color. The intensity of the color reflects the amount of beta-carotene in the endosperm.

target plant cells that are growing *in vitro*. Scientists can generate plant tissue cultures from various types of plant tissues, and these cultured cells will grow in either liquid cultures or on the surface of solid growth media. When grown in the presence of specific nutrients and hormones, these cultured cells will form clumps of cells called calluses, which, when transferred to other types of media, will form roots. When the rooted plantlets are mature, they are transferred to soil medium in greenhouses where they develop into normal plants.

The *biolistic method* is a physical method of introducing DNA into cells. Particles of heavy metals such as gold are coated with the DNA that will transform the cells; these particles are then fired at high speed into plant cells *in vitro*, using a device called a **gene gun**. Cells that survive the bombardment may take up the DNA-coated particles, and the DNA may migrate into the cell nucleus and integrate into a plant chromosome. Plants that grow from the bombarded cells are then selected for the desired phenotype.

Although biolistic methods are successful for a wide range of plant types, a much improved transformation rate is achieved using *Agrobacterium-mediated technology*. *Agrobacterium tumefaciens* (also called *Rhizobium radiobacter*) is a soil microbe that can infect plant cells and cause tumors.

These characteristics are conferred by a 200-kb tumor-inducing plasmid called a **Ti plasmid**. After infection with *Agrobacterium*, the Ti plasmid integrates a segment of its DNA known as transfer DNA (T-DNA) into random locations within the plant genome. (**ST Figure 5–4**). To use the Ti plasmid as a transformation vector, scientists remove the T-DNA segment and replace it with cloned DNA of the genes to be introduced into the plant cells.

In order to have the newly introduced gene expressed in the plant, the gene must be cloned next to an appropriate promoter sequence that will direct transcription in the required plant tissue. For example, the beta-carotene pathway genes introduced into Golden Rice were cloned next to a promoter that directs transcription of the genes in the rice endosperm. In addition, the transformed gene requires appropriate transcription termination signals and signal sequences that allow insertion of the encoded protein into the correct cell compartment.

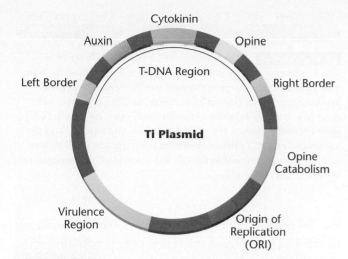

ST FIGURE 5–4 Structure of the Ti plasmid. The 250-kb Ti plasmid from *Agrobacterium tumefaciens* inserts the T-DNA portion of the plasmid into the host cell's nuclear genome and induces tumors. Genes within the virulence region code for enzymes responsible for transfer of T-DNA into the plant genome. The T-DNA region contains auxin and cytokinin genes that encode hormones responsible for cell growth and tumor formation. The opine genes encode compounds used as energy sources for the bacterium. The T-DNA region of the Ti plasmid is replaced with the gene of interest when the plasmid is used as a transformation vector.

Selectable Markers

The rates at which T-DNA successfully integrates into the plant genome and becomes appropriately expressed are low. Often, only one cell in 1000 or more will be successfully transformed. Before growing cultured plant cells into mature plants to test their phenotypes, it is important to eliminate the background of nontransformed cells. This can be done using either positive or negative selection techniques.

An example of negative selection involves use of a **marker gene** such as the hygromycin-resistance gene. This gene, together with an appropriate promoter, can be introduced into plant cells along with the gene of interest. The cells are then incubated in culture medium containing hygromycin—an antibiotic that also inhibits the growth of eukaryotic cells. Only cells that express the hygromycin-resistance gene will survive. It is then necessary to verify that the resistant cells also express the cotransformed gene. This is often done by techniques such as PCR amplification using gene-specific primers. Plants that express the gene of interest are then tested for other characteristics, including the phenotype conferred by the introduced gene of interest.

An example of positive selection involves the use of a selectable marker gene such as that encoding **phosphomannose isomerase (PMI)**. This enzyme is common in animals but is not found in most plants. It catalyzes the interconversion of mannose 6-phosphate and fructose 6-phosphate. Plant cells that express the *pmi* gene can

survive on synthetic culture medium that contains only mannose as a carbon source. Cells that are cotransformed with the *pmi* gene under control of an appropriate promoter and the gene of interest can be positively selected by growing the plant cells on a mannose-containing medium. This type of positive selection was used to create Golden Rice 2. Studies have shown that purified PMI protein is easily digested, nonallergenic, and nontoxic in mouse oral toxicity tests. A variation in positive selection involves use of a marker gene whose expression results in a visible phenotype, such as deposition of a colored pigment.

The following descriptions illustrate the methods used to engineer two GM crops: Roundup-Ready soybeans and Golden Rice 2.

Roundup-Ready® Soybeans

The Roundup-Ready soybean GM variety received market approval in the United States in 1996. It is a GM plant with resistance to the herbicide glyphosate, the active ingredient in Roundup, a commercially available broad-spectrum herbicide. Glyphosate interferes with the enzyme 5-enolpyruvylshikimate-3-phosphate synthase (EPSPS), which is present in all plants and is necessary for plant synthesis of the aromatic amino acids phenylalanine, tyrosine, and tryptophan. EPSPS is not present in mammals, which obtain aromatic amino acids from their diets.

To produce a glyphosate-resistant soybean plant, researchers cloned an *epsps* gene from the *Agrobacterium* strain CP4. This gene encodes an EPSPS enzyme that is resistant to glyphosate. They then cloned the *CP4 epsps* gene downstream of a constitutively expressed promoter from the cytomegalovirus to allow gene expression in all plant tissues. In addition, a short peptide known as a chloroplast transit peptide (in this case from petunias) was cloned onto the 5′ end of the *epsps* gene-coding sequence. This allowed newly synthesized EPSPS protein to be inserted into the soybean chloroplast (**ST Figure 5–5**). The final plasmid contained two *CP4 epsps* genes and, for the initial experiments, a *beta-glucuronidase (GUS)* gene from *E. coli*. The

pV-GMGT04   **pV-GMGT04**

E35S   ctp4   CP4 epsps   nos

ST FIGURE 5–5 Portion of plasmid pV-GMGT04 used to create Roundup-Ready soybeans. A 1365-bp fragment encoding the EPSPS enzyme from *Agrobacterium CP4* was cloned downstream from the cauliflower mosaic virus *E35S* promoter and the petunia chloroplast transit peptide signal sequence (*ctp4*). CTP4 signal sequences direct the EPSPS protein into chloroplasts, where aromatic amino acids are synthesized. The *CP4 epsps* coding region was cloned upstream of the nopaline synthase (*nos*) transcription termination and polyadenylation sequences. The *CP4 epsps* sequences encode a 455-amino-acid 46-kDa ESPSP protein.

GUS gene acted as a positive marker, as cells that expressed the plasmid after transformation could be detected by the presence of a blue precipitate. The final cell line chosen for production of Roundup-Ready soybeans did not contain the *GUS* gene.

The plasmids were introduced into cultured soybean cells using biolistic bombardment. Afterward, cells were treated with glyphosate to eliminate any nontransformed cells. (**ST Figure 5–6**). The resulting calluses were grown into plants, which were then field tested for glyphosate resistance and a large number of other parameters, including composition, toxicity, and allergenicity.

Golden Rice 2

To create Golden Rice 2, scientists cloned three genes into the T-DNA region of a Ti plasmid. The Ti plasmid, called pSYN12424, is shown in **ST Figure 5–7**. The first gene was the *carotene desaturase* (*crtI*) gene from *Erwinia uredovora*, fused between the rice *glutelin* gene promoter (*Glu*) and

ST FIGURE 5–6 Method for creating Roundup-Ready soybeans. Plasmids were loaded into the gene gun and fired at high pressure into cells growing in tissue cultures. Cells were grown in the presence of glyphosate to select those that had integrated and expressed the *epsps* gene. Surviving cells were stimulated to form calluses and to grow into plantlets.

Labels in figure: Load pV-GMGT04 plasmids into gene gun; Bombard cells with plasmids; Select transformed cells with glyphosate; Grow surviving cells into plantlets

Labels: Glu **crtI** nos Glu **psy** nos Ubi1 **pmi** nos

ST FIGURE 5–7 T-DNA region of T1 plasmid pSYN12424. The Ti plasmid used to create Golden Rice 2 contained the carotene desaturase (*crtI*) gene cloned from bacteria, the phytoene synthase (*psy*) gene cloned from maize, and the phosphomannose isomerase (*pmi*) gene cloned from *E. coli*. The *glutelin* (*Glu*) gene promoter directs transcription in rice endosperm, and the *polyubiquitin* (*Ubi1*) promoter directs transcription in all tissues. Transcription termination signals were provided by the nopaline synthase (*nos*) gene 3′ region.

the *nos* gene terminator region (*nos*). The *Glu* promoter directs transcription of the fusion gene specifically in the rice endosperm. The *nos* terminator was cloned from the *Agrobacterium tumefaciens nopaline synthase* gene and supplies the transcription termination and polyadenylation sequences required at the 3′ end of plant genes. The second gene was the *phytoene synthase* (*psy*) gene cloned from maize. The maize *psy* gene has approximately 90 percent sequence similarity to the rice *psy* gene and is involved in carotenoid synthesis in maize endosperm. This gene was also fused to the *Glu* promoter and the *nos* terminator sequences in order to obtain proper transcription initiation and termination in rice endosperm. The third gene was the selectable marker gene, *phosphomannose isomerase* (*pmi*), cloned from *E. coli*. In the Golden Rice 2 Ti plasmid, the *pmi* gene was fused to the maize *polyubiquitin* gene promoter (*Ubi1*) and the *nos* terminator sequences. The *Ubi1* promoter is a constitutive promoter, directing transcription of the *pmi* gene in all plant tissues.

To introduce the pSYN12424 plasmid into rice cells, researchers established embryonic rice cell cultures and infected them with *Agrobacterium tumefaciens* that contained pSYN12424 (**ST Figure 5–8**). The cells were then placed under selection, using culture medium containing only mannose as a carbon source. Surviving cells expressing the *pmi* gene were then stimulated to form calluses that were grown into plants. To confirm that all three genes were present in the transformed rice plants, samples were taken and analyzed by the polymerase chain reaction (PCR) using gene-specific primers. Plants that contained one integrated copy of the transgenic construct and synthesized beta-carotene in their seeds were selected for further testing.

GM Foods Controversies

GM foods may be the most contentious of all products of modern biotechnology. Advocates of GM foods state that the technologies have increased farm productivity, reduced pesticide use, preserved soils, and have the potential to feed

Ti plasmid pSYN12424

Introduce Ti plasmid into *A. tumifaciens*

Agrobacterium tumifaciens

Infect cultured cells

Select by growing on mannose medium

Grow into calluses and plants

Select plants for high endosperm color (beta-carotene)

−−   +   ++

ST FIGURE 5–8 Method for creating Golden Rice 2. Rice plant cells were transformed by pSYN12424 and selected on mannose-containing medium, as described in the text. Plants that produced high levels of beta-carotene in rice grain endosperm (++), based on the intensity of the grain's yellow color, were selected for further analysis.

growing human populations. Critics claim that GM foods are unsafe for both humans and the environment; accordingly, they are applying pressure on regulatory agencies to ban or severely limit the extent of GM food use. These campaigns have affected regulators and politicians, resulting in a patchwork of regulations throughout the world. Often the debates surrounding GM foods are highly polarized and emotional, with both sides in the debate exaggerating their points of view and selectively presenting the data. So, what are the truths behind these controversies?

One point that is important to make as we try to answer this question is that *it is not possible to make general statements about all "GM foods."* Each GM crop or organism contains different genes from different sources, attached to different expression sequences, accompanied by different marker or selection genes, inserted into the genome in different ways and in different locations. GM foods are created for different purposes and are used in ways that are both planned and unplanned. Each construction is unique and therefore needs to be assessed separately.

We will now examine two of the main GM foods controversies: those involving human health and safety, and environmental effects.

Health and Safety

GM food advocates often state that there is no evidence that GM foods currently on the market have any adverse health effects, either from the presence of toxins or from potential allergens. These conclusions are based on two observations. First, humans have consumed several types of GM foods for more than 20 years now, and no reliable reports of adverse effects have emerged. Second, the vast majority of toxicity tests in animals, which are required by government regulators prior to approval, have shown no negative effects. A few negative studies have been published, but these have been criticized as poorly executed or nonreproducible.

Critics of GM foods counter the first observation in several ways. First, as described previously, few GM foods are eaten directly by consumers. Instead, most are used as livestock feed, and the remainder form the basis of purified food ingredients. Although no adverse effects of GM foods in livestock have been detected, the processing of many food ingredients removes most, if not all, plant proteins and DNA. Hence, ingestion of GM food-derived ingredients may not be a sufficient test for health and safety. Second, GM foods critics argue that there have been few human clinical trials to directly examine the health effects of most GM foods. One notable exception is Golden Rice 2, which has undergone two small clinical trials. They also say that the toxicity studies that have been completed are performed in animals—primarily rats and mice—and most of these are short-term toxicity studies.

Supporters of GM foods answer these criticisms with several other arguments. The first argument is that short-term toxicity studies in animals are well-established methods for detecting toxins and allergens. The regulatory processes required prior to approval of any GM food demand data from animal toxicity studies. If any negative effects are detected, approval is not given. Supporters also note that several dozen long-term toxicity studies have been published that deal with GM crops such as glyphosate-resistant soybeans and Bt corn, and none of these has shown long-term negative effects on test animals. A few studies that report negative long-term effects have been criticized as poorly designed and unreliable. GM food advocates note that human clinical trials are not required for any other food derived from other genetic modification methods such as selective breeding. During standard breeding of plants and animals, genomes may be mutagenized with radiation or chemicals to enhance the possibilities of obtaining

SPECIAL TOPIC 5

a desired phenotype. This type of manipulation has the potential to introduce mutations into genes other than the ones that are directly selected. Also, plants and animals naturally exchange and shuffle DNA in ways that cannot be anticipated. These include interspecies DNA transfers, transposon integrations, and chromosome modifications. These events may result in unintended changes to the physiology of organisms—changes that could potentially be as great as those arising in GM foods.

Environmental Effects

Critics of GM foods point out that GMOs that are released into the environment have both documented and potential consequences for the environment—and hence may indirectly affect human health and safety. GM food advocates argue that these potential environmental consequences can be identified and managed. Here, we will describe two different aspects of GM foods as they may affect the natural environment and agriculture.

1. Emerging herbicide and insecticide resistance. Many published studies report that the planting of herbicide-tolerant and insect-resistant GM crops has reduced the quantities of herbicides and insecticides that are broadly applied to agricultural crops. As a result, the effects of GM crops on the environment have been assumed to be positive. However, these positive effects may be transient, as herbicide and insecticide resistance is beginning to emerge. (**ST Figure 5–9**).

   Since glyphosate-tolerant crops were introduced in the mid-1990s, more than 24 glyphosate-resistant weed species have appeared in the United States. Resistant weeds have been found in 18 other countries, and in some

ST FIGURE 5–9 Herbicide-resistant weeds. Water hemp weeds, resistant to glyphosate herbicide, growing in a field of Roundup-Ready soybeans.

cases, the presence of these weeds is affecting crop yields. One reason for the rapid rise of resistant weeds is that farmers have abandoned other weed-management practices in favor of using a single broad-spectrum herbicide. This strong selection pressure has brought the rapid evolution of weed species bearing gene variants that confer herbicide resistance. In response, biotechnology companies are developing new GM crops with tolerance to multiple herbicides. However, scientists argue that weeds will also develop resistance to the use of multiple herbicides, unless farmers vary their weed management practices and incorporate tillage, rotation, and other herbicides along with using the GM crop. Scientists point out that herbicide resistance is not limited to the use of GM crops. Weed populations will evolve resistance to any herbicide used to control them, and the speed of evolution will be affected by the extent to which the herbicide is used.

Since 1996, more than eight different species of insect pests have evolved some level of resistance to Bt insecticidal proteins. For example, in 2011 scientists reported the first cases of resistance of the western corn rootworm to Bt maize expressing the *cry3Bb1* gene, in maize fields in Iowa. In 2010, scientists from Monsanto detected large numbers of pink bollworms with resistance to the toxin expressed from the *cry-1Ac* gene in one variety of Bt cotton. In order to slow down the development of Bt resistance, several strategies are being followed. The first is to develop varieties of GM crops that express two Bt toxins simultaneously. Several of these varieties are already on the market and are replacing varieties that express only one Bt *cry* gene. The second strategy involves the use of "refuges" surrounding fields that grow Bt crops. These refuges contain non-GM crops. Insect pests grow easily within the refuges, which place no evolutionary pressure on the insects for resistance to Bt toxins. The idea is for these nonselected insects to mate with any resistant insects that appear in the Bt crop region of the field. The resulting hybrid offspring will be heterozygous for any resistance gene variant. As long as the resistance gene variant is recessive, the hybrids will be killed by eating the Bt crop. In fields that use refuges and plant GM crops containing two Bt genes, resistance to Bt toxins has been delayed or is absent. As with emerging herbicide resistance, farmers are also encouraged to combine the use of Bt crops with conventional pest control methods.

2. The spread of GM crops into non-GM crops. There have been several documented cases of GM crop plants appearing in uncultivated areas in the United States, Canada, Australia, Japan, and Europe. For example, GM sugar beet plants have been found growing in commercial top

soils. GM canola plants have been found growing in ditches and along roadways, railway tracks, and in fill soils, far from the fields in which they were grown. A 2011 study[1] found "feral" GM canola plants growing in 288 of 634 sample sites along roadways in North Dakota. Of these plants, 41 percent contained the CP4 EPSPS protein (conferring glyphosate resistance), and 39 percent contained the PAT protein (conferring resistance to the herbicide glufosinate). In addition, two of the plants (0.7 percent of the sample) expressed both proteins (resistant to both herbicides). GM plants that express both proteins have not been created by genetic modification and were assumed to have arisen by cross-fertilization of the other two GM crops. The researchers who conducted this survey were not surprised to find GM canola along transportation routes, as seeds are often spilled during shipping. More surprising was the extent of the distribution and the presence of hybridized GM canola plants.

One of the major concerns about the escape of GM crop plants from cultivation is the possibility of **outcrossing** or **gene flow**—the transfer of transgenes from GM crops into sexually compatible non-GM crops or wild plants, conferring undesired phenotypes to the other plants. Gene flow between GM crops and adjacent non-GM crops is of particular concern for farmers who want to market their crops as "GM-free" or "organic" and for farmers who grow seed for planting.

Gene flow of GM transgenes has been documented in GM and non-GM canola as well as sugar beets, and in experiments using rice, wheat, and maize. GM critics often refer to controversial studies about GM outcrossing in Oaxaca, Mexico. In the first study in 2001, it was reported that the local maize crops contained transgenes from Monsanto's Roundup-Ready and Bt insect-resistant maize. As GM crops were not approved for use in Mexico, it was thought that the transgenes came from maize that had been imported from the United States as a foodstuff, and then had been planted by farmers who were not aware that the seeds were transgenic. Over the next ten years, subsequent studies reported mixed results. In some studies, the transgenes were not detected, and in others, the same transgenes were detected. There is still no consensus about whether gene flow has occurred between the GM and non-GM maize in Mexico.

It is thought that the presence of glyphosate-resistant transgenes in wild plant populations is not likely to be an environmental risk and would confer no positive fitness benefits to the hybrids. The presence of glyphosate-resistant genes in wild populations would, however, make it more difficult to eradicate the plants. This is illustrated in a case of escaped GM bentgrass in Oregon, where it has been difficult to get rid of the plants because it is no longer possible to use the relatively safe herbicide glyphosate. The potential for environmental damage may be greater if the GM transgenes did confer an advantage—such as insect resistance or tolerance to drought or flooding.

In an attempt to limit the spread of transgenes from GM crops to non-GM crops, regulators are considering a requirement to separate the crops so that pollen would be less likely to travel between them. Each crop plant would require different isolation distances to take into account the dynamics of pollen spreading. Several other methods are being considered. For example, one proposal is to make all GM plants sterile using RNAi technology. Another is to introduce the transgenes into chloroplasts. As chloroplasts are inherited maternally, their genomes would not be transferred via pollen. All of these containment methods are in development stages and may take years to reach the market.

The Future of GM Foods

Over the last 20 years, GM foods have revealed both promise and problems. GM advocates are confident that the next generation of GM foods will show even more promising prospects—and may also address many of the problems.

Research is continuing on ways to fortify staple crops with nutrients to address diet problems in poor countries. For example, Australian scientists are adding genes to bananas that will not only provide resistance to Panama disease—a serious fungal disease that can destroy crops—but also increase the levels of beta-carotene and other nutrients, including iron. Other GM crops in the pipeline include plants engineered to resist drought, high salinity, nitrogen starvation, and low temperatures.

Scientists hope that new genome information and more precise technologies will allow them to accurately edit a plant's endogenous genes—decreasing, increasing, or eliminating expression of one or more of the plant's genes in order to create a desirable phenotype. These approaches avoid the use of transgenes and address some of the concerns about GM foods. The current techniques that researchers use to introduce genes into plant cells result in random insertions into the genome. New techniques are being devised that will allow genes to be inserted into precise locations in the genome, avoiding some of the potential unknown effects of disrupting a plant's normal genome with random integrations.

[1]Schafter, M.G. et al. 2011. *PLoS One* 6:e25736.

Researchers are also devising more creative ways to protect plants from insects and diseases. One intriguing project involves introducing into wheat a gene that encodes a pheromone that acts as a chemical alarm signal to aphids. If successful, this approach could protect the wheat plants from aphids without using toxins. Another project involves cassava, which is a staple crop for many Africans and is afflicted by two viral diseases—cassava mosaic virus and brown streak virus—that stunt growth and cause root rot (**ST Figure 5–10**). Although some varieties of cassava are resistant to these viruses, the life cycle of cassava is so long that it would be difficult to introduce resistance into other varieties using conventional breeding techniques. Scientists plan to transform plants with genes from resistant cassava. This type of cisgenic gene transfer is more comparable to traditional breeding than transgenic techniques.

In the future, GM foods will likely include additional GM animals. As described in Box 1, a transgenic Atlantic salmon variety is likely to receive marketing approval in the near future. In another project, scientists have introduced a DNA sequence into chickens that protects the birds from spreading avian influenza. The sequence encodes a hairpin RNA molecule with similarity to a normal viral RNA that binds to the viral polymerase. The presence of the hairpin RNA inhibits the activity of the viral polymerase and interferes with viral propagation. If this strategy proves useful *in vivo*, the use of these GM chickens would not only reduce

ST FIGURE 5–10 Cassava tubers infected with brown streak virus. Cassava, a major food crop in sub-Saharan Africa, is threatened by infection with the mosaic virus, which stunts plant growth, and the brown streak virus, which causes root rot.

the incidence of avian influenza in poultry production, but also reduce the transmissibility of avian influenza viruses to humans.

Although these and other GM foods show promise for increasing agricultural productivity and decreasing disease, the political pressure from anti-GM critics remains a powerful force. An understanding of the science behind these technologies will help us all to evaluate the future of GM foods.

Selected Readings and Resources

Journal Articles

Butler, D. 2012. Hyped GM maize study faces growing scrutiny. *Nature* 490: 158.

Cressey, D. 2013. A new breed. *Nature* 497: 27–29.

Domingo, J.L. 2007. Toxicity studies of genetically modified plants: A review of the published literature. *Crit. Rev. Food Sci. Nutrition* 47: 721–733.

Enserink, M. 2008. Tough lessons from Golden Rice. *Science* 320: 468–471.

Gassmann, A.J., et al. 2011. Field-evolved resistance to Bt maize by western corn rootworm. *PLoS One* 6(7): e22629.

Gilbert, N. 2013. A hard look at GM crops. *Nature* 497: 21–26.

Gonsalves, D. 2004. Transgenic papaya in Hawaii and beyond. *AgBioForum* 7: 36–40.

Oke, K.B., et al. 2013. Hybridization between genetically modified Atlantic salmon and wild brown trout reveals novel ecological interactions. *Proc. R. Soc. B.*, 280: 20131047.

Paine, J.A., et al. 2005. Improving the nutritional value of Golden Rice through increased pro-vitamin A content. *Nature Biotech.* 23(4): 482–487.

Schafer, M.G., et al. 2011. The establishment of genetically engineered canola populations in the US. *PLoS One* 6(10): e25736.

Whitty, C.J.M., et al. 2013. Africa and Asia need a rational debate on GM crops. *Nature* 497: 31–33.

Web Sites

GMO Compass: EU supported GMO database. http://www.gmo-compass.org.

Adoption of Genetically Engineered Crops in the US. U.S. Department of Agriculture, Economic Research Service. http://www.ers.usda.gov/data-products/adoption-of-genetically-engineered-crops-in-the-us.aspx#.UdmLqW3fJyI

GM Approval Databases and Information. International Service for the Acquisition of Agri-Biotech Applications. http://isaaa.org

Twenty questions on genetically modified foods. World Health Organization. http://www.who.int/foodsafety/publications/biotech/20questions/en/

Golden Rice. The International Rice Research Institute. http://irri.org/golden-rice

Review Questions

1. How do genetically modified organisms compare with organisms created through selective breeding?
2. Can current GM crops be considered as transgenic or cisgenic? Why?
3. Of the approximately 200 GM crop varieties that have been developed, only a few are widely used. What are these varieties, and how prevalent are they?
4. How does glyphosate work, and how has it been used with GM crops to increase agricultural yields?
5. Describe the mechanisms by which the Cry proteins from *Bacillus thuringiensis* act as insecticides.
6. What measures have been taken to alleviate vitamin A deficiencies in developing countries? To date, how successful have these strategies been?
7. What is Golden Rice 2, and how was it created?
8. Describe how plants can be transformed using biolistic methods. How does this method compare with *Agrobacterium tumefaciens*-mediated transformation?
9. How do positive and negative selection techniques contribute to the development of GM crops?
10. Describe how the Roundup-Ready soybean variety was developed, and what genes were used to transform the soybean plants.

Discussion Questions

1. What are the laws regulating the development, approval, and use of GM foods in your region and nationally?
2. Do you think that foods containing GM ingredients should be labeled as such? What would be the advantages and disadvantages to such a strategy?
3. One of the major objections to GM foods is that they may be harmful to human health. Do you agree or disagree, and why?

Gene Therapy

Although drug treatments can be effective in controlling symptoms of genetic disorders, the ideal outcome of medical treatment is to cure a disease. This is the goal of **gene therapy**—the delivery of therapeutic genes into a patient's cells to correct genetic disease conditions caused by a faulty gene or genes. The earliest attempts at gene therapy focused on the delivery of normal, *therapeutic* copies of a gene to be expressed in such a way as to override or negate the effects of the disease gene and thus minimize or eliminate symptoms of the genetic disease. But in recent years newer methods for inhibiting or silencing defective genes, and even approaches for targeted removal of defective genes, have increasingly emerged as potential mechanisms for gene therapy. We will introduce you to each of these approaches in this Special Topic chapter.

Gene therapy is one of the ultimate goals of **translational medicine**—taking a scientific discovery, such as the identification of a disease-causing gene, and translating the finding into an effective therapy, thus moving from the laboratory bench to a patient's bedside to treat a disease. In theory, the delivery of a therapeutic gene is rather simple, but in practice, gene therapy has been very difficult to execute. In spite of over 20 years of trials, this field has not lived up to its expectations. However, gene therapy is currently experiencing a fast-paced resurgence of sorts, with several high-profile new successes and potentially exciting new technologies sitting on the horizon. It is hoped that gene therapy will soon become part of mainstream medicine. In this Special Topic chapter we will explore how gene therapy is executed, and we will highlight selected examples of successes and failures as well as discuss new approaches to gene therapy. Finally, we will consider ethical issues regarding gene therapy.

> "The treatment of a human genetic disease by gene therapy is the ultimate application of genetic technology."

What Genetic Conditions Are Candidates for Treatment by Gene Therapy?

Two essential criteria for gene therapy are that the gene or genes involved in causing a particular disease have been identified and that the gene can be cloned or synthesized in a laboratory. As a result of the Human Genome Project, the identification of human disease genes and their specific DNA sequences has greatly increased the number of candidate genes for gene therapy trials. Almost all of the early gene therapy trials and most gene therapy approaches have focused on treating *monogenic* diseases, conditions caused by a single gene. This has been the case because theoretically it is technically easier to affect one gene than disease conditions caused by multiple genes and potentially multiple mutations. Conceptually, this approach is simple. Identify the mutant gene responsible for the genetic condition and replace or supplement it with a normal copy of the gene. As we will see below, gene therapy has proven to be much more challenging than this.

The cells affected by the genetic condition must be readily accessible for treatment by gene therapy. For example, blood disorders such as leukemia, hemophilia, and other conditions have been major targets of gene therapy because it is relatively routine to manipulate blood cells outside of the body and return them to the body in comparison to treating cells in the brain and spinal cord, skeletal or cardiac muscle, and organs with heterogeneous populations of cells such as the pancreas. Cells of the respiratory system are another example of tissues that have also been targeted for their easy access. For example, this approach has been used to treat cystic fibrosis by gene therapy, but it has been unsuccessful for many reasons.

In the past decade, every major category of genetic diseases has been targeted by gene therapy [**ST Figure 6–1(a)**]. A majority of recently approved clinical trials are for cancer treatment. Gene therapy approaches are currently being investigated for the treatment of hereditary blindness, neurological (neurodegenerative) diseases including Alzheimer disease and Parkinson disease, cardiovascular disease, a variety of cancers, and infectious diseases, such as HIV, among many other conditions, including depression and drug and alcohol addiction. Over 1700 approved gene therapy clinical trials have occurred or recently been initiated for acquired and inherited diseases [**ST Figure 6–1(b)**].

(a)

(b)

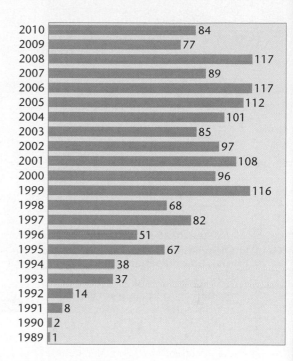

Cancer diseases (1186)
Monogenic diseases (161)
Cardiovascular disease (155)
Infectious diseases (147)
Neurological diseases (36)
Occular diseases (28)
Inflammatory diseases (13)
Others (25)
Gene marking (50)
Healthy volunteeers (42)

ST FIGURE 6–1   The current status of gene therapy worldwide. (a) Graphic representation of different genetic conditions being treated by gene therapy clinical trials worldwide. Notice that cancers are the major target for treatment. (b) Dozens of gene therapy clinical trials are approved by regulatory agencies around the world every year. Shown here is a partial representation of the number of approved trials initiated worldwide annually.

In the United States, proposed gene therapy clinical trials must first be approved by review boards at the institution where they will be carried out, and then the protocols must be approved by the Food and Drug Administration (FDA). Gene therapy trials that are funded by the National Institutes of Health also have to register with the NIH Recombinant DNA Advisory Committee.

How Are Therapeutic Genes Delivered?

In general, there are two broad approaches for delivering therapeutic genes to a patient being treated by gene therapy, *ex vivo gene therapy* and *in vivo gene therapy* (**ST Figure 6–3**). In *ex vivo* gene therapy, cells from a person with a particular genetic condition are removed, treated in a laboratory by adding either normal copies of a therapeutic gene or a DNA or RNA sequence that will inhibit expression of a defective gene, and then these cells are transplanted back into the person where the therapeutic gene will express normal copies of the required protein. Genetically altered cells treated in this manner can be transplanted back into the patient without

fear of immune system rejection because these cells were derived from the patient initially. As you will soon learn, this approach was used for the first successful gene therapy trial.

In vivo gene therapy does not involve removal of a person's cells. Instead, therapeutic DNA is introduced directly into affected cells of the body. One of the major challenges of *in vivo* gene therapy is restricting the delivery of therapeutic genes to only the intended tissues and not to all tissues throughout the body.

Viral Vectors for Gene Therapy

For both *in vitro* and *ex vivo* approaches, the key to successful gene therapy is having a delivery system to transfer genes into a patient's cells. Because of the relatively large molecular size and electrically charged properties of DNA, most human cells do not take up DNA easily. If they did, it would be possible to deliver genes simply by mixing DNA with cells in much the same way that transformation is achieved with bacterial cells. Therefore, delivering therapeutic DNA molecules into human cells is challenging. Since the early days of gene therapy, genetically engineered viruses as vectors have been the main tools for delivering therapeutic genes into human cells. Viral vectors for gene

SPECIAL TOPIC 6

BOX 1
ClinicalTrials.gov

One of the best resources on the Web for learning about ongoing clinical trials, including current gene therapy trials, is ClinicalTrials.gov. The site can easily be searched to find a wealth of resources about ongoing gene therapy trials throughout the United States that are of interest to you. To find a gene therapy clinical trial, use the "Search for Studies" box and type in the name of a disease and "gene therapy." This search string will take you to a page listing active gene therapy clinical trials, with links to detailed information about the trial.

ST FIGURE 6–2 The ClinicalTrials.gov Web site homepage.

therapy are engineered to carry therapeutic DNA as their payload so that the virus infects target cells and delivers the therapeutic DNA without causing damage to cells.

In a majority of gene therapy trials around the world, scientists have used genetically modified *retroviruses* as vectors. Recall from earlier in the text (see Chapter 10) that retroviruses (HIV is a retrovirus) contain an RNA genome that scientists use as a template for the synthesis of a complementary

DNA molecule. The first viruses used for gene therapy were from a family of murine retroviruses called Moloney murine leukemia virus. **Retroviral vectors** are created by removing replication and disease-causing genes from the virus and replacing them with a cloned human gene. After the altered RNA has been packaged into the virus, the recombinant viral vector containing the therapeutic human gene is used to infect a patient's cells. Technically, virus particles are carrying RNA

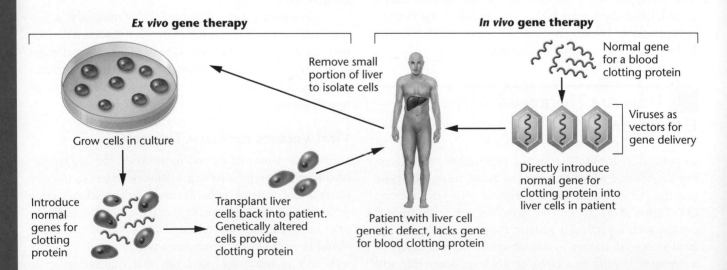

ST FIGURE 6–3 *Ex vivo* and *in vivo* gene therapy for a patient with a liver disorder. *Ex vivo* gene therapy involves isolating cells from the patient, introducing normal copies of a therapeutic gene (encoding a blood clotting protein in this example) into these cells, and then returning cells to the body where they will produce the required clotting protein. *In vivo* approaches involve introducing DNA directly into cells while they are in the body. Both approaches can also be used to deliver genes to overcome the effects of the expression of a mutant gene.

copies of the therapeutic gene. Once inside a cell, the virus cannot replicate itself, but the therapeutic RNA is reverse transcribed into DNA, which enters the nucleus of cells and *integrates* into the genome of the host cells' chromosome. If the inserted therapeutic gene is properly expressed, it produces a normal gene product that may be able to ameliorate the effects of the mutation carried by the affected individual.

One advantage of retroviral vectors is that they provide long-term expression of delivered genes because they integrate the therapeutic gene into the genome of the patient's cells. But a major problem with retroviral vectors is that they have produced severe toxicity in some cases due to *insertional mutations*. Retroviral vectors generally integrate their genome into the host-cell genome at random sites. Thus, there is the potential for retroviral integration

that randomly inactivates genes in the genome or gene-regulatory regions such as a promoter sequence. In some cases the promoter sequence of a gene therapy vector can control expression of adjacent genes in the host-cell genome—which can include activating cancer genes with devastating results, as you will soon learn.

Adenovirus vectors were used in many early gene therapy trials. An advantage of these vectors is that they are capable of carrying large therapeutic genes. But because many humans produce antibodies to adenovirus vectors they can mount immune reactions that can render the virus and its therapeutic gene ineffective or cause significant side-effects to the patient. A related virus called **adeno-associated virus (AAV)** is now widely used as a gene therapy vector [**ST Figure 6–4(a)**]. In its native form, AAV infects about

SPECIAL TOPIC 6

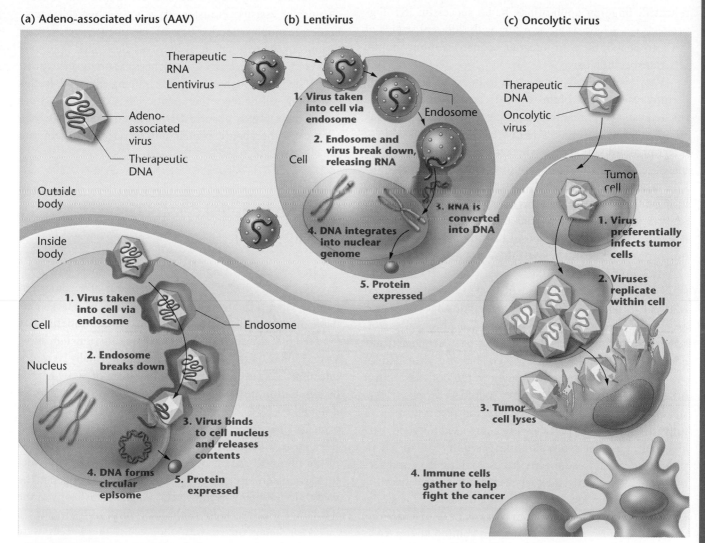

ST FIGURE 6–4   Delivering therapeutic genes. (a) Nonintegrating viruses such as modified adeno-associated virus (AAV) deliver therapeutic genes without integrating them into the genome of target cells. Delivered DNA resides as minichromosomes (episomes), but over time as cells divide, these nonintegrating hoops of DNA are gradually lost. (b) Integrating viruses include lentivirus, an RNA retrovirus that delivers therapeutic genes into the cytoplasm where reverse transcriptase converts RNA into DNA. DNA then integrates into the genome, ensuring that therapeutic DNA will be passed into daughter cells during cell division. (c) Oncolytic viruses are being used to deliver therapeutic genes to target attacks on cancer cells.

80–90 percent of humans during childhood, causing symptoms associated with the common cold. Disabled forms of AAV are popular for gene therapy because the virus is non-pathogenic, so it usually does not elicit a major response from the immune system of treated patients. AAV also does not typically integrate into the host-cell genome, so there is little risk of the insertional mutations that have plagued retroviruses, although modified forms of AAV have been used to deliver genes to specific sites on individual chromosomes. Most forms of AAV deliver genes into the host-cell nucleus where it forms small hoops of DNA called *episomes* that are expressed under the control of promoter sequences contained within the viral genome. But because therapeutic DNA delivered by AAV does not usually become incorporated into the genome, it is not replicated when host cells divide, and so the gene therapy approach may require repeated, ongoing applications to be successful [ST Figure 6–4(a)]. Scientists are working with different strains of AAV to enable them to integrate sequences into genomic DNA at specific sites.

Work with **lentivirus vectors** is an active area of gene therapy research [ST Figure 6–4(b)]. Lentivirus is a retrovirus that can accept relatively large pieces of genetic material. Another positive feature of lentivirus is that it is capable of infecting nondividing cells, whereas other viral vectors often infect cells only when they are dividing. It is still not possible to control where lentivirus integration occurs in the host-cell genome, but the virus does not appear to gravitate toward gene-regulatory regions the way that other retroviruses do. Thus the likelihood of causing insertional mutations appears to be much lower than for other vectors.

The human immunodeficiency virus (HIV) responsible for acquired immunodeficiency syndrome (AIDS) is a type of lentivirus. It may surprise you that HIV could be used as a vector for gene therapy. For any viral vector, scientists must be sure that the vector has been genetically engineered to render it inactive so that the virus cannot produce disease or spread throughout the body and infect other tissues. In the case of HIV, modified forms of HIV, strains lacking the genes necessary for reconstitution of fully functional viral particles, are being used for gene therapy trials. HIV has evolved to infect certain types of T lymphocytes (T cells) and macrophages, making it a good vector for delivering therapeutic genes into the bloodstream.

Viral vectors for gene therapy are limited by the size of the inserted therapeutic gene they are capable of accepting, about 10 kb for retroviral vectors and about 5 kb for AAV. This size presents a problem when an attempt is made to deliver very large genes or genes with complex regulatory and coding sequences. As you will learn, a major emphasis in gene therapy research is to develop safe and reliable vectors (viral and nonviral).

Researchers are even working on using *oncolytic viruses* carrying payloads of therapeutic genes [ST Figure 6–4(c)]. These viruses, such as certain forms of herpes simplex type I (HSV-1), target and destroy tumor cells and at the same time deliver therapeutic genes. Increasingly, viral vectors and nonviral vector approaches are being used to deliver therapeutic genes into *stem cells*, usually *in vitro*, and then the stem cells are either reintroduced into the patient or differentiated *in vitro* into mature cell types before being transplanted into the correct organ of a patient being treated.

Nonviral Delivery Methods

Scientists continue to experiment with various *in vivo* and *ex vivo* strategies for trying to deliver so called naked DNA into cells without the use of viral vectors. Nonviral methods that are being used to transfer genes into cells include chemically assisted transfer of genes across cell membranes, nanoparticle delivery of therapeutic genes, and fusion of cells with artificial lipid vesicles called *liposomes* that contain cloned DNA sequences. Short-term expression of genes through "gene pills" is being explored. In this concept, a pill delivers therapeutic DNA to the intestines where the DNA is absorbed by intestinal cells that then express the therapeutic protein and secrete the protein into the bloodstream.

The First Successful Gene Therapy Trial

In 1990 the FDA approved the first human gene therapy trial, which began with the treatment of a young girl named Ashanti DeSilva [ST Figure 6–5(a)], who has a heritable disorder called **severe combined immunodeficiency (SCID)**. Individuals with SCID have no functional immune system and usually die from what would normally be minor infections. Ashanti has an autosomal form of SCID caused by a mutation in the gene encoding the enzyme *adenosine deaminase (ADA)*. Her gene therapy began when clinicians isolated some of her white blood cells, called T cells [ST Figure 6–5(b)]. These cells, which are key components of the immune system, were mixed with a retroviral vector carrying an inserted copy of the normal *ADA* gene. The virus infected many of the T cells, and a normal copy of the *ADA* gene was inserted into the genome of some T cells.

After being mixed with the vector, the T cells were grown in the laboratory and analyzed to make sure that the transferred *ADA* gene was expressed (ST Figure 6–5). Then a billion or so genetically altered T cells were injected into Ashanti's bloodstream. Repeated treatments were required to produce a sufficient number of functioning T cells. In addition, Ashanti also periodically received injections of purified

ST FIGURE 6–5 The first successful gene therapy trial. (a) Ashanti DeSilva, the first person to be successfully treated by gene therapy. (b) To treat SCID using gene therapy, a cloned human *ADA* gene is transferred into a viral vector, which is then used to infect white blood cells removed from the patient. The transferred *ADA* gene is incorporated into a chromosome and becomes active. After growth to enhance their numbers, the cells are inserted back into the patient, where they produce ADA, allowing the development of an immune response.

ADA protein throughout this process. Ashanti has ADA protein expression in 25 to 30 percent of her T cells, which was enough to allow her to lead a normal life.

Subsequent gene therapy treatments for SCID have focused on using bone marrow stem cells and *in vitro* approaches to repopulate the number of ADA-producing T cells. To date, gene therapy has successfully restored the health of about 20 children affected by SCID. SCID treatment is still considered the most successful example of gene therapy so far.

Gene Therapy Setbacks

From 1990 to 1999, more than 4000 people underwent gene therapy for a variety of genetic disorders. These trials often failed and thus led to a loss of confidence in gene therapy.

In the United States, gene therapy plummeted even further in 1999 when teenager Jesse Gelsinger died while undergoing a test for the safety of a gene therapy procedure to treat a liver disease called ornithine transcarbamylase (OTC) deficiency. Large numbers of adenovirus vectors bearing the *OTC* gene were injected into his hepatic artery. His death was triggered by a massive inflammatory response to the adenovirus vector. The virus vectors were expected to target his liver, enter liver cells, and trigger the production of OTC protein. In turn, it was hoped that the OTC protein might correct his genetic defect and cure him of his liver disease.

Researchers had previously treated 18 people with the therapeutic virus, and early results from the first 17 adult patients were promising. But as the 18th patient, Jesse Gelsinger, within hours of his first treatment, developed a massive immune reaction. He developed a high fever, his lungs filled with fluid, multiple organs shut down, and he died four days later of acute respiratory failure. It was thought that Jesse's severe response to the adenovirus may have resulted from how his body reacted to a previous exposure to the virus used as the vector for this protocol.

In the aftermath of the tragedy, several government and scientific inquiries were conducted. Investigators learned that in the clinical trial scientists had not reported other adverse reactions to gene therapy and that some of the scientists were affiliated with private companies that could benefit financially from the trials. It was determined that serious side-effects seen in animal studies were not explained to patients during informed-consent discussions. The FDA subsequently scrutinized gene therapy trials across the country, halted a number of them, and shut down several gene therapy programs. Other research groups voluntarily suspended their gene therapy studies. Tighter restrictions on clinical trial protocols were imposed to correct some of the procedural problems that emerged from the Gelsinger case. Jesse's death had dealt a severe blow to the struggling field of gene therapy—a blow from which it was still reeling when a second tragedy hit.

The outlook for gene therapy brightened momentarily in 2000, when a group of French researchers reported what was hailed as the first large-scale success in gene therapy. Children with a fatal X-linked form of SCID developed functional immune systems after being treated with a retroviral vector carrying a normal gene. But elation over this study soon turned to despair, when it became clear that 5 of the 20 patients in the trial developed leukemia as a direct result of their therapy. One of these patients died as a result of the treatment, while the other four went into remission from the leukemia. In two of the children examined, their cancer cells contained the retroviral vector, inserted near or into a gene called *LMO2*. This *insertional mutagenesis* activated the *LMO2* gene, causing uncontrolled white blood cell proliferation and development of leukemia. The FDA immediately halted 27 similar gene therapy clinical trials, and once again gene therapy underwent a profound reassessment.

On a positive note, long-term survival data from trials in the UK to treat X-SCID and SCID using hematopoietic stem cells from the patients' bone marrow for gene therapy have shown that 14 of 16 children have had their immune system restored at least 9 years after the treatment. These children formerly had life expectancies of less than 20 years. Nevertheless, the above events had major negative impacts on the progress of gene therapy.

Problems with Gene Therapy Vectors

Critics of gene therapy have berated research groups for undue haste, conflicts of interest, sloppy clinical trial management, and for promising much but delivering little. Most of the problems associated with gene therapy, including the Jesse Gelsinger case and the French X-SCID trial, have been traced to the viral vectors used to transfer therapeutic genes into cells. The use of these vectors has been shown to have several serious drawbacks.

- First, integration of retroviral genomes, including the human therapeutic gene into the host cell's genome, occurs only if the host cells are replicating their DNA. In the body, only a small number of cells in any tissue are dividing and replicating their DNA.
- Second, the injection of large amounts of most viral vectors, but particularly adenovirus vectors, is capable of causing an adverse immune response in the patient, as happened in Jesse Gelsinger's case.
- Third, insertion of viral genomes into host chromosomes can activate or mutate an essential gene, as in the case of the French patients. Viral integrase, the enzyme that allows for viral genome integration into the host genome, interacts with chromatin-associated proteins, often steering integration toward transcriptionally active genes. Unfortunately, it is not yet possible to reliably target insertion of therapeutic genes into specific locations in the genome, but as we will discuss in the next section targeted gene delivery is a major area of active research.
- Fourth, AAV vectors cannot carry DNA sequences larger than about 5 kb, and retroviruses cannot carry DNA sequences much larger than 10 kb. Many human genes exceed the 5–10 kb size range.
- Finally, there is a possibility that a fully infectious virus could be created if the inactivated vector were to recombine with another unaltered viral genome already present in the host cell.

To overcome these problems, new viral vectors and strategies for transferring genes into cells are being developed in an attempt to improve the action and safety of vectors. Researchers hope that the use of new gene delivery systems will circumvent the problems inherent in earlier vectors, as well as allow regulation of both insertion sites and the levels of gene product produced from the therapeutic genes. Thus, developing safe viral and nonviral vector systems continues to be a major area of active research, as are approaches to targeted gene therapy that we will discuss later in this chapter. Fortunately, gene therapy has experienced resurgence in part because of several promising new trials and successful treatments.

Recent Successful Trials

Treating Retinal Blindness

In recent years, patients being treated for blindness have greatly benefited from gene therapy approaches. Congenital retinal blinding conditions affect about 1 in 2000 people worldwide, many of which are the result of a wide range of genetic defects. Over 165 different genes have been implicated in various forms of retinal blindness.

Successful gene therapy has been achieved in subsets of patients with *Leber congenital amaurosis (LCA)*, a degenerative disease of the retina that affects 1 in 50,000 to 1 in 100,000 infants each year and causes severe blindness. Gene therapy treatments for LCA were originally pioneered in dogs. Based on the success of these treatments, the protocols were adapted and applied to human gene therapy trials.

LCA is caused by alterations to photoreceptor cells (rods and cones), light-sensitive cells in the retina, due to 18 or more genes. One gene in particular, *RPE65*, has been the gene therapy target of choice. The protein product of the *RPE65* gene metabolizes retinol, which is a form of vitamin A that allows the rod and cone cells of the retina to detect light and transmit electrical signals to the brain. In one of the earliest trials, young adult patients with defects in the *RPE65* gene were given injections of the normal gene. Several months after a single treatment, many adult patients, while still legally blind, could detect light, and some of them could read lines of an eye chart. This treatment approach for LCA was based on injecting AAV-carrying *RPE65* at the back of the eye directly under the retina [**ST Figure 6–6(a, b)**]. The therapeutic gene enters about

15 to 20 percent of cells in the retinal pigment epithelium, the layer of cells just beneath the visual cells of the retina. Adults treated by this approach have shown substantial improvements in a variety of visual functions tests, but the greatest improvement has been demonstrated in children, all of whom have gained sufficient vision to allow them to be ambulatory. Researchers think the success in children has occurred because younger patients have not lost as many photoreceptor cells as older patients.

Over two dozen gene therapy trials have been completed or are ongoing for various forms of blindness, including age-related degenerative causes of blindness. Because of the small size of the eye and the relatively small number of cells that need to be treated, the prospects for gene therapy to become routine treatment for eye disorders appears to be very good. Retinal cells are also very long-lived; thus, AAV delivery approaches can be successful for long periods of time even if the gene does not integrate.

HIV as a Vector Shows Promise in Recent Trials

Researchers at the University of Paris and Harvard Medical School reported that two years after gene therapy treatment for **β-thalassemia**, a blood disorder involving the β-globin gene that reduces the production of hemoglobin, a young man no longer needed transfusions and appeared to be

(a)

(b)

ST FIGURE 6–6 Treatment of retinal blindness. (a) Illustration of AAV delivery of specific genes targeting individual cell types of the retina, rods, cones and the layer of retinal pigment epithelial (RPE) cells. The basic approach shown here was the delivery method used to successfully treat LCA. (b) Photoreceptor layer of a monkey retina after subretinal injection of an AAV expressing green fluorescent protein (GFP; green) in rod and cone cells demonstrating successful delivery of a transgene.

BOX 2
Glybera Is the First Commercial Gene Therapy to Be Approved in the West

In late 2012, a gene therapy product called Glybera (alipogene tiparvovec) made history when the European Medicines Agency of the European Union approved it as the first gene therapy trial to win commercial approval in the Western world. Glybera is an adenovirus-based vector system for delivering therapeutic copies of the *LPL* gene to treat patients with a rare disease called *lipoprotein lipase deficiency* (LPLD, also called familial hyperchylomicronemia). LPLD patients have high levels of triglycerides in their blood. Elevated serum triglycerides are toxic to the pancreas and cause a severe form of pancreatic inflammation called pancreatitis. Developed by Amsterdam-based company uniQure BV, it is still unclear if Glybera will be approved by the U.S. FDA. Nonetheless, the success of Glybera trials in Europe signals what many gene therapy researchers hope will be the beginning of a wave of approvals for gene therapy treatments in Europe and the United States.

healthy. A modified, disabled HIV was used to carry a copy of the normal *β-globin* gene. Although this trial resulted in activation of the growth factor gene called *HMGA2*, reminiscent of what occurred in the French X-SCID trials, activation of the transcription factor did not result in an overproduction of hematopoietic cells or create a condition of preleukemia.

In 2013, researchers at the San Raffaele Telethon Institute for Gene Therapy in Milan, Italy, reported two studies using lentivirus vectors derived from HIV in combination with hematopoietic stem cells (HSCs) to successfully treat children with either **metachromatic leukodystrophy (MLD)** or **Wiskott-Aldrich syndrome (WAS)**. Three years after the start of a trial involving a total of 16 patients, 10 patients with MLD and 6 with WAS, data from six patients analyzed 18 to 24 months after gene therapy indicated that the trials are safe and effective. These initial reports are based on studying three children from each study because these are the first patients for whom sufficient time has passed after gene therapy treatment to make significant conclusions regarding the safety and effectiveness of the trials. It took over 15 years of research to get to this point. These trials involved a team of over 70 people, including researchers and clinicians, which is indicative of the teamwork approach typical of gene therapy trials.

MLD is a neurodegenerative disorder affecting storage of enzymes in lysosomes and is caused by mutation in the arylsulfatase A (*ARSA*) gene that results in an accumulation of fats called sulfatides. These are toxic to neurons, causing progressive loss of the myelin sheath (demyelination) surrounding neurons in the brain, leading to a loss of cognitive functions and motor skills. There is no cure for MLD. Children with MLD appear healthy at birth but eventually develop MLD symptoms. In this trial, researchers used an *ex vivo* approach with a lentivirus vector to introduce a functional *ARSA* gene into bone marrow-derived HSCs from each patient and then infused treated HSCs back into patients.

In three children with MLD, gene therapy treatment halted disease progression for 18 to 24 months after therapy, as determined by magnetic resonance images of the brain and through tests of cognitive and motor skills (**ST Figure 6-7**). Because disease onset is predicted at 7 to 21 months, scientists are very encouraged by the outcomes of this trial. The trial was technically complicated because

(a) (b) (c)

ST FIGURE 6-7 Gene therapy can prevent progression of metachromatic leukodystrophy. (a) Brain magnetic resonance images (MRIs) of a MLD patient at 16 months of age prior to gene therapy. The large white patches in the center of these images show cerebrospinal fluid in the ventricles of the brain. White spots and streaks at the periphery of the brain indicate myelin. (b) MRI images of a MLD patient two years after gene therapy. The myelin content of the brain appears relatively normal. (c) MRI image of the brain from a 39-month-old MLD patient showing severe demyelination associated with MLD-related brain atrophy.

it required that HSCs travel through the bloodstream and release the ARSA protein that is taken up into neurons. A major challenge was to create enough engineered cells to produce a sufficient quantity of therapeutic ARSA protein to counteract the neurodegenerative process.

WAS is an X-linked condition caused by a mutation in the *WASP* gene that encodes a protein that functions in the cytoskeleton of platelets. WAS results in defective platelets that make patients more vulnerable to infections, frequent bleeding, autoimmune diseases, and cancer. Patients treated for WAS showed a resolution of pretreatment eczema (inflammation of the skin) typical in WAS, improved platelet counts, and decreased frequency of infections after gene therapy treatment. Genome sequencing of MLD and WAS patients treated in these trials showed no evidence of genome integration near oncogenes. Similarly, patients showed no evidence of hematopoietic stem cell overproduction, suggesting that this lentivirus delivery protocol produced a safe and stable delivery of the therapeutic genes.

Targeted Approaches to Gene Therapy

The gene therapy approaches and examples we have highlighted thus far have focused on the addition of a therapeutic gene that functions along with the defective gene. However, the removal, correction, and/or replacement of a mutated gene and silencing expression of a defective gene are two other approaches being developed. Rapid progress is being made with these approaches.

DNA-Editing Nucleases for Gene Targeting

For nearly 20 years, scientists have been working on modifications of restriction enzymes and other nucleases to engineer proteins capable of **gene targeting** or **gene editing**—replacing specific genes in the genome. The concept is to combine a nuclease with a sequence-specific DNA binding domain that can be precisely targeted for digestion. In 1996 researchers fused DNA-binding proteins with a zinc-finger motif and DNA cutting domain from the restriction enzyme *Fok*I to create enzymes called **zinc-finger nucleases (ZFNs; ST Figure 6–8)**. Recall from earlier in the text (see Chapter 17) that the zinc-finger motif is found in many transcription factors and consists of a cluster of two cysteine and two histidine residues that bind zinc atoms and interact with specific DNA sequences. By coupling zinc-finger motifs to DNA cutting portions of a polypeptide, ZFNs provide a mechanism for modifying sequences in the genome in a sequence-specific *targeted way*.

Zinc-finger arrangements in a ZFN form a loop in the polypeptide, and they dimerize to bind DNA. The DNA-binding domain of the ZFN can be engineered to attach to any sequence in the genome. Most ZFNs recognize three nucleotides in target DNA sequence. The zinc fingers bind with a spacing of 5–7 nucleotides, and the nuclease domain of the ZFN cleaves between the binding sites.

Another category of DNA-editing nucleases called **TALENs (transcription activator-like effector nucleases)** was created by adding a DNA-binding motif identified in transcription factors from plant pathogenic bacteria known as transcription activator-like effectors (TALEs) to nucleases to create TALENS. TALENS also cleave as dimers. The DNA-binding domain is a tandem array of amino acid repeats, with each TALEN repeat binding to a specific single base pair. The nuclease domain then cuts the sequence between the dimers, a stretch that spans about 13 bp.

ZFNs and TALENS have shown promise in animal models and cultured cells for gene replacement approaches that involve removing a defective gene from the genome. These enzymes can create site-specific cleavage in the genome. When coupled with certain integrases, ZFNs and TALENs may lead to gene editing by cutting out defective sequences and using recombination to introduce homologous sequences into the genome that replace defective sequences. Encouraging breakthroughs have taken place in this area using model organisms such as mice. Although this technology has not yet advanced sufficiently for reliable use in humans, there have been several promising trials.

ST FIGURE 6–8 Zinc-finger nucleases and TALENs bind and cut DNA at specific sequences.

SPECIAL TOPIC 6

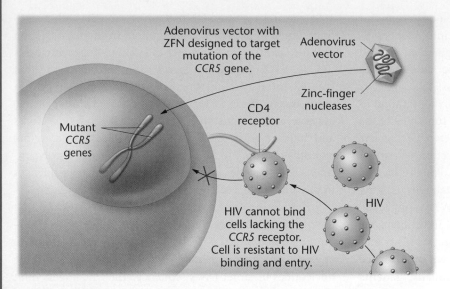

ST FIGURE 6–9 Can gene therapy be used to cure patients with HIV infections or to prevent HIV infections? One recent trial involved adenoviruses to deliver a ZFN to target disruption of the *CCR5* gene in T cells. Cells lacking the protein receptor encoded by *CCR5* are resistant to HIV binding and entry.

For example, ZFNs are actively being used in clinical trials for treating patients with HIV (**ST Figure 6–9**). Scientists are exploring ways to deliver immune system-stimulating genes that could make individuals resistant to HIV infection or cripple the virus in HIV-positive persons. In 2007, Timothy Brown, a 40-year-old HIV-positive American, had a relapse of acute myeloid leukemia and received a stem cell (bone-marrow) transplant. Because he was HIV-positive, Brown's physician selected a donor with a mutation in both copies of the *CCR5* gene, which encodes an HIV co-receptor carried on the surface of T cells to which HIV must bind to enter T cells (specifically CD4+ cells). People with naturally occurring mutations in both copies of the *CCR5* gene are resistant to most forms of HIV. Brown relapsed again and received another stem cell transplant from the *CCR5*-mutant donor. Eventually, the cancer was contained, and by 2010, levels of HIV in his body were still undetectable even though he was no longer receiving immune-suppressive treatment. Brown is generally considered to be the first person to have been cured of an HIV infection.

This example encouraged researchers to press forward with a gene therapy approach to modify the *CCR5* gene of HIV patients. In one promising trial, T cells were removed from HIV-positive men, and ZFNs were used to disrupt the *CCR5* gene. The modified cells were then reintroduced into patients. In five of six patients treated, immune-cell counts rose substantially following the therapy. What percentage of immune cells would have to be treated this way to significantly inhibit spread of the virus is not known, but initial results are very promising.

Recently, researchers working with human cells used TALENs to remove defective copies of the *COL7A1* gene, which causes recessive dystrophic epidermolysis bullosa (RDEB), an incurable and often fatal disease that causes excessive blistering of the skin, pain, and severely debilitating skin damage. Researchers at the University of Minnesota used a TALEN to cut DNA near a mutation in *COL7A1* gene in skin cells taken from an RDEB patient. These cells were then converted into a type of stem cell called induced pluripotent stem cells (iPSCs). The iPSCs were treated with therapeutic copies of the *COL7A1* gene and then differentiated into skin cells that expressed the correct protein. This is a promising result, and researchers now plan to transplant these skin cells into patients in an attempt to cure them of RDEB. Another group has recently taken a similar approach using TALENS to repair cultured cells in order to correct the mutation in Duchenne muscular dystrophy (DMD). Researchers are optimistic that this approach can soon be adapted to treat patients.

As another recent example of gene targeting, a system called *CRISPR* has shown great promise for replacing target gene sequences. During the first half of 2013, different groups used the CRISPR approach to target specific genes in human cells, mice, rats, bacteria, fruit flies, yeast, zebrafish, and other organisms. CRISPR is based on a single-stranded "guided" RNA sequence that is specific to the target gene and a protein called Cas9. Compared to TALEN approaches, guided RNAs are easier to design and synthesize. Cas9 delivers the guided RNA to the target DNA sequence, which enables the target DNA to be knocked out or replaced by a substitute sequence. Based on the rapid development of the CRISPR method, this approach may turn out to be a very valuable tool for gene therapy in the future.

RNA Silencing for Gene Inhibition

Attempts have been made to use **antisense oligonucleotides** to inhibit translation of mRNAs from defective genes, but this approach to gene therapy has generally not yet proven to be reliable. Nonetheless, the emergence of RNA interference as a powerful gene-silencing tool has reinvigorated gene therapy approaches by gene silencing. As you learned in earlier in the text (see Chapter 17), **RNA interference (RNAi)** is a form of gene-expression regulation (Figure 17–14). In animals short, double-stranded RNA molecules are delivered into cells where the enzyme Dicer chops them into 21- to 25-nt long pieces called **small interfering RNAs (siRNAs)**. siRNAs then join with an enzyme complex called the **RNA-inducing silencing complex (RISC)**, which shuttles the siRNAs to their target mRNA, where they bind by complementary base pairing. The RISC complex can block siRNA-bound mRNAs from being translated into protein or can lead to degradation of siRNA-bound mRNAs so that they cannot be translated into protein (**ST Figure 6–10**).

A main challenge to RNAi-based therapeutics so far has been *in vivo* delivery of double-stranded RNA or siRNA. RNAs degrade quickly in the body. It is also hard to get RNA to penetrate cells in the target tissue. For example, how does one deliver RNA-based therapies to cancer cells

but not to noncancerous, healthy cells? Two common delivery approaches are to inject the siRNA directly or to deliver them via a DNA plasmid vector that is taken in by cells and transcribed to make double-stranded RNA which Dicer can cleave into siRNAs. Lentivirus, liposome, and attachment of siRNAs to cholesterol and fatty acids are other approaches being used to deliver siRNAs (ST Figure 6–10).

More than a dozen clinical trials involving RNAi are underway in the United States. Several RNAi clinical trials to treat blindness are showing promising results. One RNAi strategy to treat a form of blindness called macular degeneration targets a gene called *VEGF*. The VEGF protein promotes blood vessel growth. Overexpression of this gene, causing excessive production of blood vessels in the retina,

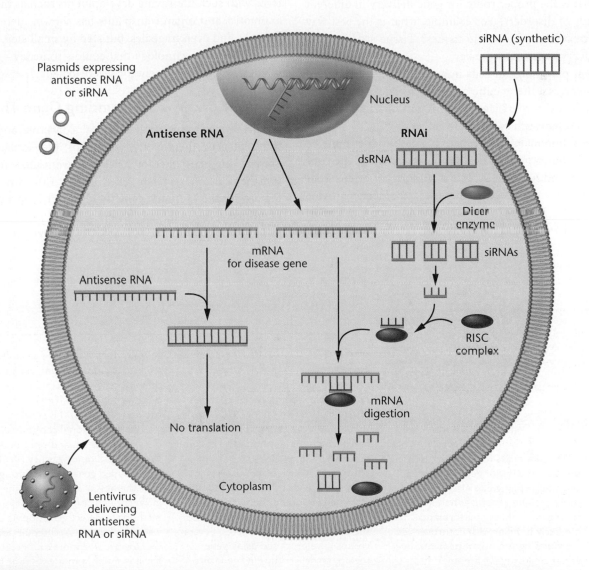

ST FIGURE 6–10 Antisense RNA and RNA interference (RNAi) approaches to silence genes for gene therapy. Antisense RNA technology and RNAi are two ways to silence gene expression and turn off disease genes. In antisense technology, an antisense RNA molecule (complementary to the sense strand of mRNA produced by a cell) binds to the mRNA expressed by the disease gene and prevents it from being translated. With RNAi technology, siRNAs are escorted by the RISC protein complex to bind to a target mRNA molecule, causing its degradation and thus preventing translation. Antisense RNA and RNAi molecules can be delivered in various ways, including direct application of synthetic RNAs, by plasmids, and via viral vectors.

leads to impaired vision and eventually blindness. Many expect that this disease will soon become the first condition to receive approval for treatment by RNAi therapy. Other disease candidates for treatment by RNAi include several different cancers, diabetes, multiple sclerosis, and arthritis.

Future Challenges and Ethical Issues

Despite the progress that we have noted thus far, many questions remain to be answered before we can hope for widespread application of the gene therapy methodology in the treatment of genetic disorders:

- What is the proper route for gene delivery in different kinds of disorders? For example, what is the best way to treat brain or muscle tissues? Tissue-specific gene delivery approaches are key.
- What percentage of cells in an organ or a tissue need to express a therapeutic gene to alleviate the effects of a genetic disorder? How can millions of cells be treated in an organ such as the brain or liver?
- What amount of a therapeutic gene product must be produced to provide lasting improvement of the condition, and how can sufficient production be ensured? Currently, many gene therapy approaches provide only short-lived delivery of the therapeutic gene and its protein.

- Will it be possible to use gene therapy to treat diseases that involve multiple genes?
- Can expression or the timing of expression of therapeutic genes be controlled in a patient so that genes can be turned on or off at a particular time or as necessary?
- Will targeted gene delivery approaches become more widely used for gene therapy trials?

For many people, the question remains whether gene therapy can ever recover from past setbacks and fulfill its promise as a cure for genetic diseases. Clinical trials for any new therapy are potentially dangerous, and often, animal studies will not accurately reflect the reaction of individual humans to the methodology leading to the delivery of new genes. However, as the history of similar struggles encountered with such life-saving developments such as the use of antibiotics and organ transplants has shown, there will be setbacks and even tragedies, but step by small step, we will move toward a technology that could—someday—provide reliable and safe treatment for severe genetic diseases.

Ethical Concerns Surrounding Gene Therapy

Gene therapy raises several ethical concerns, and many forms of gene therapy are sources of intense debate. At present, all gene therapy trials are restricted to using somatic cells as targets for gene transfer. This form of gene therapy is called **somatic gene therapy**; only one individual is affected, and the therapy is done with the permission and informed consent of the patient or family.

BOX 3
Gene Doping for Athletic Performance?

Gene therapy is intended to provide treatments or cures for genetic diseases, but the concept of gene addition or gene silencing can also apply for those seeking genetic enhancements to improve athletic performance. You are likely familiar with controversies surrounding the use of performance-enhancing drugs in amateur and professional sports. As athletes at all levels seek a competitive edge, will gene therapy as a form of "gene doping" to improve performance be far behind?

We already know that in animal models enhanced muscle function can be achieved by gene addition. For example, adding copies of the insulin-like growth factor (*IGF-1*) gene to mice improves aspects of muscle function. The kidney hormone erythropoietin (EPO) increases red blood cell production, which leads to a higher oxygen content of the blood and thus improved endurance during exercise. Synthetic forms of EPO are a banned substance in Olympic athletes. Several groups have proposed using gene therapy to deliver the *EPO* gene into athletes "naturally." As another example, transgenic mice overexpressing the peroxisome proliferator-activated receptor delta (*PPAR-δ*) gene show enhanced endurance in exercise tests.

Prior to the 2008 Olympics in Beijing, a genetics laboratory in China was offering gene-based enhancements, but it is not known if any athletes took advantage of this service.

The international community is clearly concerned, and since 2004 the World Anti-Doping Agency (WADA) has included gene doping through gene therapy as a prohibited method in sanctioned competitions. However, methods to detect gene doping are not well established. If techniques for gene therapy become more routine, many feel it is simply a matter of time before gene doping through gene therapy will be the next generation of performance-enhancement treatments. Obviously, many legal and ethical questions will arise if gene doping becomes a reality.

Two other forms of gene therapy have not been approved, primarily because of the unresolved ethical issues surrounding them. The first is called **germ-line therapy**, whereby germ cells (the cells that give rise to the gametes—i.e., sperm and eggs) or mature gametes are used as targets for gene transfer. In this approach, the transferred gene is incorporated into all the future cells of the body, including the germ cells. As a result, individuals in future generations will also be affected, without their consent. Is this kind of procedure ethical? Do we have the right to make this decision for future generations? Thus far, the concerns have outweighed the potential benefits, and such research is prohibited.

Box 3 mentioned gene doping, which is also an example of **enhancement gene therapy**, whereby people may be "enhanced" for some desired trait. This is another unapproved form of gene therapy—which is extremely controversial and is strongly opposed by many people. Should genetic technology be used to enhance human potential? For example, should it be permissible to use gene therapy to increase height, enhance athletic ability, or extend intellectual potential? Presently, the consensus is that enhancement therapy, like germ-line therapy, is an unacceptable use of gene therapy. However, there is an ongoing debate, and many issues are still unresolved. For example, the FDA now permits growth hormone produced by recombinant DNA technology to be used as a growth enhancer, in addition to its medical use for the treatment of growth-associated genetic disorders. Critics charge that the use of a gene product for enhancement will lead to the use of transferred genes for the same purpose. The outcome of these debates may affect not only the fate of individuals but the direction of our society as well.

Gene therapy is currently a fairly expensive treatment. But what is the right price for a cure? It remains to be seen how health-care insurance providers will view gene therapy. But if gene therapy treatments provide a health-care option that drastically improves the quality of life for patients for whom there are few other options, it is likely that insurance companies will reimburse patients for treatment costs.

Finally, *who* to treat by gene therapy is yet another ethically provocative consideration. In the Jesse Gelsinger case mentioned earlier, the symptoms of his OTC deficiency were minimized by a low protein diet and drug treatments. Whether it was necessary to treat Jesse by gene therapy and whether he should have ever been approved as a volunteer to test the safety of a gene therapy protocol are questions that have been widely debated.

Selected Readings and Resources

Journal Articles

Aiuti, A., et al. 2013. Lentiviral hematopoietic stem cell gene therapy in patients with Wiskott-Aldrich syndrome. *Science*, 341: 1233151.

Akst, J. 2012. Targeting DNA. *The Scientist*, 26: 36–42.

Baker, M. 2012. Gene-editing nucleases. *Nature Methods*, 9: 23–26.

Biffi, A., et al. 2013. Lentiviral hematopoietic stem cell gene therapy benefits metachromatic leukodystrophy. *Science*, 341: 1233158.

Carroll, D. 2011. Genome engineering with zinc-finger nucleases. *Genetics*, 188: 773–782.

Cartier, N., et al. 2009. Hematopoietic stem cell gene therapy with a lentiviral vector in X-linked adrenoleukodystrophy. *Science*, 326: 818–823.

Cavazzanna-Calvo, M., et al. 2010. Transfusion independence and HMGA2 activation after gene therapy of human β-thalassemia. *Nature* 467: 318–322.

Friedmann, T., Rabin, O., and Frankel, M. S. 2010. Gene doping and sport. *Science*, 327: 647–648.

Golic, K.G. 2013. RNA-guided nucleases: A new era for engineering the genomes of model and nonmodel organisms. *Genetics*, 195: 303–308.

Gorman, C., and Maron, D.F. 2014. The RNA revolution. *Scientific American*, 310:52–59.

Hacein-Bey-Abina, S., Von Kalle, C., Schmidt, M., et al. 2003. *LM02*-associated clonal T cell proliferation in two patients after gene therapy for SCID-X1. *Science*, 302: 415–419.

Jacobsen, S.G., et al. 2012. Gene therapy for Leber congenital amaurosis caused by *RPE65* mutations. *Arch. Ophthalmol.*, 130: 9–24.

Osborn, M.J., et al. 2013. TALEN-based gene correction for epidermolysis bullosa. *Molecular Therapy*, 21: 1151–1159.

Ousterout, D.G., et al. 2013. Reading frame correction by targeted genome editing restores dystrophin expression in cells from Duchene muscular dystrophy patients. *Molecular Therapy*, 4 June 2013; doi: 10.1038/mt.2013.111

Rossi, J.J., June, C.H., and Kohn, D.B. 2007. Genetic therapies against HIV. *Nature Biotechnology*, 25: 1444–1454.

Sheridan, C. 2011. Gene therapy finds its niche. *Nature Biotechnology*, 29: 121–128.

Wirth, T., Parker, N., and Ylä-Hertuttuala, S. 2013. History of gene therapy. *Gene*, 10: 162–169.

Yzer, S., et al. 2011. Gene-specific phenotypes and mechanism-based treatments in early-onset retinal dystrophies. *Retinal Physician*, July 2011.

Web Sites

All the Virology on the WWW. http://www.virology.net/garryfavwebgenether.html

American Society of Gene & Cell Therapy. http://www.asgct.org

Center for Gene Therapy – University of Iowa. http://genetherapy.genetics.uiowa.edu

ClinicalTrials.Gov. http://www.clinicaltrials.gov

Explore Research: American Cancer Society. http://www.cancer.org/research/index

Gene Therapy. http://www.nature.com/gt/index.html

Gene Therapy Clinical Trials Worldwide. http://www.abedia.com/wiley/index.html

Gene Therapy: Genetic Home Reference, National Library of Medicine. http://ghr.nlm.nih.gov/handbook/therapy

U.S. Food and Drug Administration: Cellular and Gene Therapy Research. http://www.fda.gov/BiologicsBloodVaccines/ScienceResearch/BiologicsResearchAreas/ucm124376.htm

Review Questions

1. What is gene therapy?
2. Compare and contrast *ex vivo* and *in vivo* gene therapy as approaches for delivering therapeutic genes.
3. When treating a person by gene therapy, is it necessary that the therapeutic gene becomes part of a chromosome (integration) when inserted into cells? Explain your answer.
4. Describe two ways that therapeutic genes can be delivered into cells.
5. Explain how viral vectors can be used for gene therapy and provide two examples of commonly used viral vectors. What are some of the major challenges that must be overcome to develop safer and more effective viral vectors for gene therapy?
6. During the first successful gene therapy trial in which Ashanti DeSilva was treated for SCID, did the therapeutic gene delivered to Ashanti replace the defective copy of the ADA gene? Why were white blood cells chosen as the targets for the therapeutic gene?
7. Explain an example of successful gene therapy trial. In your answer be sure to consider: a description of the disease condition that was treated, the mutation or disease gene affected, the therapeutic gene delivered, and the method of delivery use for the therapy.
8. What is targeted gene therapy or gene editing, and how does this approach differ from traditional gene therapy approaches?
9. How do ZFNs work?
10. Describe two gene-silencing techniques and explain how they may be used for gene therapy.

Discussion Questions

1. Discuss the challenges scientists face in making gene therapy a safe, reliable, and effective technique for treating human disease conditions.
2. Who should be treated by gene therapy? What criteria are used to determine if a person is a candidate for gene therapy?
3. Describe future challenges and ethical issues associated with gene therapy.

Should gene therapy be used for cosmetic purposes or to improve athletic performance?

Appendix A

SELECTED READINGS

Chapter 1 Introduction to Genetics

Amman, N. H. 2008. In defense of GM crops. *Science* 322: 1465–1466.

Bilen, J., and Bonini, N. M. 2005. *Drosophila* as a model for human neurodegenerative disease. *Annu. Rev. Genet.* 39: 153–171.

Chen, M., Shelton, A., and Ye, G. Y. 2011. Insect-resistant genetically-modified rice in China: From research to commercialization. *Ann. Rev. Entomol.* 56: 81–101.

Cohen, J. C., and Hobbs, H. H. 2013. Simple genetics for a complex disease. *Science* 340: 689–690.

Daya, S., and Berns, K. I. 2008. Gene therapy using adeno-associated virus vectors. *Clin. Microbiol. Rev.* 21: 83–93.

Ehrnhoefer, D. E., Butland, S. L., Pouladi, M. A., and Hayden, M. R. 2009. Mouse models of Huntington disease: Variations on a theme. *Dis. Models Mech.* 2: 123–129.

Gurdon, J. B. 2013. The egg and nucleus: A battle for supremacy. *Develop.* 140: 2449–2456.

McBride, S. M., Bell, A. J., and Jongens, T. A. 2012. Behavior in a *Drosophila* model of fragile X. *Results Probl. Cell Differ.* 54: 83–117.

Müller, B., and Grossnicklaus, U. 2010. Model organisms—A historical perspective. *J. Proteomics* 73: 2054–2063.

Pearson, H. 2006. What is a gene? *Nature* 441: 399–401.

Reid, J. B., and Ross, J. J. 2011. Mendel's genes: Toward a full molecular characterization. *Genetics* 189: 3–10.

Tiscornia, G., Vivas, E. L., and Belmonte, J. C. 2011. Diseases in a dish: Modeling human genetic disorders using induced pluripotent cells. *Nat. Med.* 17: 1570–1576.

Wisniewski, J-P., Frange, N., Massonneau, A., and Dumas, C. 2002. Between myth and reality: Genetically modified maize, an example of a sizeable scientific controversy. *Biochimie* 84: 1095–1103.

Zhao, Z., Tuakli-Wosornu, Y. Lagase, T. A., et al. 2006. Molecular characterization of loss-of-function mutations in *PCSK9* and identification of a compound heterozygote. *Am. J. Hum. Genet.* 79: 514–523.

Chapter 2 Mitosis and Meiosis

Alberts, B., et al. 2007. *Molecular biology of the cell,* 5th ed. New York: Garland Publ.

Bornens, M. 2012. The centrosome in cells and organisms. *Science* 335: 422–426.

Brachet, J., and Mirsky, A. E. 1961. *The cell: Meiosis and mitosis,* Vol. 3. Orlando, FL: Academic Press.

DuPraw, E. J. 1970. *DNA and chromosomes.* New York: Holt, Rinehart & Winston.

Glotzer, M. 2005. The molecular requirements for cytokinesis. *Science* 307: 1735–1739.

Glover, D. M., Gonzalez, C., and Raff, J. W. 1993. The centrosome. *Sci. Am.* (June) 268: 62–68.

Golomb, H. M., and Bahr, G. F. 1971. Scanning electron microscopic observations of surface structures of isolated human chromosomes. *Science* 171: 1024–1026.

Hartwell, L. H., and Karstan, M. B. 1994. Cell cycle control and cancer. *Science* 266: 1821–1828.

Hartwell, L. H., and Weinert, T. A. 1989. Checkpoint controls that ensure the order of cell cycle events. *Science* 246: 629–634.

Ishiguro, K., and Watanabe Y. 2007. Chromosome cohesion in mitosis and meiosis. *J. Cell Sci.* 120: 367–369.

Javerzat, J. P. 2010. Directing the centromere guardian. *Science* 327: 150–151.

Mazia, D. 1961. How cells divide. *Sci. Am.* (Jan.) 205: 101–120.

———. 1974. The cell cycle. *Sci. Am.* (Jan.) 235: 54–64.

McIntosh, J. R., and McDonald, K. L. 1989. The mitotic spindle. *Sci. Am.* (Oct.) 261: 48–56.

Nature Milestones. 2001. *Cell division.* London: Nature Publishing Group.

Watanabe Y. 2005. Shugoshin: Guardian spirit at the centromere. *Curr. Opin. Cell Biol.* 17: 590–595.

Westergaard, M., and von Wettstein, D. 1972. The synaptinemal complex. *Annu. Rev. Genet.* 6: 71–110.

Chapter 3 Mendelian Genetics

Bennett, R. L., et al. 1995. Recommendations for standardized human pedigree nomenclature. *Am. J. Hum. Genet.* 56: 745–752.

Carlson, E. A. 1987. *The gene: A critical history,* 2nd ed. Philadelphia: Saunders.

Dunn, L. C. 1965. *A short history of genetics.* New York: McGraw-Hill.

Henig, R. M. 2001. *The monk in the garden: The lost and found genius of Gregor Mendel, the father of genetics.* New York: Houghton Mifflin.

Kabeche, L., and Compton, D. A. 2013. Cyclin A regulates kinetechore microtubules to promote faithful chromosome segregation. *Nature* 502: 110–114.

Klein, J. 2000. Johann Mendel's field of dreams. *Genetics* 156: 1–6.

Miller, J. A. 1984. Mendel's peas: A matter of genius or of guile? *Sci. News* 125: 108–109.

Olby, R. C. 1985. *Origins of Mendelism,* 2nd ed. London: Constable.

Orel, V. 1996. *Gregor Mendel: The first geneticist.* Oxford: Oxford University Press.

Peters, J., ed. 1959. *Classic papers in genetics.* Englewood Cliffs, NJ: Prentice-Hall.

Schwartz, J. 2008. *In pursuit of the gene: From Darwin to DNA.* Cambridge, MA: Harvard University Press.

Sokal, R. R., and Rohlf, F. J. 1995. *Biometry,* 3rd ed. New York: W. H. Freeman.

Stern, C., and Sherwood, E. 1966. *The origins of genetics: A Mendel source book.* San Francisco: W. H. Freeman.

Stubbe, H. 1972. *History of genetics: From prehistoric times to the rediscovery of Mendel's laws.* Cambridge, MA: MIT Press.

Sturtevant, A. H. 1965. *A history of genetics.* New York: Harper & Row.

Tschermak-Seysenegg, E. 1951. The rediscovery of Mendel's work. *J. Hered.* 42: 163–172.

Welling, F. 1991. Historical study: Johann Gregor Mendel 1822–1884. *Am. J. Med. Genet.* 40: 1–25.

Chapter 4 Modification of Mendelian Ratios

Bartolomei, M. S., and Tilghman, S. M. 1997. Genomic imprinting in mammals. *Annu. Rev. Genet.* 31: 493–525.

Brink, R. A., ed. 1967. *Heritage from Mendel.* Madison: University of Wisconsin Press.

Bultman, S. J., Michaud, E. J., and Woychik, R. P. 1992. Molecular characterization of the mouse *agouti* locus. *Cell* 71: 1195–1204.

Carlson, E. A. 1987. *The gene: A critical history,* 2nd ed. Philadelphia: Saunders.

Cattanach, B. M., and Jones, J. 1994. Genetic imprinting in the mouse: Implications for gene regulation. *J. Inherit. Metab. Dis.* 17: 403–420.

Choman, A. 1998. The myoclonic epilepsy and ragged-red fiber mutation provides new insights into human mitochondrial function and genetics. *Am. J. Hum. Genet.* 62: 745–751.

Dunn, L. C. 1966. *A short history of genetics.* New York: McGraw-Hill.

Feil, R., and Khosla, S. 1999. Genomic imprinting in mammals: An interplay between chromatin and DNA methylation. *Trends Genet.* 15: 431.

Foster, M. 1965. Mammalian pigment genetics. *Adv. Genet.* 13: 311–339.

Grant, V. 1975. *Genetics of flowering plants.* New York: Columbia University Press.

Harper, P. S., et al. 1992. Anticipation in myotonic dystrophy: New light on an old problem. *Am. J. Hum. Genet.* 51: 10–16.

Howeler, C. J., et al. 1989. Anticipation in myotonic dystrophy: Fact or fiction? *Brain* 112: 779–797.

Larson, N. G., and Clayton, D. A. 1995. Molecular genetic aspects of human mitochondrial disorders. *Ann. Rev. Genet.* 29: 151–178.

Mitchell, M. B., and Mitchell, H. K. 1952. A case of maternal inheritance in *Neurospora crassa. Proc. Natl. Acad. Sci. (USA)* 38: 442–449.

Morgan, T. H. 1910. Sex-limited inheritance in *Drosophila. Science* 32: 120–122.

Nüsslein-Volhard. C. 1996. Gradients that organize embryo development. *Sci. Am.* (Aug.) 275: 54–61.

Peters, J. A., ed. 1959. *Classic papers in genetics.* Englewood Cliffs, NJ: Prentice-Hall.

Phillips, P. C. 1998. The language of gene interaction. *Genetics* 149: 1167–1171.

Race, R. R., and Sanger, R. 1975. *Blood groups in man,* 6th ed. Oxford: Blackwell.

Sager, R. 1985. Chloroplast genetics. *BioEssays* 3: 180–184.

Sapienza, C. 1990. Parental imprinting of genes. *Sci. Am.* (Oct.) 363: 52–60.

Siracusa, L. D. 1994. The *agouti* gene: Turned on to yellow. *Cell* 10: 423–428.

Taylor, R. W., and Turnbull, D. M., 2005. Mitochondrial DNA mutations in human disease. *Nature Reviews Genetics* 6: 389–402.

Wallace, D. C. 1997. Mitochondrial DNA in aging and disease. *Sci. Am.* (Aug.) 277: 40–59.

———. 1999. Mitochondrial diseases in man and mouse. *Science* 283: 1482–1488.

Wallace, D. C., et al. 1988. Familial mitochondrial encephalomyopathy (MERRF): Genetic, pathophysiological and biochemical characterization of a mitochondrial DNA disease. *Cell* 55: 601–610.

Yoshida, A. 1982. Biochemical genetics of the human blood group ABO system. *Am. J. Hum. Genet.* 34: 1–14.

Chapter 5 Chromosome Mapping in Eukaryotes

Allen, G. E. 1978. *Thomas Hunt Morgan: The man and his science.* Princeton, NJ: Princeton University Press.

Chaganti, R., Schonberg, S., and German, J. 1974. A manyfold increase in sister chromatid exchange in Bloom syndrome lymphocytes. *Proc. Natl. Acad. Sci.* 71: 4508–4512.

Creighton, H. S., and McClintock, B. 1931. A correlation of cytological and genetical crossing over in *Zea mays. Proc. Natl. Acad. Sci.* 17: 492–497.

Douglas, L., and Novitski, E. 1977. What chance did Mendel's experiments give him of noticing linkage? *Heredity* 38: 253–257.

Ellis, N. A., et al. 1995. The Bloom syndrome gene product is homologous to RecQ helicases. *Cell* 83: 655–666.

Ephrussi, B., and Weiss, M. C. 1969. Hybrid somatic cells. *Sci. Am.* (Apr.) 220: 26–35.

Latt, S. A. 1981. Sister chromatid exchange formation. *Annu. Rev. Genet.* 15: 11–56.

Lindsley, D. L., and Grell, E. H. 1972. *Genetic variations of Drosophila melanogaster.* Washington, DC: Carnegie Institute of Washington.

Morgan, T. H. 1911. An attempt to analyze the constitution of the chromosomes on the basis of sex-linked inheritance in *Drosophila. J. Exp. Zool.* 11: 365–414.

Morton, N. E. 1955. Sequential test for the detection of linkage. *Am. J. Hum. Genet.* 7: 277–318.

———. 1995. LODs—Past and present. *Genetics* 140: 7–12.

Neuffer, M. G., Jones, L., and Zober, M. 1968. *The mutants of maize.* Madison, WI: Crop Sci. Soc. of America.

Perkins, D. 1962. Crossing over and interference in a multiply marked chromosome arm of *Neurospora. Genetics* 47: 1253–1274.

Ruddle, F. H., and Kucherlapati, R. S. 1974. Hybrid cells and human genes. *Sci. Am.* (July) 231: 36–49.

Stahl, F. W. 1979. *Genetic recombination.* New York: W. H. Freeman.

Stern, C. 1936. Somatic crossing over and segregation in *Drosophila melanogaster. Genetics* 21: 625–631.

Sturtevant, A. H. 1913. The linear arrangement of six sex-linked factors in *Drosophila,* as shown by their mode of association. *J. Exp. Zool.* 14: 43–59.

———. 1965. *A history of genetics.* New York: Harper & Row.

Voeller, B. R., ed. 1968. *The chromosome theory of inheritance: Classical papers in development and heredity.* New York: Appleton-Century-Croft.

Wellcome Trust Case Control Consortium, 2007. Genome association study of 14,000 cases of seven common diseases and 3,000 shared controls. *Nature* 447: 661–676.

Wolff, S., ed. 1982. *Sister chromatid exchange.* New York: Wiley-Interscience.

Chapter 6 Genetic Analysis and Mapping in Bacteria and Bacteriophages

Adelberg, E. A. 1960. *Papers on bacterial genetics.* Boston: Little, Brown.

Benzer, S. 1962. The fine structure of the gene. *Sci. Am.* (Jan.) 206: 70–86.

Birge, E. A. 1988. *Bacterial and bacteriophage genetics—An introduction.* New York: Springer-Verlag.

Brock, T. 1990. *The emergence of bacterial genetics.* Cold Spring Harbor, NY: Cold Spring Harbor Press.

Bukhari, A. I., Shapiro, J. A., and Adhya, S. L., eds. 1977. *DNA insertion elements, plasmids, and episomes.* Cold Spring Harbor, NY: Cold Spring Harbor Press.

Cairns, J., Stent, G. S., and Watson, J. D., eds. 1966. *Phage and the origins of molecular biology.* Cold Spring Harbor, NY: Cold Spring Harbor Press.

Campbell, A. M. 1976. How viruses insert their DNA into the DNA of the host cell. *Sci. Am.* (Dec.) 235: 102–113.

Hayes, W. 1968. *The genetics of bacteria and their viruses,* 2nd ed. New York: Wiley.

Hershey, A. D., and Rotman, R. 1949. Genetic recombination between host range and plaque-type mutants of bacteriophage in single cells. *Genetics* 34: 44–71.

Hotchkiss, R. D., and Marmur, J. 1954. Double marker transformations as evidence of linked factors in deoxyribonucleate transforming agents. *Proc. Natl. Acad. Sci. (USA)* 40: 55–60.

Jacob, F., and Wollman, E. L. 1961. Viruses and genes. *Sci. Am.* (June) 204: 92–106.

Kohiyama, M., et al. 2003. Bacterial sex: Playing voyeurs 50 years later. *Science* 301: 802–803.

Kruse, H., and Sorum, H. 1994. Transfer of multiple drug resistance plasmids between bacteria of diverse origins in natural microenvironments. *Appl. Environ. Microbiol.* 60: 4015–4021.

Lederberg, J. 1986. Forty years of genetic recombination in bacteria: A fortieth anniversary reminiscence. *Nature* 324: 627–628.

Luria, S. E., and Delbruck, M. 1943. Mutations of bacteria from virus sensitivity to virus resistance. *Genetics* 28: 491–511.

Lwoff, A. 1953. Lysogeny. *Bacteriol. Rev.* 17: 269–337.

Miller, J. H. 1992. *A short course in bacterial genetics.* Cold Spring Harbor, NY: Cold Spring Harbor Press.

Miller, R. V. 1998. Bacterial gene swapping in nature. *Sci. Am.* (Jan.) 278: 66–71.

Morse, M. L., Lederberg, E. M., and Lederberg, J. 1956. Transduction in *Escherichia coli* K12. *Genetics* 41: 141–156.

Novick, R. P. 1980. Plasmids. *Sci. Am.* (Dec.) 243: 102–127.

Smith-Keary, P. F. 1989. *Molecular genetics of* Escherichia coli. New York: Guilford Press.

Stahl, F. W. 1987. Genetic recombination. *Sci. Am.* (Nov.) 256: 91–101.

Stent, G. S. 1966. *Papers on bacterial viruses,* 2nd ed. Boston: Little, Brown.

Waters, D. J., and Wildasin, K. 2006. Cancer clues from pet dogs. *Sci. Am.* (Dec.) 295: 96–101.

Wollman, E. L., Jacob, F., and Hayes, W. 1956. Conjugation and genetic recombination in *Escherichia coli* K12. *Cold Spring Harb. Symp. Quant. Biol.* 21. 141–162.

Yoshida, A. 1982. Biochemical genetics of the human blood group ABO system. *Am. J. Hum. Genet.* 34: 1–14.

Zinder, N. D. 1958. Transduction in bacteria. *Sci. Am.* (Nov.) 199: 38–46.

Chapter 7 Sex Determination and Sex Chromosomes

Amory, J. K., et al. 2000. Klinefelter's syndrome. *Lancet* 356: 333–335.

Arnold, A. P., Itoh, Y., and Melamed, E. 2008. A bird's-eye view of sex chromosome dosage compensation. *Annu. Rev. Genomics Hum. Genet.* 9: 109–127.

Court-Brown, W. M. 1968. Males with an XYY sex chromosome complement. *J. Med. Genet.* 5: 341–359.

Davidson, R., Nitowski, H., and Childs, B. 1963. Demonstration of two populations of cells in human females heterozygous for glucose-6-phosphate dehydrogenase variants. *Proc. Natl. Acad. Sci. (USA)* 50: 481–485.

Goriely, A., et al. 2012. Paternal age effect mutations and selfish spermatogonial selection: causes and consequences for human diseases. *Am J. Hum. Genet.* 90: 175–200.

Hashiyama, K., et al. 2011. *Drosophila* sex lethal gene initiates female development in germline progenitors. *Science* 333: 885–888.

Hawley, R. S. 2011. Hitting a tiny target in the dark. *Science* 331: 870–871.

Hodgkin, J. 1990. Sex determination compared in *Drosophila* and *Caenorhabditis. Nature* 344: 721–728.

Hook, E. B. 1973. Behavioral implications of the humans XYY genotype. *Science* 179: 139–150.

Hughes, J. F., et al. 2010. Chimpanzee and human Y chromosomes are remarkably divergent in structure and gene content. *Nature* 463: 536–539.

Hughes, J. F., and Rozen, S. 2012. Genomics and genetics of human and primate Y chromosomes. *Ann. Rev. Genom. Hum. Genet.* 13: 83–108.

Irish, E. E. 1996. Regulation of sex determination in maize. *BioEssays* 18: 363–369.

Jacobs, P. A., et al. 1974. A cytogenetic survey of 11,680 newborn infants. *Ann. Hum. Genet.* 37: 359–376.

Jegalian, K., and Lahn, B. T. 2001. Why the Y is so weird. *Sci. Am.* (Feb.) 284: 56–61.

Kauppi, L., et al. 2011. Distinct properties of the XY pseudoautosomal region crucial for male meiosis. *Science* 331: 916–920.

Koopman, P., et al. 1991. Male development of chromosomally female mice transgenic for *Sry. Nature* 351: 117–121.

Lahn, B. T., and Page, D. C. 1997. Functional coherence of the human Y chromosome. *Science* 278: 675–680.

Lucchesi, J. 1983. The relationship between gene dosage, gene expression, and sex in *Drosophila. Dev. Genet.* 3: 275–282.

Lyon, M. F. 1972. X-chromosome inactivation and developmental patterns in mammals. *Biol. Rev.* 47: 1–35.

Marshall Graves, J. A. 2009. Birds do it with a Z gene. *Nature* 461: 177–178.

McMillen, M. M. 1979. Differential mortality by sex in fetal and neonatal deaths. *Science* 204: 89–91.

Ng, K., Pullirsch, D., Leeb, M., and Wutz, A. 2007. Xist and the order of silencing. *EMBO Reports* 8: 34–39.

Nora, E. P., and Heard, E. 2009. X chromosome inactivation: When dosage counts. *Cell* 139: 865–868.

Penny, G. D., et al. 1996. Requirement for Xist in X chromosome inactivation. *Nature* 379: 131–137.

Pieau, C. 1996. Temperature variation and sex determination in reptiles. *BioEssays* 18: 19–26.

Quinn, A. E., et al. 2007. Temperature sex reversal implies sex gene dosage in a reptile. *Science* 316: 411.

Smith, C. A., et al. 2009. The avian Z-linked gene DMRT1 is required for male sex determination in the chicken. *Nature* 461: 267–270.

Stochholm, K., et al. 2012. Criminality in men with Klinefelter's syndrome and XYY syndrome: A cohort study. *BMJ Open* 2: 1–8.

Straub, T., and Becker, P. B. 2007. Dosage compensation: The beginning and end of a generalization. *Nat. Rev. Genet.* 8: 47–57.

Warner, D. A., and Shine, R. 2008. The adaptive significance of temperature-dependent sex determination in a reptile. *Nature* 451: 566–567.

Westergaard, M. 1958. The mechanism of sex determination in dioecious flowering plants. *Adv. Genet.* 9: 217–281.

Whitelaw, E. 2006. Unravelling the X in sex. *Dev. Cell* 11: 759–762.

Witkin, H. A., et al. 1996. Criminality in XYY and XXY men. *Science* 193: 547–555.

Xu, N., Tsai, C-L., and Lee, J. T. 2006. Transient homologous chromosome pairing marks the onset of X inactivation. *Science* 311: 1149–1152.

Chapter 8 Chromosome Mutations: Variation in Number and Arrangement

Antonarakis, S. E. 1998. Ten years of genomics, chromosome 21, and Down syndrome. *Genomics* 51: 1–16.

Ashley-Koch, A. E., et al. 1997. Examination of factors associated with instability of the *FMR1* CGG repeat. *Am. J. Hum. Genet.* 63: 776–785.

Beasley, J. O. 1942. Meiotic chromosome behavior in species, species hybrids, haploids, and induced polyploids of *Gossypium*. *Genetics* 27: 25–54.

Blakeslee, A. F. 1934. New jimson weeds from old chromosomes. *J. Hered.* 25: 80–108.

Boue, A. 1985. Cytogenetics of pregnancy wastage. *Adv. Hum. Genet.* 14: 1–58.

Carr, D. H. 1971. Genetic basis of abortion. *Ann. Rev. Genet.* 5: 65–80.

Conrad, D. F., et al. 2010. Origins and functional impact of copy number variation in the human genome. *Nature* 464: 704–710.

Croce, C. M. 1996. The *FHIT* gene at 3p14.2 is abnormal in lung cancer. *Cell* 85: 17–26.

DeArce, M. A., and Kearns, A. 1984. The fragile X syndrome: The patients and their chromosomes. *J. Med. Genet.* 21: 84–91.

Epstein, C. J. 2006. Down's syndrome: Critical genes in a critical region. *Nature* 441: 582–583.

Feldman, M., and Sears, E. R. 1981. The wild gene resources of wheat. *Sci. Am.* (Jan.) 244: 102–112.

Galitski, T., et al. 1999. Ploidy regulation of gene expression. *Science* 285: 251–254.

Gersh, M., et al. 1995. Evidence for a distinct region causing a catlike cry in patients with 5p deletions. *Am. J. Hum. Genet.* 56: 1404–1410.

Hassold, T. J., et al. 1980. Effect of maternal age on autosomal trisomies. *Ann. Hum. Genet.* (London) 44: 29–36.

Hassold, T. J., and Hunt, P. 2001. To err (meiotically) is human: The genesis of human aneuploidy. *Nat. Rev. Gen.* 2: 280–291.

Hassold, T., and Jacobs, P. A. 1984. Trisomy in man. *Annu. Rev. Genet.* 18: 69–98.

Hecht, F. 1988. Enigmatic fragile sites on human chromosomes. *Trends Genet.* 4: 121–122.

Hulse, J. H., and Spurgeon, D. 1974. *Triticale. Sci. Am.* (Aug.) 231: 72–81.

Kaiser, P. 1984. Pericentric inversions: Problems and significance for clinical genetics. *Hum. Genet.* 68: 1–47.

Lewis, E. B. 1950. The phenomenon of position effect. *Adv. Genet.* 3: 73–115.

Lewis, W. H., ed. 1980. *Polyploidy: Biological relevance.* New York: Plenum Press.

Lynch, M., and Conery, J. S. 2000. The evolutionary fate and consequences of duplicate genes. *Science* 290: 1151–1154.

Madan, K. 1995. Paracentric inversions: A review. *Hum. Genet.* 96: 503–515.

Nelson, D. L., and Gibbs, R. A. 2004. The critical region in trisomy 21. *Science* 306: 619–621.

Ohno, S. 1970. *Evolution by gene duplication.* New York: Springer-Verlag.

Oostra, B. A., and Verkerk, A. J. 1992. The fragile X syndrome: Isolation of the *FMR-1* gene and characterization of the fragile X mutation. *Chromosoma* 101: 381–387.

Patterson, D. 1987. The causes of Down syndrome. *Sci. Am.* (Aug.) 257: 52–61.

Patterson, D., and Costa, A. 2005. Down syndrome and genetics—A case of linked histories. *Nature Reviews Genetics* 6: 137–145.

Shepard, J., et al. 1983. Genetic transfer in plants through interspecific protoplast fusion. *Science* 21: 683–688.

Shepard, J. F. 1982. The regeneration of potato plants from protoplasts. *Sci. Am.* (May) 246: 154–166.

Stranger, B. E., et al. 2007. Relative impact of nucleotide and copy number variation on gene expression phenotypes. *Science* 315: 848–854.

Taylor, A. I. 1968. Autosomal trisomy syndromes: A detailed study of 27 cases of Edwards syndrome and 27 cases of Patau syndrome. *J. Med. Genet.* 5: 227–252.

Tjio, J. H., and Levan, A. 1956. The chromosome number of man. *Hereditas* 42: 1–6.

Wilkins, L. E., Brown, J. X., and Wolf, B. 1980. Psychomotor development in 65 home-reared children with cri-du-chat syndrome. *J. Pediatr.* 97: 401–405.

Chapter 9 Extranuclear Inheritance

Adams, K. L., et al. 2000. Repeated, recent and diverse transfers of a mitochondrial gene to the nucleus in flowering plants. *Nature* 408: 354–357.

Choman, A. 1998. The myoclonic epilepsy and ragged-red fiber mutation provides new insights into human mitochondrial function and genetics. *Am. J. Hum. Genet.* 62: 745–751.

Freeman, G., and Lundelius, J. W. 1982. The developmental genetics of dextrality and sinistrality in the gastropod *Lymnaea peregra. Wilhelm Roux Arch.* 191: 69–83.

Gray, M. W., Burger, G., and Lang, B. 1999. Mitochondrial evolution. *Science* 283: 1476–1481.

Green, B. R., and Burton, H. 1970. *Acetabularia* chloroplast DNA: Electron microscopic visualization. *Science* 168: 981–982.

Grivell, L. A. 1983. Mitochondrial DNA. *Sci. Am.* (Mar.) 248: 78–89.

He, Y., et al. 2010. Heteroplasmic mitochondrial DNA mutations in normal and tumour cells. *Nature* 464: 610–614.

Hiendleder, S. 2007. Mitochondrial DNA inheritance after SCNT. *Adv. Exp. Med Biol.* 591: 103–116.

Ishikawa, K. 2008. ROS-generating mitochondrial DNA mutations can regulate tumor cell metastasis. *Science* 320: 661–664.

Kuroda, R., et al. (2009). Chiral blastomere arrangement dictates zygotic left-right asymmetry pathway in snails. *Science* 462: 790–794.

Larson, N. G., and Clayton, D. A. 1995. Molecular genetic aspects of human mitochondrial disorders. *Ann. Rev. Genet.* 29: 151–178.

Margulis, L. 1970. *Origin of eukaryotic cells.* New Haven, CT: Yale University Press.

Mitchell, M. B., and Mitchell, H. K. 1952. A case of maternal inheritance in *Neurospora crassa. Proc. Natl. Acad. Sci. (USA)* 38: 442–449.

Nüsslein-Volhard, C. 1996. Gradients that organize embryo development. *Sci. Am.* (Aug.) 275: 54–61.

Preer, J. R. 1971. Extrachromosomal inheritance: Hereditary symbionts, mitochondria, chloroplasts. *Annu. Rev. Genet.* 5: 361–406.

Sager, R. 1965. Genes outside the chromosomes. *Sci. Am.* (Jan.) 212: 70–79.

———. 1985. Chloroplast genetics. *BioEssays* 3: 180–184.

Schwartz, R. M., and Dayhoff, M. O. 1978. Origins of prokaryotes, eukaryotes, mitochondria and chloroplasts. *Science* 199: 395–403.

Sonneborn, T. M. 1959. Kappa and related particles in *Paramecium. Adv. Virus Res.* 6: 229–256.

Sturtevant, A. H. 1923. Inheritance of the direction of coiling in *Limnaea. Science* 58: 269–270.

Tachibana, M., et al. 2009. Mitochondrial gene replacement in primate offspring and embryonic stem cells. *Nature* 461: 367–372.

Taylor, R. W., and Turnbull, D. M., 2005. Mitochondrial DNA mutations in human disease. *Nature Reviews Genetics* 6: 389–402.

Vafai, S. B., and Mootha, V. K. 2012. Mitochondrial disorders as windows into an ancient organelle. *Nature* 491: 374–383.

Wallace, D. C. 1997. Mitochondrial DNA in aging and disease. *Sci. Am.* (Aug.) 277: 40–59.

———. 1999. Mitochondrial diseases in man and mouse. *Science* 283: 1482–1488.

Chapter 10 DNA Structure and Analysis

Adleman, L. M. 1998. Computing with DNA. *Sci. Am.* (Aug.) 279: 54–61.

Alloway, J. L. 1933. Further observations on the use of pneumococcus extracts in effecting transformation of type *in vitro. J. Exp. Med.* 57: 265–278.

Avery, O. T., MacLeod, C. M., and McCarty, M. 1944. Studies on the chemical nature of the substance inducing transformation of pneumococcal types: Induction of transformation by a desoxyribonucleic acid fraction isolated from pneumococcus type III. *J. Exp. Med.* 79: 137–158. (Reprinted in Taylor, J. H. 1965. *Selected papers in molecular genetics.* Orlando, FL: Academic Press.)

Britten, R. J., and Kohne, D. E. 1968. Repeated sequences in DNA. *Science* 161: 529–540.

Chargaff, E. 1950. Chemical specificity of nucleic acids and mechanism for their enzymatic degradation. *Experientia* 6: 201–209.

Darnell, J. E. 1985. RNA. *Sci. Am.* (Oct.) 253: 68–87.

Dawson, M. H. 1930. The transformation of pneumococcal types: I. The interconvertibility of type-specific *S. pneumococci. J. Exp. Med.* 51: 123–147.

Dickerson, R. E., et al. 1982. The anatomy of A-, B-, and Z-DNA. *Science* 216: 475–485.

Dubos, R. J. 1976. *The professor, the Institute and DNA: Oswald T. Avery, his life and scientific achievements.* New York: Rockefeller University Press.

Felsenfeld, G. 1985. DNA. *Sci. Am.* (Oct.) 253: 58–78.

Franklin, R. E., and Gosling, R. G. 1953. Molecular configuration in sodium thymonucleate. *Nature* 171: 740–741.

Griffith, F. 1928. The significance of pneumococcal types. *J. Hyg.* 27: 113–159.

Guthrie, G. D., and Sinsheimer, R. L. 1960. Infection of protoplasts of *Escherichia coli* by subviral particles. *J. Mol. Biol.* 2: 297–305.

Hershey, A. D., and Chase, M. 1952. Independent functions of viral protein and nucleic acid in growth of bacteriophage. *J. Gen. Phys.* 36: 39–56. (Reprinted in Taylor, J. H. 1965. *Selected papers in molecular genetics.* Orlando, FL: Academic Press.)

Levene, P. A., and Simms, H. S. 1926. Nucleic acid structure as determined by electrometric titration data. *J. Biol. Chem.* 70: 327–341.

McCarty, M. 1985. *The transforming principle. Discovering that genes are made of DNA.* New York: W. W. Norton.

Olby, R. 1974. *The path to the double helix.* Seattle: University of Washington Press.

Pauling, L., and Corey, R. B. 1953. A proposed structure for the nucleic acids. *Proc. Natl. Acad. Sci. (USA)* 39: 84–97.

Rich, A., Nordheim, A., and Wang, A. H.-J. 1984. The chemistry and biology of left-handed Z-DNA. *Annu. Rev. Biochem.* 53: 791–846.

Spizizen, J. 1957. Infection of protoplasts by disrupted T2 viruses. *Proc. Natl. Acad. Sci. (USA)* 43: 694–701.

Varmus, H. 1988. Retroviruses. *Science* 240: 1427–1435.

Watson, J. D. 1968. *The double helix.* New York: Atheneum.

Watson, J. D., and Crick, F. C. 1953a. Molecular structure of nucleic acids: A structure for deoxyribose nucleic acids. *Nature* 171: 737–738.

———. 1953b. Genetic implications of the structure of deoxyribose nucleic acid. *Nature* 171: 964.

Wilkins, M. H. F., Stokes, A. R., and Wilson, H. R. 1953. Molecular structure of desoxypentose nucleic acids. *Nature* 171: 738–740.

Chapter 11 DNA Replication and Recombination

Blackburn, E. H. 1991. Structure and function of telomeres. *Nature* 350: 569–572.

DeLucia, P., and Cairns, J. 1969. Isolation of an *E. coli* strain with a mutation affecting DNA polymerase. *Nature* 224: 1164–1166.

Gilbert, D. M. 2001. Making sense of eukaryotic DNA replication origins. *Science* 294: 96–100.

Holliday, R. 1964. A mechanism for gene conversion in fungi. *Genet. Res.* 5: 282–304.

Holmes, F. L. 2001. *Meselson, Stahl, and replication of DNA: A history of the "most beautiful experiment in biology."* New Haven, CT: Yale University Press.

Kornberg, A. 1960. Biological synthesis of DNA. *Science* 131: 1503–1508.

Kornberg, A., and Baker, T. 1992. *DNA replication,* 2nd ed. New York: W. H. Freeman.

Krejci, L., et al. 2012. Homologous recombination and its regulation. *Nucleic Acids Res.* 40: 5795–5818.

Krogh, B. O., and Symington, L. S. 2004. Recombination proteins in yeast. *Annu. Rev. Genet.* 38: 233–271.

Leman, A. R., and Noguchi, E. 2013. The replication fork: Understanding the eukaryotic replication machinery and the challenges to genome duplication. *Genes (Basel)* 4: 1–32.

Luke, B., and Linguer, J. 2009. TERRA: Telomere repeat-containing RNA. *EMBO J.* 28: 2503–2510.

Meselson, M., and Stahl, F. W. 1958. The replication of DNA in *Escherichia coli. Proc. Natl. Acad. Sci. (USA)* 44: 671–682.

Okazaki, T., et al. 1979. Structure and metabolism of the RNA primer in the discontinuous replication of prokaryotic DNA. *Cold Spring Harbor Symp. Quant. Biol.* 43: 203–222.

Radman, M., and Wagner, R. 1988. The high fidelity of DNA duplication. *Sci. Am.* (Aug.) 259: 40–46.

———. 1987. Genetic recombination. *Sci. Am.* (Feb.) 256: 90–101.

Redon, S., et al. 2010. The noncoding RNA TERRA is a natural ligand of human telomerase. *Nucleic Acid Res.* 38: 5797–5806.

Shay, J. W., and Wright, W. E. 2011. Role of telomeres and telomerase in cancer. *Semin. Cancer Biol.* 21: 349–353.

Takeda, D. Y., and Dutta, A. 2005. DNA replication and progression through S phase. *Oncogene* 24: 2827–2843.

Taylor, J. H., Woods, P. S., and Hughes, W. C. 1957. The organization and duplication of chromosomes revealed by autoradiographic studies using tritium-labeled thymidine. *Proc. Natl. Acad. Sci. (USA)* 48: 122–128.

Wang, J. C. 1987. Recent studies of DNA topoisomerases. *Biochim. Biophys. Acta* 909: 1–9.

Whitehouse, H. L. K. 1982. *Genetic recombination: Understanding the mechanisms.* New York: Wiley.

Chapter 12 Chromosome Structure and DNA Sequence Organization

Angelier, N., et al. 1984. Scanning electron microscopy of amphibian lampbrush chromosomes. *Chromosoma* 89: 243–253.

Beerman, W., and Clever, U. 1964. Chromosome puffs. *Sci. Am.* (Apr.) 210: 50–58.

Carbon, J. 1984. Yeast centromeres: Structure and function. *Cell* 37: 352–353.

Chen, T. R., and Ruddle, F. H. 1971. Karyotype analysis utilizing differential stained constitutive heterochromatin of human and murine chromosomes. *Chromosoma* 34: 51–72.

DuPraw, E. J. 1970. *DNA and chromosomes.* New York: Holt, Rinehart & Winston.

Gall, J. G. 1981. Chromosome structure and the *C*-value paradox. *J. Cell Biol.* 91: 3s–14s.

Hewish, D. R., and Burgoyne, L. 1973. Chromatin substructure. The digestion of chromatin DNA at regularly spaced sites by a nuclear deoxyribonuclease. *Biochem. Biophys. Res. Comm.* 52: 504–510.

Korenberg, J. R., and Rykowski, M. C. 1988. Human genome organization: *Alu,* LINES, and the molecular organization of metaphase chromosome bands. *Cell* 53: 391–400.

Kornberg, R. D. 1975. Chromatin structure: A repeating unit of histones and DNA. *Science* 184: 868–871.

Kornberg, R. D., and Klug, A. 1981. The nucleosome. *Sci. Am.* (Feb.) 244: 52–64.

Krogh, B. O., and Symington, L. S. 2004. Recombination proteins in yeast. *Annu Rev Genet* 38: 233–271.

Lorch, Y., et al. 2006. Chromatin remodeling by nucleosome disassembly *in vitro. Proc. Nat. Acad. Sci.* 103: 3090–3093.

Luger, K., et al. 1997. Crystal structure of the nucleosome core particle at 2.8 resolution. *Nature* 389: 251–256.

Moyzis, R. K. 1991. The human telomere. *Sci. Am.* (Aug.) 265: 48–55.

Olins, A. L., and Olins, D. E. 1974. Spheroid chromatin units (*v* bodies). *Science* 183: 330–332.

———. 1978. Nucleosomes: The structural quantum in chromosomes. *Am. Sci.* 66: 704–711.

Singer, M. F. 1982. SINES and LINES: Highly repeated short and long interspersed sequences in mammalian genomes. *Cell* 28: 433–434.

Takeda, D. Y., and Dutta, A. 2005. DNA replication and progression through S phase. *Oncogene* 24: 2827–2843.

Chapter 13 The Genetic Code and Transcription

Barrell, B. G., Air, G., and Hutchinson, C. 1976. Overlapping genes in bacteriophage φX174 *Nature* 264: 34–40.

Barrell, B. G., Banker, A. T., and Drouin, J. 1979. A different genetic code in human mitochondria. *Nature* 282: 189–194.

Bass, B. L., ed. 2000. *RNA editing.* Oxford: Oxford University Press.

Brenner, S., Jacob, F., and Meselson, M. 1961. An unstable intermediate carrying information from genes to ribosomes for protein synthesis. *Nature* 190: 575–580.

Brenner, S., Stretton, A. O. W., and Kaplan, D. 1965. Genetic code: The nonsense triplets for chain termination and their suppression. *Nature* 206: 994–998.

Cattaneo, R. 1991. Different types of messenger RNA editing. *Annu. Rev. Genet.* 25: 71–88.

Cech, T. R. 1986. RNA as an enzyme. *Sci. Am.* (Nov.) 255(5): 64–75.

———. 1987. The chemistry of self-splicing RNA and RNA enzymes. *Science* 236: 1532–1539.

Chambon, P. 1981. Split genes. *Sci. Am.* (May) 244: 60–71.

Cramer, P., et al. 2000. Architecture of RNA polymerase II and implications for the transcription mechanism. *Science* 288: 640–649.

Crick, F. H. C. 1962. The genetic code. *Sci. Am.* (Oct.) 207: 66–77.

———. 1966a. The genetic code: III. *Sci. Am.* (Oct.) 215: 55–63.

———. 1966b. Codon–anticodon pairing: The wobble hypothesis. *J. Mol. Biol.* 19: 548–555.

Crick, F. H. C., Barnett, L., Brenner, S., and Watts-Tobin, R. J. 1961. General nature of the genetic code for proteins. *Nature* 192: 1227–1232.

Darnell, J. E. 1983. The processing of RNA. *Sci. Am.* (Oct.) 249: 90–100.

Dickerson, R. E. 1983. The DNA helix and how it is read. *Sci. Am.* (Dec.) 249: 94–111.

Dugaiczk, A., et al. 1978. The natural ovalbumin gene contains seven intervening sequences. *Nature* 274: 328–333.

Fiers, W., et al. 1976. Complete nucleotide sequence of bacteriophage MS2 RNA: Primary and secondary structure of the replicase gene. *Nature* 260: 500–507.

Gamow, G. 1954. Possible relation between DNA and protein structures. *Nature* 173: 318.

Hall, B. D., and Spiegelman, S. 1961. Sequence complementarity of T2-DNA and T2-specific RNA. *Proc. Natl. Acad. Sci. (USA)* 47: 137–146.

Hamkalo, B. 1985. Visualizing transcription in chromosomes. *Trends Genet.* 1: 255–260.

Khorana, H. G. 1967. Polynucleotide synthesis and the genetic code. *Harvey Lectures* 62: 79–105.

Makalowska, I., et al. 2005. Overlapping genes in vertebrate genomes. *Comput. Biol. Chem.* 29: 1–12.

Miller, O. L., Hamkalo, B., and Thomas, C. 1970. Visualization of bacterial genes in action. *Science* 169: 392–395.

Nirenberg, M. W. 1963. The genetic code: II. *Sci. Am.* (Mar.) 190: 80–94.

O'Malley, B., et al. 1979. A comparison of the sequence organization of the chicken ovalbumin and ovomucoid genes. In *Eucaryotic gene regulation*, R. Axel et al., eds., pp. 281–299. Orlando, FL: Academic Press.

Reed, R., and Maniatis, T. 1985. Intron sequences involved in lariat formation during pre-mRNA splicing. *Cell* 41: 95–105.

Rhee, H. S., and Pugh, B. F. 2012. Genome-wide structure and organization of eukaryotic pre-initiation complexes. *Nature* 483: 295–301.

Ridley, M., 2006. *Francis Crick: Discoverer of the genetic code.* New York: HarperCollins.

Roberts, J. W. 2006. RNA polymerase: A scrunching machine. *Science* 314: 1097–1098.

Sharp, P. A. 1994. Nobel lecture: Split genes and RNA splicing. *Cell* 77: 805–815.

Steitz, J. A. 1988. Snurps. *Sci. Am.* (June) 258(6): 56–63.

Volkin, E., and Astrachan, L. 1956. Phosphorus incorporation in E. coli ribonucleic acids after infection with bacteriophage T2. *Virology* 2: 149–161.

Watson, J. D. 1963. Involvement of RNA in the synthesis of proteins. *Science* 140: 17–26.

Woychik, N. A., and Jampsey, M. 2002. The RNA polymerase II machinery: Structure illuminates function. *Cell* 108: 453–464.

Chapter 14 Translation and Proteins

Anfinsen, C. B. 1973. Principles that govern the folding of protein chains. *Science* 181: 223–230.

Atkins, J. F., and Baranov, P. V. 2007. Duality in the genetic code. *Nature* 448. 1004–1005.

Bartholome, K. 1979. Genetics and biochemistry of phenylketonuria—Present state. *Hum. Genet.* 51: 241–245.

Beadle, G. W., and Tatum, E. L. 1941. Genetic control of biochemical reactions in *Neurospora*. *Proc. Natl. Acad. Sci. (USA)* 27: 499–506.

Beet, E. A. 1949. The genetics of the sickle-cell trait in a Bantu tribe. *Ann. Eugenics* 14: 279–284.

Ben-Sham, A. 2010. Crystal structure of the eukaryotic ribosome. *Science* 330: 1203–1208.

Brenner, S. 1955. Tryptophan biosynthesis in *Salmonella typhimurium*. *Proc. Natl. Acad. Sci. (USA)* 41: 862–863.

Doolittle, R. F. 1985. Proteins. *Sci. Am.* (Oct.) 253: 88–99.

Fischer, N., et al. 2010. Ribosome dynamics and tRNA movement by time-resolved electron cryomicroscopy. *Nature* 466: 329–336.

Frank, J. 1998. How the ribosome works. *Amer. Scient.* 86: 428–439.

Garrod, A. E. 1902. The incidence of alkaptonuria: A study in chemical individuality. *Lancet* 2: 1616–1620.

———. 1909. *Inborn errors of metabolism.* London: Oxford University Press. (Reprinted 1963, Oxford University Press, London.)

Garrod, S. C. 1989. Family influences on A. E. Garrod's thinking. *J. Inher. Metab. Dis.* 12: 2–8.

Ingram, V. M. 1957. Gene mutations in human hemoglobin: The chemical difference between normal and sickle-cell hemoglobin. *Nature* 180: 326–328.

Koshland, D. E. 1973. Protein shape and control. *Sci. Am.* (Oct.) 229: 52–64.

Lake, J. A. 1981. The ribosome. *Sci. Am.* (Aug.) 245: 84–97.

Lomakin, I. B., and Steitz, T. A. 2013. The initiation of mammalian protein synthesis and mRNA scanning mechanism. *Nature* 500: 307–311.

Maniatis, T., et al. 1980. The molecular genetics of human hemoglobins. *Annu. Rev. Genet.* 14: 145–178.

Neel, J. V. 1949. The inheritance of sickle-cell anemia. *Science* 110: 64–66.

Nirenberg, M. W., and Leder, P. 1964. RNA codewords and protein synthesis. *Science* 145: 1399–1407.

Nomura, M. 1984. The control of ribosome synthesis. *Sci. Am.* (Jan.) 250: 102–114.

Pauling, L., Itano, H. A., Singer, S. J., and Wells, I. C. 1949. Sickle-cell anemia: A molecular disease. *Science* 110: 543–548.

Ramakrishnan, V. 2002. Ribosome structure and the mechanism of translation. *Cell* 108: 557–572.

Rich, A., and Houkim, S. 1978. The three-dimensional structure of transfer RNA. *Sci. Am.* (Jan.) 238: 52–62.

Rich, A., Warner, J. R., and Goodman, H. M. 1963. The structure and function of polyribosomes. *Cold Spring Harbor Symp. Quant. Biol.* 28: 269–285.

Richards, F. M. 1991. The protein-folding problem. *Sci. Am.* (Jan.) 264: 54–63.

Rould, M. A., et al. 1989. Structure of *E. coli* glutaminyl-tRNA synthetase complexed with tRNA^{Gln} and ATP at 2.8 resolution. *Science* 246: 1135–1142.

Srb, A. M., and Horowitz, N. H. 1944. The ornithine cycle in *Neurospora* and its genetic control. *J. Biol. Chem.* 154: 129–139.

Warner, J., and Rich, A. 1964. The number of soluble RNA molecules on reticulocyte polyribosomes. *Proc. Natl. Acad. Sci. (USA)* 51: 1134–1141.

Wimberly, B. T., et al. 2000. Structure of the 30S ribosomal subunit. *Nature* 407: 327–333.

Yuan, J., et al. 2010. Distinct genetic code expansion strategies for selenocysteine and pyrrolysine are reflected in different aminoacyl-tRNA formation systems. *FEBS Lett*: 584: 342–349.

Yusupov, M. M., et al. 2001. Crystal structure of the ribosome at 5.5A resolution. *Science* 292: 883–896.

Chapter 15 Gene Mutation and DNA Repair

Arnheim, N., and Calabrese, P. 2009. Understanding what determines the frequency and pattern of human germline mutations. *Nature Rev. Genetics* 10: 478–488.

Cairns, J., Overbaugh, J., and Miller, S. 1988. The origin of mutants. *Nature* 335: 142–145.

Cleaver, J. E. 2005. Cancer in xeroderma pigmentosum and related disorders of DNA repair. *Nature Reviews Cancer* 5: 564–571.

Comfort, N. C. 2001. *The tangled field: Barbara McClintock's search for the patterns of genetic control.* Cambridge, MA: Harvard University Press.

Jiricny, J. 1998. Eukaryotic mismatch repair: An update. *Mutation Research* 409: 107–121.

Luria, S. E., and Delbrück, M. (1943). Mutations of bacteria from virus sensitivity to virus resistance. *Genetics* 28(6): 491–511.

Mirkin, S. M. 2007. Expandable DNA repeats and human disease. *Nature* 447: 932–940.

Mortelmans, K., and Zeigler, E. 2000. The Ames *Salmonella/microsome* mutagenicity assay. *Mutation Research* 455: 29–60.

O'Driscoll, M., and Jeggo, P. A. 2006. The role of double-strand break repair—insights from human genetics. *Nature Reviews Genetics* 7: 45–51.

O'Hare, K. 1985. The mechanism and control of *P* element transposition in *Drosophila. Trends Genet.* 1: 250–254.

Ortega-Recalde, O., et al. 2013. Whole-exome sequencing enables rapid determination of xeroderma pigmentosum molecular etiology. *PLOS One* 8: e64692.

Rosenberg, S. M. 2001. Evolving responsively: adaptive mutation. *Nature Rev. Genetics* 2: 504–515.

Chapter 16 Regulation of Gene Expression in Prokaryotes

Antson, A. A., et al. 1999. Structure of the trp RNA-binding attenuation protein, TRAP, bound to RNA. *Nature* 401: 235–242.

Beckwith, J. R., and Zipser, D., eds. 1970. *The lactose operon.* Cold Spring Harbor, NY: Cold Spring Harbor Laboratory Press.

Bertrand, K., et al. 1975. New features of the regulation of the tryptophan operon. *Science* 189: 22–26.

Breaker, Ronald R. 2008. Complex riboswitches. *Science* 319: 1795–1797.

Gilbert, W., and Müller-Hill, B. 1966. Isolation of the *lac* repressor. *Proc. Natl. Acad. Sci. (USA)* 56: 1891–1898.

———. 1967. The *lac* operator is DNA. *Proc. Natl. Acad. Sci. (USA)* 58: 2415–2421.

Jacob, F., and Monod, J. 1961. Genetic regulatory mechanisms in the synthesis of proteins. *J. Mol. Biol.* 3: 318–356.

Lewis, M., et al. 1996. Crystal structure of the lactose operon repressor and its complexes with DNA and inducer. *Science* 271: 1247–1254.

Maumita, M., et al. 2003. Riboswitches control fundamental biochemical pathways in *Bacillus subtilis* and other bacteria. *Cell* 113: 577–586.

Serganov, A. 2009. The long and the short of riboswitches. *Curr Opin Struct Biol.* 19: 251–259.

Stroynowski, I., and Yanofsky, C. 1982. Transcript secondary structures regulate transcription termination at the attenuator of *S. marcescens* tryptophan operon. *Nature* 298: 34–38.

Valbuzzi, A., and Yanofsky, C. 2001. Inhibition of the *B. subtilis*regulatory protein TRAP by the TRAP-inhibitory protein, AT. *Science* 293: 2057–2061.

Yanofsky, C. 1981. Attenuation in the control of expression of bacterial operons. *Nature* 289: 751–758.

Chapter 17 Regulation of Gene Expression in Eukaryotes

Alt, F. W., et al. 1987. Development of the primary antibody repertoire. *Science* 238: 1079–1087.

Becker, P. B., and Hörz, W. 2002. ATP-dependent nucleosome remodeling. *Annu. Rev. Biochem.* 71: 247–273.

Black, D. L. 2003. Mechanisms of alternative pre-mRNA splicing. *Annu. Rev. Biochem.* 72: 291–336.

Bumcrot, D., et al. 2006. RNAi therapeutics: a potential new class of pharmaceutical drugs. *Nature Chemical Biology* 2: 711–718.

Ecker, J. R., et al. 2012. ENCODE explained. *Nature* 489: 52–55.

Henikoff, S. 2008. Nucleosome destabilization in the epigenetic regulation of gene expression. *Nature Reviews Genetics* 9: 15–20.

Juven-Gershon, T., and Kadonaga, J. T. 2009. Regulation of gene expression via the core promoter and the basal transcriptional machinery. *Dev. Biol.* 339: 225–229.

Licatalosi, D. D., and Darnell, R. B. 2010. RNA processing and its regulation: global insights into biological networks. *Nature Rev. Genetics* 11: 75–87.

Mello, C. C., and Conte, D., Jr. 2004. Revealing the world of RNA interference. *Nature* 431: 338–342.

Newbury, S. F. 2006. Control of mRNA stability in eukaryotes. *Biochem. Soc. Trans.* 34: 30–34.

Pennacchio, L. A., et al. 2013. Enhancers: Five essential questions. *Nature Rev. Genet.* 14: 288–295.

Rana, T. M. 2007. Illuminating the silence: understanding the structure and function of small RNAs. *Nature Mol. Cell Biol.* 8: 23–34.

Weintraub, H., and Groudine, M. 1976. Chromosomal subunits in active genes have an altered conformation. *Science* 193: 848–856.

Wheeler, T. M., and Thornton, C. A. 2007. Myotonic dystrophy: RNA-mediated muscle disease. *Curr. Opin. Neurol.* 20: 572–576.

Chapter 18 Developmental Genetics

Anderson, E. R., Sandberg, R., and Lendahl, U. 2011. Notch signaling: Simplicity in design, versatility in function. *Development* 138: 3593–3612.

Davidson, E. H., and Levine, M. S. 2008. Properties of developmental gene regulatory networks. *Proc. Nat. Acad. Sci.* 115: 20063–20066.

De Leon, S. B-T., and Davidson, E. H. 2007. Gene regulation: Gene control networks in development. *Annu. Rev. Biophys. Biomol. Struct.* 36: 191–212.

Eklund, E. 2011. The role of Hox proteins in leukemogenesis: insights into key regulatory events in hematopoiesis. *Crit. Rev. Oncol.* 16: 65–76.

Feng, S., Jacobsen, S. E., and Reik, W. 2010. Epigenetic reprogramming in plant and animal development. *Science* 330: 622–627.

Goodman, F. 2002. Limb malformations and the human *HOX* genes. *Am. J. Med. Genet.* 112: 256–265.

Gramzow, L., and Theissen, G. 2010. A hitchhiker's guide to the MADS world of plants. *Genome Biol.* 11: 214.

Gridley, T. 2003. Notch signaling and inherited human diseases. *Hum. Mol. Genet.* 12: R9–R13.

Inoue, T., et al. 2005. Gene regulatory special feature: Transcriptional network underlying *Caenorhabditis elegans* vulval development. *Proc. Nat. Acad. Sci.* 102: 4972–4977.

Kestler, H. A., Wawra, C., Kracher, B., and Kuhl, M. 2008. Network modeling of signal transduction: Establishing the global view. *Bioessays* 30: 1110–1125.

Krizek, B. A., and Fletcher, J. C. 2006. Molecular mechanisms of flower development: An armchair guide. *Nat. Rev. Genet.* 6: 688–698.

Lynch, J. A., and Roth, S. 2011. The evolution of dorsal-ventral patterning mechanism in insects. *Genes Dev.* 25: 107–118.

Maeda, R. K., and Karch, F. 2006. The ABC of the BX-C: The bithorax complex explained. *Development* 133: 1413–1422.

Nüsslein-Volhard, C., and Weischaus, E. 1980. Mutations affecting segment number and polarity in *Drosophila*. *Nature* 287: 795–801.

Reyes, J. C. 2006. Chromatin modifiers that control plant development. *Curr. Opin. Plant Biol.* 9: 21–27.

Schroeder, M. D., et al. 2004. Transcriptional control in the segmentation gene network of *Drosophila*. *PLOS Biol.* 2: 1396–1410.

Schvartsman, S. Y., Coppey, M., and Berezhkovskii, A. 2008. Dynamics of maternal morphogen gradients in *Drosophila*. *Curr. Opin. Genet. Dev.* 18: 342–347.

Verakasa, A., Del Campo, M., and McGinnis, W. 2000. Developmental patterning genes and their conserved functions: From model organisms to humans. *Mol. Genet. Metabol.* 69: 85–100.

Walser, C. B., and Lipshitz, H. D. 2011. Transcript clearance during the maternal-to-zygote transition. *Curr. Opin. Genet. Dev.* 21: 431–443.

Wang, M., and Sternberg, P. W. 2001. Pattern formation during *C. elegans* vulval induction. *Curr. Top. Dev. Biol.* 51: 189–220.

Yuan, J., and Kroemer, G. 2010. Alternative cell death mechanisms in development and beyond. *Genes Dev.* 24: 2592–2602.

Chapter 19 Cancer and Regulation of the Cell Cycle

Alison, M. R., et al. 2010. Stem cells in cancer: instigators and propagators? *J. Cell Sci.* 123: 2357–2368.

Ashworth, A., and Hudson, T. J. 2013. Comparisons across cancers. *Nature* 502: 306–307.

Bernards, R., and Weinberg, R. A. 2002. A progression puzzle. *Nature* 418: 823.

Esteller, M. 2007. Cancer epigenomics: DNA methylomes and histone-modification maps. *Nature Reviews Cancer* 8: 286–297.

Futreal, P. A., et al. 2004. A census of human cancer genes. *Nature Reviews Cancer* 4: 177–183.

Gray, J. 2010. Genomics of metastasis. *Nature* 464: 989–990.

Hartwell, L. H., and Kastan, M. B. 1994. Cell cycle control and cancer. *Science* 266: 1821–1827.

Kandoth, C., et al. 2013. Mutational landscape and significance across 12 major cancer types. *Nature* 502: 333–340.

Ledford, H. 2010. The cancer genome challenge. *Nature* 464: 972–974.

Marte, B. 2013. Tumour heterogeneity. *Nature* 501: 327.

Nurse, P. 1997. Checkpoint pathways come of age. *Cell* 91: 865–867.

Varmus, H. 2006. The new era in cancer research. *Science* 312: 1162–1164.

Vazquez, J., et al. 2008. The genetics of the p53 pathway, apoptosis and cancer therapy. *Nature Reviews Drug Discov.* 7: 979–987.

Watson, I. R., et al. Emerging patterns of somatic mutations in cancer. *Nature Rev. Genet.* 14: 703–718.

Yokota, J. 2000. Tumor progression and metastasis. *Carcinogenesis* 21: 497–503.

Chapter 20 Recombinant DNA Technology

Brownlee, C. 2005. Danna and Nathans: Restriction enzymes and the boon to modern molecular biology. *Proc. Nat. Acad. Sci.* 103: 5909.

Mardis, E. R. 2008. Next-generation DNA sequencing methods. *Annu. Rev. Genomics Hum. Genet.* 9: 387–402.

Mardis, E. R. 2011. A decade's perspective on DNA sequencing technology. *Nature* 470: 198–203.

Mullis, K. B. 1990. The unusual origin of the polymerase chain reaction. *Sci. Am.* (Apr.) 262: 56–65.

Rothberg, J. M., and Leamon, J. H. 2008. The development and impact of 454 sequencing. *Nat. Biotech.* 26: 1117–1124.

Sanger, F., et al. 1977. DNA sequencing with chain-terminating inhibitors. *Proc. Natl. Acad. Sci. (USA)* 74: 5463–5467.

Shendure, J., and Ji, H. 2008. Next-generation DNA sequencing. *Nature Biotechnology* 26: 1135–1145.

Snyder, M., Du, J., and Gerstein, M. 2010. Personal genome sequencing: Current approaches and challenges. *Genes & Development* 24: 423–431.

Southern, E. 1975. Detection of specific sequences among DNA fragments separated by gel electrophoresis. *J. Mol. Biol.* 98: 503–507.

Chapter 21 Genomics, Bioinformatics, and Proteomics

Asara, J. M., et al. 2007. Protein sequences from Mastodon and *Tyrannosaurus Rex* revealed by mass spectrometry. *Science* 316: 280–285.

Amemiya, C. T., et al. 2013. The African coelacanth genome provides insights into tetrapod evolution. *Nature* 496: 311–316.

Campbell, K. L., and Hofreiter, M. 2012. New life for ancient DNA. *Scientific American* 307: 46–51.

Conrad, D. F., et al. 2010. Origins and functional impact of copy number variations in the human genome. *Nature* 464: 704–712.

Domon, B., and Aebersold, R. 2006. Mass spectrometry and protein analysis. *Science* 312: 212–217.

Doolittle, W. F. 2013. Is junk DNA bunk? A critique of ENCODE. *Proc. Natl. Acad. Sci. (USA)* 110: 5294–5300.

Green, R. E., et al. 2008. A complete Neandertal mitochondrial genome sequence determined by high-throughput sequencing. *Cell* 134: 416–426.

Green, R. E., et al. 2010. A draft sequence of the Neandertal genome. *Science* 328: 710–722.

Grice, E. A., and Segre, J. A. 2012. The human microbiome: Our second genome. *Annual Review of Genomics and Human Genetics* 13: 151–170.

Hawkins, R. D., Hon, G. C., and Ren, B. 2010. Next-generation genomics: An integrative approach. *Nature Reviews Genetics* 11: 476–486.

Hood, L., Heath, J. R., Phelps, M. E., and Lin, B. 2004. Systems biology and new technologies enable predictive and preventative medicine. *Science* 306: 640–643.

Hoskins, R. A., et al. 2007. Sequence finishing and mapping of *Drosophila melanogaster* heterochromatin. *Science* 316: 1625–1628.

Hugenholtz, P., and Tyson, G. W. 2008. Metagenomics. *Nature* 455: 481–483.

International Human Genome Sequencing Consortium. 2001. Initial sequencing and analysis of the human genome. *Nature* 409: 860–921.

International Human Genome Sequencing Consortium. 2004. Finishing the euchromatic sequence of the human genome. *Nature* 431: 931–945.

Joyce, A. R., and Palsson, B. O. 2006. The model organism as a system integrating "omics" data sets. *Nat. Rev. Mol. Cell Biol.* 7: 901–909.

Lander, E. S. 2011. Initial impact of sequencing the human genome. *Nature* 470: 187–197.

Loscalzo, J., Kohane, I., and Barabasi, A-L. 2007. Human disease classification in the postgenomic era: A complex systems approach to human pathobiology. *Molecular Systems Biology* 124: 32–42.

Lupski, J. R. 2013. Genome mosaicism—One human, multiple genomes. *Science* 341: 358–359.

Nei, M., and Rooney, A. P. 2005. Concerted and birth-and-death evolution of multigene families. *Annu. Rev. Genet.* 39: 197–218.

Nezvizhskii, A. I., Vitek, O., and Aebersold, R. 2007. Analysis and validation of proteomic data generated by tandem mass spectrometry. *Nature Methods* 4: 787–797.

Noonan, J. P., et al. 2006. Sequencing and analysis of Neanderthal DNA. *Science* 314: 1113–1118.

Pennisi, E. 2006. The dawn of Stone Age genomics. *Science* 314: 1068–1071.

Qin, J., et al. 2010. A human gun microbial gene catalogue established by metagenomic sequencing. *Nature* 464: 59–64.

Rhesus Macaque Genome Sequencing and Analysis Consortium. 2007. Evolutionary and biomedical insights from the Rhesus Macaque genome. *Science* 316: 222–234.

Schweitzer, M. H., et al. 2007. Analyses of soft tissue from *Tyrannosaurus rex* suggest the presence of protein. *Science* 316: 277–280.

Sea Urchin Genome Sequencing Consortium. 2006. The genome of the sea urchin *Stronglyocentrotus purpuratus*. *Science* 314: 941–956.

Switnoski, M., Szczerbal, I., and Nowacka, J. 2004. The dog genome map and its use in mammalian comparative genomics. *J. Appl. Physiol.* 45: 195–214.

Thalmann, O. 2012. Complete mitochondrial genomes of ancient canids suggest a European origin of domestic dogs. *Science* 342: 871–874.

The ENCODE Project Consortium. 2012. An integrated encyclopedia of DNA elements in the human genome. *Nature* 57–74. Part of ENCODE: Guidebook to the Human Genome. [A special edition of *Nature*]. *Nature* 489: 45–113.

The 1000 Genomes Project Consortium. 2010. A map of human genome variation from population-scale sequencing. *Nature* 467: 1061–1073.

The 1000 Genomes Project Consortium. 2012. An integrated map of genetic variation from 1,092 human genomes. *Nature* 492: 56–65.

The Human Microbiome Project Consortium. 2012. Structure, function and diversity of the healthy human microbiome. *Nature* 486: 207–214.

The Human Microbiome Project Consortium. 2012. A framework for human microbiome research. *Nature* 486: 215–221.

Thieman, W. J., and Palladino, M. A. 2009. *Introduction to biotechnology,* 2nd ed. San Francisco, CA: Benjamin Cummings.

Venter, J. C., et al. 2001. The sequence of the human genome. *Science* 291: 1304–1351.

Venter, J. C., et al. 2004. Environmental genome shotgun sequencing of the Sargasso Sea. *Science* 304: 6–74.

Weinstock, G. M. 2012. Genomic approaches to studying the human microbiota. *Nature* 489: 250–256.

Yooseph, S., Sutton, G., Rusch, D. B., Halpern, A. L., Williamson, S. J., et al. 2007. *The Sorcerer II* global ocean sampling expedition: Expanding the universe of protein families. *PLoS Biology* 5(3): 0432–0466.

Chapter 22 Applications and Ethics of Genetic Engineering and Biotechnology

Altshuler, D., Daly, M. J., and Lander, E. S. 2008. Genetic Mapping in Human Disease. *Science* 322: 881–888.

Anower, J., Wagner, S., McCracken, D., Wells, N., and Laible, G. 2012. Targeted microRNA expression in dairy cattle directs production of beta β-lactoglobulin-free, high-casein milk. *Proc. Natl. Acad. Sci. USA* [it] 109: 16811–16816.

Collins, F. S., and Barker, A. D. 2007. Mapping the cancer genome. *Scientific American* 296: 50–57.

Dykxhoorn, D. M., and Liberman, J. 2006. Knocking down disease with siRNAs. *Cell* 126: 231–235.

Engler, O. B., et al. 2001. Peptide vaccines against hepatitis B virus: From animal model to human studies. *Mol. Immunol.* 38: 457–465.

Fan, H. C., et al. 2012. Non-invasive prenatal measurement of the fetal genome. *Nature* 487: 320–324.

Friend, S. H., and Stoughton, R. B. 2002. The magic of microarrays. *Sci. Am.* (Feb.) 286: 44–50.

Gibson, D. G., et al. 2010. Creation of a bacterial cell controlled by a chemically synthesized genome. *Science* 329: 52–56.

Green, E. D., and Guyer, M. S. 2011. Charting a course for genomic medicine from base pairs to bedside. *Nature* 470: 204–213.

Jiang, Y. H. 2013. Detection of clinically relevant genetic variants in autism spectrum disorder by whole-genome sequencing. *Am. J. Hum. Genet.*

Knoppers, B. M., Bordet, S., and Isasi, R. M. 2006. Preimplantation genetic diagnosis: An overview of socio-ethical and legal considerations. *Annu. Rev. Genom. Hum. Genet.* 7: 201–221.

Lajoie, M. J., Kosuri, S., Mosberg, J. A., Gregg, C. J., Zhang, D., and Church, G. M. 2013. Probing the limits of genetic recoding in essential genes. *Science* 342: 361–363.

Lajoie, M. J., et al. 2013. Genomically recoding organisms expand biological functions. *Science* 342: 357–360.

Lu, S., et al. 2012. Probing meiotic recombination and aneuploidy of single sperm cells by whole-genome sequencing. *Science* 338: 1627–1630.

Maher, B. 2011. Human genetics: Genomes on prescription. *Nature* 478: 22–24.

Manolio, T. A., et al. 2009. Finding the missing heritability of complex diseases. *Nature* 461: 747–753.

Shastry, B. S. 2006. Pharmacogenetics and the concept of individualized medicine. *Pharmacogenetics Journal* 6: 16–21.

Siuti, P., Yazbek, J., and Lu, T. K. 2013. Synthetic circuits integrating logic and memory in living cells. *Nature Biotech.* 31: 448–452.

Stix, G. 2006. Owning the stuff of life. *Sci. Am.* (Feb.) 294: 76–83.

Wang, D. G., et al. 1998. Large-scale identification, mapping, and genotyping of single-nucleotide polymorphisms in the human genome. *Science* 280: 1077–1082.

Wang, J., et al. 2012. Genome-wide single-cell analysis of recombination activity and de novo mutation rates in human sperm. *Cell* 150: 402–412.

Whitelaw, C. B. A. 2004. Transgenic livestock made easy. *Trends Biotechnol.* 22(4): 257–259.

Lander, E., and Botstein, D. 1989. Mapping Mendelian factors underlying quantitative traits using RFLP linkage maps. *Genetics* 121: 185–199.

Lander, E., and Schork, N. 1994. Genetic dissection of complex traits. *Science* 265: 2037–2048.

Lynch, M., and Walsh, B. 1998. *Genetics and analysis of quantitative traits.* Sunderland, MA: Sinauer Associates.

Macy, T. F. C. 2001. Quantitative trait loci in *Drosophila*. *Nature Reviews Genetics* 2: 11–19.

Newman, H. H., Freeman, F. N., and Holzinger, K. T. 1937. *Twins: A study of heredity and environment.* Chicago: University of Chicago Press.

Paterson, A., Deverna, J., Lanini, B., and Tanksley, S. 1990. Fine mapping of quantitative traits loci using selected overlapping recombinant chromosomes in an interspecific cross of tomato. *Genetics* 124: 735–742.

Tanksley, S. D. 2004. The genetic, developmental and molecular bases of fruit size and shape variation in tomato. *Plant Cell* 16: S181–S189.

Veenma, D., et al. 2012. Copy number detection in discordant monozygotic twins of congenital diaphragmatic hernia (CDH) and esophageal atresia (EA). *Eur. J. Hum. Genet.* 20: 298 306.

Zar, J. H. 1999. *Biostatistical analysis,* 4th ed. Upper Saddle River, NJ: Prentice Hall.

Chapter 23 Quantitative Genetics and Multifactorial Traits

Browman, K. W. 2001. Review of statistical methods of QTL mapping in experimental crosses. *Lab Animal* 30: 44–52.

Cong, B., Barrero, L. S., and Tanksley, S. D. 2008. Regulatory changes in a YABBY-like transcription factor led to evolution of extreme fruit size during tomato domestication. *Nat. Genet.* 40: 800–804.

Cong, B., Liu, J., and Tanksley, S. 2002. Natural alleles at a tomato fruit size quantitative trait locus differ by heterochronic regulatory mutations. *Proc. Nat. Acad. Sci.* 99: 13606–13611.

Crow, J. F. 1993. Francis Galton: Count and measure, measure and count. *Genetics* 135: 1.

Druka, A., et al. 2010. Expression of quantitative trait loci analysis in plants. *Plant Biotech.* 8: 10–27.

Falconer, D. S., and Mackay, F. C. 1996. *Introduction to quantitative genetics,* 4th ed. Essex, UK: Longman.

Farber, S. 1980. *Identical twins reared apart.* New York: Basic Books.

Feldman, M. W., and Lewontin, R. C. 1975. The heritability hangup. *Science* 190: 1163–1166.

Frary, A., et al. 2000. *fw2.2*: A quantitative trait locus key to the evolution of tomato fruit size. *Science* 289: 85–88.

Gupta, V., et al. 2009. Genome analysis and genetic enhancement of tomato. *Crit. Rev. Biotech.* 29: 152–181.

Haley, C. 1991. Use of DNA fingerprints for the detection of major genes for quantitative traits in domestic species. *Anim. Genet.* 22: 259–277.

———. 1996. Livestock QTLs: Bringing home the bacon. *Trends Genet.* 11: 488–490.

Johnson, W. E., et al. 2010. Genetic restoration of the Florida panther. *Science* 329: 1641–1644.

Kaminsky, A. A., et al. 2009. DNA methylation profiles in monozygotic and dizygotic twins. *Nat. Genet.* 41: 240–245.

Chapter 24 Neurogenetics

Akolal, D-B, Yu, D., and Davis, R. 2011. The long-term memory trace formed in *Drosophila* α/β mushroom body neurons is abolished in long-term memory mutants. *The J. Neurosci.* 31: 5643–5647.

Bassett, A., Scherer, S. M., and Brzustowicz, L. M. 2010. Copy number variation in schizophrenia. Critical review and new perspectives on concepts of genetics and disease. *Am. J. Pschiatr.* 167: 899–914.

Bhakar, A. L. Dölen, G., and Bear, M. 2012. The pathophysiology of fragile X (and what it teaches us about synapses). *Annu. Rev. Neurosci.* 35: 417–443.

Craddock, N., and Skar, P. 2013. The genetic basis of addictive disorders. *Psychiat. Clin. North Amer.* 35: 495–519.

Cross-Disorder Group of the Psychiatric Genomics Coalition 2013. Identification of risk loci with shared effects on five major psychiatric disorders. *Lancet* 381: 1371–1379.

Ducci, F., and Goldman, D. 2012. The genetic basis of addictive disorders. *Psychiatr. Clin. North Amer.* 35: 495–519.

Ehrnhoefer, D. E., Butland, S. L., Pouladi, M. A., and Hayden, M. R. 2009. Mouse models of Huntington disease: Variations on a theme. *Dis. Models Mech.* 2: 123–129.

Ganetzky, B., 2000. Genetic analysis of ion channel dysfunction in *Drosophila*. *Kidney Intern.* 57: 766–771.

Lu, B., Al-Rahami, I., Valencia, A., et al. 2013. Identification of *NUB1* as a suppressor of mutant Huntington toxicity via enhanced protein clearance. *Nat. Neurosci.* 16: 57–66.

Lu, B., Nagappao, G., Guao, X., et al. 2013. BDNF-based synaptic repair as a disease-modifying strategy for neurodegenerative diseases. *Nat. Rev. Neurosci.* 14: 401–416.

Nielson, D. A., Utrankar, A., Reyes, J. A., et al. 2012. Epigenetics of drug abuse: Predisposition or response. *Pharmacogenomics* 13: 1149–1160.

Sullivan, P. F., Daly, M. J., and O'Donovan, M. 2012. Genetic architecture of psychiatric disorders: The emerging picture and its implications. *Nat. Rev. Genet.* 13: 537–551.

Chapter 25 Population and Evolutionary Genetics

Ansari-Lari, M. A., et al. 1997. The extent of genetic variation in the *CCR5* gene. *Nature Genetics* 16: 221–222.

Barluenga, M., Stölting, K. N., Salzburger, W., Muschick, M., and Meyer, A. 2006. Sympatric speciation in Nicaraguan crater lake cichlid fish. *Nature* 439: 719–723.

Green, R. E., et al. 2010. A draft sequence of the Neandertal genome. *Science* 328: 710–722.

Hedges, S. B., and Kumar, S. 2003. Genomic clocks and evolutionary time scales. *Trends Genet.* 19: 200–206.

Karn, M. N., and Penrose, L. S. 1951. Birth weight and gestation time in relation to maternal age, parity and infant survival. *Ann. Eugen.* 16: 147–164.

Kerr, W. E., and Wright, S. 1954. Experimental studies of the distribution of gene frequencies in very small populations of *Drosophila melanogaster. Evolution* 8: 172–177.

Knowlton, N., et al. 1993. Divergence in proteins, mitochondrial DNA, and reproductive compatibility across the Isthmus of Panama. *Science* 260: 1629–1632.

Kreitman, M. 1983. Nucleotide polymorphism at the alcohol dehydrogenase locus of *Drosophila melanogaster. Nature* 304: 412–417.

Lamb, R. S., and Irish, V. F. 2003. Functional divergence within the *APETALA3/PISTILLATA* floral homeotic gene lineages. *Proc. Natl. Acad. Sci.* 100: 6558–6563.

Leibert, F., et al. 1998. The *DCCR5* mutation conferring protection against HIV-1 in Caucasian populations has a single and recent origin in northeastern Europe. *Hum. Molec. Genet.* 7: 399–406.

Markow, T., et al. 1993. HLA polymorphism in the Havasupai: Evidence for balancing selection. *Am. J. Hum. Genet.* 53: 943–952.

Meyer, M., Kircher, J., Gansauge, M. T., et al. 2012. A high-coverage genome sequence from an archaic Denisovan individual. *Science* 338: 222–226.

Nei, M., Suzuki, Y., and Nozwa, M. 2010. The neutral theory of molecular evolution in the era of genomics. *Annu. Rev. Genomics Hum. Genet.* 11: 265–289.

Noonan, J. P., et al. 2006. Sequencing and analysis of Neanderthal genomic DNA. *Science* 314: 1113–1118.

Presgraves, D. C. 2010. The molecular evolutionary basis for species formation. *Nat. Rev. Genet.* 11: 175–180.

Prüfer, K, Racimo, F., Patterson, N., et al. 2014. The complete genome sequence of a Neanderthal from the Altai mountains. *Nature* 505: 43–49.

Rasmussen, M., et al. 2010. Ancient human genome sequence of an extinct Paleo-Eskimo. *Nature* 463: 757–762.

Reich, D., Green, R., Kircher, D., et al. 2010. Genetic history of an archaic hominin group from Denisova cave in Siberia. *Nature* 468: 1153–1160.

Reznick, D. N., and Ricklefs, R. E. 2009. Darwin's bridge between microevolution and macroevolution. *Nature* 457: 837–842.

Salzburger, W. 2009. The interaction of sexually and naturally selected traits in the adaptive radiations of cichlid fishes. *Mol. Evol.* 18: 169–185.

Schulter, D. 2009. Evidence for ecological speciation and its alternative. *Science* 323: 737–741.

Stiassny, M. L. J., and Meyer, A. 1999. Cichlids of the Rift Lakes. *Sci. Am.* (Feb.) 280: 64–69.

Vitti, J. J., Cho, M. K., Tishkoff, S. A., and Sabeti, P. C. 2012. Human evolutionary genetics: ethical and interpretative issues. *Trends Genet.* 28: 137–145.

Yi, Z., et al. 2003. A 122.5 kilobase deletion of the *P* gene underlies the high prevalence of oculocutaneous albinism type 2 in the Navajo population. *Am. J. Hum. Genet.* 72: 62–72.

Appendix B

ANSWERS TO SELECTED PROBLEMS

Chapter 1

2. Your essay should include a description of the impact of recombinant DNA technology on the following: plant and animal husbandry and production, drug development, medical advances, forensics, and understanding gene function.

4. The genotype of an organism is defined as the specific allelic or genetic constitution of an organism, or, often, the allelic composition of one or a limited number of genes under investigation. The observable feature of those genes is called the phenotype. A gene variant is called an allele. There can be many such variants in a population, but for a diploid organism, only two such alleles can exist in any given individual.

6. Genes, linear sequences of nucleotides, usually exert their influence by producing polypeptides through the process of transcription and translation. Genes are the functional units of heredity. They associate, sometimes with proteins, to form chromosomes. During the cell cycle, chromosomes, and therefore genes, are duplicated by a variety of enzymes so that daughter cells inherit copies of the parental hereditary information. Genes of eukaryotes and prokaryotes are composed of DNA.

8. The central dogma of molecular genetics refers to the relationships among DNA, RNA, and proteins. The processes of transcription and translation are integral to understanding these relationships. Because DNA and RNA are discrete chemical entities, they can be isolated, studied, and manipulated in a variety of experiments that define modern genetics.

10. Restriction enzymes (endonucleases) cut double-stranded DNA at particular base sequences. When a vector is cleaved with the same enzyme, complementary ends are created such that ends, regardless of their origin, can be combined and ligated to form intact double-stranded structures. Such recombinant forms are often useful for industrial, research, and/or pharmaceutical efforts.

12. Unique transgenic plants and animals can be patented, as ruled by the United States Supreme Court in 1980. Supporters of organismic patenting argue that it is needed to encourage innovation and allow the costs of discovery to be recovered. Capital investors assume that there is a likely chance that their investments will yield positive returns. Others argue that natural substances should not be privately owned and that once they are owned by a small number of companies, free enterprise will be stifled.

14. Model organisms are not only useful, but also necessary for understanding genes that influence human diseases. Given that many genetic/molecular systems are highly conserved across broad phylogenetic lines, what is learned in one organism is usually applied to all organisms. In addition, most model organisms have peculiarities, such as ease of growth, genetic understanding, or abundant offspring, that make their use straightforward and especially informative in genetic studies.

16. For approximately 60 years discoveries in genetics have guided our understanding of living systems, aided rational drug design, and dominated many social discussions. Genetics provides the framework for universal biological processes and helps explain species stability and diversity. Given the central focus of genetics in so many of life's processes, it is understandable why so many genetic scientists have been awarded the Nobel Prize.

18. Such groups seek to reclaim community involvement and decision-making in governmental and industrial applications of biotechnology. They consider that profit-driven motives may compromise benefits that such technology may provide. They question the safety of genetically modified organisms to human health and ecological harmony, not to mention biotechnical applications to weapons development.

Chapter 2

ANSWERS TO NOW SOLVE THIS

2-1. (a) 32 (b) 16
2-2. (a) 8 (b) 8 (c) 8
2-3. Not necessarily; if crossing over occurs in meiosis I, then the chromatids in the secondary oocyte are not identical. Once they separate during meiosis II, unlike chromatids, they reside in the ootid and the second polar body.

SOLUTIONS TO PROBLEMS AND DISCUSSION QUESTIONS

2. Compared with mitosis, which maintains chromosomal constancy, meiosis provides for a reduction in chromosome number and an opportunity for the exchange of genetic material between homologous chromosomes. In mitosis there is no change in chromosome number or kind in the two daughter cells, whereas in meiosis numerous potentially different haploid (n) cells are produced. During oogenesis, only one of the four meiotic products is functional; however, four of the four meiotic products of spermatogenesis are potentially functional.

4. Chromosomes that are homologous share many properties including *overall length, position of the centromere (metacentric, submetacentric, acrocentric, telocentric), banding patterns, type and location of genes, and autoradiographic pattern*. *Diploidy* is a term often used in conjunction with the symbol $2n$. It means that both members of a homologous pair of chromosomes are present. Haploidy refers to the presence of a single copy of each homologous chromosome (n).

8. In plants, a cell plate that was laid down during telophase becomes the middle lamella where primary and secondary layers of the cell wall are deposited. In animals, constriction of a cell membrane produces a cell furrow of daughter cells.

10. (a) *Synapsis* is the point-by-point pairing of homologous chromosomes during prophase of meiosis I.

(b) *Bivalents* are those structures formed by the synapsis of homologous chromosomes. In other words, there are two chromosomes (and four chromatids) that make up a bivalent.

(c) *Chiasmata* is the plural form of chiasma and refers to the structure, when viewed microscopically, of crossed chromatids.

(d) *Crossing over* is the exchange of genetic material between chromatids. It is a method of providing genetic variation through the breaking and rejoining of chromatids.

(e) *Chromomeres* are bands of chromatin that look different from neighboring patches along the length of a chromosome.

(f) *Sister chromatids* are "post-S phase" structures of replicated chromosomes. Sister chromatids are genetically identical (except where mutations have occurred) and are originally attached to the same centromere.

(g) *Tetrads* are synapsed homologous chromosomes thereby composed of four chromatids.

(h) *Dyads* are composed of two chromatids joined by a centromere.

(i) At anaphase II of meiosis, the centromeres divide and sister chromatids (*monads*) go to opposite poles.

12. During meiosis I chromosome number is reduced to haploid complements. This is achieved by synapsis of homologous chromosomes and their subsequent separation. It would seem to be more mechanically difficult for genetically identical daughters to form from mitosis if homologous chromosomes paired. By having chromosomes unpaired at metaphase of mitosis, only centromere division is required for daughter cells to eventually receive identical chromosomal complements.

14. First, through independent assortment of chromosomes at anaphase I of meiosis, daughter cells (secondary spermatocytes and secondary oocytes) may contain different sets of maternally and paternally derived chromosomes. Second, crossing over, which happens at a much higher frequency in meiotic cells as compared with mitotic cells, allows maternally and paternally derived chromosomes to exchange segments, thereby increasing the likelihood that daughter cells (that is, secondary spermatocytes and secondary oocytes) are genetically unique.

16. There would be 16 combinations with the addition of another chromosome pair.

18. One half of each tetrad will have a maternal homolog: $(1/2)^{10}$.

20. In angiosperms, meiosis results in the formation of microspores (male) and megaspores (female), which give rise to the haploid male and female gametophyte stage. Micro- and megagametophytes produce the pollen and the ovules, respectively. Following fertilization, the sporophyte is formed.

22. The folded-fiber model is based on each chromatid consisting of a single fiber wound like a skein of yarn. Each fiber consists of DNA and protein. A coiling process occurs during the transition of interphase chromatin into more condensed chromosomes during prophase of mitosis or meiosis. Such condensation leads to a 5000-fold contraction in the length of the DNA within each chromatid.

24. 50, 50, 50, 100, 200

26. Duplicated chromosomes A^m, A^p, B^m, B^p, C^m, and C^p will align at metaphase, with the centromeres dividing and sister chromatids going to opposite poles at anaphase.

28. As long as you have accounted for eight possible combinations in the previous problem, there would be no new ones added in this problem.

30. See the products of nondisjunction of chromosome *C* at the end of meiosis I as follows:

Two C chromosomes

A^m or A^p
B^m or B^p
no C^m or C^p

At the end of meiosis II, assuming that, as the problem states, the *C* chromosomes separate as dyads instead of monads during meiosis II, you would have monads for the A and B chromosomes, and dyads (from the cell on the left) for both *C* chromosomes as one possibility.

Meiosis II

Meiosis II

32. (a) The chromosome number in the somatic tissues of the hybrid would be the summation of the haploid numbers of each parental species: $7 + 14 = 21$.

(b) Given that no homologous chromosome pairing occurs at metaphase I, one would expect 21 univalents and random "1×0" separation of chromosomes at anaphase I.

That is, there would be a random separation of univalents to either pole at anaphase I, usually leading to inviable haploid cells and thus sterility.

34. If the polar body lacked chromosome 21, the secondary oocyte would have two dyads and the resulting zygote would have three number 21 chromsomes (Down syndrome), two coming from the mother and one coming from the father.

Chapter 3

ANSWERS TO NOW SOLVE THIS

3-1. P = checkered; p = plain.

Cross (a): $PP \times PP$ or $PP \times Pp$

Notice in cross (d) that the checkered offspring, when crossed to plain, produce only checkered F_2 progeny and in cross (g) when crossed to checkered still produce only checkered progeny. From this additional information, one can conclude that in the progeny of cross (a) there are no heterozygotes and the original cross must have been $PP \times PP$.

Cross (b): $PP \times pp$

Cross (c): Because all the offspring from this cross are plain, there is no doubt that the genotype of both parents is pp.

Genotypes of all individuals:

		Progeny	
	P_1 Cross	Checkered	Plain
(a)	$PP \times PP$	PP	
(b)	$PP \times pp$	Pp	
(c)	$pp \times pp$		pp
(d)	$PP \times pp$	Pp	
(e)	$Pp \times pp$	Pp	pp
(f)	$Pp \times Pp$	PP, Pp	pp
(g)	$PP \times Pp$	PP, Pp	

3-2. Suggested symbolism:

w = wrinkled seeds g = green cotyledons
W = round seeds G = yellow cotyledons

(a) Notice a 3:1 ratio for seed shape, therefore $Ww \times Ww$; and no green cotyledons, therefore $GG \times GG$ or $GG \times Gg$. Putting the two characteristics together gives

$WwGG \times WwGG$ or $WwGG \times WwGg$

(b) $wwGg \times WwGg$
(c) $WwGg \times WwGg$
(d) $WwGg \times wwgg$

3-3. (a)

Offspring:

Genotypes	Ratio	Phenotypes
AABBCC	(1/16)	
AABBCc	(1/16)	
AABbCC	(1/16)	
AABbCc	(1/16)	
AaBBCC	(2/16)	$A\_B\_C\_ = 12/16$
AaBBCc	(2/16)	
AaBbCC	(2/16)	
AaBbCc	(2/16)	
aaBBCC	(1/16)	
aaBBCc	(1/16)	
aaBbCC	(1/16)	$aaB\_C\_ = 4/16$
aaBbCc	(1/16)	

(b)

Offspring:

Genotypes	Ratio	Phenotypes
AaBBCC	1/8	$A\_BBC\_ = 3/8$
AaBBCc	2/8	
AaBBcc	1/8	$A\_BBcc = 1/8$
aaBBCC	1/8	$aaBBC\_ = 3/8$
aaBBCc	2/8	
aaBBcc	1/8	$aaBBcc = 1/8$

(c) There will be eight (2^n) different kinds of gametes from each of the parents and therefore a 64-box Punnett square. Doing this problem by the forked-line method helps considerably.

Simply multiply through each component to arrive at the final genotypic frequencies.

For the phenotypic frequencies, set up the problem in the following manner:

$$3/4\ B\_ \begin{cases} 3/4\ C\_ = 27/64\ A\_B\_C\_ \\ 1/4\ cc = 9/64\ A\_B\_cc \end{cases}$$

$$3/4\ A\_-1/4\ bb \begin{cases} 3/4\ C\_ \\ 1/4\ cc \end{cases} \quad etc.$$

$$1/4\ aa-3/4\ B\_ \begin{cases} 3/4\ C\_ \\ 1/4\ cc \end{cases}$$

$$1/4\ bb \begin{cases} 3/4\ C\_ \\ 1/4\ cc \end{cases}$$

3-4. One must think of this problem as a dihybrid F_2 situation with the following expectations:

Expected ratio	Observed (o)	Expected (e)
9/16	315	312.75
3/16	108	104.25
3/16	101	104.25
1/16	32	34.75

$$\chi^2 = 0.47$$

Looking at the table in the text, one can see that this χ^2 value is associated with a probability greater than 0.90 for 3 degrees of freedom (because there are now four classes in the χ^2 test). The observed and expected values do not deviate significantly.

To deal with parts (b) and (c) it is easier to see the observed values for the monohybrid ratios if the phenotypes are listed:

smooth, yellow	315
smooth, green	108
wrinkled, yellow	101
wrinkled, green	32

For the smooth: wrinkled *monohybrid component*, the smooth types total 423 (315 + 108), while the wrinkled types total 133 (101 + 32).

Expected ratio	Observed (o)	Expected (e)
3/4	423	417
1/4	133	139

The χ^2 value is 0.35, and in examining the text for 1 degree of freedom, the p value is greater than 0.50 and less than 0.90. We fail to reject the null hypothesis and are confident that the observed values do not differ significantly from the expected values.

(c) For the yellow: green portion of the problem, see that there are 416 yellow plants (315 + 101) and 140 (108 + 32) green plants.

Expected ratio	Observed (o)	Expected (e)
3/4	416	417
1/4	140	139

The χ^2 value is 0.01, and in examining the text for 1 degree of freedom, the p value is greater than 0.90. We fail to reject the null hypothesis and are confident that the observed values do not differ significantly from the expected values.

3-5. The gene is inherited as an autosomal recessive. Notice that two normal individuals II-3 and II-4 have produced a daughter (III-2) with myopia.

I-1 (*aa*), I-2 (*Aa* or *AA*), I-3 (*Aa*), I-4 (*Aa*)
II-1 (*Aa*), II-2 (*Aa*), II-3 (*Aa*), II-4 (*Aa*), II-5 (*aa*)
II-6 (*AA* or *Aa*), II-7 (*AA* or *Aa*)
III-1 (*AA* or *Aa*), III-2 (*aa*), III-3 (*AA* or *Aa*)

SOLUTIONS TO PROBLEMS AND DISCUSSION QUESTIONS

2. Your essay should include the following points: 1. Factors occur in pairs. 2. Some genes have dominant and recessive alleles. 3. Alleles segregate from each other during gamete formation. When homologous chromosomes separate from each other at anaphase I, alleles will go to opposite poles of the meiotic apparatus. 4. One gene pair separates independently from other gene pairs. Different gene pairs on the same homologous pair of chromosomes (if far apart) or on non-homologous chromosomes will separate independently from each other during meiosis.

4. Unit factors in pairs, dominance and recessiveness, segregation

6. *Pisum sativum* is easy to cultivate. It is naturally self-fertilizing, but it can be crossbred. It has several visible features (e.g., tall or short, red flowers or white flowers) that are consistent under a variety of environmental conditions, yet contrast due to genetic circumstances. Seeds could be obtained from local merchants.

8. $WWgg = 1/16$

10. Several points surface in the first sentence of this question. First, two alternatives (black and white) of one characteristic (coat color) are being described; therefore, a monohybrid condition exists. Second, which is dominant, *black* or *white*? Note that all the offspring are black; therefore, black can be considered dominant. The second sentence of the problem verifies that a monohybrid cross is involved because of the 3/4 black and 1/4 white distribution in the offspring. Referring to the appropriate figures and knowing that genes occur in pairs in diploid organisms, one can write the genotypes and the phenotypes requested in part (a) as follows: (a)

P_1:			
Phenotypes:	black	×	white
Genotypes:	*WW*		*ww*
Gametes:	Ⓦ		ⓦ
F_1:		*Ww* (black)	

F_1 × F_1:			
Phenotypes:	black	×	black
Genotypes:		*Ww* *Ww*	
Gametes:	Ⓦ ⓦ	Ⓦ ⓦ	
	(combine as in the text)		
F_2:			
Phenotypes:	black black	black	white
Genotypes:	*WW* *Ww*	*Ww*	*ww*

(b) Since *white* is a recessive gene (to *black*), each white guinea pig must be homozygous and a cross between two white guinea pigs must produce all white offspring.

white	×	white
ww		*ww*

(c) Recall the various possibilities of the genotypes capable of producing the black phenotype in the F$_2$ generation in part (a) above: *WW* and *Ww*. In Cross 1 in the problem, all black offspring are observed and the most likely parental genotypes would be as follows:

WW	×	*WW*
	or	
WW	×	*Ww*

There is the possibility that black guinea pigs of the *Ww* genotype could produce all black offspring if the sample size was such that *ww* offspring were not produced. In Cross 2, a typical 3:1 Mendelian ratio is observed, which indicates that two heterozygotes were crossed:

Ww	×	*Ww*

12. There are two characteristics presented here: body color and wing length. First, assign meaningful gene symbols.

Body color	Wing length
E = gray body color	*V* = long wings
e = ebony body color	*v* = vestigial wings

(a) P$_1$:

$$EEVV \times eevv$$

F$_1$: *EeVv* (gray, long)

F$_2$: This will be the result of a Punnett square with 16 boxes.

Phenotype	Ratio	Genotype	Ratio
gray, long	9/16	*EEVV*	1/16
		EEVv	2/16
		EeVV	2/16
		EeVv	4/16
gray, vestigial	3/16	*EEvv*	1/16
		Eevv	2/16
ebony, long	3/16	*eeVV*	1/16
		eeVv	2/16
ebony, vestigial	1/16	*eevv*	1/16

(b) P$_1$: *EEvv* × *eeVV*

F$_1$: It is important to see that the results from this cross will be exactly the same as those in part (a) above. The only difference is that the recessive genes are coming from both parents, rather than from one parent only as in (a). The F$_2$ ratio will be the same as (a) also. When you have genes on the autosomes (not X-linked), independent assortment, complete dominance, and no gene interaction (see later) in a cross involving double heterozygotes, the offspring ratio will be 9:3:3:1.

(c) P$_1$: *EEVV* × *EEVv*

F$_1$: *EEVv* (gray, long)

F$_2$: Notice that all the offspring will have gray bodies and you will get a 3:1 ratio of long to vestigial wings. You should see this before you even begin working

through the problem. Even though this cross involves two gene pairs, it will give a "monohybrid" type of ratio because one of the gene pairs is homozygous (body color) and **one** gene pair is heterozygous (wing length).

Phenotype	Ratio	Genotype	Ratio
gray, long	3/4	*EEVV*	1/4
		EEVv	2/4
gray, vestigial	1/4	*EEvv*	1/4

14.
Phenotype	Genotype
P$_1$: yellow × green	*GG* × *gg*
F$_1$: all yellow	*Gg*
F$_2$: 6022 yellow	1/4 *GG*; 2/4 *Gg*
2001 green	1/4 *gg*

$GG \times GG$ = all *GG*

$Gg \times Gg$ = 1/4 *GG*; 2/4 *Gg*; 1/4 *gg*

16.
Seed shape	Seed color
W = round	*G* = yellow
w = wrinkled	*g* = green

P$_1$:   *WWgg* × *wwGG*

F$_1$:   *WwGg* cross to *wwgg*
(which is a typical testcross)
The offspring will occur in a typical 1:1:1:1 as
1/4 *WwGg* (round, yellow)
1/4 *Wwgg* (round, green)
1/4 *wwGg* (wrinkled, yellow)
1/4 *wwgg* (wrinkled, green)

18. (a)

Expected ratio	Observed (o)	Expected (e)
3/4	882	885.75
1/4	299	295.25

$$\chi^2 = \Sigma\,(o - e)^2/e = 0.064$$

By looking at the χ^2 table with 1 degree of freedom (because there were two classes and therefore $n - 1$ or 1 degree of freedom), we find a probability (p) value between 0.9 and 0.5. We would therefore say that there is a "good fit" between the observed and expected values.

(b)

Expected ratio	Observed (o)	Expected (e)
3/4	705	696.75
1/4	224	232.25

$$\chi^2 = 0.39$$

The p value in the table for 1 degree of freedom is still between 0.9 and 0.5; however, because the χ^2 value is larger in (b) we should say that the deviations from expectation are greater. The deviation in each case can be attributed to chance.

20. Use of the $p = 0.10$ as the "critical" value for rejecting or failing to reject the null hypothesis instead of $p = 0.05$ would allow more null hypotheses to be rejected. As the critical p value is increased, it takes a smaller χ^2 value to cause rejection of the null hypothesis. It would take less difference between the expected and observed values to reject the null hypothesis; therefore, the stringency of failing to reject the null hypothesis is increased.

22. (a) There are two possibilities. Either the trait is dominant, in which case I-1 is heterozygous as are II-2 and II-3, or the trait is recessive and I-1 is homozygous

and I-2 is heterozygous. Under the condition of recessiveness, both II-1 and II-4 would be heterozygous; II-2 and II-3 are homozygous.

(b) recessive: parents *Aa, Aa*

(c) recessive: parents *Aa, Aa*

(d) recessive or dominant, not sex-linked; if recessive, parents *Aa, aa*

24. $p = [8! (3/4)^6(1/4)^2]/6!2!$

26. Most likely, the attending physician misdiagnosed the syndrome of the first child by telling the parents that the birth defects were not genetic. Given the birth of the second child with Smith-Lemli-Opitz syndrome, it is highly likely that both parents were carriers for a recessive mutant gene causing Smith-Lemli-Opitz syndrome. Under that circumstance, there is a 25 percent chance that each of their children would be affected. The probability that two children of heterozygous parents would be affected would be 0.25 × 0.25 = 0.0625, or a little over 6 percent.

28. (a) The first task is to draw out an accurate pedigree (one of several possibilities):

(b) $1/3 \times 1/4 = 1/12$

(c) The probability that neither is heterozygous is 2/3 × 3/4 = 6/12.

(d) The probability that one is heterozygous is (1/3 × 3/4) + (2/3 × 1/4) = 5/12.

Also, there are only three possibilities: both are heterozygous, neither is heterozygous, and at least one is heterozygous. You have already calculated the first two probabilities; the last is simply $1 - (1/12 + 6/12) = 5/12$.

30. (a) straight wings = w^+ curled wings = w
short bristles = b^+ long bristles = b

(b) Cross #1: $w^+/w; b^+/b$ × $w^+/w; b^+/b$
Cross #2: $w^+/w; b/b$ × $w^+/w; b/b$
Cross #3: $w/w; b/b$ × $w^+/w; b^+/b$
Cross #4: $w^+/w^+; b^+/b$ × $w^+/w^+; b^+/b$
      (one parent could be w^+/w)
Cross #5: $w/w; b^+/b$ × $w^+/w; b^+/b$

32. (a) Set I expected numbers: tall = 26.25, short = 8.75
Set II expected numbers: tall = 262.5, short = 87.5
For Set I the χ^2 value would be:
$(30 - 26.25)^2/26.25 + (5 - 8.75)^2/8.75$
  = 2.15 with p being between 0.2 and 0.05

so one would accept the null hypothesis of no significant difference between the expected and observed values.

For Set II, the χ^2 value would be 21.43 and $p < 0.001$ so one would reject the null hypothesis and assume a significant difference between the observed and expected values.

(b) In most cases, more confidence is gained as the sample size increases; however, depending on the organism or experiment, there are practical limits on sample size.

34. (a, b) Consider that if a gene is recessive, it takes two copies of the gene to produce the recessive phenotype. If, however, a gene is dominant, it takes only one copy.

36. Given that *dentinogenesis imperfecta* is inherited as a dominant allele and the man's mother had normal teeth, the man with six children must be heterozygous. Therefore, the probability that their first child will be a male with *dentinogenesis imperfecta* would be 1/2 (passage of the allele) × 1/2 (probability of child being male) = 1/4. The probability that three of their six children will have the disease is best determined by application of the following formula.

$$p = \frac{n!}{s!t!} a^s b^t$$

n= total number of events (six in this case)
s = number of times outcome a happens (three in this case)
t = number of times outcome b happens (three in this case)
a= probability of being normal in this family (1/2)
b= probability of having the disease in this family (1/2)

$$p = \frac{6!}{3!\,3!} 1/2^3 \; 1/2^3$$

The overall probability (p) would be 5/16, or about 0.31 (31%).

Chapter 4

ANSWERS TO NOW SOLVE THIS

4-1. (a) Parents: sepia × cream

Cross: $c^k c^a \times c^d c^a$ ⤵

2/4 sepia; 1/4 cream; 1/4 albino

(b) Parents: sepia × cream

($c^k c^d \times c^k c^d$ or $c^k c^d \times c^k c^a$); the cream parent could be $c^d c^d$ or $c^d c^a$.

Crosses: $c^k c^a \times c^d c^d$ ⤵

1/2 sepia; 1/2 cream*

*(if parents are assumed to be homozygous)

or $c^k c^a$ × $c^d c^a$ ⤵

1/2 sepia; 1/4 cream; 1/4 albino

(c) Parents: sepia × cream

Because the sepia guinea pig had two full color parents, which could be

$Cc^k, Cc^d,$ or Cc^a

(not CC because sepia could not be produced), its genotype could be

$c^k c^k, \quad c^k c^d, \quad$ or $c^k c^a$

Because the cream guinea pig had two sepia parents ($c^k c^d \times c^k c^d$ or $c^k c^d \times c^k c^a$), the cream parent could be $c^d c^d$ or $c^d c^a$.

Crosses:

$c^k c^k \times c^d c^d$ ⟹	all sepia
$c^k c^k \times c^d c^a$ ⟹	all sepia
$c^k c^d \times c^d c^d$ ⟹	1/2 sepia; 1/2 cream
$c^k c^d \times c^d c^a$ ⟹	1/2 sepia; 1/2 cream

$c^kc^a \times c^dc^d \implies$ 1/2 sepia; 1/2 cream

$c^kc^a \times c^dc^a \implies$ 1/2 sepia; 1/4 cream; 1/4 albino

(d) Parents: sepia × cream

Because the sepia parent had a full color parent and an albino parent ($Cc^k \times c^ac^a$), it must be c^kc^a. The cream parent had two full color parents that could be Cc^d or Cc^a; therefore, it could be c^dc^d or c^dc^a.

Crosses:

$c^kc^a \times c^dc^d \implies$ 1/2 sepia; 1/2 cream

$c^kc^a \times c^dc^a \implies$ 1/2 sepia; 1/4 cream; 1/4 albino

4-2. A = pigment; a = pigmentless (colorless); B = purple; b = red

$AaBb \times AaBb$

$\Downarrow$

$A\_B\_$ = purple

A_bb = red

$aaB\_$ = colorless

$aabb$ = colorless

4-3. For all three pedigrees, let a represent the mutant gene and A represent its normal allele.

(a) This pedigree is consistent with an X-linked recessive trait because the male would contribute an X chromosome carrying the a mutation to the aa daughter. The mother would have to be heterozygous Aa.

(b) This pedigree is consistent with an X-linked recessive trait because the mother could be Aa and transmit her a allele to her one son (a/Y) and her A allele to her other son.

(c) This pedigree is not consistent with an X-linked recessive mode of inheritance because the aa mother has an A/Y son.

SOLUTIONS TO PROBLEMS AND DISCUSSION QUESTIONS

2. Your essay should include a description of alleles that do not function independently of each other or they reduce the viability of a class of offspring. With multiple alleles, there are more than two alternatives of a given gene.

4. $Pp \times Pp$

1/4 *PP* (**lethal**)

2/4 *Pp* (platinum)

1/4 *pp* (silver)

Therefore, the ratio of surviving foxes is 2/3 platinum, 1/3 silver. The *P* allele behaves as a recessive in terms of lethality (seen only in the homozygote) but as a dominant in terms of coat color (seen in the homozygote).

6.

Blood Group (phenotype)	Genotype(s)
A	I^AI^A, I^Ai
B	I^BI^B, I^Bi
AB	I^AI^B
O	ii

I^A and I^B are codominant (notice the AB blood group) while being dominant to i.

8. The only *blood type* that would exclude a male from being the father would be AB, because no i allele is present. Because many individuals in a population could have genotypes with the i allele, one could not prove that a particular male was the father by this method.

10. The simplest explanation is that the homozygous creepers combination is lethal.

12. Three independently assorting characteristics are being dealt with: flower color (incomplete dominance), flower shape (dominant/recessive), and plant height (dominant/recessive).

Establish appropriate gene symbols:

Flower color: RR = red; Rr = pink; rr = white

Flower shape: P = personate; p = peloric

Plant height: D = tall; d = dwarf

$RRPPDD \times rrppdd$

$RrPpDd$ (pink, personate, tall)

Use *components* of the forked-line method as follows:

2/4 pink × 3/4 personate × 3/4 tall = 18/64

14. (a) This is a case of incomplete dominance in which, as shown in the third cross, the heterozygote (palomino) produces a typical 1:2:1 ratio.

$C^{ch}C^{ch}$ = chestnut

C^cC^c = cremello

$C^{ch}C^c$ = palomino

(b) The F_1 resulting from matings between cremello and chestnut horses would be expected to be all palomino. The F_2 would be expected to fall in a 1:2:1 ratio as in the third cross in part (a) above.

16. (a) In a cross of $AACC \times aacc$, the offspring are all $AaCc$ (agouti) because the C allele allows pigment to be deposited in the hair, and when it is, it will be agouti.

F_2 offspring would have the following "simplified" genotypes with the corresponding phenotypes:

$A\_C\_$ = 9/16 (agouti)

A_cc = 3/16 (colorless because cc is epistatic to A)

$aaC\_$ = 3/16 (black)

$aacc$ = 1/16 (colorless because cc is epistatic to aa)

The two colorless classes are phenotypically indistinguishable; therefore, the final ratio is 9:3:4.

(b) Results of crosses of female agouti ($A\_C\_$) × $aacc$ (males) are given in three groups:

(1) To produce an even number of agouti and colorless offspring, the female parent must have been $AACc$ so that half of the offspring are able to deposit pigment because of C; when they do, they are all agouti (having received only A from the female parent).

(2) To produce an even number of agouti and black offspring, the mother must have been Aa, and so that no colorless offspring were produced, the female must have been CC. Her genotype must have been $AaCC$.

(3) Notice that half of the offspring are colorless; therefore, the female must have been Cc. Half of the pigmented offspring are black and half are agouti; therefore, the female must have been Aa. Overall, the $AaCc$ genotype seems appropriate.

The final ratio would be

3/8 (gray)
1/8 (yellow)
4/8 (albino)

18. (a) Since this is a 9:3:3:1 ratio with no albino phenotypes, the parents must each have been double heterozygotes and incapable of producing the cc genotype.

Genotypes:

$$AaBbCC \times AaBbCC$$
or
$$AaBbCC \times AaBbCc$$

Phenotypes:

gray × gray

(b) Since there are no black offspring, there are no combinations in the parents that can produce aa. The 4/16 proportion indicates that the C locus is heterozygous in both parents.

If the parents are

$$AABbCc \times AaBbCc$$
or
$$AABbCc \times AABbCc$$

then the results would follow the pattern given.

Phenotypes: gray × gray

(c) Notice that 16/64 or 1/4 of the offspring are albino; therefore, the parents are both heterozygous at the C locus. Second, notice that without considering the C locus, there is a 27:9:9:3 ratio that reduces to a 9:3:3:1 ratio.

Given this information, the genotypes must be

$$AaBbCc \times AaBbCc$$
Phenotypes: gray × gray

(d) Genotypes: aaBbCc × aabbCc
Phenotypes: black × cream

(e) Genotypes: aaBbCc × aaBbcc
Phenotypes: black × albino

20. The initial cross must have been

$$AABB \times aabb$$

There are two gene pairs involved.
(a) A_B_ = 9/16 (tall)
A_bb = 3/16 (dwarf)
aaB_ = 3/16 (dwarf)
aabb = 1/16 (dwarf)
(b) There are three different classes of dwarf plants. Within each of the 3/16 classes there are two types:
A_bb = 3/16 (dwarf)
    = 1/3 AAbb and 2/3 Aabb
and
aaB_ = 3/16 (dwarf)
    = 1/3 aaBB and 2/3 aaBb

Therefore, the true breeding dwarf plants would be the following:

AAbb, aaBB, and aabb
and they would constitute 3/7 of the dwarf group.

22.
Cross #1 = (c)
Cross #2 = (d)
Cross #3 = (b)
Cross #4 = (e)
Cross #5 = (a)

24. The mating is $X^{RG}X^{rg}; I^A i \times X^{RG}Y; I^A i$

The final product of the independent probabilities is

$$1/2 \times 1 \times 1/4 = 1/8$$

26. Assuming that the parents are homozygous, the crosses would be as follows. Notice that the X symbol may remain to remind us that the sd gene is on the X chromosome. It is extremely important that one account for both the mutant genes and each of their wild-type alleles.

P_1: $X^{sd}X^{sd}; e^+/e^+ \times X^+/Y; e/e$

F_1:

$1/2\ X^+X^{sd}; e^+/e$ (female, normal)

$1/2\ X^{sd}/Y; e^+/e$ (male, scalloped)

F_2:

Phenotypes:

3/16 normal females
3/16 normal males
1/16 ebony females
1/16 ebony males
3/16 scalloped females
3/16 scalloped males
1/16 scalloped, ebony females
1/16 scalloped, ebony males

Forked-line method:

P_1: $X^{sd}X^{sd}; e^+/e^+ \times X^+/Y; e/e$

F_1: $1/2\ X^+X^{sd}; e^+/e$ (female, normal)
       $1/2\ X^{sd}/Y; e^+/e$ (male, scalloped)

F_2:

	Wings	Color	
1/4	females, normal	3/4 normal	3/16
		1/4 ebony	1/16
1/4	females, scalloped	3/4 normal	3/16
		1/4 ebony	1/16
1/4	males, normal	3/4 normal	3/16
		1/4 ebony	1/16
1/4	males, scalloped	3/4 normal	3/16
		1/4 ebony	1/16

28. (a) P_1: $X^v X^v; +/+ \times X^+/Y; b^r/b^r$

F_1:
$1/2\ X^+X^v; +/b^r$ (female, normal)
$1/2\ X^v/Y; +/b^r$ (male, vermilion)

F_2:

3/16 = females, normal

1/16 = females, brown eyes
3/16 = females, vermilion eyes
1/16 = females, white eyes
3/16 = males, normal
1/16 = males, brown eyes
3/16 = males, vermilion eyes
1/16 = males, white eyes

(b) P_1: X^+X^+; $b^r/b^r \times X^v/Y$; $+/+$ ⟶

F_1:

$1/2\ X^+X^v$; $+/b^r$ (female, normal)
$1/2\ X^+/Y$; $+/b^r$ (male, normal)

F_2:

6/16 = females, normal
2/16 = females, brown eyes
3/16 = males, normal
1/16 = males, brown eyes
3/16 = males, vermilion eyes
1/16 = males, white eyes

(c) P_1: X^vX^v; $b^r/b^r \times X^+/Y$; $+/+$ ⟶

F_1: $1/2\ X^+X^v$; $+/b^r$ (female, normal)
$1/2\ X^v/Y$; $+/b^r$ (male, vermilion)

F_2:

3/16 = females, normal
1/16 = females, brown eyes
3/16 = females, vermilion eyes
1/16 = females, white eyes
3/16 = males, normal
1/16 = males, brown eyes
3/16 = males, vermilion eyes
1/16 = males, white eyes

30. (a, b) The condition is *recessive*. In the second cross, note that the father is not shaded, yet the daughter (II-4) is. If the condition is recessive, then it must also be *autosomal*.
    (c) II-1 = AA or Aa
    II-6 = AA or Aa
    II-9 = Aa

32. P_1: female: $HH \times$ male: hh
    F_1: all hen-feathering
    F_2: *1/2 females*   *1/2 males*
    1/4 HH hen-feathering   hen-feathering
    2/4 Hh hen-feathering   hen-feathering
    1/4 hh hen-feathering   cock-feathering

    All of the offspring would be hen-feathered except for 1/8 of the males, which are cock-feathered.

34. Phenotypic expression is dependent on the genome of the organism, the immediate molecular and cellular environment of the genome, and numerous interactions between a genome, the organism, and the environment.

36. (a) $AAB\_ \times aaBB$ (other configurations possible, but each must give all offspring with A and B dominant alleles)
    (b) $AaB\_ \times aaBB$ (other configurations are possible, but no bb genotypes can be produced)
    (c) $AABb \times aaBb$
    (d) $AABB \times aabb$
    (e) $AaBb \times Aabb$
    (f) $AaBb \times aabb$
    (g) $aaBb \times aaBb$
    (h) $AaBb \times AaBb$

Those genotypes that will breed true will be as follows:

$$\text{black} = AABB$$
$$\text{golden} = \text{all genotypes that are } bb$$
$$\text{brown} = aaBB$$

38. The homozygous dominant type is lethal. Polled is caused by an independently assorting dominant allele, while horned is caused by the recessive allele to polled.

40. Given the degree of outcrossing, that the gene is probably quite rare and therefore heterozygotes are uncommon, and that the frequency of transmission is high, it is likely that this form of male precocious puberty is caused by an autosomal dominant, sex-limited gene.

42. Given the following genotypes of the parents,

$$aabb = \text{crimson}$$
$$AABB = \text{white}$$

the F_1 consists of $AaBb$ genotypes with a rose phenotype.

In the F_2 the following genotypes correspond to the given phenotypes:

$AAB\_$ = white 4/16
$AaBB$ = magenta 2/16
$AaBb$ = rose 4/16
$Aabb$ = orange 2/16
$aaBB$ = yellow 1/16
$aaBb$ = pale yellow 2/16
$aabb$ = crimson 1/16

Gene interaction is occurring along with the absence of complete dominance.

44. Beatrice, Alice of Hesse, and Alice of Athlone are carriers. There is a 1/2 chance that Princess Irene is a carrier.

Chapter 5

ANSWERS TO NOW SOLVE THIS

5-1. (a)
     1/4 $AaBb$
     1/4 $Aabb$
     1/4 $aaBb$
     1/4 $aabb$
(b)
     1/4 $AaBb$
     1/4 $Aabb$
     1/4 $aaBb$
     1/4 $aabb$
(c)
     1/2 AB/ab
     1/2 ab/ab

5-2. Adding the crossover percentages together $(6.9 + 7.1)$ gives 14 percent, which would be the map distance between the two genes. The dominant genes are on one homolog while the recessive alleles are on the other homolog.

5-3. (a, b) $+ b c / a + +$

$$a - b = \frac{32 + 38 + 0 + 0}{1000} \times 100 = 7 \text{ map units}$$

$$b - c = \frac{11 + 9 + 0 + 0}{1000} \times 100 = 2 \text{ map units}$$

(c) The progeny phenotypes that are missing are $+ + c$ and $a\ b +$, which, of 1000 offspring, 1.4 ($0.07 \times 0.02 \times 1000$) would be expected. Perhaps by chance or some other unknown selective factor, they were not observed.

SOLUTIONS TO PROBLEMS AND DISCUSSION QUESTIONS

2. Your essay should include methods of detection through crosses with appropriate, distinguishable markers and that in most cases, the frequency of crossing over is directly related to the distance between genes.

4. With some qualification, especially around the centromeres and telomeres, one can say that crossing over is somewhat randomly distributed over the length of the chromosome. Two loci that are far apart are more likely to have a crossover between them than two loci that are close together.

6. If the probability of one event is

$$1/X$$

then the probability of two events occurring at the same time will be

$$1/X^2$$

8. Each cross must be set up in such a way as to reveal crossovers because it is on the basis of crossover frequency that genetic maps are developed. It is necessary that genetic heterogeneity exist so that different arrangements of genes, generated by crossing over, can be distinguished. The organism that is heterozygous must be the sex in which crossing over occurs. In other words, it would be useless to map genes in *Drosophila* if the male parent is the heterozygote since crossing over is not typical in *Drosophila* males. Lastly, the cross must be set up so that the phenotypes of the offspring readily reveal their genotypes. The best arrangement is one where a fully heterozygous organism is crossed with an organism that is fully recessive for the genes being mapped.

10. Notice that the most frequent phenotypes in the offspring, the parentals, are colored, green (88) and colorless, yellow (92). This indicates that the heterozygous parent in the testcross is coupled

$$RY/ry \times ry/ry$$

with the two dominant genes on one chromosome and the two recessives on the homolog. Because there are 20 crossover progeny among the 200, or 20/200, the map distance would be 10 map units ($20/200 \times 100$ to convert to percentages) between the *R* and *Y* loci.

12.

d	b	pr	vg	c	adp
31	48	54	67	75	83

Map Units

The expected map units between *d* and *c* would be 44, between *d* and *vg* would be 36, and between *d* and *adp* 52. However, because there is a theoretical maximum of 50 map units possible between two loci in any one cross, that distance would be below the 52 determined by simple subtraction.

14. (a) P_1: *sc s v /sc s v* $\times$ $+\ \ +\ \ + /Y$
F_1: $+\ +\ \ + /sc\ s\ v \times sc\ s\ v/Y$

(b) Using method I or II for determining the sequence of genes, examine the parental classes and compare the arrangement with the double-crossover (least frequent) classes.

$$\begin{array}{c} sc\ v\ s \\ +++ \end{array}$$

$$sc - v = \frac{150 + 156 + 10 + 14}{1000} \times 100$$

$$= 33\% \text{ (map units)}$$

$$v - s = \frac{46 + 30 + 10 + 14}{1000} \times 100$$

$$= 10\% \text{ (map units)}$$

$$sc\text{-------}v\text{------}s$$

$$33 \quad 10$$

(c, d) The coefficient of coincidence = 0.727, which indicates that there were fewer double crossovers than expected; therefore, positive chromosomal interference is present.

16. (a) P_1: $D++/+++ \times +e\,p/+e\,p$
F_1: $D++/+e\,p \times +e\,p/+e\,p$

F_2: $D++/+e\,p$	Dichaete
$+e\,p/+e\,p$	ebony, pink
$D\,e+/+e\,p$	Dichaete, ebony
$++p/+e\,p$	pink
$D+p/+e\,p$	Dichaete, pink
$+e+/+e\,p$	ebony
$D\,e\,p/+e\,p$	Dichaete, ebony, pink
$+++/+e\,p$	wild type

(b) Determine which gene is in the middle by comparing the parental classes with the double-crossover classes.

F_1:

$$D+\ +/+\ pe \times +pe/+ pe$$

$$D - p = \frac{12 + 13 + 2 + 3}{1000} \times 100$$

$$= 3.0 \text{ map units}$$

$$p - e = \frac{84 + 96 + 2 + 3}{1000} \times 100$$

$$= 18.5 \text{ map units}$$

18. $+ cu\ /\ + cu$

20. Because sister chromatids are genetically identical (with the exception of rare new mutations), crossing over between sisters provides no increase in genetic variability. Somatic crossing over would have no influence on the offspring produced.

22. (a) There would be $2^n = 8$ genotypic and phenotypic classes, and they would occur in a 1:1:1:1:1:1:1:1 ratio.

(b) There would be two classes, and they would occur in a 1:1 ratio.

(c) There are 20 map units between the *A* and *B* loci, and locus *C* assorts independently from both *A* and *B* loci.

24. In contrast to the other organisms mentioned, a single human mating pair produces relatively few offspring and the haploid number of chromosomes is relatively high (23), so there are rather small numbers of identifiable genes per chromosome. In addition, accurate medical records are often difficult to obtain, and the life cycle is relatively long.

26. Assign the following symbols:

R = red $\quad\quad$ r = yellow
O = oval $\quad\quad$ o = long
Progeny A: $Ro/rO \times rroo$ = 10 map units
Progeny B: $RO/ro \times rroo$ = 10 map units

28. Look for overlap between chromosome number in given clones and genes expressed. Note that *ENO1* is expressed in clones B, D, and E; chromosomes 1 and 5 are common to these clones. However, since *ENO1* is not expressed in clone C, which is missing chromosome 1 (and has chromosome 5), *ENO1* must be on chromosome 1.

> *MDH1*: chromosome 2
> *PEPS*: chromosome 4
> *PMG1*: chromosome 1

30. There is no crossing over in males, and if two genes are on the same chromosome, there will be complete linkage of the genes in the male gametes. In females, crossing over will produce parental and crossover gametes. What you will have is the following gametes from the females (left) and males (right):

bw^+	st^+	1/4	bw^+	st^+	1/2
bw^+	st	1/4	bw	st	1/2
bw	st^+	1/4			
bw	st	1/4			

Combining these gametes will give the ratio presented in the table of results.

32. Mapping the distance between B and m would be as follows:

$$(57 + 64)/ (226 + 218 + 57 + 64) \times 100$$

$$= 121/565 \times 100 = 21.4 \text{ map units}$$

We would conclude that the *ebony* locus is either far away from B and m (50 map units or more) or that it is on a different chromosome. In fact, *ebony* is on a different chromosome.

34. (a) Data presented in this table show an inverse correlation between recombination frequency and live-born children having various trisomies. As the frequency of crossing over decreases, the frequency of trisomy increases. While these data indicate a correlation, other factors such as intrauterine survival are also likely to play a role in determining trisomy live-born frequencies.

(b) If positive interference does spread out crossovers among and within chromosomes, then ensuring that crossovers are distributed among all the chromosomes (and all portions of chromosomes) may reduce nondisjunction and therefore be of selective advantage. This model assumes that the total number of crossovers per oocyte is limiting.

Chapter 6

ANSWERS TO NOW SOLVE THIS

6-1. *T C H R O M B A K*
All of the genes can be linked together to give a consistent map, and the ends overlap, indicating that the map is circular. The order is reversed in two of the crosses, indicating that the orientation of transfer is reversed.

6-2. Multiplying 0.031×0.012 gives 0.00037 or approximately 0.04%. From this information, one would consider no linkage between these two loci. Notice that this frequency is approximately the same as the frequency in the second experiment, where the loci are transformed independently.

6-3. For Group A, d and f are in the same complementation group (gene), while e is in a different one. Therefore, $e \times f$ = lysis.

For Group B, all three mutations are in the same gene; hence $b \times i$ = no lysis.

In Group C, j and k are in different complementation groups as are j and l. It would be impossible to determine whether l and k are in the same or different complementation group if the *rII* region had more than two cistrons. However, because only two complementation regions exist, and both are not in the same one as j, k and l must both be in the other.

SOLUTIONS TO PROBLEMS AND DISCUSSION QUESTIONS

2. Your essay should include a description of conjugation, transformation, transduction, and the potential recombination that occurs as a result of these processes.

4. (a) In an $F^+ \times F^-$ cross, the transfer of the F factor produces a recipient bacterium, which is F^+. Any gene may be transferred on an F', and the frequency of transfer is relatively low. Crosses that are Hfr $\times$ F^- produce recombinants at a higher frequency than the $F^+ \times F^-$ cross. The transfer is oriented (nonrandom), and the recipient cell remains F^-.

(b) Bacteria that are F^+ possess the F factor, while those that are F^- lack the F factor. In Hfr cells the F factor is integrated into the bacterial chromosome, and in F' bacteria, the F factor is free of the bacterial chromosome, yet it possesses a piece of the bacterial chromosome.

6. Participating bacteria typically consist of two types, prototrophs and auxotrophs. If a minimal medium is used first, the auxotrophs would be unable to grow. The transfer to minimal medium allows the detection of recombinant bacteria. Mutant bacteria would not be identifiable if participating bacteria were transferred to a complete medium.

8. The F^+ element can enter the host bacterial chromosome and, upon returning to its independent state, may pick up a piece of a bacterial chromosome. When combined with a bacterium with a complete chromosome, a partial diploid, or merozygote, is formed.

10. During transformation, incoming DNA forms a complex with the host chromosome leading to a double helix that contains one host DNA strand and one incoming DNA

strand. Since these two single strands are different in base sequence (otherwise genetic recombination would not occur), the term *heteroduplex* seems appropriate. After one round of replication, the heteroduplex DNA is resolved into a double-stranded structure identical to the host's original DNA and one double-stranded mutant DNA.

12. A *plaque* results when bacteria in a "lawn" are infected by a phage and the progeny of the phage destroy (lyse) the bacteria. A somewhat clear region is produced that is called a plaque. *Lysogeny* is a complex process whereby certain temperate phages can enter a bacterial cell and, instead of following a lytic developmental path, integrate their DNA into the bacterial chromosome. In doing so, the bacterial cell becomes lysogenic. The latent, integrated phage chromosome is called a *prophage*.

14. The *c* gene is in the middle. The map distances are as follows:

$$a \text{ to } c = (740 + 670 + 90 + 110)/10,000$$
$$= 16.1 \text{ map units}$$
$$c \text{ to } b = (160 + 140 + 90 + 110)/10,000$$
$$= 5 \text{ map units}$$

Negative interference is occurring.

16. Starting with a single bacteriophage, one lytic cycle produces 200 progeny phages; three more lytic cycles would produce $(200)^4$, or 1,600,000,000 phages.

18. Both mutant (*rII*) and wild-type strains of phage T4 can grow on *E. coli* B; however, only wild type T4 can grow on K12. Therefore, the degree of recombination between various *rII* strains can be determined by examining the number of plaques on K12 because only recombinant, wild-type, strains can grow. A greater number of T4 phage can grow on *E. coli* B.

20. Because mutant 5 failed to complement with mutations in either cistron, it probably represents a major alteration in the gene such that both cistrons are altered. A deletion that overlaps both cistrons could cause such a major alteration.

22.

Combination	Complementation
1, 2	−
1, 3	+
2, 4	+
4, 5	−

24. Because the frequency of double transformants is quite high (compare the *trp⁺tyr⁺* transformants in A and B experiments), one may conclude that the genes are quite closely linked together. Part B in the experiment gives one the frequencies of transformations of the individual genes and the frequency of transformants receiving two pieces of DNA (2 in the data table). One must know these numbers in order to estimate the actual number of *trp⁺tyr⁺* cotransformations.

26. The concentration of the original phage suspension would be:

$$10 \times 10^6 \times 17 = 1.7 \times 10^8$$

plaque-forming units per mL or pfu/mL.

28. Since *g* cotransforms with *f*, it is likely to be in the *c b f* "linkage group" and would be expected to cotransform with each. One would not expect transformation with *a, d,* or *e*.

30. (a) No, all functional groups do not impact similarly on conjugative transfer of R27. Regions 1, 2, and 4 appear to be least influenced by mutation because transfer is at 100 percent.

(b) Regions 3, 5, 6, 8, 9, 10, 12, 13, and 14 appear to have the most impact on conjugation because when mutant, conjugation is abolished.

(c) Regions 7 and 11, when mutant, only partially abolish conjugation; therefore, they probably have less impact on conjugation than those listed in part (b).

(d) The data in this problem provide some insight into the complexity of the genetic processes involved in bacterial conjugation. The regions that have the most impact on conjugation fall into three different functional groups. In addition, notice that regions 1, 2, 4, 7, and 11, those that appear to have little, if any, impact on conjugation, are functionally related as indicated by their shading.

Chapter 7

ANSWERS TO NOW SOLVE THIS

7-1. In mammals, the scheme of sex determination is dependent on the presence of a piece of the Y chromosome. If present, a male is produced. In *Bonellia viridis*, the female proboscis produces some substance that triggers a morphological, physiological, and behavioral developmental pattern that produces males. To elucidate the mechanism, one could attempt to isolate and characterize the active substance by testing different chemical fractions of the proboscis. Second, mutant analysis usually provides critical approaches into developmental processes. Depending on characteristics of the organism, one could attempt to isolate mutants that lead to changes in male or female development. Third, by using micro-tissue transplantations, one could attempt to determine which anatomical "centers" of the embryo respond to the chemical cues of the female.

7-2. (a) Something is missing from the male-determining system of sex determination at the level of the genes, gene products, or receptors, etc. (b) The *SOX9* gene, or its product, is probably involved in male development. Perhaps it is activated by *SRY*. (c) There is probably some evolutionary relationship between the *SOX9* gene and *SRY*. There is considerable evidence that many other genes and pseudogenes are also homologous to *SRY*. (d) Normal female sexual development does not require the *SOX9* gene or gene product(s).

7-3. If one assumes that the ovarian cell was engaging in X chromosome inactivation, the ovarian cell that Rainbow donated to create CC contained an activated *black* gene and an inactivated *orange* gene (from X-inactivation). This would mean that as CC developed, her cells did not change that inactivation pattern. Therefore, unlike Rainbow, CC developed without any cells that specified orange coat color. The result is CC's black and white tiger-tabby coat. Had the inactivation pattern been reversed such that both the *black* and *orange* alleles were originally active and subsequently inactivated randomly, CC would still not have appeared identical to Rainbow because the pattern of inactivation is random and the distribution of white patches is variable.

SOLUTIONS TO PROBLEMS AND DISCUSSION QUESTIONS

2. Your essay should include various aspects of sex chromosomes that contain genes responsible for sex determination. Mention should also be made of those organisms in which autosomes play a role in concert with the sex chromosomes.

4. The term *homomorphic* refers to the situation in which both sex chromosomes have the same form. The term *heteromorphic* refers to the condition in many organisms in which there are two different forms (morphs) of chromosomes such as X and Y.

6. In XX/XO sex determination, sex is determined by the presence or absence of a chromosome, whereas in the XX/XY scheme, the Y chromosome may be sex determining. However, in some cases, the autosomes play a role in sex determination. The *Protenor* form of sex determination involves the XX/XO condition, while the *Lygaeus* mode involves the XX/XY condition.

8. Mammals possess a system of X chromosome inactivation whereby one of the two X chromosomes in females becomes a chromatin body or Barr body. If one of the two X chromosomes is randomly inactivated, the dosage of genetic information is more or less equivalent in males (XY) and females (XX).

10. The Y chromosome is male determining in humans, and it is a particular region of the Y chromosome that causes maleness, the *sex-determining region* (*SRY*). *SRY* encodes a product called the testis-determining factor (TDF), which causes the undifferentiated gonadal tissue to form testes. Individuals with the 47,XXY complement are males, while those with 45,XO are females. In *Drosophila* it is the balance between the number of X chromosomes and the number of haploid sets of autosomes that determines sex. In contrast to humans, XO *Drosophila* are males and the XXY complement is female.

12. (a) female $X^{rw}Y$ × male X^+X^+

| F₁: females: | X^+Y (normal) |
| males: | $X^{rw}X^+$ (normal) |

F₂: females:	X^+Y (normal)
	$X^{rw}Y$ (reduced wing)
males:	$X^{rw}X^+$ (normal)
	X^+X^+ (normal)

(b) female $X^{rw}X^{rw}$ × male X^+Y

| F₁: females: | $X^{rw}X^+$ (normal) |
| males: | $X^{rw}Y$ (reduced wing) |

F₂: females:	$X^{rw}X^+$ (normal)
	$X^{rw}X^{rw}$ (reduced wing)
males:	X^+Y (normal)
	$X^{rw}Y$ (reduced wing)

14. Because attached-X chromosomes have a mother-to-daughter inheritance and the father's X is transferred to the son, one would see daughters with the white-eye phenotype and sons with the miniature wing phenotype. In addition, there would be rare (<3%) metafemales (attached-X + X) with wild-type eye color. YY zygotes fail to develop into larvae.

16. Because synapsis of chromosomes in meiotic tissue is often accompanied by crossing over, it would be detrimental to sex-determining mechanisms to have sex-determining loci on the Y chromosome transferred, through crossing over, to the X chromosome.

18. Klinefelter syndrome (XXY) = 1
Turner syndrome (XO) = 0
47,XYY = 0
47,XXX = 2
48,XXXX = 3

20. Unless other markers, cytological or molecular, are available, one cannot test the Lyon hypothesis with homozygous X-linked genes.

22. Dosage compensation and the formation of Barr bodies occur only when there are two or more X chromosomes. Males normally have only one X chromosome; therefore, such mosaicism cannot occur.

24. Instead of X chromosome inactivation as seen in humans (mammals in general), male X-linked genes in *Drosophila* are transcribed at twice the rate of comparable genes on the X chromosome in *Drosophila* females.

26. Several possibilities are discussed in the text. One could account for the significant departures from a 1:1 ratio of males to females by suggesting that at anaphase I of meiosis, the Y chromosome more often goes to the pole that produces the more viable sperm cells. One could also speculate that the Y-bearing sperm has a higher likelihood of surviving in the female reproductive tract, or that the egg surface is more receptive to Y-bearing sperm. At this time the mechanism is unclear.

28. Because of the homology between the *red* and *green* genes, there exists the possibility for an irregular synapsis, which, following crossing over, would give a chromosome with only one (*green*) of the duplicated genes.

30. Since all haploids are male and half of the eggs are unfertilized, 50 percent of the offspring would be male at the start; adding the X_a/X_a types gives 25 percent more male; the remainder X_a/X_b would be female. Overall, 75 percent of the offspring would be male, and 25 percent would be female.

32. The presence of the Y chromosome provides a factor (or factors) that leads to the initial specification of maleness and the formation of testes. Subsequent expression of secondary sex characteristics must be dependent on the interaction of the normal X-linked *Tfm* allele with testosterone. Without such interaction, differentiation takes the female path. To test the dominant nature of the *Tfm* allele, one could generate a XXY male that is heterozygous for the *Tfm* allele. Should the same testicular feminization phenotype occur, the dominant nature of the *Tfm* allele would be supported. If the *Tfm* phenotype was eliminated in the heterozygote, one would have support for the model that the normal *Tfm* allele is needed to interact with testosterone.

34. (a) The figures below depict only those chromosomes relevant to the *Mm* and *Dd* genotypes. With the *MmDd* genotype, both dyads separate intact to the secondary spermatocytes and are potentially capable of fertilizing the egg. (Only one configuration of the *MmDd* genotype is presented here.)

Primary Spermatocyte

Secondary Spermatocyte

Below is the *Mm dd* genotype that leads to fragmentation of the *m*-bearing chromosome. Thus, only the *M*-bearing chromosome is available for fertilization.

Primary Spermatocyte

Secondary Spermatocyte

(b) There have been many attempts to control pest species by hampering the production or fertility of one sex. In this case, if a sex ratio distorter could be successfully integrated into a large enough pool of males, then female numbers might drop. Whether one could successfully manage a pest population with such a method remains to be tested.

36. Do sex cells respond to signals carried in body fluids (nonautonomous), or are they cell specific (autonomous)? Reciprocal transplantation tests can be used to determine the influence of the anatomical environment for cellular differentiation. Since male/female gynandromorphs could be produced in the first place, it argues for an autonomous form of sex differentiation in contrast with that seen in mammals.

Chapter 8

ANSWERS TO NOW SOLVE THIS

8-1. If the father had hemophilia, it is likely that the Turner syndrome individual inherited the X chromosome from the father and no sex chromosome from the mother. If nondisjunction occurred in the mother, during either meiosis I or meiosis II, an egg with no X chromosome can be the result.

8-2. The sterility of interspecific hybrids is often caused by a high proportion of univalents in meiosis I. As such, viable gametes are rare and the likelihood of two such gametes "meeting" is remote. Even if partial homology of chromosomes allows some pairing, sterility is usually the rule. The horticulturist may attempt to reverse the sterility by treating the sterile hybrid with colchicine. Such a treatment, if successful, may double the chromosome number, and each chromosome would then have a homolog with which to pair during meiosis.

8-3. The rare double crossovers within the boundaries of a paracentric or pericentric inversion produce only minor departures from the standard chromosomal arrangement as long as the crossovers involve the same two chromatids. With two-strand double crossovers, the second crossover negates the first. However, three-strand and four-strand double crossovers have consequences that lead to anaphase bridges as well as a high degree of genetically unbalanced gametes.

SOLUTIONS TO PROBLEMS AND DISCUSSION QUESTIONS

2. Your essay can draw from many examples discussed in the text as examples of deletions, duplications, inversions, translocations, and copy number variations.

4. haploid = 9, tetraploid = 36, trisomic = 19, monosomic = 17

6. Karyotype analysis of spontaneously aborted fetuses has shown that a significant percentage of abortuses are trisomic and every chromosome can be involved. Other forms of aneuploidy (monosomy, nullisomy) are less represented.

8. American cultivated cotton has 26 pairs of chromosomes: 13 large and 13 small. Old World cotton has 13 pairs of large chromosomes, and American wild cotton has 13 pairs of small chromosomes. It is likely that an interspecific hybridization occurred followed by chromosome doubling. These events probably produced a fertile amphidiploid (allotetraploid). Experiments have been conducted to reconstruct the origin of American cultivated cotton.

10. While there is the appearance that crossing over is suppressed in inversion "heterozygotes," the phenomenon extends from the fact that the crossover chromatids end up being abnormal in genetic content. As such, they fail to produce viable (or competitive) gametes, or they lead to zygotic or embryonic death.

12. Modern globin genes resulted from a duplication event in an ancestral gene about 500 million years ago. Mutations occurred over time and a chromosomal aberration separated the duplicated genes, leaving the eventual α cluster on chromosome 16 and the eventual β cluster on chromosome 11.

14. By having the genes in an inversion, crossover chromatids are not recovered and therefore are not passed on to future generations. Translocations offer an opportunity for new gene combinations by associations of genes from nonhomologous chromosomes. Under certain conditions, such new combinations may be of selective advantage. Meiotic conditions have evolved so that segregation of translocated chromosomes yields a relatively uniform set of gametes.

16. Given the basic chromosome set of 9 unique chromosomes (a haploid complement), other forms with the "*n* multiples" are forms of autopolyploidy. Individual organisms with 27 chromosomes (3*n*) are more likely to be sterile because there are trivalents at meiosis I, which cause a relatively high number of unbalanced gametes to be formed.

18. The cross would be as follows:

WWWW × *wwww*
(assuming that chromosomes pair
as bivalents at meiosis)

F₁: *WWww*
F₂: 1 *WW* 4 *Ww* 1 *ww*

1*WW*
4*WW*   fill in Punnett square
1*ww*   35 *W* phenotypes and 1 *w* phenotype

20. While a number of mechanisms for *bobbed* reversion have been documented, one based on meiotic recombination occurs through "unequal crossing over." When redundant chromosomal regions synapse, homologs can misalign. If crossing over occurs in the misaligned segments, one chromatid can gain chromosomal material at the expense of the other chromatid. As a chromosome gains rRNA genes, it harbors a selective advantage and produces flies that outcompete those with nonreverted *bobbed* mutations. Eventually, a stock that originally contained *bobbed Drosophila* contains what appear to be wild-type flies over time.

22. (a) In all probability, crossing over in the inversion loop of an inversion (in the heterozygous state) had produced defective, unbalanced chromatids, thus leading to stillbirths and/or malformed children. (b) It is probable that a significant proportion (perhaps 50 percent) of the children of the man will be similarly influenced by the inversion. (c) Since the karyotypic abnormality is observable, it may be possible to detect some of the abnormal chromosomes of the fetus by amniocentesis or CVS. However, depending on the type of inversion and the ability to detect minor changes in banding patterns, not all abnormal chromosomes may be detected.

24. (a) Reciprocal translocation

(b)

(c) Notice that all chromosomal segments are present and there is no apparent loss of chromosomal material. However, if the breakpoints for the translocation occurred within genes, then an abnormal phenotype may be the result. In addition, a gene's function is sometimes influenced by its position (its neighbors, in other words). If such "position effects" occur, then a different phenotype may result.

26. The symbolism t(14;21) indicates that a translocation (t) has occurred between chromosomes 14 and 21. Generally, a Down syndrome individual with a t(14;21) karyotype has 46 chromosomes.

28. Loss through nondisjunction of one of the sister chromatids during mitosis could have occurred, thereby producing two daughter cells, one 46,XX and the other 45,X0. The earlier the event occurred during embryogenesis, the greater the percentage of 45,X0 tissue is expected. The distribution of the 45,X0 tissue would be dependent on the eventual fate of cells where the nondisjunctional event occurred.

30. It is likely that mitotic nondisjunction contributed to the mosaic condition. If one of the X chromosomes failed to be included in a daughter mitotic cleavage cell, then a substantial proportion of the child's cells would be X0. Expression of Turner syndrome characteristics would depend on the percentage and location of the X0 cell population.

32. *Trisomic rescue* is a condition in which an original trisomic zygote occurs but a particular chromosome is lost. In the diagram below, two chromosomes originally came from the father (blue), and one came from the mother (gold). The one from the mother was eliminated during mitosis, leaving the two chromosomes from the father.

Monosomic rescue occurs when a chromosome is originally present in a zygote, and usually through mitotic nondisjunction, a duplicate of that chromosome occupies the cell.

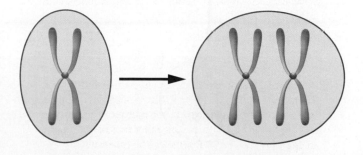

Gamete complementation occurs when a cell without either homolog of a given chromosome is fertilized by a gamete with two copies of that homolog. The resulting zygote contains two homologous chromosomes from one parent.

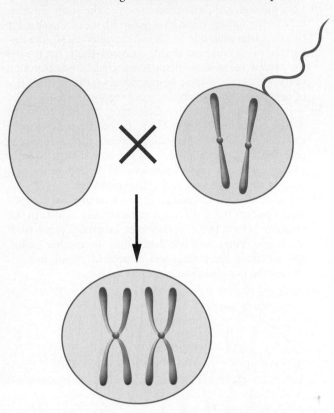

Isochromosome formation occurs when a chromosome contains two copies of one arm and has lost the homolog. Such a homolog loss can originate in mitosis or meiosis. The isochromosome compensates for the nullisomic condition. Effectively, the chromosome is "uniparental" because most the chromosomal material of a given homolog is from one parent.

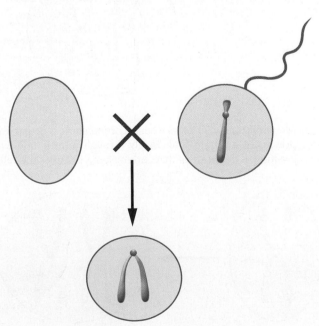

Chapter 9

ANSWERS TO NOW SOLVE THIS

9-1. The mt^+ strain is the donor of the cpDNA since the inheritance of resistance or sensitivity is dependent on the status of the mt^+ gene. In this organism, chloroplasts obtain their characteristics from the mt^+ strain, while mitochondria obtain their characteristics from the mt^- strain.

9-2. (a) neutral
(b) segregational (nuclear mutations)
(c) suppressive

9-3. In many cases, molecular components of mitochondria are recruited from the cytoplasm, having been synthesized from nuclear genes.

9-4. From an organismic standpoint, individuals with the most severe mitochondrial defects tend to be less reproductively successful. At the cellular level, mitochondria with mutations in protein-coding genes tend to be selected against. Such purifying selection tends to favor nonmutant mitochondria.

SOLUTIONS TO PROBLEMS AND DISCUSSION QUESTIONS

2. Your essay should be based on the fact that in organelle heredity, an organelle is responsible for the inheritance pattern, whereas in a maternal effect, organelles are not involved. In maternal effects, the effects persists for one generation only and is solely dependent on the genotype of the mother.

4. Because the ovule source furnishes the cytoplasm to the embryo and thus the chloroplasts, the offspring will have the same phenotype as the plant providing the ovule.
   (a) green
   (b) white
   (c) white, variegated, or green (as illustrated below)
   (d) green

6. If the two are crossed as stated in the problem, then one would expect, in the diploid zygote, the *segregational* allele to be "covered" by normal alleles from the neutral strain. On the other hand, as the nuclear genes are again "exposed" in the haploid state of the ascospores, one would expect a 1:1 ratio of normals to petites. The petite phenoytpe is caused by the nuclear, *segregational* gene.

8. The fact that all of the offspring (F_1) showed a dextral coiling pattern indicates that one of the parents (maternal parent) contains the D allele. Taking these offspring and seeing that their progeny (call these F_2) occur in a 1:1 ratio indicates that half of the offspring (F_1) are dd. In order to have these results, one of the original parents must have been Dd, while the other must have been dd.

10. Since there is no evidence for segregation patterns typical of chromosomal genes and Mendelian traits, some form of extranuclear inheritance seems possible. If the *lethargic* gene is dominant, then a maternal effect may be involved. In that case, some of the F_2 progeny would be hyperactive because maternal effects are temporary, affecting only the immediate progeny. If the lethargic condition is caused by some infective agent, then perhaps injection experiments could be used. If caused by a mitochondrial defect, then the condition would persist in all offspring of lethargic mothers, through more than one generation.

12. The endosymbiotic theory states that mitochondria and chloroplasts arose independently around 2 billion years ago from free-living protobacteria. These bacteria brought the capacity for aerobic respiration and photosynthesis to primitive eukaryotic cells. Because such organelles have prokaryotic origins, a deeper understanding of extranuclear DNA is possible.

14. Developmental phenomena that occur early are more likely to be under maternal influence than those occurring late. Anterior/posterior and dorsal/ventral orientations are among the earliest to be established, and in organisms where their study is experimentally and/or genetically approachable, they often show considerable maternal influence. Maternal-effect genes yield products that are not carried over for more than one generation, as is the case with organelle and infectious heredity. Crosses that illustrate the transient nature of a maternal effect could include the following.

Female *Aa* × male *aa* -----> all offspring of the "A" phenotype. Take a female "A" phenotype from the above cross and conduct the following mating (note that only half of the offspring from the above cross will be *aa*): *aa* × male *Aa*.

All offspring will be of the "a" phenotype because all of the offspring will reflect the *genotype* of the mother, not her *phenotype*. This cross illustrates that maternal effects last only one generation. In actual practice, the results of this cross may give a typical 1:1 ratio because the mother may be *Aa* or *aa*.

16. (a) Since mitochondrial defects are passed from mother to offspring, one would expect no defects being transferred through the grandfather. With the grandmother expressing the mitochondrial defect, one would expect adherence to a mother-to-offspring inheritance pattern throughout the pedigree. (b) Each time the defect became homozygous, a mitochondrial disease would probably appear. In the heterozygous state, heteroplasmy would probably result and a mild form of the disease might result. As defective mitochondrial are produced, typical "mother-to-offspring" transmission might follow.

18. (a) Note that to provide a meaningful pedigree, several individuals are added to the pedigree that are not listed in the table. Refer to Chapter 3 for information regarding symbols used.

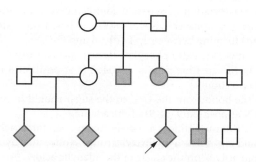

(b, c) If one looks solely at the above pedigree, one could argue that the pattern follows a typical Mendelian recessive. If that's the case, all individuals not showing the phenotype would be heterozygous. However, given that a mitochondrial DNA mutation was identified among affected family members, the pedigree is also consistent with organelle inheritance. Heteroplasmy explains variation in expression and transmission. While this may seem like an erroneous conclusion at first, consider the range of mutant mitochondria presented in the table. The maternal grandmother has 56 percent mutant mtDNA and could pass a mixed population of mitochondria to her offspring, two of which are symptomatic with percentages of mutant mtDNA above 90 percent. The two maternal cousins (of unknown sex) inherited, by chance, pools of mitochondria with relatively high frequencies (90 and 91 percent) of mutant mtDNA and are therefore symptomatic. It appears as if the threshold for phenotypic expression is 85 percent and above.

(d) Transmission of a trait by organelle heredity occurs primarily through the mother, whereas single-gene mutations (albinism) can be transmitted through either parent. In addition, because of heteroplasmy, phenotypic expression may vary and transmission patterns may complicate interpretations from pedigrees.

Chapter 10

ANSWERS TO NOW SOLVE THIS

10-1. In theory, the general design would be appropriate in that some substance, if labeled, would show up in the progeny of transformed bacteria. However, since the amount of transforming DNA is extremely small compared with the genomic DNA of the recipient bacterium and its progeny, it would be technically difficult to assay for the labeled nucleic acid. In addition, it would be necessary to know that the small stretch of DNA that caused the genetic transformation was actually labeled.

10-2. guanine = 17.5%, adenine and thymine both = 32.5%

10-3. Assuming that the value of 1.13 is statistically different from 1.00, one can conclude that rubella is a single-stranded RNA virus.

SOLUTIONS TO PROBLEMS AND DISCUSSION QUESTIONS

2. Your essay should include a description of structural aspects including sugar and base content comparisons. In addition, you should mention complementation aspects, strandedness, flexibility and conformation.

4. Griffith performed experiments with different strains of *Diplococcus pneumoniae* in which a heat-killed pathogen, when injected into a mouse with a live nonpathogenic strain, eventually led to the mouse's death. A summary of this experiment is provided in the text. Examination of the dead mouse revealed living pathogenic bacteria. Griffith suggested that the heat-killed virulent (pathogenic) bacteria transformed the avirulent (nonpathogenic) strain into a virulent strain. Avery and coworkers systematically searched for the transforming principle originating from the heat-killed pathogenic strain and determined it to be DNA. Taylor showed that transformed bacteria are capable of serving as donors of transforming DNA, indicating that the process of transformation involves a stable alteration in the genetic material (DNA).

6. Nucleic acids contain large amounts of phosphorus and no sulfur, whereas proteins contain sulfur and no phosphorus. Therefore, the radioisotopes ^{32}P and ^{35}S will selectively label nucleic acids and proteins, respectively. The Hershey and

Chase experiment was based on the premise that the substance injected into the bacterium is the substance responsible for producing the progeny phage and therefore must be the hereditary material. The experiment demonstrated that most of the ^{32}P-labeled material (DNA) was injected, while the phage ghosts (protein coats) remained outside the bacterium. Therefore, the nucleic acid must be the genetic material.

8. The early evidence would be considered indirect in that at no time was there an experiment, like transformation in bacteria, in which genetic information in one organism was transferred to another using DNA. Rather, by comparing DNA content in various cell types (sperm and somatic cells) and observing that the *action* and *absorption* spectra of ultraviolet light were correlated, DNA was considered to be the genetic material. This suggestion was supported by the fact that DNA was shown to be the genetic material in bacteria and some phages. Direct evidence for DNA being the genetic material comes from a variety of observations including gene transfer, which has been facilitated by recombinant DNA techniques.

10. The structure of deoxyadenylic acid is given below and in the text. Linkages among the three components require the removal of water (H_2O).

12. guanine: 2-amino-6-oxypurine
    cytosine: 2-oxy-4-aminopyrimidine
    thymine: 2,4-dioxy-5-methylpyrimidine
    uracil: 2,4-dioxypyrimidine

14. The following are characteristics of the Watson-Crick double-helix model for DNA:

    The base composition is such that A = T, G = C and (A + G) = (C + T). Bases are stacked, 0.34 nm (3.4 angstroms) apart, in a plectonic, antiparallel manner. There is one complete turn for each 3.4 nm that constitutes 10 bases per turn. Hydrogen bonds hold the two polynucleotide chains together, each being formed by phosphodiester linkages between the five-carbon sugars and the phosphates. There are two hydrogen bonds forming the A to T pair and three forming the G to C pair. The double helix exists as a twisted structure, approximately 20 angstroms in diameter, with a topography of major and minor grooves. The hydrophobic bases are located in the center of the molecule, while the hydrophilic phosphodiester backbone is on the outside.

16. Because in double-stranded DNA, A=T and G=C (within limits of experimental error), the data presented would have indicated a lack of pairing of these bases in favor of a single-stranded structure or some other non-hydrogen-bonded structure. Alternatively, from the data it would appear that A=C and T=G, which would negate the chance for typical hydrogen bonding since opposite charge relationships do not exist. Therefore, it is quite unlikely that a tight helical structure would form at all. In conclusion, Watson and Crick might have concluded that hydrogen bonding is not a significant factor in maintaining a double-stranded structure.

18. Three main differences between RNA and DNA are the following:
    (1) uracil in RNA replaces thymine in DNA,
    (2) ribose in RNA replaces deoxyribose in DNA, and
    (3) RNA often occurs as both single- and partially double-stranded forms, whereas DNA most often occurs in a double-stranded form.

20. The nitrogenous bases of nucleic acids (nucleosides, nucleotides, and single- and double-stranded polynucleotides) absorb UV light maximally at wavelengths of 254 to 260 nm. Using this phenomenon, one can often determine the presence and concentration of nucleic acids in a mixture. Since proteins absorb UV light maximally at 280 nm, this is a relatively simple way of dealing with mixtures of biologically important molecules. UV absorption is greater in single-stranded molecules (hyperchromic shift) as compared with double-stranded structures; therefore, one can easily determine, by applying denaturing conditions, whether a nucleic acid is in the single- or double-stranded form. In addition, A-T rich DNA denatures more readily than G-C rich DNA; therefore, one can estimate base content by denaturation kinetics.

22. A *hyperchromic effect* is the increased absorption of UV light as double-stranded DNA (or RNA for that matter) is converted to single-stranded DNA. As illustrated in the text, the change in absorption is quite significant, with a structure of higher G-C content *melting* at a higher temperature than an A-T rich nucleic acid. If one monitors the UV absorption with a spectrophotometer during the melting process, the hyperchromic shift can be observed. The T_m is the point on the profile (temperature) at which half (50 percent) of the sample is denatured.

24. The reassociation of separate complementary strands of a nucleic acid, either DNA or RNA, is based on hydrogen bonds forming between A-T (or U) and G-C.

26. As shown, the extra phosphate is not normally expected.
    (2) In the adenine ring, a nitrogen is at position 8 rather than position 9.
    (3) The bond from the C-1′ to the sugar should form with the N at position 9 (N-9) of the adenine.
    (4) The dinucleotide is a "deoxy" form; therefore, each C-2′ should not have a hydroxyl group. Notice the hydroxyl group at C-2′ on the sugar of the adenylic acid.
    (5) At the C-5 position on the thymine residue, there should be a methyl group.
    (6) There are too many bonds between the N-3–C-2 of thymine.
    (7) There are too few bonds (should be a double bond) between the C-5 and C-6 of thymine.

28. Since cytosine pairs with guanine and uracil pairs with adenine, the result would be a base substitution of G:C to A:T after two rounds of replication.

30. Fluorescence *in situ* hybridization employs fluorescently labeled DNA that hybridizes to metaphase chromosomes and interphase nuclei. A FISH survey is considered interpretable if hybridization is consistent in 70 percent or more cells examined. Results are available in one to two days after the sample is tested. Because of the relatively high likelihood of aneuploidy for chromosomes 13, 18, 21, X, and Y, they are routine candidates for analysis.

32. (a) The X-ray diffraction studies would indicate a helical structure, for it is on the basis of such data that a helical pattern is suggested. The fact that it is irregular may indicate different diameters (base pairings), additional strands in the helix, kinking, or bending.

    (b) The hyperchromic shift would indicate considerable hydrogen bonding, possibly caused by base pairing.

    (c) Such data may suggest irregular base pairing in which purines bind purines (all the bases presented are purines), thus giving the atypical dimensions.

    (d) Because of the presence of ribose, the molecule may show more flexibility, kinking, and/or folding. Although there are several situations possible for this model, the phosphates are still likely to be far apart (on the outside) because of their strong like charges. Hydrogen bonding probably exists on the inside of the molecule, and there is probably considerable flexibility, kinking, and/or bending.

34. (1) Heat application would yield a hyperchromic shift if the DNA is double stranded. One could also get a rough estimation of the GC content from the kinetics of denaturation and the degree of sequence complexity from comparative renaturation studies.

    (2) Determination of base content by hydrolysis and chromatography could be used for comparative purposes and could also provide evidence as to the strandedness of the DNA.

    (3) Antibodies for Z-DNA could be used to determine the degree of left-handed structures, if present.

    (4) Sequencing the DNA from both viruses would indicate sequence homology. In addition, through various electronic searches readily available on the Internet (Web site. *http://blast.ncbi.nlm.nih.gov/Blast.cgi*, for example), one could determine whether similar sequences exist in other viruses or in other organisms.

36. The mobility of DNA through a gel is dependent on a number of factors, including the concentration of the gel, strength of the current, ionic strength of the buffer, and the conformation of the DNA as stated in the problem. In general, superhelical/supercoiled DNA (form I) migrates the fastest, followed by linear DNA (form III). The slowest to migrate is usually the loose circle (form II).

Chapter 11

ANSWERS TO NOW SOLVE THIS

11-1. After one round of replication in the ^{14}N medium, the conservative scheme can be ruled out. After one round of replication in ^{14}N under a dispersive model, the DNA is of intermediate density, just as it is in the semiconservative model. However, in the next round of replication in ^{14}N

medium, the density of the DNA is between the intermediate and "light" densities, thus ruling out the dispersive model.

11-2. If the DNA contained parallel strands in the double helix and the polymerase would be able to accommodate such parallel strands, there would be continuous synthesis and no Okazaki fragments. Several other possibilities exist. If the DNA was replicated as single strands, the synthesis could begin at the free ends and there would be no need for Okazaki fragments.

SOLUTIONS TO PROBLEMS AND DISCUSSION QUESTIONS

2. Your essay should describe replication as the process of making a daughter nucleic acids from existing ones. Synthesis refers to the precise series of steps, components, and reactions that allow such replication to occur.

4. The Meselson and Stahl experiment has the following components. By labeling the pool of nitrogenous bases of the DNA of *E. coli* with heavy isotope ^{15}N, it would be possible to "follow" the "old" DNA. This was accomplished by growing the cells for many generations in medium containing ^{15}N. Cells were transferred to ^{14}N medium so that "new" DNA could be detected. A comparison of the density of DNA samples at various times in the experiment (initial ^{15}N culture and subsequent cultures grown in the ^{14}N medium) showed that after one round of replication in the ^{14}N medium, the DNA was half as dense (intermediate) as the DNA from bacteria grown only in the ^{15}N medium. In a sample taken after two rounds of replication in the ^{14}N medium, half of the DNA was of the intermediate density and the other half was as dense as DNA containing only ^{14}N DNA.

6. The *in vitro* replication requires a DNA template, a divalent cation (Mg^{2+}), and all four of the deoxyribonucleoside triphosphates: dATP, dCTP, dTTP, and dGTP. The lowercase "d" refers to the deoxyribose sugar.

8. Because *base composition* can be similar without reflecting sequence similarity, the least stringent test was the comparison of base composition. By comparing *nearest-neighbor frequencies*, Kornberg determined that there is a very high likelihood that the product is of the same base sequence as the template.

10. An exposed 3'-OH group is necessary for the attachment of the next nucleotide. The 3'-OH group is eventually removed in the form of water, and a covalent bond is formed to the 5'-phosphate of the added nucleotide.

12. All three enzymes share several common properties. First, none can *initiate* DNA synthesis on a template, but all can *elongate* an existing DNA strand assuming there is a template strand. Polymerization of nucleotides occurs in the 5' to 3' direction where each 5' phosphate is added to the 3' end of the growing polynucleotide.

    All three enzymes are large, complex proteins with a molecular weight in excess of 100,000 daltons, and each has 3' to 5' exonuclease activity. Refer to the text.

    DNA polymerase I:
    5' − 3' exonuclease activity
    present in large amounts
    relatively stable
    removal of RNA primer

DNA polymerase II:
    possibly involved in repair function

DNA polymerase III:
    essential for replication
    complex molecule

14. Given a stretch of double-stranded DNA, one could initiate synthesis at a given point and either replicate strands in one direction only (unidirectional) or in both directions (bidirectional) as shown below. Notice that in the text the synthesis of complementary strands occurs in a *continuous* 5′>3′ mode on the leading strand in the direction of the replication fork, and in a *discontinuous* 5′>3′ mode on the lagging strand opposite the direction of the replication fork. Such discontinuous replication forms Okazaki fragments.

16. (a) *Okazaki fragments* are relatively short (1000 to 2000 bases in prokaryotes) DNA fragments that are synthesized in a discontinuous fashion on the lagging strand during DNA replication. Such fragments appear to be necessary because template DNA is not available for 5′>3′ synthesis until some degree of continuous DNA synthesis occurs on the leading strand in the direction of the replication fork. The isolation of such fragments provides support for the scheme of replication shown in the text.

    (b) DNA *ligase* is required to form phosphodiester linkages in gaps, which are generated when DNA polymerase I removes RNA primer and meets newly synthesized DNA ahead of it. The discontinuous DNA strands are ligated together into a single continuous strand.

    (c) *Primer* RNA is formed by RNA primase to serve as an initiation point for the production of DNA strands on a DNA template. None of the DNA polymerases are capable of initiating synthesis without a free 3′ hydroxyl group. The primer RNA provides that group and thus can be used by DNA polymerase III.

18. Eukaryotic DNA is replicated in a manner that is very similar to that of *E. coli*. Synthesis is bidirectional and continuous on one strand and discontinuous on the other, and the requirements of synthesis (four deoxyribonucleoside triphosphates, divalent cation, template, and primer) are the same. Okazaki fragments of eukaryotes are about one-tenth the size of those in bacteria.

    Because there is a much greater amount of DNA to be replicated and DNA replication is slower, there are multiple initiation sites for replication in eukaryotes (and increased DNA polymerase per cell) in contrast to the single replication origin in prokaryotes. Replication occurs at different sites during different intervals of the S phase.

20. (a) no repair from DNA polymerase I and/or DNA polymerase III (b) no DNA ligase activity (c) no primase activity (d) only DNA polymerase I activity (e) no DNA gyrase activity

22. *Gene conversion* is likely to be a consequence of genetic recombination in which nonreciprocal recombination yields products in which it appears that one allele is "converted" to another. Gene conversion is now considered a result of heteroduplex formation, which is accompanied by mismatched bases. When these mismatches are corrected, the "conversion" occurs.

24. Telomerase activity is present in germ-line tissue to maintain telomere length from one generation to the next. In other words, telomeres cannot shorten indefinitely without eventually eroding genetic information.

26. If replication is conservative, the first autoradiographs (metaphase I) would have label distributed only on one side (chromatid) of the metaphase chromosome as shown below.

28. It is possible that the alien organism contains DNA that

Conservative Replication

G1 Chromosome   Metaphase chromosome

S phase

Metaphase chromosome

Key
Labeled chromatid
Unlabeled chromatid

has parallel strands or only one DNA strand. In either case, the telomere problem would occur at one end of the chromosome. Since prokaryotic DNA is generally circular, therefore having no free ends, the alien organism is most likely a eukaryote.

30. One could use a DNA strand that is stripped of its nucleosomes to determine whether Okazaki fragments are dependent on nucleosome periodicity. Since such an experiment would be *in vitro,* it may not represent a natural setting.

32. In strain *A*, DNA synthesis is reduced at both 30 and 42°C, indicating that strain *A* is temperature sensitive. In addition, strain *A* is sensitive to novobiocin. Therefore, strain *A* is *gyr^{ts}*. Strain *B* is resistant to novobiocin but temperature sensitive, and is therefore *gyr^{ts,r}*. Strain *C* is sensitive to novobiocin but not temperature sensitive, and is therefore wild type. Strain *D* is resistant to novobiocin and not temperature sensitive and is therefore *gyr^r*.

34.

Initial Labeled Base	Labeled Base after Spleen Phosphodiesterase Digestion	
	ANTIPARALLEL	PARALLEL
G	A, T	C, T
C	G, A, G	G, A
T	C, T, G	C, T, A, G
A	T, C, A, T	T, C, A, G

One can determine which model occurs in nature by comparing the pattern in which the labeled phosphate is shifted following spleen phosphodiesterase digestion. Focus your attention on the antiparallel model and notice that the frequency of which "C" (for example) is the 5′ neighbor of "G" is not necessarily the same as the frequency of which "G" is the 5′ neighbor of "C." However, in the parallel model (b), the frequency of which "C" is the 5′ neighbor of "G" is the same as the frequency of which "G" is the 5′ neighbor of "C." By examining such "digestion frequencies," it can be determined that DNA exists in the opposite polarity.

Chapter 12

ANSWERS TO NOW SOLVE THIS

12-1. By having a circular chromosome, there are no free ends to present the problem of linear chromosomes, namely, complete replication of terminal sequences.

12-2. Since eukaryotic chromosomes are "multirepliconic" in that there are multiple replication forks along their lengths, one would expect to see multiple clusters of radioactivity if labeled for a short period of time.

12-3. Volume of the nucleus $= 4/3\pi r^3$

$$= 4/3 \times 3.14 \times (5 \times 10^3 \text{ nm})^3$$

$$= 5.23 \times 10^{11} \text{ nm}^3$$

Volume of the chromosome $= \pi r^2 \times$ length

$$= 3.14 \times 5.5 \text{ nm} \times 5.5 \text{ nm} \times (2 \times 10^9 \text{ nm})$$

$$= 1.9 \times 10^{11} \text{ nm}^3$$

Therefore, the percentage of the volume of the nucleus occupied by the chromatin is

$$= (1.9 \times 10^{11} \text{ nm}^3/5.23 \times 10^{11} \text{ nm}^3) \times 100$$

$$= \text{about } 36.3\%$$

SOLUTIONS TO PROBLEMS AND DISCUSSION QUESTIONS

2. Your essay should include a description of overall chromosomal configuration, such as linearity or circularity, as well as association with chromosomal proteins. In addition, it should describe higher level structures such as condensation in the case of eukaryotic chromosomes.

4. Polytene chromosomes are formed from numerous DNA replications, pairing of homologs, and absence of strand separation or cytoplasmic division. Each chromosome contains about 1000–5000 DNA strands in parallel register. They appear in specific tissues, such as salivary glands, of many dipterans such as *Drosophila*. They appear as comparatively long, wide fibers with sharp light and dark sections (bands) along their length. Such bands (chromomeres) are useful in chromosome identification, etc.

6. Lampbrush chromosomes are typically present in vertebrate oocytes. They are also found in spermatocytes of some insects. They are found as diplotene-stage structures and are active uncoiled versions of condensed meiotic chromosomes.

8. Digestion of chromatin with endonucleases, such as micrococcal nuclease, gives DNA fragments of approximately 200 base pairs or multiples of such segments. X-ray diffraction data indicate a regular spacing of DNA in chromatin. Regularly spaced bead-like structures (nucleosomes) were identified by electron microscopy.

10. As chromosome condensation occurs, a 300 Å fiber is formed. It appears to be composed of 5 or 6 nucleosomes coiled together. Such a structure is called a solenoid. These fibers form a series of loops that further condense into the chromatin fiber, which are then coiled into chromosome arms making up each chromatid.

12. (a) Since there are 200 base pairs per nucleosome (as defined in this problem) and 10^9 base pairs, there would be 5×10^6 nucleosomes. (b) Since there are 5×10^6 nucleosomes and nine histones (including H1) per nucleosome, there must be $9(5 \times 10^6)$ histone molecules: 4.5×10^7. (c) Since there are 10^9 base pairs present and each base pair is 3.4 Å, the overall length of the DNA is 3.4×10^9 Å. Dividing this value by the packing ratio (50) gives 6.8×10^7 Å.

14. One base pair occupies 0.34 nm; therefore, the equation would be as follows:

$$52 \text{ μm}/(0.34 \text{ nm/bp}) \times 1000 \text{ nm/μm}$$
$$= 152,941 \text{ base pairs}$$

16. Long interspersed elements (LINEs) are repetitive transposable DNA sequences in humans. The most prominent family, designated **L1**, is about 6.4 kb each and is represented about 100,000 times. LINEs are often referred to as retrotransposons because their mechanism of transposition resembles that used by retroviruses.

18. First, the methylation patterns displayed by a particular disease must be stable and not change dramatically over time. Second, because DNA methylation patterns differ among individuals, specific patterns must be disease specific and not individual specific. Third, because disease-related changes in DNA methylation patterns often involve hundreds of genes, appropriate interpretation of pattern specifics requires expertise that is presently beyond our capabilities. However, some progress is being made.

20. Cancer cells undergo a variety of changes in histone acetylation compared to normal cells. Overacetylation (hyperacetylation) is often associated with increased gene activity. By introducing HDAC inhibitors, the attempt is to generally decrease gene activity. While the mode of action of HDAC inhibitors is obscure, they are thought to act by promoting cell-cycle arrest by reducing the output of a relatively small number of genes.

22. The intimate relationships among histones, nucleosomes, and DNA in chromatin clearly account for structural remodeling of chromosomes as the cell cycle proceeds from interphase to metaphase. That nucleosomes are associated with chromatin during periods of gene activity begs the question as to the possible roles they play in influencing not only chromosome structure but also gene function. The findings that natural chemical modification of nucleosomal components, as indicated in the question, increases gene activity suggests that changes in the binding of nucleosomes to DNA (in this case due to methylation) enable genes to be more accessible to factors that promote gene function. In addition, the finding that heterochromatin containing fewer genes and more repressed genes, is undermethylated further supports the suggestion that histone modification is functionally related to changes in gene activity.

24. Assuming a random distribution, dividing 3×10^9 base pairs by 10^6 gives approximately 3000 base pairs or 3 kbp between *Alu* sequences.

26. The distribution of microsatellites varies in a taxon-related manner. Microsatellites are more common within genes of yeast and fungi and quite infrequent in genes of mammals. There appears to be a general decrease in within-gene microsatellites in more recently evolved organisms.

28. In every case, the child includes at least one locus from the father and one from the mother, which is expected if the alleged father is indeed the real father. Without information as to the frequency of each marker in the general population, it is difficult to draw definitive conclusions.

Chapter 13

ANSWERS TO NOW SOLVE THIS

13-1. (a) The way to determine the fraction of each triplet that will occur with a random incorporation system is to determine the likelihood that each base will occur in each position of the codon (first, second, third) and then multiply the individual probabilities (fractions) for a final probability (fraction).

$$GGG = 3/4 \times 3/4 \times 3/4 = 27/64$$
$$GGC = 3/4 \times 3/4 \times 1/4 = 9/64$$
$$GCG = 3/4 \times 1/4 \times 3/4 = 9/64$$
$$CGG = 1/4 \times 3/4 \times 3/4 = 9/64$$

$$CCG = 1/4 \times 1/4 \times 3/4 = 3/64$$
$$CGC = 1/4 \times 3/4 \times 1/4 = 3/64$$
$$GCC = 3/4 \times 1/4 \times 1/4 = 3/64$$
$$CCC = 1/4 \times 1/4 \times 1/4 = 1/64$$

(b) Glycine:
GGG and one G_2C (adds up to 36/64)
Alanine:
one G_2C and one C_2G (adds up to 12/64)
Arginine:
one G_2C and one C_2G (adds up to 12/64)
Proline:
one C_2G and CCC (adds up to 4/64)
(c) With the wobble hypothesis, variation can occur in the third position of each codon.
Glycine: GGG, GGC
Alanine: CGG, GCC, CGC, GCG
Arginine: GCG, GCC, CGC, CGG
Proline: CCC, CCG

13-2. Assume that you have introduced a copolymer (ACACA-CAC . . .) to a cell-free protein-synthesizing system. There are two possibilities for establishing the reading frames: ACA, if one starts at the first base; and CAC, if one starts at the second base. These would code for two different amino

acids (ACA = threonine; CAC = histidine) and would produce repeating polypeptides that would alternate *thr-his-thr-his* . . . or *his-thr-his-thr* . . .

Because of a triplet code, a trinucleotide sequence will, once initiated, remain in the same reading frame and produce the same code all along the sequence regardless of the initiation site.

Given the sequence CUACUACUACUA, notice the different reading frames producing three different sequences, each containing the same amino acid.

Codons:	CUA	CUA	CUA	CUA...
Amino acids:	leu	leu	leu	leu...
	UAC	UAC	UAC	UAC...
	tyr	tyr	tyr	tyr...
	ACU	ACU	ACU	ACU...
	thr	thr	thr	thr...

If a tetranucleotide is used, such as ACGUACGUACGU...

Codons:	ACG	UAC	GUA	CGU	ACG
Amino acids:	thr	tyr	val	arg	thr
	CGU	ACG	UAC	GUA	CGU
	arg	thr	tyr	val	arg
	GUA	CGU	ACG	UAC	GUA
	val	arg	thr	tyr	val
	UAC	GUA	CGU	ACG	UAC
	tyr	val	arg	thr	tyr

Notice that the sequences are the same except that the starting amino acid changes.

13-3. Apply complementary bases, substituting U for T:
(a)
Sequence 1:   3'-GAAAAAACGGUA-5'
Sequence 2:   3'-UGUAGUUAUUGA-5'
Sequence 3:   3'-AUGUUCCCAAGA-5'
(b)
Sequence 1:   met-ala-lys-lys
Sequence 2:   ser-tyr-(termination)
Sequence 3:   arg-thr-leu-val

(c) Apply complementary bases:

3'-GAAAAAACGGTA-5'

SOLUTIONS TO PROBLEMS AND DISCUSSION QUESTIONS

2. Your essay should include a description of the nature and structure of the genetic code, the enzymes and logistics of transcription and the chemical nature of polymerization.

4. The UUACUUACUUAC tetranucleotide sequence will produce the following triplets depending on the initiation point: UUA = leu; UAC = tyr; ACU = thr; CUU = leu. Notice that because of the degenerate code, two codons correspond to the amino acid leucine.

The UAUCUAUCUAUC tetranucleotide sequence will produce the following triplets depending on the initiation point: UAU = tyr; AUC = ile; UCU = ser; CUA = leu. Notice that in this case, degeneracy is not revealed, and all the codons produce unique amino acids.

6. Given that AGG = arg, then information from the AG copolymer indicates that AGA also codes for arg and GAG must therefore code for glu. Coupling this information with that of the AAG copolymer, GAA must also code for glu, and AAG must code for lys.

8.

Original		Substitutions
threonine	----->	*alanine*
_AC(U, C, A, or G)		_GC(U, C, A, or G)
glycine	----->	*serine*
_GG(U or C)		_AG(U or C)
isoleucine	----->	*valine*
_AU(U, C, or A)		_GU(U, C, or A)

10. Polynucleotide phosphorylase generally functions in the degradation of RNA; however, in an *in vitro* environment, with high concentrations of the ribonucleoside diphosphates, the direction of the reaction can be forced toward polymerization. *In vivo*, the concentration of ribonucleoside diphosphates is low and the degradative process is favored.

12. Applying the coding dictionary, the following sequences are "decoded":

> Sequence 1: met-pro-asp-tyr-ser-(term)
> Sequence 2: met-pro-asp-(term)

The 12th base (a uracil) is deleted from Sequence #1, thereby causing a frameshift mutation, which introduced a terminating triplet UAA.

14.

G G A gly	G G U gly	
U G A **term**	G G C gly	
C G A **arg**	G G A gly	
A G A **arg**	G G G gly	
G U A **val**	U G U **cys**	
G C A **ala**	C G U **arg**	
G A A **glu**	A G U **ser**	
G G U gly	G U U **val**	
G G C gly	G C U **ala**	
G G A gly	G A U **asp**	

16. The number of codons for each particular amino acid (synonyms) is directly related to the frequency of amino acid incorporation stated in the problem.

18. First, DNA, the genetic material, is located in the nucleus of a eukaryotic cell, whereas protein synthesis occurs in the cytoplasm. DNA, therefore, does not directly participate in protein synthesis. Second, RNA, which is chemically similar to DNA, is synthesized in the nucleus of eukaryotic cells. Much of the RNA migrates to the cytoplasm, the site of protein synthesis. Third, there is generally a direct correlation between the amounts of RNA and protein in a cell. More direct support was derived from experiments showing that an RNA other than that found in ribosomes was involved in protein synthesis; shortly after phage infection, an RNA species is produced that is complementary to phage DNA.

20. Ribonucleoside triphosphates and a DNA template in the presence of RNA polymerase and a divalent cation (Mg^{2+}) produce a ribonucleoside monophosphate polymer, DNA, and pyrophosphate (diphosphate). Equimolar amounts of precursor ribonucleoside triphosphates and product ribonucleoside monophosphates and pyrophosphates (diphosphates) are formed. In *E. coli*, transcription and translation can occur simultaneously. Ribosomes add to the 5' end nascent mRNA and progress to the 3' end during translation.

22. The immediate product of transcription of an RNA destined to become a mRNA often involves modification of the 5' end to which a 7-methylguanosine cap is added. In addition, a stretch of as many as 250 adenylic acid residues is often added to the 3' end after removal of a AAUAAA sequence. The vast majority of eukaryotic pre-mRNAs also contain intervening sequences that are removed, often in a variety of combinations, during the maturation process. In some organisms, RNA editing occurs in one of two ways: substitution editing where nucleotides are altered and insertion/deletion editing that changes the total number of bases.

Processing location	Example
5' end	-addition of 7-mG
3' end	-poly-A addition
internal	-removal of internal sequences
	-RNA editing
	-substitution
	-insertion/deletion

24. Substitution editing occurs when individual nucleotide bases are altered. It is very common in mitochondrial and chloroplast RNAs as well as some nuclear-derived eukaryotic RNAs. Apolipoprotein B occurs in a long and short form, even though a single gene encodes both forms. The initial transcript is edited, which generates a stop codon that terminates the polypeptide at about half its length. The other category is insertion/deletion editing. The parasite that causes African sleeping sickness uses insertion/deletion editing of its mitochondrial RNAs in forming the initiation codon that then places the remaining sequence in a proper reading frame.

26. (a) The first two bases in the triplet code are common to more codons than the last base. If fewer amino acids were used in earlier times, perhaps the first two bases were primarily involved.

(b) Interestingly, all the amino acids mentioned as primitive use guanine as the first base in each codon. We might therefore suppose that the GNN configuration was the starting point of the present-day code. Within the GNN format, the second base is used to distinguish among the amino acids mentioned as primitive.

(c) It is interesting to note that what are considered as the most primitive amino acids are GNN coded, while the later-arriving amino acids are U(U, A, G)(U, C) coded. It would seem that some phenomenon could explain the differences in codon structure between primitive and late-arriving amino acids. It is likely that the addition of new amino acids to the codon field was a slow and mutation-prone process. Did the addition of late-arriving amino acids displace earlier codon assignments, or were some of the late-arriving amino acids able to make use of codons that originally did not code for an amino acid? If this is the case, fewer and more restricted codon assignments would be available for late-arriving amino acids. Notice that each of the late-arriving amino acids has the same starting nucleotide as the present-day stop codons. Is it possible that what were once stop codons were used for late-arriving amino acids because this would be less disruptive to protein synthesis than displacing assignments at the time of their introduction? Much is left to be discovered regarding the structure of the genetic code.

28. Proline: C_3 and one of the C_2A triplets
Histidine: one of the C_2A triplets
Threonine: one C_2A triplet and one A_2C triplet
Glutamine: one of the A_2C triplets
Asparagine: one of the A_2C triplets
Lysine: A_3

30. (a, b) Use the code table to determine the number of triplets that code each amino acid; then construct a graph.
(c) There appears to be a weak correlation between the relative frequency of amino acid usage and the number of triplets for each.
(d) To continue to investigate this issue, one might examine additional amino acids in a similar manner. In addition, different phylogenetic groups use code synonyms differently. It may be possible to find situations in which the relationships are more extreme. One might also examine more proteins to determine whether such a weak correlation is stronger with different proteins.

32. The advantage would be that if sequence homologies can be identified for a variety of HIV isolates, then perhaps a single or a few vaccines could be developed for the multitude of subtypes that infect various parts of the world. In other words, the wider the match of a vaccine to circulating infectives is, the more likely the efficacy. On the other hand, the more finely aligned a vaccine is to the target, the more likely it is that new or previously undiscovered variants will escape vaccination attempts.

Chapter 14

ANSWERS TO NOW SOLVE THIS

14-1. One can conclude that the amino acid is not involved in recognition of the codon.

14-2.

trp-8	trp-2	trp-3	trp-1

Precursor – – ⟶ AA – – ⟶ IGP – – ⟶ I – – ⟶ TRY

14-3. With the codes for valine being GUU, GUC, GUA, and GUG, single base changes from glutamic acid's GAA and GAG can cause the glu>>>val switch. The normal glutamic acid is a negatively charged amino acid, whereas valine carries no net charge and lysine is positively charged. Given these significant charge changes, one would predict some, if not considerable, influence on protein structure and function. Such changes could stem from internal changes in folding or interactions with other molecules in the RBC, especially other hemoglobin molecules.

SOLUTIONS TO PROBLEMS AND DISCUSSION QUESTIONS

2. When involved in protein synthesis, a ribosome will contain the following components: mRNA, charged tRNA, large and small ribosomal subunits, elongation and perhaps initiation factors, peptidyl transferase, GTP, Mg^{2+}, nascent proteins, and possibly GTP-dependent release factors. Together, these compoments order and form peptide bonds between adjacent amino acids, thereby forming proteins.

4. It was reasoned that there would not be sufficient affinity between amino acids and nucleic acids to account for protein synthesis. For example, acidic amino acids would not be attracted to nucleic acids. With an adaptor molecule, specific hydrogen bonding could occur between nucleic acids, and specific covalent bonding could occur between an amino acid and a nucleic acid tRNA.

6. Since there are three nucleotides that code for each amino acid, there would be 423 code letters (nucleotides), 426 including a termination codon. This assumes that other features, such as the poly-A tail, the 5' cap, and noncoding leader sequences, are omitted.

8. An amino acid in the presence of ATP, Mg^{2+}, and a specific aminoacyl synthetase produces an amino acid-AMP enzyme complex ($+ PP_i$). This complex interacts with a specific tRNA to produce the aminoacyl tRNA.

10. Isoaccepting tRNAs are those tRNAs that recognize and accept only one type of amino acid. In some way, each of the 20 different aminoacyl tRNA synthetases must be able to recognize either the base composition and/or tertiary structure of each of the isoaccepting tRNA species. Otherwise, the fidelity of translation would be severely compromised. The most direct solution to the problem would be to have each synthetase recognize each anticodon. Another reasonable consideration might involve the variable loop, which, in conjunction with the anticodon, might enable such specificity. In reality, several characteristics of each tRNA are involved: one or more of the anticodon bases, portions of the acceptor arm, and a particular base that lies near the CCA terminus.

12. Both phenylalanine and tyrosine can be obtained from the diet. Most natural proteins contain these amino acids.

14. When an expectant mother returns to consumption of phenylalanine in her diet, she subjects her baby to higher than normal levels of phenylalanine throughout its development. Since increased phenylalanine is toxic, many (approximately 90 percent) newborns are severely and irreversibly retarded at birth. Expectant mothers (who are genetically phenylketonurics) should return to a low-phenylalanine intake during pregnancy.

16.

18. The electrophoretic mobility of a protein is based on a variety of factors, primarily the net charge of the protein and, to some extent, the conformation in the electrophoretic environment. Both are based on the type and sequence (primary structure) of the component amino acids of a protein. The interactions (hydrogen bonds) of the components of the peptide bonds, hydrophobic, hydrophilic, and covalent interactions (as well as others) are all dependent on the original sequence of amino acids and take part in determining the final conformation of a protein. A change in the electrophoretic mobility of a protein would therefore indicate that the amino acid sequence had been changed.

20. Sickle cell anemia is called a *molecular* disease because it is well understood at the molecular level; there is a base change in DNA, which leads to an amino acid change in the β chain of hemoglobin. It is a *genetic* disease in that it is inherited from one generation to the next. It is not contagious, as might be the case of a disease caused by a microorganism. Diseases caused by microorganisms may not necessarily follow family blood lines, whereas genetic diseases do.

22. It is possible for an amino acid to change without changing the electrophoretic mobility of a protein under standard conditions. If the amino acid is substituted with an amino acid of like charge and similar structure, there is a chance that factors that influence electrophoretic mobility (primarily net charge) will not be altered. Other techniques such as chromatography of digested peptides may detect subtle amino acid differences.

24. All of the substitutions involve one base change.

26. *Colinearity* refers to the sequential arrangement of subunits, amino acids, and nitrogenous bases in proteins and DNA, respectively. Sequencing of genes and products in MS2 phages and studies on mutations in the A subunit of the *tryptophan synthetase* gene indicate a colinear relationship.

28. *Primary*: the linear arrangement or sequence of amino acids. This sequence determines the higher level structures.

Secondary: α-helix and β-pleated sheet structures generated by hydrogen bonds between components of the peptide bond.

Tertiary: folding that occurs as a result of interactions between the amino acid side chains. These interactions include, but are not limited to, the following: covalent disulfide bonds between cysteine residues, interactions of hydrophilic side chains with water, and interactions of hydrophobic side chains with each other.

Quaternary: the association of two (dimer) or more polypeptide chains. Called *oligomeric*, such a protein is made up of more than one protein chain.

30. Enzymes function to regulate catabolic and anabolic activities of cells. They influence (lower) the *energy of activation*, thus allowing chemical reactions to occur under conditions that are compatible with living systems. Enzymes possess active sites and/or other domains that are sensitive to the environment. The active site is considered to be a crevice, or pit, which binds reactants, thus enhancing their interaction. The other domains mentioned above may influence the conformation and, therefore, the function of the active site.

32. Even though three gene pairs are involved, notice that because of the pattern of mutations, each cross may be treated as monohybrid (a) or dihybrid (b, c).

(a) F_1: *AABbCC* = speckled

F_2: 3 *AAB_CC* = speckled
1 *AAbbCC* = yellow

(b) F_1: *AABbCc* = speckled

F_2: 9 *AAB_C_* = speckled
3 *AAB_cc* = green
3 *AAbbC_* = yellow $\Big\}$4
1 *AAbbcc* = yellow

(c) F_1: *AaBBCc* = speckled

F_2: 9 *A_BBC_* = speckled
3 *A_BBcc* = green
3 *aaBBC_* = colorless $\Big\}$4
1 *aaBBcc* = colorless

34. A cross of the following nature would satisfy the data:

$$AABBCC \times aabbcc$$

Offspring in the F_2:

27 *A_B_C_* = purple
9 *A_B_cc* = pink
9 *A_bbC_* = rose
9 *aaB_C_* = orange
3 *A_bbcc* = pink
3 *aaB_cc* = pink
3 *aabbC_* = rose
1 *aabbcc* = pink

The above hypothesis could be tested by conducting a backcross as given below:

$$AaBbCc \times aabbcc$$

The cross should give a
4 (pink):2 (rose):1 (orange):1 (purple) ratio

36.

38. (a) It would appear that the gene is inherited as a dominant because to be recessive, all three individuals from outside the blood line would have to be heterozygous, an unlikely event. In addition, one would expect a mutation in a tRNA synthetase to have considerable negative impact on glycine-bearing protein synthesis.

(b) On the other hand, because affected individuals in the pedigree are heterozygous, sufficient glycyl tRNA synthetase activity must be present to provide vital functions.

(c) Mutational and physiological perturbations, especially when occurring early in development, often cause neuropathologies. This is because of the highly sensitive nature of nerve cell development, and perhaps because axons are typically quite long, reduction of synthesis of glycine-bearing proteins inhibits the required widespread distribution of such proteins within axons.

Chapter 15

ANSWERS TO NOW SOLVE THIS

15-1. The phenotypic influence of any base change is dependent on a number of factors, including its location in coding or noncoding regions, its potential in dominance or recessiveness, and its interaction with other base sequences in the genome. If a base change is located in a noncoding region, there may be no influence on the phenotype. However, some noncoding regions in a traditional sense may influence other genes and/or gene products. If a mutation that occurs in a coding region acts as a full recessive, there should be no influence on the phenotype. If mutant gene acts as a dominant, then there would be an influence on the phenotype. Some genes interact with other genes in a variety of ways that would be difficult to predict without additional information.

15-2. If a gene is incompletely penetrant, it may be present in a population and only express itself under certain conditions. It is unlikely that the gene for hemophilia behaved in this manner. If a gene's expression is suppressed by another mutation in an individual, it is possible that offspring may inherit a given gene and not inherit its suppressor. Such offspring would have hemophilia. It is possible that the mutation in Queen Victoria's family was new, arising in the father. Lastly, it is possible that the mother was heterozygous, and by chance, no other individuals in her family were unlucky enough to receive the mutant gene.

15-3. Any agent that inhibits DNA replication, either directly or indirectly, through mutation and/or DNA cross linking, will suppress the cell cycle and may be useful in cancer therapy. Since guanine alkylation often leads to mismatched bases, they can often be repaired by a variety of mismatched repair mechanisms. However, DNA cross linking can be repaired by recombinational mechanisms. Thus, for such agents to be successful in cancer therapy, suppressors of DNA repair systems are often used in conjunction with certain cancer drugs.

15-4. Ethylmethane sulfonate (EMS) alkylates the keto groups at the sixth position of guanine and at the fourth position of thymine. In each case, base-pairing affinities are altered and transition mutations result. Altered bases are not readily repaired, and once the transition to normal bases occurs through replication, such mutations avoid repair altogether.

SOLUTIONS TO PROBLEMS AND DISCUSSION QUESTIONS

2. Your essay should include a brief description of the genomic differences between diploid and haploid organisms and, with the exception of phenomena such as cell death, disease, and cancer mutational circumstances are attributable to both groups of organisms.

4. When conducting genetic screens, one assumes that all the cells of an organism are genetically identical. Therefore, the organism responds to the screen enabling detection of the mutation. Since a somatic mutation first appears in a single cell, it is highly unlikely that the organism will be sufficiently altered to respond to a screen because none of the other cells in that organism will have the same mutation.

6. A gene is likely to be the product of perhaps a billion or so years of evolution. Each gene and its product function in an environment that has also evolved, or coevolved. A coordinated output of each gene product is required for life. Deviations from the norm, caused by mutation, are likely to be disruptive because of the complex and interactive environment in which each gene product must function. However, on occasion a beneficial variation occurs.

8. A *conditional* mutation is one that produces a wild-type phenotype under one environmental condition and a mutant phenotype under a different condition. A conditional *lethal* is a gene that under one environmental condition leads to premature death of the organism.

10. All three of the agents are mutagenic because they cause base substitutions. Deaminating agents oxidatively deaminate bases such that cytosine is converted to uracil and adenine is converted to hypoxanthine. Uracil pairs with adenine, and hypoxanthine pairs with cytosine. Alkylating agents donate an alkyl group to the amino or keto groups of nucleotides, thus altering base-pairing affinities. 6-ethyl guanine acts like adenine, thereby pairing with thymine. Base analogs such as 5-bromouracil and 2-amino purine are incorporated as thymine and adenine, respectively, yet they base-pair with guanine and cytosine, respectively.

12. X rays are of higher energy and shorter wavelength than UV light. They have greater penetrating ability and can create more disruption of DNA.

14. *Photoreactivation* can lead to repair of UV-induced damage. An enzyme, the photoreactivation enzyme, will absorb a photon of light to cleave thymine dimers. *Excision repair* involves the products of several genes, DNA polymerase I and DNA ligase, to clip out the UV-induced dimer, fill in, and join the phosphodiester backbone in the resulting gap. The excision repair process can be activated by damage that distorts the DNA helix. *Recombinational repair* is a system that responds to DNA that has escaped other repair mechanisms at the time of replication. If a gap is created on one of the newly synthesized strands, a "rescue operation or SOS response" allows the gap to be filled. Many different gene products are involved in this repair process: *recA* and *lexA*. In SOS repair, the proofreading by DNA polymerase III is suppressed, and this therefore is called an "error-prone system."

16. There are numerous regions upstream from coding regions in a gene that are sensitive to mutation. Many mutations upset the regions that signal transcription factor and/or polymerase binding, thereby influencing transcription. Mutations within introns may affect intron splicing or other factors that determine mRNA stability or translation.

18. *Xeroderma pigmentosum* is a form of human skin cancer caused by perhaps several rare autosomal genes, which interfere with the repair of damaged DNA. Studies with heterokaryons provided evidence for complementation, indicating that there may be as many as seven different genes involved. The photoreactivation repair enzyme appears to be involved. Since cancer is caused by mutations in several types of genes, interfering with DNA repair can enhance the occurrence of these types of mutations.

20. It is possible that through the reduction of certain environmental agents that cause mutations, mutation rates might be reduced. On the other hand, certain industrial and medical activities actually concentrate mutagens (radioactive agents and hazardous chemicals). Unless human populations are protected from such agents, mutation rates might actually increase. If one asks about the accumulation of mutations (not rates) in human populations as a result of improved living conditions and medical care, then it is likely that as the environment becomes less harsh (through improvements), more mutations will be tolerated as selection pressure decreases. In addition, as individuals live longer and have children at a later age, some studies indicate that older males accumulate more gametic mutations.

22. Transposons cause changes in DNA in a variety of ways, including massive chromosomal alterations. In most cases, changes in DNA are harmful to organisms, while in rare cases, an evolutionary advantage occurs because the new genetic variation confers a selective advantage.

24.
XP1	XP4	XP5
XP2		XP6
XP3		XP7

The groupings (complementation groups) indicate that at least three "genes" form products necessary for unscheduled DNA synthesis. All of the cell lines that are in the same complementation group are defective in the same product.

26. Approximately 78 percent of humans' radiation exposure comes from natural sources. While diagnostic X rays do contribute about 10 percent of the exposure, other forms of man-made forms of radiation contribute only a relatively small amount. That's not to say that man-made radiation exposure is not a factor in causing mutations; rather, it is not a major factor.

28. Since Betazoids have a 4-letter genetic code and the gene is 3332 nucleotides long, the protein involved must be 833 amino acids in length.

(*mr-1*) Codon 829 specifies an amino that is very close to the end (carboxyl) of the gene. While a nonsense mutation would terminate translation prematurely, the protein would only be shortened by five amino acids. Thus, the protein's ability to fold and perform its cellular function must not be seriously altered. Because of the direction of translation (5′ to 3′ on the mRNA) the carboxyl terminal amino acids in a protein are the last to be included in folding priorities and are sometimes less significant in determining protein function.

(*mr-2*) Since the phenotype is mild, this amino acid change does not completely inactivate the protein, but it does change its activity to some extent. Perhaps the substitution causes the protein to fold in a slightly aberrant manner, allowing it to have some residual function but preventing it from functioning entirely normally. In addition, even if the protein folds similar to the wild-type protein, charge or structural differences in the protein's active site may be only mildly influenced.

(*mr-3*) This deletion contains a total of 68 nucleotides, which account for 17 amino acids. Since Betazoids' codons contain four nucleotides, the mRNA reading frames are maintained subsequent to the deletion. Protein function significantly depends on the relative positions of secondary levels of structure: α-helices and β-sheets. If the deleted section is a "benign" linker between more significant protein domains, then perhaps the protein can tolerate the loss of some amino acids in a part of the protein without completely losing its function.

(*mr-4*) The amino acid specified by codon 192 must be critical to the function of the protein. Altering this amino acid must disrupt a critical region of the protein, thus causing it to lose most or all of its activity. If the protein is an enzyme, this amino acid could be located in its active site and be critical for the ability of the enzyme to bind and/or influence its substrate. One might expect that the amino acid alteration is rather radical such as one sees in the generation of sickle-cell anemia. HbS is caused by the substitution of a valine (no net charge) for glutamic acid (negatively charged).

(*mr-5*) A deletion of 11 base pairs, a number that is not divisible by four, will shift the reading frames subsequent to its location. Even though this deletion is smaller than the deletion discussed above (83–150) and is located in the same region, it causes a reading frame shift. In addition, some or all of the amino acids that are added downstream from the mutation may be different from those in the normal protein. All will not likely change because of synonyms in the code. There is also the possibility that a nonsense triplet may be introduced in the "out-of-phase" region, thus causing premature chain termination. Because this mutation occurs early in the gene, most of the protein will be affected. This may well explain the severe insensitive phenotype.

30. It is probable that the IS occupied or interrupted the normal function of a controlling region related to the *galactose* genes, which are in an operon with one controlling upstream element.

32. (a) Nonsense mutation in coding regions: shortened product somewhat less than 375 amino acids depending on where the chain termination occurred. (b) Insertion in Exon 1, causing frameshift: a variety of amino acid substitutions and possible chain termination downstream. (c) Insertion in Exon 7, causing frameshift: a variety of amino acid substitutions and possible chain termination downstream involving less of the protein than the insertion in Exon 1. (d) Missense mutation: an amino acid substitution. (e) Deletion in Exon 2, causing frameshift: depending on the size of the deletion, a few too many amino acids may be missing. The frameshift would cause additional amino acid changes and possible termination. (f) Deletion in Exon 2, in frame: amino acids missing from Exon 2 without additional changes in the protein. (g) Large deletion covering Exons 2 and 3: significant loss of amino acids toward the N-terminal side of the protein.

Chapter 16

ANSWERS TO NOW SOLVE THIS

16-1. (a) Due to the deletion of a base early in the *lac Z* gene, there will be "frameshift" of all the reading frames downstream from the deletion, thereby altering many amino acids. It is likely that either premature chain termination of translation will occur (from the introduction of a nonsense triplet in a reading frame) or the normal chain termination will be ignored. Regardless, a mutant condition for the *Z* gene will be likely. If such a cell is placed on a lactose medium, it will be incapable of growth because β-galactosidase is not available. (b) If the deletion occurs early in the *A* gene, one might expect impaired function of the *A* gene product, but it will not influence the use of lactose as a carbon source.

16-2. (a) With no lactose and no glucose, the operon is off because the *lac* repressor is bound to the operator and although CAP is bound to its binding site, it will not override the action of the repressor.

(b) With lactose added to the medium, the *lac* repressor is inactivated and the operon is transcribing the structural genes. With no glucose, the CAP is bound to its binding site, thus enhancing transcription.

(c) With no lactose present in the medium, the *lac* repressor is bound to the operator region, and since glucose inhibits adenyl cyclase, the CAP protein will not interact with its binding site. The operon is therefore "off."

(d) With lactose present, the *lac* repressor is inactivated; however, since glucose is also present, CAP will not interact with its binding site. Under this condition transcription is severely diminished, and the operon can be considered to be "off."

SOLUTIONS TO PROBLEMS AND DISCUSSION QUESTIONS

2. Your essay should include a description of the evolutionary advantages of the efficient response to environmental resources and challenges (antibiotics, for example) when such resources are present. Having related functions in operons provides for coordinated responses.

4. In an *inducible system*, the repressor that normally interacts with the operator to inhibit transcription is inactivated by an *inducer*, thus permitting transcription. In a *repressible system*, a normally inactive repressor is *activated* by a *co-repressor*, thus enabling it (the activated repressor) to bind to the operator to inhibit transcription. Because the interaction of the protein (repressor) has a negative influence on transcription, the systems described here are forms of *negative control*.

6. $I^+O^+Z^+$ = Because of the function of the active repressor from the I^+ gene, and no lactose to influence its function, there will be **no enzyme made**.

$I^+O^cZ^+$ = There will be a **functional enzyme made** because the constitutive operator is in *cis* with a Z gene. The lactose in the medium will have no influence because of the constitutive operator. The repressor cannot bind to the mutant operator.

$I^-O^+Z^-$ = There will be a **nonfunctional enzyme made** because with I^- the system is constitutive, but the Z gene is mutant. The absence of lactose in the medium will have no influence because of the nonfunctional repressor. The mutant repressor cannot bind to the operator.

$I^-O^+Z^-$ = There will be a **nonfunctional enzyme made** because with I^- the system is constitutive, but the Z gene is mutant. The lactose in the medium will have no influence because of the nonfunctional repressor. The mutant repressor cannot bind to the operator.

$I^-O^+Z^+/F'I^+$ = There will be **no enzyme made** because in the absence of lactose, the repressor product of the I^+ gene will bind to the operator and inhibit transcription.

$I^+O^cZ^+/F'O^+$ = Because there is a constitutive operator in *cis* with a normal Z gene, there will be a **functional enzyme made**. The lactose in the medium will have no influence because of the mutant operator.

$I^+O^+Z^-/F'I^+O^+Z^+$ = Because there is lactose in the medium, the repressor protein will not bind to the operator and transcription will occur. The presence of a normal Z gene allows a **functional and nonfunctional enzyme to be made**. The repressor protein is diffusible, working in trans.

$I^-O^+Z^-/F'I^+O^+Z^+$ = Because there is no lactose in the medium, the repressor protein (from I^+) will repress the operators and there will be **no enzyme made**.

$I^sO^+Z^+/F'O^+$ = With the product of I^s there is binding of the repressor to the operator and therefore **no enzyme made**. The lack of lactose in the medium is of no consequence because the mutant repressor is insensitive to lactose.

$I^+O^cZ^+/F'O^+Z^+$ = The arrangement of the constitutive operator (O^c) with the Z gene will cause a **functional enzyme to be made**.

8. A single *E. coli* cell contains very few molecules of the *lac* repressor. However, the *lac* I^q mutation causes a 10 × increase in repressor protein production, thus facilitating its isolation. With the use of dialysis against a radioactive gratuitous inducer (IPTG), Gilbert and Müller-Hill were able to identify the repressor protein in certain extracts of *lac* I^q cells. The material that bound the labeled IPTG was purified and shown to be heat labile and have other characteristics of protein. Extracts of *lac* I^- cells did not bind the labeled IPTG.

10. (a) Because activated CAP is a component of the cooperative binding of RNA polymerase to the *lac* promoter, absence of a functional *crp* would compromise the positive control exhibited by CAP.

(b) Without a CAP binding site there would be a reduction in the inducibility of the *lac* operon.

12. Attenuation functions to reduce the synthesis of tryptophan when it is in full supply. It does so by reducing transcription of the *tryptophan* operon. The same phenomenon is observed when tryptophan activates the repressor to shut off transcription of the *tryptophan* operon.

14. Neelaredoxin appears to be a protein that defends anaerobic and perhaps aerobic organisms from oxidative stress brought on by the metabolism of oxygen. The generation of oxygen free radicals (creates the oxidative stress) is dependent on several molecular species including O_2 and H_2O_2. Apparently, relatively high levels of neelaredoxin are produced at all times (*constitutively expressed*) even when potential inducers of gene expression are not added to the system. Additional neelaredoxin gene expression is not responsive (*induced*) as a result of O_2 and H_2O_2 treatment.

16. When arabinose is present in the medium, the structural genes for the *arabinose* operon are transcribed. If the structural genes for the *lac* operon replaced the structural genes for the *ara* operon, then in the presence of arabinose, the *lac* structural genes would be transcribed and β-galactosidase would be produced at induced levels.

18. Because a repressor stops transcription, one would consider this system, as described here, as being under negative control.

20. The system is *inducible*. C codes for the **structural gene**. B must be the **promoter**. The A locus is the **operator**, and the D locus is the **repressor** gene.

22. The first two sentences in the problem indicate an inducible system where oil stimulates the production of a protein, which turns on (positive control) genes to metabolize oil. The different results in strains #2 and #4 suggest a *cis*-acting system. Because the operon by itself (when mutant as in strain #3) gives constitutive synthesis of the structural genes, *cis*-acting system is also supported. The *cis*-acting element is most likely part of the operon.

24. If one could develop an assay for the other gene products under SOS control, with a *lexA⁻* strain the other gene products should be present at induced levels.

26. (a) The simplest model for the action of R and D in *Chlamydia* would be to have the repressor element (R) become ineffective in binding the *cis*-acting element (D) when heat-shocked. This could happen in two ways. Either the supercoiled DNA alters its conformation and becomes ineffective at binding R, or the D-binding efficiency of the R protein is altered by heat. In either case, the genes for infectivity are transcribed in the presence of the heat shock.

   (b) The most straightforward comparison between the heat shock R and D system in *Chlamydia* and the heat-shock sigma factor in *E. coli* would be where the R-D system is inactivated in *Chlamydia* and a sigma factor is activated by heat in *E. coli*.

Chapter 17

ANSWERS TO NOW SOLVE THIS

17-1. Cancer cells often originate under the influence of mutations in tumor-suppressor genes or proto-oncogenes. Should hypermethylation occur in one of many DNA repair genes, the frequency of mutation would increase because the DNA repair system is compromised. The resulting increase in mutations might occur in tumor-suppressor genes or proto-oncogenes.

17-2. General transcription factors associate with a promoter to stimulate transcription of a specific gene. Some *trans*-acting elements, when bound to enhancers, interact with coactivators to enhance transcription by forming an enhanceosome that stimulates transcription initiation. Transcription can be repressed when certain proteins bind to silencer DNA elements and generate repressive chromatin structures. The same molecule may bind to a different chromosomal regulatory site (enhancer or silencer), depending on the molecular environment of a given tissue type.

17-3. Mutations in the *tra* gene of *Drosophila* can dramatically alter development such that a normal female is produced if the TRA protein is present and a male develops when the TRA protein is absent. A null *tra* allele would produce males because of male-specific splicing while a constitutively active *tra* gene would produce females.

SOLUTIONS TO PROBLEMS AND DISCUSSION QUESTIONS

2. Your essay should include an approximation of the percentage of regulatory elements/transcription products in the human genome, the binding sites of regulatory proteins and the general architecture of regulatory elements within chromatin.

4. Chromatin is remodeled when there are significant changes in chromatin organization. Such remodeling involves changes in DNA methylation and interaction of DNA with histones in nucleosomes. Nucleosome remodeling complexes alter nucleosome structure and position by a number of processes, including histone modification and the action of enhancers/silencers.

6. When DNA is transcriptionally active, it is in a less condensed state and as such, more open to DNase digestion.

8. In general, chromatin is remodeled when there are significant changes in chromatin organization. Such remodeling involves changes in DNA methylation and interaction of DNA with histones in nucleosomes. Nucleosome remodeling complexes alter nucleosome structure and position by a number of processes, including histone modification.

10. In general, activators and repressors change the relationship of RNAP II to the transcription complex. DNA loops are thought to bring distant enhancer or silencer elements into proximity with promoter regions of the genes under their regulation.

12. Generally, one determines the influence of various regulatory elements by removing necessary elements or adding extra elements. In addition, examining the outcome of mutations within such elements often provides insight as to function. Assay systems determine the relative levels of gene expression after such alterations.

14. RNA interference begins with a double-stranded RNA being processed by a protein called Dicer that, in combination with RISC, generates short interfering RNA (siRNA). Unwinding of siRNA produces an antisense strand that combines with a protein to cleave mRNA complementary sequences. Short RNAs called microRNAs pair with the 3′ untranslated regions of mRNAs and block their translation.

16. Inr, BRE, DPE, and MTE sequences are double-stranded DNA elements located in the transcription start site (Inr), immediately upstream or downstream from the TATA box (BRE), or downstream (DPE, MTE) from the transcription site (+18 to +27 and +28 to +33, respectively).

18. Given that DNA methylation plays a role in gene expression in mammals, any change in DNA methylation, plus or minus, can potentially have a negative impact on progeny development. In addition, since $m^5C \ggg$ thymine, transitions are likely to cause mutations in coding regions of DNA; when methylation patterns change, new sites for mutation arise. Should mutations occur at a higher rate in previously unmethylated sites (genes), embryonic development is likely to be affected.

20. Since there are multiple routes that lead to cancer, one would expect complex regulatory systems to be involved. More specifically, while in some cases, downregulation of a gene, such as an oncogene, may be a reasonable cancer therapy, downregulation of a tumor-suppressor gene would be undesirable in therapy.

22. Below is a sketch of several RNA polymerase molecules (filled circles) in what might be a transcription factory. This diagram shows eight RNAP II molecules being transcribed. Nascent transcripts are shown projecting from the RNAP II molecules. For simplicity, only one promoter is shown and one structural gene is shown.

24. Since mRNA stability is directly related to the likelihood of translation, one could use a number of different constructs as shown below and test for luciferase activity in the assay system described in the problem.

5′ cap	3′ tail	mRNA (no cap, no tail)
−	−	+
+	−	+
−	+	+
+	−	−
−	+	−

26. When splice specificity is lost, one might observe several classes of altered RNAs: (1) a variety of nonspecific variants producing RNA pools with many lengths and combinations of exons and introns, (2) incomplete splicing where introns and exons are erroneously included or excluded in the mRNA product, and (3) a variety of nonsense products, which result in premature RNA decay or truncated protein products. It is presently unknown as to whether cancer-specific splices initiate or result from tumorigenesis. Given the complexity of cancer induction and the maintenance of the transformed cellular state, gene products that are significant in regulating the cell cycle may certainly be influenced by alternative splicing and thus contribute to cancer.

28. Steroid hormones interact, through receptor molecules, with DNA to regulate genes. In doing so, genes responsible for uncontrolled cell growth may be influenced. If Tamoxifen blocked the manner in which estrogen influenced DNA, it might be effective against ER-positive breast cancer. In actuality, Tamoxifen is an antagonist of the estrogen receptor.

30. 1. Devise some way, through enzymatic or RNA action, to eliminate or mask the nuclear location signal. 2. Block the active site of the receptor. 3. Block the interaction of the transcription factor and the DNA promoter site.

Chapter 18

ANSWERS TO NOW SOLVE THIS

18-1. It is possible that your screen was more inclusive; that is, it identified more subtle alterations than the screen of others. In addition, your screen may have included some

zygotic effect mutations, which were dependent on the action of maternal-effect genes. You may have identified several different mutations (multiple alleles) in some of the same genes.

18-2. Because in *ftz/ftz* embryos, the engrailed product is absent and in *en/en* embryos, *ftz* expression is normal, one can conclude that the *ftz* gene product regulates, either directly or indirectly, *en*. Because the *ftz* gene is expressed normally in *en/en* embryos, the product of the *engrailed* gene does not regulate expression of *ftz*.

SOLUTIONS TO PROBLEMS AND DISCUSSION QUESTIONS

2. Your essay should include a description and examples of differential gene activity, homeotic genes, vulval development, and a typical signaling pathway such as Notch.

4. The fact that nuclei from almost any source remain transcriptionally and translationally active substantiates the fact that the genetic code and the ancillary processes of transcription and translation are compatible throughout the animal and plant kingdoms. Because the egg represents an isolated, "closed" system that can be mechanically, environmentally, and to some extent biochemically manipulated, various conditions may develop that allow one to study facets of gene regulation. For instance, the influence of transcriptional enhancers and suppressors may be studied along with factors that impact translational and post-translational processes. Combinations of injected nuclei may reveal nuclear-nuclear interactions, which could not normally be studied by other methods.

6. (a) Genes that control early development are often dependent on the deposition of their products (mRNA, transcription factors, various structural proteins, etc.) in the egg by the mother. When observable, these are maternal-effect genes. (b) They are made in the early oocyte or nurse cells during oogenesis. (c) Such maternal-effect genes control early developmental events such as defining anterior-posterior polarity. Such products are placed in eggs during oogenesis and are activated immediately after fertilization. (d) A variety of phenotypes are possible, and they are often revealed in the offspring of females. Maternal effects reveal the genotype of the mother.

8. The three main classes of zygotic genes are (1) *gap* genes, which specify adjacent segments; (2) *pair-rule* genes, which specify every other segment and a part of each segment; and (3) *segment polarity* genes, which specify homologous parts of each segment.

10. There are several somewhat indirect methods for determining the transcriptional activity of a given gene in different cell types. First, if protein products of a given gene are present in different cell types, it can be assumed that the responsible gene is being transcribed. Second, if one is able to actually observe, microscopically, gene activity, as is the case in some specialized chromosomes (polytene chromosomes), gene activity can be inferred by the presence of localized chromosomal puffs. A more direct and common practice to assess transcription of particular genes is to use labeled probes. If a labeled probe can be obtained that contains base sequences that are complementary to the transcribed RNA, then such probes will hybridize to that RNA if present in different tissues. This technique is called *in situ* hybridization and is a powerful tool.

12. A dominant gain-of-function mutation is one that changes the specificity or expression pattern of a gene or gene product. The "gain-of-function" *Antp* mutation causes the wild-type *Antennapedia* gene to be expressed in the eye-antenna disc and mutant flies have legs on the head in place of antenna.

14. Because of the regulatory nature of *homeotic* genes in fundamental cellular activities of determination and differentiation, it would be difficult to ignore their possible impact on oncogenesis. Homeotic genes encode DNA binding domains, which influence gene expression; any factor that influences gene expression may, under some circumstances, influence cell-cycle control.

However attractive this model, there have been no homeotic transformations noted in mammary glands, so the typical expression of mutant homeotic genes in insects is not revealed in mammary tissue, according to Lewis (2000). A substantial number of experiments will be needed to establish a functional link between homeotic gene mutation and cancer induction. Mutagenesis and transgenesis experiments are likely to be most productive in establishing a cause-effect relationship.

16. First, it would be interesting to know whether inhibitors of mitochondrial-ribosomal translation would interfere with germ-cell formation. Second, one should know what types of mRNAs are being translated with these ribosomes.

18. Given the information in the problem, it is likely that this gene normally controls the expression of *BX-C* genes in all body segments. The wild-type product of *esc* stored in the egg may be required to interpret the information correctly stored in the egg.

20. Three classes of flower homeotic genes specify various floral organs. Class A group gives rise to petals. B and C genes control stamen formation, and C genes regulate carpels.

22. Since *her-1⁻* mutations cause males to develop into hermaphrodites, and *tra-1⁻* mutations cause hermaphrodites to develop into males, one may hypothesize that the *her-1⁺* gene produces a product that suppresses hermaphrodite development, while the *tra-1⁺* gene product is needed for hermaphrodite development.

24. If the *her-1⁺* product acts as a negative regulator, then when the gene is mutant, suppression over *tra-1⁺* is lost and hermaphroditism would be the result. This hypothesis fits the information provided. The double mutant should be male because even though there is no suppression from *her-1*, there is no *tra-1⁺* product to support hermaphrodite development.

26. (a) The patterns somewhat follow expectations in that genes involved in photosynthesis appear to be most active in the leaf and flower. In addition, high levels of protein synthesis in the root are expected. Since pollen and seeds would be called upon early in development, it would seem reasonable to have such tissues show strong expression of transcriptional regulators.

(b) Two factors may be driving the expression of photosynthetic gene expression in flowers and seeds. First, since development in plants is more continuous or sequential, genes may not necessarily be shut off when their products are not in demand. Second, perhaps various posttranscriptional modifications redirect the function of photosynthetic gene products. In other words, alternative uses for such gene products may have evolved in plants much like that observed in some animal tissues.

(c) Having a global view of gene expression in an organism and its various tissues and organs allows one to estimate the relative contribution a particular gene may have in development. Since developmental and transcriptional networks are common in development, it is helpful to know the context in which a particular gene may function. Lastly, the only way in which development will be understood at the molecular level is to have a broad view of classes and clusters of gene activity.

Chapter 19

ANSWERS TO NOW SOLVE THIS

19-1. Several approaches are used to combat CML. One includes the use of a tyrosine kinase inhibitor that binds competitively to the ATP binding site of ABL kinase, thereby inhibiting phosphorylation of BCR-ABL and preventing the activation of additional signaling pathways. In addition, real-time quantitative reverse transcription-polymerase chain reaction (Q-RT-PCR) allows one to monitor the drug responses of cell populations in patients so that less toxic and more effective treatments are possible. Being able to distinguish leukemic cells from healthy cells allows one not only to target therapy to specific cell populations, but also to quantify responses to therapy. Because such cells produce a hybrid protein, it may be possible to develop a therapy, perhaps an immunotherapy, based on the uniqueness of the BCR/ABL protein.

19-2. *p53* is a tumor-suppressor gene that protects cells from multiplying with damaged DNA. It is present in its mutant state in more than 50 percent of all tumors. Since the immediate control of a critical and universal cell-cycle checkpoint is mediated by *p53*, mutation will influence a wide range of cell types. *p53*'s action is not limited to specific cell types.

19-3. Cancer is a complex alteration in normal cell-cycle controls. Even if a major "cancer-causing" gene is transmitted, other genes, often new mutations, are usually necessary in order to drive a cell toward tumor formation. Full expression of the cancer phenotype is likely to be the result of an interplay among a variety of genes and therefore show variable penetrance and expressivity.

19-4. Unfortunately, it is common to spend enormous amounts of money dealing with diseases after they occur rather than concentrating on disease prevention. Too often, pressure from special interest groups or lack of political will retard advances in education and prevention. Obviously, it is less expensive, both in terms of human suffering and money, to seek preventive measures for as many diseases as possible. However, having gained some understanding of the mechanisms of disease, in this case cancer, it must also be stated that no matter what preventive measures are taken it will be impossible to completely eliminate disease from the human population. It is extremely important, however, that we increase efforts to educate and protect the human population from as many hazardous environmental agents as possible. A balanced, multipronged approach seems appropriate.

SOLUTIONS TO PROBLEMS AND DISCUSSION QUESTIONS

2. Your essay should include describe the general influence of genetics in cancer. Since epigenetic factors alter gene output, it is likely that such factors could cause cancer.

4. Kinases regulate other proteins by adding phosphate groups. Cyclins bind to the kinases, switching them on and off. CDK4 binds to cyclin D, moving cells from G1 to S. At the G2/mitosis border, a CDK1 (cyclin-dependent kinase) combines with another cyclin (cyclin B). Phosphorylation occurs, bringing about a series of changes in the nuclear membrane via caldesmon, cytoskeleton, and histone H1.

6. To say that a particular trait is inherited conveys the assumption that when a particular genetic circumstance is present, it will be revealed in the phenotype. When one discusses an inherited predisposition, one usually refers to situations where a particular phenotype is expressed in families in some consistent pattern. However, the phenotype may not always be expressed or may manifest itself in different ways. In retinoblastoma, the gene is inherited as an autosomal dominant, and those that inherit the mutant *RB* allele are predisposed to develop eye tumors. However, approximately 10 percent of the people known to inherit the gene do not actually express it, and in some cases expression involves only one eye, rather than two.

8. Apoptosis, or programmed cell death, is a genetically controlled process that leads to death of a cell. It is a natural process involved in morphogenesis and a protective mechanism against cancer formation. During apoptosis, nuclear DNA becomes fragmented, cellular structures are disrupted, and the cells are dissolved. Caspases are involved in the initiation and progress of apoptosis.

10. The nonphosphorylated form of pRB binds to transcription factors such as E2F, causing inactivation and suppression of the cell cycle. Phosphorylation of pRB activates the cell cycle by releasing transcription factors (E2F) to advance the cell cycle. With the phosphorylation site inactivated in the PSM-RB form, phosphorylation cannot occur, thereby leaving the cell cycle in a suppressed state.

12. Various kinases can be activated by breaks in DNA. One kinase, called ATM, and/or a kinase called Chk2 phosphorylates BRCA1 and p53. The activated p53 arrests replication during the S phase to facilitate DNA repair. The activated BRCA1 protein, in conjunction with BRCA2, mRAD51, and other nuclear proteins, is involved in repairing the DNA.

14. Mutations that produce oncogenes alter gene expression either directly or indirectly and act in a dominant capacity. Proto-oncogenes are those that normally function to promote or maintain cell division. In the mutant state (oncogenes), they induce or maintain uncontrolled cell division; that is, there is a gain of function. Generally, this gain of function takes the form of increased or abnormally continuous gene output. On the other hand, loss of function is generally attributed to mutations in tumor-suppressor genes, which function to halt passage through the cell cycle. When such genes are mutant, they have lost their capacity to halt the cell cycle. Such mutations are generally recessive.

16. To encourage infected cells to undergo growth and division, viruses often encode genes that stimulate growth and division. Many viruses either inactivate tumor-suppressor genes of the host or bring in genes that stimulate cell growth and division. By inactivating tumor-suppressor genes, the normal breaking mechanism of the cell cycle is destroyed.

18. Normal cells are often capable of withstanding mutational assault because they have checkpoints and DNA repair mechanisms in place. When such mechanisms fail, cancer may be a result. Through mutation, such protective mechanisms are compromised in cancer cells, and as a result they show higher than normal rates of mutation, chromosomal abnormalities, and genomic instability.

20. Epigenetic effects can be caused by DNA methylation and/or histone modifications, including acetylation and/or phosphorylation. As such, they can silence or activate chromosomes (X chromosome, for example) or certain chromosomal regions and be responsible for parental imprinting or influencing gene activity in heterochromatin. Patterns of nucleotide demethylation and hypermethylation are often different when cancer cells are compared to normal cells.

22. No, she will still have the general population risk of about 10 percent. In addition, it is possible that genetic tests will not detect all breast cancer mutations.

24. Proteases in general and serine proteases, specifically, are considered tumor-promoting agents because they degrade proteins, especially those in the extracellular matrix. When such proteolysis occurs, cellular invasion and metastasis are encouraged. Consistent with this observation are numerous observations that metastatic tumor cells are associated with higher than normal amounts of protease expression. Inhibitors of serine proteases are often tested for their anticancer efficacy.

26. (a) Since a normal p53 protein is very helpful in preventing cancer, loss of p53 synthesis through hypermethylation of such a promoter would decrease p53 concentration and thus be detrimental. (b) If one has comparison blood from an individual before he or she has cancer, the origin of a cancer might contain cancer-related DNA that could be detected in the blood. Since blood is relatively easy to obtain, this would be an extremely useful diagnostic tool.

28. As with many forms of cancer, a single gene alteration is not the only requirement. The authors (Bose et al.) state "but only infrequently do the cells acquire the additional changes necessary to produce leukemia in humans." Some studies indicate that variations (often deletions) in the region of the breakpoints may bring about cancer-related genetic change.

30. (a) The mRNA triplet for Gln is CAG(A). The mRNA triplet that specifies a stop is one of three: UAA, UAG, or UGA. The strand of DNA that codes for the CAG(A) would be the following: 3′-GTC(T)-5′. Therefore, if the G mutated to an A (transition), then the DNA strand would be 3′-ATC(T)-5′, which would cause a UAG(A) triplet to be produced, and this would cause the stop.

(b) It is likely to be a tumor-suppressor gene because loss of function causes predisposition to cancer.

(c) Some women may carry genes (perhaps mutant) that "spare" for the *BRCA1* gene product. Some women may have immune systems that recognize and destroy precancerous cells, or they may have mutations in breast signal transduction genes so that cell division suppression occurs in the absence of *BRCA1*.

32. Various alterations in gene activity related to hyper- and hypomethylation have been associated with numerous cancers. Hypermethylation usually leads to a suppression of gene activity. *Hormonal response genes* often synthesize

receptors that respond to a variety of hormones such as androgens, retinoic acid, and estrogens. For example, prostate cancer is often associated with suppressed *ESR1* and *ESR2* activity, both of which are estrogen receptors.

Cell-cycle control genes are involved in both upregulation and downregulation of the cell cycle as they influence cyclins and cyclin-dependent kinases. The cyclin-dependent kinase inhibitor *CDKN2A*, when hypermethylated, fails to inhibit cyclin-dependent kinase and thereby contributes to cancer progression.

A number of *tumor cell invasion genes* have been described, some of which interfere with intercellular adhesion. When such genes are suppressed through hypermethylation, cadherin–catenin adherence mechanisms are compromised, which can influence cell-to-cell contacts.

One of the most common causes of cancer is a breakdown in *DNA repair* mechanisms. Hypermethylation suppresses the genes that normally supply DNA repair components.

Proper *signal transduction* is required to maintain cell–cell adherence and response to extracellular signals. For example, when *CD44*, an integral membrane protein that is involved in matrix adhesion and signal transduction, is hypermethylated, cells cannot maintain proper cell–cell contact and communication, without which cell-cycle control is compromised.

Chapter 20

ANSWERS TO NOW SOLVE THIS

20-1. (a) Bacteria that have been transformed with the recombinant plasmid will be resistant to tetracycline, and therefore tetracycline should be added to the medium.

(b) Colonies that grow on a tetracycline medium only should contain the insert. Those bacteria that do not grow on the ampicillin medium probably contain the *Drosophila* DNA insert.

(c) Resistance to both antibiotics by a transformed bacterium could be explained in several ways. First, if cleavage with the *Pst*I was incomplete, then no change in biological properties of the uncut plasmids would be expected. Also, it is possible that the cut ends of the plasmid were ligated together in the original form with no insert.

20-2. The genomic clone probably contained a number of introns that were removed from the mRNA during processing. The cDNA was parepared from mRNA.

20-3. Using the human nucleotide sequence, one can produce a probe to screen the library of the African okapi. Second, one can use the amino acid sequence and the genetic code to generate a complementary DNA probe for screening of the library. The probe is used, through hybridization, to identify the DNA that is complementary to the probe and can allow one to identify the library clone containing the DNA of interest. Cells with the desired clone are then picked from the original plate and the plasmid is isolated from the cells.

SOLUTIONS TO PROBLEMS AND DISCUSSION QUESTIONS

2. Your essay should include an appreciation for the relative ease in which sections of DNA can be inserted into various vectors and the amplification and isolation of such DNA. You should also include the possibilities of modifying recombinant molecules.

4. Even though the human gene coding for insulin contains a number of introns, a cDNA generated from insulin mRNA is free of introns. Plasmids containing insulin genes (from cDNA) are free of introns, so no processing issue surfaces.

6. This segment contains the palindromic sequence of GGATCC, which is recognized by the restriction enzyme *Bam*HI. The double-stranded sequence is the following:

GGATCC
CCTAGG

8. Plasmids were the first to be used as cloning vectors, and they are still routinely used to clone relatively small fragments of DNA. Because of their small size, they are relatively easy to separate from the host bacterial chromosome, and they have relatively few restriction sites. They can be engineered fairly easily (i.e., polylinkers and reporter genes added). For cloning larger pieces of DNA such as entire eukaryotic genes, cosmids are often used. For instance, when modifications are made in the bacterial virus lambda (λ), relatively large inserts of about 20 kb can be cloned. This is an important advantage when one needs to clone a large gene or generate a genomic library from a eukaryote. In addition, some cosmids will only accept inserts of a limited size, which means that small, perhaps, less meaningful fragments will not be cloned unnecessarily. Both plasmids and cosmids suffer from the limitation that they can only use bacteria as hosts. BACs are artificial bacterial chromosomes that can be engineered for certain qualities.

YACs (yeast artificial chromosomes) contain telomeres, an origin of replication, and a centromere and are extensively used to clone DNA in yeast. With selectable markers (TRP1 and URA3) and a cluster of restriction sites, DNA inserts ranging from 100 kb to 1000 kb can be cloned and inserted into yeast. Since yeast, being a eukaryote, undergoes many of the typical RNA and protein processing steps of other, more complex eukaryotes, the advantages are numerous when working with eukaryotic genes.

10. No. The tumor-inducing plasmid (Ti) that is used to produce genetically modified plants is specific for the bacterium *Agrobacterium tumifaciens,* which causes tumors in many plant species. There is no danger that this tumor-inducing plasmid will cause tumors in humans.

12. The total number of molecules after 15 cycles would be 16,384, or $(2)^{14}$.

14. A cDNA library provides DNAs from RNA transcripts and is, therefore, useful in identifying what are likely to be functional DNAs. If one desires an examination of noncoding as well as coding regions, a genomic library would be more useful.

16. Several factors may contribute to the lack of representation of the 5′ end of the mRNA. One has to deal with the possibility that the reverse transcriptase may not completely synthesize the DNA from the RNA template. The other reason may be that the 3′ end of the copied DNA tends to fold back on itself, thus providing a primer for the DNA polymerase. Additional preparation of the cDNA requires some digestion at the folded region. Since this folded region corresponds to the 5′ end of the mRNA, some of the message is often lost.

18. Assuming that one has knowledge of the amino acid sequence of the protein product or the nucleotide sequence of the target nucleic acid, a degenerate set of DNA strands can be prepared for cloning into an appropriate vector or amplified by PCR. A variety of labeling techniques can then be used, through hybridization, to identify complementary base sequences contained in the genomic library. One must know at least a portion of the amino acid sequence of the protein product or its nucleic acid sequence in order for the procedure to be applied. Some problems can occur through degeneracy in the genetic code (not allowing construction of an appropriate probe), the possible existence of pseudogenes in the library (hybridizations with inappropriate related fragments in the library), and variability of DNA sequences in the library due to introns (causing poor or background hybridization). To overcome some of these problems, one can construct a variety of relatively small probes of different types that take into account the degeneracy in the code. By varying the conditions of hybridization (salt and temperature), one can reduce undesired hybridizations.

20. (a) Heating to 90–95°C denatures the double-stranded DNA so that it dissociates into single strands. It usually takes about five minutes, depending on the length and GC content of the DNA.

(b) Lowering the temperature to 50–70°C allows the primers to bind to the denatured DNA.

(c) Bringing the temperature to 70–75°C allows the heat-stable DNA polymerase an opportunity to extend the primers by adding nucleotides to the 3′ ends of each growing strand. Each PCR is designed with specific temperatures (not ranges) based on the characteristics of the DNAs (template and primers).

22. ddNTPs are analogs of the "normal" deoxyribonucleotide triphosphates (dNTPs), but they lack a 3′-hydroxyl group. As DNA synthesis occurs, the DNA polymerase occasionally inserts a ddNTP into a growing DNA strand. Since there is no 3′-hydroxyl group, chain elongation cannot take place, and resulting fragments are formed, which can be separated by electrophoresis. Where the ddNTP was incorporated, the length of each strand and, therefore, the position of the particular ddNTP and established and used to eventually provide the base sequence of the DNA.

24. FISH involves the hybridization of a labeled probe to a complementary stretch of DNA in a chromosome. As such, it can be used to locate a specific DNA sequence (often a gene or gene fragment) in a chromosome. Spectral karyotyping uses FISH to detect individual chromosomes, a distinct advantage in identifying chromosomal abnormalities.

26. If a transgene integrates into a coding or regulatory region, it will likely cause a mutation. Any random integration may also alter the function of endogenous DNA.

28. Reporter genes, surface traits, and various probes are often used to determine the integration of a transgene.

30. $T_m(°C) = 81.5 + 0.41(\%GC) - (675/N) = 81.5 + 0.41(33.3) - (675/21) =$ about 63°C. Subtracting 5°C gives us a good starting point of about 58°C for PCR with this primer. Notice that as the % of GC and length increase, the $T_m(°C)$ increases. GC pairs contain three hydrogen bonds rather than two as between AT pairs.

32. (a) As the percent dT increases, the required annealing temperature decreases.

(b) Because random sequence primers contain G and C bases, the annealing temperatures need to be adjusted.

(c) One could isolate RNAs from each side, trap the mRNAs using oligo(dT), and analyse the mRNAs using quantitative PCR.

34. By examining previous equations, it is clear that a variety of factors influence T_m and, therefore, annealing of primers with DNA. Primers with different percentages of GC and/or length will have different annealing temperatures. To factor these variables into a single T_m given a number of other factors (divalent and monovalent cation concentrations, primer and target concentrations) has, to date, been a complex problem that is often unresolvable.

Chapter 21

ANSWERS TO NOW SOLVE THIS

21-1. (a) To annotate a gene, one identifies gene-regulatory sequences found upstream of genes (promoters, enhancers, and silencers), downstream elements (termination sequences), and in-frame triplet nucleotides that are part of the coding region of the gene. In addition, 5′ and 3′ splice sites that are used to distinguish exons from introns as well as polyadenylation sites are also used in annotation.

(b) Similarity to other annotated sequences often provides insight as to a sequence's function and may serve to substantiate a particular genetic assignment. Direct sequencing of cDNAs from various tissues and developmental stages aids in verification.

(c) Taking an average of 20,000 for the estimated number of genes in the human genome and computing the percentage represented by 3141 gives 15.7 percent. It appears as if chromosome 1 is gene rich.

21-2. Since structural and chemical factors determine the function of a protein, it is likely to have several proteins share a considerable amino acid sequence identity, but not be functionally identical. Since the *in vivo* function of such a protein is determined by secondary and tertiary structures, as well as local surface chemistries in active or functional sites, the nonidentical sequences may have considerable influence on function. Note that the query matches to different site positions within the target proteins. A number of other factors suggesting different functions include associations with other molecules (cytoplasmic, membrane, or extracellular), chemical nature and position of binding domains, posttranslational modification, signal sequences, and so on.

21-3. Because blood is relatively easy to obtain in a pure state, its components can be analyzed without fear of tissue-site contamination. Second, blood is intimately exposed to virtually all cells of the body and may therefore carry chemical markers to certain abnormal cells it represents. Theoretically, it is an ideal probe into the human body. However, when blood is removed from the body, its proteome changes, and those changes are dependent on a number of environmental factors. Thus, what might be a valid diagnostic for one condition might not be so for other conditions. In addition, the serum proteome is subject to change depending on the genetic, physiologic, and environmental state of the patient. Age and sex are additional variables that must be considered. Validation of a plasma proteome for a particular cancer would be strengthened by demonstrating that the stage of development of the cancer correlates with a commensurate change in the proteome in a relatively large, statistically significant pool of patients. Second, the types of changes in the proteome should be reproducible and, at least until complexities are clarified, involve tumorigenic proteins. It would be helpful to have comparisons with archived samples of each individual at a disease-free time.

SOLUTIONS TO PROBLEMS AND DISCUSSION QUESTIONS

2. Your essay should include a description of traditional recombinant DNA technology involving cutting and splicing genes, as well as modern methods of synthesizing genes of interest, PCR amplification, microarray analysis, etc.

4. Whole-genome shotgun sequencing involves randomly cutting the genome into numerous smaller segments. Overlapping sequences are used to identify segments that were once contiguous, eventually producing the entire sequence. Difficulties in alignment often occur in repetitive regions of the genome. Map-based sequencing relies on known landmarks (genes, nucleotide polymorphisms, etc.) to orient the alignment of cloned fragments that have been sequenced. Compared to whole-genome sequencing, the map-based approach is somewhat cumbersome and time consuming. Whole-genome sequencing has become the most common method for assembling genomes, with map-based cloning being used to resolve the problems often encountered during whole-genome sequencing.

6. The main goals of the Human Genome Project are to establish, categorize, and analyze functions for human genes. As stated in the text:

> To analyze genetic variations between humans, including the identification of single-nucleotide polymorphisms (SNPs)

> To map and sequence the genomes of several model organisms used in experimental genetics, including *E. coli*, *S. cerevisiae*, *C. elegans*, *D. melanogaster*, and *M. musculus* (the mouse)

> To develop new sequencing technologies, such as high-throughput computer-automated sequencers, to facilitate genome analysis

> To disseminate genome information, both among scientists and the general public

8. One initial approach to annotating a sequence is to compare the newly sequenced genomic DNA to the known sequences already stored in various databases. The National Center for Biotechnology Information (NCBI) provides access to BLAST (Basic Local Alignment Search Tool) software, which directs searches through databanks of DNA and protein sequences. A segment of DNA can be compared to sequences in major databases such as GenBank to identify matches that align in whole or in part. One might seek similarities to a sequence on chromosome 11 in a mouse and find that or similar sequences in a number of taxa. BLAST will compute a similarity score or identity value to indicate the degree to which two sequences are similar. BLAST is one of many sequence alignment algorithms (RNA-RNA, protein-protein, etc.) that may sacrifice sensitivity for speed.

10. The human genome is composed of over 3 billion nucleotides in which about 2 percent code for genes. Genes are unevenly distributed over chromosomes, with clusters of gene-rich regions separated by gene-poor ones (deserts). Human genes tend to be larger and contain more and larger introns than in invertebrates such as *Drosophila*. It is estimated that at least half of the genes generate products by alternative splicing. Hundreds of genes have been transferred from bacteria into vertebrates. Duplicated regions are common, which may facilitate chromosomal rearrangement. The human genome appears to contain approximately 20,000 protein-coding genes. However, there is still uncertainty as to the total number.

12. Because many repetitive regions of the genome are not directly involved in production of a phenotype, they tend to be isolated from selection and show considerable variation in redundancy. Length variation in such repeats is unique among individuals (except for identical twins) and, with various detection methods, provides the basis for DNA fingerprinting. Single-nucleotide polymorphisms also occur frequently in the genome and can be used to distinguish individuals.

14. The Personal Genome Project (PGP) provides individual sequences of diploid genomes, and results of such projects indicate that the HGP may underestimate genome variation by as much as fivefold. Genome variation between individuals may be 0.5 percent rather than the 0.1 percent estimated from the HGP. Since the PGP provides sequence information on individuals, fundamental questions about human diversity and evolution may be more answerable.

16. A number of new subdisciplines of molecular biology will provide the infrastructure for major advances in our understanding of living systems. The following terms identify specific areas within that infrastructure:

> proteomics—proteins in a cell or tissue
> metabolomics—enzymatic pathways
> glycomics—carbohydrates of a cell or tissue
> toxicogenomics—toxic chemicals
> metagenomics—environmental issues
> pharmacogenomics—customized medicine
> transcriptomics—expressed genes

Many other "-omics" are likely in the future.

18. Most microarrays, known also as gene chips, consist of a glass slide that is coated, using a robotic system, with single-stranded DNA molecules. Some microarrays are coated with single-stranded sequences of expressed sequenced tags or DNA sequences that are complementary to gene transcripts. A single microarray can have as many as 20,000 different spots of DNA, each containing a unique sequence. Researchers use microarrays to compare patterns of gene expression in tissues under different conditions or to compare gene-expression patterns in normal and diseased tissues. In addition, microarrays can be used to identify pathogens. Microarray databases allow investigators to compare any given pattern to others worldwide.

20. Increased protein production from approximately 20,000 genes is probably related to alternative splicing and various posttranslational processing schemes. In addition, a particular DNA segment may be read in a variety of ways and in two directions.

22. While the β-globin gene family is a relatively large (60 kb) sequence and restriction analyses show that it is composed of six genes, one is a pseudogene and therefore does not produce a product. The five functional genes each contain two similarly sized introns, which, when included with non-coding flanking regions (5′ and 3′) and spacer DNA between genes, account for the 95 percent mentioned in the question.

24. (a) arm of human, wing of bird, fin of whale (b) Homologous proteins may have similar functions; however, this is not always the case. (c) If proteins evolved by convergent evolution, they may have similar function but not share homology.

26. The position of the homologous track is pivotal in determining the 3D structure of a protein. It is the 3D structure, facilitated by chaperones, with its particular surface chemistry that specifies function.

28. (a, b) With WES, one may get lucky and find an issue within a gene that has relevance. Given the multitude of genetic variations among individuals, this might be similar to finding a needle in a haystack. Many significant genomic functions are regulated outside the exon pool. Introns and mitochondria are highly variable among individuals, but may contribute significantly among individuals.

Chapter 22

ANSWERS TO NOW SOLVE THIS

22-1. Antigens are usually quite large molecules, and in the process of digestion, they are sometimes broken down into smaller molecules, thus becoming ineffective in stimulating the immune system. Some individuals are allergic to the food they eat, testifying to the fact that all antigens are not completely degraded or modified by digestion. In some cases, ingested antigens do indeed stimulate the immune system (e.g., oral polio vaccine) and provide a route for immunization. Localized (intestinal) immunity can sometimes be stimulated by oral introduction of antigens, and in some cases, this can offer immunity to ingested pathogens.

22-2. The child in question is a carrier of the deletion in the β-globin gene, just as the parents are carriers. Its genotype is therefore $\beta^A\beta^0$.

22-3. It will hybridize by base complementation to the normal DNA sequence.

SOLUTIONS TO PROBLEMS AND DISCUSSION QUESTIONS

2. Your essay should include a description of genomic applications that relate to agriculture, health and welfare, scientific exploration and appreciation of the earth's flora and fauna, etc. In addition, areas of patent protection, personal privacy, and potential agricultural and environmental hazards should be addressed.

4. In general, bacteria do not process eukaryotic proteins in the same manner as eukaryotes. Transgenic eukaryotes are more likely to correctly process eukaryotic proteins, thus increasing the likelihood of their normal biological activity.

6. (a) Both the saline and column extracts of Lkt50 appear to be capable of inducing at least 50 percent neutralization of toxicity when injected into rabbits.

(b) First, the immunogen must be stably incorporated into the host plant hereditary material, and the host must express only that immunogen. During feeding, the immunogen must be transported across the intestinal wall unaltered or altered in such a way as to stimulate the desired immune response. There must be guarantees that potentially harmful by-products of transgenesis have not been produced. In other words, broad ecological and environmental issues must be addressed to prevent a transgenic plant from becoming an unintended vector for harm to the environment or any organisms feeding on the plant (directly or indirectly).

8. Even though you have developed a method for screening seven of the mutations described, it is possible that negative results can occur when the person carries the gene for CF. In other words, the specific probes (or allele-specific oligonucleotides) that have been developed will not necessarily be useful for screening all mutant alleles. In addition, the cost-effectiveness of such a screening proposal would need to be considered.

10. Since both mutations occur in the CF gene, children who possess both alleles will suffer from CF. With both parents heterozygous, each child born will have a 25 percent chance of developing CF.

12. Using restriction enzyme analysis to detect point mutations in humans is a tedious trial-and-error process. Given the size of the human genome in terms of base sequences and the relatively low number of unique restriction enzymes, the likelihood of matching a specific point mutation, separate from other normal sequence variations, to a desired gene is low.

14. Genome-wide association studies involve scanning the genomes of thousands of unrelated individuals with a particular disease and comparing them with the genomes of individuals who do not have the disease. GWAS attempt to identify genes that influence disease risk.

16. In the case of haplo-insufficient mutations, gene therapy holds promise; however, in "gain-of-function" mutations, in all probability the mutant gene's activity or product must be compromised. RNAi strategies may apply more effectively. Addition of a normal gene probably will not help unless it can compete out the mutant gene product.

18. Certainly, information provided to physicians and patients about genetic testing is a strong point in favor of wide distribution. It would probably be helpful for companies involved in genetic testing to also participate by providing information peculiar to their operations. It would be necessary, however, that any individual results from tests would be held in strict confidence. It would be helpful if pooled statistical data would be available to the public in terms of frequencies of false positives and negatives, as well as population and/or geographical distributions.

20. It is a personal decision to have one's genome sequenced, but in doing so one must be armed with information as to the expected variability of the genome and the possibility of false positives. A publically available genome might lead to employment bias, changes in personal relationships, and so on.

22. Raw genomic information is difficult to interpret. 23andMe now provides only ancestry information and has stopped giving health-related data. In November 2013, the FDA warned 23andMe to stop marketing its genomic service.

24. *Sample size:* Is the sample size sufficiently robust to minimize spurious correlations? *Epigenetic factors:* Since the genome is strongly influenced by epigenetic factors, how might this influence a study based on SNPs? *Environmental factors:* Have samples been compiled in such a way as to negate significant differences in environmental exposure? *Genetic background:* Since the entire genome is not compared, what suppressors and/or modifiers that mask or enhance the expression of certain genes are present, but missed? What emergent properties are present in the entire allelic architecture? *Population stratification:* Might there be allelic frequency differences peculiar to the case population as compared with the control group? Such population frequency differences may result from differences in ancestry, depending on the composition of the cases and the controls.

26. There are several reasons why CF mice do not exhibit airway symptoms similar to humans with CF. First, the distribution of cell types, CFTR presence, and chloride/sodium handling differ in the upper and lower airways of mice and humans. Second, mice tend not to suffer from airway bacterial infections that severely influence human pathology. A complete review of this topic is available in Grubb and Boucher, 1999, *Physiological Reviews,* vol. 71, 5193–5214.

Chapter 23

ANSWERS TO NOW SOLVE THIS

23-1. (a) Since 1/256 of the F_2 plants are 20 cm and 1/256 are 40 cm, there must be four gene pairs involved in determining flower size.

(b) Since there are nine size classes, one can conduct the following backcross: $AaBbCcDd \times AABBCCDD$. The frequency distribution in the backcross would be:

$$1/16 = 40 \text{ cm}$$
$$4/16 = 37.5 \text{ cm}$$
$$6/16 = 35 \text{ cm}$$
$$4/16 = 32.5 \text{ cm}$$
$$1/16 = 30 \text{ cm}$$

23-2. (a) Taking the sum of the values and dividing by the number in the sample gives the following means:

mean sheep fiber length = 7.7 cm
mean fleece weight = 6.4 kg

The variance for each is:

variance sheep fiber length = 6.097
variance fleece weight = 3.12

The standard deviation is the square root of the variance:

sheep fiber length = 2.469
fleece weight = 1.766

(b, c) The covariance for the two traits is 30.36/7, or 4.34, while the correlation coefficient is +0.998.

(d) There is a very high correlation between fleece weight and fiber length, and it is likely that this correlation is not by chance. Even though correlation does not mean cause and effect, it would seem logical that as you increased fiber length, you would also increase fleece weight. It is probably safe to say that the increase in fleece weight is directly related to an increase in fiber length.

23-3. *Monozygotic twins* are derived from a single fertilized egg and are thus genetically identical to each other. They provide a method for determining the influence of genetics and environment on certain traits. *Dizygotic twins* arise from two eggs fertilized by two sperm cells. They have the same genetic relationship as siblings. The role of genetics and the role of the environment can be studied by comparing the expression of traits in monozygotic and dizygotic twins. The higher concordance value for monozygotic twins indicates a significant genetic component for a given trait. Notice that for traits including blood type, eye color, and mental retardation, there is a fairly significant difference between MZ and DZ groups. However, for measles, the difference is not as significant, indicating a greater role of the environment. Hair color has a significant genetic component, as do idiopathic epilepsy, schizophrenia, diabetes, allergies, cleft lip, and club foot. The genetic component of mammary cancer is present but minimal according to these data.

SOLUTIONS TO PROBLEMS AND DISCUSSION QUESTIONS

2. Your essay should include a description of various ratios typical of Mendelian genetics as compared with the more blending, continuously varying expressions of neo-Mendelian modes of inheritance. It should contrast discontinuous inheritance and continuous patterns.

4. (a) Because a dihybrid result has been identified, there are two loci involved in the production of color. There are two alleles at each locus, for a total of four alleles.

(b, c) Because the description of red, medium red, and so on gives us no indication of a *quantity* of color in any form of units, we would not be able to actually quantify a unit amount for each change in color. We can say that each gene (additive allele) provides an equal unit amount to the phenotype, and the colors differ from each other in multiples of that unit amount. The number of additive alleles needed to produce each phenotype is as follows:

1/16 = dark red	= AABB
4/16 = medium-dark red	= 2AABb
	2AaBB
6/16 = medium red	= AAbb
	4AaBb
	aaBB
4/16 = light red	= 2aaBb
	2Aabb
1/16 = white	= aabb

(d)

F_1 = all light red
F_2 = 1/4 medium red
  2/4 light red
  1/4 white

6. (a, b) See that where four gene pairs act additively, the proportion of one of the extreme phenotypes to the total number of offspring is 1/256. The same may be said for the other extreme type. The extreme types in this

problem are the 12-cm and 36-cm plants. From this observation one would suggest that there are four gene pairs involved.

(c) If there are four gene pairs, there are nine ($2n + 1$) phenotypic categories and eight increments between these categories. Since there is a difference of 24 cm between the extremes, 24 cm/8 = 3 cm for each increment (each of the additive alleles).

(d) Because the parents are inbred, it is expected that they are fully homozygous. An example:

$$AABBccdd \times aabbCCDD$$

(e) Since the *aabbccdd* genotype gives a height of 12 cm and each uppercase allele adds 3 cm to the height, there are many possibilities for an 18 cm plant:

AAbbccdd,
AaBbccdd,
aaBbCcdd, etc.

Any plant with seven uppercase letters will be 33 cm tall:

AABBCCDd,
AABBCcDD,
AABbCCDD, for example.

8. For height, notice that average differences between MZ twins reared together (1.7 cm) and MZ twins reared apart (1.8 cm) are similar (meaning little environmental influence) and considerably less than differences of DZ twins (4.4 cm) or sibs (4.5) reared together. These data indicate that genetics plays a major role in determining height.

However, for weight, notice that MZ twins reared together have a much smaller (1.9 kg) difference than MZ twins reared apart, indicating that the environment has a considerable impact on weight. By comparing the weight differences of MZ twins reared apart with DZ twins and sibs reared together, one can conclude that the environment has almost as much an influence on weight as genetics.

For ridge count, the differences between MZ twins reared together and those reared apart are small. For the data in the table, it would appear that ridge count and height have the highest heritability values.

10. Many traits, especially those we view as quantitative, are likely to be determined by a polygenic mode with possible environmental influences. The following are some common examples: height, general body structure, skin color, and perhaps most common behavioral traits, including intelligence.

12. (a) *For back fat:*

Broad-sense heritability = H^2 = 12.2/30.6 = 0.398
Narrow-sense heritability = h^2 = 8.44/30.6 = 0.276

For body length:

Broad-sense heritability = H^2 = 26.4/52.4 = 0.504
Narrow-sense heritability = h^2 = 11.7/52.4 = 0.223

(b) Selection for back fat would produce more response.

14. (a) For vitamin A: $h_A^2 = 0.097$
For cholesterol: $h_A^2 = 0.223$

(b) Cholesterol content should be influenced to a greater extent by selection.

16. $h^2 = (7.5 - 8.5/6.0 - 8.5) = 0.4$ (realized heritability)
18. $h^2 = 0.3 = (M2 - 60/80 - 60)$ $M2 = 66$ g

20. (a, b) In many instances, a trait may be clustered in families, yet traditional mapping procedures may not be applicable because the trait might be influenced by a number of genes. In general, researchers look for associations to particular DNA sequences (molecular markers). When the trait cosegregates with a particular marker and it statistically associates with that trait above chance, a likely QTL has been identified. Markers such as RFLPs, SNPs, and microsatellites are often used because they are highly variable, relatively easy to assess, and present in all individuals.

22. The solution to these types of problems rests on determining the ratio of individuals expressing the extreme phenotype to the total number of individuals. In this case, 8:2028 is equal to 1:253, which is close to 1:256. If there are three gene pairs, the ratio is 1:64; four gene pairs, 1:256; or five gene pairs, 1:1024. Therefore, these data indicate that four gene pairs influence size in these guinea pigs.

24. (a, b) Because there are nine phenotypic classes in the F_2, four gene pairs must be involved. The genotypes of the parents could be symbolized as $AABBCCDD \times aabbccdd$, and the F_1 as $AaBbCcDd$.

26. $6 \times 5 \times 4 \times 3 \times 2 \times 1/(2 \times 1)(4 \times 3 \times 2 \times 1) = 15$ of a total of 64.

28. (a) The average response to selection (in mm) would be the sum of the differences between the control and offspring, divided by 3: (2.17 + 3.79 + 4.06)/3 = 3.34 mm.

(b) One computes realized heritability by the following formula:

$$h^2 = \frac{M2 - M}{M1 - M}$$

where M represents the mean size (control), $M1$ represents the selected parents, and $M2$ represents the size in offspring.
For 1997:

$$h^2 = (32.21 - 30.04)/(34.13 - 30.04) = 0.53$$

For 1998:

$$h^2 = (31.90 - 28.11)/(31.98 - 28.11) = 0.98$$

For 1999:

$$h^2 = (33.74 - 29.68)/(31.81 - 29.68) = 1.91$$

The overall realized heritability would be the average of all three heritability values, or 1.14.

(c) A key factor in determining response to selection is the genetic variability available to respond to selection. The greater the genetic variability, the greater the response. Another key factor in rapid response to selection often relates to the number of loci involved. If there are few loci, each with large phenotypic effects controlling a trait, response to selection is usually high. Finally, if flower size is not genetically correlated with other floral traits, size alone may not be subject to strong stabilizing selection, which would reduce genetic variation. Therefore, whereas other floral traits may show low response to selection, size alone may be more responsive.

(d) With high heritability, one expects a high genetic contribution to phenotypic variation. Genetic variability that provides rapid adjustments to changing environments is an evolutionary advantage. Therefore, in general, one would expect that high heritability would contribute to high evolutionary potential.

Chapter 24

ANSWERS TO NOW SOLVE THIS

24-1. One of the easiest ways to determine whether a genetic basis exists for a given abnormality is to cross the abnormal fly to a normal fly. If the trait is determined by a dominant gene, that trait should appear in the offspring—probably half of them if the gene was in the heterozygous state. If the gene is recessive and homozygous, then one may not see expression in the offspring of the first cross. However, if one crosses the F_1, the trait might appear in approximately 1/4 of the offspring. Such ratios would not be expected if the trait is polygenic, which generates complexities in any study. Modifications of these patterns would be expected if the mode of inheritance were X-linked or showed other modifications of typical Mendelian ratios. One might hypothesize that the trait influences the nervous, cuticular, or muscular system.

24-2. The presence of normal might to some extent soften or dilute the influence of mutant *HD* human genes.

SOLUTIONS TO PROBLEMS AND DISCUSSION QUESTIONS

2. Your essay should include an overall discussion of the anatomy and chemistry of synapses and neurotransmitters as well as examples of affected diseases: Alzheimer disease, Angelman syndrome, autism, etc.

4. Concordance for traits such as addictive behavior in monozygotic and dizygotic twins has been applied to many types of behaviors. Monozygotic twins are genetically identical, whereas dizygotic twins are genetically like siblings. Since members of each set of twins are likely to be reared under similar environmental conditions, it is possible to get some estimate of the genetic contribution to a given behavior. A higher rate of concordance for monozygotic twins compared with dizygotic twins often indicates a genetic component to a trait. Although such studies suggest that a genetic component exists, they do not reveal the precise genetic basis of pathological gambling.

8. Usually, if traits that are considered to be homozygous (the pure breeds of dogs) fail to breed true, it is likely that the trait is determined by conditioning or complex genetic factors that have minor influences. Such breeds of dogs, although being highly selected, are not homozygous for all genes. Even though the dogs are considered to be pure breeds, it is likely that alleles are segregating and combining in various ways to produce the variations noted. There may also be different interactions with environmental stimuli from subtle genetic variations.

10. One might compare gene expression through microarray analysis between space-reared flies with a control population on earth. By comparing behavioral (metabolic, mating, feeding, walking, flying) rituals between the two populations (space and earth), one might be able to correlate genetic expression profiles and determine which genes are most likely to respond to which behavioral alteration.

While a number of parameters would be interesting to study in this way, one might concentrate the study on genes known to influence muscle and nerve function in flies and humans. A second study might focus on the immune system since it is known that there are surprisingly high genetic correlations between the immune response of flies and mammals (Hoffmann, 2003). Since it is known that microgravity negatively influences the human immune system (reduces mitogenic activity of T cells), a comparison of the gene-expression profiles of the immune-response system would also be worthy of study. The behavioral side of the experiment would focus on determining whether changes in gravitational stress alter behavior (inactivity, muscle and nerve use) to a point where the immune response is altered. Coupling the two studies, gene-expression profiles associated with behavioral and the immune response might provide insight into a number of significant problems that humans encounter in space flight and thereby be justifiable and relatively inexpensive.

12. Genome-wide association (GWA) studies make use of millions of SNPs in an attempt to find associations to a given trait such as schizophrenia. Such studies indicate that no single gene or allele is a defining contributor to this disorder.

14. Data in the table indicate that females (*Gasterosteus aculeatus*) spend more time with males having the optimal MHC constitution than with those that do not. As with other organisms, it appears that genetic diversity for the MHC is a selective advantage. Since immunological functions are associated with the MHC complex, mate selection mechanisms that support the maintenance of such diversity seem reasonable from an evolutionary viewpoint.

16. DNA hypermethylation generally leads to a downregulation of a given section of DNA. In the case of the *FMR1* gene, such hypermethylation is associated with the expression of the fragile-X syndrome.

Chapter 25

ANSWERS TO NOW SOLVE THIS

25-1. Calculate p and q, then apply the equation $p^2 + 2pq + q^2$ to determine genotypic frequencies in the next generation.

$$p = \text{frequency of A}$$
$$= 0.2 + 0.3$$
$$= 0.5$$
$$q = 1 - p = 0.5$$
$$\text{Frequency of } AA = p^2$$
$$= (0.5)^2$$
$$= 0.25, \text{ or } 25\%$$
$$\text{Frequency of } Aa = 2pq$$
$$= 2(0.5)(0.5)$$
$$= 0.5, \text{ or } 50\%$$
$$\text{Frequency of } aa = q^2$$
$$= (0.5)^2$$
$$= 0.25, \text{ or } 25\%$$

The initial population was not in equilibrium; however, after one generation of mating under the Hardy–Weinberg conditions, the population is in equilibrium and will continue to be so (and not change) until one or more of the Hardy–Weinberg conditions is not met.

25-2. (a) Children: frequency of *M* allele: $p = 0.25 + 0.25 = 0.5$; frequency of *N* allele: $q = 0.25 + 0.25 = 0.5$. Adults: frequency of *M* allele: $p = 0.3 + 0.2 = 0.5$; frequency of *N* allele: $q = 0.3 + 0.2 = 0.5$.

(b, c) The allelic frequencies are the same; however, the genotypic frequencies appear to not be in equilibrium for the adult population.

25-3. Given that the recessive allele *a* is present in the homozygous state (q^2) at a frequency of 0.0001, the value of *q* is 0.01 and $p = 0.99$.

(a) *q* is 0.01
(b) $p = 1 - q$ or 0.99
(c) $2pq = 2(0.01)(0.99) = 0.0198$ (or about 1/50)
(d) $2pq \times 2pq = 0.0198 \times 0.0198 = 0.000392$ (or about 1/255)

25-4. The overall probability of the couple producing a CF child is $98/2500 \times 2/3 \times 1/4 = 0.00653$, or about 1/153.

SOLUTIONS TO PROBLEMS AND DISCUSSION QUESTIONS

2. Your essay should include a discussion of the original sources of variation coming from mutation and that migration can cause gene frequencies to change in a population if the immigrants have different gene frequencies compared to the host population. You should also describe selection as resulting from the biased passage of gametes and offspring to the next generation.

4. The classification of organisms into different species is based on evidence (morphological, genetic, ecological, etc.) that they are reproductively isolated. That is, there must be evidence that gene flow does not occur among the groups being called different species. Classifications above the species level (genus, family, etc.) are not based on such empirical data. Indeed, classification above the species level is somewhat arbitrary and based on traditions that extend far beyond DNA sequence information. In addition, recall that DNA sequence divergence is not always directly proportional to morphological, behavioral, or ecological divergence. Although the genus classifications provided in this problem seem to be invalid, other factors, well beyond simple DNA sequence comparison, must be considered in classification practices. As more information is gained on the meaning of DNA sequence differences in comparison to morphological factors, many phylogenetic relationships will be reconsidered, and it is possible that adjustments will be needed in some classification schemes.

6.

$q^2 = 37/125 = 0.296$
$q = 0.544$
$p = 1 - q$
$p = 0.456$

The frequencies of the genotypes are determined by applying the formula $p^2 + 2pq + q^2$ as follows:

Frequency of $AA = p^2$
$= (0.456)^2$
$= 0.208$, or 20.8%
Frequency of $Aa = 2pq$
$= 2(0.456)(0.544)$
$= 0.496$, or 49.6%

Frequency of $aa = q^2$
$= (0.544)^2$
$= 0.296$, or 29.6%

8. In order for the Hardy–Weinberg equations to apply, the population must be in Hardy–Weinberg equilibrium.

10. (a) For the CCR5 analysis, first determine *p* and *q*. Since one has the frequencies of all the genotypes, one can add 0.6 and 0.351/2 to provide *p* (= 0.7755); *q* will be 0.049 and 0.351/2 = 0.2245

The equilibrium values will be as follows:

Frequency of $l/l = p^2 = (0.7755)^2 = 0.6014$, or 60.14%
Frequency of $l/\Delta32 = 2pq = 2(0.7755)(0.2245) = 0.3482$, or 34.82%
Frequency of $\Delta32/\Delta32 = q^2 = (0.2245)^2 = 0.0504$, or 5.04%

Comparing these equilibrium values with the observed values strongly suggests that the observed values are drawn from a population in Hardy–Weinberg equilibrium.

(b) For the *AS* (sickle-cell) analysis, first determine *p* and *q*. Since one has the frequencies of all the genotypes, one can add 0.756 and 0.242/2 to provide *p* (= 0.877); *q* will be $1 - 0.877$, or 0.123

The equilibrium values will be as follows:

Frequency of $AA = p^2 = (0.877)^2 = 0.7691$, or 76.91%
Frequency of $AS = 2pq = 2(0.877)(0.123) = 0.2157$, or 21.57%
Frequency of $SS = q^2 = (0.123)^2 = 0.0151$, or 1.51%

Comparing these equilibrium values with the observed values suggests that the observed values may be drawn from a population that is not in equilibrium. Notice that there are more heterozygotes than predicted, and fewer *SS* types in the population. Since data are given in percentages, χ^2 values can not be computed.

12. The following formula calculates the frequency of an allele in the next generation for any selection scenario, given the frequencies of *a* and *A* in this generation and the fitness of all three genotypes; $q_{g+1} = [w_{Aa}p_gq_g + w_{aa}q_g^2]/[w_{AA}p_g^2 + w_{Aa}2p_gq_g + w_{aa}q_g^2]$, where q_{g+1} is the frequency of the *a* allele in the next generation, q_g is the frequency of the *a* allele in this generation, p_g is the frequency of the *A* allele in this generation, and each "*w*" represents the fitness of its respective genotype.

(a) $q_{g+1} = [0.9(0.7)(0.3) + 0.8(0.3)2]/[1(0.7)_2 + 0.9(2)(0.7)(0.3) + 0.8(0.3)_2]$
$q_{g+1} = 0.278$ $p_{g+1} = 0.722$
(b) $q_{g+1} = 0.289$ $p_{g+1} = 0.711$
(c) $q_{g+1} = 0.298$ $p_{g+1} = 0.702$
(d) $q_{g+1} = 0.319$ $p_{g+1} = 0.681$

14. Because a dominant lethal gene is highly selected against, it is unlikely that it will exist at too high a frequency, if at all. However, if the gene shows incomplete penetrance or late age of onset (after reproductive age), it may remain in a population.

16. The frequency of an allele is determined by a number of factors, including the fitness it confers, mutation rate, and input from migration. There is no tendency for a gene to reach any artificial frequency such as 0.5. In fact, you have seen that rare alleles tend to remain rare even when they are dominant—unless there is very strong selection for the allele. The distribution of a gene among individuals is determined by mating (population size, inbreeding, etc.) and environmental factors (selection, etc.). A population is in Hardy–Weinberg equilibrium when the distribution of genotypes occurs at or around the $p^2 + 2pq + q^2 = 1$ expression. Equilibrium does not mean 25 percent AA, 50 percent Aa, and 25 percent aa. This confusion often stems from the 1:2:1 (or 3:1) ratio seen in Mendelian crosses.

18. The frequency of mutation is 2/100,000, or 2×10^{-5}.

20. The presence of selectively neutral alleles and genetic adaptations to varied environments contribute significantly to genetic variation in natural populations.

22. The frequency of the b allele after one generation of corn borers fed on Bt corn would be computed as follows:

$$q' = q(1 - sq)/1 - sq^2$$
$$q' = 0.98[1 - (0.9)(0.98)]/1 - [(0.9)(0.98)(0.98)]$$
$$q' - 0.852 \text{ and } p' - 0.148$$

24. Note that the value of 0.2 comes from the fact that 10 sheep out of 50, or 20 percent, are being introduced, and there are no cc alleles in the introduced population, so $p_m = 1.0$.

$$p_i' = (1 - 0.2)(0.75) + (0.2)(1.0)$$
$$p_i' = 0.8$$

26. Somatic gene therapy, like any therapy, allows some individuals to live more normal lives than those not the receiving therapy. As such, the ability of these individuals to contribute to the gene pool increases the likelihood that less fit alleles will enter and be maintained in the gene pool. This is a normal consequence of therapy, genetic or not, and in the face of disease control and prevention, societies have generally accepted this consequence. Germ-line therapy could, if successful, lead to limited, isolated, and infrequent removal of an allele from a gene lineage. However, given the present state of the science, its impact on the course of human evolution will be diluted and negated by a host of other factors that afflict humankind.

28. Reproductive isolating mechanisms are grouped into prezygotic and postzygotic and include the following:

- geographic or ecological
- seasonal or temporal
- behavioral
- mechanical
- physiological
- hybrid inviability or weakness
- developmental hybrid sterility
- segregational hybrid sterility
- F_2 breakdown

30. In small populations, large fluctuations in gene frequency occur because random gametic sampling may not include all the genetic variation in the parents. The same phenomenon occurs in molecular populations. Two factors can cause the extinction of a particular mutation in small populations. First, sampling error may allow fixation of one form and the elimination of others. If an advantageous mutation occurs, it must be included in the next replicative round in order to be maintained in subsequent generations. If the founding population is small, it is possible that the advantageous mutation might not be represented. Second,

although the previous statements also hold for deleterious mutations, if a deleterious mutation becomes fixed, it can lead to extinction of that population.

32. All of the amino acid substitutions (Ala – Gly, Val – Leu, Asp – Asn, Met – Leu) require only one nucleotide change. The last change from Pro (CC–) – Lys (AAA,G) requires two changes (the minimal mutational distance).

34. (a, b) The pattern of genetic distances through time indicates that from the present to about 25,000 years ago, modern humans and Cro-Magnons show an approximately constant number of differences. Conversely, there is an abrupt increase in genetic distance seen in comparing modern humans and Cro-Magnons with Neanderthals. The results indicate a clear discontinuity between modern humans, Cro-Magnons, and Neanderthals with respect to genetic variation in the mitochondrial DNAs sampled.

Special Topic 1

REVIEW QUESTION ANSWERS

2. In general, periodic methylation occurs at CpG-rich regions and promoter sequences. When a gene is imprinted by methylation, it remains transcriptionally silent. In a mammalian embryo, imprinting may silence only the paternal set of chromosomes, for example.

4. Reversible histone modifications influence the structure of chromatin by altering the accessibility of nucleosomes to the transcriptional machinery. These chromatin alterations "open" or "close" genes for transcription.

6. Imprinting usually involves certain genes, restricted in number, that are altered by passage through meiosis. A maternally derived imprint or a paternally derived imprint may occur. Imprinted alleles are transcriptionally silent in all cells of the organism, whereas epigenetic modifications (methylation) can be reactivated by environmental signals.

8. In addition to functioning in cellular signaling, microRNAs play a significant role in the developing embryo. MiRNAs are involved with RNA silencing through RISCs that act as repressors of gene expression. They do so by making mRNAs less likely to be translated.

DISCUSSION QUESTION ANSWERS

2. While data are scant, some studies have shown that children born after in vitro fertilization are at risk for low to very low birth weight that may have resulted from abnormal imprinting. There also appears to be an increased risk of the ART child having Beckwith-Wiedemann syndrome. Given these data, it would seem reasonable that such information should be provided to prospective parents of an ART child. Each couple would need to reach a decision based on available science and their own value and belief sets.

4. Plant miRNAs are known to downregulate gene expression and some foods are the source of miRNAs that circulate in body fluids of humans. Given this information, it has been suggested that as yet poorly understood environmental factors may play a significant role in the regulation of gene function in humans. At this point it might be premature to design a dietary regimen based on such a frail understanding of the role of plant miRNAs in humans.

Special Topic 2

REVIEW QUESTION ANSWERS

2. Since RNA can both serve in information storage and transfer and catalyze reactions, it has been hypothesized that RNA was the precursor to molecular life-like events. In addition, RNAs are components of many primitive yet biologically significant reactions.

4. DNA methylation provides a defense to the integration of foreign DNA into the bacterial chromosome, whereas *CRISPR* loci transcribe crRNAs that guide nucleases to invading complementary DNAs in order to destroy them.

6. Through a series of transcriptive and Dicer-related activities, siRNAs are formed that are complementary to centromeric DNA. A RITS silencing complex forms that leads to methylation, thus triggering heterochromatin formation. At this point, the evolution of such a complex process of heterchromatin formation is not well understood.

8. Interestingly, extracellular RNA is a heterogeneous group composed of mRNAs and miRNAs that, in association with proteins, are secreted from cells in vesicles. These vesicles may serve for protection or signaling.

DISCUSSION QUESTION ANSWERS

2. Negative or positive regulation depends on whether the ribosome binding site is masked or available. When repression occurs, the RBS is masked by sRNA. When positive regulation occurs, sRNA pairing unmasks the RBS.

4. In bacteria and Archaea, foreign DNA can be inserted into *CRISPR* loci in the genome, which brings about transcription of crRNAs that guide nucleases to invading complementary DNAs. In addition, foreign DNA can be digested by restriction endonucleases. One form of eukaryotic genome protection involves piRNAs that are pivotal in silencing transposons, mobile DNA sequences that change position. Associated with Piwi proteins, certain proteins (such as RNA-induced silencing complexes [RISC]) target transposon-derived RNAs and their complementary sequences. This process represses transposon transcription by promoting DNA methylation of transposon DNA. A broadly functioning protective mechanism involves siRNA in association with RISC and Dicer, an RNAse III protein.

6. Even though a particular species of mRNA may be fairly uniformly distributed throughout a cell, it does not follow that it is uniformly translated. It is likely that different domains reside in cells that contain different translational signals. Anterior-posterior protein gradients are known to be present in *Drosophila* eggs. If a mRNA finds itself in a particular molecular environment, it may be destined for translation, whereas that same mRNA in another part of a cell may not have the environmental stimulation necessary for translation.

Special Topic 3

REVIEW QUESTION ANSWERS

2. With the development of the polymerase chain reaction, trace samples of DNA can be used, commonly in forensic applications. STRs are like VNTRs, but the repeat portion is shorter, between two and nine base pairs, repeated from 7 to 40 times. A core set of STR loci, about 13, is most often used in forensic applications.

4. Since males typically contain a Y chromosome (exceptions include transgender and mosaic individuals), gender separation of a mixed tissue sample is easily achieved by Y chromosome profiling. In addition, STR profiling is possible for over 200 loci; however, because of the relative stability of DNA in the Y chromosome, it is difficult to differentiate between DNA from fathers and sons or male siblings.

6. Like Y-chromosome DNA, mtDNA is very stable because it undergoes very little, if any, recombination. Since there is a high copy number of mitochondria in cells, it is especially useful in situations where samples are small, old, or degraded, which is often the case in catastrophes.

8. The Combined DNA Index System (CODIS) is a collection of DNA databases and analytical tools of both state and federal governments, maintained by the FBI. As of 2013, it contained more than 11 million DNA profiles. DNA profiles are collected from convicted offenders, forensic investigations, and in some states, those suspected of crimes as well as from unidentified human remains and missing persons (in cases where DNA is available).

10. The prosecutor's fallacy attempts to equate guilt with a numerical probability produced by a single piece of evidence. Just because a match occurs between a crime scene and a suspect, it does not mean that the suspect is guilty. Human error, contamination, or evidence tampering all contribute to the complexities of interpreting DNA profiling data.

DISCUSSION QUESTION ANSWERS

2. To gain information as to laws and regulations in various states, one could navigate to "Welcome to the DNA Laws Database" within the National Conference of State Legislatures website. There, one can select a particular state for its laws and regulations regarding DNA collection and profiling. In general, one will see that most states contain descriptions of the following topics:
   (a) various DNA databases used
   (b) methods of DNA collection
   (c) post-conviction DNA collection of felons
   (d) oversight and advisory committees
   (e) convicted offender statutes

4. Somatic mosaicism and chimerism involve a mixture of cell types, the origin of which may involve a variety of embryonic events, some of which are understood. Since a single individual may contain a mixed population of cells, a DNA sample taken from one tissue site may not match a DNA sample taken from another site. This can lead to a conflicted set of results when it comes to matching a DNA sample to a sample of DNA from a crime scene. Taking DNA samples from various sites on an individual may be useful in mitigating such confusion. In addition, in STR DNA profiling, mosaicism may present itself at the electrophoresis/analysis stage by additional peaks or peak height imbalances.

Special Topic 4

REVIEW QUESTION ANSWERS

2. Herceptin is used in the treatment of breast cancer that targets the epidermal growth factor receptor 2 (*HER-2*) gene located on chromosome 17. Overexpression of this gene

occurs in about 25 percent of invasive breast cancer cases. Herceptin is a monoclonal antibody that binds specifically to inhibit the HER-2 receptor.

4. Cytochrome P450 is composed of a family of enzymes that are encoded by 57 different genes. Certain variants of cytochrome P450 metabolize drugs slowly and can lead to harmful accumulations of a drug. Other variants cause drugs to be eliminated quickly, which can lead to drug ineffectiveness. A pivotal gene, *CYP2D6*, influences the metabolism of approximately 25 percent of all drugs, while *VKORC1* influences the response to warfarin, an anticoagulant drug.

6. Recently, large-scale genomic sequencing has shown that each tumor is genetically unique. With such information, it is often possible to provide a personalized diagnosis and possibly apply personalized treatments. One such example is the use of Herceptin for the treatment of breast cancer; another is the use of Erbitux and Vectibix to inhibit epidermal growth factor receptors that are commonly expressed in cancer cells.

8. Using the search function in the PharmGKB database one can find a number of references that discuss the variants of *CYP2D6* and tamoxifen. For example, according to Hertz et al. (Hertz, D. et al. 2012. *The Oncologist.* 17(5): 2011-0418), tamoxifen efficacy is dependent on the highly polymorphic cytochrome P450 gene (*CYP2D6*). Depending on a particular variant genotype, tamoxifen treatment outcome is highly inconsistent. The entire Hertz et al. paper is available through the PharmGKB database and provides a complete and detailed description of the interactions of *CYP2D6* variants and tamoxifen.

DISCUSSION QUESTION ANSWERS

2. Given the obvious progress that has occurred in recent years, it is highly likely that more personalized therapies will be developed in the near future. There are several bridges that must be crossed before one can claim universal use and acceptance. First, it will be necessary to close the gap between data collection and interpretation of complex interactions. Second, personalized medicines are dependent on the development of effective therapies that have few side effects and a reasonable cost. Finally, given the complexity of living systems, there will likely be diseases for which therapies will be difficult to develop. In addition, hopefully, incentives will be sufficient for entities to develop therapies for rare, financially less-rewarding diseases.

4. At present, genetic discrimination does exist; however, recent developments in health care laws seek to minimize such discrimination by medical insurance companies. It remains to be seen whether genetic discrimination in the workplace continues.

Special Topic 5

REVIEW QUESTION ANSWERS

2. Genetic engineering allows genetic material to be transferred within and between species and to alter expression levels of genes. A transgenic organism is one that involves the transfer of genetic material between different species, whereas the term cisgenic is sometimes used in cases where gene transfers occur within a species.

4. Herbicide-tolerant plants make up approximately 70 percent of all GM plants, the majority of which confer tolerance to the herbicide glyphosate. Glyphosate interferes with the enzyme 5-enolpyruvylshikimate-3-phosphate synthetase, which is present in all plants and is required for the synthesis of aromatic amino acids phenylalanine, tyrosine, and tryptophan.

6. The first iteration of Golden Rice involved the introduction of phytoene synthetase originating from the daffodil plant and carotene desaturase from a bacterium engineered into the rice plant. Resulting rice grains were yellow in color due to the production of beta-carotene. Later versions of Golden Rice 2 involved the introduction of similar genes from maize thus leading to a much higher production of beta-carotene. At present, Golden Rice 2 is being tested in preparation for use in Bangladesh and the Philippines.

8. The biolistic method of gene introduction achieves DNA transfer by coating the transforming DNA in a heavy metal to form particles that are fired at high speed into plant cells using a gene gun. The introduced DNA may migrate into the cell nucleus and integrate into a plant chromosome.

10. Roundup-Ready soybeans received market approval almost ten years ago. This GM plant is resistant to the herbicide glyphosate, a broad-spectrum herbicide, because glyphosate interferes with the enzyme 5-enolpyruvylshikimate-3-phosphate synthetase, which is necessary for the plant to synthesize the aromatic amino acids phenylalanine, tyrosine, and tryptophan. The *epsps* gene was cloned from *Agrobacterium* strain CP4 and introduced into soybeans using biolistic bombardment.

DISCUSSION QUESTION ANSWERS

2. There are many positions taken and bills filed in various states to address the question of GM food labeling. Generally, many feel a "right to know" would allow consumers to make educated choices about the food they consume. They would consider it an advantage to be able to judge the safety of a given food if they had information about the possibility that it contains GM components. Others wonder about the usefulness of a GM label if there is little information provided as to how the food has been modified. Of what value would it be to know that food was genetically modified if the science and specifics about the modifications were not included? How much background knowledge would be needed by the consumer to be able to interpret such information?

Special Topic 6

REVIEW QUESTION ANSWERS

2. In *ex vivo* gene therapy, a potential genetic correction takes place in cells that have been removed from the patient. *In vivo* gene therapy treats cells of the body through the introduction of DNA into the patient.

4. In many cases, therapeutic DNA hitches a ride with genetically engineered viruses, such as retrovirus or adenovirus vectors. Nonviral delivery methods may use chemical assistance to cross cell membranes, nanoparticles, or cell fusion with artificial vesicles.

6. White blood cells, T cells in this case, were used because they are key players in the mounting of an immune response, which Ashanti was incapable of developing. A

normal copy of the *ADA* gene was engineered into a retroviral vector, which then infected many of her T cells. Those cells that expressed the *ADA* gene were then injected into Ashanti's blood stream, and some of them populated her bone marrow. At the time of Ashanti's treatment, targeted gene therapy was not possible, so integration of the *ADA* gene into Ashanti's genome probably did not replace her defective gene.

8. To some extent, targeted gene therapy is designed to alleviate one of the major pitfalls of gene therapy, random DNA integration. In addition, recent research holds promise for approaches of targeted removal and even the silencing of defective genes. DNA editing makes use of nucleases and zinc-finger arrangements to remove defective genes from the genome.

10. One method of gene inhibition follows from the use of RNA interference (RNAi) whereby double-stranded RNA molecules are delivered into cells, and the enzyme Dicer cleaves them into relatively short pieces of RNA (siRNA). siRNA can form a complex with enzymes that target mRNA. Another approach to silence genes involves the use of antisense RNA in which RNA is introduced that is complementary to a strand of mRNA, thus blocking its translation.

DISCUSSION QUESTION ANSWERS

2. Generally, gene therapy is an accepted procedure, given appropriate conditions, for the relief of genetic disease states. Since it is a fairly expensive medical approach, considerable debate attends its use. It remains to be seen whether insurance companies will embrace what might be considered experimental treatments. Use of gene therapy to enhance the competitive status of individuals (genetic enhancement or gene doping) is presently viewed as cheating by most organizations and the public. It is unlikely that germ-line therapy will be viewed favorably by the public or scientific communities; however, this and other issues mentioned here will be the subject of considerable future debate.

Glossary

abortive transduction An event in which transducing DNA fails to be incorporated into the recipient chromosome. See also *transduction*.

accession number An identifying number or code assigned to a nucleotide or amino acid sequence for entry and cataloging in a database.

acentric chromosome Chromosome or chromosome fragment with no centromere.

acridine dyes A class of organic compounds that bind to DNA and intercalate into the double-stranded structure, producing local disruptions of base pairing. These disruptions result in nucleotide additions or deletions in the next round of replication.

acrocentric chromosome Chromosome with the centromere located very close to one end. Human chromosomes 13, 14, 15, 21, and 22 are acrocentric.

active site The substrate-binding site of an enzyme; in other proteins, the portion whose structural integrity is required for function.

adaptation A heritable component of the phenotype that confers an advantage in survival and reproductive success. The process by which organisms adapt to current environmental conditions.

additive genes See *polygenic inheritance*.

additive variance Genetic variance attributed to the substitution of one allele for another at a given locus. This variance can be used to predict the rate of response to phenotypic selection in quantitative traits.

A-DNA An alternative form of right-handed, double-helical DNA. Its helix is more tightly coiled than the more common B-DNA, with 11 base pairs per full turn. In the A form, the bases in the helix are displaced laterally and tilted in relation to the longitudinal axis. It is not yet clear whether this form has biological significance. See *B-DNA*.

adeno-associated virus (AAV) A virus that commonly infects humans, typically without pathogenic consequences. Modified versions of AAV can be used in gene therapy to deliver therapeutic genes *in vivo* and *in vitro*.

albinism A condition caused by the lack of melanin production in the iris, hair, and skin. In humans, it is most often inherited as an autosomal recessive trait.

alkaptonuria An autosomal recessive condition in humans caused by lack of the enzyme homogentisic acid oxidase. Urine of homozygous individuals turns dark upon standing because of oxidation of excreted homogentisic acid. The cartilage of homozygous adults blackens from deposition of a pigment derived from homogentisic acid. Affected individuals often develop arthritic conditions.

allele One of the possible alternative forms of a gene, often distinguished from other alleles by phenotypic effects.

allele-specific oligonucleotide (ASO) Short nucleotide chains, synthesized in the laboratory, usually 15–20 bp in length, that under carefully controlled conditions will hybridize only to a perfectly matching complementary sequence.

allelic exclusion In a plasma cell heterozygous for an immunoglobulin gene, the selective action of only one allele.

allelism test See *complementation test*.

allolactose A lactose derivative that acts as the inducer for the *lac* operon.

allopatric speciation Process of speciation associated with geographic isolation.

allopolyploid Polyploid condition formed by the union of two or more distinct chromosome sets with a subsequent doubling of chromosome number.

allosteric effect Conformational change in the active site of a protein brought about by interaction with an effector molecule.

allotetraploid An allopolyploid containing two genomes derived from different species.

allozyme An allelic form of a protein that can be distinguished from other forms by electrophoresis.

alternative splicing Generation of different protein molecules from the same pre-mRNA by incorporation of a different set and order of exons into the mRNA product.

***Alu* sequence** A DNA sequence of approximately 300 bp found interspersed within the genomes of primates that is cleaved by the restriction enzyme *Alu*I. In humans, 300,000–600,000 copies are dispersed throughout the genome and constitute some 3–6 percent of the genome. See also *short interspersed elements*.

amber codon The codon UAG, which does not code for an amino acid but for chain termination. One of the stop codons.

Ames test A bacterial assay developed by Bruce Ames to detect mutagenic compounds; it assesses reversion to histidine independence in the bacterium *Salmonella typhimurium*.

amino acids Aminocarboxylic acids comprising the subunits covalently linked to form proteins.

aminoacyl tRNA A covalently linked combination of an amino acid and a tRNA molecule. Also referred to as a charged tRNA.

amniocentesis A procedure in which fluid and fetal cells are withdrawn from the amnion, a membrane surrounding the fetus; used for genetic testing of the fetus.

amphidiploid See *allotetraploid*.

anabolism The metabolic synthesis of complex molecules from less complex precursors.

analog A chemical compound that differs structurally from a similar compound but whose chemical behavior is the same. See also *base analog*.

anaphase Stage of mitosis or meiosis in which chromosomes begin moving to opposite poles of the cell.

anaphase I The stage in the first meiotic division during which members of homologous pairs of chromosomes separate from one another.

aneuploidy A condition in which the chromosome number is not an exact multiple of the haploid set.

annotation Analysis of genomic nucleotide sequence data to identify the protein-coding genes, the non-protein-coding genes, and the regulatory sequences and function(s) of each gene.

antibody Protein (immunoglobulin) produced in response to an antigenic stimulus with the capacity to bind specifically to an antigen.

anticipation See *genetic anticipation*.

anticodon In a tRNA molecule, the nucleotide triplet that binds to its complementary codon triplet in an mRNA molecule.

antigen A molecule, often a cell-surface protein, that is capable of eliciting the formation of antibodies.

antiparallel A term describing molecules in parallel alignment but running in opposite directions. Most commonly used to describe the opposite orientations of the two strands of a DNA molecule.

antisense oligonucleotide A short, single-stranded DNA or RNA molecule complementary to a specific sequence.

antisense RNA An RNA molecule (synthesized *in vivo* or *in vitro*) with a ribonucleotide sequence that is complementary to part of an mRNA molecule.

apoptosis A genetically controlled program of cell death, activated as part of normal development or as a result of cell damage.

Argonaute A family of proteins found within the RNA-induced silencing complex (RISC) with endonuclease activity associated with the destruction of target mRNAs.

artificial selection See *selection*.

ascospore A meiotic spore produced in certain fungi.

ascus In fungi, the sac enclosing the four or eight ascospores.

asexual reproduction Production of offspring in the absence of any sexual process.

assortative mating Nonrandom mating between males and females of a species. Positive assortative mating selects mates with the same genotype; negative selects mates with opposite genotypes.

ATP Adenosine triphosphate, a nucleotide that is the main energy source in cells.

attached-X chromosome Two conjoined X chromosomes that share a single centromere and thus migrate together during cell division.

attenuator A nucleotide sequence between the promoter and the structural gene of some bacterial operons that regulates the transit of RNA polymerase, reducing transcription of the related structural gene.

autism spectrum disorder (ASD) A range of symptoms and neurodevelopmental disorders characterized by specific social, cognitive, and communication behaviors or deficits.

autogamy A process of self-fertilization resulting in homozygosis.

autoimmune disease The production of antibodies that results from an immune response to one's own molecules, cells, or tissues. Such a response results from the inability of the immune system to distinguish self from nonself. Diseases such as arthritis, scleroderma, systemic lupus erythematosus, and juvenile-onset diabetes are autoimmune diseases.

autoinducer A signaling molecule produced by prokaryotes that provides a population of cells with cellular population density information through a quorum sensing pathway.

autonomously replicating sequences (ARS) Origins of DNA replication, about 100 nucleotides in length, found in yeast chromosomes. ARS elements are also present in organelle DNA.

autopolyploidy Polyploid condition resulting from the duplication of one diploid set of chromosomes.

autoradiography Production of a photographic image by radioactive decay. Used to localize radioactively labeled compounds within cells and tissues or to identify radioactive probes in various blotting techniques. See also *Southern blotting*.

autosomes Chromosomes other than the sex chromosomes. In humans, there are 22 pairs of autosomes.

autotetraploid An autopolyploid condition composed of four copies of the same genome.

auxotroph A mutant microorganism or cell line that through mutation has lost the ability to synthesize one or more substances required for growth.

backcross A cross between an F₁ heterozygote and one of the P₁ parents (or an organism with a genotype identical to one of the parents).

bacteriophage A virus that infects bacteria, using it as the host for reproduction (also, *phage*).

balanced lethals Recessive, nonallelic lethal genes, each carried on different homologous chromosomes. When organisms carrying balanced lethal genes are interbred, only organisms with genotypes identical to the parents (heterozygotes) survive.

balanced polymorphism Maintenance of two alleles in a population by natural selection because the heterozygote is more fit than either homozygote.

balanced translocation carrier An individual with a chromosomal translocation in which there has been an exchange of genetic information with no associated extra or missing genetic material.

balancer chromosome A chromosome containing one or more inversions that suppress crossing over with its homolog and which carries a dominant marker that is usually lethal when homozygous.

Barr body Densely staining DNA-positive mass seen in the somatic nuclei of mammalian females. Discovered by Murray Barr, this body represents an inactivated X chromosome.

base analog A purine or pyrimidine base that differs structurally from one normally used in biological systems but whose chemical behavior is the same. For example, 5-bromouracil, which "looks like" thymidine, substitutes for it, and after incorporation into a DNA or RNA molecule, can be detected because of its increased mass. See also *analog*.

base pair See *nucleotide pair*.

base substitution A single base change in a DNA molecule that produces a mutation. There are two types of substitutions: *transitions*, in which a purine is substituted for a purine, or a pyrimidine for a pyrimidine; and *transversions*, in which a purine is substituted for a pyrimidine or vice versa.

B-DNA The conformation of DNA most often found in cells and which serves as the basis of the Watson-Crick double-helical model. There are 10 base pairs per full turn of its right-handed helix, with the nucleotides stacked 0.34 nm apart. The helix has a diameter of 2.0 nm.

β-galactosidase A bacterial enzyme, encoded by the *lacZ* gene, that converts lactose into galactose and glucose.

β-globin Polypeptide subunit of hemoglobin. A combination of two alpha and two beta chains comprise hemoglobin.

β-thalassemia Inherited blood disorder caused by a reduction or absence of β-hemoglobin subunits.

bidirectional replication A mechanism of DNA replication in which two replication forks move in opposite directions from a common origin.

biodiversity The genetic diversity present in populations and species of plants and animals.

bioinformatics A field that focuses on the design and use of software and computational methods for the storage, analysis, and management of biological information such as nucleotide or amino acid sequences.

biometry The application of statistics and statistical methods to biological problems.

biotechnology Commercial and/or industrial processes that utilize biological organisms or products.

bivalents Synapsed homologous chromosomes in the first prophase of meiosis.

BLAST (Basic Local Alignment Search Tool) Any of a family of search engines designed to compare or query nucleotide or amino acid sequences against sequences in databases. BLAST also calculates the statistical significance of the matches.

Bombay phenotype A rare variant of the ABO antigen system in which affected individuals do not have A or B antigens and thus appear to have blood type O, even though their genotype may carry unexpressed alleles for the A and/or B antigens.

bottleneck See *population bottleneck.*

bovine spongiform encephalopathy (BSE) A fatal, degenerative brain disease of cattle (transmissible to humans and other animals) caused by prion infection. Also known as mad cow disease.

BrdU (5-bromodeoxyuridine) A mutagenically active analog of thymidine in which the methyl group at the 5′ position in thymine is replaced by bromine; also abbreviated BUdR.

broad heritability That proportion of total phenotypic variance in a population that can be attributed to genotypic differences.

buoyant density A property of particles (and molecules) that depends on their actual density, as determined by partial specific volume and degree of hydration. It provides the basis for density-gradient separation of molecules or particles.

CAAT box A highly conserved DNA sequence found in the untranslated promoter region of eukaryotic genes. This sequence is recognized by transcription factors.

cancer stem cells Tumor-forming cells in a cancer that can give rise to all the cell types in a particular form of cancer. These cells have the properties of normal stem cells: self-renewal and ability to differentiate into multiple cell types.

CAP Catabolite activator protein; a protein that binds cAMP and regulates the activation of inducible operons.

capillary electrophoresis A group of analytical methods that separates large and small charged molecules in a capillary tube by their size to charge ratio. Detection and analysis of separated components takes place in the capillary usually by use of ultraviolet (UV) light.

carcinogen A physical or chemical agent that causes cancer.

carrier An individual heterozygous for a recessive trait.

catabolism A metabolic reaction in which complex molecules are broken down into simpler forms, often accompanied by the release of energy.

catabolite activator protein See *CAP.*

catabolite repression The selective inactivation of an operon by a metabolic product of the enzymes encoded by the operon.

***cdc* mutation** A class of *cell division cycle* (*cdc*) mutations in yeasts that affect the timing of and progression through the cell cycle.

cDNA (complementary DNA) DNA synthesized from an RNA template by the enzyme reverse transcriptase.

cDNA library A collection of cloned cDNA sequences.

cell cycle The sequence of growth phases in a cell; divided into G1 (gap 1), S (DNA synthesis), G2 (gap 2), and M (mitosis). A cell may temporarily or permanently withdraw from the cell cycle, in which case it is said to enter the G0 stage.

cell-free extract A preparation of the soluble fraction of cells, made by lysing cells and removing the particulate matter, such as nuclei, membranes, and organelles. Often used to carry out the synthesis of proteins by the addition of specific, exogenous mRNA molecules.

CEN The DNA region of centromeres critical to their function. In yeasts, fragments of chromosomal DNA, about 120 bp in length, that when inserted into plasmids confer the ability to segregate during mitosis.

centimorgan (cM) A unit of distance between genes on chromosomes representing 1 percent crossing over between two genes. Equivalent to 1 map unit (mu).

central dogma The classical concept that genetic information flow progresses from DNA to RNA to proteins. Although exceptions are now known, this idea is central to an understanding of gene function.

centric fusion See *Robertsonian translocation.*

centriole A cytoplasmic organelle composed of nine groups of microtubules, generally arranged in triplets. Centrioles function in the generation of cilia and flagella and serve as foci for the spindles in cell division.

centromere The specialized heterochromatic chromosomal region at which sister chromatids remain attached after replication, and the site to which spindle fibers attach to the chromosome during cell division. Location of the centromere determines the shape of the chromosome during the anaphase portion of cell division. Also known as the primary constriction.

centrosome Region of the cytoplasm containing a pair of centrioles.

CFTR The protein (cystic fibrosis transmembrane conductance regulator) encoded by the *CFTR* gene. The protein regulates the movement of chloride ions across the plasma membrane of epithelial cells. Mutations in *CFTR* lead to cystic fibrosis.

chaperone A protein that regulates the folding of a polypeptide into the three-dimensional shape of a functional protein.

character An observable phenotypic attribute of an organism.

charon phages A group of genetically modified lambda phages designed to be used as vectors (carriers) for cloning foreign DNA. Named after the ferryman in Greek mythology who carried the souls of the dead across the River Styx.

chemotaxis Movement of a cell or organism in response to a chemical gradient.

chiasma (pl., chiasmata) The crossed strands of nonsister chromatids seen in diplotene of the first meiotic division. Regarded as the cytological evidence for exchange of chromosomal material, or crossing over.

ChIP on chip A technique that combines chromatin immunoprecipitation (ChIP) with microarrays (chips) to identify and localize DNA sites that bind DNA-binding proteins of interest. These sites may be enhancers, promoters, transcription initiation sites, or other functional DNA regions.

chi-square (χ^2) analysis Statistical test to determine whether or not an observed set of data is equivalent to a theoretical expectation.

chloroplast A self-replicating cytoplasmic organelle containing chlorophyll. The site of photosynthesis.

chorionic villus sampling (CVS) A technique of prenatal diagnosis in which chorionic fetal cells are retrieved and used to detect cytogenetic and biochemical defects in the embryo.

chromatid One of the longitudinal subunits of a replicated chromosome.

chromatin The complex of DNA, RNA, histones, and nonhistone proteins that make up uncoiled chromosomes, characteristic of the eukaryotic interphase nucleus.

chromatin immunoprecipitation (ChIP) An analytical method used to identify DNA-binding proteins that bind to DNA sequences of interest. In ChIP, antibodies to specific proteins are used to isolate DNA sequences that bind these proteins. See also *ChIP-on-chip*.

chromatin remodeling   A process in which the structure of chromatin is altered by a protein complex, resulting in changes in the transcriptional state of genes in the altered region.

chromatography   Technique for the separation of a mixture of solubilized molecules by their differential migration over a substrate.

chromocenter   In polytene chromosomes, an aggregation of centromeres and heterochromatic elements where the chromosomes appear to be attached together.

chromomere   A coiled, beadlike region of a chromosome, most easily visualized during cell division. The aligned chromomeres of polytene chromosomes are responsible for their distinctive banding pattern.

chromosomal aberration   Any duplication, deletion, or rearrangement of the otherwise diploid chromosomal content of an organism.

chromosomal mutation   The process resulting in the duplication, deletion, or rearrangements of the diploid chromosomal content of an organism. See also *chromosomal aberration*.

chromosomal polymorphism   Possession of alternative structures or arrangements of a chromosome among members of a population.

chromosome   In prokaryotes, a DNA molecule containing the organism's genome; in eukaryotes, a DNA molecule complexed with RNA and proteins to form a threadlike structure containing genetic information arranged in a linear sequence; a structure that is visible during mitosis and meiosis.

chromosome banding   Technique for the differential staining of mitotic or meiotic chromosomes to produce a characteristic banding pattern; or selective staining of certain chromosomal regions such as centromeres, the nucleolus organizer regions, and GC- or AT-rich regions. Not to be confused with the banding pattern present in polytene chromosomes, which is produced by the alignment of chromomeres.

chromosome map   A diagram showing the location of genes on chromosomes.

chromosome puff   A localized uncoiling and swelling in a polytene chromosome, usually regarded as a sign of active transcription.

chromosome theory of inheritance   The idea put forward independently by Walter Sutton and Theodor Boveri that chromosomes are the carriers of genes and the basis for the Mendelian mechanisms of segregation and independent assortment.

chromosome walking   A method for analyzing long stretches of DNA. The end of a cloned segment of DNA is subcloned and used as a probe to identify other clones that overlap the first clone.

circular RNAs (circRNAs)   RNAs with a circular single-stranded conformation. Some of these act as "molecular sponges" that bind to and block the action of microRNAs that modulate gene expression.

***cis*-acting sequence**   A DNA sequence that regulates the expression of a gene located on the same chromosome. This contrasts with a *trans*-acting element where regulation is under the control of a sequence on the homologous chromosome. See also *trans-acting element*.

***cis* configuration**   The arrangement of two genes (or two mutant sites within a gene) on the same homolog, such as

$$\frac{a^1 \quad a^2}{+ \quad +}$$

This contrasts with a *trans* arrangement, where the mutant alleles are located on opposite homologs. See also *trans configuration*.

***cis–trans* test**   A genetic test to determine whether two mutations are located within the same cistron (or gene).

cistron   That portion of a DNA molecule (a gene) that encodes a single-polypeptide chain; defined by a genetic test as a region within which two mutations cannot complement each other.

cline   A gradient of genotype or phenotype distributed over a geographic range.

clonal selection theory   Proposed explanation in immunology that antibody diversity precedes exposure to the antigen and that the antigen functions to select the cells containing its specific antibody to undergo proliferation.

clone   Identical molecules, cells, or organisms derived from a single ancestor by asexual or parasexual methods; for example, a DNA segment that has been inserted into a plasmid or chromosome of a phage or a bacterium and replicated to produce many copies, or an organism with a genetic composition identical to that used in its production.

codominance   Condition in which the phenotypic effects of a gene's alleles are fully and simultaneously expressed in the heterozygote.

codon   A triplet of messenger RNA (mRNA) nucleotides that specifies a particular amino acid or a start or stop signal in the genetic code. Sixty-one codons specify the amino acids used in proteins, and three codons, called stop codons (UAG, UAA, UGA), signal termination of growth of the polypeptide chain. One codon (AUG) acts as a start codon in addition to specifying an amino acid.

coefficient of coincidence   A ratio of the observed number of double crossovers divided by the expected number of such crossovers.

coefficient of inbreeding   The probability that two alleles present in a zygote are descended from a common ancestor.

coefficient of selection (s)   A measurement of the reproductive disadvantage of a given genotype in a population. For example, for genotype *aa* if only 99 of 100 individuals reproduce, then the selection coefficient is 0.01.

cohesin   A protein complex that holds sister chromatids together during mitosis and meiosis and facilitates attachments of spindle fibers to kinetochores.

colchicine   An alkaloid compound that inhibits spindle formation during cell division. In the preparation of karyotypes, it is used for collecting a large population of cells inhibited at the metaphase stage of mitosis.

colinearity   The linear relationship between the nucleotide sequence in a gene (or the RNA transcribed from it) and the order of amino acids in the polypeptide chain specified by the gene.

Combined DNA Index System (CODIS)   A standardized set of 13 short tandem repeat (STR) DNA sequences used by law enforcement and government agencies in preparing DNA profiles.

comparative genomic hybridization (CGH)   A microarray-based method for the analysis of copy number variations in genomic DNA or in specific cell types, such as tumor cells.

competence   In bacteria, the transient state or condition during which the cell can bind and internalize exogenous DNA molecules, making transformation possible.

complementarity   Chemical affinity between nitrogenous bases of nucleic acid strands as a result of hydrogen bonding. Responsible for the base pairing between the strands of the DNA double helix and between DNA and RNA strands during gene expression in cells and during the use of molecular hybridization techniques.

complementation test A genetic test to determine whether two mutations occur within the same gene (cistron). If two mutations are introduced into a cell simultaneously and produce a wild-type phenotype (i.e., they complement each other), they are often nonallelic. If a mutant phenotype is produced, the mutations are noncomplementing and are often allelic.

complete linkage A condition in which two genes are located so close to each other that no recombination occurs between them.

complexity (X) The total number of nucleotides or nucleotide pairs in a population of nucleic acid molecules as determined by reassociation kinetics.

complex locus A gene within which a set of functionally related pseudoalleles can be identified by recombinational analysis (e.g., the *bithorax* locus in *Drosophila*).

complex trait A trait whose phenotype is determined by the interaction of multiple genes and environmental factors.

concatemer A chain or linear series of subunits linked together. The process of forming a concatemer is called concatenation (e.g., multiple units of a phage genome produced during replication).

concordance Pairs or groups of individuals with identical phenotypes. In twin studies, a condition in which both twins exhibit or fail to exhibit a trait under investigation.

conditional knockout A type of gene knockout in which the gene targeted for interruption or knockout can be turned on or off under different experimental conditions. The CRE-lox system is one common method for creating conditional knockouts.

conditional mutation A mutation expressed only under a certain condition; that is, a wild-type phenotype is expressed under certain (permissive) conditions and a mutant phenotype under other (restrictive) conditions.

conjugation Temporary fusion of two single-celled organisms for the sexual transfer of genetic material.

consanguineous Related by a common ancestor within the previous few generations.

consensus sequence The sequence of nucleotides in DNA or amino acids in proteins most often present in a particular gene or protein.

conservation genetics The branch of genetics concerned with the preservation and maintenance of genetic diversity and existing species of plants and animals in their natural environments.

contig A continuous DNA sequence reconstructed from overlapping DNA sequences derived by cloning or sequence analysis.

continuous variation Phenotype variation in which quantitative traits range from one phenotypic extreme to another in an overlapping or continuous fashion.

copy number variant (CNV) Any DNA segments larger than 1 kb that are repeated a variable number of times in the genome.

core enzyme The subunits of an enzyme necessary for catalytic activity. For DNA polymerase III, the core enzyme consists of three subunits: alpha, beta, and theta that confer catalytic activity to the holoenzyme.

cosmid A vector designed to allow cloning of large segments of foreign DNA. Cosmids are composed of the *cos* sites of phage inserted into a plasmid. In cloning, the recombinant DNA molecules are packaged into phage protein coats, and after infection of bacterial cells, the recombinant molecule replicates and can be maintained as a plasmid.

coupling conformation See *cis configuration*.

covalent bond A nonionic chemical bond, formed by the sharing of electrons.

CpG island A short region of regulatory DNA found upstream of genes that contain unmethylated stretches of sequence with a high frequency of C and G nucleotides.

Creutzfeldt–Jakob disease (CJD) A progressive degenerative and fatal disease of the brain and nervous system caused by mutations that lead to aberrant forms of the encoded protein (prions). CJD is inherited as an autosomal dominant trait.

cri-du-chat syndrome A clinical syndrome produced by a deletion of a portion of the short arm of chromosome 5 in humans. Afflicted infants have a distinctive cry that sounds like a cat.

CRISPR Regions of the prokaryotic genome that contain Clusters of Regularly Interspersed Short Palindromic Repeats. Following insertion of foreign DNA into CRISPR loci, transcription from these regions produces CRISPR RNAs, which guide nucleases to invading complementary DNAs to destroy them.

CRISPR/Cas The adaptive immunity mechanism present in many prokaryotes, which utilizes CRISPR RNAs to guide Cas nucleases to invading complementary DNAs and destroy them. The CRISPR/Cas mechanism has also been exploited to introduce specific mutations in eukaryotic genomes.

crossing over The exchange of chromosomal material (parts of chromosomal arms) between homologous chromosomes by breakage and reunion. The exchange of material between nonsister chromatids during meiosis is the basis of genetic recombination.

cross-reacting material (CRM) A nonfunctional enzyme produced by a mutant gene, yet recognized by antibodies made against the normal enzyme.

crRNA biogenesis One of the steps in the CRISPR/Cas mechanism in which RNAs are transcribed and processed by Cas proteins.

C-terminal amino acid In a peptide chain, the terminal amino acid that carries a free carboxyl group.

C terminus In a polypeptide, the end that carries a free carboxyl group on the last amino acid. By convention, the structural formula of polypeptides is written with the C terminus at the right.

C value The haploid amount of DNA present in a genome.

C value paradox The apparent paradox that there is no relationship between the size of the genome and the evolutionary complexity of species. For example, the C value (haploid genome size) of amphibians varies by a factor of 100.

cyclic adenosine monophosphate (cAMP) An important regulatory molecule in both prokaryotic and eukaryotic organisms.

cyclins In eukaryotic cells, a class of proteins that are synthesized and degraded in synchrony with the cell cycle and regulate passage through stages of the cycle.

cytogenetics A branch of biology in which the techniques of both cytology and genetics are used in genetic investigations.

cytokinesis The division or separation of the cytoplasm during mitosis or meiosis.

cytoplasmic inheritance Non-Mendelian form of inheritance in which genetic information is transmitted through the cytoplasm rather than the nucleus, usually by DNA-containing, self-replicating cytoplasmic organelles such as mitochondria and chloroplasts.

cytoskeleton An internal array of microtubules, microfilaments, and intermediate filaments that confers shape and motility to a eukaryotic cell.

dalton (Da) A unit of mass equal to that of the hydrogen atom, which is 1.67×10^{-24} gram. A unit used in designating molecular weights.

Darwinian fitness See *fitness*.

Database of Genomic Variants (DGV) A catalog of structural variants present in the human genome including copy number variations and inversions.

deficiency A chromosomal mutation, also referred to as a deletion, involving the loss of chromosomal material.

degenerate code In the genetic code, representation of a given amino acid by more than one codon.

deletion A chromosomal mutation, also referred to as a deficiency, involving the loss of chromosomal material. See also *deficiency*.

deme A local interbreeding population.

denatured DNA DNA molecules that have separated into single strands.

de novo Newly arising; synthesized from less complex precursors rather than being produced by modification of an existing molecule.

density gradient centrifugation A method of separating macromolecular mixtures by the use of centrifugal force and solutions of varying density. In buoyant density gradient centrifugation using cesium chloride, the centrifugal field produces a density gradient in a cesium solution through which a mixture of macromolecules such as DNA will migrate until each component reaches a point equal to its own density. Sometimes referred to as equilibrium sedimentation centrifugation.

deoxyribonuclease (DNase) A class of enzymes that breaks down DNA into oligonucleotide fragments by introducing single-stranded or double-stranded breaks into the double helix.

deoxyribonucleic acid (DNA) A macromolecule usually consisting of nucleotide polymers comprising antiparallel chains in which the sugar residues are deoxyribose and which are held together by hydrogen bonds. The primary carrier of genetic information.

deoxyribose The five-carbon sugar associated with the deoxyribonucleotides in DNA.

dermatoglyphics The study of the surface ridges of the skin, especially of the hands and feet.

determination Establishment of a specific pattern of gene activity and developmental fate for a given cell, usually prior to any manifestation of the cell's future phenotype.

diakinesis The final stage of meiotic prophase I, in which the chromosomes become tightly coiled and compacted and move toward the periphery of the nucleus.

dicentric chromosome A chromosome having two centromeres, which can be pulled in opposite directions during anaphase of cell division.

Dicer An enzyme (a ribonuclease) that cleaves double-stranded RNA (dsRNA) and pre-micro RNA (miRNA) to form small interfering RNA (siRNA) molecules about 20–25 nucleotides long that serve as guide molecules for the degradation of mRNA molecules with sequences complementary to the siRNA.

dideoxynucleotide A nucleotide containing a deoxyribose sugar lacking a hydroxyl group. It stops further chain elongation when incorporated into a growing polynucleotide and is used in the Sanger method of DNA sequencing.

dideoxynucleotide chain-terminating sequencing See *Sanger sequencing*.

differentiation The complex process of change by which cells and tissues attain their adult structure and functional capacity.

dihybrid cross A genetic cross involving two characters in which the parents possess different forms of each character (e.g., yellow, round × green, wrinkled peas).

diploid (2n) A condition in which each chromosome exists in pairs; having two of each chromosome.

diplotene The stage of meiotic prophase I immediately following pachytene. In diplotene, the sister chromatids begin to separate, and chiasmata become visible. These cross-like overlaps move toward the ends of the chromatids (terminalization) as this stage proceeds.

directed mutagenesis See *gene targeting*.

directional selection A selective force that changes the frequency of an allele in a given direction, either toward fixation or toward elimination.

discontinuous replication of DNA The synthesis of DNA in discontinuous fragments on the lagging strand during replication. The fragments, known as Okazaki fragments, are subsequently joined by DNA ligase to form a continuous strand.

discontinuous variation Pattern of variation for a trait whose phenotypes fall into two or more distinct classes.

discordance In twin studies, a situation where one twin expresses a trait but the other does not.

disjunction The separation of chromosomes during the anaphase stage of cell division.

disruptive selection Simultaneous selection for phenotypic extremes in a population, usually resulting in the production of two phenotypically discontinuous strains.

dizygotic twins Twins produced from separate fertilization events; two ova fertilized independently. Also known as fraternal twins.

DNA See *deoxyribonucleic acid*.

DNA cloning vectors See *vector*.

DNA fingerprinting A molecular method for identifying an individual member of a population or species. A unique pattern of DNA fragments is obtained by restriction enzyme digestion followed by Southern blot hybridization using minisatellite probes. See also *DNA profiling; STR sequences*.

DNA footprinting A technique for identifying a DNA sequence that binds to a particular protein, based on the idea that the phosphodiester bonds in the region covered by the protein are protected from digestion by deoxyribonucleases.

DNA gyrase One of a class of enzymes known as topoisomerases that converts closed circular DNA to a negatively supercoiled form prior to replication, transcription, or recombination. The enzyme acts during DNA replication to reduce molecular tension caused by supercoiling.

DNA helicase An enzyme that participates in DNA replication by unwinding the double helix near the replication fork.

DNA knockout technology See *gene knockout*.

DNA ligase An enzyme that forms a covalent bond between the 5′ end of one polynucleotide chain and the end of another polynucleotide chain. It is also called polynucleotide-joining enzyme.

DNA microarray An ordered arrangement of DNA sequences or oligonucleotides on a substrate (often glass). Microarrays are used in quantitative assays of DNA–DNA or DNA–RNA binding to measure profiles of gene expression (for example, during development or to compare the differences in gene expression between normal and cancer cells).

DNA polymerase An enzyme that catalyzes the synthesis of DNA from deoxyribonucleotides utilizing a template DNA molecule.

DNA profiling A method for identification of individuals that uses variations in the length of short tandem repeating DNA sequences (STRs) that are widely distributed in the genome.

DNase See *deoxyribonuclease*.

DNase I A nuclease that preferentially cleaves DNA at phosphodiester bonds adjacent to pyrimidine nucleotides. DNase I can act on single- and double-stranded DNA and on DNA in chromatin.

dominance The expression of a trait in the heterozygous condition.

dominant negative mutation A mutation whose gene product acts in opposition to the normal gene product, usually by binding to it to form dimers.

dosage compensation A genetic mechanism that equalizes the levels of expression of genes at loci on the X chromosome. In mammals, this is accomplished by random inactivation of one X chromosome, leading to Barr body formation.

double crossover Two separate events of chromosome breakage and exchange occurring within the same tetrad.

double helix The model for DNA structure proposed by James Watson and Francis Crick, in which two antiparallel hydrogen-bonded polynucleotide chains are wound into a right-handed helical configuration 2 nm in diameter, with 10 base pairs per full turn.

driver mutation A mutation in a cancer cell that contributes to tumor progression.

Drosha A nuclear RNA-specific nuclease involved in the maturation of microRNAs. It removes 5′ and 3′ non-self-complementary regions of a primary miRNA to produce a pre-miRNA.

Duchenne muscular dystrophy An X-linked recessive genetic disorder caused by a mutation in the gene for dystrophin, a protein found in muscle cells. Affected males show a progressive weakness and wasting of muscle tissue. Death ensues by about age 20 caused by respiratory infection or cardiac failure.

duplication A chromosomal aberration in which a segment of the chromosome is repeated.

dyad The products of tetrad separation or disjunction at meiotic prophase I. Each dyad consists of two sister chromatids joined at the centromere.

dystrophin A protein that attaches to the inside of the muscle cell plasma membrane and stabilizes the membrane during muscle contraction. Mutations in the gene-encoding dystrophin cause Duchenne and Becker muscular dystrophy. See *Duchenne muscular dystrophy*.

effective population size In a population, the number of individuals with an equal probability of contributing gametes to the next generation.

effector molecule A small biologically active molecule that regulates the activity of a protein by binding to a specific receptor site on the protein.

electrophoresis A technique that separates a mixture of molecules by their differential migration through a stationary medium (such as a gel) under the influence of an electrical field.

electroporation A technique that uses an electric pulse to move polar molecules across the plasma membrane into the cell.

ELSI (Ethical, Legal, Social Implications) A program established by the National Human Genome Research Institute in 1990 as part of the Human Genome Project to sponsor research on the ethical, legal, and social implications of genomic research and its impact on individuals and social institutions.

embryonic stem cells Cells derived from the inner cell mass of early blastocyst mammalian embryos. These cells are pluripotent, meaning they can differentiate into any of the embryonic or adult cell types characteristic of the organism.

Encyclopedia of DNA Elements (ENCODE) Project A worldwide consortium of researchers using experimental approaches and bioinformatics to identify and analyze functional elements of the genome (such as transcriptional start sites, promoters, and enhancers) that regulate expression of human genes.

endocytosis The uptake by a cell of fluids, macromolecules, or particles by pinocytosis, phagocytosis, or receptor-mediated endocytosis.

endogenous siRNAs (endo-siRNAs) Short interfering RNAs derived from endogenous sources such as bi-directional transcription of repetitive sequences (centromeres and transposons); these RNAs are processed by Dicer.

endomitosis An increased DNA content in multiples of the haploid amount occurring in the absence of nuclear or cytoplasmic division. Polytene chromosomes are formed by endomitosis.

endonuclease An enzyme that hydrolyzes internal phosphodiester bonds in a single- or double-stranded polynucleotide chain.

endoplasmic reticulum (ER) A membranous organelle system in the cytoplasm of eukaryotic cells. In rough ER, the outer surface of the membranes is ribosome-studded; in smooth ER, it is not.

endopolyploidy The increase in chromosome sets within somatic nuclei that results from endomitotic replication.

endosymbiont theory The proposal that self-replicating cellular organelles such as mitochondria and chloroplasts were originally free-living prokaryotic organisms that entered into a symbiotic relationship with eukaryotic cells.

enhancement gene therapy Gene therapy for the purpose of enhancing a desired trait and not for disease treatment or prevention.

enhancer A DNA sequence that enhances transcription and the expression of structural genes. Enhancers can act over a distance of thousands of base pairs and can be located upstream, downstream, or internal to the gene they affect, differentiating them from promoters.

environment The complex of geographic, climatic, and biotic factors within which an organism lives.

enzyme A protein or complex of proteins that catalyzes a specific biochemical reaction by lowering the energy of activation that would otherwise required to initiate the reaction.

epidermal growth-factor receptor A cell-surface receptor for proteins belonging to the family of epidermal growth factors. Binding of a growth factor to the receptor stimulates a signal transduction pathway. In humans, this receptor protein is encoded by the *HER* gene, and mutant alleles are associated with cancer.

epigenesis The idea that an organism or organ arises through the sequential appearance and development of new structures, in contrast to preformationism, which holds that development is the result of the assembly of structures already present in the egg.

epigenetics The study of the effects of reversible chemical modifications to DNA and/or histones on the pattern of gene expression. Epigenetic modifications do not alter the nucleotide sequence of DNA.

episome In bacterial cells, a circular genetic element that can replicate independently of the bacterial chromosome or integrate into and replicate as part of the chromosome.

epistasis Nonreciprocal interaction between nonallelic genes such that one gene influences or interferes with the expression of another gene, leading to a specific phenotype.

epitope That portion of a macromolecule or cell that acts to elicit an antibody response; an antigenic determinant. A complex molecule or cell can contain several such sites.

equational division A division stage where the number of centromeres is not reduced by half but where each chromosome is split into longitudinal halves that are distributed into two daughter nuclei. Chromosome division in mitosis and the second meiotic division are examples of equational divisions. See also *reductional division*.

equatorial plate   See *metaphase plate.*

euchromatin   Chromatin or chromosomal regions that are lightly staining and relatively uncoiled during the interphase portion of the cell cycle. Euchromatic regions contain most of the structural genes.

eugenics   A movement advocating the improvement of the human species by selective breeding. Positive eugenics refers to the promotion of breeding between people thought to possess favorable genes, and negative eugenics refers to the discouragement of breeding among those thought to have undesirable traits.

eukaryotes   Organisms having true nuclei and membranous organelles and whose cells divide by mitosis and meiosis.

euphenics   Medical or genetic intervention to reduce the impact of defective genotypes.

euploid   A cell with a chromosome number that is an exact multiple of the haploid number.

evolution   Descent with modification. The emergence of new kinds of plants and animals from preexisting types.

excision repair   Removal of damaged DNA segments followed by repair. Excision can include the removal of individual bases (base repair) or of a stretch of damaged nucleotides (nucleotide repair).

exome sequencing   A DNA sequencing method in which only the protein-coding regions (exons) of the genome are sequenced.

exon   The DNA segments of a gene that contain the sequences that, through transcription and translation, are eventually represented in the final polypeptide product.

exonuclease   An enzyme that breaks down nucleic acid molecules by breaking the phosphodiester bonds at the 3'- or 5'-terminal nucleotides.

expressed sequence tag (EST)   All or part of the nucleotide sequence of a cDNA clone. ESTs are used as markers in the construction of genetic maps.

expression vector   Plasmids or phages carrying promoter regions designed to cause expression of inserted DNA sequences.

expressivity   The degree to which a phenotype for a given trait is expressed.

extracellular RNAs (exRNAs)   Several types of RNAs (such as mRNAs and microRNAs) with diverse functions that are secreted in association with proteins or within vesicles for protection from RNAses.

extranuclear inheritance   Transmission of traits by genetic information contained in the DNA of cytoplasmic organelles such as mitochondria and chloroplasts.

5-methylcytosine   A methylated cytosine base that represents an epigenetic modification that alters gene expression.

F$^-$ cell   A bacterial cell that contains a fertility factor and that acts as a donor in bacterial conjugation.

F$^+$ cell   A bacterial cell that does not contain a fertility factor and that acts as a recipient in bacterial conjugation.

F factor   An episomal plasmid in bacterial cells that confers the ability to act as a donor in conjugation.

F' factor   A fertility factor that contains a portion of the bacterial chromosome.

F$_1$ generation   First filial generation; the progeny resulting from the first cross in a series.

F$_2$ generation   Second filial generation; the progeny resulting from a cross of the F$_1$ generation.

F pilus   On bacterial cells possessing an F factor, a filament-like projection that plays a role in conjugation.

familial trait   A trait transmitted through and expressed by members of a family. Usually used to describe a trait that runs in families, but whose precise mode of inheritance is not clear.

fate map   A diagram showing the location of embryonic cells whose developmental fate is known.

fertility factor   See *F factor.*

fetal cell sorting   A noninvasive method of prenatal diagnosis that recovers and tests fetal cells from the maternal circulation.

filial generations   See *F$_1$, F$_2$ generations.*

fingerprint   The unique pattern of ridges and whorls on the tip of a human finger. Also, the pattern obtained by enzymatically cleaving a protein or nucleic acid and subjecting the digest to two-dimensional chromatography or electrophoresis. See also *DNA fingerprinting.*

FISH   See *fluorescence* in situ *hybridization.*

fitness   A measure of the relative survival and reproductive success of a given individual or genotype.

fixation   In population genetics, a condition in which all members of a population are homozygous for a given allele.

fluctuation test   A statistical test developed by Salvador Luria and Max Delbrück demonstrating that bacterial mutations arise spontaneously, in contrast to being induced by selective agents.

fluorescence *in situ* hybridization (FISH)   A method of *in situ* hybridization that utilizes probes labeled with a fluorescent tag, causing the site of hybridization to fluoresce when viewed using ultraviolet light.

flush–crash cycle   A period of rapid population growth followed by a drastic reduction in population size.

f-met   See *formylmethionine.*

folded-fiber model   A model of eukaryotic chromosome organization in which each sister chromatid consists of a single chromatin fiber composed of double-stranded DNA and proteins wound together like a tightly coiled skein of yarn.

footprinting   See *DNA footprinting.*

forensic DNA fingerprinting   In law enforcement, the use of a standard set of short tandem repeats (STRs) to identify an individual. Also known as DNA typing. See also *DNA profiling.*

forensic science   The use of laboratory scientific methods to obtain data used in criminal and civil law cases.

formylmethionine (f-met)   A molecule derived from the amino acid methionine by attachment of a formyl group to its terminal amino group. This is the first monomer used in the synthesis of all bacterial polypeptides. Also known as *N*-formyl methionine.

forward genetics   The classical approach used to identify a gene controlling a phenotypic trait in the absence of knowledge of the gene's location in the genome or its DNA sequence. Accomplished by isolating mutant alleles and mapping the gene's location, most traditionally using recombination analysis. Once mapped, the gene may be cloned and further studied at the molecular level. An approach contrasted with *reverse genetics.*

founder effect   A form of genetic drift. The establishment of a population by a small number of individuals whose genotypes carry only a fraction of the different alleles present in the parental population.

fragile site   A heritable gap, or nonstaining region, of a chromosome that can be induced to generate chromosome breaks.

fragile-X syndrome   A human genetic disorder caused by the expansion of a CGG trinucleotide repeat and a fragile site at Xq27.3 within the *FMR-1* gene. Fragile-X syndrome is the most common form of mental retardation in males. Affected males have distinctive facial features and are mentally retarded. Carrier females lack physical symptoms but as a group have higher rates of mental retardation than normal individuals.

frameshift mutation A mutational event leading to the insertion or deletion (indels) of a number of base pairs in a gene that is not a multiple of three. This shifts the codon reading frame in all codons that follow the mutational site.

fraternal twins See *dizygotic twins*.

G1 checkpoint A point in the G1 phase of the cell cycle when a cell becomes committed to initiating DNA synthesis and continuing the cycle or withdrawing into the G0 resting stage.

G0 A nondividing but metabolically active state (G-zero) that cells may enter from the G1 phase of the cell cycle.

gain-of-function mutation A type of mutation in which the gene product takes on a new function and produces a phenotype different from that of the normal allele and from any loss of function alleles.

gamete A specialized reproductive cell with a haploid number of chromosomes.

gap genes Genes expressed in contiguous domains along the anterior–posterior axis of the *Drosophila* embryo that regulate the process of segmentation in each domain.

GC box In eukaryotes, a region in a promoter containing a 5′-GGGCGG-3′ sequence, which is a binding site for transcriptional regulatory proteins.

gene The fundamental physical unit of heredity, whose existence can be confirmed by allelic variants and which occupies a specific chromosomal locus. A DNA sequence coding for a single polypeptide or an RNA molecule.

gene amplification The process by which gene sequences are selected and differentially replicated either extrachromosomally or intrachromosomally.

gene chip See *DNA microarray*.

gene conversion A meiotic event in heterozygotes by which one allele of a gene directs the conversion of the other allele of the gene into its own form.

gene duplication An event leading to the production of a tandem repeat of a gene sequence during replication.

gene family A number of closely related genes derived from a common ancestral gene by duplication and sequence divergence over evolutionary time.

gene flow The exchange of genes between two populations; brought about by the dispersal of gametes resulting from the migration of individuals between populations.

gene frequency The percentage of alleles of a given type in a population.

gene interaction Production of novel phenotypes by the interaction of alleles of different genes.

gene knockout Generation of a *null mutation* in a gene that is subsequently introduced into an organism using transgenic techniques, causing a loss of function in the targeted gene. Often used in mice. See also *gene targeting*.

gene mutation See *point mutation*.

gene pool The total of all alleles possessed by the reproductive members of a population.

gene redundancy The presence of several genes in an organism's genome that all have variations of the same function.

gene targeting A transgenic technique used to create and introduce a specifically altered gene into an organism. In mice, gene targeting often involves the induction of a specific mutation in a cloned gene that is subsequently introduced into the genome of a gamete involved in fertilization. The organism produced is bred to produce adults homozygous for the mutation, for example, the creation of a *gene knockout*.

gene therapy A therapeutic approach for providing a normal copy of a gene, replacement of a defective gene, or supplementing a gene for treating or curing a genetic disorder.

generalized transduction The transfer of a gene from a bacterial host to a bacterial recipient in a process mediated by a bacteriophage. See also *specialized transduction*.

genetically modified organism (GMO) A plant or animal whose genome carries a gene transferred from another species by recombinant DNA technology and expressed to produce a gene product and a novel phenotype.

genetic anticipation The phenomenon in which the severity of symptoms in genetic disorders increases from generation to generation and the age of onset decreases from generation to generation. It is caused by the expansion of trinucleotide repeats within or near a gene and was first observed in myotonic dystrophy.

genetic background The impact of the collective genome of an organism on the expression of a gene under investigation.

genetic code The deoxynucleotide triplets that encode the 20 amino acids or specify initiation or termination of translation.

genetic counseling Analysis of risk for genetic defects in a family and the presentation of options available to avoid or ameliorate possible risks.

genetic drift Random variation in allele frequency from generation to generation, most often observed in small populations.

genetic engineering The technique of altering the genetic constitution of cells or individuals by the selective removal, insertion, or modification of individual genes or gene sets.

genetic equilibrium A condition in which allele frequencies in a population are neither increasing nor decreasing from generation to generation.

genetic erosion The loss of genetic diversity from a population or a species.

genetic fine structure analysis Recombinational analysis that provides intragenic mapping information at the level of individual nucleotides.

genetic load Average number of recessive lethal genes carried in the heterozygous condition by an individual in a population.

genetic polymorphism The stable coexistence of two or more distinct genotypes for a given trait in a population. When the frequencies of two alleles for such a trait are in equilibrium, the condition is called a balanced polymorphism.

Genetic Testing Registry (GTR) A centralized, online database, sponsored by the U.S. government to provide information about the scientific basis and availability of genetic tests.

genetic variability A measure of the tendency of the genotypes of individuals in a population to vary from one another. Genetic variability can be measured by determining the rate of mutation of specific genes.

genetics The branch of biology concerned with study of inherited variation. More specifically, the study of the origin, transmission, and expression of genetic information.

genome The set of hereditary information encoded in the DNA of an organism, including both the protein-coding and non–protein-coding sequences.

genome-wide association studies (GWAS) Analysis of genetic variation across an entire genome, searching for linkage (associations) between variations in DNA sequences and a genome region encoding a specific phenotype.

genomic imprinting The process by which the expression of an allele depends on whether it has been inherited from a male or a female parent. Also referred to as parental imprinting.

genomic library A collection of clones that contains all the DNA sequences of an organism's genome.

genomics A subdiscipline of genetics created by the union of classical and molecular biology with the goal of sequencing and understanding genes, gene interaction, genetic elements, as well as the structure and evolution of genomes.

genotype The allelic or genetic constitution of an organism; often, the allelic composition of one or a limited number of genes under investigation.

germ line An embryonic cell lineage that will form the reproductive cells (eggs and sperm).

germ-line therapy Gene therapy involving germ cells or mature gametes as targets for gene transfer.

germ plasm Hereditary material transmitted from generation to generation.

GMO See *genetically modified organism (GMO)*.

Goldberg–Hogness box A short nucleotide sequence 20–30 bp upstream from the initiation site of eukaryotic genes to which RNA polymerase II binds. The consensus sequence is TATAAAA. Also known as a TATA box.

gynandromorphy An individual composed of cells with both male and female genotypes.

gyrase See *DNA gyrase*.

haploid (*n*) A cell or an organism having one member of each pair of homologous chromosomes. Also referred to as the gametic chromosome number.

haploinsufficiency In a diploid organism, a condition in which an individual possesses only one functional copy of a gene with the other inactivated by mutation. The amount of protein produced by the single copy is insufficient to produce a normal phenotype, leading to an abnormal phenotype. In humans, this condition is present in many autosomal dominant disorders.

haplotype A set of alleles from closely linked loci carried by an individual that are inherited as a unit.

HapMap Project An international effort by geneticists to identify haplotypes (closely linked genetic markers on a single chromosome) shared by certain individuals as a way of facilitating efforts to identify, map, and isolate genes associated with disease or disease susceptibility.

Hardy–Weinberg law The principle that genotype frequencies will remain in equilibrium in an infinitely large, randomly mating population in the absence of mutation, migration, and selection.

heat shock A transient genetic response following exposure of cells or organisms to elevated temperatures. The response includes activation of a small number of loci, inactivation of some previously active loci, and selective translation of heat-shock mRNA.

helicase See *DNA helicase*.

helix–turn–helix (HTH) motif In DNA-binding proteins, the structure of a region in which a turn of four amino acids contains two helices at right angles to each other.

hemizygous Having a gene present in a single dose in an otherwise diploid cell. Usually applied to genes on the X chromosome in heterogametic males.

hemoglobin (Hb) An iron-containing, oxygen-carrying multimeric protein occurring chiefly in the red blood cells of vertebrates.

hemophilia An X-linked trait in humans that is associated with defective blood-clotting mechanisms.

heredity Transmission of traits from one generation to another.

heritability A relative measure of the degree to which observed phenotypic differences for a trait are genetic.

heterochromatin The heavily staining, late-replicating regions of chromosomes that are prematurely condensed in interphase.

heteroduplex A double-stranded nucleic acid molecule in which each polynucleotide chain has a different origin. It may be produced as an intermediate in a recombinational event or by the *in vitro* reannealing of single-stranded complementary molecules.

heterogametic sex The sex that produces gametes containing unlike sex chromosomes. In mammals, the male is the heterogametic sex.

heterogeneous nuclear RNA (hnRNA) The collection of RNA transcripts in the nucleus, consisting of precursors to and processing intermediates for rRNA, mRNA, and tRNA. Also includes RNA transcripts that will not be transported to the cytoplasm, such as snRNA.

heterokaryon A somatic cell containing nuclei from two different sources.

heterozygote An individual with different alleles at one or more loci. Such individuals will produce unlike gametes and therefore will not breed true.

Hfr Strains of bacteria exhibiting a high frequency of recombination. These strains have a chromosomally integrated F factor that is able to mobilize and transfer part of the chromosome to a recipient F⁻ cell.

high-throughput DNA sequencing A collection of DNA sequencing methods that outperform the standard (Sanger) method of DNA sequencing by a factor of 100–1000 and reduce sequencing costs by more than 99 percent. Also called *next-generation sequencing*.

histocompatibility antigens See *HLA*.

histone code Chemical modifications of amino acids in histone tails (the free ends of histone molecules, projecting from nucleosomes). These modifications influence DNA–histone interactions and promote or repress transcription.

histone methyltransferase An enzyme that catalyzes the addition of methyl groups to histone proteins.

histones Positively charged proteins complexed with DNA in the nucleus. They are rich in the basic amino acids arginine and lysine, and function in coiling DNA to form nucleosomes.

HLA Cell-surface proteins produced by histocompatibility loci and involved in the acceptance or rejection of tissue and organ grafts and transplants.

hnRNA See *heterogeneous nuclear RNA*.

Holliday structure In DNA recombination, an intermediate stage seen in transmission electron microscope images as an X-shaped structure showing four single-stranded DNA regions.

holoenzyme For proteins with multiple subunits, the complex formed by the union of all subunits necessary for all functions of the enzyme.

homeobox A sequence of 180 nucleotides that encodes a sequence of 60 amino acids called a *homeodomain*, which is part of a DNA-binding protein that acts as a transcription factor.

homeotic mutation A mutation that causes a tissue normally determined to form a specific organ or body part to alter its pathway of differentiation and form another structure.

homogametic sex The sex that produces gametes with identical sex-chromosome content; in mammals, the female is homogametic.

homologous chromosomes Chromosomes that synapse or pair during meiosis and that are identical with respect to their genetic loci and centromere placement.

homozygote An individual with identical alleles for a gene or genes of interest. These individuals will produce identical gametes (with respect to the gene or genes in question) and will therefore breed true.

horizontal gene transfer The nonreproductive transfer of genetic information from one organism to another, across species and higher taxa (even domains). This mode is contrasted with vertical gene transfer, which is the transfer of genetic information from parent to offspring. In some species of bacteria and archaea, up to 5 percent of the genome may have originally been acquired through horizontal gene transfer.

H substance The carbohydrate group present on the surface of red blood cells to which the A and/or B antigen may be added. When unmodified, it results in blood type O.

hot spots Genome regions where mutations are observed with a high frequency. These include a predisposition toward single-nucleotide substitutions or unequal crossing over.

human immunodeficiency virus (HIV) An RNA-containing human retrovirus associated with the onset and progression of acquired immunodeficiency syndrome (AIDS).

hybrid An individual produced by crossing parents from two different genetic strains.

hybrid vigor The general superiority of a hybrid over a purebred.

hydrogen bond A weak electrostatic attraction between a hydrogen atom covalently bonded to an oxygen or a nitrogen atom and an atom that contains an unshared electron pair.

hypervariable regions The regions of antibody molecules that attach to antigens. These regions have a high degree of diversity in amino acid content.

identical twins See *monozygotic twins*.

Ig See *immunoglobulin*.

immunoglobulin (Ig) The class of serum proteins having the properties of antibodies.

imprinting See *genomic imprinting*.

inborn error of metabolism A genetically controlled biochemical disorder; usually an enzyme defect that produces a clinical syndrome.

inbreeding Mating between closely related organisms.

inbreeding depression A decrease in viability, vigor, or growth in progeny after several generations of inbreeding.

incomplete dominance Expressing a heterozygous phenotype that is distinct from the phenotype of either homozygous parent. Also called *partial dominance*.

independent assortment The independent behavior of each pair of homologous chromosomes during their segregation in meiosis I. The random distribution of maternal and paternal homologs into gametes.

inducer An effector molecule that activates transcription.

inducible enzyme system An enzyme system under the control of an inducer, a regulatory molecule that acts to block a repressor and allow transcription.

initiation codon The nucleotide triplet AUG that in an mRNA molecule codes for incorporation of the amino acid methionine as the first amino acid in a polypeptide chain.

insertion sequence See *IS element*.

***in situ* hybridization** A cytological technique for pinpointing the chromosomal location of DNA sequences complementary to a given nucleic acid or polynucleotide.

interference (*I*) A measure of the degree to which one crossover affects the incidence of another crossover in an adjacent region of the same chromatid. Negative interference increases the chance of another crossover; positive interference reduces the probability of a second crossover event.

interphase In the cell cycle, the interval between divisions.

intervening sequence See *intron*.

intron Any segment of DNA that lies between coding regions in a gene. Introns are transcribed but are spliced out of the RNA product and are not represented in the polypeptide encoded by the gene.

inversion A chromosomal aberration in which a chromosomal segment has been reversed.

inversion loop The chromosomal configuration resulting from the synapsis of homologous chromosomes, one of which carries an inversion.

in vitro Literally, *in glass*; outside the living organism; occurring in an artificial environment.

***in vitro* evolution** A form of directed evolution using small, stepwise changes to a nucleic acid that occurs outside a cell and mimics natural selection.

in vivo Literally, *in the living*; occurring within the living body of an organism.

IS element A mobile DNA segment that is transposable to any of a number of sites in the genome.

isoagglutinogen An antigen present on the surface of cells that is capable of inducing the formation of an antibody (e.g., the A and B antigens on the surface of human red blood cells).

isochromosome An aberrant chromosome with two identical arms and homologous loci.

isolating mechanism Any barrier to the exchange of genes between different populations of a species. In general, isolation can be classified as spatial, environmental, or reproductive.

isotopes Alternative forms of atoms with identical chemical properties that have the same atomic number but differ in the number of neutrons (and thus their mass) contained in the nucleus.

isozyme Any of two or more distinct forms of an enzyme with identical or nearly identical chemical properties but differ in some property such as net electrical charge, pH optima, number and type of subunits, or substrate concentration.

kappa (κ) particles DNA-containing cytoplasmic particles found in certain strains of *Paramecium aurelia* capable of releasing a toxin, paramecin, that kills other, sensitive strains.

K-RAS A plasma membrane-associated protein encoded by the *KRAS* gene. This protein is important in cellular signal transduction events. Mutant alleles of *KRAS* are oncogenes present in many forms of cancer.

karyokinesis The process of nuclear division.

karyotype The chromosome complement of a cell or an individual. An arrangement of metaphase chromosomes in a sequence according to length and centromere position.

kilobase (kb) A unit of length consisting of 1000 nucleotides.

kinetochore A fibrous structure with a size of about 400 nm, located within the centromere. It is the site of microtubule attachment during cell division.

Klinefelter syndrome A genetic disorder in human males caused by the presence of one or more additional X chromosomes. Klinefelter males are usually XXY instead of XY. This syndrome can include enlarged breasts, small testes, sterility, and mild mental retardation.

knockout mice Mice created by a process in which a normal gene is cloned, inactivated by the insertion of a marker (such as an antibiotic resistance gene), and transferred to embryonic stem cells, where the altered gene will replace the normal gene (in some cells). These cells are injected into a blastomere embryo, producing a mouse that is then bred to yield mice homozygous for the mutated gene. See also *gene targeting*.

Kozak sequence   A short nucleotide sequence adjacent to the initiation codon that is recognized as the translational start site in eukaryotic mRNA.

***lac* repressor protein**   A protein that binds to the operator in the *lac* operon and blocks transcription.

lagging strand   During DNA replication, the strand synthesized in a discontinuous fashion, in the direction opposite of the replication fork. See also *Okazaki fragment*.

lampbrush chromosomes   Meiotic chromosomes characterized by extended lateral loops that reach maximum extension during diplotene. Although most intensively studied in amphibians, these structures occur in meiotic cells of organisms ranging from insects to humans.

lariat structure   A structure formed during pre-mRNA processing by formation of a 5′ to 3′ bond in an intron, leading to removal of that intron from an mRNA molecule.

leader sequence   That portion of an mRNA molecule from the 5′ end to the initiating codon, often containing regulatory or ribosome binding sites.

leading strand   During DNA replication, the strand synthesized continuously in the direction of the replication fork.

leptotene   The initial stage of meiotic prophase I, during which the replicated chromosomes become visible; they are often arranged with one or both ends gathered at one spot on the inner nuclear membrane (the so-called bouquet configuration).

lethal gene   A gene whose expression results in premature death of the organism at some stage of its life cycle.

leucine zipper   In DNA-binding proteins, a structural motif characterized by a stretch in which every seventh amino acid residue is leucine, with adjacent regions containing positively charged amino acids. Leucine zippers on two polypeptides may interact to form a dimer that binds to DNA.

linkage   The condition in which genes are present on the same chromosome, causing them to be inherited as a unit, provided that they are not separated by crossing over during meiosis.

linking number   The number of times that two strands of a closed, circular DNA duplex cross over each other.

locus (pl., loci)   The place on a chromosome where a particular gene is located.

lod score (LOD)   A statistical method used to determine whether two loci are linked or unlinked. A lod (log of the odds) score of 4 indicates that linkage is 10,000 times more likely than nonlinkage. By convention, lod scores of 3–4 are signs of linkage.

long interspersed elements (LINEs)   Long, repetitive sequences found interspersed in the genomes of higher organisms.

long noncoding RNAs (lncRNAs)   RNAs longer than 200 nt that are noncoding transcripts and have various functions including epigenetic modification of DNA and regulation of gene specific transcription.

long terminal repeat (LTR)   A sequence of several hundred base pairs found at both ends of a retroviral DNA.

loss-of-function mutation   Mutations that produce alleles encoding proteins with reduced or no function.

Lyon hypothesis   The proposal that there is random inactivation of the maternal or paternal X chromosome in somatic cells of mammalian females early in development. All daughter cells will have the same X chromosome inactivated as in the cell they descended from, producing a mosaic pattern of expression of X chromosome genes.

lysis   The disintegration of a cell brought about by the rupture of its membrane.

lysogenic bacterium   A bacterial cell carrying the DNA of a temperate bacteriophage integrated into its chromosome.

lysogeny   The process by which the DNA of an infecting phage becomes repressed and integrated into the chromosome of the bacterial cell it infects.

lytic phase   The condition in which a bacteriophage invades, reproduces, and lyses the bacterial cell. Lysogenic bacteria may be induced to enter the lytic phase.

major histocompatibility (MHC) loci   Loci encoding antigenic determinants responsible for tissue specificity. The HLA complex of humans and the H2 complex of mice are located within the MHC complex. See also *HLA*.

mapping functions   A mathematical formula that relates map distances to recombination frequencies.

map unit   A measure of the genetic distance between two genes, corresponding to a recombination frequency of 1 percent. See also *centimorgan*.

maternal effect   Phenotypic effects in offspring attributable to genetic information in the oocyte derived from the maternal genome.

maternal influence   See *maternal effect*.

maternal inheritance   The transmission of traits strictly through the maternal parent, usually due to DNA found in mitochondria or chloroplasts.

mean ($\bar{X}$)   The arithmetic average.

median   In a set of data points, the point below and above which there are equal numbers of other data points.

meiosis   The process of cell division in gametogenesis or sporogenesis during which the diploid number of chromosomes is reduced to the haploid number.

melting profile (T_m)   The temperature at which a population of double-stranded nucleic acid molecules is half-dissociated into single strands.

merozygote   A partially diploid bacterial cell containing, in addition to its own chromosome, a chromosome fragment introduced into the cell by transformation, transduction, or conjugation.

messenger RNA (mRNA)   An RNA molecule transcribed from DNA and translated into the amino acid sequence of a polypeptide.

metabolism   The collective chemical processes by which living cells are created and maintained. In particular, the chemical basis of generating and utilizing energy in living organisms.

metacentric chromosome   A chromosome with a centrally located centromere and therefore chromosome arms of equal lengths.

metachromatic leukodystrophy (MLD)   Inherited neurodegenerative disorder affecting storage of enzymes in lysosomes caused by mutation in the arylsulfatase A (*ARSA*) gene. Accumulation of the ARSA enzyme is toxic to neurons, causing progressive loss of the myelin sheath (demyelination) surrounding neurons in the brain leading to a loss of cognitive functions and motor skills.

metafemale   In *Drosophila*, a poorly developed female of low viability with a ratio of X chromosomes to sets of autosomes that exceeds 1.0. Previously called a *superfemale*.

metagenomics   The study of DNA recovered from organisms collected from the environment as opposed to those grown as laboratory cultures. Often used for estimating the diversity of organisms in an environmental sample.

metamale In *Drosophila*, a poorly developed male of low viability with a ratio of X chromosomes to sets of autosomes that is below 0.5. Previously called a *supermale*.

metaphase The stage of cell division in which condensed chromosomes lie in a central plane between the two poles of the cell and during which the chromosomes become attached to the spindle fibers.

metaphase plate The structure formed when mitotic or meiotic chromosomes collect at the equator of the cell during metaphase.

metastasis The process by which cancer cells spread from the primary tumor and establish malignant tumors in other parts of the body.

methylation Enzymatic transfer of methyl groups from S-adenosylmethionine to biological molecules, including phospholipids, proteins, RNA, and DNA. Methylation of DNA is associated with the regulation of gene expression and with epigenetic phenomena such as imprinting.

MHC See *major histocompatibility (MHC) loci*.

microarray See *DNA microarray*.

microRNA Single-stranded RNA molecules approximately 20–23 nucleotides in length that regulate gene expression by participating in the degradation of mRNA.

microsatellite A short, highly polymorphic DNA sequence of 1–4 base pairs, widely distributed in the genome, that are used as molecular markers in a variety of methods. Also called *simple sequence repeats (SSRs)*.

migration coefficient A measure of the proportion of migrant genes entering the population per generation.

minimal medium A medium containing only the essential nutrients needed to support the growth and reproduction of wild-type strains of an organism. Usually comprised of inorganic components that include a carbon and nitrogen source.

minisatellite Series of short tandem repeat sequences (STRs) 10–100 nucleotides in length that occur frequently throughout the genome of eukaryotes. Because the number of repeats at each locus is variable, the loci are known as variable number tandem repeats (VNTRs). Used in the preparation of DNA fingerprints and DNA profiles. See also *variable number tandem repeats (VNTRs)*; *STR sequences*.

mismatch repair A form of excision repair of DNA in which the repair mechanism is able to distinguish between the strand with the error and the strand that is correct.

missense mutation A mutation that changes a codon to that of another amino acid and thus results in an amino acid substitution in the translated protein. Such changes can make the protein nonfunctional.

mitochondrial DNA (mtDNA) Double-stranded, self-replicating circular DNA found in mitochondria that encodes mitochondrial ribosomal RNAs, transfer RNAs, and proteins used in oxidative respiratory functions of the organelle.

mitochondrial swapping The exchange of defective mitochondria in an egg with normal mitochondria to correct a mitochondrial genetic disorder. This is accomplished by transferring the nucleus from an egg with defective mitochondria into a nondefective egg that has had its nucleus removed. The reconstructed egg is fertilized via *in vitro* fertilization and implanted for development.

mitochondrion The so-called power house of the cell—a self-reproducing, DNA-containing, cytoplasmic organelle in eukaryotes involved in generating the high-energy compound ATP.

mitogen A substance that stimulates mitosis in nondividing cells.

mitosis A form of cell division producing two progeny cells identical genetically to the parental cell—that is, the production of two cells from one, each having the same chromosome complement as the parent cell.

mode In a set of data, the value occurring with the greatest frequency.

model genetic organism An experimental organism conducive to research whose genetics is intensively studied on the premise that the findings can be applied to other organisms; for example, the fruit fly (*Drosophila melanogaster*) and the mouse (*Mus musculus*) are model organisms used to study the causes and development of human genetic diseases.

molecular clock In evolutionary studies, a method that counts the number of differences in DNA or protein sequences as a way of measuring the time elapsed since two species diverged from a common ancestor.

monohybrid cross A genetic cross involving only one character (e.g., $AA \times aa$).

monophyletic group A taxon (group of organisms) consisting of an ancestor and all its descendants.

monosomic An aneuploid condition in which one member of a chromosome pair is missing; having a chromosome number of $2n - 1$.

monozygotic twins Twins produced from a single fertilization event; the first division of the zygote produces two cells, each of which develops into an embryo. Also known as *identical twins*.

mRNA See *messenger RNA*.

mtDNA See *mitochondrial DNA*.

multigene family A set of genes descended from a common ancestral gene usually by duplication and subsequent sequence divergence. The globin genes are an example of a multigene family.

multiple alleles In a population of organisms, the presence of three or more alleles of the same gene.

multiple factor inheritance See *polygenic inheritance*.

mu (μ) bacteriophage A phage group in which the genetic material behaves like an insertion sequence (i.e., capable of insertion, excision, transposition, inactivation of host genes, and induction of chromosomal rearrangements).

mutagen Any agent that causes an increase in the rate of mutation.

mutant A cell or organism carrying one or more mutant alleles.

mutation The process that produces an alteration in DNA or chromosome structure; in genes, the source of new alleles.

mutation rate The frequency with which mutations take place at a given locus or in a population.

muton In fine structure analysis of the gene, the smallest unit of mutation, corresponding to a single base.

myotonic dystrophy An inherited progressive neuromuscular disorder characterized by muscle weakness and myotonia (inability of muscles to relax after contraction).

natural selection Differential reproduction among members of a species owing to variable fitness conferred by genotypic differences.

neutral mutation A mutation with no perceived immediate adaptive significance or phenotypic effect.

next-generation sequencing (NGS) technologies See *high-throughput DNA sequencing*.

nonautonomous transposon A transposable element that lacks a functional transposase gene.

noncoding RNAs (ncRNAs) RNAs that do not encode polypeptides.

noncrossover gamete A gamete whose chromosomes have undergone no genetic recombination.

nondisjunction A cell division error in which homologous chromosomes (in meiosis) or the sister chromatids (in mitosis) fail to separate and migrate to opposite poles; responsible for defects such as monosomy and trisomy.

noninvasive prenatal genetic diagnosis (NIPGD) A noninvasive method of fetal genotyping that uses a maternal blood sample to analyze thousands of fetal loci using fetal cells or fetal DNA fragments present in the maternal blood.

nonsense codons The nucleotide triplets (UGA, UAG, and UAA) in an mRNA molecule that signal the termination of translation.

nonsense mutation A mutation that changes a codon specifying an amino acid into a termination codon, leading to premature termination during translation of mRNA.

NOR See *nucleolar organizer region*.

normal distribution A probability function that approximates the distribution of random variables. The normal curve, also known as a Gaussian or bell-shaped curve, is the graphic display of a normal distribution.

northern blot An analytic technique in which RNA molecules are separated by electrophoresis and transferred by capillary action to a nylon or nitrocellulose membrane. Specific RNA molecules can then be identified by hybridization to a labeled nucleic acid probe.

N-terminal amino acid In a peptide chain, the terminal amino acid that carries a free amino group.

N terminus The free amino group of the first amino acid in a polypeptide. By convention, the structural formula of polypeptides is written with the N terminus at the left.

nuclease An enzyme that breaks covalent bonds in nucleic acid molecules.

nucleoid The DNA-containing region within the cytoplasm in prokaryotic cells.

nucleolar organizer region (NOR) A chromosomal region containing the genes for ribosomal RNA (rRNA); most often found in physical association with the *nucleolus*.

nucleolus The nuclear site of ribosome biosynthesis and assembly; associated with or formed in association with the DNA comprising the *nucleolar organizer region*.

nucleoside In nucleic acid chemical nomenclature, a purine or pyrimidine base covalently linked to a ribose or deoxyribose sugar molecule.

nucleosome In eukaryotes, a complex consisting of four pairs of histone molecules wrapped by two turns of a DNA molecule. The major structure associated with the organization of chromatin in the nucleus.

nucleotide In nucleic acid chemical nomenclature, a nucleoside covalently linked to one or more phosphate groups. Nucleotides containing a single phosphate linked to the 5′ carbon of the ribose or deoxyribose are the building blocks of nucleic acids.

nucleotide pair The base-paired nucleotides (A with T or G with C) on opposite strands of a DNA molecule that are hydrogen-bonded to each other.

nucleus The membrane-bound cytoplasmic organelle of eukaryotic cells that contains the chromosomes and nucleolus.

null allele A mutant allele that produces no functional gene product. Usually inherited as a recessive trait.

null hypothesis (H$_0$) Used in statistical tests, the hypothesis that there is no real difference between the observed and expected datasets. Statistical methods such as chi-square analysis are used to test the probability associated with this hypothesis.

nullisomic Term describing an individual with a chromosomal aberration in which both members of a chromosome pair are missing.

nutrigenomics The study of how food and components of food affect gene expression.

Okazaki fragment The short, discontinuous strands of DNA produced on the lagging strand during DNA synthesis.

oligonucleotide A linear sequence of about 10–20 nucleotides connected by 5′-3′ phosphodiester bonds.

oncogene A gene whose activity promotes uncontrolled proliferation in eukaryotic cells. Usually a mutant gene derived from a *proto-oncogene*.

Online Mendelian Inheritance in Man (OMIM) A database listing all known genetic disorders and disorders with genetic components. It also contains a listing of all known human genes and links genes to genetic disorders.

open reading frame (ORF) A nucleotide sequence organized as triplets that encodes the amino acid sequence of a polypeptide, including an initiation codon and a termination codon.

operator region In bacterial DNA, a region that interacts with a specific repressor protein to regulate the expression of an adjacent gene or gene set.

operon A genetic unit consisting of one or more structural genes encoding polypeptides, and an adjacent operator gene that regulates the transcriptional activity of the structural gene or genes.

origin of replication (*ori*) Sites where DNA replication begins along the length of a chromosome.

orthologs Genes with sequence similarity found in two or more related species that arose from a single gene in a common ancestor.

outbreeding depression Reduction in fitness in the offspring produced by mating genetically diverse parents. It is thought to result from a lowered adaptation to local environmental conditions.

overdominance The phenomenon in which heterozygotes have a phenotype that is more extreme than either homozygous genotype.

overlapping code A hypothetical genetic code in which any given triplet is shared by more than one adjacent codon.

pachytene The stage in meiotic prophase I when the synapsed homologous chromosomes split longitudinally (except at the centromere), producing a group of four chromatids called a tetrad.

pair-rule genes Genes expressed as stripes around the blastoderm embryo during development of the *Drosophila* embryo.

palindrome In genetics, a sequence of DNA base pairs that reads the same backwards or forward. Because strands run antiparallel to one another in DNA, the base sequences on the two strands read the same backwards and forward when read from the 5′ end. For example:

5′-G A A T T C-3′
3′-C T T A A G-5′

Palindromic sequences are noteworthy as recognition and cleavage sites for restriction endonucleases.

paracentric inversion A chromosomal inversion that does not include the region containing the centromere.

paralogs Two or more genes in the same species derived by duplication and subsequent divergence from a single ancestral gene.

parental gamete See *noncrossover gamete*.

parthenogenesis Development of an egg without fertilization.

partial diploids See *merozygote*.

partial dominance See *incomplete dominance*.

patroclinous inheritance A form of genetic transmission in which the offspring have the phenotype of the father.

pedigree   In human genetics, a diagram showing the ancestral relationships and transmission of genetic traits over several generations in a family.

P element   In *Drosophila*, a transposable DNA element responsible for hybrid dysgenesis.

penetrance   The frequency, expressed as a percentage, with which individuals of a given genotype manifest at least some degree of a specific mutant phenotype associated with a trait.

peptide bond   The covalent bond between the amino group of one amino acid and the carboxyl group of another amino acid.

pericentric inversion   A chromosomal inversion that involves both arms of the chromosome and thus the centromere.

Personal Genome Project   A project to enroll 100,000 individuals to share their genome sequence, personal information, and medical history with researchers and the general public to increase understanding of the contribution of genetic and environmental factors to genetic traits.

phage   See *bacteriophage*.

pharmacogenomics   The study of how genetic variation influences the action of pharmaceutical drugs in individuals.

PharmGKB database   A repository for genetic, molecular, cellular, and genomic information about individuals who have participated in clinical pharmacogenomic research studies. It is designed to assist researchers in studying how genetic variation among individuals contributes to differences in drug reactions among members of a population.

phenotype   The overt appearance of a genetically controlled trait.

phenylketonuria (PKU)   A hereditary condition in humans associated with the inability to metabolize the amino acid phenylalanine due to the loss of activity of the enzyme phenylalanine hydroxylase.

Philadelphia chromosome   The product of a reciprocal translocation in humans that contains the short arm of chromosome 9, carrying the *C-ABL* oncogene, and the long arm of chromosome 22, carrying the *BCR* gene.

phosphodiester bond   In nucleic acids, covalent bonds by which a phosphate group links adjacent nucleotides, extending from the 5′ carbon of one pentose sugar (ribose or deoxyribose) to the 3′ carbon of the pentose sugar in the neighboring nucleotide. Phosphodiester bonds create the backbone of nucleic acid molecules.

photoreactivation enzyme (PRE)   An exonuclease that catalyzes the light-activated excision of ultraviolet-induced thymine dimers from DNA.

photoreactivation repair   Light-induced repair of damage caused by exposure to ultraviolet light. Associated with an intracellular enzyme system.

phyletic evolution   The gradual transformation of one species into another over time; so-called vertical evolution.

pilus   A filamentlike projection from the surface of a bacterial cell. Often associated with cells possessing F factors.

piRNAs (Piwi-interacting RNAs)   Short dsRNA sequences processed by a Dicer-independent mechanism and associated with PIWI proteins. Participate in transcriptional, posttranscriptional, and epigenetic mechanisms to silence transposons and repetitive sequences in germ cells.

plaque   On an otherwise opaque bacterial lawn, a clear area caused by the growth and reproduction of a single bacteriophage.

plasmid   An extrachromosomal, circular DNA molecule that replicates independently of the host chromosome.

pleiotropy   Condition in which a single mutation causes multiple phenotypic effects.

ploidy   A term referring to the basic chromosome set or to multiples of that set.

pluripotent   See *totipotent*.

point mutation   A mutation that can be mapped to a single locus. At the molecular level, a mutation that results in the substitution of one nucleotide for another. Also called a *gene mutation*.

polar body   Produced in females at the first and second meiotic division of gametogenesis, a discarded cell that contains one of the nuclei of the division process, but almost no cytoplasm as a result of an unequal cytokinesis.

polycistronic mRNA   A messenger RNA molecule that encodes the amino acid sequence of two or more polypeptide chains in adjacent structural genes.

polygenic inheritance   The transmission of a phenotypic trait whose expression depends on the additive effect of a number of genes.

polylinker   A segment of DNA engineered to contain multiple sites for restriction enzyme digestion. Polylinkers are usually found in engineered vectors such as plasmids.

polymerase chain reaction (PCR)   A method for amplifying DNA segments that depends on repeated cycles of denaturation, primer annealing, and DNA polymerase–directed DNA synthesis.

polymerases   Enzymes that catalyze the formation of DNA and RNA from deoxynucleotides and ribonucleotides, respectively.

polymorphism   The existence of two or more discontinuous, segregating phenotypes in a population.

polynucleotide   A linear sequence of 20 or more nucleotides, joined by 5′-3′ phosphodiester bonds. See also *oligonucleotide*.

polypeptide   A molecule composed of amino acids linked together by covalent peptide bonds. This term is used to denote the amino acid chain before it assumes its functional three dimensional configuration and is called a protein.

polyploid   A cell or individual having more than two haploid sets of chromosomes.

polyribosome   See *polysome*.

polysome   A structure composed of two or more ribosomes associated with an mRNA engaged in translation. Also called a *polyribosome*.

polytene chromosome   Literally, a many-stranded chromosome; one that has undergone numerous rounds of DNA replication without separation of the replicated strands, which remain in exact parallel register. The result is a giant chromosome with aligned chromomeres displaying a characteristic banding pattern, often studied in *Drosophila* larval salivary gland cells.

population   A local group of actually or potentially interbreeding individuals belonging to the same species.

population bottleneck   A drastic reduction in population size and consequent loss of genetic diversity, followed by an increase in population size. The rebuilt population has a gene pool with reduced diversity caused by genetic drift.

positional cloning   The identification and subsequent cloning of a gene without knowledge of its polypeptide product or function. The process uses cosegregation of mutant phenotypes with DNA markers to identify the chromosome containing the gene; the position of the gene is identified by establishing linkage with additional markers.

position effect   Change in expression of a gene associated with a change in the gene's location within the genome.

posttranscriptional modification   Changes made to pre-mRNA molecules during conversion to mature mRNA. These include the addition of a methylated cap at the 5′ end and a poly-A tail at the 3′ end, excision of introns, and exon splicing.

posttranslational modification The processing or modification of the translated polypeptide chain by enzymatic cleavage, addition of phosphate groups, carbohydrate chains, or lipids.

postzygotic isolation mechanism A factor that prevents or reduces inbreeding by acting after fertilization to produce nonviable, sterile hybrids or hybrids of lowered fitness.

preadaptive mutation A mutational event that later becomes of adaptive significance.

preformationism See *epigenesis*.

preimplantation genetic diagnosis (PGD) The removal and genetic analysis of unfertilized oocytes, polar bodies, or single cells from an early embryo (3–5 days old).

prezygotic isolation mechanism A factor that reduces inbreeding by preventing courtship, mating, or fertilization.

Pribnow box In prokaryotic genes, a 6-bp sequence to which the sigma (σ) subunit of RNA polymerase binds, upstream from the beginning of transcription. The consensus sequence for this box is TATAAT.

primary miRNAs (pri-miRNAs) Transcriptional product of a microRNA gene containing a 5′ methylated cap, a 3′ polyadenylated tail, and a hairpin structure derived from self-complementary sequences.

primary protein structure The sequence of amino acids in a polypeptide chain.

primary sex ratio Ratio of males to females at fertilization, often expressed in decimal form (e.g., 1.06).

primer In nucleic acids, a short length of RNA or single-stranded DNA required for initiating synthesis directed by polymerases.

primordial germ cells (PCGs) Precursor cells in the early embryo that migrate into gonads and develop to form gametes.

prion An infectious pathogenic agent devoid of nucleic acid and composed of a protein, PrP, with a molecular weight of 27,000–30,000 Da. Prions are known to cause scrapie, a degenerative neurological disease in sheep; bovine spongiform encephalopathy (BSE, or mad cow disease) in cattle; and similar diseases in humans, including kuru and Creutzfeldt–Jakob disease.

probability A way of expressing the mathematical likelihood that a particular event will occur or has occurred.

proband An individual who is the focus of a genetic study leading to the construction of a pedigree tracking the inheritance of a genetically determined trait of interest. Formerly known as a *propositus*.

probe A macromolecule such as DNA or RNA that has been labeled and can be detected by an assay such as autoradiography or fluorescence microscopy. Probes are used to identify target molecules, genes, or gene products.

processivity The ability of an enzyme to carry out consecutive reactions before dissociating from its substrate. In the case of DNA polymerase III, processivity is the number of nucleotides added to a template strand before the enzyme falls off the template.

product law In statistics, the law holding that the probability of two independent events occurring simultaneously is equal to the product of their independent probabilities.

progeny The offspring produced from a mating.

prokaryotes Organisms lacking nuclear membranes and true chromosomes. Bacteria and blue–green algae are examples of prokaryotic organisms.

promoter element An upstream regulatory region of a gene to which RNA polymerase binds prior to the initiation of transcription.

proofreading A molecular mechanism for scanning and correcting errors in replication, transcription, or translation.

prophage A bacteriophage genome integrated into a bacterial chromosome that is replicated along with the bacterial chromosome. Bacterial cells carrying prophages are said to be *lysogenic* and to be capable of entering the *lytic cycle*, whereby phage particles are produced.

propositus (female, proposita) See *proband*.

protein A molecule composed of one or more polypeptides, each composed of amino acids covalently linked together. Proteins demonstrate *primary*, *secondary*, *tertiary*, and often, *quaternary structure*.

protein domain Amino acid sequences with specific conformations and functions that are structurally and functionally distinct from other regions of the same protein.

proteome The entire set of proteins expressed by a cell, tissue, or organism at a given time.

proteomics The study of the expressed proteins present in a cell at a given time.

proto-oncogene A gene that functions to initiate, facilitate, or maintain cell growth and division. Proto-oncogenes can be converted to *oncogenes* by mutation.

protoplast A bacterial or plant cell with the cell wall removed. Sometimes called a *spheroplast*.

prototroph A strain (usually of a microorganism) that is capable of growth on a defined, minimal medium. Wild-type strains are usually regarded as prototrophs and contrasted with *auxotrophs*.

pseudoalleles Genes that behave as alleles to one another by complementation but can be separated from one another by recombination.

pseudoautosomal region A region on the human Y chromosome that is also represented on the X chromosome. Genes found in this region of the Y chromosome have a pattern of inheritance that is indistinguishable from genes on autosomes.

pseudodominance The expression of a recessive allele on one homolog owing to the deletion of the dominant allele on the other homolog.

pseudogene A nonfunctional gene with sequence homology to a known structural gene present elsewhere in the genome. It differs from the functional version by insertions or deletions and by the presence of flanking direct-repeat sequences of 10–20 nucleotides.

puff See *chromosome puff*.

punctuated equilibrium A pattern in the fossil record of long periods of species stability, punctuated with brief periods of species divergence.

pyrosequencing A high-throughput method of DNA sequencing that determines the sequence of a single-stranded DNA molecule by synthesis of a complementary strand. During synthesis, the sequence is determined by the chemiluminescent detection of pyrophosphate release that accompanies nucleotide incorporation into a newly synthesized strand of DNA.

quantitative inheritance See *polygenic inheritance*.

quantitative real-time PCR (qPCR) A variation of PCR (polymerase chain reaction) that uses fluorescent probes to quantitate the amount of DNA or RNA product present after each round of amplification.

quantitative trait loci (QTLs) Two or more genes that act on a single polygenic trait in a quantitative way.

quantum speciation Formation of a new species within a single or a few generations by a combination of selection and drift.

quaternary protein structure Types and modes of interaction between two or more polypeptide chains within a protein molecule.

quorum sensing A mechanism used to regulate gene expression in response to changes in cellular population density.

race A genotypically or geographically distinct subgroup within a species.

rad A unit of absorbed dose of radiation with an energy equal to 100 ergs per gram of irradiated tissue.

radioactive isotope An unstable isotope with an altered number of neutrons that emits ionizing radiation during decay as it is transformed to a stable atomic configuration. See also *isotopes*.

random amplified polymorphic DNA (RAPD) A PCR method that uses random primers about 10 nucleotides in length to amplify unknown DNA sequences.

random mating Mating between individuals without regard to genotype.

reactive oxygen species (ROS) Ions or molecules formed by incomplete reduction of oxygen. They include hydroxyl radicals, superoxides, and peroxides. ROS cause oxidative damage to DNA and other macromolecules.

reading frame A linear sequence of codons in a nucleic acid.

reannealing Formation of double-stranded DNA molecules from denatured single strands.

recessive An allele whose potential phenotypic expression is overridden in the heterozygous condition by a dominant allele.

reciprocal cross A pair of crosses in which the genotype of the female in one is present as the genotype of the male in the other, and vice versa.

reciprocal translocation A chromosomal aberration in which nonhomologous chromosomes exchange parts.

recombinant DNA technology A collection of methods used to create DNA molecules by *in vitro* ligation of DNA from two different organisms, and the replication and recovery of such recombinant DNA molecules.

recombinant gamete A gamete containing a new combination of alleles produced by crossing over during meiosis.

recombination The process that leads to the formation of new allele combinations on chromosomes.

recon A term utilized in fine structure analysis studies to denote the smallest intragenic units between which recombination can occur. Corresponds to a single base.

reductional division The chromosome division that halves the number of centromeres and thus reduces the chromosome number by half. The first division of meiosis is a reductional division, producing haploid cells. See also *equational division*.

redundant genes Gene sequences present in more than one copy per haploid genome (e.g., ribosomal genes).

regulatory site A DNA sequence that functions in the control of expression of other genes, usually by interaction with another molecule.

rem Radiation equivalent in humans; the dosage of radiation that will cause the same biological effect as one roentgen of X rays.

renaturation The process by which a denatured protein or nucleic acid returns to its normal three-dimensional structure.

repetitive DNA sequence A DNA sequence present in many copies in the haploid genome.

replicating form (RF) Double-stranded nucleic acid molecules present as an intermediate during the reproduction of certain RNA-containing viruses.

replication The process whereby DNA is duplicated.

replication fork The Y-shaped region of a chromosome at the site of DNA replication.

replicon The unit of DNA replication, beginning with DNA sequences necessary for the initiation of DNA replication. In bacteria, the entire chromosome is a replicon.

replisome The complex of proteins, including DNA polymerase, that assembles at the bacterial replication fork to synthesize DNA.

repressible enzyme system An enzyme or group of enzymes whose synthesis is regulated by the intracellular concentration of certain metabolites.

repressor A protein that binds to a regulatory sequence adjacent to a gene and blocks transcription of the gene.

reproductive isolation Absence of interbreeding between populations, subspecies, or species. Reproductive isolation can be brought about by extrinsic factors, such as behavior, or intrinsic barriers, such as hybrid inviability.

rescue experiment An experimental approach that involves transferring a gene or protein to cells of an organism to restore a particular phenotype or function. Often used in experiments when a gene has been mutated. Investigators add back the relevant gene to try and rescue the phenotype and thus provide functional evidence for the gene being studied.

resistance transfer factor (RTF) A component of R plasmids that confers the ability to transfer the R plasmid between bacterial cells by conjugation.

restriction endonuclease A bacterial nuclease that recognizes specific nucleotide sequences in a DNA molecule, often a *palindrome*, and cleaves or nicks the DNA at those sites. It provides bacteria with a defense against invading viral DNA and is widely used in the construction of *recombinant DNA molecules*.

restriction fragment length polymorphism (RFLP) Variation in the length of DNA fragments generated by restriction endonucleases. These variations are caused by mutations that create or abolish cutting sites for restriction enzymes. RFLPs are inherited in a codominant fashion and are extremely useful as genetic markers.

restriction site A DNA sequence, often palindromic, recognized by a restriction endonuclease. The enzyme binds to and cleaves DNA at the restriction site.

restrictive transduction See *specialized transduction*.

retrotransposon Mobile genetic elements that are major components of many eukaryotic genomes, which are copied by means of an RNA intermediate and inserted at a distant chromosomal site.

retroviral vectors Gene delivery vectors derived from retroviruses. Often used in gene therapy.

retrovirus A type of virus that uses RNA as its genetic material and employs the enzyme reverse transcriptase during its life cycle.

reverse genetics An experimental approach used to discover gene function after the gene has been identified, isolated, cloned, and sequenced. The cloned gene may be knocked out (e.g., by *gene targeting*) or have its expression altered (e.g., by *RNA interference* or *transgenic overexpression*) and the resulting phenotype studied. An approach contrasted with *forward genetics*.

reverse transcriptase A polymerase that uses RNA as a template to transcribe a single-stranded DNA molecule as a product.

reversion A mutation that restores the wild-type phenotype.

R factor (R plasmid) A bacterial plasmid that carries antibiotic resistance genes. Most R plasmids have two components: an r-determinant which carries the antibiotic resistance genes and the resistance transfer factor (RTF).

RFLP See *restriction fragment length polymorphism*.

Rh factor   An antigenic system first described in the rhesus monkey. Recessive *r/r* individuals produce no Rh antigens and are Rh negative, while *R/R* and *R/r* individuals have Rh antigens on the surface of their red blood cells and are classified as Rh positive. This is the genetic basis of the immunological incompatibility disease called erythroblastosis fetalis (hemolytic disease of the newborn).

ribonucleic acid (RNA)   A nucleic acid similar to DNA but characterized by the pentose sugar ribose, the pyrimidine uracil, and the single-stranded nature of the polynucleotide chain. Several forms are recognized, including ribosomal RNA, messenger RNA, transfer RNA, and a variety of small regulatory RNA molecules.

ribonucleoprotein (RNP) particles   A collection of small, stable RNA molecules complexed with one or more proteins. RNPs are found in the nucleus, cytoplasm, and mitochondria; they have a variety of functions, including RNA splicing, transport, posttranscriptional regulation of mRNA, and protein export.

ribose   The five-carbon sugar associated with ribonucleosides and ribonucleotides associated with RNA.

ribosomal RNA (rRNA)   The RNA molecules that are the structural components of the ribosomal subunits. In prokaryotes, these are the 16*S*, 23*S*, and 5*S* molecules; in eukaryotes, they are the 18*S*, 28*S*, and 5*S* molecules. See also *Svedberg coefficient (S)*.

ribosome   A ribonucleoprotein organelle consisting of two subunits, each containing RNA and protein molecules. Ribosomes are the site of translation of mRNA codons into the amino acid sequence of a polypeptide chain.

riboswitch   An RNA-based intracellular sensor that binds to a small ligand, such as a metabolite, modulating control of gene expression.

ribozymes   RNAs that catalyze specific biochemical reactions.

RNA   See *ribonucleic acid*.

RNA editing   Alteration of the nucleotide sequence of an mRNA molecule after transcription and before translation. There are two main types of editing: substitution editing, which changes individual nucleotides, and insertion/deletion editing, in which individual nucleotides are added or deleted.

RNA interference (RNAi)   Inhibition of gene expression in which a protein complex (RNA-induced silencing complex, or RISC) containing a partially complementary RNA strand binds to an mRNA, leading to degradation or reduced translation of the mRNA.

RNA polymerase   An enzyme that catalyzes the formation of an RNA polynucleotide strand using the base sequence of a DNA molecule as a template.

RNA World Hypothesis   A hypothesis describing life based on RNA acting in informational (genomes) and catalytic (ribozymes) roles that predates current life forms that utilize DNA genomes and protein catalysts.

RNA-binding proteins (RBPs)   Proteins that bind to RNAs and have various activities such as influencing RNA translation, splicing, stability, localization, and degradation.

RNA-directed RNA polymerase (RdRP)   An enzyme that directs the synthesis of a complementary RNA strand from an RNA template.

RNA-induced gene silencing   A mechanism by which small noncoding RNAs and the RNA-induced silencing complex (RISC) negatively regulate transcription or the translation of mRNA transcripts.

RNA-induced silencing complex (RISC)   A protein complex containing an Argonaute family protein with endonuclease activity. siRNAs and miRNAs guide RISC to complementary mRNAs to cleave them.

RNA-induced transcriptional silencing (RITS)   A mechanism by which small noncoding RNAs direct a protein complex (containing an Argonaute family protein and a histone methyltransferase) to bind to complementary DNA sequences where nearby histones are methylated, silencing transcription at this locus.

RNase   A class of enzymes that hydrolyzes RNA.

Robertsonian translocation   A chromosomal aberration created by breaks in the short arms of two acrocentric chromosomes followed by fusion of the long arms of these chromosomes at the centromere. Also called *centric fusion*.

roentgen (R)   A unit of measure of radiation emission, corresponding to the amount that generates 2.083×10^9 ion pairs in one cubic centimeter of air at 0°C and an atmospheric pressure of 760 mm of mercury.

rolling circle model   A model of DNA replication in which the growing point, or replication fork, rolls around a circular template strand; in each pass around the circle, the newly synthesized strand displaces the strand from the previous replication, producing a series of contiguous copies of the template strand.

rRNA   See *ribosomal RNA*.

RTF   See *resistance transfer factor*.

S_1 nuclease   A deoxyribonuclease that cuts and degrades single-stranded molecules of DNA.

Sanger sequencing   DNA sequencing by synthesis of DNA chains that are randomly terminated by incorporation of a nucleotide analog (dideoxynucleotides) followed by sequence determination by analysis of resulting fragment lengths in each reaction.

satellite DNA   DNA that forms a minor band when genomic DNA is centrifuged in a cesium salt gradient. This DNA usually consists of short sequences repeated many times in the genome.

SCE   See *sister chromatid exchange*.

secondary protein structure   The α-helical or β-pleated-sheet formations in a polypeptide, dependent on hydrogen bonding between certain amino acids.

secondary sex ratio   The ratio of males to females at birth, usually expressed in decimal form (e.g., 1.05).

secretor   An individual who secretes soluble forms of the blood group antigens A and/or B in saliva and other body fluids. This condition is caused by a dominant autosomal gene independent of the *ABO* locus.

sedimentation coefficient (S)   See *Svedberg coefficient unit*.

segment polarity genes   Genes that regulate the spatial pattern of differentiation within each segment of the developing *Drosophila* embryo.

segregation   The separation of maternal and paternal homologs of each homologous chromosome pair into gametes during meiosis.

selection   The changes that occur in the frequency of alleles and genotypes in populations as a result of differential reproduction.

selection coefficient (s)   A quantitative measure of the relative fitness of one genotype compared with another. See *coefficient of selection*.

selfing   In plant genetics, the fertilization of a plant's ovules by pollen produced by the same plant. Reproduction by self-fertilization.

semiconservative replication   A mode of DNA replication in which a double-stranded molecule replicates in such a way that the daughter molecules are each composed of one parental (old) and one newly synthesized strand.

semisterility   A condition in which a percentage of all zygotes are inviable.

severe combined immunodeficiency (SCID) A collection of genetic disorders characterized by a lack of immune system response; both cell-mediated and antibody-mediated responses are missing.

sex chromatin body See *Barr body.*

sex chromosome A chromosome, such as the X or Y in humans, which is involved in sex determination.

sexduction Transmission of chromosomal genes from a donor bacterium to a recipient cell by means of the F factor.

sex-influenced inheritance Phenotypic expression conditioned by the sex of the individual. A heterozygote may express one phenotype in one sex and an alternate phenotype in the other sex (e.g., pattern baldness in humans).

sex-limited inheritance A trait that is expressed in only one sex even though the trait may not be X-linked or Y-linked.

sex ratio See *primary sex ratio; secondary sex ratio.*

sexual reproduction Reproduction through the fusion of gametes, which are the haploid products of meiosis.

Shine–Dalgarno sequence The nucleotides AGGAGG that serve as a ribosome-binding site in the leader sequence of prokaryotic genes. The 16S RNA of the small ribosomal subunit contains a complementary sequence to which the mRNA binds.

short interspersed elements (SINEs) Repetitive sequences found in the genomes of higher organisms. The 300-bp *Alu* sequence is a SINE element.

short tandem repeats See *STR sequences.*

shotgun cloning The cloning of random fragments of genomic DNA into a vector (a plasmid or phage), usually to produce a library from which clones of specific interest can be selected for use, as in sequencing.

shugoshins A class of proteins involved in maintaining cohesion of the centromeres of sister chromatids during mitosis and meiosis.

sibling species Species that are morphologically similar but reproductively isolated from one another.

sickle-cell anemia A human genetic disorder caused by an autosomal recessive allele, often fatal in the homozygous condition if untreated. Caused by a nucleotide substitution that alters one amino acid in the β chain of globin.

sickle-cell trait The phenotype exhibited by individuals heterozygous for the sickle-cell allele.

sigma (σ) factor In RNA polymerase, a polypeptide subunit that recognizes the DNA binding site for the initiation of transcription.

signal transduction An intercellular or intracellular molecular pathway by which an external signal is converted into a functional biological response.

single molecule sequencing A high-throughput sequencing by synthesis involving direct sequencing of single DNA or RNA molecules without the need for amplification by PCR before sequencing.

single-nucleotide polymorphism (SNP) A variation in one nucleotide pair in DNA, as detected during genomic analysis. Present in at least 1 percent of a population, a SNP is useful as a genetic marker.

single-stranded binding proteins (SSBs) In DNA replication, proteins that bind to and stabilize the single-stranded regions of DNA that result from the action of unwinding proteins.

siRNAs Small (or short) interfering RNAs. Short 20–25 nucleotide double-stranded RNA sequences with two 3′ overhanging nucleotides; processed by Dicer and participate in transcriptional and/or posttranscriptional mechanisms of gene regulation.

sister chromatid exchange (SCE) A crossing over event in meiotic or mitotic cells involving the reciprocal exchange of chromosomal material between sister chromatids joined by a common centromere. Such exchanges can be detected cytologically after BrdU incorporation into the replicating chromosomes.

site-directed mutagenesis A process that uses a synthetic oligonucleotide containing a mutant base or sequence as a primer for inducing a mutation at a specific site in a cloned gene.

sliding clamp loader A component of the DNA polymerase III holoenzyme consisting of five subunits that attach a circular protein complex to the polymerase in an ATP-dependent reaction.

sliding DNA clamp A component of the DNA polymerase III holoenzyme composed of multiple copies of the beta subunit that forms a circular structure attached to the polymerase, which promotes processivity

small noncoding RNAs (sncRNAs) Any of a number of short RNAs that are noncoding transcripts that associate with the RNA-induced silencing complex (RISC) to regulate transcription or to regulate mRNAs posttranscriptionally.

small nuclear RNA (snRNA) Abundant species of small RNA molecules ranging in size from 90 to 400 nucleotides that in association with proteins form RNP particles known as snRNPs or *snurps*. Located in the nucleoplasm, snRNAs have been implicated in the processing of pre-mRNA and may have a range of cleavage and ligation functions.

SNP See *single-nucleotide polymorphism.*

snurps See *small nuclear RNA.*

solenoid structure A feature of eukaryotic chromatin conformation generated by nucleosome supercoiling.

somatic cell genetics The use of cultured somatic cells to investigate genetic phenomena by means of parasexual techniques involving the fusion of cells from different organisms.

somatic cells All cells other than the germ cells or gametes in an organism.

somatic gene therapy Gene therapy involving somatic cells as targets for gene transfer.

somatic mutation A nonheritable mutation occurring in a somatic cell.

somatic pairing The pairing of homologous chromosomes in somatic cells.

SOS response The induction of enzymes for repairing damaged DNA in *Escherichia coli.* The response involves activation of an enzyme that cleaves a repressor, activating a series of genes involved in DNA repair.

Southern blotting Developed by Edwin Southern, a technique in which DNA fragments produced by restriction enzyme digestion are separated by electrophoresis and transferred by capillary action to a nylon or nitrocellulose membrane. Specific DNA fragments can be identified by hybridization to a complementary radioactively labeled nucleic acid probe using the technique of *autoradiography.*

spacer DNA DNA sequences found between genes. Usually, these are repetitive DNA segments.

specialized transduction Genetic transfer of specific host genes by transducing phages. See also *generalized transduction.*

speciation The process by which new species of plants and animals arise.

species A group of actually or potentially interbreeding individuals that is reproductively isolated from other such groups.

spectral karyotype A display of all the chromosomes in an organism as a karyotype with each chromosome stained in a different color.

spheroplast See *protoplast*.

spindle fibers Cytoplasmic fibrils formed during cell division that attach to and are involved with separation of chromatids at the anaphase stage of mitosis and meiosis as well as their movement toward opposite poles in the cell.

spliceosome The nuclear macromolecule complex within which splicing reactions occur to remove introns from pre-mRNAs.

spontaneous mutation A mutation that is not induced by a mutagenic agent.

spore A unicellular body or cell encased in a protective coat. Produced by some bacteria, plants, and invertebrates, spores are capable of surviving in unfavorable environmental conditions and give rise to a new individual upon germination. In plants, spores are the haploid products of meiosis.

Src A protein kinase that phosphorylates many target proteins to regulate their activity, for example, regulating the activity of the RNA-binding protein ZBP1.

sRNA Small noncoding RNA in prokaryotes that regulates gene expression by binding to mRNAs to influence translation or by binding to proteins and modifying their function.

SRY The sex-determining region of the Y chromosome, found near the chromosome's pseudoautosomal boundary. Accumulated evidence indicates that a gene in this region encodes the testis-determining factor (TDF).

stabilizing selection Preferential reproduction of individuals with genotypes close to the mean for the population. A selective elimination of genotypes at both extremes.

standard deviation (SD) A quantitative measure of the amount of variation present in a sample of measurements from a population calculated as the square root of the variance.

standard error (SE) A quantitative measure of the amount of variation around the mean in a sample of measurements from a population.

strain A group of organisms with common ancestry having physiological or morphological characteristics of interest for genetic analysis or domestication.

STR sequences Short tandem repeats 2–9 base pairs long found within minisatellites. These sequences are used to prepare DNA profiles in forensics, paternity identification, and other applications.

structural gene A gene that encodes the amino acid sequence of a polypeptide chain.

sublethal gene A mutation causing lowered viability, with death before maturity in less than 50 percent of the individuals carrying the gene.

submetacentric chromosome A chromosome with the centromere placed so that one arm of the chromosome is slightly longer than the other.

subspecies A morphologically or geographically distinct interbreeding population of a species.

sum law The law that holds that the probability of one of two mutually exclusive outcomes occurring, where that outcome can be achieved by two or more events, is equal to the sum of their individual probabilities.

supercoiled DNA A DNA configuration in which the helix is coiled upon itself. Supercoils can exist in stable forms only when the ends of the DNA are not free, as in a covalently closed circular DNA molecule.

superfemale See *metafemale*.

supermale See *metamale*.

suppressor mutation A mutation that acts to completely or partially restore the function lost by a mutation at another site.

Svedberg coefficient unit (S) A unit of measure for the rate at which particles (molecules) sediment in a centrifugal field. This rate is a function of several physicochemical properties, including size and shape. A rate of 1×10^{-13} sec is defined as one Svedberg coefficient unit.

symbiont An organism coexisting in a mutually beneficial relationship with another organism.

sympatric speciation Speciation occurring in populations that inhabit, at least in part, the same geographic range.

synapsis The pairing of homologous chromosomes at meiosis.

synaptonemal complex (SC) A sub-microscopic structure consisting of a tripartite nucleoprotein ribbon that forms between the paired homologous chromosomes in the pachytene stage of the first meiotic division.

syndrome A group of characteristics or symptoms associated with a disease or an abnormality. An affected individual may express a number of these characteristics but not necessarily all of them.

synkaryon The fusion of two gametic or somatic nuclei. Also, in somatic cell genetics, the product of nuclear fusion.

syntenic test In somatic cell genetics, a method for determining whether two genes are on the same chromosome.

synthetic biology A scientific discipline that combines science and engineering to research the complexity of living systems and to construct biological-based systems that do not exist in nature.

synthetic genome A genome assembled from chemically synthesized DNA fragments that is transferred to a host cell without a genome.

systems biology A scientific discipline that identifies and analyzes gene and protein networks to gain an understanding of intracellular regulation of metabolism, intra- and intercellular communication, and complex interactions within, between, and among cells.

TATA box See *Goldberg–Hogness box*.

tautomeric shift A reversible isomerization in a molecule, brought about by a shift in the location of a hydrogen atom. In nucleic acids, tautomeric shifts in the bases of nucleotides can cause changes in other bases at replication and are a source of mutations.

TDF (testis-determining factor) The product of the *SRY* gene on the Y chromosome; it controls the switch point for the development of the indifferent gonad into a testis.

telocentric chromosome A chromosome in which the centromere is located at its very end.

telomerase The enzyme that adds short, tandemly repeated DNA sequences to the ends of eukaryotic chromosomes.

telomere repeat-containing RNA (TERRA) Large noncoding RNA molecules transcribed from telomere repeats that are an integral part of telomeric heterochromatin.

telomere The heterochromatic terminal region of a chromosome.

telophase The stage of cell division in which the daughter chromosomes have reached the opposite poles of the cell and reverse the stages characteristic of prophase, re-forming the nuclear envelopes and uncoiling the chromosomes. Telophase ends during cytokinesis, which divides the cytoplasm and splits the parental cell into two daughter cells.

telophase I The stage in the first meiotic division when duplicated chromosomes reach the poles of the dividing cell.

temperate phage A bacteriophage that can become a prophage, integrating its DNA into the chromosome of the host bacterial cell and making the latter lysogenic.

temperature-sensitive mutation A conditional mutation that produces a mutant phenotype at one temperature and a wild-type phenotype at another.

template The single-stranded DNA or RNA molecule that specifies the sequence of a complementary nucleotide strand synthesized by DNA or RNA polymerase.

terminalization The movement of chiasmata toward the ends of chromosomes during the diplotene stage of the first meiotic division.

tertiary protein structure The three-dimensional conformation of a polypeptide chain in space, specified by the polypeptide's *primary structure*. The tertiary structure achieves a state of maximum thermodynamic stability.

testcross A cross between an individual whose genotype at one or more loci may be unknown and an individual who is homozygous recessive for the gene or genes in question.

tetrad The four chromatids that make up paired homologs in the prophase of the first meiotic division. In eukaryotes with a predominant haploid stage (some algae and fungi), a tetrad denotes the four haploid cells produced by a single meiotic division.

tetrad analysis A method that analyzes gene linkage and recombination in organisms with a predominant haploid phase in their life cycle. See also *tetrad*.

tetranucleotide hypothesis An early theory of DNA structure proposing that the molecule was composed of repeating units, each consisting of the four nucleotides represented by adenine, thymine, cytosine, and guanine.

theta (θ) structure An intermediate configuration in the bidirectional replication of circular DNA molecules. At about midway through the cycle of replication, the intermediate resembles the Greek letter theta.

third-generation sequencing (TGS) DNA sequencing technologies based largely on methods for sequencing individual molecules of single-stranded DNA.

thymine dimer In a polynucleotide strand, a lesion consisting of two adjacent thymine bases that become joined by a covalent bond. Usually caused by exposure to ultraviolet light, this lesion inhibits DNA replication.

Ti plasmid A bacterial plasmid used as a vector to transfer foreign DNA to plant cells.

T_m See *melting profile*.

topoisomerase A class of enzymes that converts DNA from one topological form to another. During replication, a topoisomerase, *DNA gyrase*, facilitates DNA replication by reducing molecular tension caused by supercoiling upstream from the *replication fork*.

totipotent The capacity of a cell or an embryo part to differentiate into all cell types characteristic of an adult. This capacity is usually progressively restricted during development. Used interchangeably with *pluripotent*.

trait Any detectable phenotypic variation of a particular inherited character.

***trans*-acting element** A gene product (usually a diffusible protein or an RNA molecule) that acts to regulate the expression of a target gene.

***trans* configuration** An arrangement in which two mutant alleles are on opposite homologs, such as

$$\frac{a^1 \quad +}{+ \quad a^2}$$

in contrast to a *cis arrangement*, in which the alleles are located on the same homolog.

transcription Transfer of genetic information from DNA by the synthesis of a complementary RNA molecule using one strand of the DNA as a template.

transcription activator-like effector nucleases (TALENs) Artificial DNA cleaving enzymes created by combining DNA-binding motifs (transcription activator-like effectors or TALEs) from plant pathogenic bacteria to a DNA-cutting domain from a nuclease. This method can produce restriction enzymes for any DNA sequence.

transcription factor A DNA-binding protein that binds to specific sequences adjacent to or within the promoter region of a gene; regulates gene transcription.

transcriptome The set of mRNA molecules present in a cell at any given time.

transdetermination Change in developmental fate of a cell or group of cells.

transduction Virally mediated bacterial recombination. Also used to describe the transfer of eukaryotic genes mediated by a retrovirus.

transfer RNA (tRNA) A small ribonucleic acid molecule with an essential role in *translation*. tRNAs contain: (1) a three-base segment (anticodon) that recognizes a codon in mRNA; (2) a binding site for the specific amino acid corresponding to the anticodon; and (3) recognition sites for interaction with ribosomes and with the enzyme that links the tRNA to its specific amino acid.

transformation Heritable change in a cell or an organism brought about by exogenous DNA. Known to occur naturally and also used in *recombinant DNA* studies.

transgenic animals Genetically engineered animals that express or overexpress an inserted gene of interest (a transgene). Sometimes called "knock-in" animals. See also *transgenic organism*.

transgenic organism An organism whose genome has been modified by the introduction of external DNA sequences into the germ line.

transition mutation A mutational event in which one purine is replaced by another or one pyrimidine is replaced by another.

translation The derivation of the amino acid sequence of a polypeptide from the base sequence of an mRNA molecule in association with a ribosome and tRNAs.

translational medicine Also called translational genetics. Refers to moving research discoveries in genetics and other disciplines from the laboratory bench to the bedside to improve human health by disease prevention and the treatment of diseases.

translocation A chromosomal mutation associated with the reciprocal or nonreciprocal transfer of a chromosomal segment from one chromosome to another. Also denotes the movement of mRNA through the ribosome during translation.

transmission genetics The field of genetics concerned with heredity and the mechanisms by which genes are transferred from parent to offspring.

transposable element A DNA segment that moves to other sites in the genome, essentially independent of sequence homology. Usually, such elements are flanked at each end by short inverted repeats of 20–40 base pairs. Insertion into a structural gene can produce a mutant phenotype. Insertion and excision of transposable elements depend on two enzymes, transposase and resolvase. Such elements have been identified in both prokaryotes and eukaryotes.

transversion mutation A mutational event in which a purine is replaced by a pyrimidine or a pyrimidine is replaced by a purine.

trinucleotide repeat A tandemly repeated cluster of three nucleotides (such as CTG) within or near a gene. Certain diseases (myotonic dystrophy, Huntington disease) are caused by expansion in copy number of such repeats.

triploidy The condition in which a cell or an organism possesses three haploid sets of chromosomes.

trisomy The condition in which a cell or an organism possesses two copies of each chromosome except for one, which is present in three copies (designated $2n + 1$).

tRNA See *transfer RNA*.

true single molecule sequencing See *single molecule sequencing*.

tumor-suppressor gene A gene that encodes a product that normally functions to suppress cell division. Mutations in tumor-suppressor genes result in the activation of cell division and tumor formation.

Turner syndrome A genetic condition in human females caused by a 45,X genotype. Such individuals are phenotypically female but are sterile.

unequal crossing over A crossover between two improperly aligned homologs, producing one homolog with three copies of a region and the other with one copy of that region.

unique DNA DNA sequences that are present only once per genome.

universal code A genetic code used by all life forms. Some exceptions are found in mitochondria, ciliates, and mycoplasmas.

unwinding proteins Nuclear proteins that act during DNA replication to destabilize and unwind the DNA helix ahead of the replicating fork.

variable number tandem repeats (VNTRs) Short, repeated DNA sequences (of 2–20 nucleotides) present as tandem repeats between two restriction enzyme sites. Variation in the number of repeats creates DNA fragments of differing lengths following restriction enzyme digestion. Used in early versions of *DNA fingerprinting*.

variable region (V) Portion of an immunoglobulin molecule that exhibits many amino acid sequence differences between antibodies of differing specificities.

variance (s^2) A statistical measure of the variation of values from a central value, calculated as the square of the standard deviation.

variegation Patches of differing phenotypes, such as color, in a tissue.

vector In recombinant DNA, an agent such as a phage or plasmid into which a foreign DNA segment will be inserted and used to transform host cells.

vertical gene transfer The transfer of genetic information from parents to offspring generation after generation.

viability The ability of individuals in a given phenotypic class to survive as compared to another class (usually wild type).

virulence factors Molecules produced by pathogens, such as some viruses and bacteria, that enable them to colonize a host, evade and/or suppress the host's immune system, and cause a disease in the host.

virulent phage A bacteriophage that infects, replicates within, and lyses bacterial cells, releasing new phage particles.

VNTRs See *variable number tandem repeats*.

western blot An analytical technique in which proteins are separated by gel electrophoresis and transferred by capillary action to a nylon membrane or nitrocellulose sheet. A specific protein can be identified through hybridization to a labeled antibody.

whole genome shotgun cloning See *shotgun cloning*.

wild type The most commonly observed phenotype or genotype, designated as the norm or standard.

Wiskott-Aldrich syndrome (WAS) X-linked condition caused by a mutation in the *WASP* gene that encodes a protein that localizes to the cytoskeleton of platelets. WAS produces defective platelets that make patients more vulnerable to infections, frequent bleeding, autoimmune diseases, and cancer.

wobble hypothesis An idea proposed by Francis Crick, stating that the third base in an anticodon can align in several ways to allow it to recognize more than one base in the codons of mRNA.

W, Z chromosomes The sex chromosomes in species where the female is the heterogametic sex (WZ).

X chromosome The sex chromosome present in species where females are the homogametic sex (XX).

X chromosome inactivation In mammalian females, the random transcriptional silencing of the maternally or paternally derived X chromosome. This event, which occurs early in development, is a mechanism of dosage compensation, and all progeny cells inactivate the same X chromosome. See also *Barr body*; *Lyon hypothesis*; *XIST*.

XIST A locus in the X chromosome inactivation center that controls inactivation of the X chromosome in mammalian females.

X-linkage The pattern of inheritance resulting from genes located on the X chromosome.

X-ray crystallography A technique for determining the three-dimensional structure of molecules by analyzing X-ray diffraction patterns produced by bombarding crystals of the molecule under study with X rays.

YAC A cloning vector in the form of a yeast artificial chromosome, constructed using chromosomal components including telomeres (from a ciliate) and centromeres, origin of replication, and marker genes from yeast. YACs are used to clone long stretches of eukaryotic DNA.

Y chromosome The sex chromosome in species where the male is heterogametic (XY).

Y-linkage Mode of inheritance shown by genes located on the Y chromosome.

Z-DNA An alternative "zig-zag" structure of DNA in which the two antiparallel polynucleotide chains form a left-handed double helix. Implicated in regulation of gene expression.

zein Principal storage protein of maize endosperm, consisting of two major proteins with molecular weights of 19,000 and 21,000 Da.

zinc finger A class of DNA-binding domains seen in proteins. They have a characteristic pattern of cysteine and histidine residues that complex with zinc ions, throwing intermediate amino acid residues into a series of loops or fingers.

zinc-finger nucleases (ZFNs) Sequence-specific DNA cleaving enzymes consisting of a zinc-finger motif (a cluster of two cysteine and two histidine residues that bind zinc atoms). ZFNs provide a mechanism for modifying sequences in the genome in a sequence-specific targeted way. See also *zinc finger*.

zip code Sequences found in many mRNAs that serve as binding sites for RNA-binding proteins that influence transcript localization within the cell and translational control.

zip code binding protein 1 (ZBP1) One of a family of highly conserved RNA-binding proteins that play important roles in the localization, stability, and translational control of mRNAs.

zygote The diploid cell produced by the fusion of haploid gametic nuclei.

zygotene A stage of meiotic prophase I in which the homologous chromosomes synapse and pair along their entire length, forming bivalents. The synaptonemal complex forms at this stage.

Credits

PHOTO CREDITS

Cover Dr. Gopal Murti/Science Source

FM FM-1: Jacek Lasa/Alamy

Chapter 1: Introduction to Genetics CO1: Sinclair Stammers/Science Source; CO2: Mark Smith/Science Source; CO3: Alberto Salguero; F1-1: N. Hartsoeker/National Library of Medicine; F1-2: Photo Researchers, Inc./Science Source; F1-3: Biphoto Associates/Photo Researchers, Inc/Science Source; F1-4: Dr. Alexey Khodjakov/Photo Researchers, Inc./Science Source; F1-6-1: Science Source/Photo Researchers, Inc; F1-6-2: Science Source/Photo Researchers, Inc; F1-10: Eye of Science/Photo Researchers, Inc./Science Source; F1-11: Roslin Institute/The Roslin Institute, The University of Edinburgh; F1-13(a): John Paul Endress/Pearson Education Corporate Digital Archive/Pearson Education; F1-13(b): Hermann Eisenbeiss/Photo Researchers, Inc./Science Source; F1-14(a): Jeremy Burgess/Photo Researchers, Inc./Science Source; F1-14(b): David McCarty/Photo Researchers, Inc./Science Source.

Chapter 2: Mitosis and Meiosis CO: Andrew S. Bajer; F2-2: CNRI/SPL/Science Source; F2-4: David Ward; F2-7(a-e): Andrew S. Bajer; F2-7(f.1): Andrew S. Bajer; F2-7(f.2): Andrew S. Bajer; F2-14(a): Biphoto Associates/Science Source; F2-14(b): Andrew Syred/Science Source; F2-14(c): Photo Researchers, Inc./Science Source.

Chapter 3: Mendelian Genetics CO: National Library of Medicine; F3-UN6-1 Elenamiv/Shutterstock; F3-UNF3-7 Jenny Dean/Rex Features; F3-14: Martin Shields/Alamy; F3-UN6-2 PLUS ONE.

Chapter 4: Extensions of Mendelian Genetics CO: Juniors Bildarchiv/Alamy; F4-1(a): John Kaprielian/Photo Researchers; F4-4-1: The Jackson Laboratory; F4-4-2: The Jackson Laboratory; F4-9: RoJo Images/Shutterstock; F4-12-2: Herman Eisenbeiss/Science Source; F4-12-3: Herman Eisenbeiss/Science Source; F4-14(a): Prisma Bildagentur AG/Alamy; F4-15: Hans Reinhard/Photoshot; F4-16: Debra P. Hershkowitz/Photoshot; F4-17-1: Tanya Wolff; F4-17-2: Joel C. Eissenberg/Washington University Press; F4-17-3, F4-18: Tanya Wolff; F4-19(a): Jane Burton/Photoshot; F4-19(b): William S. Klug; F4-UN-2: Ralph Somes; F4-UN-2. J. James Bitgood; F4-UN-4: J. James Bitgood; F4-UN-5(a): Shout It Out Design/Shutterstock; F4-UN-5(b): Zuzule/Shutterstock; F4-UN-5(c): Julia Remezova/Shutterstock.

Chapter 5: Chromosome Mapping in Eukaryotes CO: James Kezer/Stanley Sessions; F5-16: Sheldon Wolff.

Chapter 6: Genetic Analysis and Mapping in Bacteria and Bacteriophages CO: Photo Researchers/Science Source; F6-2: Pearson Education; F6-11-1: Gopal Murti/Photo Researchers/Science Source; F6-13-1: M. Wurtz/Photo Researchers/Science Source; F6-15-2: Christine Case; F6-18: Dr. William S. Klug.

Chapter 7: Sex Determination and Sex Chromosomes CO: Wessex Reg. Genetics Centre/Wellcome Images/Wellcome Institute Library;F7-1-2: Biophoto Associates/Photo Researchers; F7-2-2: Artem Solovev/Fotolia; F7-3(a): Maria Gallegos;F7-5(a,b): Greenwood Genetic Center (GGC); F7-6(a,b): Catherine G.Palmer; F7-8(a,b): Michael Abbey/Photo Researchers/Science Source; F7-10(a): Sari O'Neal/Shutterstock; F7-10(b): William S. Klug; F7-UN-1: AP Images.

Chapter 8: Chromosome Mutations: Variation in Number and Arrangement CO: National Institutes of Health; F8-2: Arco Images GmbH/Alamy; F8-3-1: Greenwood Genetic Center (GGC); F8-3-2: Design Pics/Alamy; F8-5: David D. Weaver/Indiana University; F8-9: National Cotton Council of America; F8-12-1: Douglas B. Chapman; F8-12-2: Cri Du Chat Syndrome Support Group; F8-14: Mary Lilly/Carnegie Institution for Science; F8-18-2: Jorge Yunis; F8-19: Christine J Harrison.

Chapter 9: Extranuclear Inheritance CO: Super-resolution microscopy reveals that mammalian mitochondrial nucleoids have a uniform size and frequently contain a single copy of mtDNA. Kukat C, Wurm CA, Spåhr H, Falkenberg M, Larsson NG, Jakobs S.; Proc Natl Acad Sci U S A. 2011 Aug 16;108(33):13534-99.1b:Ryushi Abura; F9-1-2: Aida Ricciardiello/Shutterstock; F9-2-1: Dartmouth College Electron Microscope Facility; F9-3: Jackelyn Valle; F9-4: Ronald A. Butow; F9-6: David Kolodnar; F9-7: Don W. Fawcett/Science Source/Photo Researchers; F9-9(a,b): Alan Pestronk/Washington University Press; F9-10-2: Koteshwar Rao/Flickr Open/Getty Images; F9-11-1: Kuroda Laboratory; F9-12: Uwe Irion.

Chapter 10: DNA Structure and Analysis CO: Fundamental Photographs; F10-4-2: Science Source/Photo Researchers; F10-11: M. H. F. Wilkins; F10-18: Ventana Medical Systems

Chapter 11: DNA Replication and Recombination CO: Science Source/Photo Researchers; F11-5(a,b): Copyright Clearance Center; F11-14: D. S. Hogness; F11-15: Harold Weintraub; F11-18-1: David Dressler.

Chapter 12: DNA Organization in Chromosomes CO: Don. W. Fawcett/Science Source; F12-1(a): Science Source; F12-1(b): William Klug; F12-2: Biology Pics/Science Source/Photo Researchers; F12-3: Gopal Murti/Science Source/Photo Researchers; F12-5-1: Harald Eggert; F12-5-2: H.EGGBERT,A;GORTCHAKOV,H.SAUM-WEBE; JCS 2004 AUG 15;117(PT18):4253-64/The Company of Biologists, Ltd; F12-6-2: John Ellison; F12-7(a): Science Source/Photo Researchers; F12-7(b): William Klug; F12-8: Oscar L Miller, Jr; F12-11, F12-12: David Adler; F12-16: William S. Klug.

Chapter 13: The Genetic Code and Transcription CO: Science Source/Photo Researchers; F13-11-1: Bert O'Malley; F13-15-1:Copyright Clearance Center

Chapter 14: Translation and Proteins CO: Copyright Clearance Center; 14-9(a): Cold Spring Harbor Laboratory Archives; F14-9(b): E. V. Kiseleva; F14-13: Sebastian Kaulitzki/Shutterstock; F14-19: Science Source/Photo Researchers.

Chapter 15: Gene Mutation, DNA Repair, and Transposition CO: M.G. Neuffer; F15-15: Hadj/Sipa/Newscom; 15-UNF-3(a,b): T.K Starr/Copyright Clearance Center.

Chapter 17: Regulation of Gene Expression in Eukaryotes CO: T. Cremer, I. Solovei, and F. Habermann, Biozentrum(LMU); F17-15(b): Klaus Boller/Science Source.

Chapter 18: Developmental Genetics CO: Edward B. Lewis, California Institute of Technology; F18-1(a): F. Rudolf Turner; F18-1(b): Georg Halder; F18-6: Stephen Paddock; F18-8(a,b): Peter A.

Lawrence; F18-9: Stephen Paddock; F18-10: British Dental Journal/ Macmillan Publishers Ltd; F18-11: Mike J. Owen/Elsevier Science; F18-12(a,b): F. Rudolf Turner/Indiana University – Indiana Memorial Union; F18-16: Custom Medical Stock; F18-17: Elliot M. Meyerowitz; F18-18(a,b): Max-Planck-Institut fur Entwicklungsbiologie; F18-20 (a–d): Elliot M. Meyerowitz; F18-25(a): Darwin Dale/Science Source; F18-25(b): Tanya Wolff/Washington University School of Medicine; F18-26(a): Urs Kloter/Georg Halder; F18-27(a): Walter J. Gehring; F18-UN-02: Nature/12414/Reactivating head regrowth in a regeneration-deficient planarian species/10.1038/S.-Y. Liu, C. Selck, B. Friedrich, R. Lutz, M. Vila-Farré, A. Dahl

Chapter 19: Cancer and Regulation of the Cell Cycle
CO: SPL/Science Source; F19-1(a,b): Hesed M. Padilla-Nash/Antonio Fargiano/National Institute of Health Genetics; F19-2-2: Elizabeth Cook; F19-3ab: Manfred Schwab; F19-8(a): Dr. Gopal Murti/ Science Source.

Chapter 20: Recombinant DNA Techology
CO: Tom Fielder; F20-3: Gopal Murti/Science Source; F20-5(b): Gabridge/ Custom Medical Stock Photo; F20-10: NIH/CMSP/Custom Medical Stock; F20-12(a,b): Proceedings of the National Academy of Sciences; F20-13: American Society for Cell Biology; F20-14: B.D. Olson and G.B. Downes; F20-20(a): Tom Fielder; F20-20(b): Michael A. Palladino; F20-22(a): Eye of Science/Science Source; F20-22(b): Photograph courtesy of Ralph Brinster. University of Pennsylvania School of Veterinary Medicine.

Chapter 21: Genomics, Bioinformatics, and Proteomics
F21-10(a): iStock collections/Getty Images; F21-19(a): Oxford Journals; F21-19(b): Copyright Clearance Center

Chapter 22: Applications and Ethics of Genetic Engineering and Biotechnology
CO: Nature/Synthetic genomes/The next step for the synthetic genome/Monya Baker/Harris Wang; F22-1(a): SIU Biomed Com/Custom Medical Stock Photo; F22-4: GloFish; 22-5(c.1): J. Craig Venter; F22-5(c.2): D.G. Gibson/Copyright Clearance Center; F22-6: Monya Baker/Nature/Synthetic genomes: The next step for the synthetic genome; F22-13: Affymetrix Inc; F22-14(c): National Cancer Institute; F22-15(a,b): Frederik Wilkman; F22-16-2: Cancer Genetics Branch/National Human Genome Research Institute/National Institutes of Health; F22-17(a): Ash Ali Zadeh/Nature Magazine; F22-18-1: Janice Haney Carr/Centers for Disease Control and Prevention; F22-18-2: Affymetrix; F22-19-1: Sebastian Kaulitzki/ Shutterstock; F22-19-2: C.D. Humphrey/T.G. Ksiazek/Centers for Disease Control and Prevention; F22-19-3: Janice Haney Carr/Centers for Disease Control and Prevention; F22-19-4: C.D. Humphrey/ T.G. Ksiazek/Centers for Disease Control and Prevention; F22-19-5: Affymetrix; F22-19-6: Lorence.

Chapter 23: Quantitative Genetics and Multifactorial Traits
CO: 2009fotofriends/Shutterstock; F23-9(a,b): Steven D. Tanksley/Copyright Clearance Center; F23-UN-2: Nature's Image/ Science Source

Chapter 24: Neurogenetics
CO: Daisy Daisy/Shutterstock; F24-10: Developmental Neurobiology/Cellular bases of behavioral plasticity: Establishing and modifying synaptic circuits in theDrosophila genetic system/Jeffrey Rohrbough,Diane K. O'Dowd,Richard A. Baines,Kendal Broadie.

Chapter 25: Population and Evolutionary Genetics
CO: Simon Booth/Science Source; F25-7: Nature Magazine; F25-14(a): Courtesy of Murray Brilliant, "A 122.5 kilobase deletion of P gene underlies the high prevalence of oculocutaneous albinism type 2 in the Navajo population." From: American Journal Human Genetics 72:62–72, Figure 1, 65. Published by University of Chicago Press; F25-14(b): Courtesy of Murray Brilliant, "A 122.5 kilobase deletion

of P gene underlies the high prevalence of oculocutaneous albinism type 2 in the Navajo population." From: American Journal Human Genetics 72: 62–72, Figure 3, p. 67. Published by University of Chicago Press; F25-15: Courtesy of Murray Brilliant, "A 122.5 kilobase deletion of P gene underlies the high prevalence of oculocutaneous albinism type 2 in the Navajo population." From: American Journal Human Genetics 72: 62–72, Figure 3, p. 67. Published by University of Chicago Press; F25-17: Smithsonian Institution (Reproductions); F25-19(a): Niels Poulsen DK/Alamy; F25-19(b): National Ciklid Society.

Special Topics in Modern Genetics, Epigenetics
ST 1-8: Environmental Health Perspectives.

Special Topics in Modern Genetics, Emerging Roles of RNA
ST 2-10-1: Brosnan and Voinnet, 2011 Current Opinions in Plant Biology (Fig 1B) Original experiment: Brosnan et al 2007 PNAS; ST 2-10-2: Brosnan and Voinnet, 2011 Current Opinions in Plant Biology (Fig 1B) Original experiment: Brosnan et al 2007 PNAS; ST 2-11-1: Nature/Cell biology: Silenced RNA on the move/ Ralf Dahm and Michael Kiebler.

Special Topics in Modern Genetics, Genomics and Personalized Medicine
ST 4-2(a,b): Dako Denmark A/S

Special Topics in Modern Genetics, Genetically Modified Foods
ST 5-1: PASCAL PAVANI/AFP/Getty Images; ST 5-3: Isagani Serrano/International Rice Research Institute ; ST 5-6-1: Helios Gene Gun from Biorad Corp; ST 5-8-2: Nature Biotechnology/Improving the nutritional value of Golden Rice through increased pro-vitamin A content/Jacqueline A Paine,Catherine A Shipton,Sunandha Chaggar,Rhian M Howells,Mike J Kennedy et al.; ST 5-9: Bob Hartzle, Department of Agronomy, Iowa State University; ST 5-10: NY Times; ST5-UN-1: AquaBounty Technologies Inc; ST5-UN-2 Science Photo Library; ST5-UN-3: APS/Dennis Gonsalves, Savarni Tripathi, James B. Carr, and Jon Y. Suzuki USDA/ ARS Pacific Basin Agricultural Research.

Special Topics in Modern Genetics, Gene Therapy
ST 6-5(a): Van de Silva; ST 6-6(b): Luk Vandenberghe; ST 6-7-2: Alessandra Biffi/Copyright Clearance Center

TEXT CREDITS

Chapter 1: Introduction to Genetics
Fig 1.01 N. Hartsoeker. Essay de dioptrique Paris. (Washington: National Library of Medicine, 1694), p. 230.

Chapter 5: Chromosome Mapping in Eukaryotes
p 126 Reprinted by permission from Macmillan Publishers Ltd: Nature, "Molecular Structure of Nucleic Acids: A Structure for Deoxyribose Nucleic Acid" by F.H.C. Crick and J.D. Watson, Nature, Vol. 171, No. 4356, pp. 737–38. Copyright ©1953. www.nature.com p 108 Source: A. H. STURTEVANT, A HISTORY OF GENETICS, New York, Harper & Row [1965], pg. 47

Chapter 6: Genetic Analysis and Mapping in Bacteria and Bacteriophages
Table 6.2 Data derived from Hershey, A.D. and R. Rotman, "Genetic Rocombination between host-range and plague-type mutants of bacteriophage in single bacteriological cells," Genetics 34 (1949): 44-71.

Chapter 7: Sex Determination and Sex Chromosomes Table 7.1 Compiled from data presented in Hook, 1973, Tables 1–8. Copyright 1973 by the American Association for the Advancement of Science. **p 181** Source: Hashiyama, K., Shigenobu, S. and Kobayashi, S. 2009. Expression of genes involved in sumoylation in the Drosophila germline. Gene Expression Patterns 9(1): 50–53.

Chapter 8: Chromosome Mutations: Variation in Number and Arrangement p 299 Sébastien Malinge, Shai Izraeli, and John D. "Crispino. Insights into the manifestations, outcomes, and mechanisms of leukemogenesis in Down syndrome," Blood. March 19, 2009 vol. 113 no. 12: 2619-2628.

Chapter 10: DNA Structure and Analysis Table 10.3 Data from Chargaff, Erwin. 1950. Chemical Specificity of nucleic acids and mechanism of their enzymatic degradation. Experientia 6: 201-209. **p 248** Reprinted by permission from Macmillan Publishers Ltd: Nature, "Molecular Structure of Nucleic Acids: A Structure for Deoxyribose Nucleic Acid" by F.H.C. Crick and J.D. Watson, Nature, Vol. 171, No. 4356, pp. 737–38. Copyright © 1953. www.nature.com **p 235** Source: Oswald T. Avery, Colin M. MacLeod, and Maclyn McCarty, STUDIES ON THE CHEMICAL NATURE OF THE SUBSTANCE INDUCING TRANSFORMATION OF PNEUMOCOCCAL TYPES INDUCTION OF TRANSFORMATION BY A DESOXYRIBONUCLEIC ACID FRACTION ISOLATED FROM PNEUMOCOCCUS TYPE III, February 1, 1944//JEM vol. 79 no. 2 137-158, The Rockefeller University Press, p. 156. **p 236** Oswald T. Avery, Colin M. MacLeod, and Maclyn McCarty, STUDIES ON THE CHEMICAL NATURE OF THE SUBSTANCE INDUCING TRANSFORMATION OF PNEUMOCOCCAL TYPES INDUCTION OF TRANSFORMATION BY A DESOXYRIBONUCLEIC ACID FRACTION ISOLATED FROM PNEUMOCOCCUS TYPE III, February 1, 1944//JEM vol. 79 no. 2 137-158, The Rockefeller University Press, p. 155 **p 244** J. D. Watson and F. H. C. Crick, A Structure for Deoxyribose Nucleic Acid, April 25, 1953 (2), Nature (3), 171, 737-738. **p 249** Source: J. D. Watson and F. H. C. Crick, A Structure for Deoxyribose Nucleic Acid, April 25, 1953 (2), Nature (3), 171, 737-738

Chapter 11: DNA Replication and Recombination Table 11.1 Source: Kornberg, Arthur. 1960. Biologic Synthesis of DNA. Science: 1503-1508.

Chapter 12 DNA Organization in Chromosomes p306 Source: Renzo Lucchini, Ralf Erik Wellinger, and José M. Sogo. Nucleosome positioning at the replication fork, The EMBO Journal. Volume 20, Issue 24, pp 6937–7343.

Chapter 13: The Genetic Code and Transcription Table 13.1 Source: After Nirenberg, M.W. and J.H. Matthaei. 1961. The dependence of cell-free protein synthesis in e. coli in nautrally occurring or synthetic polyribonucleotides. Proceedings of the National Academy of Science 77: 1588-1602. **Table 13.6** Source: Volkin, E. and L. Astrachan. 1956. Intracellular distrobution of labelled RNA after phage infection of E. coli. Virology 2: 433-437.; Volkin, E., L. Astrachan, and J.L. Countryman. 1958. Metabolism of RNA phosphorous in E. coli infected with bacteriophage T7. Virology 6: 545-555.

Chapter 15: Gene Mutation, DNA Repair, and Transposition Table 15.2 Source: After Luria, S.E. and M. Delbrück. 1943. Mutations of bacteria from virus sensitivity to virus resistance. Genetics 28: 491-511.

Chapter 17: Regulation of Gene Expression in Eukaryotes p 435 Hidetoshi Hasuwa et al. "MiR-200b and miR-429 Function in Mouse Ovulation and Are Essential for Female Fertility" Science 341, 71 (2013). Reprinted with permission from AAAS.

Chapter 18: Developmental Genetics Table 18.4 Gerhart, J. 1999. 1998 Warkany lecture: Signaling pathways in development. Teratology 60: 226 239. **p 501** Adapted by permission from Macmillan Publishers Ltd: Nature Genetics, "A gene expression map of Arabidopsis thaliana development," by M. Schmid. Nature Genetics, 37: 501-506, fig. 4, p. 504. Copyright 2005, www.nature.com/ng. **p 463** Based on Wawersik, S. and Maas, R.L. 2000. Vertebrate eye development as modelled in Drosophila. Hum. Mol. Genet. 9:917–925, Table 1, p. 921.

Chapter 19: Cancer and Regulation of the Cell Cycle Fig 19.02 Data from Vogelstein, B. et al. 2013. Cancer Genome Landscapes. Science 339: 1546-1558. **p488** Based on Y Miki et al. 1994. A strong candidate for the breast and ovarian cancer susceptibility gene BRCA1. Science 266: 66–71. © AAAS.

Chapter 20: Recombinant DNA Technology Fig 20.17 From "Gene reading steps up a gear. Third-generation sequencing machines promise to make their mark one molecule at a time," By Heidi Ledford. NATURE, Vol 470 (Fed 2011) p. 155. Reprinted with permission. **Fig 20.21** From "The Mouse Ascending: perspectives for human-disease models" By Nadia Rosenthal and Steve Brown. NATURE CELL BIOLOGY, Vol 9 (issue 9) (Sept 2007). Reprinted with permission. **Fig 20.18** Based on Boyle, N.R., and Gill, R.T. (2012) Tools for genome-wide strain design and construction. Current Opinion in Biotechnology. Volume 23, Issue 5, October 2012, Pages 666–671

Chapter 21: Genomics, Bioinformatics, and Proteomics Fig 21.09 SOURCE: From Fields S (2007) "Molecular biology. Site-seeing by sequencing," Science 316: 1441-1442..Reprinted with permission from AAAS. **Fig 21.12** Adapted by permission from Miller et al. NATURE'Sequencing the nuclear genome of the extinct woolly mammoth.', NATURE, 456: 387-390. fig 2 pg 388. **Fig 21.13** from Human Genome at Ten, Nature, 464, April 2010, pg. 671. Reprinted with permission. **Fig 21.24** SOURCE: From J M Asara et al 2007 Protein sequences from Mastadon and Tyrannosaurus rex revealed by mass spectrometry. Science 316: 280-285, Fig. 3, p. 283 Reprinted with permission from AAAS. **Fig 21.25** "Human disease classification in the postgenomic era: A complex systems approach to human pathobiology. Joseph Loscalzo, Isaac Kohane, Albert-Laszlo Barabasi, From MOLECULAR SYSTEMS BIOLOGY, October 7, 2007. Copyright © 2007 EMBO and Nature Publishing Group" **Table 21.2** Source: Adapted from Palladino, M. A. Understanding the Human Genome Project, 2nd ed. Benjamin Cummings, 2006.

Chapter 22: Applications and Ethics of Genetic Engineering and Biotechnology Fig 22.03 P. Rainard. 'Tackling mastitis in dairy cows.' NATURE BIOTECHNOLOGY, 23.4, pp. 430-432. Reprinted with permission. **Fig 22.05a** From Itaya, M. A synthetic DNA transplant. Nature Biotechnology, 28(7):687-689, 2010. Panel A from figure 1, p. 688. (c) 2010 MacMillan Publisher's Ltd. Reprinted with permission. **Fig 22.05b** SOURCE: From Gibson, D. G. et al. Creation of a bacterial cell controlled by a chemically synthesized genome. Science 329: 52-56, 2010. Panel B from figure 1, p. 53. Reprinted with permission from AAAS **Fig 22.08** From Bianchi, D.W., 2012. Fatal Gene's in mother's blood. NATURE 487: 304-305. Reprinted with permission. **Fig 22.20** "SOURCE: Voight et al. 'Twelve type 2 diabetes susceptibility loci idenitified through large scale association analysis.' NATURE GENETICS 42.7, pp. 579–89 (c) 2010 MacMillan Publisher's Ltd. **p 601** Petukhova et al., Genome-wide association study in alopecia areata implicates both innate and adaptive immunity. Nature 466: 113-117, 2010. P. 113, figure 1. (c) 2010 MacMillan Publisher's Ltd. **p 577** Source: J. Craig Venter [7.30.07], CHANGING ONE SPECIES TO ANOTHER. **p 602** Source: Modified from Lee et al. 2001. Infect. and Immunity 69: 5786–5793.

Chapter 23: Quantitative Genetics and Multifactorial Traits

Fig 23.08 Figure from: Mackay, T. 2001. Quantitative trait loci in Drosophila. Nature Reviews Genetics 2: 11-20, their Fig. 3, p. 13. Reprinted with permission. **Table 23.5** "Reproduced with permission of Annual Review of Genetics, Volume 27 by Annual Reviews, http://www.annualreviews.org". Copyright © 2003, Annual Reviews

Chapter 24: Neurogenetics

Fig 24.03 Marieb, Elaine. N. and Hoehn, Katjia, Human Anatomy and Physiology, 9/e.(c) 2013, pp 409, 422. Reprinted and Electronically reproduced with the permission of Pearson Education, Inc., Upper Saddle River, New Jersey. **Fig 24.04** Marieb, Elaine. N. and Hoehn, Katjia, Human Anatomy and Physiology, 9/e.(c) 2013, pp 409, 422. Reprinted and Electronically reproduced with the permission of Pearson Education, Inc., Upper Saddle River, New Jersey. **Fig 24.05** From Brunner, H.G., et al., 1993. Abnormal behavior associated with a point mutation in the structural gene for monoamine oxidase A. Science 262: 578-580, their Figure 1, page 579. Reprinted with permission from AAAS **Fig 24.11** From Plomin, R, et al. 1994. The genetic basis of complex human behavior. Science 264: 1733-1739, their Figure 1 (left), page 1734 Reprinted with permission from AAAS **Fig 24.14** Cross-disorder Group of the Psychiatric Genomics Consortium. 2013. Genetic relationship between five psychiatric disorders estimated from genome-wide SNPs. Nature Genetic 45:(9): pp. 984–994, their Figure 1. Reprinted with permission. **Fig 24.15** From: Goldman, D., et al. 2005. The genetics of addictions: uncovering the genes. Nature Reviews Genetics 6: 521-531, their Figure 2a, page 525. Reprinted with permission. **Fig 24.10** Adapted from B. Riley and K.S. Kendler, 2006. "Molecular genetics studies of schizophrenia," European Journal of Human Genetics, 14: 669-680, fig. 1, p. 670. Reprinted with permission. **Fig 24.13** From: Shi, et al. 2009. Common variants on chromosome 6p22.1 are associated with schizophrenia. Nature 460: 753-757; their Figure 1, p. 756. Reprinted with permission. **p 637** From Pavlopoulos, E., et al. 2013. Molecular mechanism for age-related memory loss: the histone-binding protein RbAp48. Science Translational Medicine 5:1-12. Reprinted from permission of AAAS. **Table 24.5** Source: Adapted from Macmillan Publishers Ltd: Nature Reviews Genetics, "Drosophila: Genetics Meets Behavior," by M.B. Sokolowski. Nature Reviews Genetics 2:879–890, table 1, p. 882. **Table 24.6** Source: Crespi, B, et al., 2010. Comparative genomics of autism and schizophrenia. Proceedings of the National Academy of Science 107: 1736–1741; their Table 1, page 1737.

Chapter 25: Population and Evolutionary Genetics

Fig 25.02 Adapted from 'Nucleotide polymorphism at the alcohol dehydrogenase locus of the Drosophila melanogaster,' NATURE, 304 (4): 412-417, table 1, p. 413 (c) 1983 MacMillan Publisher's Ltd. Reprinted with permission. **Fig 25.21** Fitch, W.M. and Margoliash, E. 'Construction of phylogenetic trees.' SCIENCE 279: 279–284, Figure 2. (c) 1967 AAAS. Reprinted with permission of the AAAS. **Fig 25.22** 'The Natural Theory in the Genomic Era.' ANNUAL REVIEW GENOMICS HUMAN GENETICS: 11, 265-289, fig 1, pg 271. Reprinted with permission. **Fig 25.23** From Noonan, J.P. et al. 'Sequencing and analysis of Neanderthal genomic DNA.' SCIENCE 314: 1113–1118. Reprinted with permission from AAAS.

Special Topics in Modern Genetics, Emerging Roles of RNA

Fig ST 2.02 based on http://mcb.illinois.edu/faculty/profile/cvanderp/**Fig ST 2.06** Verdel et al RNAi-Mediated Targeting of Heterochromatin by the RITS Comple, 2004, Science Figure 5 pp 672–676. Reprinted with permission from AAAS. **Fig ST 2.07** Wang et. al. Signaling Pathways that Control Cell Proliferation. Cold Spring Harbor. Perspectives of Biology March 1, 2013;5. Reprinted with permission. **Fig ST 2.08** Gene Regulation: Long RNAs wire up cancer growth, Schmitt and Chang 2013, Nature Fig 1 (August 29, 2013), 536-537. Reprinted with permission. **Fig ST 2.09** Hentze and Preiss, 'Circular RNAs: Splicing Enigma Variations. EMBO Press. Copyright © 2013, European Molecular Biology Organization. Reprinted with permission. **Fig ST 2.11b** Dahm, Ralf and Michael Kiebler. Silenced RNA on the Move. Nature, (November 21, 2005), Vol. 438. Reprinted with permission.

Special Topics in Modern Genetics, DNA Forensics

Fig ST 3.03 (c) 2014 Thermo Fisher Scientific Inc. Used under permission. **Fig ST 3.05** (c) 2011 Life Technologies Corp. Reprinted with permission. **ST Table 3.2** Reprinted with Permission from Butler, J.M., et al. 2003. Allele frequencies for 15 autosomal STR loci on U.S. Caucasian, African American, and Hispanic populations. Journal of Forensic Science 48(4):908-911.

Special Topics in Modern Genetics, Genomics and Personalized Medicine

Fig ST 4.01 "Personalized Medicine Coalition. The Case for Personalized Medicine: 3rd ed, fig.2 Copyright © 2011 Personalized Medical Coalition **Fig ST 4.03**"Source: "Pharmacogenomics: Bench to Bedside", by R. Weinshilboum and L. Wang, from Nature Reviews Drug Discovery,3. Copyright © 2004 by Macmillan Publishers Ltd. Reprinted with permission. **ST Table 4.2** With kind permission of Springer Science+Business media: APPS Pharmsci 2(1): Article 4, "Pharmacogenomics: The Promise of Personalized Medicine," 2000, Mancinelli, L., Table 1, Copyright 2000 **ST Table 4.3** Gene Reviews at http://www.ncbi.nlm.nih.gov/bookshelf/br.fcgi?book=gene.

Special Topics in Modern Genetics, Genetically Modified Foods

ST Table 5.1 Information from the International Service for the Acquisition of Agri-Biotech Applications, www.isaaa.org.

Special Topics in Modern Genetics, Gene Therapy

Fig ST 6.01a The Journal of Gene Medicine, Wiley and Sons. **Fig ST 6.03** THIEMAN, WILLIAM J.; PALLADINO, MICHAEL A., INTRODUCTION TO BIOTECHNOLOGY, 3rd Ed ©2013, pp.280, 282. Reprinted and Electronically reproduced by permission of Pearson Education, Inc., Upper Saddle River, New Jersey. **Fig ST 6.04** Reprinted with permission of The Scientist from "Targeting DNA" July, 2002. **Fig ST 6.09** Reprinted with permission of The Scientist from "Targeting DNA" July, 2002. **Fig ST 6.10** "THIEMAN, WILLIAM J.; PALLADINO, MICHAEL A., INTRODUCTION TO BIOTECHNOLOGY, 3rd Ed"" ©2013, pp.280, 282. Reprinted and Electronically reproduced by permission of Pearson Education, Inc., Upper Saddle River, New Jersey." **Fig ST 6.01** French institute prepares for gene-therapy push. Nature 481:423-424, p. 42. Nature by Nature Publishing Group. Reproduced with permission of Nature Publishing Group in the format Republish in a book via Copyright Clearance Center.

Index

A

A site, in translation, 342
2-Amino-purine (2-AP), 375
ABO blood groups, 74–75
  and albinism in humans, 79
  A and B antigens, 74–75
  Bombay phenotype, 75–76, 80–81
Abortive transcription, 325
Abortive transduction, 150
Absorption spectrum, 239
Acceptor and donor sequences, 329
Accession number, 528
Acentric chromatids, 204
Acetaldehyde, in alcoholism, 642
Acetylation, 297
  histone, 676
Achondroplasia, 378, 399, 659
Acrocentric chromosomes, 19
Actin, 18, 359
Action spectrum (UV light), 239
Activator (Ac)-dissociation (Ds) system,
    387–388
Activator (Ac) elements, 386–387
Activators, 424
  interaction with general transcription
    factors at promoter, 425–427
Active center, 325
Active site, 359–360
Acute transforming retroviruses, 483
Adaptation hypothesis, 135
Adaptive mutations, vs. random mutations,
    371–372
ADAR (adenosine deaminase acting on RNA)
    enzymes, 330
Addiction, 641–642
Additive allele, 606
Additive variance, 612
Adduct-forming agents, mutations from, 376
Adelberg, Edward, 141–142
Adenine (A), 6, 240, 244–246
  adenine-thymine base pairs, 247
Adenine methylase, 380
Adenoma, 471
Adenomatous polyposis (APC) gene, 471, 482
Adenosine triphosphate (ATP), 18, 242
Adenosine-uracil rich element (ARE), 432
Adenoviruses, in gene therapy, 741–742
Adenyl cyclase, 403
Adjacent segregation, 205–206
A-DNA, 249
Adverse drug reactions, 715–716
Aerobic respiration, mitochondrial mutations
    in Neurospora, 217–218
Aflatoxin, 484
Africa, human origins in, 668–669
Agarose gel, 254
  in electrophoresis, 504
  in Southern blotting, 506
Age of Genetics, 12
Age of onset, gene expression, 93

Aging
  age-related cancers and, 471
  memory loss and, 637–638
  mitochondrial mutations and, 222–223
  telomeres and, 283
agouti gene, 77
Agricultural biotechnology, 574–576. *See also*
    Genetically modified food
Agrobacterium tumefaciens–mediated
    transformation, 729–730
AIDS. *See* Human immunodeficiency virus
    (HIV) infection
Albinism, 60, 78
  ABO blood group and, 79
  in Native American population, 660–661
Alcohol dehydrogenase locus (Adh), in
    Drosophila, 648
Alcoholism, 641–642
Alignment, DNA sequence, 524
Aliquot, 149
Alkaptonuria, 347–348
ALK/EML4 fusion gene, 713
Alkylating agents, mutations from, 375–376
Alleles, 43
  additive, 606–607
  alteration of phenotypes, 71–72
  calculating frequency for X-linked traits,
    655
  calculating frequency in population,
    650–655
  codominance, 73–74
  defined, 5, 20
  frequency in a population, 650–655
  incomplete (partial) dominance, 72–73
  lethal, 76–77
  migration and gene flow altering
    frequencies, 659–660
  multiple, 74–76
  from mutation, 658–659
  natural selection driving allele frequency
    change, 655–658
  nonadditive, 607
  symbols for, 72
Allele-specific oligonucleotides, 583–584
Allopolyploidy, 195–196, 197–198
Allosteric repressor, 399
Allotetraploidy, 197
Alloway, J. Lionel, 234
Alpha (α) chains, hemoglobin, 353
Alpha (α) helix, 356
Alpha (α) subunit, of DNA polymerase III
    holoenzyme, 268
α1-antitrypsin, 572
α-globin gene, 550–551
Alphoid family, 301
Alternate segregation, 205
Alternative lengthening of telomeres (ALT),
    283
Alternative splicing, 180, 329, 428–431, 535
  and human diseases, 430

  of mRNA, 429–431
  sex determination in Drosophila, 430–431
Alu element, 390
Alu family, 302
Alzheimer disease, 359, 637
Ames test, 385
Amino acids, 354
  coding dictionary, 316–318
  colinearity and, 353
  linkage of, 354
  results and interpretation of mixed
    copolymer experiment, 312–313
  structure of, 354, 355
  triple-binding assay and, 313–315
  types of, 354, 355
Amino group, 354
  conversion to keto group, in deamination, 374
Aminoacyl tRNA, 341
Aminoacyl tRNA synthetases, 220, 340
Aminoacyladenylic acid, 340–341
Aminoacylation, of tRNA, 340
Amniocentesis, 194, 580–581
Amphidiploidy, 197–198
AmpliChip CYP450 assay, 716
Amplicon, 174
Amtzen, C. J., 158
Anabolism, 360
Anaphase, in mitosis, 24–25
Anaphase I, in meiosis, 29
Anaphase II, in meiosis, 30
Anaplastic lymphoma kinase (ALK), 713
Aneuploidy, 189–195
  defined, 189
  human, 195
  monosomy, 189–190
  trisomy, 190–195
Angelman syndrome, 94
Angiosperms, diploid sporophyte and haploid
    gametophyte stages, 34
Animals
  cloning of, 8
  as model organisms. *See* Model organisms
  monosomy in, 189–190
  transgenic. *See* Transgenic animals
  trisomy in, 190
Annealing, 491
  in polymerase chain reaction, 501
Annotations, 528–529
  hallmark characteristics of gene sequence,
    529–531
Antennapedia genes, 452
Antibiotic-resistant bacteria, 159
Antibodies, 436
Anticodon, 313, 338
Anticodon loop, 340
Anticodon-codon base-pairing rules, 317
Antigen recognition, 436
Antigens, 436
  ABO blood groups in humans, 74–77
Antiparallel strands, 245, 270–271